S A U N D E R S

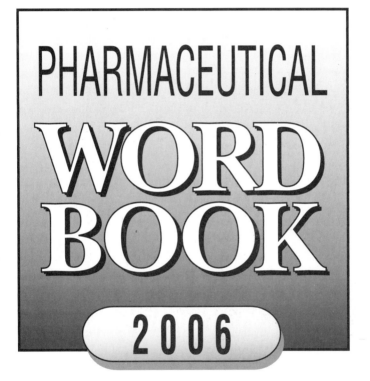

PHARMACEUTICAL WORD BOOK

2006

ELLEN DRAKE, CMT
RANDY DRAKE, MS

SAUNDERS

PHARMACEUTICAL WORD BOOK

2006

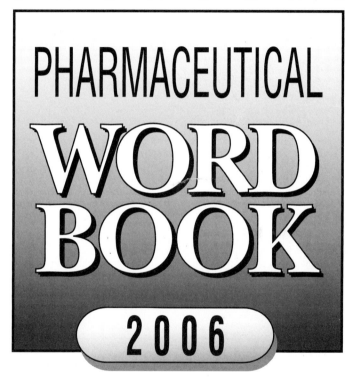

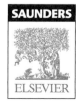

SAUNDERS

ELSEVIER

SAUNDERS
ELSEVIER

11830 Westline Industrial Drive
St. Louis, Missouri 63146

SAUNDERS PHARMACEUTICAL WORD BOOK 2006   ISBN-13: 978-1-4160-0295-6
         ISBN-10:   1-4160-0295-2

Copyright © 2006, Elsevier Inc.

Notice

Knowledge and best practice in this field are constantly changing. As new research and experience broaden our knowledge, changes in practice, treatment, and drug therapy may become necessary or appropriate. Readers are advised to check the most current information provided (i) on procedures featured or (ii) by the manufacturer of each product to be administered, to verify the recommended dose or formula, the method and duration of administration, and contraindications. It is the responsibility of the practitioner, relying on his or her own experience and knowledge of the patient, to make diagnoses, to determine dosages and the best treatment for each individual patient, and to take all appropriate safety precautions. To the fullest extent of the law, neither the Publisher nor the Authors assume any liability for any injury and/or damage to persons or property arising out or related to any use of the material contained in this book.

The Publisher

Previous editions copyrighted 2005, 2004, 2003, 2002, 2001, 2000, 1999, 1998, 1997, 1996, 1995, 1994, 1992

ISSN: 1072-7779

ISBN-13: 978-1-4160-0295-6

ISBN-10: 1-4160-0295-2

Working together to grow libraries in developing countries

www.elsevier.com | www.bookaid.org | www.sabre.org

ELSEVIER   BOOK AID International   Sabre Foundation

Printed in the United States of America

Last digit is the print number: 9   8   7   6   5   4   3   2   1

Contents

Preface

Saunders Pharmaceutical Word Book has been compiled primarily with the medical transcriptionist in mind, although it will also appeal to nurses, coders, ward clerks, quality assurance personnel, pharmacy technicians, students of all allied health professions—anyone who has a need for a quick, easy-to-use drug reference that gives more information than just the spelling. Even physicians may find it useful to get quick information on medications their patients may be using for conditions outside their specialty. The "Notes on Using the Text" explains the variety of information this book contains as well as how to find that information.

We think you will find this fourteenth edition more complete and more valuable than ever; however, no book is ever perfect. We keep our database current by adding new entries and updating the current entries as new information becomes available. Although we have tried to be as accurate and comprehensive as possible, we certainly welcome your comments regarding additions, inconsistencies, or inaccuracies. Please send them to us via e-mail at the address below, or via regular mail to Elsevier Saunders, 11830 Westline Industrial Drive, St. Louis, MO 63146-3313. We welcome your suggestions.

Authors' e-mail address:
   authors@spwb.com
Authors' web site:
   spwb.com

ELLEN DRAKE, CMT
RANDY DRAKE, MS
Atlanta, Georgia

Notes on Using the Text

The purpose of the *Saunders Pharmaceutical Word Book* is to provide the medical transcriptionist (as well as medical record administrators and technicians, coders, nurses, ward clerks, court reporters, legal secretaries, medical assistants, allied health students, physicians, and even pharmacists) a quick, easy-to-use reference that gives not only the correct spellings and capitalizations of drugs, but the designated uses of those drugs, the cross-referencing of brand names to generics, and the usual methods of administration (e.g., capsule, IV, cream). The indication of the preferred nonproprietary (generic) names and the agencies adopting these names (e.g., USAN, USP) should be particularly useful to those writing for publication. The reader will also find various trademarked or proprietary names (e.g., Spansule, Dosepak) that are not drugs but are closely associated with the packaging or administration of drugs.

There are four different ways to refer to drugs. One of these ways is not the name of the drug itself but the class to which it belongs—aminoglycosides, for example. Inexperienced transcriptionists sometimes confuse these classes with the names of drugs. We have included some 200 drug classes in the main list, with a brief description of the therapeutic use and/or method of action common to drugs in the class. Beyond a class description, each drug has three names. The first is the *chemical name*, which describes its chemical composition and how the molecules are arranged. It is often long and complex, sometimes containing numbers, Greek letters, italicized letters, and hyphens between elements. This name is rarely used in dictation except in research hospitals and sometimes in the laboratory section when the blood or urine is examined for traces of the drug. The second name for a drug is the *nonproprietary* or *generic name*. This is a name chosen by the discovering manufacturer or agency and submitted to a nomenclature committee (the United States Adopted Names Council, for example). The name is simpler than the chemical name but often reflects the chemical entity. It is arrived at by using guidelines provided by the nomenclature committee—beta-blockers must end in "olol," for example—and must be unique. There is increasing emphasis on the adoption of the same nonproprietary name by various nomenclature committees worldwide (see the list on page xiii). The third name for a drug is the *trade* or *brand name*. There may be several trade names for the same generic drug, each marketed by a different company. These are the ones that are highly advertised, and sometimes have unusual capitalization. An interesting article on the naming of drugs is "Pharmaceutical Nomenclature: The Lawless Language" in *Perspectives on the Medical Transcription Profession*.[1] *Understanding Pharmacology*[2] also discusses the naming of drugs.

We have included many foreign names of drugs for our Canadian friends, and also because we have so many visitors to the United States from other countries (and they get sick, too). The international and British spellings of generic drugs are cross-referenced to the American spellings, and vice versa. Occasionally there will

The general format for a *brand name* entry is:

Entry Ⓒ form(s) ℞/OTC *designated use* [generics] dosages 🔊 sound-alike(s)

| #1 | #2 | #3 | #4 | #5 | #6 | #7 | #8 |

1. The drug name (in bold), which almost always starts with a capital letter.
2. If a brand is not marketed in the U.S., an icon designates the country where it is available. Canadian brands are designated by Ⓒ.
3. The form of administration; e.g., tablets, capsules, syrup. (Sometimes these words are slurred by the dictator, causing confusion regarding the name.)
4. The ℞ or OTC status. A few drugs may be either ℞ or OTC depending on strength or various state laws.
5. The designated use in italics as for generics. These are more complete or less complete as supplied by the individual drug companies.
6. The brackets that follow contain the generic names of the active ingredients to which the reader may refer for further information.
7. Dosage information follows the generics. For multi-ingredient drugs, a bullet separates the dosages of each ingredient, listed in the same order as the generics. For example,

    Ser-Ap-Es tablets ℞ *antihypertensive; vasodilator; diuretic* [hydrochlorothiazide; reserpine; hydralazine HCl] 15●0.1●25 mg

shows a three-ingredient product containing 15 mg hydrochlorothiazide, 0.1 mg reserpine, and 25 mg hydralazine HCl.

Some drugs may have more than one strength, indicated by a comma in the dosage field:

    Norpace capsules ℞ *antiarrhythmic* [disopyramide phosphate] 100, 150 mg

A semicolon in the dosage field separates either different products listed together, such as:

    Pred Mild; Pred Forte eye drop suspension ℞ *corticosteroidal anti-inflammatory* [prednisolone acetate] 0.12%; 1%

Or different delivery forms:

    Phenergan tablets, suppositories, injection ℞ *antihistamine; sedative; antiemetic; motion sickness relief* [promethazine HCl] 25, 50 mg; 12.5, 25, 50 mg; 25, 50 mg/mL

(Note that all three delivery forms of Phenergan come in multiple strengths.)

Liquid delivery forms show the strength per usual dose where appropriate. Thus injectables and drops are usually shown per milliliter (mL), with oral liquids and syrups shown per 5 mL or 15 mL.

The ⩒ symbol indicates that dosage information has not been supplied by the manufacturer for one or more ingredients.

The ⩳ symbol is used when a value *cannot* be given because the generic entry refers to multiple ingredients.

8. Sound-alike drugs follow the "ear" icon.

The general format of a *generic* entry is:

entry council(s) *designated use* [other references] dosages 👂 sound-alike(s)

| #1 | #2 | #3 | #4 | #5 | #6 |

1. The name of the drug (in bold).
2. The various agencies that have approved the name, shown in small caps, which may be any or all of the following (listed according to appearance in the book):

   USAN — United States Adopted Name Council
   USP — United States Pharmacopeial Convention
   NF — National Formulary
   FDA — U.S. Food and Drug Administration
   INN — International Nonproprietary Name (a project of the World Health Organization)
   BAN — British Approved Name
   JAN — Japanese Accepted Name
   DCF — Dénomination Commune Française (French)

3. The indications, sometimes referred to as the drug's "designated use," "approved use," or "therapeutic action." This is provided only for official FDA-approved names or other names for the same substance (e.g., the British name of an official U.S. generic). This entry is always in italic.

4. The entry in brackets is one of four cross-references:

   see: refers the reader to the "official" name(s).

   now: for an older generic name no longer used, refers reader to the current official name(s).

   also: a substance that has two or more different names, each officially recognized by one of the above groups, will cross-reference the other name(s).

   q.v. Latin for quod vide; which see. Used exclusively for abbreviations, it invites the reader to turn to the reference in parentheses.

   If there is more than one cross reference, alternate names will follow the order of the above agency list; i.e., U.S. names, then international names, then British, Japanese, and French names. The first cross-reference will always be to the approved U.S. name, unless the entry itself is the U.S. name.

5. Dosage information, including the delivery form(s), is given for medications that may be dispensed generically. No dosage information appears for drugs dispensed only under the brand name, or for those containing multiple ingredients. Some drugs may be available in more than one strength, indicated by a comma in the dosage field:

   erythromycin stearate USP, BAN *macrolide antibiotic* 250, 500 mg oral

   A semicolon in the dosage field separates different delivery forms, such as:

   nitroglycerin USP *coronary vasodilator; antianginal; antihypertensive* [also: glyceryl trinitrate] 0.3, 0.4, 0.6 mg sublingual; 2.5, 6.5, 9 mg oral; 5 mg/mL injection; 0.1, 0.2, 0.4, 0.6 mg/hr. transdermal; 2% topical

   (Note that some delivery forms come in multiple strengths.)

6. Sound-alike drugs follow the "ear" icon.

The general format for a *brand name* entry is:

Entry ⒸⒶⓃ form(s) Ṛ/OTC *designated use* [generics] dosages ② sound-alike(s)

| #1 | #2 | #3 | #4 | #5 | #6 | #7 | #8 |

1. The drug name (in bold), which almost always starts with a capital letter.
2. If a brand is not marketed in the U.S., an icon designates the country where it is available. Canadian brands are designated by ⒸⒶⓃ.
3. The form of administration; e.g., tablets, capsules, syrup. (Sometimes these words are slurred by the dictator, causing confusion regarding the name.)
4. The Ṛ or OTC status. A few drugs may be either Ṛ or OTC depending on strength or various state laws.
5. The designated use in italics as for generics. These are more complete or less complete as supplied by the individual drug companies.
6. The brackets that follow contain the generic names of the active ingredients to which the reader may refer for further information.
7. Dosage information follows the generics. For multi-ingredient drugs, a bullet separates the dosages of each ingredient, listed in the same order as the generics. For example,

> **Ser-Ap-Es** tablets Ṛ *antihypertensive; vasodilator; diuretic* [hydrochlorothiazide; reserpine; hydralazine HCl] 15•0.1•25 mg

shows a three-ingredient product containing 15 mg hydrochlorothiazide, 0.1 mg reserpine, and 25 mg hydralazine HCl.

Some drugs may have more than one strength, indicated by a comma in the dosage field:

> **Norpace** capsules Ṛ *antiarrhythmic* [disopyramide phosphate] 100, 150 mg

A semicolon in the dosage field separates either different products listed together, such as:

> **Pred Mild; Pred Forte** eye drop suspension Ṛ *corticosteroidal anti-inflammatory* [prednisolone acetate] 0.12%; 1%

Or different delivery forms:

> **Phenergan** tablets, suppositories, injection Ṛ *antihistamine; sedative; antiemetic; motion sickness relief* [promethazine HCl] 25, 50 mg; 12.5, 25, 50 mg; 25, 50 mg/mL

(Note that all three delivery forms of Phenergan come in multiple strengths.)

Liquid delivery forms show the strength per usual dose where appropriate. Thus injectables and drops are usually shown per milliliter (mL), with oral liquids and syrups shown per 5 mL or 15 mL.

The ⒈ symbol indicates that dosage information has not been supplied by the manufacturer for one or more ingredients.

The ⒌ symbol is used when a value *cannot* be given because the generic entry refers to multiple ingredients.

8. Sound-alike drugs follow the "ear" icon.

Experimental, Investigational, and Orphan Drugs

Before a drug can be advertised or sold in the United States, it must first be approved for marketing by the U.S. Food and Drug Administration. With a few exceptions, FDA approval is contingent solely upon the manufacturer demonstrating that the proposed drug is both safe and effective.

To provide such proof, the manufacturer undertakes a series of tests. Preclinical (before human) research is done through computer simulation, then *in vitro* (L. "in glass," meaning laboratory) tests, then in animals. In most cases neither the public nor the general medical community hears about "experimental drugs" in this stage of testing. Neither are they listed in this reference.

If safety and efficacy are successfully demonstrated during the preclinical stage, an Investigational New Drug (IND) application is filed with the FDA. There are three phases of clinical trials, designated Phase I, Phase II, and Phase III. After each phase, the FDA will review the findings and approve or deny further testing.

Phase I trials involve 20 to 100 patients, primarily to establish safety. Phase II trials may involve several hundred patients for up to two years. The goal in this phase is to determine the drug's effectiveness for the proposed indication. Phase III trials, which routinely last up to four years and involve several thousand patients, determine the optimum effective, but safe, dosage. The manufacturer will then file a New Drug Application (NDA) with the FDA, requesting final marketing approval. Only 20% of drugs entering Phase I trials will ultimately be approved for marketing, at an average cost of $359 million and 8½ years in testing.[3]

An orphan drug is a drug or biological product for the diagnosis, treatment, or prevention of a rare disease or condition. A rare disease is one that affects less than 200,000 persons or for which there is no reasonable expectation that the cost of development and testing will be recovered through U.S. sales of the product. Federal subsidies are provided to the manufacturer or sponsor for the development of orphan drugs. Applications for orphan status are made through the FDA, and may be made during drug development or after marketing approval.

A Brief Note on the Transcription of Drugs

Many references are available describing several acceptable ways to transcribe drug information when dictated. We offer the following only as brief guidelines.

Although some institutions favor capitalizing every drug, others promote not capitalizing any drug, and yet others put drugs in all capital letters, the generally accepted style today for the transcription of medical reports for hospital and doctors' office charts (see the American Medical Association *Manual of Style*[4] for publications) is to capitalize the initial letter of brand name drugs and lowercase generic name drugs. The institution may also designate that brand name drugs with unusual capitalization may be typed with initial capital letter only, or typed using the manufacturer's scheme.

In general, commas are omitted between the drug name, the dosage, and the instructions for purposes of simplification. Items in a series may be separated by either commas (if no internal commas are used) or semicolons. A simple series might be typed thus:

Procardia, nitroglycerin sublingual, and Tolinase

or

Procardia 10 mg three times a day, nitroglycerin 0.4 mg p.r.n., and Tolinase 250 mg twice a day.

or

Procardia 10 mg t.i.d., nitroglycerin 0.4 mg p.r.n., and Tolinase 250 mg b.i.d.

A more complex or lengthy list of medications, or a list with internal commas, may require the use of semicolons to separate the items in a series. For example,

Procardia 10 mg, one t.i.d.; nitroglycerin 0.4 mg p.r.n., to take one with onset of pain, a second in five minutes, and a third five minutes later, if no relief to go immediately to the ER; Tolinase 250 mg, one b.i.d.; and Coumadin 2.5 mg on Mondays, Wednesdays, and Fridays, and 5 mg on Tuesdays, Thursdays, and Saturdays...

Note that the "one" following Procardia 10 mg and Tolinase 250 mg is not necessary, but many doctors dictate something like this; when they do, it is acceptable to place a comma after the dosage. In addition, when two numbers are adjacent to each other, write out one number and use a numeral for the other.

The typing of chemicals with superscripts or subscripts, italics, small capitals, and Greek letters often presents a problem to the medical transcriptionist. In general, Greek letters are written out (alpha-, beta-, gamma-, etc.). Italics and small capitals are written as standard letters followed by a hyphen (dl-alpha-tocopherol, L-dopa).

When typing nonproprietary (generic) isotope names, element symbols should be included with the name. It may appear to be redundant, but it is the correct form. Therefore, we would type sodium pertechnetate Tc 99m, iodohippurate sodium I 131, or sodium iodide I 125. Occasionally the physician may simply dictate isotopes such as Tc 99m, iodine 131 or I 131, or sodium iodide I 125, and unless he is indicating a trademarked name, it should be typed with a space, no hyphen, and no superscript. This reference indicates proper capitalization, spacing, and hyphenation of isotope entries.

Other combinations of letters and numbers are usually written without spaces or hyphens (OKT1, OKT3, T101, SC1), but this is a complex subject and is dealt with extensively in the AMA *Manual of Style*.

[1] Dirckx, John, M.D.: "Pharmaceutical Nomenclature: The Lawless Language," *Perspectives on the Medical Transcription Profession*, Vol. 1, No. 4. Modesto: Health Professions Institute, 1991, p. 9.

[2] Turley, Susan M.: *Understanding Pharmacology for Health Professionals*–2nd ed.. Upper Saddle River, NJ: Prentice-Hall, 1999.

[3] *FDA Consumer*, January, 1995. www.fda.gov/fdac/special/newdrug/ndd_toc.html

[4] American Medical Association: *Manual of Style*, 9th ed. Baltimore: Williams & Wilkins, 1997.

PHARMACEUTICAL

WORD BOOK

2006

a-(3-aminophthalimido) glutaramide *investigational (orphan) agent for lupus nephritis*

A (vitamin A) [q.v.]

A and D ointment OTC *moisturizer; emollient* [fish liver oil (vitamins A and D); cholecalciferol; lanolin]

A and D Medicated ointment OTC *diaper rash treatment* [zinc oxide; vitamins A and D]

A + D (ara-C, daunorubicin) *chemotherapy protocol*

A1cNOW fingerstick test kit for home use R̸ *in vitro diagnostic aid for glycosylated hemoglobin levels*

A-200 shampoo concentrate OTC *pediculicide for lice* [pyrethrins; piperonyl butoxide] 0.33%•4%

AA (ara-C, Adriamycin) *chemotherapy protocol*

AA (arachadonic acid) [q.v.]

abacavir succinate USAN *antiviral nucleoside reverse transcriptase inhibitor for HIV infection*

abacavir sulfate USAN *antiviral nucleoside reverse transcriptase inhibitor for HIV infection*

abafilcon A USAN *hydrophilic contact lens material*

abamectin USAN, INN *antiparasitic*

abanoquil INN, BAN

abaperidone INN

abarelix USAN *GnRH antagonist to suppress LH and FSH, leading to the cessation of testosterone production (medical castration, androgen ablation); treatment for prostate cancer; investigational for uterine fibroids, endometriosis, and precocious puberty*

Abarelix-Depot-M (name changed to Plenaxis upon marketing release in 2004)

abatacept *investigational (NDA filed) selective T-cell co-stimulation modulator for rheumatoid arthritis*

abavca & perthon *investigational (Phase I/II) plant derivative combination for HIV and AIDS*

Abbokinase powder for IV or intracoronary artery infusion R̸ *thrombolytic enzymes for pulmonary embolism or coronary artery thrombosis* [urokinase] 250 000 IU/vial

Abbokinase Open-Cath powder for catheter clearance (discontinued 2003) R̸ *thrombolytic enzymes* [urokinase] 5000 IU/mL

Abbo-Pac (trademarked packaging form) *unit dose package*

Abbott TestPack Plus hCG-Urine Plus test kit for professional use *in vitro diagnostic aid; urine pregnancy test* [monoclonal antibody-based enzyme immunoassay]

ABC (Adriamycin, BCNU, cyclophosphamide) *chemotherapy protocol*

ABC to Z tablets OTC *vitamin/mineral/iron supplement* [multiple vitamins & minerals; ferrous fumarate; folic acid; biotin] ±•18 mg•0.4 mg•30 μg

abciximab USAN, INN *glycoprotein (GP) IIb/IIIa receptor antagonist; antithrombotic monoclonal antibody; antiplatelet agent for PTCA and acute arterial occlusive disorders*

ABCM (Adriamycin, bleomycin, cyclophosphamide, mitomycin) *chemotherapy protocol*

ABD (Adriamycin, bleomycin, DTIC) *chemotherapy protocol*

ABDIC (Adriamycin, bleomycin, DIC, [CCNU, prednisone]) *chemotherapy protocol*

ABDV (Adriamycin, bleomycin, DTIC, vinblastine) *chemotherapy protocol*

ABE (antitoxin botulism equine) [see: botulism equine antitoxin, trivalent]

abecarnil INN *investigational anxiolytic*

Abelcet suspension for IV infusion R̸ *systemic polyene antifungal for aspergillosis and other resistant fungal infections (orphan)* [amphotericin B lipid complex (ABLC)] 100 mg/20 mL

Abelmoschus moschatus *medicinal herb* [see: ambrette]

Abenol ⓒᴬᴺ *suppositories* OTC *analgesic; antipyretic* [acetaminophen] 120, 325, 650 mg

abetimus INN

abetimus sodium USAN *investigational (NDA filed, orphan) oligonucleotide immunosuppressant for systemic lupus erythematosus–associated nephritis*

Abilify *tablets, oral solution* ℞ *antipsychotic for schizophrenia and manic episodes of a bipolar disorder* [aripiprazole] 5, 10, 15, 20, 30 mg; 5 mg/5 mL

Abilitat (name changed to **Abilify** upon marketing release in 2002)

ABLC [see: TLC ABLC]

ABLC (**amphotericin B lipid complex**) [q.v.]

ablukast USAN, INN *antiasthmatic; leukotriene antagonist*

ablukast sodium USAN *antiasthmatic; leukotriene antagonist*

Abolic *a veterinary steroid abused as a street drug*

abortifacients *a class of agents that stimulate uterine contractions sufficient to produce uterine evacuation*

ABP (**Adriamycin, bleomycin, prednisone**) *chemotherapy protocol*

ABPP (**aminobromophenylpyrimidinone**) [see: bropirimine]

Abraxane *suspension of albumin-bound microspheres for IV infusion* ℞ *antineoplastic for metastatic breast cancer* [paclitaxel; human albumin] 100•900 mg/dose

Abreva *cream* OTC *antiviral for cold sores and fever blisters* [docosanol] 10%

abrineurin USAN *treatment for amyotrophic lateral sclerosis (ALS)*

Abrus precatorius *medicinal herb* [see: precatory bean]

absinthe; absinthites; absinthium *medicinal herb* [see: wormwood]

absorbable cellulose cotton [see: cellulose, oxidized]

absorbable collagen sponge [see: collagen sponge, absorbable]

absorbable dusting powder [see: dusting powder, absorbable]

absorbable gelatin film [see: gelatin film, absorbable]

absorbable gelatin powder [see: gelatin powder, absorbable]

absorbable gelatin sponge [see: gelatin sponge, absorbable]

absorbable surgical suture [see: suture, absorbable surgical]

Absorbase OTC *ointment base* [water-in-oil emulsion of cholesterolized petrolatum and purified water]

absorbent gauze [see: gauze, absorbent]

Absorbine Antifungal Foot *aerosol powder* OTC *antifungal* [miconazole nitrate; alcohol 10%] 2%

Absorbine Arthritis Strength Liquid with Capsaicin *topical liquid* OTC *analgesic; counterirritant* [menthol; capsaicin] 4%•0.025%

Absorbine Athlete's Foot *cream* OTC *antifungal* [tolnaftate] 1%

Absorbine Footcare *spray liquid* OTC *antifungal* [tolnaftate] 1%

Absorbine Jr. *liniment* OTC *analgesic; counterirritant* [menthol] 1.27%, 4%

Absorbine Jr. Extra Strength *topical liquid* OTC *analgesic; counterirritant* [menthol] 4%

abunidazole INN

ABV (**actimomycin D, bleomycin, vincristine**) *chemotherapy protocol*

ABV (**Adriamycin, bleomycin, vinblastine**) *chemotherapy protocol for Kaposi sarcoma*

ABV (**Adriamycin, bleomycin, vincristine**) *chemotherapy protocol for Kaposi sarcoma*

ABVD (**Adriamycin, bleomycin, vinblastine, dacarbazine**) *chemotherapy protocol for Hodgkin lymphoma*

ABVD/MOPP (**alternating cycles of ABVD and MOPP**) *chemotherapy protocol*

AC (**Adriamycin, carmustine**) *chemotherapy protocol*

AC (**Adriamycin, CCNU**) *chemotherapy protocol*

AC (Adriamycin, cisplatin) *chemotherapy protocol for bone sarcoma*

AC; A-C (Adriamycin, cyclophosphamide) *chemotherapy protocol for breast cancer and pediatric neuroblastoma*

AC/paclitaxel, sequential (Adriamycin, cyclophosphamide; paclitaxel) *chemotherapy protocol for breast cancer*

ACA125 *investigational (orphan) agent for epithelial ovarian cancer*

acacia NF, JAN *suspending agent; emollient; demulcent*

acacia (Acacia senegal; A. verek) gum *medicinal herb for colds, cough, periodontal disease, and wound healing*

acadesine USAN, INN, BAN *platelet aggregation inhibitor*

acamprosate INN

acamprosate calcium *GABA/taurine analogue for the treatment of alcoholism*

acamylophenine [see: camylofin]

Acanthopanax senticosus medicinal herb [see: Siberian ginseng]

acaprazine INN

acarbose USAN, INN, BAN *antidiabetic agent for type 2 diabetes; alpha-glucosidase inhibitor that delays the digestion of dietary carbohydrates*

ACAT (acylCoA transferase) inhibitors *a class of antihyperlipidemics that lower serum cholesterol levels*

Accolate film-coated tablets ℞ *leukotriene receptor antagonist (LTRA) for prevention and chronic treatment of asthma* [zafirlukast] 10, 20 mg

Accu-Chek Advantage reagent strips for home use *in vitro diagnostic aid for blood glucose*

AccuHist DM Pediatric oral drops OTC *decongestant; antihistamine; antitussive* [pseudoephedrine HCl; brompheniramine maleate; dextromethorphan hydrobromide] 15•1•4 mg/mL

AccuHist DM Pediatric syrup OTC *decongestant; antihistamine; antitussive; expectorant* [pseudoephedrine HCl; brompheniramine maleate; dextromethorphan hydrobromide; guaifenesin] 30•2•5•50 mg/5 mL

AccuHist LA sustained-release caplets ℞ *decongestant; antihistamine; anticholinergic* [phenylephrine HCl; chlorpheniramine maleate; hyoscyamine sulfate; atropine sulfate; scopolamine hydrobromide] 20•8•0.19•0.04•0.01 mg

AccuHist PDX oral drops ℞ *decongestant; antihistamine; antitussive* [pseudoephedrine HCl; brompheniramine maleate; dextromethorphan hydrobromide] 12.5•1•3 mg/mL

AccuHist PDX syrup ℞ *decongestant; antihistamine; antitussive; expectorant* [phenylephrine HCl; brompheniramine maleate; dextromethorphan hydrobromide; guaifenesin] 5•2•5•50 mg/5 mL

AccuHist Pediatric oral drops (discontinued 2004) OTC *decongestant; antihistamine* [pseudoephedrine HCl; brompheniramine maleate] 12.5•1 mg/mL

AccuNeb solution for inhalation ℞ *sympathomimetic bronchodilator for children 2–12 years* [albuterol sulfate] 0.63, 1.25 mg/3 mL

Accu-Pak (trademarked packaging form) *unit dose blister pack*

Accupep HPF powder OTC *enteral nutritional therapy for GI impairment*

Accupril film-coated tablets ℞ *antihypertensive; angiotensin-converting enzyme (ACE) inhibitor; adjunctive treatment for CHF* [quinapril HCl] 5, 10, 20, 40 mg

Accurbron syrup ℞ *antiasthmatic; bronchodilator* [theophylline; alcohol 7.5%] 150 mg/15 mL ⊠ Accutane

Accuretic film-coated tablets ℞ *antihypertensive; angiotensin-converting enzyme (ACE) inhibitor; diuretic* [quinapril HCl; hydrochlorothiazide] 10•12.5, 20•12.5, 20•25 mg

Accutane capsules ℞ *keratolytic for severe recalcitrant cystic acne; investigational (Phase III) for neuroblastoma* [isotretinoin] 10, 20, 40 mg ⊠ Accurbron

Accuzyme ointment, spray ℞ *proteolytic enzyme for debridement of necrotic tissue; vulnerary* [papain; urea] 830 000 IU/g•10%

ACD solution (acid citrate dextrose; anticoagulant citrate dextrose) [see: anticoagulant citrate dextrose solution]

ACD whole blood [see: blood, whole]

ACe (Adriamycin, cyclophosphamide) *chemotherapy protocol for breast cancer*

ACE (Adriamycin, cyclophosphamide, etoposide) *chemotherapy protocol for small cell lung cancer (SCLC)* [also: CAE]

ACE inhibitors (angiotensin-converting enzyme inhibitors) [q.v.]

acebrochol INN, DCF

aceburic acid INN, DCF

acebutolol USAN, INN, BAN *antihypertensive; antianginal; antiarrhythmic; antiadrenergic (β-receptor)* [also: acebutolol HCl]

acebutolol HCl JAN *antihypertensive; antianginal; antiarrhythmic for premature ventricular contractions (PVCs); antiadrenergic (β-blocker)* [also: acebutolol] 200, 400 mg oral

acecainide INN *antiarrhythmic* [also: acecainide HCl]

acecainide HCl USAN *antiarrhythmic* [also: acecainide]

acecarbromal INN *CNS depressant; sedative; hypnotic*

aceclidine USAN, INN *cholinergic*

aceclofenac INN, BAN

acedapsone USAN, INN, BAN *antimalarial; antibacterial; leprostatic*

acediasulfone sodium INN, DCF

acedoben INN

acefluranol INN, BAN

acefurtiamine INN

acefylline clofibrol INN

acefylline piperazine INN, DCF [also: acepifylline]

aceglaton JAN [also: aceglatone]

aceglatone INN [also: aceglaton]

aceglutamide INN *antiulcerative* [also: aceglutamide aluminum]

aceglutamide aluminum USAN, JAN *antiulcerative* [also: aceglutamide]

ACEIs (angiotensin-converting enzyme inhibitors) [q.v.]

Acel-Imune IM injection (discontinued 2001) ℞ *immunization against diphtheria, tetanus and pertussis* [diphtheria & tetanus toxoids & acellular pertussis (DTaP) vaccine] 7.5 LfU•5 LfU•300 HAU per 0.5 mL

acellular pertussis vaccine [see: diphtheria & tetanus toxoids & acellular pertussis (DTaP) vaccine, adsorbed]

Acel-P Ⓒᴬᴺ suspension for IM injection (discontinued 2001) ℞ *active immunization against pertussis* [pertussis vaccine, acellular adsorbed] 300 HAU/0.5 mL

acemannan USAN, INN *hydrogel wound dressing*

acemetacin INN, BAN, JAN

acemethadone [see: methadyl acetate]

aceneuramic acid INN

acenocoumarin [see: acenocoumarol]

acenocoumarol NF, INN [also: nicoumalone]

Aceon tablets ℞ *antihypertensive; angiotensin-converting enzyme (ACE) inhibitor* [perindopril erbumine] 2, 4, 8 mg

aceperone INN

Acephen suppositories OTC *analgesic; antipyretic* [acetaminophen] 120, 325, 650 mg

acephenazine dimaleate [see: acetophenazine maleate]

acepifylline BAN [also: acefylline piperazine]

acepromazine INN, BAN *veterinary sedative* [also: acepromazine maleate]

acepromazine maleate USAN *veterinary sedative* [also: acepromazine]

aceprometazine INN, DCF

acequinoline INN, DCF

acerola (Malpighia glabra; M. punicifolia) *fruit natural dietary source of vitamin C*

acesulfame INN, BAN

Aceta tablets, elixir OTC *analgesic; antipyretic* [acetaminophen] 325, 500 mg; 120 mg/5 mL

Aceta with Codeine tablets ℞ *narcotic analgesic; antitussive* [codeine phosphate; acetaminophen] 30•300 mg

Acetadote IV injection ℞ *antidote to severe acetaminophen overdose (orphan)* [acetylcysteine] 20% in 30 mL single-dose vials

Aceta-Gesic tablets OTC *analgesic; antihistaminic sleep aid* [acetaminophen; phenyltoloxamine citrate] 325•30 mg

p-**acetamidobenzoic acid** [see: acedoben]

6-acetamidohexanoic acid [see: acexamic acid]

4-acetamidophenyl acetate [see: diacetamate]

acetaminocaproic acid [see: acexamic acid]

acetaminophen USP *analgesic; antipyretic* [also: paracetamol] 80, 325, 500, 650 mg, 100 mg/mL, 120, 160 mg/5 mL, 500/15 mL oral; 120, 300, 325, 650 mg suppository

acetaminophen & caffeine & butalbital *analgesic; barbiturate sedative* 325•40•50, 500•40•50 mg oral

acetaminophen & caffeine & butalbital & codeine phosphate *analgesic; barbiturate sedative; narcotic antitussive* 325•40•50•30 mg oral

acetaminophen & codeine *narcotic analgesic; narcotic antitussive* 300•15, 300•30, 300•60 mg oral; 30•12 mg/5 mL oral

acetaminophen & hydrocodone bitartrate *analgesic; narcotic antitussive* 325•5, 325•10, 500•2.5, 500•10, 650•7.5, 650•10, 750•7.5, 750•10 mg oral; 167•2.5 mg/5 mL oral

acetaminophen & isometheptene mucate & dichloralphenazone *cerebral vasoconstrictor and analgesic for vascular and tension headaches; "possibly effective" for migraine headaches* 325•65•100 mg oral

acetaminophen & oxycodone HCl *narcotic analgesic* 325•7.5, 325•10, 500•7.5, 650•10 mg oral

acetaminophen & pentazocine HCl *narcotic analgesic* 650•25 mg oral

acetaminophenol [see: acetaminophen]

acetaminosalol INN, DCF

acetanilid (or acetanilide) NF

acetannin [see: acetyltannic acid]

acetarsol INN, BAN, DCF [also: acetarsone]

acetarsone NF [also: acetarsol]

acetarsone salt of arecoline [see: drocarbil]

Acetasol ear drops ℞ *antibacterial; antifungal* [acetic acid] 2%

Acetasol HC ear drops ℞ *corticosteroidal anti-inflammatory; antibacterial; antifungal* [hydrocortisone; acetic acid] 1%•2%

acetazolamide USP, INN, BAN, JAN *carbonic anhydrase inhibitor; diuretic; anticonvulsant; antiglaucoma; treatment for acute mountain sickness* 125, 250 mg oral; 500 mg injection

acetazolamide sodium USP, JAN *carbonic anhydrase inhibitor; diuretic; anticonvulsant; antiglaucoma; treatment for acute mountain sickness*

acetcarbromal [see: acecarbromal]

acet-dia-mer-sulfonamide (sulfacetamide, sulfadiazine & sulfamerazine) [q.v.]

acetergamine INN

Acetest reagent tablets for professional use *in vitro diagnostic aid for acetone (ketones) in the urine or blood*

acetiamine INN

acetic acid NF, JAN *acidifying agent* 0.25%

acetic acid, aluminum salt [see: aluminum acetate]

acetic acid, calcium salt [see: calcium acetate]

acetic acid, diluted NF *bladder irrigant*

acetic acid, ethyl ester [see: ethyl acetate]

acetic acid, glacial USP, INN *acidifying agent*

acetic acid, potassium salt [see: potassium acetate]

acetic acid, sodium salt trihydrate [see: sodium acetate]

acetic acid, zinc salt dihydrate [see: zinc acetate]

acetic acid & hydrocortisone *acidifying agent; corticosteroid; anti-inflammatory* 2%•1% otic solution

acetic acid 5-nitrofurfurylidenehydrazide [see: nihydrazone]

aceticyl [see: aspirin]

acetilum acidulatum [see: aspirin]

acetiromate INN

acetohexamide USAN, USP, INN, BAN, JAN *sulfonylurea antidiabetic* 250, 500 mg oral

acetohydroxamic acid (AHA) USAN, USP, INN *urease enzyme inhibitor for chronic urea-splitting urinary infections*

acetol [see: aspirin]

acetomenaphthone BAN

acetomeroctol

acetone NF *solvent; antiseptic*

acetophen [see: aspirin]

acetophenazine INN *antipsychotic* [also: acetophenazine maleate]

acetophenazine maleate USAN, USP *antipsychotic* [also: acetophenazine]

p-acetophenetidide (*withdrawn from market*) [see: phenacetin]

acetophenetidin (*withdrawn from market*) [now: phenacetin]

acetorphan *investigational enkephalinase inhibitor for acute diarrhea, opioid withdrawal, and gastroesophageal reflux disease (GERD)*

acetorphine INN, BAN *enkephalinase inhibitor for acute diarrhea; investigational for opioid withdrawal and GERD*

acetosal [see: aspirin]

acetosalic acid [see: aspirin]

acetosalin [see: aspirin]

acetosulfone sodium USAN *antibacterial; leprostatic* [also: sulfadiasulfone sodium]

acetoxyphenylmercury [see: phenylmercuric acetate]

acetoxythymoxamine [see: moxisylyte]

acetphenarsine [see: acetarsone]

acetphenetidin (*withdrawn from market*) [now: phenacetin]

acetphenolisatin [see: oxyphenisatin acetate]

acetrizoate sodium USP [also: sodium acetrizoate]

acetrizoic acid USP

acetryptine INN

acetsalicylamide [see: salacetamide]

acet-theocin sodium [see: theophylline sodium acetate]

aceturate USAN, INN *combining name for radicals or groups*

acetyl adalin [see: acetylcarbromal]

N-acetyl cysteine (NAC) *natural source of cysteine; promotes an increase in the endogenous antioxidant glutathione*

acetyl sulfisoxazole [see: sulfisoxazole acetyl]

l-acetyl-α-methadol (LAAM) [see: levomethadyl acetate]

p-acetylaminobenzaldehyde thiosemicarbazone [see: thioacetazone; thiacetazone]

acetylaminobenzene [see: acetanilid]

N-acetyl-p-aminophenol (APAP; NAPA) [see: acetaminophen]

acetylaniline [see: acetanilid]

acetylated polyvinyl alcohol *viscosity-increasing agent*

acetyl-bromo-diethylacetylcarbamide [see: acecarbromal]

acetylcarbromal [see: acecarbromal]

acetylcholine chloride USP, INN, BAN, JAN *cardiac depressant; cholinergic; miotic; peripheral vasodilator*

acetylcholinesterase (AChE) inhibitors *a class of drugs that alter acetylcholine neurotransmitters, used as a cognition adjuvant in Alzheimer dementia* [also called: cholinesterase inhibitors]

acetylcysteine (N-acetylcysteine) USAN, USP, INN, BAN *mucolytic inhaler; antidote to severe acetaminophen overdose (orphan)* [also: N-acetyl-L-cysteine; NAC] 10%, 20% oral

acetylcysteine sodium *mucolytic inhaler* 10%, 20% inhalation

acetyldigitoxin (α-acetyldigitoxin)
NF, INN

acetyldihydrocodeinone [see: thebacon]

N-acetyl-DL-leucine [see: acetylleucine]

acetylin [see: aspirin]

acetylkitasamycin JAN antibacterial
[also: kitasamycin; kitasamycin tartrate]

acetyl-L-carnitine (ALC; ALCAR)
natural protector of neurologic and cardiac function; biologically active amino
acid that transports fatty acids into the
cellular mitochondria for increased energy
output; acetylated form of L-carnitine

N-acetyl-L-cysteine JAN mucolytic
inhaler [also: acetylcysteine]

N-acetyl-L-cysteine salicylate [see:
salnacedin]

acetylleucine (N-acetyl-DL-leucine)
INN

acetylmethadol INN, DCF narcotic
analgesic [also: methadyl acetate]

acetyloleandomycin [see: troleandomycin]

2-acetyloxybenzoic acid [see: aspirin]

acetylpheneturide JAN [also: pheneturide]

acetylphenylisatin [see: oxyphenisatin acetate]

N-acetyl-procainamide (NAPA)
[see: acecainide HCl]

acetylpropylorvinol [see: acetorphine]

acetylresorcinol [see: resorcinol monoacetate]

acetylsal [see: aspirin]

N-acetylsalicylamide [see: salacetamide]

acetylsalicylate aluminum [see: aspirin aluminum]

acetylsalicylic acid (ASA) [now: aspirin]

acetylsalicylic acid, phenacetin &
caffeine [see: APC]

acetylspiramycin JAN macrolide antibiotic [also: spiramycin]

acetylsulfamethoxazole JAN broad-spectrum sulfonamide bacteriostatic
[also: sulfamethoxazole; sulphamethoxazole; sulfamethoxazole sodium]

N¹-acetylsulfanilamide [see: sulfacetamide]

acetyltannic acid USP

acetyltannin [see: acetyltannic acid]

acevaltrate INN

acexamic acid INN, DCF

ACFUCY (actinomycin D, fluoro-uracil, cyclophosphamide) chemotherapy protocol

AChE (acetylcholinesterase) inhibitors [q.v.]

Achillea millefolium medicinal herb
[see: yarrow]

aciclovir INN, JAN antiviral [also: acyclovir]

acid acriflavine [see: acriflavine HCl]

acid citrate dextrose (ACD) [see: anti-coagulant citrate dextrose solution]

acid histamine phosphate [see: histamine phosphate]

Acid Jelly OTC antibacterial; acidity
modifier [acetic acid; oxyquinoline
sulfate; ricinoleic acid; glycerin]
0.921%•0.025%•0.7%•5%

Acid Mantle OTC cream base

acid sphingomyelinase investigational
(orphan) agent for Niemann-Pick disease type B

acid trypaflavine [see: acriflavine HCl]

acidogen [see: glutamic acid HCl]

acidol HCl [see: betaine HCl]

acidophilus (Lactobacillus acidophilus) natural bacteria for replenishment of normal flora in the gastrointestinal tract and vagina; not generally
regarded as safe and effective as an
antidiarrheal

acidulated phosphate fluoride
(sodium fluoride & hydrofluoric
acid) dental caries prophylactic

acidum acetylsalicylicum [see: aspirin]

Acid-X tablets OTC analgesic; antipyretic; antacid [acetaminophen; calcium carbonate] 500•250 mg

acifran USAN, INN antihyperlipoproteinemic

aciglumin [see: glutamic acid HCl]

Aci-jel vaginal jelly (discontinued
2005) OTC antibacterial; acidity modifier [acetic acid; oxyquinoline sulfate;

ricinoleic acid; glycerin] 0.921% • 0.025% • 0.7% • 5%

acinitrazole BAN *veterinary antibacterial* [also: nithiamide; aminitrozole]

Aciphex enteric-coated delayed-release tablets ℞ *proton pump inhibitor for duodenal ulcers, erosive or ulcerative gastroesophageal reflux disease (GERD), H. pylori infection, and other gastroesophageal disorders* [rabeprazole sodium] 20 mg ② AcuTect

acipimox INN, BAN

acistrate INN *combining name for radicals or groups*

acitemate INN

acitretin USAN, INN, BAN *systemic antipsoriatic; retinoic acid analogue*

acivicin USAN, INN *antineoplastic*

ackee (Blighia sapida) fruit *medicinal herb for colds, fever, edema, and epilepsy; not generally regarded as safe and effective as seeds and unripened fruit are highly toxic*

aclacinomycin A [now: aclarubicin]

aclantate INN

Aclaro emulsion ℞ *hyperpigmentation bleaching agent* [hydroquinone] 4%

aclarubicin USAN, INN, BAN *antibiotic antineoplastic* [also: aclarubicin HCl]

aclarubicin HCl JAN *antibiotic antineoplastic* [also: aclarubicin]

aclatonium napadisilate INN, BAN, JAN

Aclophen long-acting tablets (discontinued 2002) ℞ *decongestant; antihistamine; analgesic* [phenylephrine HCl; chlorpheniramine maleate; acetaminophen] 40 • 8 • 500 mg

Aclovate ointment, cream ℞ *corticosteroidal anti-inflammatory* [alclometasone dipropionate] 0.05%

ACM (Adriamycin, cyclophosphamide, methotrexate) *chemotherapy protocol*

A.C.N. tablets OTC *vitamin supplement* [vitamins A, B₃, and C] 25 000 IU • 25 mg • 250 mg

Acne Lotion 10 OTC *antibacterial and exfoliant for acne* [colloidal sulfur] 10%

Acne-5 lotion, mask (discontinued 2003) OTC *keratolytic for acne* [benzoyl peroxide] 5%

Acne-10 lotion (discontinued 2003) OTC *keratolytic for acne* [benzoyl peroxide] 10%

Acno lotion OTC *acne treatment* [sulfur] 3%

Acno Cleanser topical liquid OTC *cleanser for acne* [isopropyl alcohol] 60%

Acnomel; Adult Acnomel cream OTC *acne treatment* [sulfur; resorcinol; alcohol] 8% • 2% • 11%

Acnotex lotion OTC *acne treatment* [sulfur; resorcinol; isopropyl alcohol] 8% • 2% • 20%

ACNU (1-(4-amino-2-methyl-5-pyrimidnyl)-methyl-3-(2-chloroethyl)-3-nitrosourea) [see: nimustin]

acodazole INN *antineoplastic* [also: acodazole HCl]

acodazole HCl USAN *antineoplastic* [also: acodazole]

Acomplia ℞ *investigational (NDA filed) selective cannabinoid CB-1 blocker for smoking cessation, weight loss, increasing HDL, increasing insulin sensitivity, and decreasing C-reactive protein (CRP) levels* [rimonabant]

aconiazide INN *investigational (orphan) agent for tuberculosis*

aconite (Aconitum napellus) plant and root *medicinal herb for fever, hypertension, and neuralgia; not generally regarded as safe and effective as it is highly toxic*

aconitine USP

ACOP (Adriamycin, cyclophosphamide, Oncovin, prednisone) *chemotherapy protocol*

ACOPP; A-COPP (Adriamycin, cyclophosphamide, Oncovin, procarbazine, prednisone) *chemotherapy protocol*

acortan [see: corticotropin]

Acorus calamus *medicinal herb* [see: calamus]

Acova IV infusion ℞ *anticoagulant for thrombosis due to heparin-induced* thrombocytopenia (HIT); investigational (Phase II) for myocardial infarction [argatroban] 1 mg/mL

acoxatrine INN

9-acridinamine monohydrochloride [see: aminacrine HCl]

acridinyl anisidide [see: amsacrine]

acridinylamine methanesulfon anisidide (AMSA) [see: amsacrine]

acridorex INN

acrids a class of agents that have a pungent taste or cause heat and irritation when applied to the skin

acriflavine NF

acriflavine HCl NF [also: acriflavinium chloride]

acriflavinium chloride INN [also: acriflavine HCl]

acrihellin INN

acrinol JAN [also: ethacridine lactate; ethacridine]

acrisorcin USAN, USP, INN antifungal

acrivastine USAN, INN, BAN antihistamine

acrocinonide INN, DCF

acronine USAN, INN antineoplastic

acrosoxacin BAN antibacterial [also: rosoxacin]

AcryDerm Strands wound dressing high-exudate absorbent dressing for cavitated wounds

ACT oral rinse OTC dental caries preventative [sodium fluoride; alcohol 7%] 0.05%

ACT (actinomycin) [see: cactinomycin; dactinomycin]

ACT (activated cellular therapy) [q.v.]

Actaea alba; A. pachypoda; A. rubra medicinal herb [see: white cohosh]

Actaea racemosa medicinal herb [see: black cohosh]

actagardin INN

Actagen tablets, syrup (discontinued 2002) OTC decongestant; antihistamine [pseudoephedrine HCl; triprolidine HCl] 60•2.5 mg; 30•1.25 mg/5 mL

Actagen-C Cough syrup (discontinued 2002) R narcotic antitussive; decongestant; antihistamine [codeine phosphate; pseudoephedrine HCl; triprolidine HCl] 10•30•2 mg/5 mL

actaplanin USAN, INN, BAN veterinary growth stimulant

actarit INN

ACTH powder for IM or subcu injection (discontinued 2002) R corticosteroid; anti-inflammatory [corticotropin] 40 U/vial

ACTH (adrenocorticotropic hormone) [see: corticotropin]

ACTH-80 subcu or IM injection (discontinued 2002) R corticosteroid; anti-inflammatory [corticotropin repository] 80 U/mL

Acthar powder for IM or subcu injection (discontinued 2002) R corticosteroid; anti-inflammatory [corticotropin] 25, 40 U/vial

Acthar Gel [see: H.P. Acthar Gel]

ActHIB powder for injection R infant (2–18 months) vaccine for Haemophilus influenzae type b (HIB) and invasive diseases (15–18 months) caused by HIB [Hemophilus b conjugate vaccine; tetanus toxoid] 10•24 μg/0.5 mL

ActHIB/Tripedia IM injection R pediatric vaccine for children younger than 5 months old [Hemophilus b conjugate vaccine; diphtheria & tetanus toxoids & acellular pertussis (DTaP) vaccine] 10 μg•6.7 LfU•5 LfU•46.8 μg per 0.5 mL

Acthrel IV infusion R diagnostic aid for adrenocorticotropic hormone (ACTH)-dependent Cushing syndrome (orphan) [corticorelin ovine triflutate] 100 μg

ActiBath effervescent tablets OTC moisturizer; emollient [colloidal oatmeal] 20%

Actical Plus ⓒⒶⓃ tablets OTC dietary supplement [calcium citrate; multiple minerals; vitamin D₃] 135 mg• ≛ •40 IU

Acticin cream R pediculicide for lice; scabicide [permethrin] 5%

Acticort 100 lotion R corticosteroidal anti-inflammatory [hydrocortisone] 1%

Actidose with Sorbitol oral suspension OTC *adsorbent antidote for poisoning; reduces intestinal transit time* [activated charcoal; sorbitol] 25•⸱²⸱ g/120 mL; 50•⸱²⸱ g/240 mL

Actidose-Aqua oral suspension OTC *adsorbent antidote for poisoning* [activated charcoal] 25 g/120 mL, 50 g/240 mL

Actifed Allergy daytime caplets + nighttime caplets (discontinued 2002) OTC *decongestant; (antihistamine/sleep aid added at night)* [pseudoephedrine HCl; (diphenhydramine HCl added at night)] 30 mg; 30•25 mg ⊡ Actidil

Actifed Cold & Allergy tablets OTC *decongestant; antihistamine* [pseudoephedrine HCl; triprolidine HCl] 60•2.5 mg ⊡ Actidil

Actifed Cold & Sinus caplets OTC *decongestant; antihistamine; analgesic* [pseudoephedrine HCl; chlorpheniramine maleate; acetaminophen] 30•2•500 mg

Actifed Plus caplets, tablets (discontinued 2002) OTC *decongestant; antihistamine; analgesic* [pseudoephedrine HCl; triprolidine HCl; acetaminophen] 30•1.25•500 mg ⊡ Actidil

Actifed Sinus daytime caplets + nighttime caplets (discontinued 2002) OTC *decongestant; analgesic; (antihistamine/sleep aid added at night)* [pseudoephedrine HCl; acetaminophen; (diphenhydramine HCl added at night)] 30•325 mg; 30•500•25 mg ⊡ Actidil

Actigall capsules ℞ *naturally occurring bile acid; gallstone preventative and dissolving agent* [ursodiol] 300 mg

Actimid ℞ *investigational (orphan) agent for lupus nephritis* [a-(3-aminophthalimido) glutaramide]

Actimmune subcu injection ℞ *immunoregulator for chronic granulomatous disease (orphan) and severe congenital osteopetrosis (orphan); investigational (orphan) for renal cell carcinoma; investigational (Phase III) for multi-drug-resistant pulmonary tuberculosis* [interferon gamma-1b] 100 μg (2 million IU) per 0.5 mL

actinium *element (Ac)*

actinomycin C BAN *antibiotic antineoplastic* [also: cactinomycin] ⊡ Achromycin; Aureomycin

actinomycin D JAN *antibiotic antineoplastic* [also: dactinomycin] ⊡ Achromycin; Aureomycin

actinoquinol INN *ultraviolet screen* [also: actinoquinol sodium]

actinoquinol sodium USAN *ultraviolet screen* [also: actinoquinol]

actinospectocin [see: spectinomycin]

Actiq "lollipops" ℞ *oral transmucosal narcotic analgesic for breakthrough pain in cancer patients* [fentanyl citrate] 200, 400, 600, 800, 1200, 1600 μg

Actisite periodontal fiber (discontinued 2004) ℞ *oral antibiotic for periodontitis* [tetracycline] 12.7 mg/23 cm

actisomide USAN, INN *antiarrhythmic*

Activase powder for IV infusion ℞ *tissue plasminogen activator (tPA) for acute myocardial infarction, acute ischemic stroke, or pulmonary embolism; investigational (orphan) for intraventricular hemorrhage with intracerebral hemorrhage* [alteplase] 50, 100 mg/vial (29, 58 million IU/vial)

Activase Cathflo [see: Cathflo Activase]

activated attapulgite [see: attapulgite, activated]

activated carbon

activated cellular therapy (ACT) *investigational (Phase II) agent for AIDS*

activated charcoal [see: charcoal, activated]

activated 7-dehydrocholesterol [see: cholecalciferol]

activated ergosterol [see: ergocalciferol]

activated prothrombin complex BAN

Activella tablets (in packs of 28) ℞ *hormone replacement therapy for postmenopausal symptoms* [estradiol; norethindrone acetate] 1•0.5 mg

actodigin USAN, INN *cardiotonic*

Actonel film-coated tablets ℞ *bisphosphonate bone resorption inhibitor for osteoporosis and Paget disease* [risedronate sodium] 5, 30, 35 mg ⑨
atenolol

Actonel with Calcium weekly dosepak (7 tablets) ℞ *bisphosphonate bone resorption inhibitor for osteoporosis and Paget disease; calcium supplement* [risedronate sodium; calcium] 35•0 mg × 1 tablet; 0•500 mg × 6 tablets

Actoplus Met tablets ℞ *investigational (NDA filed) combination antidiabetic agent to increase cellular response to insulin without increasing insulin secretion* [pioglitazone HCl; metformin HCl]

Actos tablets ℞ *thiazolidinedione (TZD) antidiabetic; increases cellular response to insulin without increasing insulin secretion* [pioglitazone HCl] 15, 30, 45 mg

Act-O-Vial (trademarked packaging form) *vial system*

ACU-dyne ointment, perineal wash concentrate, prep solution, skin cleanser, prep swabs, swabsticks OTC *broad-spectrum antimicrobial* [povidone-iodine]

ACU-dyne Douche concentrate OTC *antiseptic/germicidal; vaginal cleanser and deodorizer* [povidone-iodine]

Acular; Acular LS; Acular PF eye drops ℞ *nonsteroidal anti-inflammatory drug (NSAID) for allergic conjunctivitis, cataract extraction, or corneal refractive surgery* [ketorolac tromethamine] 0.5%; 0.4%; 0.5%

AcuTect ℞ *radiopharmaceutical diagnostic aid for acute venous thrombosis* [technetium Tc 99m apcitide] ② Aciphex

Acutrim 16 Hour; Acutrim Late Day; Acutrim II precision-release tablets (discontinued 2001) OTC *diet aid* [phenylpropanolamine HCl] 75 mg

AcuTrim Diet chewing gum (discontinued 2001) OTC *diet aid* [phenylpropanolamine HCl] 75 mg

acycloguanosine [see: acyclovir]

acyclovir USAN, USP, BAN *oral antiviral for herpes simplex virus type 2 (HSV-2, genital herpes), herpes zoster (shingles), and adult-onset varicella (chickenpox); prophylaxis of viral infections in immunocompromised patients* [also: aciclovir] 200, 400, 800 mg oral; 200/5 mL oral

acyclovir redox [see: redox-acyclovir]

acyclovir sodium USAN *parenteral antiviral for herpes simplex virus types 1 and 2 (HSV-1 and HSV-2), herpes simplex encephalitis, and neonatal HSV infections; prophylaxis of viral infections in immunocompromised patients* 50 mg/mL injection

acylCoA transferase (ACAT) inhibitors *a class of antihyperlipidemics that lower serum cholesterol levels*

acylpyrin [see: aspirin]

Aczone gel ℞ *antibacterial for acne* [dapsone] 5%

AD (Adriamycin, dacarbazine) *chemotherapy protocol for soft tissue sarcoma*

ad5CMV-p53 [see: adenoviral p53 gene]

ADA (adenosine deaminase) [see: pegademase bovine; pegademase]

Adacel IM injection ℞ *active immunizing agent for diphtheria, tetanus and pertussis* [diphtheria & tetanus toxoids & acellular pertussis (DTaP) vaccine, adsorbed] 2 LfU•5 LfU•2.5 µg per 0.5 mL dose

adafenoxate INN

Adagen IM injection ℞ *adenosine deaminase (ADA) enzyme replacement for severe combined immunodeficiency disease (orphan)* [pegademase bovine] 250 U/mL

Adalat capsules ℞ *antianginal; antihypertensive; calcium channel blocker* [nifedipine] 10, 20 mg

Adalat CC film-coated sustained-release tablets ℞ *antianginal; antihypertensive; calcium channel blocker* [nifedipine] 30, 60, 90 mg

Adalat XL ⓒ extended-release tablets ℞ *antianginal; antihypertensive; cal-*

cium channel blocker [nifedipine] 20, 30, 60 mg

adalimumab INN *recombinant human immunoglobulin G1 (IgG1); tumor necrosis factor-α (TNF-α) blocker; disease-modifying antirheumatic drug (DMARD) for moderate to severe rheumatoid arthritis*

adamantanamine [see: amantadine]

adamantanamine HCl [see: amantadine HCl]

adamexine INN

adapalene USAN, INN, BAN *synthetic retinoid analogue for topical treatment of acne*

Adapettes solution OTC *rewetting solution for hard contact lenses*

Adapettes Especially for Sensitive Eyes solution OTC *rewetting solution for soft contact lenses*

adaprolol maleate USAN *ophthalmic antihypertensive (β-blocker)*

adatanserin INN *anxiolytic; antidepressant* [also: adatanserin HCl]

adatanserin HCl USAN *anxiolytic; antidepressant* [also: adatanserin]

AdatoSil 5000 intraocular injection Ŗ *retinal tamponade for retinal detachment* [polydimethylsiloxane] 10, 15 mL

Adavite tablets OTC *vitamin supplement* [multiple vitamins; folic acid; biotin] ≐•400•35 μg

Adavite-M tablets OTC *vitamin/mineral/iron supplement* [multiple vitamins & minerals; iron; folic acid; biotin] ≐•27 mg•0.4 mg•30 μg

ADBC (Adriamycin, DTIC, bleomycin, CCNU) *chemotherapy protocol*

ADC with Fluoride pediatric oral drops Ŗ *vitamin supplement; dental caries preventative* [vitamins A, C, and D; fluoride] 1500 IU•35 mg•400 IU•0.5 mg per mL

Adderall tablets Ŗ *CNS stimulant for attention-deficit hyperactivity disorder (ADHD), narcolepsy, and obesity* [amphetamine aspartate; amphetamine sulfate; dextroamphetamine sulfate; dextroamphetamine saccha-rate] 5, 7.5, 10, 12.5, 15, 20, 30 mg total amphetamines (25% of each)

Adderall XR capsules containing extended-release spheres Ŗ *CNS stimulant for attention-deficit hyperactivity disorder (ADHD); once-daily doseform* [amphetamine aspartate; amphetamine sulfate; dextroamphetamine sulfate; dextroamphetamine saccharate] 5, 10, 15, 20, 25, 30 mg total amphetamines (25% of each)

adder's mouth *medicinal herb* [see: chickweed]

adder's tongue (Erythronium americanum) bulb and leaves *medicinal herb used as an emetic, antiscrofulous agent, and emollient*

ADD-Vantage (trademarked delivery system) *intravenous drug admixture system*

ADE (ara-C, daunorubicin, etoposide) *chemotherapy protocol*

Adeflor M tablets (discontinued 2004) Ŗ *pediatric vitamin deficiency and dental caries prevention* [multiple vitamins; fluoride; calcium; iron] ≐•1•250•30 mg

adefovir dipivoxil USAN *nucleotide analogue reverse transcriptase inhibitor for chronic hepatitis B virus (HBV) infection*

ADEKs chewable tablets OTC *vitamin/mineral supplement* [multiple vitamins & minerals; folic acid; biotin] ≐•200•50 μg

ADEKs pediatric drops OTC *vitamin/mineral supplement* [multiple vitamins & minerals; biotin] ≐•15 μg

adelmidrol INN

ademetionine INN

adenazole [see: tocladesine]

adenine USP, JAN *amino acid*

adenine arabinoside (ara-A) [see: vidarabine]

adeno-associated viral vector containing the gene for human coagulation Factor IX *investigational (orphan) agent for moderate to severe hemophilia*

adeno-associated viral-based vector cystic fibrosis gene therapy *investigational (orphan) for cystic fibrosis*

Adenocard IV injection ℞ *antiarrhythmic* [adenosine] 3 mg/mL

Adenoscan IV infusion ℞ *cardiac diagnostic aid; cardiac stressor; adjunct to thallium 201 myocardial perfusion scintigraphy* [adenosine] 3 mg/mL

adenosine USAN, BAN *antiarrhythmic for paroxysmal supraventricular tachycardia; diagnostic aid; investigational (orphan) for brain tumors* 3 mg/mL injection

adenosine deaminase (ADA) [see: pegademase bovine; pegademase]

adenosine monophosphate (AMP) [see: adenosine phosphate]

adenosine phosphate USAN, INN, BAN *nutrient; treatment for varicose veins and herpes infections* 25 mg/mL IM injection

adenosine triphosphate (ATP) disodium JAN

S-adenosyl-L-methionine (SAMe) *natural amino acid derivative used to treat depression and protect the liver from toxic overload; regenerates liver function and restores hepatic glutathione levels when taken with vitamins B_6, B_{12}, and folic acid*

adenoviral p53 gene *investigational (Phase III) gene therapy for head and neck cancer* [also: p53 adenoviral gene]

adenovirus-based vector Factor VIII complementary DNA to somatic cells *investigational (orphan) agent for hemophilia A*

adenovirus-mediated herpes simplex virus-thymidine kinase gene *investigational (orphan) agent for malignant glioma*

5′-adenylic acid [see: adenosine phosphate]

adepsine oil [see: mineral oil]

adhesive bandage [see: bandage, adhesive]

adhesive tape [see: tape, adhesive]

adibendan INN

A-DIC (Adriamycin, dacarbazine) *chemotherapy protocol*

adicillin INN, BAN

adimolol INN

adinazolam USAN, INN, BAN *antidepressant; sedative*

adinazolam mesylate USAN *antidepressant*

Adipex-P capsules, tablets ℞ *anorexiant; CNS stimulant* [phentermine HCl] 37.5 mg

adiphenine INN *smooth muscle relaxant* [also: adiphenine HCl]

adiphenine HCl USAN *smooth muscle relaxant* [also: adiphenine]

adipiodone INN, JAN *parenteral radiopaque contrast medium* [also: iodipamide]

adipiodone meglumine JAN *parenteral radiopaque contrast medium (49.42% iodine)* [also: iodipamide meglumine]

Adipost slow-release capsules (discontinued 2001) ℞ *anorexiant; CNS stimulant* [phendimetrazine tartrate] 105 mg

aditeren INN

aditoprim INN

Adlone injection ℞ *corticosteroid; anti-inflammatory* [methylprednisolone acetate] 40, 80 mg/mL

adnephrine [see: epinephrine]

ADOAP (Adriamycin, Oncovin, ara-C, prednisone) *chemotherapy protocol*

Adolph's Salt Substitute OTC *salt substitute* [potassium chloride] 64 mEq K/5 g; 35 mEq K/5 g

ADOP (Adriamycin, Oncovin, prednisone) *chemotherapy protocol*

adosopine INN

Adoxa film-coated tablets ℞ *tetracycline antibiotic* [doxycycline monohydrate] 50, 75, 100 mg

adozelesin USAN, INN *antineoplastic*

Adprin-B coated tablets OTC *analgesic; antipyretic; anti-inflammatory; antirheumatic* [aspirin (buffered with calcium carbonate, magnesium oxide, and magnesium carbonate)] 325, 500 mg

ADR (Adriamycin) [see: Adriamycin; doxorubicin HCl]

adrafinil INN

adrenal [see: epinephrine]

adrenal cortical steroids *a class of steroid hormones that stimulate the adrenal cortex*

Adrenalin Chloride nose drops, nasal spray ℞ *nasal decongestant* [epinephrine HCl] 0.1%

Adrenalin Chloride solution for inhalation ℞ *sympathomimetic bronchodilator* [epinephrine HCl] 1:100, 1:1000

Adrenalin Chloride subcu, IV, IM or intracardiac injection ℞ *sympathomimetic bronchodilator for bronchial asthma, bronchospasm, and COPD; vasopressor for shock* [epinephrine HCl] 1:1000 (1 mg/mL)

adrenaline BAN *vasoconstrictor; sympathomimetic bronchodilator; topical antiglaucoma agent; vasopressor for shock* [also: epinephrine] ② adrenalone

adrenaline bitartrate [see: epinephrine bitartrate]

adrenaline HCl [see: epinephrine HCl]

adrenalone USAN, INN *ophthalmic adrenergic* ② adrenaline

adrenamine [see: epinephrine]

adrenergic agonists *a class of bronchodilators that relax the bronchial muscles, reducing bronchospasm; a class of cardiac agents that increase myocardial contractility, causing a vasopressor effect to counteract shock (inadequate tissue perfusion)* [also called: sympathomimetics]

adrenine [see: epinephrine]

adrenochromazone [see: carbazochrome salicylate]

adrenochrome [see: carbazochrome salicylate]

adrenochrome guanylhydrazone mesilate JAN

adrenochrome monoaminoguanidine sodium methylsulfonate [see: adrenochrome guanylhydrazone mesilate]

adrenochrome monosemicarbazone sodium salicylate [see: carbazochrome salicylate]

adrenocorticotrophin [see: corticotropin]

adrenocorticotropic hormone (ACTH) [see: corticotropin]

adrenone [see: adrenalone]

Adria + BCNU (Adriamycin, BCNU) *chemotherapy protocol*

Adria-L-PAM (Adriamycin, L-phenylalanine mustard) *chemotherapy protocol*

Adriamycin PFS (preservative-free solution) IV injection ℞ *anthracycline antibiotic antineoplastic* [doxorubicin HCl] 2 mg/mL

Adriamycin RDF (rapid dissolution formula) powder for IV injection ℞ *anthracycline antibiotic antineoplastic* [doxorubicin HCl] 10, 20, 50, 150 mg/vial

Adria-Oncoline Chemo-Pin (trademarked delivery system)

adrogolide INN

adrogolide HCl USAN *dopamine D_1 receptor agonist for Parkinson disease*

Adrucil IV injection ℞ *antimetabolite antineoplastic for colorectal (orphan), esophageal (orphan), breast, stomach, and pancreatic cancers; investigational (orphan) for glioblastoma multiforme* [fluorouracil] 50 mg/mL

ADS (azodisal sodium) [now: olsalazine sodium]

adsorbed diphtheria toxoid [see: diphtheria toxoid, adsorbed]

Adsorbocarpine eye drops ℞ *antiglaucoma agent; direct-acting miotic* [pilocarpine HCl] 1%, 2%, 4%

Adsorbonac eye drops OTC *corneal edema-reducing agent* [sodium chloride (hypertonic saline solution)] 2%, 5%

ADT (trademarked dosage form) *alternate-day therapy*

Adult Acnomel [see: Acnomel]

Advair Diskus (powder for inhalation) ℞ *bronchodilator and corticosteroidal anti-inflammatory combination for asthma and chronic obstructive pulmonary disease (COPD)* [salmeterol xinafoate; fluticasone propionate] 50•100, 50•250, 50•500 μg

Advance test stick for home use *in vitro diagnostic aid; urine pregnancy test*

Advanced Care Cholesterol Test kit for home use *in vitro diagnostic aid for cholesterol in the blood*

"Advanced Formula" products [see under product name]

Advanced-RF Natal Care tablets ℞ *vitamin/mineral/calcium/iron supplement; stool softener* [multiple vitamins & minerals; calcium; iron; folic acid; docusate sodium] ±•200•90•1•50 mg

Advantage 24 vaginal gel OTC *spermicidal contraceptive (for use with a diaphragm)* [nonoxynol 9] 3.5%

Advate powder for injection ℞ *antihemophilic for the prevention and control of bleeding in hemophilia A* [antihemophilic factor VIII, recombinant (rAHF; rFVIII)] 250, 500, 1000, 1500 U/vial

Advera oral liquid OTC *enteral nutritional therapy for HIV and AIDS patients* [lactose-free formula] 240 mL

Advexin ℞ *investigational (Phase III) gene therapy for head and neck cancer* [p53 adenoviral gene]

Advicor caplets ℞ *combination antihyperlipidemic for hypercholesterolemia and hypertriglyceridemia* [lovastatin; extended-release niacin] 20•500, 20•1000 mg

Advil tablets, Liqui-Gels (soft liquid-filled gelatin capsules) OTC *analgesic; antiarthritic; antipyretic; nonsteroidal anti-inflammatory drug (NSAID)* [ibuprofen] 200 mg ⑦ Avail

Advil, Children's chewable tablets, oral suspension OTC *analgesic; antipyretic; nonsteroidal anti-inflammatory drug (NSAID)* [ibuprofen] 50 mg; 100 mg/5 mL

Advil, Junior Strength chewable tablets OTC *analgesic; antiarthritic; antipyretic; nonsteroidal anti-inflammatory drug (NSAID)* [ibuprofen] 100 mg

Advil Allergy Sinus tablets OTC *decongestant; antihistamine; analgesic; antipyretic* [pseudoephedrine HCl; chlorpheniramine maleate; ibuprofen] 30•2•200 mg

Advil Cold, Children's oral suspension OTC *pediatric decongestant, analgesic, and antipyretic* [pseudoephedrine HCl; ibuprofen] 15•100 mg/5 mL

Advil Cold & Sinus Liqui-gels (liquid-filled gelcaps), caplets OTC *decongestant; analgesic; antipyretic* [pseudoephedrine HCl; ibuprofen] 30•200 mg

Advil Flu & Body Ache caplets OTC *decongestant; analgesic; antipyretic* [pseudoephedrine HCl; ibuprofen] 30•200 mg

Advil Migraine liquid-filled capsules OTC *analgesic; antipyretic; nonsteroidal anti-inflammatory drug (NSAID)* [ibuprofen] 200 mg

Advil Pediatric Drops oral suspension OTC *analgesic; antipyretic; nonsteroidal anti-inflammatory drug (NSAID)* [ibuprofen] 100 mg/2.5 mL

AE-941 *investigational (Phase III) shark cartilage–based angiogenesis inhibitor for osteoarthritis, rheumatoid arthritis, and various cancers; investigational (orphan) for renal cell carcinoma*

AEDs (anti-epileptic drugs) [see: anticonvulsants]

A-E-R pads OTC *astringent* [hamamelis water] 50%

Aerius ⓒ tablets ℞ *nonsedating antihistamine for allergic rhinitis* [desloratadine] 5 mg

Aeroaid spray OTC *antiseptic; antibacterial; antifungal* [thimerosal; alcohol 72%] 1:1000

AeroBid; AeroBid-M oral inhalation aerosol ℞ *corticosteroidal anti-inflammatory for chronic asthma* [flunisolide] 250 μg/dose

AeroCaine aerosol solution OTC *local anesthetic* [benzocaine; benzethonium chloride] 13.6%•0.5%

AeroChamber (trademarked form) *aerosol holding chamber*

Aerodine aerosol (discontinued 2004) OTC *broad-spectrum antimicrobial* [povidone-iodine]

Aerofreeze spray OTC *vapo-coolant anesthetic/analgesic* [trichloromonofluoromethane; dichlorodifluoromethane]

AeroHist Plus extended-release caplets ℞ *decongestant; antihistamine; anticholinergic to dry mucosal secretions* [phenylephrine HCl; chlorpheniramine maleate; methscopolamine nitrate] 20•8•2.5 mg

AeroKid syrup ℞ *decongestant; antihistamine; anticholinergic to dry mucosal secretions* [phenylephrine HCl; chlorpheniramine maleate; methscopolamine nitrate] 10•4•125 mg/5 mL

Aerolate Sr.; Aerolate Jr.; Aerolate III timed-action capsules ℞ *antiasthmatic; bronchodilator* [theophylline] 260 mg; 130 mg; 65 mg

Aerolizer (trademarked delivery system) *oral inhaler for encapsulated dry powder*

Aeropin *investigational (orphan) for cystic fibrosis* [heparin, 2-0-desulfated]

Aeroseb-Dex aerosol spray ℞ *corticosteroidal anti-inflammatory* [dexamethasone] 0.01%

aerosol OT [see: docusate sodium]

aerosolized pooled immune globulin [see: globulin, aerosolized pooled immune]

AeroTherm aerosol solution (discontinued 2004) OTC *local anesthetic* [benzocaine; benzethonium chloride] 13.6%•0.5%

Aerotrol (trademarked form) *inhalation aerosol*

AeroZoin spray OTC *skin protectant* [benzoin; isopropyl alcohol 44.8%] 30%

AERx ℞ *investigational (Phase III) insulin inhalation system for diabetes management* [morphine sulfate]

Aesculus hippocastanum; A. californica; A. glabra *medicinal herb* [see: horse chestnut]

Aethusa cynapium *medicinal herb* [see: dog poison]

aethylis chloridum [see: ethyl chloride]

afalanine INN

Afeditab CR extended-release tablets ℞ *antianginal; antihypertensive; calcium channel blocker* [nifedipine] 30, 60 mg

Affinitac ℞ *investigational (Phase III) antisense agent for lung cancer*

afloqualone INN, JAN

AFM (Adriamycin, fluorouracil, methotrexate [with leucovorin rescue]) *chemotherapy protocol*

afovirsen INN *antisense antiviral*

afovirsen sodium USAN *antisense antiviral; investigational for genital warts*

African ginger *medicinal herb* [see: ginger]

African pepper; African red pepper *medicinal herb* [see: cayenne]

Afrin extended-release tablets (discontinued 2002) OTC *nasal decongestant* [pseudoephedrine sulfate] 120 mg ⚕ aspirin

Afrin 12-Hour Original nasal spray, pump spray OTC *nasal decongestant* [oxymetazoline HCl] 0.05% ⚕ aspirin

Afrin Children's Nose Drops (discontinued 2002) OTC *pediatric nasal decongestant* [oxymetazoline HCl] 0.025% ⚕ aspirin

Afrin Children's Pump Mist nasal spray OTC *nasal decongestant* [phenylephrine HCl] 0.25%

Afrin Moisturizing Saline Mist solution OTC *nasal moisturizer* [sodium chloride (saline solution)] 0.64% ⚕ aspirin

Afrin No-Drip 12-Hour; Afrin No-Drip 12-Hour Extra Moisturizing; Afrin No-Drip 12-Hour Severe Congestion with Menthol nasal spray OTC *nasal decongestant* [oxymetazoline HCl] 0.05%

Afrin Severe Congestion with Menthol nasal spray OTC *nasal decongestant* [oxymetazoline HCl] 0.05%

Afrin Sinus nasal spray OTC *nasal decongestant* [oxymetazoline HCl] 0.05% ⚕ aspirin

Afrin Sinus with Vapornase; Afrin No-Drip Sinus with Vapornase nasal spray OTC *nasal decongestant* [oxymetazoline HCl] 0.05%

Aftate for Athlete's Foot spray powder, spray liquid OTC *antifungal* [tolnaftate] 1%

Aftate for Jock Itch spray powder OTC *topical antifungal* [tolnaftate] 1%

afurolol INN

A/G Pro tablets OTC *dietary supplement* [protein hydrolysate; multiple vitamins & minerals; multiple amino acids] 542•≛ mg

agalsidase alfa USAN *investigational (NDA filed, orphan) enzyme replacement therapy for Fabry disease*

agalsidase beta *enzyme replacement therapy for Fabry disease (orphan)*

aganodine INN

agar NF, JAN *suspending agent*

agar-agar [see: agar]

Agathosma betulina medicinal herb [see: buchu]

agave *(Agave americana)* plant *medicinal herb used as an antiseptic, diuretic, and laxative and for jaundice and liver disease, pulmonary tuberculosis, and syphilis; also used to combat putrefactive bacteria in the stomach and intestines*

age cross-link breakers *a class of investigational antiaging compounds that break age-mediated bonds between proteins*

Agenerase capsules, oral solution ℞ *protease inhibitor antiviral for HIV infection* [amprenavir; vitamin E] 50 mg•36 IU; 15 mg•46 IU per mL

Aggrastat IV infusion ℞ *GP IIb/IIIa platelet aggregation inhibitor for acute coronary syndrome, unstable angina, myocardial infarction, and cardiac surgery* [tirofiban HCl] 50, 250 μg/mL

aggregated albumin [see: albumin, aggregated]

aggregated radio-iodinated I 131 serum albumin [see: albumin, aggregated iodinated I 131 serum]

Aggrenox dual-release capsules ℞ *platelet aggregation inhibitor for stroke* [dipyridamole (extended release); aspirin (immediate release)] 200•25 mg

Agilect ℞ *investigational (NDA filed) once-daily monoamine oxidase B (MAO-B) inhibitor for Parkinson disease* [rasagiline mesylate]

aglepristone INN

agofollin [see: estradiol]

Agoral oral liquid OTC *stimulant laxative* [sennosides] 25 mg/15 mL ② Argyrol

agrimony *(Agrimonia eupatoria)* plant *medicinal herb for diarrhea, gastroenteritis, jaundice, kidney stones, liver disorders, mucous membrane inflammation with discharge; also used topically as an astringent and antiseptic*

agrimony, hemp *medicinal herb* [see: hemp agrimony]

Agropyron repens medicinal herb [see: couch grass]

Agrylin capsules ℞ *thrombolytic and antiplatelet agent for essential thrombocytopenia (orphan); investigational (orphan) for thrombocytosis and polycythemia vera* [anagrelide HCl] 0.5, 1 mg

ague tree *medicinal herb* [see: sassafras]

agurin [see: theobromine sodium acetate]

AHA (acetohydroxamic acid) [q.v.]

AHA (alpha hydroxy acids) [see: glycolic acid]

AH-chew chewable tablets, oral suspension ℞ *decongestant; antihistamine; anticholinergic to dry mucosal secretions* [phenylephrine HCl; chlorpheniramine maleate; methscopolamine nitrate] 10•2•1.25 mg; 11•2•1.5 mg/5 mL

AH-chew D chewable tablets ℞ *nasal decongestant* [phenylephrine HCl] 10 mg

AHF (antihemophilic factor) [q.v.]

AHG (antihemophilic globulin) [see: antihemophilic factor]

A-Hydrocort IV or IM injection ℞ *corticosteroid; anti-inflammatory* [hydrocortisone sodium succinate] 100, 250, 500, 1000 mg/vial

AIDS vaccine (several different compounds are included in this general category; e.g., gp120, rgp160, rgp160 MN, rp24) *investigational (Phase I–III) antiviral for HIV and AIDS treatment and prophylaxis* [also: gp120; rgp160; rp24]

AIDSVax ℞ *investigational (Phase III) bivalent HIV vaccine* [gp120 antigens]

AIIRAs (angiotensin II receptor antagonists) [q.v.]

air, compressed [see: air, medical]

air, medical USP *medicinal gas*

Airet solution for inhalation ℞ *sympathomimetic bronchodilator* [albuterol sulfate] 0.083%

Airomir ⒸⒶⓃ *pressurized metered-dose inhaler (pMDI) with a CFC-free propellant sympathomimetic bronchodilator* [salbutamol sulfate] 100 μg/dose

Airozin ℞ *investigational leukotriene synthesis inhibitor for asthma*

AI-RSA *investigational (orphan) agent for autoimmune uveitis*

ajmaline JAN

Akarpine eye drops ℞ *antiglaucoma agent; direct-acting miotic* [pilocarpine HCl] 1%, 2%, 4%

AKBeta eye drops ℞ *antiglaucoma agent (β-blocker)* [levobunolol HCl] 0.25%, 0.5%

AK-Chlor eye drops, ophthalmic ointment ℞ *antibiotic* [chloramphenicol] 5 mg/mL; 10 mg/g

AK-Cide eye drop suspension, ophthalmic ointment (discontinued 2004) ℞ *corticosteroidal anti-inflammatory; antibiotic* [prednisolone acetate; sulfacetamide sodium] 0.5%•10%

AK-Con eye drops ℞ *decongestant; vasoconstrictor* [naphazoline HCl] 0.1%

AK-Dex eye drops (discontinued 2004) ℞ *corticosteroidal anti-inflammatory* [dexamethasone sodium phosphate] 0.1%

AK-Dilate eye drops ℞ *decongestant; vasoconstrictor; mydriatic* [phenylephrine HCl] 2.5%, 10%

AK-Fluor antecubital venous injection ℞ *ophthalmic diagnostic agent* [fluorescein] 10%, 25%

Akineton IV or IM injection ℞ *anticholinergic; antiparkinsonian* [biperiden lactate] 5 mg/mL

Akineton tablets ℞ *anticholinergic; antiparkinsonian* [biperiden HCl] 2 mg

aklomide USAN, INN, BAN *coccidiostat for poultry*

AK-NaCl eye drops, ophthalmic ointment OTC *corneal edema-reducing agent* [sodium chloride (hypertonic saline solution)] 5%

AK-Nefrin eye drops (discontinued 2003) OTC *ophthalmic decongestant* [phenylephrine HCl] 0.12%

Akne-Mycin ointment ℞ *antibiotic for acne* [erythromycin] 2% ⍰ Ak-Mycin

Akne-Mycin topical solution (discontinued 2003) ℞ *antibiotic for acne* [erythromycin] 2% ⍰ Ak-Mycin

AK-Pentolate eye drops ℞ *mydriatic; cycloplegic* [cyclopentolate HCl] 1%

AK-Poly-Bac ophthalmic ointment ℞ *antibiotic* [polymyxin B sulfate; bacitracin zinc] 10 000•500 U/g

AK-Pred eye drops ℞ *corticosteroidal anti-inflammatory* [prednisolone sodium phosphate] 0.125%, 1%

AKPro eye drops ℞ *antiglaucoma agent* [dipivefrin HCl] 0.1%

AK-Rinse ophthalmic solution OTC *extraocular irrigating solution* [sterile isotonic solution]

AK-Spore eye drops ℞ *antibiotic* [polymyxin B sulfate; neomycin sulfate; gramicidin] 10 000 U•1.75 mg•0.025 mg per mL

AK-Spore ophthalmic ointment ℞ *antibiotic* [polymyxin B sulfate; neomycin sulfate; bacitracin zinc] 10 000 U•5 mg•400 U per g

AK-Spore H.C. ear drops, otic suspension (discontinued 2004) ℞ *corticosteroidal anti-inflammatory; antibiotic* [hydrocortisone; neomycin sulfate; polymyxin B sulfate] 1%•5 mg•10 000 U per mL

AK-Spore H.C. ophthalmic ointment ℞ *corticosteroidal anti-inflammatory; antibiotic* [hydrocortisone; neomycin sulfate; bacitracin zinc; polymyxin B sulfate] 1%•0.35%•400 U/g•10 000 U/g

AK-Sulf eye drops, ophthalmic ointment ℞ *antibiotic* [sulfacetamide sodium] 10%

AKTob eye drops ℞ *antibiotic* [tobramycin] 0.3%

AK-Tracin ophthalmic ointment ℞ *antibiotic* [bacitracin] 500 U/g

AK-Trol eye drop suspension (discontinued 2004) ℞ *corticosteroidal anti-inflammatory; antibiotic* [dexamethasone; neomycin sulfate; polymyxin B sulfate] 0.1%•0.35%•10 000 U/mL

AK-Trol ophthalmic ointment ℞ *corticosteroidal anti-inflammatory; antibiotic* [dexamethasone; neomycin sulfate; polymyxin B sulfate] 0.1%•0.35%•10 000 U/g

Akwa Tears eye drops OTC *moisturizer/lubricant* [polyvinyl alcohol] 1.4%

Akwa Tears ophthalmic ointment OTC *moisturizer/lubricant* [white petrolatum; mineral oil]

ALA (alpha lipoic acid) *natural antioxidant* [q.v.]

ALA; 5-ALA HCl [see: aminolevulinic acid HCl]

alacepril INN, JAN

Alacol DM syrup ℞ *pediatric decongestant, antihistamine, and expectorant* [phenylephrine HCl; brompheniramine maleate; dextromethorphan hydrobromide] 5•2•10 mg/5 mL

Ala-Cort cream, lotion ℞ *topical corticosteroidal anti-inflammatory* [hydrocortisone] 1%

Alacramyn ℞ *investigational (orphan) antitoxin for scorpion stings* [centruroides immune Fab 2]

alafosfalin INN, BAN

Alamag oral suspension OTC *antacid* [aluminum hydroxide; magnesium hydroxide] 225•200 mg/5 mL ☒ Alma-Mag

Alamag Plus oral suspension OTC *antacid; antiflatulent* [aluminum hydroxide; magnesium hydroxide; simethicone] 225•200•25 mg/5 mL

Alamast eye drops ℞ *mast cell stabilizer for allergic conjunctivitis* [pemirolast potassium] 0.1%

alamecin USAN *antibacterial*

alanine (L-alanine) USAN, USP, INN *nonessential amino acid; symbols: Ala, A*

alanine nitrogen mustard [see: melphalan]

alanosine INN

alaproclate USAN, INN *antidepressant*

Ala-Quin cream ℞ *corticosteroidal anti-inflammatory; antifungal; antibacterial* [hydrocortisone; clioquinol] 0.5%•3%

Ala-Scalp lotion ℞ *corticosteroidal anti-inflammatory* [hydrocortisone] 2%

AlaSTAT lab test for professional use *test for allergic reaction to latex*

Alasulf vaginal cream ℞ *broad-spectrum antibiotic; antiseptic; vulnerary* [sulfanilamide; aminacrine HCl; allantoin] 15%•0.2%•2%

alatrofloxacin mesylate USAN *broad-spectrum fluoroquinolone antibiotic*

Alavert orally disintegrating tablets OTC *nonsedating antihistamine for allergic rhinitis and chronic idiopathic urticaria* [loratadine] 10 mg

Alavert Children's syrup OTC *nonsedating antihistamine for allergic rhinitis and chronic idiopathic urticaria* [loratadine] 5 mg/5 mL

Alavert D-12 Hour, Allergy & Sinus extended-release tablets OTC *nonsedating antihistamine; decongestant* [loratadine; pseudoephedrine HCl] 5•120 mg

alazanine triclofenate INN

Albalon eye drops ℞ *topical ophthalmic decongestant and vasoconstrictor and lubricant* [naphazoline HCl; polyvinyl alcohol] 0.1%•1.4%

Albamycin capsules (discontinued 2004) ℞ *bacteriostatic antibiotic* [novobiocin sodium] 250 mg

Albay subcu or IM injection ℞ *venom sensitivity testing (subcu); venom desensitization therapy (IM)* [extracts of honeybee, yellow jacket, yellow hornet, white-faced hornet, mixed vespid, and wasp venom]

albendazole USAN, INN, BAN *anthelmintic for neurocysticercosis (tapeworm) and cestode-induced hydatid cyst disease (orphan)*

albendazole oxide INN, BAN

Albenza Tiltab (film-coated tablets) ℞ *anthelmintic for neurocysticercosis (tapeworm) and cestode-induced hydatid cyst disease (orphan)* [albendazole]

Alberta Lens, The ℞ *contact lens* [sulfocon B]

Albright solution (sodium citrate and citric acid) *urine alkalizer; compounding agent*

albucid [see: sulfacetamide]

albumin, aggregated USAN *lung imaging aid (with technetium Tc 99m)*

albumin, aggregated iodinated I 131 serum USAN, USP *radioactive agent*

albumin, chromated Cr 51 serum USAN *radioactive agent*

albumin, human USP *blood volume expander for shock, burns, and hypoproteinemia* 5%, 25% injection

albumin, iodinated (¹²⁵I) human serum INN *radioactive agent; blood volume test* [also: albumin, iodinated I 125 serum]

albumin, iodinated (¹³¹I) human serum INN, JAN *radioactive agent; intrathecal imaging agent; blood volume test* [also: albumin, iodinated I 131 serum]

albumin, iodinated I 125 USP *radioactive agent; blood volume test*

albumin, iodinated I 125 serum USAN, USP *radioactive agent; blood volume test* [also: iodinated (¹²⁵I) human serum albumin]

albumin, iodinated I 131 USP *radioactive agent; intrathecal imaging agent; blood volume test*

albumin, iodinated I 131 serum USAN, USP *radioactive agent; intrathecal imaging agent; blood volume test* [also: iodinated (¹³¹I) human serum albumin]

albumin, normal human serum [now: albumin, human]

Albuminar-5; Albuminar-25 IV infusion ℞ *blood volume expander for shock, burns, and hypoproteinemia* [human albumin] 5%; 25%

Albunex injection ℞ *ultrasound heart imaging agent; investigational (Phase III) diagnostic aid for infertility due to obstructed fallopian tubes* [human albumin, sonicated] 5%

Albustix reagent strips for professional use *in vitro diagnostic aid for albumin (protein) in the urine*

Albutein 5%; Albutein 25% IV infusion ℞ *blood volume expander for shock, burns, and hypoproteinemia* [human albumin] 5%; 25%

albuterol USAN, USP *sympathomimetic bronchodilator; investigational (orphan) to prevent paralysis caused by spinal cord injury* [also: salbutamol] 42, 90 μg inhalation

Albuterol HFA inhalation aerosol with a CFC-free propellant ℞ *sympathomimetic bronchodilator* [albuterol] 90 μg/dose

albuterol sulfate USAN, USP *sympathomimetic bronchodilator* [also: salbutamol sulfate] 2, 4 mg oral; 2 mg/5 mL oral; 0.083%, 0.5% inhalation

albutoin USAN, INN *anticonvulsant*

ALC (acetyl-L-carnitine) [q.v.]

Alcaine Drop-Tainers (eye drops) ℞ *topical ophthalmic anesthetic* [proparacaine HCl] 0.5%

alcanna *medicinal herb* [see: henna (Alkanna)]

ALCAR (acetyl-L-carnitine) [q.v.]

Alcare foam OTC *topical antiseptic* [ethyl alcohol] 62%

Alchemilla xanthochlora; A. vulgaris *medicinal herb* [see: lady's mantle]

alclofenac USAN, INN, BAN, JAN *anti-inflammatory*

alclometasone INN, BAN *topical corticosteroidal anti-inflammatory* [also: alclometasone dipropionate]

alclometasone dipropionate USAN, USP, JAN *topical corticosteroidal anti-inflammatory* [also: alclometasone] 0.05% topical

alcloxa USAN, INN *astringent; keratolytic* [also: aluminum chlorohydroxy allantoinate]

Alco-Gel OTC *topical antiseptic for instant sanitation of hands* [ethyl alcohol] 60% ☑ aloe gel

alcohol USP *topical anti-infective/anti-septic; astringent; solvent; a widely abused "legal street drug" used to produce euphoria* [also: ethanol]

alcohol, dehydrated USP *antidote* [also: ethanol, dehydrated]

alcohol, diluted NF *solvent*

alcohol, rubbing USP, INN *rubefacient*

5% Alcohol and 5% Dextrose in Water; 10% Alcohol and 5% Dextrose in Water IV infusion ℞ *for caloric replacement and rehydration* [dextrose; alcohol] 5%•5%; 10%•5%

Alcon Saline Especially for Sensitive Eyes solution OTC *rinsing/storage solution for soft contact lenses* [sodium chloride (preserved saline solution)]

Alconefrin nose drops, nasal spray (discontinued 2002) OTC *nasal decongestant* [phenylephrine HCl] 0.25%, 0.5%

Alconefrin 12 nose drops (discontinued 2002) OTC *nasal decongestant* [phenylephrine HCl] 0.16%

Alcortin gel ℞ *corticosteroidal anti-inflammatory* [hydrocortisone] 2%

alcuronium chloride USAN, INN, BAN, JAN *skeletal muscle relaxant*

Aldactazide tablets ℞ *antihypertensive; diuretic* [spironolactone; hydrochlorothiazide] 25•25, 50•50 mg ⑨ Aldactone

Aldactone tablets ℞ *antihypertensive; potassium-sparing diuretic* [spironolactone] 25, 50, 100 mg ⑨ Aldactazide

Aldara cream ℞ *immunomodulator for external genital and perianal warts (condylomata acuminata), actinic keratoses, and superficial basal cell carcinoma (sBCC)* [imiquimod] 5% in 250 mg single-use packets

alder, spotted *medicinal herb* [see: witch hazel]

alder, striped *medicinal herb* [see: winterberry; witch hazel]

alder buckthorn; European black alder *medicinal herb* [see: buckthorn]

alderlin [see: pronethalol]

aldesleukin USAN, INN, BAN *immuno-stimulant; biological response modifier;* *antineoplastic for metastatic melanoma and renal cell carcinoma (orphan); investigational (Phase III, orphan) for immunodeficiency diseases and acute myelogenous leukemia (AML); investigational (Phase II) for non-Hodgkin lymphoma*

aldesulfone sodium INN, DCF *antibacterial; leprostatic* [also: sulfoxone sodium]

aldioxa USAN, INN, JAN *astringent; keratolytic*

Aldoclor-150; Aldoclor-250 film-coated tablets ℞ *antihypertensive* [chlorothiazide; methyldopa] 150•250 mg; 250•250 mg

aldocorten [see: aldosterone]

Aldomet film-coated tablets, oral suspension (discontinued 2002) ℞ *antihypertensive* [methyldopa] 125, 250, 500 mg; 250 mg/5 mL

Aldomet; Aldomet Ester HCl IV injection ℞ *antihypertensive* [methyldopate HCl] 50 mg/mL

Aldoril 15; Aldoril 25; Aldoril D30; Aldoril D50 film-coated tablets ℞ *antihypertensive; diuretic* [hydrochlorothiazide; methyldopa] 15•250 mg; 25•250 mg; 30•500 mg; 50•500 mg ⑨ Elavil; Eldepryl; Enovil; Equanil; Mellaril

aldosterone INN, BAN, DCF

Aldurazyme powder for IV infusion ℞ *enzyme replacement therapy for mucopolysaccharidosis I (MPS I) (orphan)* [laronidase] 2.9 mg/vial

Alec ℞ *investigational (orphan) agent to prevent or treat neonatal respiratory distress syndrome* [colfosceril palmitate; phosphatidylglycerol]

alefacept USAN *immunosuppressant; recombinant human LFA-3/IgG1 (leukocyte function–associated antigen, type 3/immunoglobulin G1) fusion protein for chronic plaque psoriasis*

alemcinal USAN, INN *motilin agonist to stimulate gastrointestinal peristaltic action*

alemtuzumab *humanized monoclonal antibody (huMAb) immunosuppressant for chronic lymphocytic leukemia (orphan); investigational (Phase II) for* *non-Hodgkin lymphoma, organ transplants, and multiple sclerosis*

alendronate sodium USAN *bisphosphonate bone resorption inhibitor for Paget disease and corticosteroid-induced or age-related osteoporosis in men and women; investigational (orphan) for bone manifestations of Gaucher disease and pediatric osteogenesis imperfecta*

alendronic acid INN, BAN

Alenic Alka chewable tablets OTC *antacid* [aluminum hydroxide; magnesium trisilicate] 80•20 mg

Alenic Alka oral liquid OTC *antacid* [aluminum hydroxide; magnesium carbonate] 31.7•137.3 mg/5 mL

Alenic Alka, Extra Strength chewable tablets OTC *antacid* [aluminum hydroxide; magnesium carbonate] 160•105 mg

alentemol INN *antipsychotic; dopamine agonist* [also: alentemol hydrobromide]

alentemol hydrobromide USAN *antipsychotic; dopamine agonist* [also: alentemol]

alepride INN

Alertec Ⓒⁿ tablets ℞ *analeptic for excessive daytime sleepiness of narcolepsy* [modafinil] 100 mg

Alesse tablets (in packs of 28) ℞ *monophasic oral contraceptive* [levonorgestrel; ethinyl estradiol] 100•20 μg

alestramustine INN

aletamine HCl USAN *antidepressant* [also: alfetamine]

Aletris farinosa medicinal herb [see: star grass]

Aleurites moluccana; A. cordata medicinal herb [see: tung seed]

Aleve tablets, capsules, gelcaps OTC *analgesic; antiarthritic; antipyretic; nonsteroidal anti-inflammatory drug (NSAID)* [naproxen sodium] 220 mg (=200 mg base)

Aleve Cold & Sinus; Aleve Sinus & Headache extended-release caplets OTC *decongestant; analgesic; antipyretic* [pseudoephedrine HCl; naproxen sodium] 120•220 mg

alexidine USAN, INN *antibacterial*

alexitol sodium INN, BAN

alexomycin USAN *veterinary growth promoter for poultry and swine*

alfacalcidol (1α-hydroxycholecalciferol; 1α-hydroxyvitamin D₃) INN, BAN, JAN *vitamin D precursor (converted to calcifediol in the body); calcium regulator for treatment of hypocalcemia and osteodystrophy from chronic renal dialysis*

alfadex INN

alfadolone INN, DCF [also: alphadolone]

alfalfa (Medicago sativa) leaves and flowers *medicinal herb for anemia, appetite stimulation, arthritis, atherosclerosis, blood cleansing, diabetes, hemorrhages, kidney cleansing, lowering cholesterol levels, nausea, pituitary disorders, and peptic ulcers*

alfaprostol USAN, INN, BAN *veterinary prostaglandin*

alfaxalone INN, JAN, DCF [also: alphaxalone]

Alfenta IV or IM injection ℞ *narcotic analgesic; primary anesthetic for surgery* [alfentanil HCl] 500 μg/mL

alfentanil INN, BAN *narcotic analgesic* [also: alfentanil HCl]

alfentanil HCl USAN *narcotic analgesic; primary anesthetic for surgery* [also: alfentanil] 500 μg/mL injection

Alferon LDO (low dose oral) ℞ *investigational (Phase I/II) cytokine for HIV, AIDS, and ARC* [interferon alfa-n3]

Alferon N intralesional injection ℞ *immunomodulator and antiviral for condylomata acuminata; investigational (Phase III) cytokine for HIV, AIDS, ARC, and hepatitis C* [interferon alfa-n3] 5 million IU/mL

alfetamine INN *antidepressant* [also: aletamine HCl]

alfetamine HCl [see: aletamine HCl]

alfuzosin INN, BAN *alpha₁-adrenergic blocker for hypertension and benign prostatic hyperplasia (BPH)* [also: alfuzosin HCl]

Alfuzosin tablets ℞ *anti-inflammatory for benign prostatic hyperplasia (BPH)* [leflunomide]

alfuzosin HCl USAN *alpha$_1$-adrenergic blocker for hypertension and benign prostatic hyperplasia (BPH)* [also: alfuzosin]

algeldrate USAN, INN *antacid*

algestone INN *anti-inflammatory* [also: algestone acetonide]

algestone acetonide USAN, BAN *anti-inflammatory* [also: algestone]

algestone acetophenide USAN *progestin*

algin [see: sodium alginate]

alginic acid NF, BAN *tablet binder and emulsifying agent*

alginic acid, sodium salt [see: sodium alginate]

alglucerase USAN, INN, BAN *glucocerebrosidase enzyme replacement for Gaucher disease type I (orphan); investigational (orphan) for types II and III*

alibendol INN, DCF

alicaforsen sodium USAN, INN *anti-inflammatory; antisense inhibitor of intercellular adhesion molecule 1 (ICAM-1); investigational (Phase III) injection for Crohn disease; investigational (Phase II) suppository for ulcerative colitis; investigational (Phase II) topical treatment of psoriasis*

aliconazole INN

alidine dihydrochloride [see: anileridine]

alidine phosphate [see: anileridine]

alifedrine INN

aliflurane USAN, INN *inhalation anesthetic*

alimadol INN

alimemazine INN *phenothiazine antihistamine; antipruritic* [also: trimeprazine tartrate; trimeprazine; alimemazine tartrate]

alimemazine tartrate JAN *phenothiazine antihistamine; antipruritic* [also: trimeprazine tartrate; trimeprazine; alimemazine; trimeprazine]

Alimentum ready-to-use oral liquid OTC *hypoallergenic infant food* [casein protein formula]

Alimentum Advance ready-to-use oral liquid OTC *hypoallergenic infant food with omega-3 and omega-6 fatty acids* [casein protein formula; iron; docosahexaenoic acid (DHA); arachidonic acid (AA)]

Alimta powder for IV infusion ℞ *folic acid antagonist; antineoplastic for malignant pleural mesothelioma (MPM) and non–small cell lung cancer (NSCLC)* [pemetrexed disodium] 500 mg/dose

Alinia tablets, powder for oral suspension ℞ *antiprotozoal for pediatric diarrhea due to* Cryptosporidium parvum *and* Giardia lamblia *infections* [nitazoxanide] 500 mg; 100 mg/5 mL

alinidine INN, BAN

alipamide USAN, INN, BAN *diuretic; antihypertensive*

alisactide [see: alsactide]

alisobumal [see: butalbital]

Alista cream ℞ *investigational (Phase III) treatment for female sexual arousal disorder* [alprostadil]

alitame USAN *sweetener*

alitretinoin USAN, INN *retinoic acid for topical treatment of cutaneous lesions of AIDS-related Kaposi sarcoma (orphan); investigational (Phase III, orphan) oral treatment for Kaposi sarcoma and acute promyelocytic leukemia (APL)*

alizapride INN

Alka-Mints chewable tablets OTC *antacid* [calcium carbonate] 850 mg

Alkanna tinctoria *medicinal herb* [see: henna]

Alka-Seltzer effervescent tablets OTC *antacid; analgesic* [sodium bicarbonate; citric acid; aspirin; phenylalanine] 1700•1000•325•9 mg

Alka-Seltzer, Extra Strength effervescent tablets OTC *antacid; analgesic* [sodium bicarbonate; citric acid; aspirin] 1985•1000•500 mg

Alka-Seltzer, Gold effervescent tablets OTC *antacid* [sodium bicarbonate; citric acid; potassium bicarbonate] 958•832•312 mg

Alka-Seltzer, Original effervescent tablets OTC *antacid; analgesic* [sodium

bicarbonate; citric acid; aspirin]
1916•1000•325 mg

Alka-Seltzer Plus Allergy Liqui-Gels
(liquid-filled gelcaps) (discontinued
2002) OTC *decongestant; antihistamine; analgesic* [pseudoephedrine
HCl; chlorpheniramine maleate;
acetaminophen] 30•2•250 mg

Alka-Seltzer Plus Children's Cold
effervescent tablets (discontinued
2002) OTC *antitussive; decongestant;
antihistamine* [dextromethorphan
hydrobromide; phenylpropanolamine bitartrate; chlorpheniramine
maleate] 5•10•1 mg

Alka-Seltzer Plus Cold & Cough
Liqui-Gels (liquid-filled gelcaps) OTC
*antitussive; decongestant; antihista-
mine; analgesic* [dextromethorphan
hydrobromide; pseudoephedrine
HCl; chlorpheniramine maleate;
acetaminophen] 10•30•2•325 mg

**Alka-Seltzer Plus Cold & Cough
Medicine** effervescent tablets OTC
antitussive; decongestant; antihistamine
[dextromethorphan hydrobromide;
phenylephrine HCl; chlorpheniramine maleate] 10•5•2 mg

Alka-Seltzer Plus Cold Medicine
effervescent tablets OTC *decongestant;
antihistamine; analgesic* [phenyleph-
rine HCl; chlorpheniramine maleate; acetaminophen] 5•2•250 mg

Alka-Seltzer Plus Cold Medicine
Liqui-Gels (liquid-filled gelcaps) OTC
decongestant; antihistamine; analgesic
[pseudoephedrine HCl; chlorpheniramine maleate; acetaminophen] 30•
2•325 mg

**Alka-Seltzer Plus Cold Medicine;
Alka-Seltzer Plus Cold Tablets**
for oral solution (discontinued 2001)
OTC *decongestant; antihistamine; analgesic; antipyretic* [phenylpropanol-
amine bitartrate; brompheniramine
maleate; aspirin] 20•2•325 mg;
24.08•2•325 mg

Alka-Seltzer Plus Cold & Sinus
effervescent tablets OTC *decongestant;*

analgesic; antipyretic [phenylephrine
HCl; aspirin] 5•250 mg

Alka-Seltzer Plus Cold & Sinus
Liqui-Gels (liquid-filled gelcaps) OTC
decongestant; analgesic [pseudoephed-
rine HCl; acetaminophen] 30•325 mg

**Alka-Seltzer Plus Flu & Body
Aches Non-Drowsy** Liqui-Gels
(name changed to **Alka-Seltzer
Plus Flu Medicine** in 2002)

Alka-Seltzer Plus Flu Medicine
effervescent tablets OTC *antitussive;
antihistamine; analgesic* [dextromethorphan
orphan hydrobromide; chlorpheniramine maleate; aspirin] 15•2•500 mg

Alka-Seltzer Plus Flu Medicine
Liqui-Gels (liquid-filled gelcaps) OTC
antitussive; decongestant; analgesic
[dextromethorphan hydrobromide;
pseudoephedrine HCl; acetamino-
phen] 10•30•325 mg

Alka-Seltzer Plus Night-Time Cold
Liqi-Gels (liquid-filled gelcaps) OTC
*antitussive; decongestant; antihista-
mine; analgesic* [dextromethorphan
hydrobromide; pseudoephedrine
HCl; doxylamine succinate; aceta-
minophen] 10•30•6.25•250 mg

Alka-Seltzer Plus Night-Time Cold
tablets (discontinued 2002) OTC
*antitussive; decongestant; antihistamine;
analgesic; antipyretic* [dextromethor-
phan hydrobromide; phenylpropanolamine bitartrate; doxylamine succinate; aspirin] 10•20•6.25•500 mg

**Alka-Seltzer Plus Night-Time Cold
Medicine** effervescent tablets OTC
antitussive; decongestant; antihistamine
[dextromethorphan hydrobromide;
phenylephrine HCl; doxylamine
succinate] 10•5•6.25 mg

Alka-Seltzer Plus Nose & Throat
effervescent tablets OTC *antitussive;
antihistamine; analgesic* [dextrometh-
orphan hydrobromide; chlorpheniramine maleate; acetaminophen] 10•
2•250 mg

Alka-Seltzer Plus Sinus tablets (discontinued 2002) OTC *decongestant;*

analgesic; antipyretic [phenylpropanol-
amine bitartrate; aspirin] 20•325 mg

Alka-Seltzer with Aspirin effervescent tablets OTC antacid; analgesic
[sodium bicarbonate; citric acid;
aspirin] 1900•1000•325, 1900•
1000•500 mg

**alkavervir (Veratrum viride alka-
loids)**

Alkavite extended-release tablets OTC
vitamin/mineral supplement for alcohol-
related deficiencies [multiple vitamins
& minerals; calcium carbonate; iron
sulfate; folic acid; biotin] ±•68.5•
60•1•0.03 mg

Alkeran film-coated tablets, powder
for IV infusion ℞ nitrogen mustard-
type alkylating antineoplastic for multiple myeloma (orphan) and ovarian
cancer; investigational (orphan) for
metastatic melanoma [melphalan] 2
mg; 50 mg

Alkets chewable tablets (discontinued
2005) OTC antacid [calcium carbon-
ate] 500, 750 mg

alkyl aryl sulfonate surfactant/wetting
agent

alkylade investigational (Phase III)
AGT inhibitor for brain cancer

alkylamines a class of antihistamines

**alkylbenzyldimethylammonium
chloride** [see: benzalkonium chloride]

**alkyldimethylbenzylammonium
chloride** [see: benzalkonium chloride]

alkylpolyaminoethylglycine JAN

alkylpolyaminoethylglycine HCl JAN

All Clear; All Clear AR eye drops
OTC decongestant; vasoconstrictor
[naphazoline HCl] 0.012%; 0.03%

allantoin USAN, BAN topical vulnerary;
investigational (orphan) for skin blistering and erosions associated with inherited epidermolysis bullosa

Allbee C-800 film-coated tablets OTC
vitamin supplement [multiple B vitamins; vitamins C and E] ±•800•45
mg

Allbee C-800 plus Iron film-coated
tablets OTC vitamin/iron supplement
[ferrous fumarate; multiple B vita-

mins; vitamins C and E; folic acid]
27 mg•±•800 mg•45 IU•0.4 mg

Allbee with C caplets OTC vitamin
supplement [multiple B vitamins;
vitamin C] ±•300 mg

Allbee-T tablets OTC vitamin supplement [multiple B vitamins; vitamin
C] ±•500 mg

Allegra film-coated tablets, capsules ℞
nonsedating antihistamine for allergic
rhinitis and chronic idiopathic urticaria
[fexofenadine HCl] 30, 60, 180 mg;
60 mg

Allegra 24 Hour ⓒᴬᴺ extended-release
tablets OTC nonsedating antihistamine
for allergic rhinitis [fexofenadine HCl]
120 mg

Allegra-D 12-Hour extended-release
film-coated tablets ℞ decongestant;
nonsedating antihistamine [pseudo-
ephedrine HCl; fexofenadine HCl]
120•60, 240•180 mg

allegron [see: nortriptyline]

Allent sustained-release capsules ℞
decongestant; antihistamine [pseudo-
ephedrine HCl; brompheniramine
maleate] 120•12 mg

Aller-Chlor tablets, syrup OTC antihistamine [chlorpheniramine maleate] 4
mg; 2 mg/5 mL

Allercon tablets (discontinued 2002)
OTC decongestant; antihistamine [pseu-
doephedrine HCl; triprolidine HCl]
60•2.5 mg

Allercreme Skin lotion (discontinued
2004) OTC moisturizer; emollient

Allercreme Ultra Emollient cream
(discontinued 2004) OTC moisturizer;
emollient

Allerest eye drops OTC topical ophthalmic decongestant and vasoconstrictor
[naphazoline HCl] 0.012%

Allerest tablets OTC decongestant; antihistamine [pseudoephedrine HCl;
chlorpheniramine maleate] 30•2 mg

Allerest, Children's chewable tablets
(discontinued 2001) OTC pediatric
decongestant and antihistamine [phen-
ylpropanolamine HCl; chlorpheniramine maleate] 9.4•1 mg

Allerest 12 Hour nasal spray (discontinued 2002) oTc *nasal decongestant* [oxymetazoline HCl] 0.05%

Allerest 12 Hour sustained-release caplets (discontinued 2001) oTc *decongestant; antihistamine* [phenyl-propanolamine HCl; chlorpheniramine maleate] 75•12 mg

Allerest Allergy & Sinus Relief tablets oTc *decongestant; analgesic* [pseudoephedrine HCl; acetaminophen] 30•325 mg

Allerest Headache; Allerest Sinus Pain Formula tablets (discontinued 2002) oTc *decongestant; antihistamine; analgesic* [pseudoephedrine HCl; chlorpheniramine maleate; acetaminophen] 30•2•325 mg; 30•2•500 mg

Allerest No Drowsiness tablets, caplets (discontinued 2002) oTc *decongestant; analgesic* [pseudoephedrine HCl; acetaminophen] 30•500 mg; 30•325 mg

Allerfrim film-coated tablets, syrup oTc *decongestant; antihistamine* [pseudoephedrine HCl; triprolidine HCl] 60•2.5 mg; 60•2.5 mg/10 mL

Allerfrim with Codeine syrup (discontinued 2002) R *narcotic antitussive; decongestant; antihistamine* [codeine phosphate; pseudoephedrine HCl; triprolidine HCl] 10•30•1.25 mg/5 mL

Allergan Enzymatic tablets oTc *enzymatic cleaner for soft contact lenses* [papain] 🔲 allergen; Auralgan

Allergan Hydrocare [see: Hydrocare]

Allergen Ear Drops R *topical local anesthetic; analgesic* [benzocaine; antipyrine] 1.4%•5.4%

allergenic extracts *a class of agents derived from various biological sources containing antigens that possess immunologic activity*

allergenic extracts (aqueous, glycerinated, or alum-precipitated) *over 900 allergens available for diagnosis of and desensitization to specific allergies*

Allergy tablets oTc *antihistamine* [chlorpheniramine maleate] 4 mg

Allergy Drops eye drops oTc *topical ophthalmic decongestant and vasoconstrictor* [naphazoline HCl] 0.012%; 0.03%

Allergy Relief tablets oTc *antihistamine* [chlorpheniramine maleate] 4 mg

AllerMax caplets, oral liquid oTc *antihistamine; sleep aid* [diphenhydramine HCl] 50 mg; 12.5 mg/5 mL

AllerMax Allergy & Cough Formula oral liquid (discontinued 2002) oTc *antihistamine* [diphenhydramine HCl] 6.25 mg/5 mL

Allermed capsules (discontinued 2002) oTc *nasal decongestant* [pseudoephedrine HCl] 60 mg

Allerphed syrup (discontinued 2002) oTc *decongestant; antihistamine* [pseudoephedrine HCl; triprolidine HCl] 30•1.25 mg/5 mL

AlleRx pediatric oral suspension R *decongestant; antihistamine* [phenylephrine tannate; chlorpheniramine tannate; pyrilamine tannate] 5•2•12.5 mg/5 mL

AlleRx Dose Pack controlled-release tablets (AM and PM) R AM: *decongestant, anticholinergic;* PM: *antihistamine, anticholinergic* [AM: pseudoephedrine HCl, methscopolamine nitrate; PM: chlorpheniramine maleate, methscopolamine nitrate] AM: 120•2.5 mg; PM: 8•2.5 mg

AlleRx-D controlled-release caplets R *decongestant; anticholinergic to dry mucosal secretions* [pseudoephedrine HCl; methscopolamine nitrate] 120•2.5 mg

alletorphine BAN, INN

Allfen sustained-release tablets (discontinued 2004) R *expectorant* [guaifenesin] 1000 mg

Allfen Jr. tablets R *expectorant* [guaifenesin] 400 mg

Allfen-DM sustained-release tablets R *antitussive; expectorant* [dextromethorphan hydrobromide; guaifenesin] 55•1000 mg

all-heal *medicinal herb* [see: mistletoe; valerian]

Allium cepa *medicinal herb* [see: onion]

Allium porrum *medicinal herb* [see: leek]

Allium sativum *medicinal herb* [see: garlic]

All-Nite Children's Cold/Cough Relief oral liquid OTC *antitussive; decongestant; antihistamine* [dextromethorphan hydrobromide; pseudoephedrine HCl; chlorpheniramine maleate] 15•30•2 mg/15 mL

All-Nite Cold Formula oral liquid (name changed to **All-Nite Liquid** in 2002)

All-Nite Liquid OTC *antitussive; decongestant; antihistamine; analgesic* [dextromethorphan hydrobromide; pseudoephedrine HCl; doxylamine succinate; acetaminophen; alcohol 10%] 30•60•12.5•1000 mg/30 mL

allobarbital USAN, INN *hypnotic*

allobarbitone [see: allobarbital]

alloclamide INN, DCF

allocupreide sodium INN, DCF

allomethadione INN, DCF [also: aloxidone]

allopurinol USAN, USP, INN, BAN, JAN *xanthine oxidase inhibitor for gout and hyperuricemia; antineoplastic adjunct for reducing uric acid levels following chemotherapy for leukemia, lymphoma, and solid-tumor malignancies (orphan)* 100, 300 mg oral

allopurinol riboside *investigational (orphan) agent for Chagas disease and for cutaneous and visceral leishmaniasis*

allopurinol sodium *antineoplastic adjunct for reducing uric acid levels following chemotherapy for leukemia, lymphoma, and solid tumor malignancies (orphan); investigational (orphan) for ex vivo preservation of organs for transplant* 500 mg injection

Allpyral subcu or IM injection ℞ *allergenic sensitivity testing (subcu); allergenic desensitization therapy (IM)* [allergenic extracts, alum-precipitated]

allspice (*Eugenia pimenta*; *Pimenta dioica*; *P. officinalis*) unripe fruit and leaves *medicinal herb for diarrhea and gas; also used as a purgative and tonic*

all-*trans*-retinoic acid [see: tretinoin]

allyl isothiocyanate USAN, USP

allylamines *a class of antifungals*

allylbarbituric acid [now: butalbital]

allylestrenol INN, JAN [also: allyloestrenol]

allyl-isobutylbarbituric acid [see: butalbital]

allylisopropylmalonylurea [see: aprobarbital]

4-allyl-2-methoxyphenol [see: eugenol]

N-allylnoretorphine [see: alletorphine]

N-allylnoroxymorphone HCl [see: naloxone HCl]

allyloestrenol BAN [also: allylestrenol]

allylprodine INN, BAN, DCF

5-allyl-5-*sec*-butylbarbituric acid [see: talbutal]

allylthiourea INN

allypropymal [see: aprobarbital]

Almacone chewable tablets, oral liquid OTC *antacid; antiflatulent* [aluminum hydroxide; magnesium hydroxide; simethicone] 200•200•20 mg; 200•200•20 mg/5 mL

Almacone II oral liquid OTC *antacid; antiflatulent* [aluminum hydroxide; magnesium hydroxide; simethicone] 400•400•40 mg/5 mL

almadrate sulfate USAN, INN *antacid*

almagate USAN, INN *antacid*

almagodrate INN

almasilate INN, BAN

Almebex Plus B$_{12}$ oral liquid OTC *vitamin supplement* [multiple B vitamins]

almecillin INN

almestrone INN

alminoprofen INN, JAN

almitrine INN, BAN *respiratory stimulant* [also: almitrine mesylate]

almitrine mesylate USAN *respiratory stimulant* [also: almitrine]

almokalant INN *investigational antiarrhythmic*

almond (*Prunus amygdalus*) kernels *medicinal herb used as a demulcent, emollient, and pectoral*

almond oil NF *emollient and perfume; oleaginous vehicle*

Almora tablets OTC *magnesium supplement* [magnesium gluconate dihydride] 500 mg (27 mg Mg)

almotriptan USAN, INN *vascular serotonin 5-HT$_{1B/1D/1F}$ receptor agonist for the acute treatment of migraine*

almotriptan malate USAN *vascular serotonin 5-HT$_{1B/1D/1F}$ receptor agonist for the acute treatment of migraine*

almoxatone INN

alnespirone INN

alniditan dihydrochloride USAN *serotonin 5-HT$_{1D}$ agonist for migraine*

Alnus glutinosa medicinal herb [see: black alder]

Alocril eye drops R *mast cell stabilizer for allergic conjunctivitis* [nedocromil sodium] 2%

aloe USP ☒ Alco-Gel

aloe (*Aloe vera* and over 500 other **species**) leaves and juice *medicinal herb for burns, hemorrhoids, insect bites, and scalds; also used as a deodorant and to aid digestion and limit scarring; not generally regarded as safe and effective as a cathartic*

Aloe Grande lotion OTC *moisturizer; emollient; skin protectant* [vitamins A and E; aloe] 3333.3•50•$\frac{2}{1}$ U/g

Aloe Vesta lotion OTC *emollient/protectant* [dimethicone; aloe vera gel] 3%•$\frac{2}{1}$

Aloe Vesta Perineal solution OTC *emollient/protectant* [propylene glycol; aloe vera gel]

alofilcon A USAN *hydrophilic contact lens material*

aloin BAN

ALOMAD (Adriamycin, Leukeran, Oncovin, methotrexate, actinomycin D, dacarbazine) *chemotherapy protocol* ☒ Alomide

Alomide Drop-Tainers (eye drops) R *topical antiallergic for vernal keratoconjunctivitis* (orphan) [lodoxamide tromethamine] 0.1% ☒ ALOMAD

alonacic INN

alonimid USAN, INN *sedative; hypnotic*

Alophen enteric-coated tablets OTC *stimulant laxative* [bisacodyl] 5 mg

Aloprim powder for IV infusion R *antineoplastic adjunct for reducing uric acid levels following chemotherapy for leukemia, lymphoma, and solid-tumor malignancies* (orphan); *investigational* (orphan) *for ex vivo preservation of organs for transplant* [allopurinol] 500 mg

Alor 5/500 tablets R *narcotic analgesic* [hydrocodone bitartrate; aspirin] 5• 500 mg

Alora transdermal patch R *estrogen replacement therapy for the treatment of postmenopausal symptoms and prevention of postmenopausal osteoporosis* [estradiol] 25, 50, 75, 100 μg/day

aloracetam INN

alosetron INN, BAN *antiemetic; 5-HT$_3$ receptor antagonist for irritable bowel syndrome* [also: alosetron HCl]

alosetron HCl USAN *antiemetic; 5-HT$_3$ receptor antagonist for irritable bowel syndrome (IBS)* (base=89%) [also: alosetron]

alovudine USAN, INN *antiviral*

Aloxi IV injection R *antiemetic for chemotherapy-induced nausea and vomiting (CINV)* [palonosetron HCl] 0.25 mg/5 mL

aloxidone BAN [also: allomethadione]

aloxiprin INN, BAN, DCF

aloxistatin INN

Aloysiatriphylla spp. medicinal herb [see: lemon verbena]

alozafone INN

alpertine USAN, INN *antipsychotic*

alpha amylase (α-amylase) USAN *anti-inflammatory*

alpha hydroxy acids (AHA) [see: glycolic acid]

alpha interferon-2A [see: interferon alfa-2A]

alpha interferon-2B [see: interferon alfa-2B]

alpha interferon-N1 [see: interferon alfa-N1]

alpha interferon-N3 [see: interferon alfa-N3]

Alpha Keri Moisturizing Soap bar (discontinued 2004) OTC *therapeutic skin cleanser*

Alpha Keri Spray (discontinued 2004) OTC *bath emollient*

Alpha Keri Therapeutic Bath Oil OTC *bath emollient*

alpha lipoic acid (ALA) *natural antioxidant that is both fat- and water-soluble and readily crosses cell membranes; used in the treatment of AIDS, diabetes, liver ailments, oxidative stress injuries, and various cancers*

d-**alpha tocopherol** *(relative potency: 100%)* [see: vitamin E]

dl-**alpha tocopherol** *(relative potency: 74%)* [see: vitamin E]

d-**alpha tocopheryl acetate** *(relative potency: 91%)* [see: vitamin E]

dl-**alpha tocopheryl acetate** *(relative potency: 67%)* [see: vitamin E]

d-**alpha tocopheryl acid succinate** *(relative potency: 81%)* [see: vitamin E]

dl-**alpha tocopheryl acid succinate** *(relative potency: 60%)* [see: vitamin E]

alpha₁ PI (alpha₁-proteinase inhibitor) [q.v.]

alpha₁-adrenergic blockers *a class of agents that block the alpha₁ adrenergic receptors, used for the treatment of hypertension and benign prostatic hyperplasia (BPH)* also called: antiadrenergics

alpha₁-antitrypsin (AAT), recombinant *investigational (orphan) for alpha₁-antitrypsin deficiency in the ZZ phenotype population*

alpha₁-antitrypsin, transgenic human *investigational (Phase II, orphan) for cystic fibrosis*

alpha₁-proteinase inhibitor (alpha₁ PI) *enzyme replacement therapy for hereditary alpha₁ PI deficiency, which leads to progressive panacinar emphysema (orphan)*

alphacemethadone [see: alphacetylmethadol]

alphacetylmethadol BAN, INN, DCF

alpha-chymotrypsin [see: chymotrypsin]

alpha-cypermethrin BAN

α-D-galactopyranose [see: galactose]

alpha-D-galactosidase *digestive enzyme*

alphadolone BAN [also: alfadolone]

alpha-estradiol [see: estradiol]

alpha-estradiol benzoate [see: estradiol benzoate]

alpha-ethyltryptamine (alpha-EtT) *a hallucinogenic street drug chemically related to MDMA* [see also: MDMA; alpha-methyltryptamine]

alphafilcon A USAN *hydrophilic contact lens material*

alpha-galactosidase A [see: agalsidase alfa; agalsidase beta]

agalsidase beta & ceramide trihexosidase (CTH) *investigational (orphan) enzyme replacement therapy for Fabry disease*

Alphagan eye drops (discontinued 2004) ℞ *selective α₂ agonist for open-angle glaucoma and ocular hypertension; investigational (orphan) for anterior ischemic optic neuropathy* [brimonidine tartrate] 0.2%

Alphagan P eye drops ℞ *selective α₂ agonist for open-angle glaucoma and ocular hypertension; investigational (orphan) for anterior ischemic optic neuropathy* [brimonidine tartrate] 0.15%

alpha-hypophamine [see: oxytocin]

alpha-L-iduronidase [now: laronidase]

alpha-melanocyte stimulating hormone *investigational (orphan) agent for the prevention and treatment of acute renal failure due to ischemia*

alphameprodine INN, BAN, DCF

alphamethadol INN, BAN, DCF

alpha-methyldopa [now: methyldopa]

alpha-methyltryptamine (alpha-MeT) *a hallucinogenic street drug chemically related to MDMA* [see also: MDMA; alpha-ethyltryptamine]

Alphanate powder for IV injection ℞ *antihemophilic; investigational (orphan) for von Willebrand disease* [antihemophilic factor concentrate, solvent/detergent treated]

AlphaNine SD powder for IV injection ℞ *antihemophilic for factor IX* deficiency (hemophilia B; Christmas disease) (orphan) [factor IX, solvent/detergent treated]

alpha-phenoxyethyl penicillin, potassium [see: phenethicillin potassium]

alphaprodine INN, BAN [also: alphaprodine HCl]

alphaprodine HCl USP [also: alphaprodine]

alphasone acetophenide [now: algestone acetonide]

Alphatrex cream (discontinued 2004) ℞ corticosteroidal anti-inflammatory [betamethasone dipropionate] 0.05%

Alphatrex ointment, lotion (discontinued 2003) ℞ corticosteroidal anti-inflammatory [betamethasone dipropionate] 0.05%

alphaxalone BAN [also: alfaxalone]

alpidem USAN, INN, BAN anxiolytic

Alpinia officinarum; A. galanga medicinal herb [see: galangal]

Alpinia oxyphylla; A. fructus medicinal herb [see: bitter cardamom]

Alpinia speciosa medicinal herb for edema, fungal infections, hypertension, and thrombosis

alpiropride INN

alprafenone INN

alprazolam USAN, USP, INN, BAN, JAN benzodiazepine anxiolytic; sedative; treatment for panic disorders and agoraphobia 0.25, 0.5, 1, 2 mg oral

Alprazolam Intensol oral drops ℞ benzodiazepine anxiolytic; sedative [alprazolam] 1 mg/mL

alprenolol INN, BAN antiadrenergic (β-receptor) [also: alprenolol HCl]

alprenolol HCl USAN, JAN antiadrenergic (β-receptor) [also: alprenolol]

alprenoxime HCl USAN antiglaucoma agent

alprostadil USAN, USP, INN, BAN, JAN vasodilator for erectile dysfunction; platelet aggregation inhibitor; investigational (orphan) for peripheral arterial occlusive disease; investigational (Phase III) topical treatment for female sexual arousal disorder

alprostadil, liposomal investigational (Phase III) for erectile dysfunction; investigational (orphan) for acute respiratory distress and ischemic ulcerations due to peripheral artery disease

alprostadil alfadex BAN

Alredase ℞ investigational (NDA filed) aldose reductase inhibitor for diabetic neuropathy [tolrestat]

alrestatin INN aldose reductase enzyme inhibitor [also: alrestatin sodium]

alrestatin sodium USAN aldose reductase enzyme inhibitor [also: alrestatin]

Alrex eye drop suspension ℞ corticosteroidal anti-inflammatory [loteprednol etabonate] 0.2%

alsactide INN

alseroxylon JAN antihypertensive; rauwolfia derivative

ALT-711 investigational (Phase II) anti-aging compound; reverses collagen cross-linkage formed by advanced glycation end-products (AGE)

Altace capsules ℞ angiotensin-converting enzyme (ACE) inhibitor for hypertension, myocardial infarction, CHF, and stroke [ramipril] 1.25, 2.5, 5, 10 mg

altanserin INN serotonin antagonist [also: altanserin tartrate]

altanserin tartrate USAN serotonin antagonist [also: altanserin]

altapizone INN

Altarussin syrup OTC expectorant [guaifenesin] 100 mg/5 mL

Altaryl Children's Allergy oral liquid OTC antihistamine; sleep aid [diphenhydramine HCl] 12.5 mg/5 mL

alteconazole INN

alteplase USAN, INN, BAN, JAN tissue plasminogen activator (tPA) for acute myocardial infarction, acute ischemic stroke, or pulmonary embolism; investigational (orphan) for intraventricular hemorrhage with intracerebral hemorrhage

alteratives a class of agents that produce gradual beneficial changes in the body, usually by improving nutrition, without having any marked specific effect

ALternaGEL oral liquid OTC *antacid* [aluminum hydroxide gel] 600 mg/ 5 mL

Althaea officinalis *medicinal herb* [see: marsh mallow]

althiazide USAN *antihypertensive* [also: altizide]

Alti-Amiodarone ⓒ tablets ℞ *antiarrhythmic* [amiodarone HCl] 200 mg

Alti-Amoxi Clav ⓒ tablets ℞ *aminopenicillin antibiotic* [amoxicillin; clavulanic acid] 250•125, 500•125 mg

Alti-Clindamycin ⓒ capsules ℞ *lincosamide antibiotic* [clindamycin HCl] 150, 300 mg

Alti-Clobazam ⓒ tablets ℞ *minor tranquilizer and anxiolytic; adjunct to anticonvulsant therapy* [clobazam] 10 mg

Alti-Dexamethasone ⓒ tablets ℞ *corticosteroid; anti-inflammatory* [dexamethasone] 0.5, 0.75, 4 mg

Alti-Doxazosin ⓒ tablets ℞ *antihypertensive (α-blocker)* [doxazosin mesylate] 1, 2, 4 mg

Alti-Famotidine ⓒ film-coated tablets ℞ *histamine H_2 antagonist for gastric and duodenal ulcers* [famotidine] 20, 40 mg

Alti-Flunisolide ⓒ nasal spray ℞ *corticosteroidal anti-inflammatory for chronic asthma and rhinitis* [flunisolide] 0.025% (25 μg/metered dose)

Alti-Fluoxetine ⓒ capsules ℞ *selective serotonin reuptake inhibitor (SSRI) for depression, obsessive-compulsive disorder (OCD), and bulimia nervosa* [fluoxetine HCl] 10, 20 mg

Alti-Ipratropium ⓒ nasal spray, solution for inhalation ℞ *anticholinergic bronchodilator for bronchospasm; antisecretory for rhinorrhea* [ipratropium bromide] 0.03%; 0.0125%, 0.025%

Alti-Metformin HCl ⓒ film-coated tablets ℞ *biguanide antidiabetic* [metformin HCl] 500, 850 mg

Alti-MPA ⓒ tablets ℞ *progestin for secondary amenorrhea, abnormal uterine bleeding, and endometrial hyperplasia* [medroxyprogesterone acetate] 2.5, 5, 10 mg

Altinac cream (discontinued 2004) ℞ *keratolytic for acne* [tretinoin] 0.025%, 0.05%, 0.1%

altinicline INN

altinicline maleate USAN *investigational (Phase II) nicotinic acetylcholine receptor agonist for Parkinson disease*

Alti-Nortriptylene Hydrochloride ⓒ capsules ℞ *tricyclic antidepressant* [nortriptyline HCl] 10, 25 mg

Alti-Ticlopidine ⓒ film-coated tablets ℞ *platelet aggregation inhibitor for stroke* [ticlopidine HCl] 250 mg

Alti-Timolol ⓒ eye drops ℞ *topical antiglaucoma agent (β-blocker)* [timolol maleate] 0.25%, 0.5%

altizide INN, DCF *antihypertensive* [also: althiazide]

Alti-Zopiclone ⓒ tablets ℞ *sedative; hypnotic* [zopiclone] 7.5 mg

Altocor (name changed to **Altoprev** in 2004)

Altoprev extended-release tablets ℞ *HMG-CoA reductase inhibitor for hyperlipidemia and atherosclerosis; also for primary prevention of coronary heart disease* [lovastatin] 10, 20, 40, 60 mg

altoqualine INN

Altracin *investigational (orphan) antibiotic for pseudomembranous enterocolitis* [bacitracin]

altrenogest USAN, INN, BAN *veterinary progestin*

altretamine USAN, INN, BAN *antineoplastic for advanced ovarian adenocarcinoma (orphan)*

altumomab USAN, INN *radiodiagnostic monoclonal antibody for colorectal carcinoma; anticarcinoembryonic antigen (anti-CEA)* [also: indium In 111 altumomab pentetate]

altumomab pentetate USAN *monoclonal antibody conjugate* [also: indium In 111 altumomab pentetate]

Alu-Cap capsules OTC *antacid* [aluminum hydroxide gel] 400 mg

Aludrox oral suspension OTC *antacid; antiflatulent* [aluminum hydroxide; magnesium hydroxide; simethicone] 307•103•⸮ mg/5 mL

alukalin [see: kaolin]

alum, ammonium USP *topical astringent*

alum, potassium USP *topical astringent* [also: aluminum potassium sulfate]

alum root (*Geranium maculatum*) *medicinal herb used as an astringent, hemostatic, and antiseptic*

Alumadrine tablets (discontinued 2001) ℞ *decongestant; antihistamine; analgesic* [phenylpropanolamine HCl; chlorpheniramine maleate; acetaminophen] 25•4•500 mg

alumina & magnesia USP *antacid*

aluminopara-aminosalicylate calcium (alumino *p*-aminosalicylate calcium) JAN

aluminosilicic acid, magnesium salt hydrate [see: silodrate]

aluminum *element (Al)*

aluminum, micronized *astringent*

aluminum acetate USP *topical astringent; Burow solution*

aluminum aminoacetate [see: dihydroxyaluminum aminoacetate]

aluminum ammonium sulfate dodecahydrate [see: alum, ammonium]

aluminum bismuth oxide [see: bismuth aluminate]

aluminum carbonate, basic USAN, USP *antacid*

aluminum chlorhydroxide [now: aluminum chlorohydrate]

aluminum chlorhydroxide alcohol soluble complex [now: aluminum chlorohydrex]

aluminum chloride USP *topical astringent for hyperhidrosis* 20% topical

aluminum chloride, basic [see: aluminum sesquichlorohydrate]

aluminum chloride hexahydrate [see: aluminum chloride]

aluminum chloride hydroxide hydrate [see: aluminum chlorohydrate]

aluminum chlorohydrate USAN *anhidrotic*

aluminum chlorohydrex USAN *topical astringent*

aluminum chlorohydrol propylene glycol complex [now: aluminum chlorohydrex]

aluminum chlorohydroxy allantoinate JAN *astringent; keratolytic* [also: alcloxa]

aluminum clofibrate INN, BAN, JAN

aluminum dihydroxyaminoacetate [see: dihydroxyaluminum aminoacetate]

aluminum flufenamate JAN

aluminum glycinate, basic [see: dihydroxyaluminum aminoacetate]

aluminum hydroxide gel USP *antacid* 320, 450, 600 mg/5 mL oral

aluminum hydroxide gel, dried USP, JAN *antacid*

aluminum hydroxide glycine [see: dihydroxyaluminum aminoacetate]

aluminum hydroxide hydrate [see: algeldrate]

aluminum hydroxychloride [now: aluminum chlorohydrate]

aluminum magnesium carbonate hydroxide dihydrate [see: almagate]

aluminum magnesium hydroxide carbonate hydrate [see: hydrotalcite]

aluminum magnesium hydroxide oxide sulfate [see: almadrate sulfate]

aluminum magnesium hydroxide oxide sulfate hydrate [see: almadrate sulfate]

aluminum magnesium hydroxide sulfate [see: magaldrate]

aluminum magnesium hydroxide sulfate hydrate [see: magaldrate]

aluminum monostearate NF, JAN

aluminum oxide

Aluminum Paste ointment OTC *occlusive skin protectant* [metallic aluminum] 10%

aluminum phosphate gel USP *antacid* (*disapproved for use as an antacid in 1989*)

aluminum potassium sulfate JAN *topical astringent* [also: alum, potassium]

aluminum potassium sulfate dodecahydrate [see: alum, potassium]

aluminum sesquichlorohydrate USAN *anhidrotic*

aluminum silicate, natural JAN

aluminum silicate, synthetic JAN

aluminum sodium carbonate hydroxide [see: dihydroxyaluminum sodium carbonate]

aluminum subacetate USP *topical astringent*

aluminum sulfate USP *anhidrotic*

aluminum sulfate hydrate [see: aluminum sulfate]

aluminum zirconium glycine tetrachloro hydrate complex [see: aluminum zirconium tetrachlorohydrex gly]

aluminum zirconium glycine trichloro hydrate complex [see: aluminum zirconium trichlorohydrex gly]

aluminum zirconium octachlorohydrate USP *anhidrotic*

aluminum zirconium octachlorohydrex gly USP *anhidrotic*

aluminum zirconium pentachlorohydrate USP *anhidrotic*

aluminum zirconium pentachlorohydrex gly USP *anhidrotic*

aluminum zirconium tetrachlorohydrate USP *anhidrotic*

aluminum zirconium tetrachlorohydrex gly USAN, USP *anhidrotic*

aluminum zirconium trichlorohydrate USP *anhidrotic*

aluminum zirconium trichlorohydrex gly USAN, USP *anhidrotic*

Alupent inhalation aerosol powder, solution for inhalation ℞ *sympathomimetic bronchodilator* [metaproterenol sulfate] 0.65 mg/dose; 0.4%, 0.6%, 5%

Alupent syrup (discontinued 2001) ℞ *sympathomimetic bronchodilator* [metaproterenol sulfate] 10 mg/5 mL

Alurate elixir (discontinued 2004) ℞ *sedative; hypnotic* [aprobarbital] 40 mg/5 mL

Alustra cream ℞ *hyperpigmentation bleaching agent* [hydroquinone; tretinoin (in a base containing glycolic acid and vitamins C and E)] 4%•0.1% ⊡ Lustra

alusulf INN

Alu-Tab film-coated tablets OTC *antacid* [aluminum hydroxide gel] 500 mg

ALVAC-120TMG *investigational (Phase II) vaccine for HIV* [also: VCP 205]

alvameline INN

alverine INN, BAN *anticholinergic* [also: alverine citrate]

alverine citrate USAN, NF *anticholinergic* [also: alverine]

Alvesco (approved in Europe) ℞ *investigational (NDA filed) inhaled corticosteroid for persistent asthma* [ciclesonide]

alvimopan *investigational (NDA filed) narcotic analgesic; opioid receptor antagonist*

alvircept sudotox USAN, INN *antiviral; investigational (Phase II) for AIDS*

Alwextin ℞ *investigational (orphan) topical vulnerary for skin blistering and erosions associated with inherited epidermolysis bullosa* [allantoin]

Alzhemed ℞ *investigational (Phase III) amyloid protein–binding agent for Alzheimer disease*

AM Caps ⊛ OTC *vitamin supplement* [multiple vitamins; folic acid; biotin] ±•0.2•0.15 mg

amabevan [see: carbarsone]

amacetam HCl [now: pramiracetam HCl]

amacetam sulfate [now: pramiracetam sulfate]

amadinone INN *progestin* [also: amadinone acetate]

amadinone acetate USAN *progestin* [also: amadinone]

amafolone INN, BAN

amalgucin

Amanita muscaria **mushrooms** *a species that produces muscarine and ibotenic acid, a psychotropic substance ingested as a street drug*

amanozine INN

amantadine INN, BAN *antiviral for influenza A virus; dopaminergic antiparkinson agent* [also: amantadine HCl]

amantadine HCl USAN, USP, JAN *antiviral for influenza A infections; dopamin-*

ergic antiparkinson agent [also: amantadine] 100 mg oral; 50 mg/5 mL oral

amantanium bromide INN

amantocillin INN

amara; amargo *medicinal herb* [see: quassia]

amaranth (*Amnaranthus* spp.) leaves and flowers *medicinal herb for diarrhea, dysentery, excessive menstruation, and nosebleeds*

amaranth (FD&C Red No. 2) USP

amargo; amara *medicinal herb* [see: quassia]

amarsan [see: acetarsone]

Amaryl tablets ℞ *once-daily sulfonylurea antidiabetic* [glimepiride] 1, 2, 4 mg ⊘ Reminyl

ambamustine INN

ambasilide INN *investigational antiarrhythmic*

ambazone INN, BAN, DCF

ambenonium chloride USP, INN, BAN, JAN *anticholinesterase muscle stimulant*

ambenoxan INN, BAN

Ambenyl Cough syrup (discontinued 2002) ℞ *narcotic antitussive; antihistamine* [codeine phosphate; bromodiphenhydramine HCl; alcohol 5%] 10•12.5 mg/5 mL ⊘ Aventyl

Ambenyl-D oral liquid (discontinued 2002) OTC *antitussive; decongestant; expectorant* [dextromethorphan hydrobromide; pseudoephedrine HCl; guaifenesin; alcohol 9.5%] 10•30•100 mg/5 mL

amber; amber touch-and-heal *medicinal herb* [see: St. John wort]

Ambi 10 bar OTC *therapeutic skin cleanser*

Ambi 10 cream (discontinued 2003) OTC *keratolytic for acne* [benzoyl peroxide] 10%

Ambi 60/580 caplets ℞ *decongestant; expectorant* [pseudoephedrine HCl; guaifenesin] 60•580 mg

Ambi 60/580/30 extended-release caplets ℞ *decongestant; expectorant; antitussive* [pseudoephedrine HCl;

guaifenesin; dextromethorphan hydrobromide] 60•580•30 mg

Ambi 600; Ambi 800; Ambi 1000; Ambi 1200 sustained-release caplets (discontinued 2004) ℞ *expectorant* [guaifenesin] 600 mg; 800 mg; 1000 mg; 1200 mg

Ambi 1000/55 extended-release tablets ℞ *expectorant; antitussive* [guaifenesin; dextromethorphan hydrobromide] 1000•55 mg

Ambi Skin Tone cream (discontinued 2003) OTC *hyperpigmentation bleaching agent* [hydroquinone (in a sunscreen base)]

ambicromil INN, BAN *prophylactic antiallergic* [also: probicromil calcium]

ambicromil calcium [see: probicromil calcium]

Ambien film-coated tablets ℞ *imidazopyridine sedative and hypnotic* [zolpidem tartrate] 5, 10 mg

Ambien CR controlled-release bilayered tablets ℞ *imidazopyridine sedative and hypnotic* [zolpidem tartrate] 6.25, 12.5 mg

AmBisome powder for IV infusion ℞ *systemic polyene antifungal for cryptococcal meningitis, visceral leishmaniasis, and histoplasmosis (orphan)* [amphotericin B lipid complex (ABLC)] 50 mg/vial

ambomycin USAN, INN *antineoplastic*

ambrette (*Abelmoschus moschatus*) seeds and oil *medicinal herb for gastric cancer, gonorrhea, hysteria, and respiratory disorders; also used as a fragrance in cosmetics and a flavoring in alcoholic beverages, bitters, and coffees; not generally regarded as safe and effective for medicinal uses*

ambroxol INN [also: ambroxol HCl]

ambroxol HCl JAN [also: ambroxol]

ambruticin USAN, INN *antifungal*

ambucaine INN, DCF

ambucetamide INN, BAN

ambuphylline USAN *diuretic; smooth muscle relaxant* [also: bufylline]

ambuside USAN, INN, BAN *diuretic*

ambuterol [see: mabuterol]

ambutonium bromide BAN
ambutoxate [see: ambucaine]
amcinafal USAN, INN *anti-inflammatory*
amcinafide USAN, INN *anti-inflammatory*
amcinonide USAN, USP, INN, BAN, JAN
topical corticosteroidal anti-inflammatory 0.1% topical
Amcort IM injection ℞ *corticosteroid; anti-inflammatory* [triamcinolone diacetate] 40 mg/mL
amdinocillin USAN, USP *aminopenicillin antibiotic* [also: mecillinam]
amdinocillin pivoxil USAN *antibacterial* [also: pivmecillinam; pivmecillinam HCl]
amdoxovir USAN *investigational (Phase II) nucleoside analog antiviral for HIV-1 and hepatitis B infections*
Amdray IV infusion, oral solution, capsules ℞ *investigational (Phase III) P-glycoprotein (P-gp) inhibitor for multi-drug–resistant (MDR) cancers, including acute myelogenous leukemia (AML), multiple myeloma, and ovarian cancer* [valspodar]
ameban [see: carbarsone]
amebarsone [see: carbarsone]
amebicides *a class of drugs that kill amoebae*
amebucort INN
amechol [see: methacholine chloride]
amedalin INN *antidepressant* [also: amedalin HCl]
amedalin HCl USAN *antidepressant* [also: amedalin]
amediplase INN
ameltolide USAN, INN, BAN *anticonvulsant*
Amen tablets (discontinued 2004) ℞ *synthetic progestin for secondary amenorrhea, abnormal uterine bleeding, and endometrial hyperplasia* [medroxyprogesterone acetate] 10 mg
amenozine [see: amanozine]
Amerge film-coated tablets ℞ *vascular serotonin 5-HT$_{1D}$ receptor agonist for the acute treatment of migraine* [naratriptan HCl] 1, 2.5 mg

Americaine ointment, anorectal ointment, aerosol spray OTC *topical local anesthetic* [benzocaine] 20%
Americaine Anesthetic Lubricant gel ℞ *anesthetic lubricant for upper GI procedures* [benzocaine] 20%
Americaine First Aid ointment OTC *topical local anesthetic* [benzocaine] 20%
Americaine Otic ear drops (discontinued 2004) ℞ *local anesthetic* [benzocaine] 20%
American angelica *medicinal herb* [see: angelica]
American aspen *medicinal herb* [see: poplar]
American centaury (Sabatia angularis) plant *medicinal herb used as a bitter tonic, emmenagogue, febrifuge, and vermifuge*
American elder *medicinal herb* [see: elderberry]
American elm *medicinal herb* [see: slippery elm]
American foxglove *medicinal herb* [see: feverweed]
American ginseng (Panax quinquefolia) *medicinal herb* [see: ginseng]
American hellebore (Veratrum viride) [see: hellebore]
American ivy (Parthenocissus quinquefolia) bark and twigs *medicinal herb used as an alterative, astringent, and expectorant*
American nightshade *medicinal herb* [see: pokeweed]
American pepper; American red pepper *medicinal herb* [see: cayenne]
American saffron *medicinal herb* [see: safflower]
American valerian *medicinal herb* [see: lady's slipper]
American vegetable tallow tree; American vegetable wax *medicinal herb* [see: bayberry]
American woodbine *medicinal herb* [see: American ivy]
Americet tablets ℞ *analgesic; barbiturate sedative* [aspirin; caffeine; butalbital] 325•40•50 mg

americium *element (Am)*

Amerifed oral liquid OTC *pediatric decongestant and antihistamine* [pseudoephedrine HCl; chlorpheniramine maleate] 80•4 mg/5 mL

Amerigel lotion, ointment OTC *emollient; diaper rash treatment*

Amerituss AD oral liquid ℞ *pediatric decongestant, antihistamine, and expectorant* [phenylephrine HCl; chlorpheniramine maleate; dextromethorphan hydrobromide] 10•3•15 mg/5 mL

amesergide USAN, INN *serotonin antagonist; investigational antidepressant*

ametantrone INN *antineoplastic* [also: ametantrone acetate]

ametantrone acetate USAN *antineoplastic* [also: ametantrone]

ametazole BAN [also: betazole HCl; betazole]

A•Methapred powder for injection ℞ *corticosteroid; anti-inflammatory; immunosuppressant* [methylprednisolone sodium succinate] 40, 125, 500, 1000 mg/vial

amethocaine BAN *topical anesthetic* [also: tetracaine]

amethocaine HCl BAN *local anesthetic* [also: tetracaine HCl]

amethopterin [now: methotrexate]

Amevive powder for IV or IM injection ℞ *immunosuppressant for chronic plaque psoriasis* [alefacept] 7.5 mg/dose IV, 15 mg/dose IM

amezepine INN

amezinium metilsulfate INN, JAN

amfebutamone INN *aminoketone antidepressant; non-nicotine aid to smoking cessation* [also: bupropion HCl; bupropion]

amfebutamone HCl [see: bupropion HCl]

amfecloral INN, BAN *anorectic* [also: amphecloral]

amfenac INN, BAN *anti-inflammatory* [also: amfenac sodium]

amfenac sodium USAN, JAN *anti-inflammatory* [also: amfenac]

amfepentorex INN, DCF

amfepramone INN, DCF *anorexiant* [also: diethylpropion HCl; diethylpropion]

amfepramone HCl *anorexiant* [see: diethylpropion HCl]

amfetamine INN *CNS stimulant* [also: amphetamine sulfate; amphetamine]

amfetaminil INN

amfilcon A USAN *hydrophilic contact lens material*

amflutizole USAN, INN *gout suppressant*

amfodyne [see: imidecyl iodine]

amfomycin INN, DCF *antibacterial* [also: amphomycin]

amfonelic acid USAN, INN, BAN *CNS stimulant*

AMG 531 *investigational (Phase III, orphan) platelet growth factor for immune thrombocytopenic purpura*

AMG 706 *investigational (Phase II) multikinase inhibitor (MKI) for advanced gastrointestinal stromal tumors (GISTs)*

Amgenal Cough syrup (discontinued 2002) ℞ *narcotic antitussive; antihistamine* [codeine phosphate; bromodiphenhydramine HCl] 10•12.5 mg/5 mL

amibiarson [see: carbarsone]

Amicar tablets, syrup, IV infusion ℞ *systemic hemostatic to control excessive bleeding* [aminocaproic acid] 500, 1000 mg; 250 mg/mL; 250 mg/mL ⊘ Amikin

amicarbalide INN, BAN

amicibone INN

amicloral USAN *veterinary food additive*

amicycline USAN, INN *antibacterial*

amidantel INN, BAN

amidapsone USAN, INN *antiviral for poultry*

Amidate IV injection ℞ *rapid-acting nonbarbiturate general anesthetic* [etomidate] 2 mg/mL

amidefrine mesilate INN *adrenergic* [also: amidephrine mesylate; amidephrine]

amidephrine BAN *adrenergic* [also: amidephrine mesylate; amidefrine mesilate]

amidephrine mesylate USAN *adrenergic* [also: amidefrine mesilate; amidephrine]

amidofebrin [see: aminopyrine]

amidol [see: dimepheptanol]

amidone HCl [see: methadone HCl]

amidopyrazoline [see: aminopyrine]

amidopyrine [now: aminopyrine]

amidotrizoate sodium [see: diatrizoate sodium]

amidotrizoic acid JAN *radiopaque contrast medium* [also: diatrizoic acid]

amiflamine INN

amifloverine INN, DCF

amifloxacin USAN, INN, BAN *broadspectrum fluoroquinolone antibiotic*

amifloxacin mesylate USAN *broadspectrum fluoroquinolone antibiotic*

amifostine USAN, INN, BAN *chemoprotective agent for cisplatin and paclitaxel chemotherapy (orphan); investigational (orphan) for cyclophosphamide; treatment for moderate to severe xerostomia following postoperative radiation therapy (orphan)*

Amigesic film-coated tablets, film-coated caplets, capsules ℞ *analgesic; antipyretic; anti-inflammatory; antirheumatic* [salsalate] 500 mg; 750 mg; 500 mg

amiglumide INN

amikacin USP, INN, BAN *aminoglycoside antibiotic; investigational (Phase II) liposomal formulation for complicated urinary tract infections and AIDS-related Mycobacterial infection*

amikacin sulfate USAN, USP, JAN *aminoglycoside antibiotic* 50, 250 mg/mL injection

amikhelline INN

Amikin IV or IM injection, pediatric injection ℞ *aminoglycoside antibiotic* [amikacin sulfate] 250 mg/mL; 50 mg/mL ☑ Amicar

amilomer INN

amiloride INN, BAN *antihypertensive; potassium-sparing diuretic* [also: amiloride HCl]

amiloride HCl USAN, USP *antihypertensive; potassium-sparing diuretic;* investigational (orphan) inhalant for cystic fibrosis [also: amiloride]

amiloxate USAN *ultraviolet B sunscreen*

aminacrine BAN *topical anti-infective/antiseptic* [also: aminacrine HCl; aminoacridine]

aminacrine HCl USAN *vaginal antibacterial and antiseptic* [also: aminoacridine; aminacrine]

aminarsone [see: carbarsone]

amindocate INN

amine resin [see: polyamine-methylene resin]

amineptine INN

Aminess 5.2% IV infusion ℞ *nutritional therapy for renal failure* [multiple essential amino acids]

Aminess N film-coated tablets ℞ *nutritional therapy for dialysis patients* [multiple essential amino acids]

aminicotin [see: niacinamide]

aminitrozole INN *veterinary antibacterial* [also: nithiamide; acinitrazole]

2-amino-2-deoxyglucose [see: glucosamine]

aminoacetic acid JAN *nonessential amino acid; urologic irrigant; symbols: Gly, G* [also: glycine]

aminoacridine INN *topical anti-infective/antiseptic* [also: aminacrine HCl; aminacrine]

aminoacridine HCl [see: aminacrine HCl]

9-aminoacridine monohydrochloride [see: aminacrine HCl]

***p*-aminobenzenearsonic acid** [see: arsanilic acid]

***p*-aminobenzenesulfonamide** [see: sulfanilamide]

***p*-aminobenzene-sulfonylacetylimide** [see: sulfacetamide]

aminobenzoate potassium USP *water-soluble vitamin; analgesic; "possibly effective" for scleroderma and other skin diseases and Peyronie disease* 500 mg oral

aminobenzoate sodium USP *analgesic*

***p*-aminobenzoic acid** [see: aminobenzoic acid]

aminobenzoic acid (4-aminobenzoic acid) USP *water-soluble vitamin; ultraviolet screen*

aminobenzylpenicillin [see: ampicillin]

γ-amino-β-hydroxybutyric acid JAN

aminobromophenylpyrimidinone (ABPP) [see: bropirimine]

γ-aminobutyric acid (GABA) JAN *inhibitory neurotransmitter*

aminocaproic acid USAN, USP, INN, BAN *systemic hemostatic; investigational (orphan) topical treatment for traumatic hyphema of the eye* [also: ε-aminocaproic acid] 250 mg oral; 250 mg/mL oral; 250 mg/mL injection

ε-aminocaproic acid JAN *systemic hemostatic* [also: aminocaproic acid]

aminocardol [see: aminophylline]

Amino-Cerv pH 5.5 vaginal cream ℞ *emollient; antifungal; anti-inflammatory* [urea; sodium propionate; methionine; cystine; inositol] 8.34%•0.5%•0.83%•0.35%•0.83%

aminodeoxykanamycin [see: bekanamycin]

2-aminoethanethiol [see: cysteamine]

2-aminoethanethiol HCl [see: cysteamine HCl]

2-aminoethanol [see: monoethanolamine]

aminoethyl nitrate (2-aminoethyl nitrate) INN, DCF

amino-ethyl-propanol [see: ambuphylline]

aminoethylsulfonic acid JAN [also: taurine]

aminoform [see: methenamine]

2-aminoglutaramic acid [see: glutamine]

aminoglutethimide USP, INN, BAN *adrenal steroid inhibitor; antisteroidal antineoplastic*

aminoglycosides *a class of bactericidal antibiotics effective against gram-negative organisms* [also called: "mycins"]

aminoguanidine monohydrochloride [see: pimagedine HCl]

6-aminohexanoic acid [see: aminocaproic acid]

aminohippurate sodium USP *diagnostic aid for renal function* [also: p-aminohippurate sodium] 20% injection

p-aminohippurate sodium JAN *renal function test* [also: aminohippurate sodium]

aminohippuric acid (p-aminohippuric acid) USP

aminohydroxypropylidene diphosphonate (APD) [see: pamidronate disodium]

aminoisobutanol [see: ambuphylline]

3-(4′-aminoisoindoline-1′-one)-1-piperidine-2,6-dione *investigational (orphan) for multiple myeloma*

aminoisometradine [see: methionine]

aminoketones *a class of oral antidepressants*

5-aminolevulinic acid HCl (5-ALA HCl) USAN *photosensitizer for photodynamic therapy of precancerous actinic keratoses of the face and scalp (for use with the BLU-U Blue Light Photodynamic Therapy Illuminator)*

aminometradine INN, BAN

Amino-Min-D capsules OTC *dietary supplement* [calcium carbonate; multiple minerals; vitamin D] 250 mg• ≜ •100 IU

aminonat [see: protein hydrolysate]

Amino-Opti-C sustained-release tablets OTC *vitamin C supplement with multiple bioflavonoids* [vitamin C; rose hips; lemon bioflavonoids; rutin; hesperidin] 1000• ≜ •250• ≜ • ≜ mg

aminopenicillins *a subclass of penicillins (q.v.)*

aminopentamide sulfate [see: dimevamide]

aminophenazone INN [also: aminopyrine]

aminophenazone cyclamate INN

p-aminophenylarsonic acid [see: arsanilic acid]

aminophylline USP, INN, BAN, JAN *smooth muscle relaxant; bronchodilator* 100, 200 mg oral; 105 mg/5 mL oral; 250 mg/10 mL injection; 250, 500 suppositories

aminopromazine INN, DCF [also: proquamezine]

aminopterin sodium INN, BAN, DCF *investigational (Phase II) antifolate for breast and ovarian cancer*

4-aminopyridine [see: fampridine]

aminopyrine NF, JAN [also: aminophenazone]

aminoquin naphthoate [see: pamaquine naphthoate]

aminoquinol INN

aminoquinoline [see: aminoquinol]

4-aminoquinoline [see: chloroquine phosphate]

8-aminoquinoline [see: primaquine phosphate]

aminoquinuride INN

aminorex USAN, INN, BAN *anorectic*

aminosalicylate calcium USP [also: calcium para-aminosalicylate]

aminosalicylate potassium USP

aminosalicylate sodium (*p*-aminosalicylate sodium) USP *bacteriostatic; tuberculosis retreatment agent; investigational (orphan) for Crohn disease*

aminosalicylic acid (4-aminosalicylic acid) USP *antibacterial; tuberculostatic (orphan); investigational (orphan) for ulcerative colitis*

5-aminosalicylic acid (5-ASA) [see: mesalamine]

aminosalyle sodium [see: aminosalicylate sodium]

aminosidine *investigational (orphan) agent for tuberculosis,* Mycobacterium avium *complex (MAC), and visceral leishmaniasis*

aminosidine sulfate [see: paromomycin sulfate]

21-aminosteroids *a class of potent antioxidants that can protect against oxygen radical–mediated lipid peroxidation and progressive neuronal degeneration following brain or spinal trauma, subarachnoid hemorrhage, or stroke* [also called: lazaroids]

aminosuccinic acid [see: aspartic acid]

Aminosyn 3.5% (5%, 7%, 8.5%, 10%); Aminosyn (pH6) 10%; Aminosyn II 3.5% (5%, 7%, 8.5%, 10%, 15%); **Aminosyn-PF 7% (10%)** IV infusion ℞ *total parenteral nutrition (except 3.5%); peripheral parenteral nutrition (all)* [multiple essential and nonessential amino acids]

Aminosyn 3.5% M; Aminosyn II 3.5% M IV infusion ℞ *peripheral parenteral nutrition* [multiple essential and nonessential amino acids; electrolytes]

Aminosyn 7% (8.5%) with Electrolytes; Aminosyn II 7% (8.5%, 10%) with Electrolytes IV infusion ℞ *total parenteral nutrition; peripheral parenteral nutrition* [multiple essential and nonessential amino acids; electrolytes]

Aminosyn II 3.5% in 5% (25%) Dextrose; Aminosyn II 4.25% in 10% (20%, 25%) Dextrose; Aminosyn II 5% in 25% Dextrose IV infusion ℞ *total parenteral nutrition (except 3.5% in 5%); peripheral parenteral nutrition (not 20% and 25%)* [multiple essential and nonessential amino acids; dextrose]

Aminosyn II 3.5% M in 5% Dextrose; Aminosyn II 4.25% M in 10% Dextrose IV infusion ℞ *total parenteral nutrition (4.25% in 10% only); peripheral parenteral nutrition (both)* [multiple essential and nonessential amino acids; electrolytes; dextrose]

Aminosyn-HBC 7% IV infusion ℞ *nutritional therapy for high metabolic stress* [multiple branched-chain essential and nonessential amino acids; electrolytes]

Aminosyn-RF 5.2% IV infusion ℞ *nutritional therapy for renal failure* [multiple essential amino acids]

aminothiazole INN

aminotrate phosphate [see: trolnitrate phosphate]

aminoxaphen [see: aminorex]

Aminoxin enteric-coated tablets OTC *vitamin B_6 supplement* [pyridoxal-5′-phosphate] 20 mg

aminoxytriphene INN

aminoxytropine tropate HCl [see: atropine oxide HCl]

Amio-Aqueous ℞ *investigational (orphan) antiarrhythmic for incessant ventricular tachycardia* [amiodarone]

amiodarone USAN, INN, BAN *investigational (orphan) ventricular antiarrhythmic for incessant ventricular tachycardia*

amiodarone HCl *ventricular antiarrhythmic for acute ventricular tachycardia and fibrillation (orphan)* 200 mg oral; 50 mg/mL injection

amiperone INN

amiphenazole INN, BAN

amipizone INN

amipramidine [see: amiloride HCl]

amiprilose INN *synthetic monosaccharide anti-inflammatory* [also: amiprilose HCl]

amiprilose HCl USAN *investigational (NDA filed) synthetic monosaccharide anti-inflammatory for rheumatoid arthritis* [also: amiprilose]

amiquinsin INN *antihypertensive* [also: amiquinsin HCl]

amiquinsin HCl USAN *antihypertensive* [also: amiquinsin]

amisometradine NF, INN, BAN

amisulpride INN

amiterol INN

Ami-Tex LA long-acting tablets (discontinued 2002) ℞ *decongestant; expectorant* [phenylpropanolamine HCl; guaifenesin] 75•400 mg

amithiozone [see: thioacetazone; thiacetazone]

amitivir USAN, INN *influenza vaccine*

Amitone chewable tablets (discontinued 2005) OTC *antacid* [calcium carbonate] 350 mg

amitraz USAN, INN, BAN *scabicide*

amitriptyline (AMT) INN, BAN *tricyclic antidepressant* [also: amitriptyline HCl] 💬 nortriptyline

amitriptyline HCl USP, JAN *tricyclic antidepressant* [also: amitriptyline] 10, 25, 50, 75, 100, 150 mg oral

amitriptylinoxide INN

amixetrine INN, DCF

AmLactin cream, lotion OTC *moisturizer; emollient* [ammonium lactate] 12%

AmLactin AP cream OTC *local anesthetic; moisturizer; emollient* [pramoxine HCl; lactic acid] 1%•12%

amlexanox USAN, INN, JAN *antiallergic; anti-inflammatory for aphthous ulcers*

amlintide USAN *antidiabetic for type 1 diabetes*

amlodipine INN, BAN *antianginal; antihypertensive; calcium channel blocker* [also: amlodipine besylate]

amlodipine besylate USAN *antianginal; antihypertensive; calcium channel blocker* [also: amlodipine]

amlodipine maleate USAN *antianginal; antihypertensive*

ammi (Ammi majus; A. visnaga) dried ripe fruits *medicinal herb for angina, bronchial asthma, diabetes, diuresis, kidney and bladder stones, psoriasis, respiratory diseases, and vitiligo*

ammoidin [see: methoxsalen]

[^{13}N]ammonia [see: ammonia N 13]

ammonia [see: ammonia spirit, aromatic]

ammonia N 13 USAN, USP *radioactive diagnostic aid for cardiac and liver imaging*

ammonia solution, strong NF *solvent; source of ammonia* [also: ammonia water]

ammonia spirit, aromatic USP *respiratory stimulant*

ammonia water JAN *solvent; source of ammonia* [also: ammonia solution, strong]

ammoniated mercury [see: mercury, ammoniated]

ammonio methacrylate copolymer NF *coating agent*

ammonium alum [see: alum, ammonium]

ammonium benzoate USP

ammonium carbonate NF *source of ammonia*

ammonium chloride USP, JAN *urinary acidifier; diuretic; expectorant* 486,

500 mg oral; 5 mEq/mL (26.75%) injection

ammonium 2-hydroxypropanoate [see: ammonium lactate]

ammonium ichthosulfonate [see: ichthammol]

ammonium lactate (lactic acid neutralized with ammonium hydroxide) USAN *antipruritic; emollient for xerosis* 12% topical

ammonium mandelate USP

ammonium molybdate USP *dietary molybdenum supplement* 25 μg/mL injection

ammonium molybdate tetrahydrate [see: ammonium molybdate]

ammonium phosphate NF *pharmaceutic aid*

ammonium salicylate NF

ammonium tetrathiomolybdate *investigational (orphan) for Wilson disease*

ammonium valerate NF

Ammonul IV infusion ℞ *adjunctive therapy (rescue agent) to prevent and treat hyperammonemia due to urea cycle enzymopathy (orphan)* [sodium benzoate; sodium phenylacetate] 10%•10%

ammophyllin [see: aminophylline]

Amnaranthus **spp.** *medicinal herb* [see: amaranth]

Amnesteem capsules ℞ *keratolytic for severe recalcitrant cystic acne* [isotretinoin] 10, 20, 40 mg

AMO Endosol; AMO Endosol Extra ophthalmic solution ℞ *intraocular irrigating solution* [sodium chloride (balanced saline solution)]

AMO Vitrax intraocular injection ℞ *viscoelastic agent for ophthalmic surgery* [hyaluronate sodium] 30 mg/mL

amobarbital USP, INN, JAN *sedative; hypnotic; anticonvulsant; also abused as a street drug* [also: amylobarbitone]

amobarbital sodium USP, JAN *hypnotic; sedative; anticonvulsant; also abused as a street drug*

amocaine chloride [see: amolanone HCl]

amocarzine INN

Amoclan powder for oral suspension ℞ *aminopenicillin antibiotic plus synergist* [amoxicillin; clavulanate potassium] 200•28.5, 400•57 mg/5 mL

amodiaquine USP, INN, BAN *antiprotozoal*

amodiaquine HCl USP *antimalarial*

amogastrin INN, JAN

amolanone INN

amolanone HCl [see: amolanone]

amonafide INN *investigational antineoplastic*

amoproxan INN, DCF

amopyroquine INN

amorolfine USAN, INN, BAN *antimycotic*

Amorphophallus konjac *medicinal herb* [see: glucomannan]

Amosan powder OTC *oral antibacterial* [sodium peroxyborate monohydrate]

amoscanate INN

amosulalol INN [also: amosulalol HCl]

amosulalol HCl JAN [also: amosulalol]

amotriphene [see: aminoxytriphene]

amoxapine USAN, USP, INN, BAN, JAN *tricyclic antidepressant* 25, 50, 100, 150 mg oral ⊠ amoxicillin; Amoxil

amoxecaine INN

amoxicillin USAN, USP, JAN *aminopenicillin antibiotic* [also: amoxicilline; amoxycillin] 125, 200, 250, 400, 500, 875 mg oral; 125, 200, 250, 400 mg/5 mL oral ⊠ amoxapine

amoxicillin & clavulanate potassium *aminopenicillin antibiotic plus synergist* 200•28.5, 400•57, 500•125, 875•125 mg oral; 200•28.5, 400•57, 600•42.9 mg/5 mL oral

amoxicillin sodium USAN *aminopenicillin antibiotic*

amoxicillin trihydrate [see: amoxicillin]

amoxicilline INN *aminopenicillin antibiotic* [also: amoxicillin; amoxycillin]

Amoxil capsules, film-coated caplets, chewable tablets, powder for oral suspension, pediatric drops ℞ *aminopenicillin antibiotic* [amoxicillin] 500 mg; 500, 875 mg; 200, 400 mg; 125, 200, 250, 400 mg/5 mL; 50 mg/mL ⊠ amoxapine

amoxycillin BAN *aminopenicillin antibiotic* [also: amoxicillin; amoxicilline]

amoxydramine camsilate INN [also: amoxydramine camsylate]

amoxydramine camsylate DCF [also: amoxydramine camsilate]

AMP; A₅MP (adenosine monophosphate) [see: adenosine phosphate]

amperozide INN, BAN *investigational antipsychotic for schizophrenia*

Amphadase solution for injection ℞ *adjuvant to increase the absorption and dispersion of injected drugs, hypodermoclysis, and subcutaneous urography; investigational (NDA filed) agent to clear vitreous hemorrhage; also used for diabetic retinopathy* [hyaluronidase (bovine)] 150 U/mL

amphecloral USAN *anorectic* [also: amfecloral]

amphenidone INN

amphetamine BAN *CNS stimulant; widely abused as a street drug, which causes strong psychic dependence* [also: amphetamine sulfate; amfetamine]

d-**amphetamine** [see: dextroamphetamine]

(+)-amphetamine [see: dextroamphetamine]

l-**amphetamine** [see: levamphetamine]

(–)-amphetamine [see: levamphetamine]

amphetamine aspartate *CNS stimulant*

amphetamine complex (resin complex of amphetamine & dextroamphetamine) [q.v.]

amphetamine phosphate, dextro [see: dextroamphetamine phosphate]

Amphetamine Salt Combo tablets ℞ *CNS stimulant mixture for attention-deficit hyperactivity disorder (ADHD)* [amphetamine aspartate; amphetamine sulfate; dextroamphetamine sulfate; dextroamphetamine saccharate] 5, 10, 20, 30 mg total amphetamines (1.25, 2.5, 5, 7.5 mg of each)

amphetamine succinate, levo [see: levamphetamine succinate]

amphetamine sulfate USP *CNS stimulant; widely abused as a street drug,* which causes strong psychic dependence [also: amfetamine; amphetamine]

amphetamine sulfate, dextro [see: dextroamphetamine sulfate]

amphetamines *a class of CNS stimulants that includes amphetamine, dextroamphetamine, levamphetamine, methamphetamine, and their salts*

amphetamines, mixed (equal parts amphetamine aspartate, amphetamine sulfate, dextroamphetamine sulfate, and dextroamphetamine saccharate) *CNS stimulant for attention-deficit hyperactivity disorder (ADHD), narcolepsy, and obesity; also abused as a street drug, which causes strong psychic dependence* [5, 10, 20, 30 mg oral]

Amphocin powder for IV infusion ℞ *systemic polyene antifungal* [amphotericin B deoxycholate] 50 mg/vial

amphocortrin [see: amphomycin]

Amphojel oral suspension (discontinued 2004) OTC *antacid* [aluminum hydroxide gel] 320 mg/5 mL 🔁 Amphocil

Amphojel tablets OTC *antacid* [aluminum hydroxide gel] 300, 600 mg 🔁 Amphocil

amphomycin USAN, BAN *antibacterial* [also: amfomycin]

amphotalide INN, DCF

Amphotec powder for IV infusion ℞ *systemic polyene antifungal for invasive aspergillosis* [amphotericin B cholesteryl sulfate] 50, 100 mg/vial

amphotericin B USP, INN, BAN, JAN *polyene antifungal*

amphotericin B cholesteryl *systemic polyene antifungal for invasive aspergillosis*

amphotericin B deoxycholate *systemic polyene antifungal* 50 mg injection

amphotericin B lipid complex (ABLC) *systemic polyene antifungal for meningitis, leishmaniasis, histoplasmosis, and other invasive infections (orphan)*

ampicillin USAN, USP, INN, BAN, JAN *aminopenicillin antibiotic* 250, 500 mg oral

ampicillin sodium USAN, USP, JAN *aminopenicillin antibiotic* 250, 500 mg, 1, 2 g injection

ampicillin sodium & sulbactam sodium *aminopenicillin antibiotic plus synergist* 1•0.5, 2•1 g injection

ampiroxicam INN, BAN

Amplicor Chlamydia test kit for professional use *in vitro diagnostic aid for Chlamydia trachomatis* [DNA amplification test]

Amplicor HIV-1 Monitor test kit for professional use *in vitro diagnostic aid for HIV-1 in blood* [polymerase chain reaction (PCR) test]

Amplicor MTB test kit for professional use *in vitro diagnostic aid for Mycobacterium tuberculosis* [polymerase chain reaction (PCR) test]

Ampligen Ṛ *investigational (Phase III, orphan) RNA synthesis inhibitor and immunomodulator for HIV, renal cell carcinoma, metastatic melanoma, and chronic fatigue syndrome* [poly I: poly C12U]

amprenavir USAN, INN *protease inhibitor antiviral for HIV infection*

amprocidum [see: amprolium]

amprolium USP, INN, BAN *coccidiostat for poultry*

amprotropine phosphate

ampyrimine INN

ampyzine INN *CNS stimulant* [also: ampyzine sulfate]

ampyzine sulfate USAN *CNS stimulant* [also: ampyzine]

amquinate USAN, INN *antimalarial*

amrinone INN, BAN *cardiotonic* [also: inamrinone (USAN changed 2000)]

amrinone lactate [now: inamrinone lactate]

amrubicin INN

AMSA; *m*-AMSA (acridinylamine methanesulfon anisidide) [see: amsacrine]

amsacrine USAN, INN, BAN *investigational (NDA filed, orphan) antineo-*

plastic for acute adult leukemias (AML, APL, and ALL) and lymphomas

Amsidyl Ṛ *investigational (NDA filed, orphan) antineoplastic for acute adult leukemias (AML, APL, and ALL) and lymphomas* [amsacrine]

amsonate INN, BAN *combining name for radicals or groups*

AMT (amitriptyline HCl) [q.v.]

amtolmetin guacil INN

Amvaz tablets Ṛ *antianginal; antihypertensive; calcium channel blocker* [amlodipine] 2.5, 5, 10 mg

Amvisc; Amvisc Plus intraocular injection Ṛ *viscoelastic agent for ophthalmic surgery* [hyaluronate sodium] 12 mg/mL; 16 mg/mL

amyl alcohol, tertiary [see: amylene hydrate]

amyl nitrite USP, JAN *vasodilator; antianginal; also abused as a euphoric street drug and sexual stimulant* 0.3 mL inhalant

amylase *digestive enzyme (digests carbohydrates)* [100 IU/mg in pancrelipase; 25 IU/mg in pancreatin]

amylase [see: alpha amylase]

amylene hydrate NF *solvent*

amylin [see: amlintide]

amylmetacresol INN, BAN

amylobarbitone BAN *sedative; hypnotic; anticonvulsant* [also: amobarbital]

amylocaine BAN

amylopectin sulfate, sodium salt [see: sodium amylosulfate]

amylosulfate sodium [see: sodium amylosulfate]

Amytal Sodium powder for injection Ṛ *sedative; hypnotic; anxiolytic; anticonvulsant; also abused as a street drug* [amobarbital sodium]

anabolic steroids *a class of hormones derived from or closely related to testosterone that increase anabolic (tissue-building) and decrease catabolic (tissue-depleting) processes*

Anacin caplets, tablets OTC *analgesic; antipyretic; anti-inflammatory* [aspirin; caffeine] 400•32 mg; 400•32, 500•32 mg ☑ Unisom; Unasyn

Anacin Aspirin Free tablets, caplets, gelcaps OTC *analgesic; antipyretic* [acetaminophen] 500 mg ☒ Unisom; Unasyn

Anacin P.M., Aspirin Free film-coated caplets OTC *antihistaminic sleep aid; analgesic* [diphenhydramine HCl; acetaminophen] 25•500 mg ☒ Unisom; Unasyn

Anadrol-50 tablets ℞ *anabolic steroid for anemia; also abused as a street drug* [oxymetholone] 50 mg

anafebrina [see: aminopyrine]

Anafranil capsules ℞ *tricyclic antidepressant for obsessive-compulsive disorders* [clomipramine HCl] 25, 50, 75 mg ☒ enalapril

anagestone INN *progestin* [also: anagestone acetate]

anagestone acetate USAN *progestin* [also: anagestone]

anagrelide INN *antithrombotic/antiplatelet agent* [also: anagrelide HCl]

anagrelide HCl USAN *antithrombotic/ antiplatelet agent for essential thrombocythemia (orphan); investigational (orphan) for thrombocytosis and polycythemia vera* [also: anagrelide] 0.5, 1 mg oral

Ana-Guard subcu or IM injection (discontinued 2001) ℞ *sympathomimetic bronchodilator for emergency treatment of anaphylaxis; vasopressor for shock* [epinephrine] 1:1000

anakinra USAN, INN *interleukin-1 receptor antagonist (IL-1ra); nonsteroidal anti-inflammatory for inflammatory bowel disease and rheumatoid arthritis (RA); investigational (Phase II, orphan) for juvenile rheumatoid arthritis (JRA) and graft vs. host disease (GVHD)*

Ana-Kit (discontinued 2002) ℞ *emergency treatment of anaphylaxis* [epinephrine; chlorpheniramine maleate; alcohol; tourniquet] 1:100 000•2 mg

analeptics *a class of central nervous system stimulants used to maintain or improve alertness*

Analgesia Creme OTC *topical analgesic* [trolamine salicylate] 10%

Analgesic Balm OTC *analgesic; counterirritant* [methyl salicylate; menthol]

analgesics *a class of drugs that relieve pain or reduce sensitivity to pain without causing loss of consciousness*

analgesine [see: antipyrine]

Analpram-HC anorectal cream ℞ *corticosteroidal anti-inflammatory; local anesthetic* [hydrocortisone acetate; pramoxine] 1%•1%, 2.5%•1% ☒ Analbalm

AnaMantle HC cream ℞ *corticosteroidal anti-inflammatory; local anesthetic* [hydrocortisone acetate; lidocaine] 0.5%•3%

Anamine syrup (discontinued 2002) ℞ *decongestant; antihistamine* [pseudoephedrine HCl; chlorpheniramine maleate] 30•2 mg/5 mL

Anamine T.D. sustained-release capsules (discontinued 2002) ℞ *decongestant; antihistamine* [pseudoephedrine HCl; chlorpheniramine maleate] 120•8 mg

Anamirta cocculus; A. paniculata *medicinal herb* [see: levant berry]

ananain *investigational (orphan) proteolytic enzymes for debridement of severe burns*

Ananas comosus *medicinal herb* [see: pineapple]

Anandron ⓒ tablets (also approved in Europe and Latin America) ℞ *antiandrogen antineoplastic adjunct to surgical or chemical castration for metastatic prostate cancer* [nilutamide] 50, 100 mg

Anaphalis margaritacea; Gnaphalium polycephalum; G. uliginosum *medicinal herb* [see: everlasting]

anaphrodisiacs *a class of agents that reduce sexual desire or potency*

Anaplex oral liquid (discontinued 2002) ℞ *decongestant; antihistamine* [pseudoephedrine HCl; chlorpheniramine maleate] 30•2 mg/5 mL

Anaplex HD oral liquid ℞ *narcotic antitussive; decongestant; antihistamine*

[hydrocodone bitartrate; pseudoephedrine HCl; brompheniramine
maleate] 3.4•60•4 mg/10 mL

Anaplex-DM oral liquid ℞ *antitussive;
decongestant; antihistamine* [dextro-
methorphan hydrobromide; pseudoephedrine HCl; brompheniramine
maleate] 30•60•4 mg/5 mL

Anaprox; Anaprox DS film-coated
tablets ℞ *analgesic; antiarthritic; nonsteroidal anti-inflammatory drug (NSAID)*
[naproxen sodium] 275 mg (=250 mg
base); 550 mg (=500 mg base)

anarel [see: guanadrel sulfate]

anaritide INN, BAN *antihypertensive;
diuretic* [also: anaritide acetate]

anaritide acetate USAN *antihypertensive;
diuretic; investigational (orphan) for
acute renal failure and renal transplants*

Anaspaz tablets ℞ *GI/GU antispasmodic; antiparkinsonian; anticholinergic "drying agent" for allergic rhinitis
and hyperhidrosis* [hyoscyamine sul-
fate] 0.125 mg

anastrozole USAN, INN, BAN *aromatase
inhibitor; estrogen antagonist; antineoplastic for advanced breast cancer*

Anatrast rectal paste ℞ *radiopaque
contrast medium for defecography* [bar-
ium sulfate] 100%

Anatrofin *brand name for stenbolone
acetate, an anabolic steroid abused as a
street drug*

anatumomab mafenatox INN

Anatuss film-coated tablets (discontinued 2002) ℞ *antitussive; decongestant;
expectorant; analgesic* [dextromethor-
phan hydrobromide; phenylpropanolamine HCl; guaifenesin; aceta-
minophen] 15•25•100•325 mg

Anatuss syrup (discontinued 2002)
OTC *antitussive; decongestant; expectorant* [dextromethorphan hydrobromide; phenylpropanolamine HCl;
guaifenesin] 15•25•100 mg/5 mL

Anatuss DM tablets, syrup (discontinued 2002) OTC *antitussive; decongestant; expectorant* [dextromethorphan
hydrobromide; pseudoephedrine

HCl; guaifenesin] 20•60•400 mg;
10•30•100 mg/5 mL

Anatuss LA long-acting tablets (discontinued 2002) ℞ *decongestant;
expectorant* [pseudoephedrine HCl;
guaifenesin] 120•400 mg

Anavar *brand name for oxandrolone, an
anabolic steroid abused as a street drug*

anaxirone INN

anayodin [see: chiniofon]

anazocine INN

anazolene sodium USAN, INN *blood
volume and cardiac output test* [also:
sodium anoxynaphthonate]

Anbesol topical liquid, gel OTC *mucous
membrane anesthetic; antipruritic/
counterirritant; antiseptic* [benzocaine;
phenol; alcohol 70%] 6.3%•0.5%

Anbesol, Baby gel OTC *topical oral
anesthetic* [benzocaine] 7.5%

Anbesol, Maximum Strength topical
liquid, gel OTC *mucous membrane anesthetic* [benzocaine; alcohol 60%] 20%

ancarolol INN

Ancef powder or frozen premix for IV
or IM injection ℞ *cephalosporin antibiotic* [cefazolin sodium] 0.5, 1, 5, 10 g

ancestim USAN, INN *recombinant-
methionyl human stem cell factor (r-
metHuSCF); hematopoietic growth
factor; investigational (NDA filed,
orphan) myelosuppressive and myeloablative therapy for non-Hodgkin
lymphoma, breast and ovarian cancer,
and multiple myeloma*

Ancet topical liquid OTC *soap-free therapeutic skin cleanser*

anchusa *medicinal herb* [see: henna
(Alkanna)]

ancitabine INN [also: ancitabine HCl]

ancitabine HCl JAN [also: ancitabine]

Ancobon capsules ℞ *systemic antifungal*
[flucytosine] 250, 500 mg ⚕ Oncovin

ancrod USAN, INN, BAN *anticoagulant
enzyme derived from the venom of the
Malayan pit viper; investigational
(orphan) for cardiopulmonary bypass in
heparin-intolerant patients*

Andehist pediatric oral drops (discontinued 2004) ℞ *decongestant; antihis-*

tamine [pseudoephedrine HCl; carbinoxamine maleate] 15•2 mg/mL

Andehist syrup (discontinued 2004) ℞ *decongestant; antihistamine* [pseudoephedrine HCl; brompheniramine maleate] 60•4 mg/5 mL

Andehist DM NR pediatric oral drops ℞ *antitussive; decongestant; antihistamine* [dextromethorphan hydrobromide; pseudoephedrine HCl; carbinoxamine maleate] 4•15•1 mg/mL

Andehist-DM syrup (discontinued 2004) ℞ *antitussive; decongestant; antihistamine* [dextromethorphan hydrobromide; pseudoephedrine HCl; brompheniramine maleate] 15•60•4 mg/5 mL

andolast INN

andrachne *(Andrachne aspera; A. cordifolia; A. phyllanthoides)* root *medicinal herb for eye inflammation; not generally regarded as safe and effective*

Andro 100; Andro 200 [see: depAndro 100; depAndro 200]

Andro L.A. 200 IM injection (discontinued 2001) ℞ *androgen replacement for delayed puberty or breast cancer* [testosterone enanthate] 200 mg/mL

Androcur *investigational (orphan) antiandrogen for severe hirsutism* [cyproterone acetate]

Androderm transdermal patch (for nonscrotal area) ℞ *hormone replacement therapy for male hypogonadism; investigational (Phase III) for AIDS-wasting syndrome* [testosterone] 2.5, 5 mg/day (12.2, 24.3 mg total)

AndroGel single-use packets, metered-dose pump ℞ *hormone replacement for male hypogonadism; investigational (orphan) for AIDS-wasting syndrome* [testosterone; alcohol 67%] 1% (25, 50 mg/pkt.; 12.5 mg/pump)

Androgel-DHT ℞ *investigational (Phase III) transdermal testosterone replacement in elderly men; investigational (Phase II, orphan) for AIDS-wasting syndrome* [dihydrotestosterone]

androgens *a class of sex hormones responsible for the development of the male sex organs and secondary sex characteristics*

Androgyn [see: depAndrogyn]

Android capsules (discontinued 2005) ℞ *androgen for hypogonadism or testosterone deficiency in men, delayed puberty in boys, and metastatic breast cancer in women; also abused as a street drug* [methyltestosterone] 10 mg

Android-10; Android-25 tablets (discontinued 2001) ℞ *androgen for hypogonadism or testosterone deficiency in men, delayed puberty in boys, and metastatic breast cancer in women* [methyltestosterone] 10 mg; 25 mg

Andropogon citratus *medicinal herb* [see: lemongrass]

Andropository-200 IM injection (discontinued 2001) ℞ *androgen replacement for delayed puberty or breast cancer* [testosterone enanthate] 200 mg/mL

androstanazole [now: stanozolol]

androstane [see: androstanolone; stanolone]

androstanolone INN *investigational (orphan) for AIDS-wasting syndrome* [also: stanolone]

androtest P [see: testosterone propionate]

Androvite tablets OTC *vitamin/mineral/iron supplement* [multiple vitamins & minerals; iron; folic acid; biotin] ± • 3•0.06• ⁒ mg

anecortave INN *angiostatic steroid for neovascularization of the eye to preserve vision in patients with wet age-related macular degeneration* [also: anecortave acetate]

anecortave acetate USAN *investigational (NDA filed) angiostatic steroid for neovascularization of the eye to preserve vision in patients with wet age-related macular degeneration* [also: anecortave]

Anectine IV or IM injection, Flo-Pack (powder for injection) ℞ *muscle relax-*

ant; anesthesia adjunct [succinylcholine chloride] 20 mg/mL; 500, 1000 mg

Anemagen gelcaps (discontinued 2004) ℞ hematinic; vitamin/iron supplement [multiple vitamins; ferrous fumarate] ± • 200 mg

Anemagen OB gelcaps ℞ vitamin/calcium/iron supplement [multiple vitamins; calcium; ferrous fumarate; folic acid] ± • 200 • 27 • 1 mg

Anemone patens medicinal herb [see: pasque flower]

Anergan 50 IM injection (discontinued 2002) ℞ antihistamine; sedative; antiemetic; motion sickness relief [promethazine HCl] 50 mg/mL

anertan [see: testosterone propionate]

Anestacon jelly ℞ mucous membrane anesthetic [lidocaine HCl] 2%

anesthesin [see: benzocaine]

anesthetics a class of agents that abolish the sensation of pain

anesthrone [see: benzocaine]

anethaine [see: tetracaine HCl]

anethole NF flavoring agent

anetholtrithion JAN

Anethum foeniculum medicinal herb [see: fennel]

Anethum graveolens medicinal herb [see: dill]

aneurine HCl [see: thiamine HCl]

Anexsia; Anexsia 5/500; Anexsia 7.5/650; Anexsia 10/660 tablets ℞ narcotic analgesic [hydrocodone bitartrate; acetaminophen] 5 • 325, 7.5 • 325 mg; 5 • 500 mg; 7.5 • 650 mg; 10 • 660 mg

angelica (*Angelica atropurpurea*) root medicinal herb for appetite stimulation, bronchial disorders, colds, colic, cough, exhaustion, gas, heartburn, and rheumatism; also used as a tonic

Angelica levisticum medicinal herb [see: lovage]

Angelica polymorpha; A. sinensis; A. dahurica medicinal herb [see: dong quai]

Angiomax powder for IV injection ℞ anticoagulant thrombin inhibitor for patients with unstable angina undergo-

ing percutaneous transluminal coronary angioplasty (PTCA) [bivalirudin] 250 mg/vial

angiotensin 1-7 investigational (orphan) agent for myelodysplastic syndrome and neutropenia due to bone marrow transplantation

angiotensin II INN

angiotensin II receptor antagonists (AIIRAs) a class of antihypertensives that reduce the vasoconstricting effects of angiotensin II by blocking the angiotensin II receptor sites in the vascular smooth muscles [compare to: angiotensin-converting enzyme inhibitors]

angiotensin amide USAN, NF, BAN vasoconstrictor [also: angiotensinamide]

angiotensinamide INN vasoconstrictor [also: angiotensin amide]

angiotensin-converting enzyme inhibitors (ACEIs) a class of antihypertensives that reduce the vasoconstricting effects of angiotensin II by blocking the enzyme (kininase II) that converts angiotensin I to angiotensin II [compare to: angiotensin II receptor antagonists]

anhidrotics a class of agents that reduce or suppress perspiration [also called: anidrotics; antihydrotics]

anhydrohydroxyprogesterone [now: ethisterone]

anhydrous lanolin [see: lanolin, anhydrous]

anidoxime USAN, INN, BAN analgesic

anidrotics a class of agents that reduce or suppress perspiration [also called: anhidrotics; antihydrotics]

anidulafungin USAN, INN antifungal for Candida, Aspergillus, and Pneumocystis infections; investigational (Phase III) for esophageal candidiasis

anilamate INN

anileridine USP, INN, BAN narcotic analgesic

anileridine HCl USP narcotic analgesic

anilopam INN analgesic [also: anilopam HCl]

anilopam HCl USAN analgesic [also: anilopam]

Animal Shapes chewable tablets OTC *vitamin supplement* [multiple vitamins; folic acid] ± •0.3 mg

Animal Shapes + Iron chewable tablets OTC *vitamin/iron supplement* [multiple vitamins; iron; folic acid] ± •15•0.3 mg

Animi-3 capsules OTC *dietary supplement* [omega-3 fatty acids (source of DHA and EPA); vitamins B_6 and B_{12}; folic acid] 500 (350+35)•12.5•0.5•1 mg

anion exchange resin [see: polyamine-methylene resin]

anipamil INN

aniracetam USAN, INN *mental performance enhancer*

anirolac USAN, INN *anti-inflammatory; analgesic*

anisacril INN

anisatil USAN *combining name for radicals or groups*

anise (Pimpinella anisum) oil and seeds *medicinal herb for colic, convulsions, cough, gas, intestinal cleansing, iron-deficiency anemia, mucous discharge, promoting expectoration, and psoriasis; also used as an antibacterial, antimicrobial, and antiseptic*

anise oil NF

anise root; sweet anise *medicinal herb* [see: sweet cicely]

anisindione NF, INN, BAN *indanedione-derivative anticoagulant*

anisopirol INN

anisopyradamine [see: pyrilamine maleate]

anisotropine methylbromide USAN, JAN *anticholinergic; peptic ulcer adjunct* [also: octatropine methylbromide] 50 mg oral

anisoylated plasminogen streptokinase activator complex (APSAC) [see: anistreplase]

anisperimus INN

anistreplase USAN, INN, BAN *fibrinolytic; thrombolytic enzyme for acute myocardial infarction*

Anisum officinarum; A. vulgare *medicinal herb* [see: anise]

anitrazafen USAN, INN *topical anti-inflammatory*

anodynes *a class of agents that lessen or relieve pain*

anodynine [see: antipyrine]

anodynon [see: ethyl chloride]

anorectics *a class of central nervous system stimulants that suppress the appetite* [also called: anorexiants; anorexigenics]

anorexiants *a class of central nervous system stimulants that suppress the appetite* [also called: anorectics; anorexigenics]

anorexigenics *a class of central nervous system stimulants that suppress the appetite* [also called: anorexiants; anorectics]

anovlar [see: norethindrone & ethinyl estradiol]

anoxomer USAN *antioxidant; food additive*

anoxynaphthonate sodium [see: anazolene sodium]

anpirtoline INN

Ansaid film-coated tablets Ṛ *antiarthritic; nonsteroidal anti-inflammatory drug (NSAID)* [flurbiprofen] 50, 100 mg ▣ NSAID

ansamycin [see: rifabutin]

ansoxetine INN

Answer One-Step; Answer Plus; Answer Quick & Simple test kit for home use *in vitro diagnostic aid; urine pregnancy test*

Answer Ovulation test kit for home use *in vitro diagnostic aid to predict ovulation time*

Antabuse tablets Ṛ *deterrent to alcohol consumption* [disulfiram] 250 mg

Antacid chewable tablets OTC *antacid* [calcium carbonate] 500, 750 mg

Antacid oral suspension OTC *antacid* [aluminum hydroxide; magnesium hydroxide] 225•200 mg/5 mL

antacids *a class of drugs that neutralize gastric acid*

antafenite INN

Antagon subcu injection (discontinued 2004) Ṛ *gonadotropin-releasing hor-*

mone (GnRH) antagonist for infertility [ganirelix acetate] 250 µg/0.5 mL

Antara capsules ℞ *antihyperlipidemic for primary hypercholesterolemia (types IIa and IIb hyperlipidemia), hypertriglyceridemia (types IV and V hyperlipidemia), and mixed dyslipidemia; also used for hyperuricemia* [fenofibrate] 43, 87, 130 mg

antastan [see: antazoline HCl]

antazoline INN, BAN [also: antazoline HCl]

antazoline HCl USP [also: antazoline]

antazoline phosphate USP *antihistamine*

antazoline phosphate & naphazoline HCl *topical ocular antihistamine and decongestant* 0.5%•0.05%

antazonite INN

Antegren (name changed to **Tysabri** upon marketing release in 2004)

antelmycin INN *anthelmintic* [also: anthelmycin]

anterior pituitary

anthelmintics *a class of drugs effective against parasitic infections* [also called: vermicides; vermifuges]

anthelmycin USAN *anthelmintic* [also: antelmycin]

Anthemis nobilis medicinal herb [see: chamomile]

anthiolimine INN

Anthoxanthum odoratum medicinal herb [see: sweet vernal grass]

anthracyclines *a class of antibiotic antineoplastics*

Anthra-Derm ointment ℞ *topical antipsoriatic* [anthralin] 0.1%, 0.25%, 0.5%, 1%

anthralin USP *topical antipsoriatic* [also: dithranol] 1% topical

anthramycin USAN *antineoplastic* [also: antramycin]

anthraquinone of cascara [see: cascara sagrada]

anthrax test [see: Rapid Anthrax Test]

anthrax vaccine, adsorbed (AVA) *active bacterin derived from an attenuated strain of* Bacillus anthracis

Anthriscus cerefolium medicinal herb [see: chervil]

anti pan T lymphocyte monoclonal antibodies (MAb) *investigational (orphan) agent for in vivo and ex vivo treatment of bone marrow transplants* [also: anti-T lymphocyte immunotoxin XMMLY-H65-RTA]

anti-A blood grouping serum USP *in vitro blood testing*

antiadrenergics *a class of agents that block the alpha$_1$ adrenergic receptors, used for the treatment of hypertension and benign prostatic hyperplasia (BPH)* also called: alpha$_1$-adrenergic blockers

antiadrenergics *a class of cardiovascular drugs that block the passage of impulses through the sympathetic nervous system* [also called: sympatholytics]

antiandrogens *a class of hormonal antineoplastics*

antib [see: thioacetazone; thiacetazone]

anti-B blood grouping serum USP *in vitro blood testing*

antibason [see: methylthiouracil]

AntibiŌtic ear drops, otic suspension ℞ *topical corticosteroidal anti-inflammatory; antibiotic* [hydrocortisone; neomycin sulfate; polymyxin B sulfate] 1%•5 mg•10 000 U per mL

Antibiotic Ear Solution ℞ *topical corticosteroidal anti-inflammatory; antibiotic* [hydrocortisone; neomycin sulfate; polymyxin B sulfate] 1%•5 mg•10 000 U per mL

Antibiotic Ear Suspension ℞ *topical corticosteroidal anti-inflammatory; antibiotic* [hydrocortisone; neomycin sulfate; polymyxin B sulfate] 1%•5 mg•10 000 U per mL

antibiotics *a class of agents that destroy or arrest the growth of micro-organisms*

antibromics *a class of agents that mask undesirable or offensive odors* [also called: deodorants]

anti-C blood grouping serum [see: blood grouping serum, anti-C]

anti-c blood grouping serum [see: blood grouping serum, anti-c]

anti-CD3 [see: muromonab-CD3]

anti-CD23 kappa monoclonal antibodies (MAb) to immunoglobu-

lin G1 (IgG1) *investigational (orphan) agent for chronic lymphocytic leukemia*

anti-CD45 monoclonal antibodies (MAb) *investigational (orphan) agent to prevent acute graft rejection of human organ transplants*

anti-CEA sheep-human chimeric monoclonal antibodies (MAb) radiolabeled with iodine I 131 *investigational (orphan) agent for pancreatic cancer*

anticholinergics *a class of agents that block parasympathetic nerve impulses, producing antiemetic, antinausea, and antispasmodic effects; also used to dry mucosal secretions*

anticoagulant citrate dextrose (ACD) solution USP *anticoagulant for storage of whole blood and during cardiac surgery*

anticoagulant citrate phosphate dextrose adenine solution USP *anticoagulant for storage of whole blood*

anticoagulant citrate phosphate dextrose solution USP *anticoagulant for storage of whole blood*

anticoagulant heparin solution USP *anticoagulant for storage of whole blood*

anticoagulant sodium citrate solution USP *anticoagulant for plasma and for blood for fractionation*

anticoagulants *a class of therapeutic agents that inhibit or inactivate blood clotting factors*

anticonvulsants *a class of drugs that prevent seizures by suppressing abnormal neuronal discharges in the central nervous system [also called: anti-epileptic drugs (AEDs)]*

Anticort ℞ *investigational anti-aging and anticancer agent; investigational (Phase II) for HIV infection [procaine HCl]*

anticytomegalovirus monoclonal antibodies (MAb) *investigational (orphan) agent to prevent or treat cytomegalovirus infections due to bone marrow transplants, organ transplants, or AIDS*

anti-D antibodies [see: $Rh_O(D)$ immune globulin]

antidopaminergics *a class of antiemetic drugs*

antidotes *a class of drugs that counteract the effects of toxic doses of other drugs or toxic substances*

anti-E blood grouping serum [see: blood grouping serum, anti-E]

anti-e blood grouping serum [see: blood grouping serum, anti-e]

antiemetics *a class of agents that prevent or alleviate nausea and vomiting [also called: antinauseants]*

antiendotoxin monoclonal antibodies (MAb) E5 [now: edobacomab]

antienite INN

antiepilepsirine [now: ilepcimide]

anti-epileptic drugs (AEDs) *a class of drugs that prevent seizures by suppressing abnormal neuronal discharges in the central nervous system [also called: anticonvulsants]*

antiestrogen [see: tamoxifen citrate]

antiestrogens *a class of hormonal antineoplastics*

antifebriles *a class of agents that relieve or reduce fever [also called: antipyretics; antithermics; febricides; febrifuges]*

antifebrin [see: acetanilide]

antifolic acid [see: methotrexate]

antiformin, dental JAN [also: sodium hypochlorite, diluted]

antigen-presenting cells pulsed with tumor immunoglobulin idiotype *investigational (orphan) agent for multiple myeloma*

antihemophilic factor (AHF; FVIII) USP *systemic hemostatic; antihemophilic for von Willebrand disease (orphan)*

Antihemophilic Factor (Porcine) Hyate:C *powder for IV injection* ℞ *antihemophilic to correct coagulation deficiency [antihemophilic factor VIII:C] 400–700 porcine units/vial*

antihemophilic factor, human [now: antihemophilic factor]

antihemophilic factor, recombinant (rFVIII) *antihemophilic for treatment*

of hemophilia A and presurgical pro-
phylaxis for hemophiliacs (orphan)

antihemophilic factor A [see: antihemophilic factor]

antihemophilic factor B [see: factor
IX complex]

antihemophilic globulin (AHG)
[see: antihemophilic factor]

antihemophilic human plasma [now:
plasma, antihemophilic human]

antihemophilic plasma, human
[now: plasma, antihemophilic human]

antiheparin [see: protamine sulfate]

Antihist-1 tablets (discontinued 2002)
OTC *antihistamine* [clemastine fuma-
rate] 1.34 mg

antihistamines *a class of drugs that*
counteract the effect of histamine

Antihist-D tablets (discontinued 2001)
OTC *decongestant; antihistamine* [phen-
ylpropanolamine HCl (extended
release); clemastine fumarate (immediate release)] 75•1.34 mg

antihydrotics *a class of agents that*
reduce or suppress perspiration [also
called: anhidrotics; anidrotics]

antihyperlipidemic agents *a class of*
drugs that lower serum lipid levels [also
called: antilipemics]

anti-inhibitor coagulant complex
antihemophilic

anti-interferon-gamma Fab from
goats *investigational (orphan) immu-*
nologic for corneal allograft rejection

Anti-Itch cream OTC *poison ivy treat-*
ment [diphenhydramine HCl; zinc
acetate] 2%•0.1%

Anti-Itch gel OTC *poison ivy treatment*
[camphor; alcohol 37%] 0.45%

antilipemics *a class of drugs that lower*
serum lipid levels [also called: antihy-
perlipidemics]

Antilirium IV or IM injection ℞ *cho-*
linergic to reverse anticholinergic over-
dose; investigational (orphan) for
Friedreich and other inherited ataxias
[physostigmine salicylate] 1 mg/mL

antilithics *a class of agents that prevent*
the formation of stone or calculus [see
also: litholytics]

antilymphocyte immunoglobulin
BAN

antimelanoma antibody XMMME-
001-DTPA 111 indium *investiga-*
tional (orphan) imaging aid for systemic
and nodal melanoma metastasis

antimelanoma antibody XMMME-
001-RTA *investigational (orphan)*
agent for melanoma

Antiminth oral suspension (discontinued 2004) OTC *anthelmintic for ascari-*
asis (roundworm) and enterobiasis (pin-
worm) [pyrantel pamoate] 50 mg/mL

antimony *element (Sb)*

antimony potassium tartrate USP
antischistosomal

antimony sodium tartrate USP, JAN
antischistosomal

antimony sodium thioglycollate USP

antimony sulfide [see: antimony
trisulfide colloid]

antimony trisulfide colloid USAN
pharmaceutic aid

antimonyl potassium tartrate [see:
antimony potassium tartrate]

antimuscarinics *a class of anticholiner-*
gic agents

antinauseants *a class of agents that pre-*
vent or alleviate nausea and vomiting
[also called: antiemetics]

antineoplastics *a class of chemothera-*
peutic agents capable of selective action
on neoplastic (abnormally proliferating)
tissues

antineoplastons *a class of naturally*
occurring peptides that suppress cancer
oncogenes and stimulate the body's can-
cer suppressor genes

Antiox capsules OTC *vitamin supple-*
ment [vitamins C and E; beta caro-
tene] 120 mg•100 IU•25 mg

anti-pellagra vitamin [see: niacin]

antiperiodics *a class of agents that pre-*
vent periodic or intermittent recurrence
of symptoms, as in malaria

anti-pernicious anemia principle
[see: cyanocobalamin]

antiphlogistics *a class of agents that*
reduce inflammation and fever

antipsychotics *a class of psychotropic agents that are used to treat schizophrenia and other psychiatric illnesses; further classified as conventional (typical) antipsychotics and novel (atypical) antipsychotics* [q.v.]

antipyretics *a class of agents that relieve or reduce fever* [also called: antifebriles; antithermics; febricides; febrifuges]

antipyrine USP, JAN *analgesic; investigational (orphan) diagnostic agent to determine hepatic drug metabolizing activity* [also: phenazone]

N-antipyrinylnicotinamide [see: nifenazone]

antirabies serum (ARS) USP *passive immunizing agent*

anti-Rh antibodies [see: $Rh_O(D)$ immune globulin]

anti-Rh typing serums [now: blood grouping serums]

antiscorbutic vitamin [see: ascorbic acid]

antiscorbutics *a class of agents that are sources of vitamin C and are effective in the prevention or relief of scurvy*

antiscrofulous herbs *a class of agents that counteract scrofuloderma (tuberculous cervical lymphadenitis)*

antisense 20-mer phosphorothiolate oligonucleotide *investigational (orphan) agent for renal cell carcinoma*

antisense drugs *a class of antiviral drugs that interfere with the replication of viral protein*

antiseptics *a class of agents that inhibit the growth and development of microorganisms, usually on a body surface, without necessarily killing them* [see also: disinfectants; germicides]

Antispas IM injection ℞ *GI antispasmodic* [dicyclomine HCl] 10 mg/mL

Antispasmodic elixir ℞ *GI antispasmodic; anticholinergic; sedative* [atropine sulfate; scopolamine hydrobromide; hyoscyamine sulfate; phenobarbital] 0.0194•0.0065• 0.1037•16.2 mg/5 mL

antispasmodics *a class of agents that relieve spasms or cramps, usually of gastrointestinal tract or blood vessels*

antisterility vitamin [see: vitamin E]

anti-T lymphocyte immunotoxin XMMLY-H65-RTA *investigational (orphan) agent for in vivo and ex vivo treatment of bone marrow transplants* [also: anti pan T lymphocyte monoclonal antibody]

anti-tac, humanized; SMART antitac [now: dacliximab]

anti-tap-72 immunotoxin *investigational (orphan) for metastatic colorectal adenocarcinoma*

antithermics *a class of agents that relieve or reduce fever* [also called: antifebriles; antipyretics; febricides; febrifuges]

antithrombin III (AT-III) INN, BAN *agent for thrombosis and pulmonary emboli of congenital AT-III deficiency (orphan); investigational (Phase III, orphan) for heparin resistance in patients undergoing coronary artery bypass grafts and other surgical procedures*

antithrombin III, human [see: antithrombin III]

antithrombin III, recombinant human (rhATIII) [see: antithrombin III]

antithrombin III concentrate IV [see: antithrombin III]

antithymocyte globulin (ATG) *treatment for aplastic anemia; passive immunizing agent to prevent allograft rejection of renal transplants (orphan); investigational (orphan) for other solid organ and bone marrow transplants; investigational (orphan) for myelodysplastic syndrome (MDS)* [also: lymphocyte immune globulin (LIG)]

antithymocyte serum [see: antithymocyte globulin]

anti-TNF (tumor necrosis factor) monoclonal antibodies (MAb) [now: nerelimomab]

antitoxin botulism equine (ABE) [see: botulism equine antitoxin, trivalent]

antitoxins *a class of drugs used for passive immunization that consist of antibodies which combine with toxins to neutralize them*

α₁-antitrypsin [see: alpha₁-antitrypsin]

antituberculous agents *a class of antibiotics, divided into primary and retreatment agents*

Anti-Tuss syrup (discontinued 2004) OTC *expectorant* [guaifenesin; alcohol 3.5%] 100 mg/5 mL

antitussives *a class of drugs that prevent or relieve cough*

antivenin (Crotalidae) polyvalent USP *passive immunizing agent for pit viper (rattlesnake, copperhead, and cottonmouth moccasin) bites*

antivenin (Crotalidae) polyvalent immune Fab (equine) *investigational (orphan) treatment for pit viper (rattlesnake, copperhead, and cottonmouth moccasin) bites*

antivenin (Crotalidae) polyvalent immune Fab (ovine) *treatment for pit viper (rattlesnake, copperhead, and cottonmouth moccasin) bites (orphan)*

antivenin (Crotalidae) purified (avian) *investigational (orphan) treatment for pit viper (rattlesnake, copperhead, and cottonmouth moccasin) bites*

antivenin (*Latrodectus mactans*) USP *passive immunizing agent for black widow spider bites* 6000 U/vial

antivenin (*Micrurus fulvius*) USP *passive immunizing agent for coral snake bites*

antivenins *a class of drugs used for passive immunization against or treatment for venomous bites and stings*

Antivert; Antivert/25; Antivert/50 tablets ℞ *anticholinergic; antihistamine; antivertigo agent; motion sickness preventative* [meclizine HCl] 12.5 mg; 25 mg; 50 mg

Antivipmyn ℞ *investigational (orphan) treatment for pit viper (rattlesnake, copperhead, and cottonmouth moccasin) bites* [antivenin (Crotalidae) polyvalent immune Fab (equine)]

antivirals *a class of drugs effective against viral infections*

antixerophthalmic vitamin [see: vitamin A]

Antizol injection ℞ *alcohol dehydrogenase inhibitor for methanol or ethylene glycol poisoning* (orphan) [fomepizole] 1 g/mL

antler (deer and elk) *natural remedy for aging, energy, hormone balancing, impotence, infertility, and longevity*

antrafenine INN

antramycin INN *antineoplastic* [also: anthramycin]

Antril ℞ *nonsteroidal anti-inflammatory drug (NSAID) for inflammatory bowel disease; investigational (orphan) for juvenile rheumatoid arthritis and graft vs. host disease* [anakinra]

Antrin ℞ *investigational photodynamic therapy for peripheral vascular and cardiovascular atherosclerosis* [motexafin lutetium]

Antrizine tablets ℞ *anticholinergic; antihistamine; antivertigo agent; motion sickness preventative* [meclizine HCl] 12.5 mg

Antrocol elixir ℞ *GI anticholinergic; sedative* [atropine sulfate; phenobarbital] 0.195•16 mg/5 mL

Antrypol (available only from the Centers for Disease Control) ℞ *antiparasitic for African trypanosomiasis and onchocerciasis* [suramin sodium]

antrypol [see: suramin sodium]

Anturane tablets, capsules ℞ *uricosuric for gout* [sulfinpyrazone] 100 mg; 200 mg ⊡ Artane

Anucort HC rectal suppositories ℞ *corticosteroidal anti-inflammatory* [hydrocortisone acetate] 25 mg

Anumed rectal suppositories OTC *temporary relief of hemorrhoidal symptoms* [bismuth subgallate; bismuth resorcin compound; benzyl benzoate; zinc oxide; peruvian balsam] 2.25%•1.75%•1.2%•11%•1.8%

Anumed HC rectal suppositories ℞ *corticosteroidal anti-inflammatory* [hydrocortisone acetate] 10 mg

Anusol anorectal ointment OTC *local anesthetic; astringent* [pramoxine HCl; zinc oxide] 1%•12.5% ⑨ Aplisol

Anusol rectal suppositories OTC *emollient* [topical starch] 51%

Anusol-HC anorectal cream ℞ *topical corticosteroidal anti-inflammatory* [hydrocortisone] 2.5%

Anusol-HC rectal suppositories ℞ *corticosteroidal anti-inflammatory* [hydrocortisone acetate] 25 mg

Anusol-HC 1 ointment ℞ *topical corticosteroidal anti-inflammatory* [hydrocortisone acetate] 1%

Anuzinc ⒸⒶⓃ anorectal ointment, suppositories ℞ *astringent* [zinc sulfate] 0.5%; 10 mg

Anzemet film-coated tablets, IV injection ℞ *serotonin 5-HT₃ receptor antagonist; antiemetic for nausea following chemotherapy, radiation, or surgery* [dolasetron mesylate] 50, 100 mg; 20 mg/mL

AOPA (ara-C, Oncovin, prednisone, asparaginase) *chemotherapy protocol*

AOPE (Adriamycin, Oncovin, prednisone, etoposide) *chemotherapy protocol*

Aosept + Aodisc solution + tablet OTC *two-step chemical disinfecting system for soft contact lenses* [hydrogen peroxide based] 3%

AP (Adriamycin, Platinol) *chemotherapy protocol for ovarian and endometrial cancer*

AP-1903 *investigational (orphan) agent for graft-versus-host disease*

Apacet chewable tablets, drops OTC *analgesic; antipyretic* [acetaminophen] 80 mg; 100 mg/mL

apafant USAN, INN *platelet activating factor antagonist for allergies, asthma, and acute pancreatitis*

apalcillin sodium USAN, INN *antibacterial*

APAP (N-acetyl-p-aminophenol) [see: acetaminophen]

APAP Plus tablets OTC *analgesic; antipyretic* [acetaminophen; caffeine] 500•65 mg

Apatate chewable tablets, oral liquid (discontinued 2004) OTC *vitamin supplement* [vitamins B₁, B₆, and B₁₂] 15•0.5•0.025 mg; 15•0.5•0.025 mg/5 mL

Apatate with Fluoride oral liquid ℞ *pediatric vitamin supplement and dental caries preventative* [vitamins B₁, B₆, and B₁₂; fluoride] 15•0.5•0.025•0.5 mg/5 mL

apaxifylline USAN, INN *selective adenosine A₁ antagonist for cognitive deficits*

apazone USAN *anti-inflammatory* [also: azapropazone]

APC (AMSA, prednisone, chlorambucil) *chemotherapy protocol*

APC (aspirin, phenacetin & caffeine) [q.v.]

apcitide [see: technetium Tc 99m apcitide]

APD (aminohydroxypropylidene diphosphonate) [see: pamidronate disodium]

APE (Adriamycin, Platinol, etoposide) *chemotherapy protocol*

APE (aminophylline, phenobarbital, ephedrine)

APE (ara-C, Platinol, etoposide) *chemotherapy protocol*

aperients *a class of agents that have a mild purgative or laxative effect* [see also: aperitives]

aperitives *a class of agents that stimulate the appetite or have a mild purgative or laxative effect* [see also: aperients]

Apetil oral liquid OTC *vitamin/mineral supplement* [multiple B vitamins; multiple minerals]

ApexiCon ointment ℞ *corticosteroidal anti-inflammatory* [diflorasone diacetate] 0.05%

ApexiCon E cream ℞ *corticosteroidal anti-inflammatory; emollient* [diflorasone diacetate] 0.05%

aphrodisiacs *a class of agents that arouse or increase sexual desire or potency*

Aphrodyne tablets ℞ *alpha₂-adrenergic blocker for impotence and orthostatic hypotension; sympatholytic; mydriatic; may have aphrodisiac activity; no FDA-sanctioned indications* [yohimbine HCl] 5.4 mg

Aphthasol oral paste ℞ *anti-inflammatory for aphthous ulcers* [amlexanox] 5%

apicillin [see: ampicillin]

apicycline INN

Apidra subcu injection ℞ *human insulin analogue; rapid-onset, short-acting antidiabetic* [insulin glulisine (rDNA)] 100 IU/mL

apiquel fumarate [see: aminorex]

Apium graveolens medicinal herb [see: celery]

A.P.L. powder for IM injection (discontinued 2004) ℞ *hormone for prepubertal cryptorchidism and hypogonadism; ovulation stimulant* [chorionic gonadotropin] 500, 1000, 2000 U/mL

APL 400-020 V-Beta DNA vaccine *investigational (orphan) agent for cutaneous T-cell lymphoma*

Apligraf ℞ *living skin construct for diabetic foot ulcers and pressure sores* [graftskin]

Aplisol intradermal injection *tuberculosis skin test* [tuberculin purified protein derivative (PPD)] 5 U/0.1 mL ⓘ Anusol; Apresoline

Aplitest single-use intradermal puncture test device (discontinued 2002) *tuberculosis skin test* [tuberculin purified protein derivative (PPD)] 5 U

aplonidine HCl [see: apraclonidine HCl]

APO (Adriamycin, prednisone, Oncovin) *chemotherapy protocol*

Apo-Acetaminophen ⓒ tablets, film-coated caplets OTC *analgesic; antipyretic* [acetaminophen] 325, 500 mg

Apo-Acyclovir ⓒ tablets ℞ *antiviral for herpes infections* [acyclovir] 200, 400, 800 mg

Apo-Amitriptyline ⓒ film-coated tablets ℞ *tricyclic antidepressant* [amitriptyline HCl] 10, 25, 50, 75 mg

Apo-Amoxi ⓒ capsules, oral suspension ℞ *aminopenicillin antibiotic* [amoxicillin trihydrate] 250, 500 mg; 125, 250 mg/5 mL

Apo-Atenolol ⓒ tablets ℞ *antihypertensive; antianginal; antiadrenergic (β-blocker)* [atenolol] 50, 100 mg

Apo-Beclomethasone ⓒ nasal spray ℞ *corticosteroidal anti-inflammatory for chronic asthma and rhinitis* [beclomethasone dipropionate] 50 μg/spray

Apo-Benzydamine ⓒ oral rinse ℞ *topical analgesic and anti-inflammatory* [benzydamine HCl] 0.15%

Apo-Butorphanol ⓒ nasal spray ℞ *narcotic agonist-antagonist analgesic; antimigraine agent* [butorphanol tartrate] 10 mg/mL

Apo-Carbamazepine CR ⓒ controlled-release tablets ℞ *twice-daily anticonvulsant; antipsychotic* [carbamazepine] 100, 200, 400 mg

Apo-Cefaclor ⓒ capsules, oral suspension ℞ *cephalosporin antibiotic* [cefaclor] 250, 500 mg; 125, 250, 375 mg/5 mL

Apo-Cefadroxil ⓒ capsules ℞ *cephalosporin antibiotic* [cefadroxil] 500 mg

Apo-Cetirizine ⓒ tablets OTC *antihistamine* [cetirizine HCl] 10 mg

Apo-Chlorhexidine ⓒ oral rinse ℞ *antimicrobial; gingivitis treatment* [chlorhexidine gluconate] 0.12%

Apo-Cimetidine ⓒ film-coated tablets, oral liquid ℞ *histamine H₂ antagonist for gastric and duodenal ulcers and gastric hypersecretory conditions* [cimetidine] 200, 300, 400, 600, 800 mg; 300 mg/5 mL

Apo-Clonazepam ⓒ tablets ℞ *anticonvulsant* [clonazepam] 0.5, 2 mg

Apo-Cromolyn ⓒ nasal spray ℞ *anti-inflammatory/mast cell stabilizer for the prophylaxis of allergic rhinitis* [cromolyn sodium (sodium cromoglycate)] 2% (5.2 mg/dose)

Apo-Cromolyn ⓒ Sterules (solution for nebulization) ℞ *anti-inflammatory/mast cell stabilizer for the prophylaxis of asthma and bronchospasm* [cro-

molyn sodium (sodium cromoglycate)] 1% (20 mg/2 mL dose)

Apocynum androsaemifolium *medicinal
herb* [see: dogbane]

Apo-Desmopressin Ⓐ nasal spray ℞
*posterior pituitary hormone; antidi-
uretic for nocturnal enuresis* [desmo-
pressin acetate] 10 μg/dose

Apo-Diazepam Ⓐ tablets ℞ *benzodiazepine sedative; anxiolytic; anticonvulsant; skeletal muscle relaxant*
[diazepam] 2, 5, 10 mg

Apo-Diclo Rapide Ⓐ tablets ℞ *analgesic; antiarthritic; nonsteroidal anti-
inflammatory drug (NSAID)* [diclo-
fenac potassium] 50 mg

Apo-Diltiaz Ⓐ IV injection ℞ *calcium
channel blocker for atrial fibrillation or
paroxysmal supraventricular tachycardia (PSVT)* [diltiazem HCl] 5 mg/mL

Apo-Diltiaz Ⓐ tablets ℞ *antianginal;
antihypertensive; antiarrhythmic; calcium channel blocker* [diltiazem HCl]
30, 60 mg

Apo-Diltiaz CD Ⓐ (once daily) sustained-release capsules ℞ *antihypertensive; antianginal; antiarrhythmic;
calcium channel blocker* [diltiazem
HCl] 120, 180, 240, 300 mg

Apo-Diltiaz SR Ⓐ (twice daily) sustained-release capsules ℞ *antihypertensive; antianginal; antiarrhythmic;
calcium channel blocker* [diltiazem
HCl] 60, 90, 120 mg

Apo-Dipivefrin Ⓐ eye drops ℞ *topical
antiglaucoma agent* [dipivefrin HCl]
0.1%

Apo-Divalproex Ⓐ enteric-coated
tablets ℞ *anticonvulsant* [divalproex
sodium] 125, 250, 500 mg

apodol [see: anileridine HCl]

Apo-Domperidone Ⓐ film-coated
tablets ℞ *antiemetic for diabetic gastroparesis and chronic gastritis* [dom-
peridone maleate] 10 mg

Apo-Doxazosin Ⓐ tablets ℞ *antihypertensive (α-blocker); treatment for
benign prostatic hyperplasia* [doxazosin
mesylate] 1, 2, 4 mg

Apo-Etodolac Ⓐ capsules ℞ *nonsteroidal anti-inflammatory drug; analgesic;
antiarthritic* [etodolac] 200, 300 mg

Apo-Fluconazole Ⓐ tablets ℞ *broad-
spectrum antifungal* [fluconazole] 50,
100, 200 mg

Apo-Flunisolide Ⓐ metered dose
nasal spray ℞ *corticosteroidal anti-
inflammatory for seasonal or perennial
rhinitis* [flunisolide] 25 μg/dose

Apo-Fluphenazine Ⓐ tablets ℞ *conventional (typical) phenothiazine antipsychotic for schizophrenia and psychotic
disorders* [fluphenazine HCl] 1, 2, 5 mg

Apo-Fluphenazine Decanoate Ⓐ
injection ℞ *conventional (typical) phenothiazine antipsychotic for schizophrenia and psychotic disorders; used for
prolonged parenteral neuroleptic therapy*
[fluphenazine decanoate] 25 mg/mL

Apo-Flutamide Ⓐ tablets ℞ *antiandrogen antineoplastic* [flutamide] 250 mg

Apo-Furosemide Ⓐ tablets ℞ *antihypertensive; loop diuretic* [furosemide]
20, 40, 80 mg

Apo-Gemfibrozil Ⓐ capsules, tablets
℞ *antihyperlipidemic for hypertriglyceridemia and coronary heart disease*
[gemfibrozil] 300 mg; 600 mg

Apo-Glyburide Ⓐ tablets ℞ *sulfonylurea antidiabetic* [glyburide] 2.5, 5 mg

Apo-Haloperidol LA Ⓐ long-acting
IM injection ℞ *conventional (typical)
butyrophenone antipsychotic; antispas-
modic/antidyskinetic for Tourette syndrome; treatment for severe pediatric
behavioral disorders such as aggression,
combativeness, hyperexcitability, and
poor impulse control* [haloperidol dec-
anoate] 50, 100 mg/mL

Apo-Hydro Ⓐ tablets ℞ *antihypertensive; diuretic* [hydrochlorothiazide]
25, 50, 100 mg

Apo-Ipravent Ⓐ Sterules (solution for
nebulization), solution for inhalation
℞ *anticholinergic bronchodilator for
bronchospasm; antisecretory for rhinorrhea* [ipratropium bromide] 250 μg/mL

Apo-Ketoconazole CAN tablets Ŗ *systemic antifungal* [ketoconazole] 200 mg

Apo-Ketorolac CAN tablets, IM or IV injection Ŗ *analgesic; nonsteroidal anti-inflammatory drug (NSAID)* [ketorolac tromethamine] 10 mg; 30 mg/mL

Apokinon (French name for U.S. product Apokyn)

Apokyn subcu injection Ŗ *dopamine agonist for hypomobility episodes of late-stage Parkinson disease (orphan)* [apomorphine HCl] 10 mg/mL

Apo-Lactulose CAN oral/rectal solution Ŗ *hyperosmotic laxative* [lactulose] 10 g/15 mL

Apo-Levobunolol CAN eye drops Ŗ *topical antiglaucoma agent (β-blocker)* [levobunolol HCl] 0.25%, 0.5%

Apo-Lithium CAN capsules Ŗ *antipsychotic for manic episodes* [lithium carbonate] 150, 300 mg

Apo-Lorazepam CAN tablets Ŗ *benzodiazepine anxiolytic* [lorazepam] 0.5, 1, 2 mg

Apo-Loxapine CAN film-coated tablets Ŗ *conventional (typical) dibenzoxazepine antipsychotic for schizophrenia* [loxapine succinate] 5, 10, 25, 50 mg

Apo-Methoprazine CAN tablets Ŗ *CNS depressant; neuroleptic* [methotrimeprazine maleate] 2, 5, 25, 50 mg

Apo-Metoprolol CAN tablets Ŗ *antihypertensive; antianginal; antiadrenergic (β-blocker)* [metoprolol tartrate] 50, 100 mg

Apo-Metoprolol L CAN film-coated caplets Ŗ *antihypertensive; antianginal; antiadrenergic (β-blocker)* [metoprolol tartrate] 50, 100 mg

Apo-Moclobemide CAN film-coated tablets Ŗ *antidepressant; MAO inhibitor* [moclobemide] 100, 150 mg

apomorphine BAN *dopamine D₁ agonist* [also: apomorphine HCl]

apomorphine HCl USP *dopamine D₁ agonist for hypomobility episodes of late-stage Parkinson disease (orphan);*

investigational (NDA filed) for erectile dysfunction [also: apomorphine]

Apo-Nabumetone CAN tablets Ŗ *antiarthritic; nonsteroidal anti-inflammatory drug (NSAID)* [nabumetone] 500 mg

Apo-Naproxen CAN tablets Ŗ *analgesic; antiarthritic; nonsteroidal anti-inflammatory drug* [naproxen] 125, 250, 375, 500 mg

Apo-Naproxen SR CAN sustained-release tablets Ŗ *analgesic; antiarthritic; nonsteroidal anti-inflammatory drug (NSAID)* [naproxen] 750 mg

Apo-Nefazodone CAN tablets Ŗ *antidepressant* [nefazodone HCl] 50, 100, 150, 200 mg

Apo-Norflox CAN tablets Ŗ *broad-spectrum fluoroquinolone antibiotic* [norfloxacin] 400 mg

Apo-Oflox CAN film-coated tablets Ŗ *broad-spectrum fluoroquinolone antibiotic* [ofloxacin] 200, 300, 400 mg

Apo-Orciprenaline CAN syrup Ŗ *sympathomimetic bronchodilator* [orciprenaline sulfate] 10 mg/5 mL

Apo-Oxazepam CAN tablets Ŗ *benzodiazepine anxiolytic* [oxazepam] 10, 15, 30 mg

Apo-Pen VK CAN tablets, powder for oral solution Ŗ *natural penicillin antibiotic* [penicillin V potassium] 300 mg; 125, 300 mg/5 mL

Apo-Perphenazine CAN film-coated tablets Ŗ *conventional (typical) phenothiazine antipsychotic for schizophrenia and psychotic disorders; treatment for nausea and vomiting* [perphenazine] 4, 8, 16 mg

Apo-Pravastatin CAN tablets Ŗ *HMG-CoA reductase inhibitor for hyperlipidemia and hypertriglyceridemia* [pravastatin sodium] 10, 20, 40 mg

Apo-Prednisone CAN tablets Ŗ *corticosteroid; anti-inflammatory* [prednisone] 1, 5, 50 mg

Apo-Prochlorazine CAN tablets Ŗ *conventional (typical) phenothiazine antipsychotic for schizophrenia; anxiolytic; antiemetic for nausea and vomiting; also used for acute treatment of*

migraine headaches [prochlorperazine maleate] 5, 10 mg

Apo-Propafenone Ⓒ🅰🅝 film-coated tablets ℞ *antiarrhythmic* [propafenone HCl] 150, 300 mg

Apo-Ranitidine Ⓒ🅰🅝 film-coated tablets OTC *histamine H₂ antagonist for episodic heartburn* [ranitidine HCl] 75 mg

Apo-Ranitidine Ⓒ🅰🅝 film-coated tablets ℞ *histamine H₂ antagonist for gastric and duodenal ulcers* [ranitidine HCl] 150, 300 mg

Apo-Salvent Ⓒ🅰🅝 inhaler ℞ *sympathomimetic bronchodilator* [salbutamol] 100 μg/dose

Apo-Salvent Ⓒ🅰🅝 tablets, solution for nebulization ℞ *sympathomimetic bronchodilator* [salbutamol sulfate] 2, 4 mg; 1, 2 mg/mL

Apo-Sertraline Ⓒ🅰🅝 capsules ℞ *selective serotonin reuptake inhibitor (SSRI) for depression, obsessive-compulsive disorder (OCD), and panic disorder* [sertraline HCl] 25, 50, 100 mg

Apo-Temazepam Ⓒ🅰🅝 capsules ℞ *benzodiazepine sedative; hypnotic* [temazepam] 15, 30 mg

Apo-Terazosin Ⓒ🅰🅝 tablets ℞ *antihypertensive (α-blocker); treatment for benign prostatic hyperplasia (BPH)* [terazosin HCl] 1, 2, 5, 10 mg

Apo-Terbinafine Ⓒ🅰🅝 tablets ℞ *systemic allylamine antifungal* [terbinafine HCl] 250 mg

Apo-Thioridazine Ⓒ🅰🅝 film-coated tablets ℞ *conventional (typical) phenothiazine antipsychotic for schizophrenia; sedative; also used for agitation or psychosis due to Alzheimer or other dementias* [thioridazine HCl] 10, 25 mg

Apo-Ticlopidine Ⓒ🅰🅝 film-coated tablets ℞ *platelet aggregation inhibitor for stroke* [ticlopidine HCl] 250 mg

Apo-Trifluoperazine Ⓒ🅰🅝 film-coated tablets ℞ *conventional (typical) phenothiazine antipsychotic for schizophrenia; anxiolytic for nonpsychotic anxiety* [trifluoperazine HCl] 1, 2, 5, 10, 20 mg

Apo-Valproic Ⓒ🅰🅝 capsules, syrup ℞ *anticonvulsant* [valproic acid] 250 mg; 250 mg/5 mL

apovincamine INN

Apo-Warfarin Ⓒ🅰🅝 tablets ℞ *coumarin-derivative anticoagulant* [warfarin sodium] 1, 2, 2.5, 4, 5, 10 mg

Appedrine tablets (discontinued 2001) OTC *nonprescription diet aid; vitamin/mineral supplement* [phenylpropanolamine HCl; multiple vitamins & minerals; folic acid] 25●±● 0.4 mg ② aprindine; ephedrine

appetizers *a class of agents that stimulate the appetite* [see also: aperitives]

APPG (aqueous penicillin G procaine) [see: penicillin G procaine]

apple *(Pyrus malus)* fruit *medicinal herb for constipation and diarrhea, dysentery, fever, heart ailments, scurvy, and warts*

apple, ground *medicinal herb* [see: chamomile]

apple, hog; Indian apple; May apple *medicinal herb* [see: mandrake]

Appli-Kit (trademarked form) *ointment and adhesive dosage covers*

Appli-Ruler (trademarked name) OTC *dose-determining pads*

Appli-Tape (trademarked name) OTC *dosage covers*

Apra ℞ *investigational (Phase II, orphan) antineoplastic for soft tissue sarcomas and malignant mesothelioma* [CT-2584 mesylate (code name—generic name not yet assigned)]

Apra oral liquid OTC *analgesic; antipyretic* [acetaminophen] 160 mg/5 mL

apraclonidine INN, BAN *topical adrenergic for glaucoma* [also: apraclonidine HCl]

apraclonidine HCl USAN *topical adrenergic for glaucoma* [also: apraclonidine]

apramycin USAN, INN, BAN *antibacterial*

aprepitant USAN *neurokinin NK₁ receptor antagonist; antiemetic for chemotherapy*

Apresazide 25/25; Apresazide 50/50; Apresazide 100/50 capsules ℞ *antihypertensive; vasodilator; diuretic* [hydralazine HCl; hydrochlorothiazide] 25•25 mg; 50•50 mg; 100•50 mg

Apresoline tablets ℞ *antihypertensive; vasodilator* [hydralazine HCl] 10, 25, 50, 100 mg

Apri tablets (in packs of 28) ℞ *monophasic oral contraceptive* [desogestrel; ethinyl estradiol] 0.15 mg•30 μg

apricot *(Prunus armeniaca)* fruit, seeds, and kernel oil *medicinal herb for asthma, constipation, cough, eye inflammation, hemorrhage, infertility, spasm, and vaginal infections; not generally regarded as safe and effective as apricot kernel ingestion causes cyanide poisoning*

apricot kernel water JAN

aprikalim INN *investigational antianginal*

aprindine USAN, INN, BAN *antiarrhythmic* ⊡ Appedrine; ephedrine

aprindine HCl USAN, JAN *antiarrhythmic*

aprobarbital NF, INN, DCF *sedative*

Aprodine tablets, syrup OTC *decongestant; antihistamine* [pseudoephedrine HCl; triprolidine HCl] 60•2.5 mg; 60•2.5 mg/10 mL

Aprodine with Codeine syrup (discontinued 2002) ℞ *narcotic antitussive; decongestant; antihistamine* [codeine phosphate; pseudoephedrine HCl; triprolidine HCl] 10•30•1.25 mg/5 mL

aprofene INN

aprosulate sodium INN

aprotinin USAN, INN, BAN, JAN *systemic hemostatic for coronary artery bypass graft (CABG) surgery (orphan); protease inhibitor*

A.P.S. (aspirin, phenacetin & salicylamide) [q.v.]

APSAC (anisoylated plasminogen streptokinase activator complex) [see: anistreplase]

aptazapine INN *antidepressant* [also: aptazapine maleate]

aptazapine maleate USAN *antidepressant* [also: aptazapine]

aptiganel HCl USAN *investigational (Phase III) NMDA ion channel blocker for stroke and traumatic brain injury*

Aptivus softgels ℞ *antiviral protease inhibitor (PI) for HIV infection; must use with ritonavir* [tipranavir disodium] 250 mg

aptocaine INN, BAN, DCF

Aptosyn ℞ *investigational (NDA filed, orphan) apoptosis modulator for adenomatous polyposis coli (APC); investigational (Phase III) for lung cancer* [exisulind]

apyron [see: magnesium salicylate]

AquaBalm cream OTC *moisturizer; emollient*

Aqua-Ban enteric-coated tablets OTC *diuretic* [ammonium chloride; caffeine] 325•100 mg

Aqua-Ban, Maximum Strength tablets OTC *diuretic* [pamabrom] 50 mg

Aqua-Ban Plus enteric-coated tablets OTC *diuretic; iron supplement* [ammonium chloride; caffeine; ferrous sulfate] 650•200•6 mg

Aquabase OTC *ointment base*

Aquacare cream, lotion OTC *moisturizer; emollient; keratolytic* [urea] 10%

Aquachloral Supprettes (suppositories) ℞ *nonbarbiturate sedative and hypnotic* [chloral hydrate] 324, 648 mg

aquaday [see: menadione]

aquakay [see: menadione]

AquaMEPHYTON IM or subcu injection ℞ *coagulant to correct anticoagulant-induced prothrombin deficiency; vitamin K supplement* [phytonadione] 2, 10 mg/mL

Aquanil lotion OTC *moisturizer; emollient*

Aquanil Cleanser lotion OTC *soap-free therapeutic skin cleanser*

Aquaphilic OTC *ointment base*

Aquaphilic with Carbamide OTC *ointment base* [urea] 10%, 20%

Aquaphor OTC *ointment base*

Aquaphyllin syrup (discontinued 2004) ℞ *antiasthmatic; bronchodilator* [theophylline] 80 mg/15 mL

AquaSite eye drops (discontinued 2004) OTC *ophthalmic moisturizer/lubricant* [polyethylene glycol 400] 0.2%

Aquasol A IM injection ℞ *vitamin deficiency therapy* [vitamin A] 50 000 IU/mL

Aquatab C extended-release tablets ℞ *antitussive; decongestant; expectorant* [dextromethorphan hydrobromide; pseudoephedrine HCl; guaifenesin] 60•60•1200 mg

Aquatab D extended-release tablets ℞ *decongestant; expectorant* [pseudoephedrine HCl; guaifenesin] 75• 1200 mg

Aquatab D Dose Pack sustained-release tablets ℞ *decongestant; expectorant* [pseudoephedrine HCl; guaifenesin] 60•600 mg

Aquatab DM tablets, syrup ℞ *antitussive; expectorant* [dextromethorphan hydrobromide; guaifenesin] 60•1200 mg; 10•200 mg/5 mL

AquaTar gel (discontinued 2003) OTC *antipsoriatic; antiseborrheic* [coal tar extract] 2.5%

Aquatensen tablets ℞ *diuretic; antihypertensive* [methyclothiazide] 5 mg

Aquavit-E drops ℞ *vitamin supplement* [vitamin E (as *dl*-alpha tocopheryl acetate)] 15 IU/0.3 mL

aqueous penicillin G procaine (APPG) [see: penicillin G procaine]

Aquilegia vulgaris medicinal herb [see: columbine]

aquinone [see: menadione]

ara-A (adenine arabinoside) [see: vidarabine]

ara-AC (azacytosine arabinoside) [see: fazarabine]

arabinofuranosylcytosine [see: cytarabine]

arabinogalactans *a class of dietary fiber used as an immune booster; stimulates macrophages, increases levels of natural killer (NK) cells, interferon-gamma (IFN-γ), tumor necrosis factor-alpha (TNF-α), and interleukin-1 beta (IL-1 β)* [see also: larch]

arabinoluranosylcytosine HCl [see: cytarabine HCl]

arabinosyl cytosine [see: cytarabine]

ara-C (cytosine arabinoside) [see: cytarabine] ℞ ERYC

ara-C + 6-TG (ara-C, thioguanine) *chemotherapy protocol*

ara-C + ADR (ara-C, Adriamycin) *chemotherapy protocol*

ara-C + DNR + PRED + MP (ara-C, daunorubicin, prednisolone, mercaptopurine) *chemotherapy protocol*

ARAC-DNR (ara-C, daunorubicin) *chemotherapy protocol for acute myelocytic leukemia (AML)*

arachadonic acid (AA) *natural omega-6 fatty acid*

arachis oil [see: peanut oil]

ara-C-HU (ara-C, hydroxyurea) *chemotherapy protocol*

ara-cytidine [see: cytarabine]

Aralast powder for IV infusion ℞ *enzyme replacement therapy for hereditary alpha₁-proteinase inhibitor deficiency, which leads to progressive panacinar emphysema* [alpha$_1$-proteinase inhibitor] ≥ 16 mg/mL (400, 800 mg/vial)

Aralen HCl IM injection ℞ *antimalarial; amebicide* [chloroquine HCl] 50 mg/mL ℞ Arlidin

Aralen Phosphate film-coated tablets ℞ *antimalarial; amebicide* [chloroquine phosphate] 500 mg

Aralia racemosa medicinal herb [see: spikenard]

Aralia spp. medicinal herb [see: ginseng]

Aramine IV, subcu or IM injection ℞ *vasopressor for acute hypotensive shock, anaphylaxis, or traumatic shock* [metaraminol bitartrate] 10 mg/mL

Aranelle tablets (in packs of 28) ℞ *triphasic oral contraceptive* [norethindrone; ethinyl estradiol]
Phase 1 (7 days): 500•35 μg;
Phase 2 (9 days): 1000•35 μg;
Phase 3 (5 days): 500•35 μg

Aranesp IV or subcu injection, prefilled syringes ℞ *hematopoietic; recombinant erythropoietin analogue for anemia associated with chronic renal failure* [darbepoetin alfa] 25, 40, 60,

100, 200, 300, 500 µg/mL; 25, 40, 60, 100, 150, 200, 300, 500 µg/dose

aranidipine INN

aranotin USAN, INN *antiviral*

araprofen INN

Arava film-coated tablets ℞ *antiinflammatory for rheumatoid arthritis (RA)* [leflunomide] 10, 20, 100 mg

ARBs (angiotensin II receptor blockers) [see: angiotensin II receptor antagonists]

arbaprostil USAN, INN *gastric antisecretory*

arbekacin INN

arberry *medicinal herb* [see: uva ursi]

arbutamine INN, BAN *cardiac stressor for diagnosis of coronary artery disease* [also: arbutamine HCl]

arbutamine HCl USAN *cardiac stressor for diagnosis of coronary artery disease* [also: arbutamine]

Arbutus uva ursi *medicinal herb* [see: uva ursi]

archangel *medicinal herb* [see: angelica]

arcitumomab USAN *investigational (orphan) imaging agent for detection of recurrent or metastatic thyroid cancers; investigational (Phase III) for lung cancer*

arclofenin USAN, INN *hepatic function test*

Arcobee with C caplets OTC *vitamin supplement* [multiple B vitamins; vitamin C] ≛•300 mg

Arco-Lase chewable tablets (discontinued 2002) OTC *digestive enzymes* [amylase; protease; lipase; cellulase] 30•6•25•2 mg

Arco-Lase Plus tablets (discontinued 2002) ℞ *digestive enzymes; GI antispasmodic; sedative* [amylase; protease; lipase; cellulase; hyoscyamine sulfate; atropine sulfate; phenobarbital] 30•6•25•2•0.1•0.02•7.5 mg

Arcoxia tablets *investigational (NDA filed) COX-2 inhibitor for osteoarthritis, rheumatoid arthritis, musculoskeletal pain, and gout* [etoricoxib] 60, 90, 10 mg

Arctium lappa; A. majus; A. minus *medicinal herb* [see: burdock]

Arctostaphylos uva ursi *medicinal herb* [see: uva ursi]

ardacin INN

ardeparin sodium USAN, INN *a low molecular weight heparin–type anticoagulant and antithrombotic for the prevention of deep vein thrombosis (DVT) following knee replacement surgery*

Arduan powder for IV injection (discontinued 2004) ℞ *nondepolarizing neuromuscular blocking agent; muscle relaxant; adjunct to general anesthesia* [pipecuronium bromide] 10 mg/vial

arecoline acetarsone salt [see: drocarbil]

arecoline hydrobromide NF

Aredia powder for IV infusion ℞ *bisphosphonate bone resorption inhibitor for Paget disease, hypercalcemia of malignancy, breast cancer, and multiple myeloma* [pamidronate disodium] 30, 90 mg

Arestin sustained-release microspheres for subgingival injection ℞ *antibiotic for periodontitis* [minocycline HCl] 1 mg

arfalasin INN

arfendazam INN

argatroban USAN, INN, JAN *anticoagulant for heparin-induced thrombocytopenia (HIT) and thrombosis syndrome (HITTS); prevention of HIT or HITTS in percutaneous coronary intervention (PCI)* 1 mg/mL injection

Argesic cream (discontinued 2004) OTC *analgesic; counterirritant* [methyl salicylate; trolamine]

Argesic-SA tablets ℞ *analgesic; antiinflammatory* [salsalate] 500 mg

argimesna INN

Arginaid Extra oral liquid OTC *enteral nutritional treatment for wound healing* [whey protein–based]

L-argininamide [see: iseganan HCl]

arginine (L-arginine) USP, INN *nonessential amino acid; ammonia detoxicant; diagnostic aid for pituitary function; symbols: Arg, R*

arginine butanoate [see: arginine butyrate]

arginine butyrate (L-arginine butyrate) USAN *investigational (orphan) for beta-hemoglobinopathies, beta-thalassemia, and sickle cell disease*

arginine glutamate (L-arginine L-glutamate) USAN, BAN, JAN *ammonia detoxicant*

arginine HCl USAN, USP, JAN *ammonia detoxicant; pituitary (growth hormone) function diagnostic aid*

L-arginine monohydrochloride [see: arginine HCl]

8-L-arginine vasopressin [see: vasopressin]

8-arginineoxytocin [see: argiprestocin]

8-L-argininevasopressin tannate [see: argipressin tannate]

argipressin INN, BAN *antidiuretic* [also: argipressin tannate]

argipressin tannate USAN *antidiuretic* [also: argipressin]

argiprestocin INN

argon *element (Ar)*

argyn [see: silver protein, mild]

Aricept tablets ℞ *reversible acetylcholinesterase (AChE) inhibitor; cognition adjuvant for Alzheimer dementia; also used for vascular dementia and memory improvement in multiple sclerosis patients* [donepezil HCl] 5, 10 mg ⊉ Erycette

Aricept ODT (orally disintegrating tablets) ℞ *reversible acetylcholinesterase (AChE) inhibitor; cognition adjuvant for Alzheimer dementia; also used for vascular dementia and memory improvement in multiple sclerosis patients* [donepezil HCl] 5, 10 mg

Ariflo tablets ℞ *investigational (NDA filed) pulmonary anti-inflammatory for COPD* [cilomilast] 15 mg

arildone USAN, INN *antiviral*

Arimidex film-coated tablets ℞ *aromatase inhibitor; estrogen antagonist; antineoplastic for breast cancer* [anastrozole] 1 mg

aripiprazole USAN *quinolinone antipsychotic for schizophrenia and manic epi-* sodes of a bipolar disorder; dopamine D_2 and serotonin 5-HT$_1$ and 5-HT$_2$ agonist

Aristocort ointment, cream ℞ *topical corticosteroidal anti-inflammatory* [triamcinolone acetonide] 0.1%, 0.5%; 0.025%, 0.1%, 0.5%

Aristocort tablets ℞ *corticosteroid; anti-inflammatory* [triamcinolone] 1, 2, 4, 8 mg

Aristocort A ointment, cream ℞ *topical corticosteroidal anti-inflammatory* [triamcinolone acetonide in a water-washable base] 0.1%; 0.025%, 0.1%, 0.5%

Aristocort Forte IM injection (discontinued 2004) ℞ *corticosteroid; anti-inflammatory* [triamcinolone diacetate] 40 mg/mL

Aristocort Intralesional injection ℞ *corticosteroid; anti-inflammatory* [triamcinolone diacetate] 25 mg/mL

Aristolochia clematitis medicinal herb [see: birthwort]

Aristospan Intra-articular injection ℞ *corticosteroid; anti-inflammatory* [triamcinolone hexacetonide] 20 mg/mL

Aristospan Intralesional injection ℞ *corticosteroid; anti-inflammatory* [triamcinolone hexacetonide] 5 mg/mL

Arixtra subcu injection in prefilled syringes ℞ *selective factor Xa inhibitor; antithrombotic for prevention of deep vein thrombosis (DVT) and acute pulmonary embolism following orthopedic surgery* [fondaparinux sodium] 2.5 mg/0.5 mL, 5 mg/0.4 mL, 7.5 mg/0.6 mL, 10 mg/0.8 mL

A.R.M. (Allergy Relief Medicine) caplets (discontinued 2001) OTC *decongestant; antihistamine* [phenylpropanolamine HCl; chlorpheniramine maleate] 25•4 mg

Arm-A-Med (trademarked packaging form) *single-dose plastic vial*

Arm-A-Vial (trademarked packaging form) *single-dose plastic vial*

Armoracia rusticana; A. lapathiofolia medicinal herb [see: horseradish]

Armour Thyroid tablets ℞ *thyroid replacement therapy for hypothyroidism or thyroid cancer* [thyroid, desiccated (porcine)] 15, 30, 60, 90, 120, 180, 240, 300 mg

arnica (*Arnica montana; A. cordifolia; A. fulgens*) flowers *medicinal herb used as a topical counterirritant and vulnerary for acne, bruises, rashes, and other dermal lesions; not generally regarded as safe and effective taken internally as it is highly toxic*

arnolol INN

arofylline USAN *phosphodiesterase IV inhibitor for asthma*

Aromasin tablets ℞ *aromatase inhibitor; antihormonal antineoplastic for advanced breast cancer in postmenopausal women (orphan)* [exemestane] 25 mg

aromatase inhibitors *a class of antihormonal antineoplastics which block the conversion of androgens to estrogens, effectively depriving hormone-dependent tumors of estrogen in postmenopausal women*

aromatic ammonia spirit [see: ammonia spirit, aromatic]

aromatic cascara fluidextract [see: cascara fluidextract, aromatic]

aromatic cascara sagrada [see: cascara fluidextract, aromatic]

aromatic elixir NF *flavored and sweetened vehicle*

aromatics *a class of agents that have an agreeable odor and stimulating qualities; also, substances with a specific molecular structure in organic chemistry*

aronixil INN

arotinolol INN [also: arotinolol HCl]

arotinolol HCl JAN [also: arotinolol]

arprinocid USAN, INN, BAN *coccidiostat*

arpromidine INN

arrow wood; Indian arrow wood; Indian arrow *medicinal herb* [see: wahoo]

ARS (antirabies serum) [q.v.]

arsambide [see: carbarsone]

arsanilic acid INN, BAN *investigational (Phase I/II, orphan) immunomodulator for AIDS*

arseclor [see: dichlorophenarsine HCl]

arsenic *element (As)*

arsenic acid, sodium salt [see: sodium arsenate]

arsenic trioxide (AsO₃) JAN *antineoplastic for acute promyelocytic leukemia (orphan); investigational (NDA filed) for renal cell carcinoma; investigational (orphan) for multiple myeloma and myelodysplastic syndromes*

arsenobenzene [see: arsphenamine]

arsenobenzol [see: arsphenamine]

arsenphenolamine [see: arsphenamine]

Arsobal (available only from the Centers for Disease Control) ℞ *investigational anti-infective for trypanosomiasis* [melarsoprol]

arsphenamine USP

arsthinenol DCF [also: arsthinol]

arsthinol INN [also: arsthinenol]

Artane tablets, elixir, Sequels (sustained-release capsules) (discontinued 2001) ℞ *anticholinergic; antiparkinsonian* [trihexyphenidyl HCl] 2, 5 mg; 2 mg/5 mL; 5 mg ② Anturane

arteflene USAN, INN *antimalarial*

artegraft USAN *arterial prosthetic aid*

artemether INN

Artemisia absinthium *medicinal herb* [see: wormwood]

Artemisia dracunculus *medicinal herb* [see: tarragon]

Artemisia vulgaris *medicinal herb* [see: mugwort]

artemisinin INN *natural herbal drug for malaria*

artemotil INN

artenimol INN

arterenol [see: norepinephrine bitartrate]

artesunate INN *antimalarial; investigational (NDA filed, orphan) rectal suppositories for emergency treatment of malaria*

Artha-G tablets OTC *analgesic; anti-inflammatory* [salsalate] 750 mg

ArthriCare, Double Ice gel OTC *analgesic; counterirritant* [menthol; camphor] 4%•3.1%

ArthriCare, Odor Free rub OTC *analgesic; counterirritant* [menthol;

methyl nicotinate; capsaicin]
1.25%•0.25%•0.025%

ArthriCare Triple Medicated gel
OTC *analgesic; counterirritant* [methyl
salicylate; menthol; methyl nicotin-
ate] 30%•1.5%•0.7%

**"Arthritis Formula"; "Arthritis
Strength"** products [see under product name]

Arthritis Hot Creme OTC *analgesic;
counterirritant* [methyl salicylate;
menthol] 15%•10%

Arthritis Pain Formula caplets OTC
*analgesic; antipyretic; anti-inflamma-
tory; antirheumatic* [aspirin (buffered
with magnesium hydroxide and aluminum hydroxide)] 500 mg

Arthropan IM injection R̸ *analgesic;
antipyretic; anti-inflammatory; antirheumatic* [choline salicylate] 870 mg/5 mL

Arthrotec film-coated tablets R̸ *antiarthritic NSAID with a coating to protect gastric mucosa* [diclofenac sodium
(enteric-coated core); misoprostol
(coating)] 50•0.2, 75•0.2 mg

articaine INN *amide local anesthetic for
dentistry* [also: carticaine]

articaine HCl USAN *amide local anesthetic for dentistry* [also: articaine;
carticaine]

artichoke (*Cynara scolymus*) flower
heads *medicinal herb for albuminuria,
bile stimulation, diabetes, diuresis, dyspepsia, jaundice, liver diseases, and
postoperative anemia*

Articoat bandages OTC *antimicrobial
dressings*

Articulose L.A. IM injection R̸ *corticosteroid; anti-inflammatory* [triam-
cinolone diacetate] 40 mg/mL

Artificial Tears eye drops OTC *ocular
moisturizer/lubricant*

Artificial Tears ophthalmic ointment
OTC *ocular moisturizer/lubricant* [white
petrolatum; mineral oil; lanolin]

Artificial Tears Plus eye drops OTC
ophthalmic moisturizer/lubricant [poly-
vinyl alcohol] 1.4%

artilide INN *antiarrhythmic* [also: artilide fumarate]

artilide fumarate USAN *antiarrhythmic*
[also: artilide]

Arzol Silver Nitrate applicators R̸
antiseptic [silver nitrate; potassium
nitrate] 75%•25%

arzoxifene INN *selective estrogen receptor modulator (SERM) for breast cancer, uterine fibroids, endometriosis, and
dysfunctional uterine bleeding* [also:
arzoxifene HCl]

arzoxifene HCl USAN *selective estrogen
receptor modulator (SERM) for breast
cancer, uterine fibroids, endometriosis,
and dysfunctional uterine bleeding*
[also: arzoxifene]

[74]As [see: sodium arsenate As 74]

5-ASA (5-aminosalicylic acid) [see:
mesalamine]

ASA (acetylsalicylic acid) [see: aspi-
rin]

Asacol delayed-release tablets R̸ *anti-
inflammatory for active ulcerative colitis, proctosigmoiditis, and proctitis*
[mesalamine (5-aminosalicylic acid)]
400 mg

asafetida; asafoetida (*Ferula assafoetida; F. foetida; F. rubricaulis*) gum
resin from dried roots and rhizomes
*medicinal herb for abdominal tumors,
amenorrhea, asthma, colic, convulsions, corns and calluses, edema; also
used as an expectorant; not generally
regarded as safe and effective in children
as it may induce methemoglobinemia*

asafoetida *medicinal herb* [see: asafetida]

Asarum canadense *medicinal herb* [see:
wild ginger]

ASC Lotionized topical liquid OTC
medicated cleanser for acne [triclosan]
0.3%

Asclepias geminata *medicinal herb* [see:
gymnema]

Asclepias syriaca *medicinal herb* [see:
milkweed]

Asclepias tuberosa *medicinal herb* [see:
pleurisy root]

Ascocaps capsules OTC *vitamin C supplement* [ascorbic acid] 500 mg

Ascomp with Codeine capsules R̸
narcotic analgesic; barbiturate sedative

[codeine phosphate; aspirin; caffeine; butalbital] 30•325•40•50 mg

Ascor L injection ℞ *vitamin C supplement* [ascorbic acid] 500 mg/mL

ascorbic acid (L-ascorbic acid; vitamin C) USP, INN, BAN, JAN *water-soluble vitamin; antiscorbutic; urinary acidifier; topical sunscreen* 250, 500, 1000, 1500 mg oral; 240 mg/tsp. oral; 500 mg/5 mL oral; 500 mg/mL injection

L-**ascorbic acid, monosodium salt** [see: sodium ascorbate]

L-**ascorbic acid 6-palmitate** [see: ascorbyl palmitate]

ascorbyl gamolenate INN, BAN

ascorbyl palmitate NF *antioxidant*

Ascriptin; Ascriptin A/D coated tablets OTC *analgesic; antipyretic; antiinflammatory; antirheumatic* [aspirin (buffered with magnesium hydroxide, aluminum hydroxide, and calcium carbonate)] 325, 500 mg; 325 mg

Asendin tablets ℞ *tricyclic antidepressant* [amoxapine] 25, 50, 100, 150 mg

aseptichrome [see: merbromin]

Aseptone 1; Aseptone 2; Aseptone 5; Aseptone QUAT ⓖ solution OTC *antiseptic; disinfectant; germicide*

ash, bitter *medicinal herb* [see: quassia; wahoo]

ash, mountain; American mountain ash; European mountain ash *medicinal herb* [see: mountain ash]

ash, poison *medicinal herb* [see: fringe tree]

ASHAP; A-SHAP (Adriamycin, Solu-Medrol, high-dose ara-C, Platinol) *chemotherapy protocol*

Asimina triloba *medicinal herb* [see: pawpaw]

Aslera ℞ *investigational (Phase III) treatment for systemic lupus erythematosus (SLE)* [prasterone]

Asmalix elixir ℞ *antiasthmatic; bronchodilator* [theophylline] 80 mg/15 mL

Asmanex Twisthaler (powder for oral inhalation) ℞ *corticosteroidal antiinflammatory for chronic asthma* [mometasone furoate] 200 μg/dose

AsO₃ (arsenic trioxide) [q.v.]

asobamast INN, BAN

asocainol INN

Aspalathus linearis; A. contaminata; Borbonia pinifolia *medicinal herb* [see: red bush tea]

asparaginase (L-asparaginase) USAN, JAN *antineoplastic for acute lymphocytic leukemia* [also: colaspase]

asparagine (L-asparagine) *nonessential amino acid; symbols: Asn, N*

L-**asparagine amidohydrolase** [see: asparaginase]

asparagus (*Asparagus officinalis***)** roots, seeds *medicinal herb for acne, constipation, contraception, edema, neuritis, parasites, rheumatism, stimulating hair growth, and toothache*

aspartame USAN, NF, INN, BAN *sweetener*

L-**aspartate potassium** JAN

aspartic acid (L-aspartic acid) USAN, INN *nonessential amino acid; symbols: Asp, D*

L-**aspartic acid insulin** [see: insulin aspart]

aspartocin USAN, INN *antibacterial*

A-Spas S/L sublingual tablets ℞ *GI/GU antispasmodic; anticholinergic* [hyoscyamine sulfate] 0.125 mg

aspen, European *medicinal herb* [see: black poplar]

aspen poplar; American aspen; quaking aspen *medicinal herb* [see: poplar]

Aspercreme cream OTC *analgesic* [trolamine salicylate] 10%

Aspercreme Rub lotion OTC *analgesic* [trolamine salicylate] 10%

Aspergillus oryase **proteinase** [see: asperkinase]

Aspergum chewing gum tablets OTC *analgesic; antipyretic; anti-inflammatory; antirheumatic* [aspirin] 227.5 mg

asperkinase

asperlin USAN *antibacterial; antineoplastic*

Asperula odorata *medicinal herb* [see: sweet woodruff]

aspidium (*Dryopteris filix-mas***)** plant *medicinal herb for bloody nose, menorrhagia, worm infections including tape-*

*worm and ringworm, and wound heal-
ing; not generally regarded as safe and
effective for internal use as it is highly
toxic*

aspidosperma USP

aspirin USP, BAN, JAN *analgesic; antipyretic; anti-inflammatory; antirheumatic*
325, 500, 650, 975 mg oral; 120, 200,
300, 600 mg suppositories ☑ Afrin

aspirin, buffered USP *analgesic; antipyretic; anti-inflammatory; antirheumatic*
325 mg oral

aspirin aluminum NF, JAN

aspirin & butalbital & caffeine *analgesic; barbiturate sedative* 325•50•40
mg oral

aspirin & codeine phosphate *antipyretic; analgesic; narcotic antitussive*
15•325 mg oral

**aspirin & codeine phosphate & car-
isoprodol** *narcotic analgesic; skeletal
muscle relaxant* 325•16•200 mg oral

aspirin DL-lysine JAN

Aspirin Free Excedrin caplets, geltabs OTC *analgesic; antipyretic* [aceta-
minophen; caffeine] 500•65 mg

**Aspirin with Codeine No. 2, No. 3,
and No. 4** tablets ℞ *narcotic antitussive; analgesic* [codeine phosphate;
aspirin] 15•325 mg; 30•325 mg;
60•325 mg

ASPIRINcheck urine test kit for professional use *in vitro diagnostic aid for
antiplatelet metabolites of aspirin*

Aspirin-Free Pain Relief tablets, caplets OTC *analgesic; antipyretic* [aceta-
minophen] 325, 500 mg; 500 mg

Aspirol (trademarked delivery form)
crushable ampule for inhalation

aspogen [see: dihydroxyaluminum
aminoacetate]

aspoxicillin INN, JAN

**Asprimox; Asprimox Extra Protec-
tion for Arthritis Pain** tablets, caplets OTC *analgesic; antipyretic; anti-
inflammatory; antirheumatic* [aspirin
(buffered with aluminum hydroxide,
magnesium hydroxide, and calcium
carbonate)] 325 mg

aspro [see: aspirin]

astatine *element (At)*

Astelin Ready-Spray nasal spray in a
metered-dose pump sprayer ℞
*peripherally selective phthalazinone
antihistamine and mast cell stabilizer
for allergic and vasomotor rhinitis* [azel-
astine HCl] 137 μg/spray

astemizole USAN, INN, BAN *antiallergic;
second-generation piperidine antihistamine*

AsthmaHaler inhalation aerosol (discontinued 2002) OTC *sympathomimetic bronchodilator* [epinephrine
bitartrate] 0.35 mg/dose

AsthmaNefrin solution for inhalation
(discontinued 2001) OTC *sympathomimetic bronchodilator* [racepineph-
rine HCl] 2.25%

astifilcon A USAN *hydrophilic contact
lens material*

Astracaine; Astracaine Forte ⓒⓐⓝ
intraoral injection ℞ *local anesthetic
for dentistry* [articaine HCl; epineph-
rine] 4%•1:200 000; 4%•1:100 000

**astragalus (*Astragalus membrana-
ceus*)** root *medicinal herb for cancer,
chronic fatigue, and Epstein-Barr syndrome; also used to strengthen the
immune system, especially after chemotherapy and HIV treatments*

Astramorph PF (preservative free) IV,
IM, or subcu injection ℞ *narcotic analgesic* [morphine sulfate] 0.5, 1 mg/mL

astringents *a class of agents that contract
tissue, reducing secretions or discharges*
[see also: hemostatics; styptics]

Astroglide vaginal gel OTC *lubricant*
[glycerin; propylene glycol]

astromicin INN *antibacterial* [also:
astromicin sulfate]

astromicin sulfate USAN, JAN *antibacterial* [also: astromicin]

AT-III (antithrombin III) [q.v.]

Atacand tablets ℞ *antihypertensive;
angiotensin II receptor antagonist;
treatment for heart failure; investigational (Phase III) for the prevention of
diabetic retinopathy* [candesartan
cilexetil] 4, 8, 16, 32 mg ☑ Ativan

Atacand HCT 16-12.5; Atacand HCT 32-12.5 tablets ℞ *antihypertensive; angiotensin II receptor antagonist; diuretic* [candesartan cilexetil; hydrochlorothiazide] 16•12.5; 32•12.5 mg

Atacand Plus ⊕ tablets ℞ *antihypertensive; angiotensin II receptor antagonist; diuretic* [candesartan cilexetil; hydrochlorothiazide] 16•12.5 mg

atamestane INN *investigational (Phase III) aromatase inhibitor for breast cancer*

ataprost INN

ataquimast INN

Atarax tablets, syrup (discontinued 2004) ℞ *anxiolytic; minor tranquilizer* [hydroxyzine HCl] 10, 25, 50, 100 mg; 10 mg/5 mL ⊘ Marax

Atarax 100 tablets (discontinued 2004) ℞ *anxiolytic; minor tranquilizer; antihistamine for allergic pruritus* [hydroxyzine HCl] 100 mg ⊘ Marax

atarvet [see: acepromazine]

atazanavir sulfate *antiviral; azapeptide protease inhibitor for HIV-1 infection*

atenolol USAN, INN, BAN, JAN *antihypertensive; antiadrenergic (β-receptor)* 25, 50, 100 mg oral ⊘ Actonel; timolol

atevirdine INN *antiviral* [also: atevirdine mesylate]

atevirdine mesylate USAN *antiviral; investigational (Phase II/III) non-nucleoside reverse transcriptase inhibitor (NNRTI) for HIV and AIDS* [also: atevirdine]

ATG (antithymocyte globulin) [q.v.]

Atgam IV infusion ℞ *treatment for aplastic anemia; immunizing agent to prevent allograft rejection of renal transplants; investigational (orphan) for organ and bone marrow transplants* [antithymocyte globulin, equine] 50 mg/mL

athyromazole [see: carbimazole]

atipamezole USAN, INN, BAN *α₂-receptor antagonist*

atiprimod dihydrochloride USAN *immunomodulator; anti-inflammatory; antiarthritic*

atiprimod dimaleate USAN *immunomodulator; anti-inflammatory; antiarthritic*

atiprosin INN *antihypertensive* [also: atiprosin maleate]

atiprosin maleate USAN *antihypertensive* [also: atiprosin]

Ativan IV or IM injection ℞ *benzodiazepine anxiolytic; preanesthetic sedative; anticonvulsant* [lorazepam] 2, 4 mg/mL ⊘ Atacand; Adapin; Avitene

Ativan tablets (discontinued 2003) ℞ *benzodiazepine anxiolytic; sedative* [lorazepam] 0.5, 1, 2 mg ⊘ Adapin; Avitene

atizoram USAN, INN

atlaﬁlcon A USAN *hydrophilic contact lens material*

ATnativ ℞ *investigational (orphan) agent for congenital AT-III deficiency in patients undergoing surgical or obstetrical procedures* [antithrombin III]

atolide USAN, INN *anticonvulsant*

Atolone tablets ℞ *corticosteroid; anti-inflammatory* [triamcinolone] 4 mg

atomoxetine HCl *selective norepinephrine reuptake inhibitor for attention-deficit hyperactivity disorder (ADHD); investigational (orphan) for Tourette syndrome*

Atopik ℞ *investigational (Phase III) topical phosphodiesterase 4 (PDE₄) inhibitor for eczema*

atorolimumab INN

atorvastatin calcium USAN *HMG-CoA reductase inhibitor for hypercholesterolemia, dysbetalipoproteinemia, and hypertriglyceridemia; prevention of cardiovascular disease in high-risk patients*

atosiban USAN, INN *oxytocin antagonist*

atovaquone USAN, INN, BAN *antimalarial; antiprotozoal for AIDS-related Pneumocystis carinii pneumonia (orphan); investigational (orphan) for AIDS-related Toxoplasma gondii encephalitis*

ATP (adenosine triphosphate) [see: adenosine triphosphate disodium]

ATPase (adenosine triphosphatase) inhibitors *a class of gastric antisecretory agents that inhibit the ATPase "proton pump" within the gastric parietal cell*

[also called: proton pump inhibitors; substituted benzimidazoles]

atracurium besilate INN *skeletal muscle relaxant; nondepolarizing neuromuscular blocker; adjunct to anesthesia* [also: atracurium besylate]

atracurium besylate USAN, BAN *skeletal muscle relaxant; nondepolarizing neuromuscular blocker; adjunct to anesthesia* [also: atracurium besilate] 10 mg/mL injection

atrasentan HCl USAN *investigational (NDA filed) endothelin-A (EtA; ETA; ET_A) receptor antagonist to retard the progression of metastatic prostate cancer by reducing its proliferative effects in bone and prostate tissue*

atreleuton USAN *5-lipoxygenase inhibitor for asthma*

Atretol tablets (discontinued 2004) ℞ *anticonvulsant; analgesic for trigeminal neuralgia; antipsychotic* [carbamazepine] 200 mg

Atridox controlled-release gel for subgingival injection ℞ *antibiotic for periodontal disease* [doxycycline hyclate] 10%

Atrigel (trademarked delivery system) *sustained-release delivery*

Atrigel Depot (trademarked delivery system) *sustained-release subcu injection*

atrimustine INN

atrinositol INN

Atrohist Pediatric oral suspension (discontinued 2002) ℞ *pediatric decongestant and antihistamine* [phenylephrine tannate; chlorpheniramine tannate; pyrilamine tannate] 5•2•12.5 mg/5 mL

Atrohist Pediatric sustained-release capsules (discontinued 2002) ℞ *pediatric decongestant and antihistamine* [pseudoephedrine HCl; chlorpheniramine maleate] 60•4 mg

Atrohist Plus sustained-release tablets (discontinued 2001) ℞ *decongestant; antihistamine; anticholinergic* [phenylpropanolamine HCl; phenylephrine HCl; chlorpheniramine maleate; hyoscyamine sulfate; atropine sul-

fate; scopolamine hydrobromide] 50•25•8•0.19•0.04•0.01 mg

atromepine INN, DCF

Atromid-S capsules (discontinued 2002) ℞ *triglyceride-lowering antihyperlipidemic for primary dysbetalipoproteinemia (type III hyperlipidemia) and hypertriglyceridemia (types IV and V hyperlipidemia)* [clofibrate] 500 mg (1 g available in Canada)

Atropa belladonna medicinal herb [see: belladonna]

AtroPen auto-injector (automatic IM injection device) ℞ *antidote for organophosphorous or carbamate insecticides* [atropine sulfate] 0.5, 1, 2 mg/0.7 mL dose

atropine USP, BAN *anticholinergic*

Atropine Care eye drops (discontinued 2004) ℞ *mydriatic; cycloplegic* [atropine sulfate] 1%

atropine methonitrate INN, BAN *anticholinergic* [also: methylatropine nitrate]

atropine methylnitrate [see: methylatropine nitrate]

atropine oxide INN *anticholinergic* [also: atropine oxide HCl]

atropine oxide HCl USAN *anticholinergic* [also: atropine oxide]

atropine propionate [see: prampine]

atropine sulfate USP, JAN *GI/GU antispasmodic; antiparkinsonian; bronchodilator; cycloplegic; mydriatic; antidote to insecticide poisoning* [also: atropine sulphate] 0.4, 0.6 mg oral; 1%, 2% eye drops; 0.05, 0.1, 0.3, 0.4, 0.5, 0.8, 1 mg/mL injection

atropine sulphate BAN *GI/GU antispasmodic; antiparkinsonian; bronchodilator; cycloplegic; mydriatic* [also: atropine sulfate]

Atropine-1 eye drops ℞ *mydriatic; cycloplegic* [atropine sulfate] 1%

Atropisol Dropperettes (eye drops) (discontinued 2003) ℞ *cycloplegic; mydriatic* [atropine sulfate] 1%

Atrosept sugar-coated tablets ℞ *urinary antibiotic; analgesic; antispasmodic; acidifier* [methenamine;

phenyl salicylate; atropine sulfate; methylene blue; hyoscyamine sulfate; benzoic acid] 40.8•18.1•0.03•5.4•0.03•4.5 mg

Atrovent nasal spray, inhalation aerosol ℞ *anticholinergic bronchodilator for bronchospasm; antisecretory for rhinorrhea* [ipratropium bromide] 0.03%, 0.06%; 18 μg/dose ☑ Trovan

Atrovent solution for inhalation (discontinued 2005) ℞ *anticholinergic bronchodilator for bronchospasm; antisecretory for rhinorrhea* [ipratropium bromide] 0.02% ☑ Trovan

Atrovent HFA inhalation aerosol with a CFC-free propellant ℞ *bronchodilator for bronchospasm due to chronic obstructive pulmonary disease (COPD)* [ipratropium bromide] 17 μg/dose

A/T/S topical solution, gel ℞ *antibiotic for acne* [erythromycin; alcohol 66%–92%] 2%

Attain oral liquid OTC *enteral nutritional therapy* [lactose-free formula]

attapulgite, activated USP *suspending agent; GI adsorbent*

Attenuvax powder for subcu injection ℞ *measles vaccine* [measles virus vaccine, live attenuated] 0.5 mL

Atuss DM syrup ℞ *antitussive; decongestant; antihistamine* [dextromethorphan hydrobromide; phenylephrine HCl; chlorpheniramine maleate] 30•20•4 mg/10 mL

Atuss EX syrup (discontinued 2004) ℞ *narcotic antitussive; expectorant* [hydrocodone bitartrate; potassium guaiacolsulfonate] 5•240 mg/10 mL

Atuss G syrup ℞ *narcotic antitussive; decongestant; expectorant* [hydrocodone bitartrate; phenylephrine HCl; guaifenesin] 4•20•200 mg/10 mL

Atuss HC; Atuss HD; Atuss MS oral liquid ℞ *narcotic antitussive; decongestant; antihistamine* [hydrocodone bitartrate; phenylephrine HCl; chlorpheniramine maleate] 2.5•10•2 mg/5 mL; 2.5•10•4 mg/5 mL; 5•10•2 mg/5 mL

Atuss-12 DM extended-release oral suspension ℞ *antitussive; decongestant; antihistamine* [dextromethorphan polistirex; pseudoephedrine polistirex; chlorpheniramine polistirex] 30•30•6 mg/5 mL

Atuss-12 DX extended-release oral suspension ℞ *antitussive; expectorant* [dextromethorphan hydrobromide; guaifenesin] 30•200 mg/5 mL

"atypical" antipsychotics [see: novel antipsychotics]

¹⁹⁸Au [see: gold Au 198]

augmented betamethasone dipropionate *topical corticosteroid*

Augmentin film-coated tablets, chewable tablets, powder for oral suspension ℞ *aminopenicillin antibiotic plus synergist* [amoxicillin; clavulanate potassium] 250•125, 500•125, 875•125 mg; 125•31.25, 200•28.5, 250•62.5, 400•57 mg; 125•31.25, 200•28.5, 250•62.5, 400•57 mg/5 mL

Augmentin ES-600 powder for oral suspension ℞ *aminopenicillin antibiotic plus synergist* [amoxicillin; clavulanate potassium] 600•43.9 mg/5 mL

Augmentin XR extended-release film-coated tablets ℞ *aminopenicillin antibiotic plus synergist* [amoxicillin; clavulanic acid] 1000•62.5 mg

augmerosen investigational (NDA filed, orphan) antineoplastic for malignant melanoma; investigational (Phase III, orphan) for multiple myeloma and chronic lymphocytic leukemia (CLL)

Auralgan Otic ear drops ℞ *local anesthetic; analgesic* [benzocaine; antipyrine] 1.4%•5.4% ☑ Allergan; allergen

auranofin USAN, INN, BAN, JAN *antirheumatic (29% gold)*

aureoquin [now: quinetolate]

Auriculin investigational (orphan) for acute renal failure and renal transplants [anaritide acetate]

Auro Ear Drops OTC *agent to emulsify and disperse ear wax* [carbamide peroxide] 6.5%

Auro-Dri ear drops OTC *antibacterial; antifungal* [boric acid] 2.75%

Auroguard Otic ear drops ℞ *local anesthetic; analgesic* [benzocaine; antipyrine] 1.4%•5.4%

Aurolate IM injection ℞ *antirheumatic* [gold sodium thiomalate] 50 mg/mL

aurolin [see: gold sodium thiosulfate]

auropin [see: gold sodium thiosulfate]

aurosan [see: gold sodium thiosulfate]

aurothioglucose USP *antirheumatic (50% gold)*

aurothioglycanide INN, DCF

aurothiomalate disodium [see: gold sodium thiomalate]

aurothiomalate sodium [see: gold sodium thiomalate]

Auroto Otic ear drops (discontinued 2004) ℞ *local anesthetic; analgesic* [antipyrine; benzocaine] 1.4%•5.4%

Australian tea tree *medicinal herb* [see: tea tree oil]

Autohaler (delivery form) *breath-activated metered-dose inhaler*

auto-injector (delivery device) *automatic IM injection device*

autologous cell (AC) vaccine *investigational (Phase III, orphan) therapeutic vaccine for adjuvant treatment of ovarian cancer*

autolymphocyte therapy (ALT) *investigational (orphan) for metastatic renal cell carcinoma*

Autoplex T IV injection or drip ℞ *antihemophilic to correct factor VIII deficiency and coagulation deficiency* [anti-inhibitor coagulant complex, heat treated] (each bottle is labeled with dosage)

autoprothrombin I [see: factor VII]

autoprothrombin II [see: factor IX]

autumn crocus (Colchicum autumnale; C. speciosum; C. vernum) plant and corm *medicinal herb for edema, gonorrhea, gout, prostate enlargement, and rheumatism; not generally regarded as safe and effective as it is highly toxic because of its colchicine content*

AV (Adriamycin, vincristine) *chemotherapy protocol*

AVA (anthrax vaccine, adsorbed) [q.v.]

Avage cream ℞ *retinoid pro-drug; adjuvant treatment for facial wrinkles, hyper- and hypopigmentation, and benign lentigines* [tazarotene] 0.1%

Avail tablets OTC *vitamin/mineral/iron supplement* [multiple vitamins & minerals; iron; folic acid] ≛•18•0.4 mg ⧉ Advil

Avalide tablets ℞ *antihypertensive; angiotensin II receptor antagonist; diuretic* [irbesartan; hydrochlorothiazide] 150•12.5, 300•12.5, 300•25 mg

Avandamet film-coated tablets ℞ *antidiabetic combination for type 2 diabetes* [rosiglitazone maleate; metformin HCl] 1•500, 2•500, 2•1000, 4•500, 4•1000 mg

Avandia film-coated tablets ℞ *thiazolidinedione (TZD) antidiabetic; increases cellular response to insulin without increasing insulin secretion* [rosiglitazone maleate] 2, 4, 8 mg

Avapro tablets ℞ *angiotensin II receptor antagonist for hypertension; treatment to delay the progression of diabetic nephropathy* [irbesartan] 75, 150, 300 mg

Avar cleanser, gel ℞ *acne treatment* [sulfacetamide sodium; sulfur] 10%•5%

Avar Green gel ℞ *acne treatment; tinted for "color correction"* [sulfacetamide sodium; sulfur] 10%•5%

avasimibe USAN, INN *acylCoA transferase (ACAT) inhibitor for hyperlipidemia and atherosclerosis*

Avastin IV infusion ℞ *antineoplastic; angiogenesis inhibitor for metastatic colorectal cancer; investigational (Phase III) for metastatic breast cancer, cervical cancer, non–small cell lung cancer (NSCLC), and renal cell carcinoma* [bevacizumab] 25 mg/mL

Avaxim ⊕ prefilled syringe for IM injection ℞ *immunization against hepatitis A virus (HAV)* [hepatitis A vaccine, inactivated] 0.5 mL

AVC vaginal cream, vaginal inserts (discontinued 2001) ℞ *broad-spectrum antibiotic* [sulfanilamide] 15%; 1.05 g

Aveeno lotion OTC *moisturizer; emollient* [colloidal oatmeal] 1%

Aveeno Anti-Itch cream, lotion (discontinued 2003) OTC *poison ivy treatment* [calamine; pramoxine HCl; camphor] 3%•1%•0.3%

Aveeno Cleansing bar OTC *soap-free therapeutic skin cleanser* [colloidal oatmeal] 51%

Aveeno Cleansing for Acne-Prone Skin bar OTC *medicated cleanser for acne* [salicylic acid; colloidal oatmeal]

Aveeno Moisturizing cream OTC *moisturizer; emollient* [colloidal oatmeal] 1%

Aveeno Oilated Bath packets OTC *bath emollient* [colloidal oatmeal; mineral oil] 43%• ⍰

Aveeno Regular Bath packets OTC *bath emollient* [colloidal oatmeal] 100%

Aveeno Shave gel OTC *moisturizer; emollient* [oatmeal flour]

Aveeno Shower & Bath oil OTC *bath emollient* [colloidal oatmeal] 5%

Avelox film-coated tablets, IV infusion ℞ *broad-spectrum fluoroquinolone antibiotic* [moxifloxacin HCl] 400 mg; 400 mg/bag

Avena sativa medicinal herb [see: oats]

Aventyl HCl oral solution (discontinued 2005) ℞ *tricyclic antidepressant* [nortriptyline HCl] 10 mg/5 mL ⍰ Ambenyl; Bentyl

Aventyl HCl Pulvules (capsules) ℞ *tricyclic antidepressant* [nortriptyline HCl] 10, 25 mg ⍰ Ambenyl; Bentyl

avertin [see: tribromoethanol]

Aviane tablets (in packs of 28) ℞ *monophasic oral contraceptive* [levonorgestrel; ethinyl estradiol] 0.1 mg•20 μg

avicatonin INN

Avicine ℞ *investigational (Phase III) theraccine for cervical and pancreatic cancer; investigational (Phase II) for prostate and advanced colorectal cancers* [CTP-37 (code name—generic name not yet assigned)]

avilamycin USAN, INN, BAN *antibacterial*

avinar [see: uredepa]

Avinza dual-release (immediate- plus extended-release) capsules ℞ *once-daily narcotic analgesic for treatment of chronic pain* [morphine sulfate] 30, 60, 90, 120 mg

Avita cream, gel ℞ *keratolytic for acne* [tretinoin] 0.025% ⍰ Evista

Avitene Hemostat nonwoven web ℞ *topical hemostatic aid for surgery* [microfibrillar collagen hemostat] ⍰ Ativan

avitriptan fumarate USAN *serotonin 5-HT₁ agonist for migraine*

avizafone INN, BAN

avobenzone USAN, INN *sunscreen*

avocado (*Persea americana; P. gratissima*) fruit and seed *medicinal herb for diarrhea, dysentery, inducing menstruation, lowering total cholesterol and improving overall lipid profile, promoting hair growth, and stimulating wound healing; also used as an aphrodisiac*

avocado sugar extract *natural weight-loss agent used to diminish carbohydrate cravings* [see also: D-mannoheptulose]

Avodart capsules ℞ *5α-reductase blocker for benign prostatic hyperplasia (BPH); investigational (Phase III) for prostate cancer* [dutasteride] 0.5 mg

Avolean capsules OTC *natural weight-loss agent used to diminish carbohydrate cravings* [avocado sugar extract] 50 mg

Avonex powder for IM injection (multidose vials replaced by single-use prefilled syringes in 2003)

Avonex prefilled syringes for IM injection ℞ *immunomodulator for relapsing remitting multiple sclerosis (orphan); investigational (orphan) for non-A, non-B hepatitis, Kaposi sarcoma, brain tumors, and various other cancers* [interferon beta-1a] 30 μg (6 MIU)/ 0.5 mL syringe

avoparcin USAN, INN, BAN *glycopeptide antibiotic*

AVP (actinomycin D, vincristine, Platinol) *chemotherapy protocol*

avridine USAN, INN *antiviral*

Award *hydrophilic contact lens material* [hilafilcon A]

axamozide INN

axerophthol [see: vitamin A]

Axert tablets ℞ *vascular serotonin HT$_{1B/1D/1F}$ receptor agonist for the acute treatment of migraine* [almotriptan malate] 6.25, 12.5 mg

axetil USAN, INN *combining name for radicals or groups*

Axid Pulvules (capsules); oral liquid ℞ *histamine H$_2$ antagonist for treatment of gastric and duodenal ulcers* [nizatidine] 150, 300 mg; 15 mg/mL ② Biaxin

Axid AR ("acid reducer") tablets OTC *histamine H$_2$ antagonist for heartburn* [nizatidine] 75 mg

axitirome USAN, INN *antihyperlipidemic*

Axocet caplets (discontinued 2004) ℞ *analgesic; barbiturate sedative* [acetaminophen; butalbital] 650•50 mg

Axocet capsules (discontinued 2003) ℞ *analgesic; barbiturate sedative* [acetaminophen; butalbital] 650•50 mg

Axokine ℞ *investigational (Phase III) second-generation ciliary neurotrophic factor for obesity associated with type 2 diabetes*

Aygestin tablets ℞ *progestin for amenorrhea, abnormal uterine bleeding, or endometriosis* [norethindrone acetate] 5 mg

Ayr Saline nasal mist, nose drops, nasal gel OTC *nasal moisturizer* [sodium chloride (saline solution)] 0.65%

5-AZA (5-azacitidine) [see: azacitidine]

5-aza-2'-deoxycytidine *investigational (orphan) for acute leukemia*

azabon USAN, INN *CNS stimulant*

azabuperone INN

azacitidine (5-AZA; 5-AZC) USAN, INN *demethylating antineoplastic for myelodysplastic syndrome (orphan)*

azaclorzine INN *coronary vasodilator* [also: azaclorzine HCl]

azaclorzine HCl USAN *coronary vasodilator* [also: azaclorzine]

azaconazole USAN, INN *antifungal*

azacosterol INN *avian chemosterilant* [also: azacosterol HCl]

azacosterol HCl USAN *avian chemosterilant* [also: azacosterol]

AZA-CR [see: azacitidine]

Azactam powder for IV or IM injection ℞ *monobactam bactericidal antibiotic* [aztreonam] 0.5, 1, 2 g

azacyclonol INN, BAN [also: azacyclonol HCl]

azacyclonol HCl NF [also: azacyclonol]

5-azacytosine arabinoside (ara-AC) [see: fazarabine]

5-aza-2'-deoxycytidine *investigational (orphan) for acute leukemia*

Azadirachta indica *medicinal herb* [see: neem tree]

azaftozine INN

azalanstat dihydrochloride USAN *hypolipidemic*

azaline B [now: prazarelix acetate]

azalomycin INN, BAN

azaloxan INN *antidepressant* [also: azaloxan fumarate]

azaloxan fumarate USAN *antidepressant* [also: azaloxan]

azamethiphos BAN

azamethonium bromide INN, BAN

azamulin INN

azanator INN *bronchodilator* [also: azanator maleate]

azanator maleate USAN *bronchodilator* [also: azanator]

azanidazole USAN, INN, BAN *antiprotozoal*

azaperone USAN, INN, BAN *antipsychotic*

azapetine BAN

azapetine phosphate [see: azapetine]

azaprocin INN

azapropazone INN, BAN, DCF *antiinflammatory* [also: apazone]

azaquinzole INN

azaribine USAN, INN, BAN *antipsoriatic*

azarole USAN *immunoregulator*

Azasan tablets ℞ *immunosuppressant for organ transplantation (orphan) and rheumatoid arthritis* [azathioprine] 25, 50, 75, 100 mg

azaserine USAN, INN *antifungal*

azasetron INN

azaspirium chloride INN

azaspirones *a class of anxiolytics*

azastene

azatadine INN, BAN *piperidine antihista-mine for allergic rhinitis and chronic urticaria* [also: azatadine maleate]

azatadine maleate USAN, USP *piperidine antihistamine for allergic rhinitis and chronic urticaria* [also: azatadine]

azatepa INN *antineoplastic* [also: azetepa]

azathioprine USAN, USP, INN, BAN, JAN *immunosuppressant for organ transplantation (orphan) and rheumatoid arthritis* 50 mg oral

azathioprine sodium USP *immunosuppressant for organ transplantation (orphan) and rheumatoid arthritis* 100 mg injection

5-AZC (5-azacitidine) [see: azacitidine]

Azdone tablets ℞ *narcotic analgesic* [hydrocodone bitartrate; aspirin] 5•500 mg

azdU (3′-azido-2′,3′-dideoxyuridine) [see: azidouridine]

azelaic acid USAN, INN *topical antimicrobial and keratolytic for acne and rosacea*

azelastine INN, BAN *peripherally selective phthalazinone antihistamine for allergic and vasomotor rhinitis; mast cell stabilizer; antiasthmatic* [also: azelastine HCl]

azelastine HCl USAN, JAN *peripherally selective phthalazinone antihistamine for allergic and vasomotor rhinitis; mast cell stabilizer; antiasthmatic* [also: azelastine]

Azelex cream ℞ *antimicrobial and keratolytic for inflammatory acne vulgaris* [azelaic acid] 20%

azelnidipine INN

azepexole INN, BAN

azephine [see: azapetine phosphate]

azepinamide [see: glypinamide]

azepindole USAN, INN *antidepressant*

azetepa USAN, BAN *antineoplastic* [also: azatepa]

azetirelin INN

azidamfenicol INN, BAN, DCF

3′-azido-2′,3′-dideoxyuridine (azdU) [see: azidouridine]

azidoamphenicol [see: azidamfenicol]

azidocillin INN, BAN

azidothymidine (AZT) [now: zidovudine]

azidouridine (azdU) *investigational (orphan) antiviral for HIV and AIDS*

azimexon INN

azimilide dihydrochloride USAN *investigational (NDA filed) antiarrhythmic and antifibrillatory*

azintamide INN

azinthiamide [see: azintamide]

azipramine INN *antidepressant* [also: azipramine HCl]

azipramine HCl USAN *antidepressant* [also: azipramine]

aziridinyl benzoquinone [see: diaziquone]

azithromycin USAN, USP, INN, BAN *macrolide antibiotic*

azlocillin USAN, INN, BAN *penicillin antibiotic*

azlocillin sodium USP *penicillin antibiotic*

Azmacort oral inhalation aerosol ℞ *corticosteroidal anti-inflammatory for chronic asthma* [triamcinolone acetonide] 100 μg/dose

Azo Test Strips reagent strips for home use *in vitro diagnostic aid for urinary tract infections*

azoconazole [now: azaconazole]

azodisal sodium (ADS) [now: olsalazine sodium]

"azoles" *a class of fungicides that include all with generic names ending in "azole," such clotrimazole, fluconazole, etc.*

azolimine USAN, INN *diuretic* ⊘ Azulfidine

Azoline ℞ *investigational (Phase III) oral triazole antifungal for fungal infections of the skin, hair, nails, and oral and genital mucosa*

Azopt eye drop suspension ℞ *carbonic anhydrase inhibitor for glaucoma* [brinzolamide] 1%

azosemide USAN, INN, JAN *diuretic*

Azo-Standard tablets OTC *urinary analgesic* [phenazopyridine HCl] 95 mg

Azostix reagent strips for professional use *in vitro diagnostic aid to estimate the amount of BUN in whole blood*

Azo-Sulfisoxazole tablets ℞ *urinary anti-infective; urinary analgesic* [sulfisoxazole; phenazopyridine HCl] 500•50 mg

azotomycin USAN, INN *antibiotic antineoplastic*

azovan blue BAN *blood volume test* [also: Evans blue]

azovan sodium [see: Evans blue]

AZT (azidothymidine) [now: zidovudine]

Aztec controlled release ℞ *investigational (Phase III) antiviral for early HIV and AIDS* [zidovudine]

aztreonam USAN, USP, INN, BAN, JAN *monobactam bactericidal antibiotic; investigational (orphan) inhalation therapy for cystic fibrosis*

azulene sulfonate sodium JAN [also: sodium gualenate]

Azulfidine tablets ℞ *broad-spectrum bacteriostatic; anti-inflammatory for ulcerative colitis* [sulfasalazine] 500 mg ② Silvadene

Azulfidine EN-tabs enteric-coated delayed-release tablets ℞ *broad-spectrum bacteriostatic; anti-inflammatory for ulcerative colitis, rheumatoid arthritis (RA), and juvenile rheumatoid arthritis (JRA)* [sulfasalazine] 500 mg

azumolene INN *skeletal muscle relaxant* [also: azumolene sodium]

azumolene sodium USAN *skeletal muscle relaxant* [also: azumolene]

azure A carbacrylic resin [see: azuresin]

azuresin NF, BAN

1,4-B (1,4-butanediol) *a precursor to gamma hydroxybutyrate (GHB); a formerly legal alternative to GHB, now also illegal (Schedule I)* [see: gamma hydroxybutyrate (GHB)]

B Complex + C timed-release tablets OTC *vitamin supplement* [multiple B vitamins; vitamin C] ≛•500 mg

B Complex with C and B-12 injection ℞ *parenteral vitamin supplement* [multiple vitamins]

B Complex-50 sustained-release tablets OTC *vitamin supplement* [multiple B vitamins; folic acid; biotin] ≛• 400•50 μg

B Complex-150 sustained-release tablets OTC *vitamin supplement* [multiple B vitamins; folic acid; biotin] ≛• 400•150 μg

B & O Supprettes No. 15A; B & O Supprettes No. 16A suppositories ℞ *narcotic analgesic* [belladonna extract; opium] 16.2•30 mg; 16.2•60 mg

B vitamins [see: vitamin B]

B₁ (vitamin B₁) [see: thiamine HCl]

B₂ (vitamin B₂) [see: riboflavin]

B₃ (vitamin B₃) [see: niacin; niacinamide]

B₅ (vitamin B₅) [see: calcium pantothenate]

B₆ (vitamin B₆) [see: pyridoxine HCl]

B₈ (vitamin B₈) [see: adenosine phosphate]

B₁₂ (vitamin B₁₂) [see: cyanocobalamin]

B₁₂ₐ (vitamin B₁₂ₐ) [see: hydroxocobalamin]

B₁₂ᵦ (vitamin B₁₂ᵦ) [see: hydroxocobalamin]

B-50 tablets OTC *vitamin supplement* [multiple B vitamins; folic acid; biotin] ≛•100•50 μg

B-100 tablets, timed-release tablets OTC *vitamin supplement* [multiple B vitamins; folic acid; biotin] ≛•100• 100 μg; ≛•400•50 μg

Bᶜ (vitamin Bᶜ) [see: folic acid]

Bₜ (vitamin Bₜ) [see: carnitine]

Babee Teething lotion OTC *topical oral anesthetic; antiseptic* [benzocaine; cetalkonium chloride] 2.5%•0.02%

baby brain I *chemotherapy protocol for pediatric brain tumors* [see: COPE]

Baby Vitamin drops OTC *vitamin supplement* [multiple vitamins]

Baby Vitamin with Iron drops OTC *vitamin/iron supplement* [multiple vitamins; iron] ≟•10 mg/mL

BabyBIG powder for IV infusion ℞ *treatment for infant botulism type A or B (orphan)* [botulism immune globulin (BIG)] 100 mg/vial

Babylax [see: Fleet Babylax]

BAC (BCNU, ara-C, cyclophosphamide) *chemotherapy protocol*

BAC (benzalkonium chloride) [q.v.]

bacampicillin INN, BAN *aminopenicillin antibiotic* [also: bacampicillin HCl]

bacampicillin HCl USAN, USP, JAN *aminopenicillin antibiotic* [also: bacampicillin]

bachelor's buttons *medicinal herb* [see: cornflower; feverfew; tansy; buttercup]

Bacid capsules OTC *probiotic; dietary supplement; fever blister treatment; not generally regarded as safe and effective as an antidiarrheal* [*Lactobacillus acidophilus*] 500 million CFU ⊡ Banacid

Baciguent ointment (discontinued 2003) OTC *antibiotic* [bacitracin] 500 U/g

Baci-IM powder for IM injection ℞ *bactericidal antibiotic* [bacitracin] 50 000 U

bacillus Calmette-Guérin (BCG) vaccine [see: BCG vaccine]

bacitracin USP, INN, BAN, JAN *bactericidal antibiotic; investigational (orphan) for pseudomembranous enterocolitis* 500 U/g topical; 50 000 U/vial injection ⊡ Bacitrin; Bactrim

bacitracin zinc USP, BAN *bactericidal antibiotic*

bacitracin zinc & neomycin sulfate & polymyxin B sulfate *topical antibiotic* 400 U•5 mg•10 000 U per g ophthalmic

bacitracin zinc & polymyxin B sulfate *topical antibiotic* 500•10 000 U/g ophthalmic

bacitracins zinc complex [see: bacitracin zinc]

Backache Maximum Strength Relief film-coated caplets OTC *analgesic; antirheumatic* [magnesium salicylate] 467 mg

Back-Pack (trademarked packaging form) *unit-of-use package*

baclofen (L-baclofen) USAN, USP, INN, BAN, JAN *skeletal muscle relaxant for intractable spasticity due to spinal cord injury or disease (orphan); investigational (orphan) for dystonia* 10, 20 mg oral

bacmecillinam INN

Bacmin tablets ℞ *vitamin/mineral/iron supplement* [multiple vitamins & minerals; iron; folic acid; biotin] ≟• 27•0.8•0.15 mg

BACOD (bleomycin, Adriamycin, CCNU, Oncovin, dexamethasone) *chemotherapy protocol*

BACON (bleomycin, Adriamycin, CCNU, Oncovin, nitrogen mustard) *chemotherapy protocol*

BACOP (bleomycin, Adriamycin, cyclophosphamide, Oncovin, prednisone) *chemotherapy protocol*

BACT (BCNU, ara-C, cyclophosphamide, thioguanine) *chemotherapy protocol*

bactericidal and permeability-increasing (BPI) protein, recombinant *investigational (Phase III, orphan) treatment for gram-negative sepsis, hemorrhagic shock, and meningococcemia*

bacteriostatic sodium chloride [see: sodium chloride]

Bacteriostatic Sodium Chloride Injection ℞ *IV diluent* [sodium chloride (normal saline solution)] 0.9% (normal)

Bacti-Cleanse topical liquid OTC *soap-free therapeutic skin cleanser* [benzalkonium chloride]

Bactigen B Streptococcus-CS slide test for professional use *in vitro diag-*

nostic aid for Group B streptococcal antigens in vaginal and cervical swabs

Bactigen Meningitis Panel slide test for professional use *in vitro diagnostic aid for* H. influenzae, N. meningitidis, *and* S. pneumoniae *in various fluids* [latex agglutination test]

Bactigen N. *meningitidis* slide test for professional use (discontinued 2004) *in vitro diagnostic aid for* Neisseria meningitidis [latex agglutination test]

Bactigen Salmonella-Shigella slide test for professional use *in vitro diagnostic aid for salmonella and shigella* [latex agglutination test]

Bactine Antiseptic Anesthetic topical liquid, spray OTC *local anesthetic; antiseptic* [lidocaine HCl; benzalkonium chloride] 2.5%•0.13%

Bactine First Aid Antibiotic Plus Anesthetic ointment (discontinued 2001) OTC *antibiotic; local anesthetic* [polymyxin B sulfate; neomycin sulfate; bacitracin; diperodon HCl] 5000 U•3.5 mg•400 U•10 mg per g

Bactine Hydrocortisone; Maximum Strength Bactine cream OTC *corticosteroidal anti-inflammatory* [hydrocortisone] 0.5%; 1%

Bactine Pain Relieving Cleansing Spray OTC *local anesthetic; antiseptic* [lidocaine HCl; benzalkonium chloride] 2.5%•0.13%

Bactine Pain Relieving Cleansing Wipes OTC *local anesthetic; antiseptic* [pramoxine HCl; benzalkonium chloride] 1%•0.13%

Bactocill powder for IV or IM injection (discontinued 2002) ℞ *penicillinase-resistant penicillin antibiotic* [oxacillin sodium] 0.5, 1, 2, 4, 10 g ☐ Pathocil

BactoShield aerosol foam, solution OTC *broad-spectrum antimicrobial; germicidal* [chlorhexidine gluconate; alcohol 4%] 4%

BactoShield 2 solution OTC *broad-spectrum antimicrobial; germicidal* [chlorhexidine gluconate; alcohol 4%] 2%

Bactrim; Bactrim DS tablets ℞ *anti-infective; antibacterial* [trimethoprim; sulfamethoxazole] 80•400 mg; 160•800 mg ☐ bacitracin

Bactrim IV infusion ℞ *anti-infective; antibacterial* [trimethoprim; sulfamethoxazole] 80•400 mg/5 mL

Bactrim Pediatric oral suspension ℞ *anti-infective; antibacterial* [trimethoprim; sulfamethoxazole] 40•200 mg/5 mL

Bactroban cream ℞ in the U.S.; OTC in Canada *antibiotic* [mupirocin calcium] 2.15% (=2% base)

Bactroban ointment ℞ *antibiotic for impetigo* [mupirocin] 2%

Bactroban Nasal ointment in single-use tubes ℞ *antibiotic for iatrogenic methicillin-resistant* Staphylococcus aureus (MRSA) *infections* [mupirocin calcium] 2.15% (=2% base)

Bagshawe protocol, modified *chemotherapy protocol* [see: CHAMOCA]

bakeprofen INN

baker's yeast *natural source of protein and B-complex vitamins*

BAL (British antilewisite) [now: dimercaprol]

BAL in Oil deep IM injection ℞ *chelating agent for arsenic, gold, and mercury poisoning; adjunct to lead poisoning* [dimercaprol in peanut oil] 10% ☐ Balneol

Balacet 325 tablets ℞ *narcotic analgesic* [propoxyphene napsylate; acetaminophen] 100•325 mg

balafilcon A USAN *hydrophilic contact lens material*

balaglitazone *peroxisome proliferator–activated receptor (PPAR) gamma agonist; investigational oral insulin sensitizer for type 2 diabetes*

Balamine DM syrup, pediatric oral drops ℞ *antitussive; decongestant; antihistamine* [dextromethorphan hydrobromide; pseudoephedrine HCl; carbinoxamine maleate] 12.5•60•4 mg/5 mL; 3.5•25•2 mg/mL

balipramine BAN [also: depramine]

balm *medicinal herb* [see: lemon balm]

balm, eye; eye root *medicinal herb* [see: goldenseal]

balm, mountain *medicinal herb* [see: yerba santa]

balm, squaw; squaw mint *medicinal herb* [see: pennyroyal]

balm of Gilead (*Populus balsam-ifera; P. candicans*) buds *medicinal herb used as an antiscorbutic, balsamic, diuretic, stimulant, and vulnerary*

Balmex ointment OTC *astringent; moisturizer; emollient* [zinc oxide] 11.3%

Balmex Baby powder OTC *topical diaper rash treatment* [zinc oxide; peruvian balsam; corn starch]

Balmex Emollient lotion OTC *moisturizer; emollient*

balmony *medicinal herb* [see: turtlebloom]

Balneol Perianal Cleansing lotion OTC *emollient/protectant* [mineral oil; lanolin] ⑨ BAL in Oil

Balnetar bath oil OTC *antipsoriatic; antipruritic; emollient* [coal tar] 2.5%

balsalazide INN, BAN *gastrointestinal anti-inflammatory for ulcerative colitis* [also: balsalazide disodium]

balsalazide disodium USAN *gastrointestinal anti-inflammatory for ulcerative colitis* [also: balsalazide]

balsalazide sodium [see: balsalazide disodium]

balsalazine [see: balsalazide disodium; balsalazide]

balsam apple; balsam pear *medicinal herb* [see: bitter melon]

balsam Peru [see: peruvian balsam; balsam tree]

balsam poplar *medicinal herb* [see: balm of Gilead]

balsam tree *medicinal herb* [see: Peruvian balsam]

balsamics; balsams *a class of agents that soothe or heal; balms; also, certain resinous substances of vegetable origin*

Balsamodendron myrrha medicinal herb [see: myrrh]

balsan [see: peruvian balsam]

Baltussin syrup ℞ *narcotic antitussive; decongestant; antihistamine* [dihydrocodeine bitartrate; phenylephrine HCl; chlorpheniramine maleate] 3•20•2 mg/5 mL

Balziva tablets (in packs of 21 or 28) ℞ *monophasic oral contraceptive* [norethindrone; ethinyl estradiol] 0.4 mg•35 μg

bamaluzole INN

bambermycin INN, BAN *antibacterial antibiotic* [also: bambermycins]

bambermycins USAN *antibacterial antibiotic* [also: bambermycin]

bambuterol INN, BAN

bamethan INN, BAN *vasodilator* [also: bamethan sulfate]

bamethan sulfate USAN, JAN *vasodilator* [also: bamethan]

bamifylline INN, BAN *bronchodilator* [also: bamifylline HCl]

bamifylline HCl USAN *bronchodilator* [also: bamifylline]

bamipine INN, BAN, DCF

bamnidazole USAN, INN *antiprotozoal (Trichomonas)*

BAMON (bleomycin, Adriamycin, methotrexate, Oncovin, nitrogen mustard) *chemotherapy protocol*

Banadyne-3 solution OTC *topical oral anesthetic; analgesic; counterirritant; antiseptic* [lidocaine; menthol; alcohol 45%] 4%•1%

Banalg lotion OTC *analgesic; counterirritant* [methyl salicylate; camphor; menthol] 4.9%•2%•1%

Banalg Hospital Strength lotion OTC *analgesic; counterirritant* [methyl salicylate; menthol] 14%•3%

Bancap HC capsules ℞ *narcotic analgesic* [hydrocodone bitartrate; acetaminophen] 5•500 mg

bandage, adhesive USP *surgical aid*

bandage, gauze USP *surgical aid*

Band-Aid Plus ointment (discontinued 2003) OTC *antibiotic; anesthetic* [polymyxin B sulfate; neomycin sulfate; bacitracin zinc; pramoxine HCl] 10 000 U•3.5 mg•500 U•10 mg per g

Banflex IV or IM injection ℞ *skeletal muscle relaxant* [orphenadrine citrate] 30 mg/mL

banocide [see: diethylcarbamazine citrate]

Banophen caplets, capsules OTC *antihistamine* [diphenhydramine HCl] 25 mg

Banophen Allergy elixir OTC *antihistamine* [diphenhydramine HCl] 12.5 mg/5 mL

Banophen Decongestant capsules (discontinued 2002) OTC *decongestant; antihistamine* [pseudoephedrine HCl; diphenhydramine HCl] 60•25 mg ⑦ Barophen

Banthīne tablets (discontinued 2001) ℞ *anticholinergic; peptic ulcer treatment adjunct* [methantheline bromide] 50 mg ⑦ Brethine; Vantin

Baptisia tinctoria medicinal herb [see: wild indigo]

baquiloprim INN, BAN

Baraclude film-coated tablets, oral solution ℞ *nucleoside reverse transcriptase inhibitor (NRTI); antiviral for chronic hepatitis B virus (HBV) infection* [entecavir] 0.5, 1 mg; 0.05 mg/mL

Barbados aloe medicinal herb [see: aloe]

barbenyl [see: phenobarbital]

barberry (Berberis vulgaris) bark *medicinal herb for bacteria-associated diarrhea, blood cleansing, cough, fever, indigestion, jaundice, liver disorders, sciatica, and sore throat*

barberry, California medicinal herb [see: Oregon grape]

barbexaclone INN

Barbidonna; Barbidonna No. 2 tablets ℞ *GI antispasmodic; anticholinergic; sedative* [atropine sulfate; scopolamine hydrobromide; hyoscyamine hydrobromide; phenobarbital] 0.025•0.0074•0.1286•16 mg; 0.025•0.0074•0.1286•32 mg

barbiphenyl [see: phenobarbital]

barbital NF, INN, JAN [also: barbitone]

barbital, soluble [now: barbital sodium]

barbital sodium NF, INN [also: barbitone sodium]

barbitone BAN [also: barbital]

barbitone sodium BAN [also: barbital sodium]

barbiturates *a class of sedative/hypnotics that produce a wide range of mood alteration; also widely abused as addictive street drugs*

Barc topical liquid (discontinued 2003) OTC *pediculicide for lice* [pyrethrins; piperonyl butoxide; petroleum distillate] 0.18%•2.2%•5.52%

bardana medicinal herb [see: burdock]

Baricon powder for oral suspension ℞ *radiopaque contrast medium for gastrointestinal imaging* [barium sulfate] 98%

Baridium tablets ℞ *urinary analgesic* [phenazopyridine HCl] 100 mg

barium element (Ba)

barium hydroxide lime USP *carbon dioxide absorbent*

barium sulfate USP, JAN *oral/rectal radiopaque contrast medium for gastrointestinal imaging* 100% for oral/rectal suspension

barley (Hordeum vulgare) juice powder *medicinal herb for anemia, arthritis, blood cleansing, boils, bronchitis, cancer, metal poisoning, poor circulation, and reducing total and LDL cholesterol and increasing HDL cholesterol*

barley malt soup extract *bulk laxative*

barmastine USAN, INN *antihistamine*

BarnesHind Saline for Sensitive Eyes solution OTC *rinsing/storage solution for soft contact lenses* [sodium chloride (preserved saline solution)]

barnidipine INN

Barobag rectal suspension ℞ *radiopaque contrast medium for gastrointestinal imaging* [barium sulfate] 97%

Baro-cat oral suspension ℞ *radiopaque contrast medium for gastrointestinal imaging* [barium sulfate] 1.5%

Baros effervescent granules (discontinued 2004) ℞ *adjunct to gastrointestinal imaging* [sodium bicarbonate; tartaric acid; simethicone] 460•420•⁇ mg/g

Barosma betulina; B. cenulata; B. serratifolia medicinal herb [see: buchu]

barosmin [see: diosmin]

Barosperse powder for oral suspension ℞ *radiopaque contrast medium for gastrointestinal imaging* [barium sulfate] 95%

Barosperse, Liquid oral/rectal suspension ℞ *radiopaque contrast medium for gastrointestinal imaging* [barium sulfate] 60%

barucainide INN

BAS (benzyl analogue of serotonin) [see: benanserin HCl]

Basaljel tablets, capsules, suspension (discontinued 2002) OTC *antacid* [aluminum carbonate gel, basic] 500 mg; 500 mg; 400 mg/5 mL

base [def.] *The active part of a compound. In* naproxen sodium, *for example, the base is* naproxen. [compare to: salt]

basic aluminum acetate [see: aluminum subacetate]

basic aluminum aminoacetate [see: dihydroxyaluminum aminoacetate]

basic aluminum carbonate [see: aluminum carbonate, basic]

basic aluminum chloride [see: aluminum sesquichlorohydrate]

basic aluminum glycinate [see: dihydroxyaluminum aminoacetate]

basic bismuth carbonate [see: bismuth subcarbonate]

basic bismuth gallate [see: bismuth subgallate]

basic bismuth nitrate [see: bismuth subnitrate]

basic bismuth potassium bismutho-tartrate [see: bismuth potassium tartrate]

basic bismuth salicylate [see: bismuth subsalicylate]

basic fibroblast growth factor (bFGF) [see: ersofermin]

basic fuchsin [see: fuchsin, basic]

basic zinc acetate [see: zinc acetate, basic]

basifungin USAN, INN *antifungal*

basil (Ocimum basilicum) leaves *medicinal herb for colds, headache, indigestion, insect and snake bites, and whooping cough*

basiliximab USAN *immunosuppressant; IL-2 receptor antagonist for the prevention of acute rejection of renal transplants (orphan)*

basswood; bast tree *medicinal herb* [see: linden tree]

bastard hemp *medicinal herb* [see: hemp nettle]

bastard saffron *medicinal herb* [see: safflower]

batanopride INN *antiemetic* [also: batanopride HCl]

batanopride HCl USAN *antiemetic* [also: batanopride]

batebulast INN

batelapine INN *antipsychotic* [also: batelapine HCl]

batelapine maleate USAN *antipsychotic* [also: batelapine]

batilol INN

batimastat USAN, INN *investigational (Phase III) antineoplastic; matrix metalloproteinase (MMP) inhibitor*

batoprazine INN

batroxobin INN, JAN

batyl alcohol [see: batilol]

batylol [see: batilol]

BAVIP (bleomycin, Adriamycin, vinblastine, imidazole carboxamide, prednisone) *chemotherapy protocol*

baxitozine INN

bay; bay laurel; bay tree; Indian bay; sweet bay *medicinal herb* [see: laurel]

bay, holly; red bay; white bay *medicinal herb* [see: magnolia]

bayberry (Myrica cerifera) bark, berries, root bark *medicinal herb for cholera, diarrhea, dysentery, glands, goiter, indigestion, jaundice, excessive menstruation, scrofuloderma, and uterine hemorrhage; not generally regarded as safe and effective because of its high tannin content*

Baycol tablets (discontinued 2001 due to safety concerns) ℞ *HMG-CoA reductase inhibitor for hyperlipidemia and hypertriglyceridemia* [cerivastatin sodium] 0.2, 0.3, 0.4, 0.8 mg

Bayer Arthritis Regimen delayed-release enteric-coated tablets OTC *analgesic; antipyretic; anti-inflammatory; antirheumatic* [aspirin] 500 mg

Bayer Aspirin, Genuine; Maximum Bayer Aspirin film-coated tablets, film-coated caplets OTC *analgesic; antipyretic; anti-inflammatory; antirheumatic* [aspirin] 325 mg; 500 mg

Bayer Aspirin Regimen delayed-release enteric-coated tablets and caplets OTC *analgesic; antipyretic; anti-inflammatory; antirheumatic* [aspirin] 81, 325 mg

Bayer Back & Body Pain caplets OTC *analgesic; antipyretic; anti-inflammatory; antirheumatic* [aspirin; caffeine] 500•32.5 mg

Bayer Buffered Aspirin tablets OTC *analgesic; antipyretic; anti-inflammatory; antirheumatic* [aspirin, buffered] 325 mg

Bayer Children's Aspirin chewable tablets OTC *analgesic; antipyretic; anti-inflammatory; antirheumatic* [aspirin] 81 mg

Bayer Muscle & Joint Cream OTC *analgesic; counterirritant* [methyl salicylate; menthol; camphor] 30%•10%•4%

Bayer Plus caplets OTC *analgesic; antipyretic; anti-inflammatory; antirheumatic; antacid* [aspirin; calcium carbonate] 500•250 mg

Bayer PM Aspirin Plus Sleep Aid caplet OTC *analgesic; antipyretic; anti-inflammatory; antirheumatic; antihistaminic sleep aid* [aspirin; diphenhydramine HCl] 500•25 mg

Bayer Select Allergy Sinus, Aspirin-Free caplets (discontinued 2002) OTC *decongestant; antihistamine; analgesic; antipyretic* [pseudoephedrine HCl; chlorpheniramine maleate; acetaminophen] 30•2•500 mg

Bayer Select Backache caplets OTC *analgesic; antipyretic; anti-inflammatory; antirheumatic* [magnesium salicylate] 580 mg

Bayer Select Chest Cold caplets (discontinued 2002) OTC *antitussive; analgesic; antipyretic* [dextromethorphan hydrobromide; acetaminophen] 15•500 mg

Bayer Select Flu Relief caplets (discontinued 2002) OTC *antitussive; decongestant; antihistamine; analgesic; antipyretic* [dextromethorphan hydrobromide; pseudoephedrine HCl; chlorpheniramine maleate; acetaminophen] 15•30•2•500 mg

Bayer Select Head & Chest Cold, Aspirin-Free caplets (discontinued 2002) OTC *antitussive; decongestant; expectorant; analgesic; antipyretic* [dextromethorphan hydrobromide; pseudoephedrine HCl; guaifenesin; acetaminophen] 10•30•100•325 mg

Bayer Select Head Cold; Bayer Select Sinus Pain Relief caplets (discontinued 2002) OTC *decongestant; analgesic; antipyretic* [pseudoephedrine HCl; acetaminophen] 30•500 mg

Bayer Select Night Time Cold caplets (discontinued 2002) OTC *antitussive; decongestant; antihistamine; analgesic; antipyretic* [dextromethorphan hydrobromide; pseudoephedrine HCl; triprolidine HCl; acetaminophen] 15•30•1.25•500 mg

Bayer Timed Release, 8-Hour caplets OTC *analgesic; antipyretic; anti-inflammatory; antirheumatic* [aspirin] 650 mg

Bayer Women's Aspirin Plus Calcium caplets OTC *analgesic; antipyretic; anti-inflammatory; antirheumatic; calcium supplement* [aspirin; calcium] 81•300 mg

BayGam IM injection ℞ *immunizing agent for hepatitis A, measles, varicella, and rubella; treatment for immunoglobulin G deficiency and acquired agammaglobulinemia* [immune globulin, solvent/detergent treated] 2, 10 mL

BayHep B IM injection ℞ *hepatitis B immunizing agent* [hepatitis B immune globulin, solvent/detergent treated] 0.5, 1, 5 mL

Baypress ℞ *investigational (NDA filed) antihypertensive; calcium channel blocker* [nitrendipine]

BayRab IM injection ℞ *passive immunizing agent for use after rabies exposure* [rabies immune globulin, solvent/detergent treated] 300, 1500 IU/dose

BayRho-D Full Dose; BayRho-D Mini Dose IM injection ℞ *obstetric Rh factor immunity suppressant* [Rh$_O$(D) immune globulin, solvent/detergent treated] 300 μg; 50 μg

BayTet IM injection ℞ *passive immunizing agent for post-exposure tetanus prophylaxis in patients with incomplete or uncertain pre-exposure immunization with tetanus toxoids* [tetanus immune globulin, solvent/detergent treated] 250 U

bazedoxifene *second-generation selective estrogen receptor modulator (SERM); investigational (Phase III) for the prevention and treatment of postmenopausal osteoporosis*

bazinaprine INN

BBVP-M (BCNU, bleomycin, VePesid, prednisone, methotrexate) *chemotherapy protocol*

BC powder OTC *analgesic; antipyretic; anti-inflammatory* [aspirin; salicylamide; caffeine] 650•195•33.3 mg/pkt.

B$_c$ (vitamin B$_c$) [see: folic acid]

BC Arthritis Strength powder OTC *analgesic; antipyretic; anti-inflammatory* [aspirin; salicylamide; caffeine] 742•222•38 mg

BC Cold-Sinus Powder packets (discontinued 2001) OTC *decongestant; analgesic; antipyretic* [phenylpropanolamine HCl; aspirin] 25•650 mg

BC Cold-Sinus-Allergy Powder packets (discontinued 2001) OTC *decongestant; antihistamine; analgesic; antipyretic* [phenylpropanolamine HCl; chlorpheniramine maleate; aspirin] 25•4•650 mg

B-C with Folic Acid tablets ℞ *vitamin supplement* [multiple B vitamins; vitamin C; folic acid] ≗•500•0.5 mg

B-C with Folic Acid Plus tablets ℞ *vitamin/mineral/iron supplement* [multiple vitamins & minerals; ferrous fumarate; folic acid; biotin] ≗•27•0.8•0.15 mg

BCAA (branched-chain amino acids) [see: isoleucine; leucine; valine]

BCAD 2 powder OTC *enteral nutritional therapy for maple syrup urine disease (MSUD)*

BCAP (BCNU, cyclophosphamide, Adriamycin, prednisone) *chemotherapy protocol*

BCAVe; B-CAVe (bleomycin, CCNU, Adriamycin, Velban) *chemotherapy protocol for Hodgkin lymphoma*

B-C-Bid caplets (discontinued 2005) OTC *vitamin supplement* [multiple B vitamins; vitamin C] ≗•300 mg

BCD (bleomycin, cyclophosphamide, dactinomycin) *chemotherapy protocol*

BCG vaccine (bacillus Calmette-Guérin) USP *active bacterin for tuberculosis prevention; antineoplastic for urinary bladder cancer*

B-CHOP (bleomycin, Cytoxin, hydroxydaunomycin, Oncovin, prednisone) *chemotherapy protocol*

BCMF (bleomycin, cyclophosphamide, methotrexate, fluorouracil) *chemotherapy protocol*

BCNU (bis-chloroethyl-nitrosourea) [see: carmustine]

B-Complex elixir OTC *vitamin supplement* [multiple B vitamins]

B-Complex and B-12 tablets OTC *vitamin supplement* [multiple B vitamins; protease] ≗•10 mg

B-Complex with B-12 tablets OTC *vitamin supplement* [multiple B vitamins]

B-Complex/Vitamin C caplets OTC *vitamin supplement* [multiple B vitamins; vitamin C] ≗•300 mg

BCOP (BCNU, cyclophosphamide, Oncovin, prednisone) *chemotherapy protocol*

BCP (BCNU, cyclophosphamide, prednisone) *chemotherapy protocol*

BCVP (BCNU, cyclophosphamide, vincristine, prednisone) *chemotherapy protocol*

BCVPP (BCNU, cyclophosphamide, vinblastine, procarbazine, prednisone) *chemotherapy protocol for Hodgkin lymphoma*

B-D glucose chewable tablets OTC *glucose elevating agent* [glucose] 5 g

BDO (1,4-butanediol) *a precursor to gamma hydroxybutyrate (GHB); a formerly legal alternative to GHB, now also illegal (Schedule I)* [see: gamma hydroxybutyrate (GHB)]

B-DOPA (bleomycin, DTIC, Oncovin, prednisone, Adriamycin) *chemotherapy protocol*

BDP (beclomethasone dipropionate) [q.v.]

BEAC (BCNU, etoposide, ara-C, cyclophosphamide) *chemotherapy protocol*

BEACOPP (bleomycin, etoposide, Adriamycin, cyclophosphamide, Oncovin, procarbazine, prednisone, [filgrastim]) *chemotherapy protocol for Hodgkin lymphoma*

BEAM (BCNU, etoposide, ara-C, melphalan) *chemotherapy protocol*

bean herb *medicinal herb* [see: summer savory]

bean trefoil *medicinal herb* [see: buckbean]

Beano oral liquid, tablets OTC *digestive aid* [alpha-D-galactosidase enzyme]

bearberry *medicinal herb* [see: uva ursi]

beard, old man's *medicinal herb* [see: fringe tree; woodbine]

Bear-E-Bag Pediatric rectal suspension (discontinued 2004) ℞ *radiopaque contrast medium for gastrointestinal imaging* [barium sulfate] 95%

Bear-E-Yum CT oral suspension ℞ *radiopaque contrast medium for gastrointestinal imaging* [barium sulfate] 1.5%

Bear-E-Yum GI oral/rectal suspension ℞ *radiopaque contrast medium for gastrointestinal imaging* [barium sulfate] 60%

bear's grape *medicinal herb* [see: uva ursi]

bear's weed *medicinal herb* [see: yerba santa]

bearsfoot *medicinal herb* [see: hellebore]

Beaumont root *medicinal herb* [see: Culver root]

beaver tree *medicinal herb* [see: magnolia]

Bebulin VH powder for injection ℞ *antihemophilic for hemophilia B (orphan)* [coagulation factors II, IX, and X, heat treated]

becanthone HCl USAN *antischistosomal* [also: becantone]

becantone INN *antischistosomal* [also: becanthone HCl]

becantone HCl [see: becanthone HCl]

becaplermin USAN *recombinant platelet-derived growth factor B for chronic diabetic foot ulcers*

Because vaginal foam (discontinued 2002) OTC *spermicidal contraceptive* [nonoxynol 9] 8%

beciparcil INN

beclamide INN, BAN, DCF

becliconazole INN

beclobrate INN, BAN

Becloforte Inhaler ⒸⒶⓃ oral inhalation aerosol (discontinued 2001) ℞ *corticosteroidal anti-inflammatory for chronic asthma* [beclomethasone dipropionate] 250 µg/dose

beclometasone INN *corticosteroidal inhalant for asthma; intranasal steroid* [also: beclomethasone dipropionate; beclomethasone; beclometasone dipropionate]

beclometasone dipropionate JAN *corticosteroidal inhalant for asthma; intranasal steroid* [also: beclomethasone dipropionate; beclomethasone; beclometasone]

beclomethasone BAN *corticosteroidal anti-inflammatory for chronic asthma* [also: beclomethasone dipropionate;

beclometasone; beclometasone dipropionate]

beclomethasone dipropionate (BDP) USAN, USP *corticosteroidal anti-inflammatory for chronic asthma and rhinitis; investigational (orphan) oral treatment for intestinal graft vs. host disease* [also: beclometasone; beclomethasone; beclometasone dipropionate]

beclotiamine INN

Beclovent oral inhalation aerosol (discontinued 2001) ℞ *corticosteroidal anti-inflammatory for chronic asthma* [beclomethasone dipropionate] 42 μg/dose

Beclovent Inhaler Ⓒᴬᴺ oral inhalation aerosol (discontinued 2001) ℞ *corticosteroidal anti-inflammatory for chronic asthma* [beclomethasone dipropionate] 50 μg/dose

Beconase nasal inhalation aerosol (discontinued 2004) ℞ *corticosteroidal anti-inflammatory for seasonal or perennial rhinitis* [beclomethasone dipropionate] 42 μg/dose

Beconase AQ nasal spray ℞ *corticosteroidal anti-inflammatory for seasonal or perennial rhinitis* [beclomethasone dipropionate] 0.042% (42 μg/dose)

bectumomab USAN *monoclonal antibody; investigational (Phase III, orphan) diagnostic aid for non-Hodgkin lymphoma and AIDS-related lymphoma* [also: technetium Tc 99m bectumomab]

Bedoz Ⓒᴬᴺ injection ℞ *hematopoietic; vitamin B_{12}* [cyanocobalamin] 100 μg/mL

bedstraw (Galium aparine; G. verum) plant *medicinal herb used as an antispasmodic, aperient, diaphoretic, diuretic, and vulnerary*

bee balm *medicinal herb* [see: lemon balm]

bee pollen *natural remedy for anemia, bodily weakness, cerebral hemorrhage, colitis, constipation, enteritis, and weight loss; also used as an anti-aging agent and prenatal nutritional supplement; not generally regarded as safe and effective because of widespread allergic reactions*

bee venom (derived from Apis mellifera) *natural remedy for arthritis and multiple sclerosis, and for hyposensitization of persons highly sensitive to bee stings*

beechwood creosote [see: creosote carbonate]

beef tallow JAN

Beelith tablets OTC *dietary supplement* [vitamin B_6; magnesium oxide] 20 • 362 mg

Beepen-VK tablets, powder for oral solution (discontinued 2002) ℞ *natural penicillin antibiotic* [penicillin V potassium] 250, 500 mg; 125, 250 mg/5 mL

bee's nest plant *medicinal herb* [see: carrot]

beeswax, white JAN [also: wax, white]

beeswax, yellow JAN [also: wax, yellow]

Bee-Zee tablets OTC *vitamin/zinc supplement* [multiple vitamins; zinc] ≛ • 22.5 mg

befiperide INN

befloxatone INN

befunolol INN [also: befunolol HCl]

befunolol HCl JAN [also: befunolol]

befuraline INN

behenyl alcohol [see: docosanol]

behepan [see: cyanocobalamin]

bekanamycin INN *antibiotic* [also: bekanamycin sulfate]

bekanamycin sulfate JAN *antibiotic* [also: bekanamycin]

belarizine INN

belfosdil USAN, INN *antihypertensive; calcium channel blocker*

Belganyl (available only from the Centers for Disease Control) ℞ *antiparasitic for African trypanosomiasis and onchocerciasis* [suramin sodium]

Bellacane elixir ℞ *GI antispasmodic; anticholinergic; sedative* [atropine sulfate; scopolamine hydrobromide; hyoscyamine sulfate; phenobarbital] 0.0194 • 0.0065 • 0.1037 • 16.2 mg/ 5 mL

Bellacane tablets ℞ GI antispasmodic; anticholinergic; sedative [hyoscyamine sulfate; phenobarbital] 0.125•15 mg

Bellacane SR sustained-release tablets ℞ GI anticholinergic; sedative; analgesic [belladonna alkaloids; phenobarbital; ergotamine tartrate] 0.2•40•0.6 mg

belladonna (*Atropa belladonna*) leaves, tops, and berries *medicinal herb used as an antispasmodic, calmative, diaphoretic, diuretic, and narcotic*

belladonna extract USP GI/GU *anticholinergic/antispasmodic; antiparkinsonian* 27–33 mg/100 mL oral

Bellahist-D LA sustained-release caplets ℞ decongestant; antihistamine; anticholinergic to dry mucosal secretions [phenylephrine HCl; chlorpheniramine maleate; hyoscyamine sulfate; atropine sulfate; scopolamine hydrobromide] 20•8•0.19•0.04•0.01 mg

Bellamine tablets ℞ GI anticholinergic; sedative; analgesic [belladonna alkaloids; phenobarbital; ergotamine tartrate] 0.2•40•0.6 mg

Bell/ans tablets OTC antacid [sodium bicarbonate] 520 mg

Bellatal tablets ℞ long-acting barbiturate sedative, hypnotic, and anticonvulsant [phenobarbital] 16.2 mg

Bellergal-S tablets ℞ GI anticholinergic; sedative; analgesic [belladonna extract; phenobarbital; ergotamine tartrate] 0.2•40•0.6 mg

Bellis perennis medicinal herb [see: wild daisy]

bells, May medicinal herb [see: lily of the valley]

beloxamide USAN, INN antihyperlipoproteinemic

beloxepin USAN norepinephrine uptake inhibitor for depression

Bel-Phen-Ergot SR sustained-release tablets ℞ GI anticholinergic; sedative; analgesic [belladonna alkaloids; phenobarbital; ergotamine tartrate] 0.2•40•0.6 mg

bemarinone INN cardiotonic; positive inotropic; vasodilator [also: bemarinone HCl]

bemarinone HCl USAN cardiotonic; positive inotropic; vasodilator [also: bemarinone]

bemegride USP, INN, BAN, JAN

bemesetron USAN, INN antiemetic

bemetizide INN, BAN

Beminal 500 tablets OTC vitamin supplement [multiple B vitamins; vitamin C] ✱•500 mg ⑨ Benemid

bemitradine USAN, INN antihypertensive; diuretic

bemoradan USAN, INN cardiotonic

BEMP (**bleomycin, Eldisine, mitomycin, Platinol**) chemotherapy protocol

benactyzine INN, BAN

benactyzine HCl mild antidepressant; anticholinergic

Benadryl IV or IM injection ℞ antihistamine; motion sickness preventative; sleep aid; antiparkinsonian [diphenhydramine HCl] 50 mg/mL ⑨ Bentyl; Benylin; Caladryl

Benadryl; Benadryl 2% cream, spray OTC antihistamine [diphenhydramine HCl] 1%; 2% ⑨ Bentyl; Benylin; Caladryl

Benadryl Allergy Liqui-Gels (liquid-filled gelcaps), Kapseals (sealed capsules), Ultratabs (tablets), chewable tablets OTC antihistamine [diphenhydramine HCl] 25 mg; 25 mg; 25 mg; 12.5 mg ⑨ Bentyl; Benylin; Caladryl

Benadryl Allergy & Cold caplets OTC decongestant; antihistamine; analgesic [pseudoephedrine HCl; diphenhydramine HCl; acetaminophen] 30•12.5•500 mg

Benadryl Allergy Decongestant oral liquid (name changed to Benadryl Allergy & Sinus in 2002)

Benadryl Allergy & Sinus tablets, oral liquid OTC decongestant; antihistamine [pseudoephedrine HCl; diphenhydramine HCl] 60•25 mg; 60•25 mg/10 mL ⑨ Bentyl; Benylin; Caladryl

Benadryl Allergy & Sinus Fastmelt (orally dissolving tablets) OTC decongestant; antihistamine [pseudoephedrine

HCl; diphenhydramine citrate] 30•19 mg ▣ Bentyl; Benylin; Caladryl

Benadryl Allergy & Sinus Headache caplets, gelcaps OTC *decongestant; antihistamine; analgesic* [pseudoephedrine HCl; diphenhydramine HCl; acetaminophen] 30•12.5•500 mg ▣ Bentyl; Benylin; Caladryl

Benadryl Children's Allergy oral liquid OTC *antihistamine* [diphenhydramine HCl] 12.5 mg/5 mL ▣ Bentyl; Benylin; Caladryl

Benadryl Children's Allergy Fastmelt (orally disintegrating tablets) OTC *antihistamine* [diphenhydramine citrate] 19 mg

Benadryl Children's Allergy & Sinus oral liquid OTC *decongestant; antihistamine* [pseudoephedrine HCl; diphenhydramine HCl] 30•12.5 mg/5 mL

Benadryl Children's Allergy/Cold Fastmelt (orally dissolving tablets) OTC *decongestant; antihistamine* [pseudoephedrine HCl; diphenhydramine citrate] 30•19 mg

Benadryl Decongestant Allergy film-coated tablets OTC *decongestant; antihistamine* [pseudoephedrine HCl; diphenhydramine HCl] 60•25 mg ▣ Bentyl; Benylin; Caladryl

Benadryl Dye-Free Allergy Liqui-Gels [see: Benadryl Allergy Liqui-Gels] ▣ Bentyl; Benylin; Caladryl

Benadryl Dye-Free Allergy oral liquid (discontinued 2002) OTC *antihistamine* [diphenhydramine HCl] 6.25 mg/5 mL ▣ Bentyl; Benylin; Caladryl

Benadryl Itch Relief spray, cream, stick OTC *antihistamine; astringent* [diphenhydramine HCl; zinc acetate] 2%•0.1% ▣ Bentyl; Benylin; Caladryl

Benadryl Itch Relief, Children's spray, cream OTC *antihistamine; astringent* [diphenhydramine HCl; zinc acetate] 1%•0.1% ▣ Bentyl; Benylin; Caladryl

Benadryl Itch Stopping Gel; Benadryl Itch Stopping Gel Children's Formula OTC *antihistamine; astringent* [diphenhydramine HCl; zinc acetate] 2%•1%; 1%•1% ▣ Bentyl; Benylin; Caladryl

Benadryl Itch Stopping Spray OTC *antihistamine; astringent* [diphenhydramine HCl; zinc acetate; alcohol] 1%•0.1%•73.6%, 2%•0.1%•73.5%

Benadryl Junior ⊛ chewable tablets OTC *antihistamine* [diphenhydramine HCl] 12.5 mg

Benadryl Severe Allergy & Sinus Headache caplets OTC *decongestant; antihistamine; analgesic* [pseudoephedrine HCl; diphenhydramine HCl; acetaminophen] 30•25•500 mg

benafentrine INN

benanserin HCl

benapen [see: benethamine penicillin]

benaprizine INN *anticholinergic* [also: benapryzine HCl; benapryzine]

benapryzine BAN *anticholinergic* [also: benapryzine HCl; benaprizine]

benapryzine HCl USAN *anticholinergic* [also: benaprizine; benapryzine]

benaxibine INN

benazepril INN, BAN *antihypertensive; angiotensin-converting enzyme (ACE) inhibitor* [also: benazepril HCl]

benazepril HCl USAN *antihypertensive; angiotensin-converting enzyme (ACE) inhibitor; also used for nondiabetic neuropathy* [also: benazepril] 5, 10, 20, 40 mg oral

benazepril HCl & hydrochlorothiazide *antihypertensive; angiotensin-converting enzyme (ACE) inhibitor; diuretic* 5•6.25, 10•12.5, 20•12.5, 20•25 mg oral

benazeprilat USAN, INN *angiotensin-converting enzyme inhibitor*

bencianol INN

bencisteine INN, DCF

benclonidine INN

bencyclane INN [also: bencyclane fumarate]

bencyclane fumarate JAN [also: bencyclane]

bendacalol mesylate USAN *antihypertensive*

bendamustine INN

bendazac USAN, INN, BAN, JAN *anti-inflammatory*

bendazol INN, DCF

benderizine INN

bendrofluazide BAN *diuretic; antihypertensive* [also: bendroflumethiazide]

bendroflumethiazide USP, INN *diuretic; antihypertensive* [also: bendrofluazide]

Benefiber powder for oral solution OTC *dietary fiber supplement* [guar gum] 3 g fiber per pkt. or tbsp.

Benefix powder for IV injection ℞ *antihemophilic for factor IX deficiency (hemophilia B; Christmas disease) (orphan)* [nonacog alfa (synthetic coagulation factor IX)] 250, 500, 1000 IU

Benemid Ⓒ tablets ℞ *uricosuric for gout* [probenecid] 500 mg ☒ Beminal

benethamine penicillin INN, BAN

benexate INN

benexate HCl JAN

benfluorex INN, DCF

benfosformin INN, DCF

benfotiamine INN, JAN, DCF

benfurodil hemisuccinate INN, DCF

bengal gelatin [see: agar]

Ben-Gay, Arthritis Formula cream OTC *analgesic; counterirritant* [methyl salicylate; menthol] 30%•8%

Ben-Gay Original ointment OTC *analgesic; counterirritant* [methyl salicylate; menthol] 18.3%•16%

Ben-Gay Patch OTC *analgesic; counterirritant* [menthol] 1.4%

Ben-Gay Regular Strength cream OTC *analgesic; counterirritant* [methyl salicylate; menthol] 15%•10%

Ben-Gay SPA cream (discontinued 2004) OTC *analgesic; counterirritant* [menthol] 10%

Ben-Gay Ultra Strength cream OTC *analgesic; counterirritant* [methyl salicylate; menthol; camphor] 30%•10%•4%

Ben-Gay Vanishing Scent gel OTC *analgesic; counterirritant* [menthol; camphor] 3%• ☒

benhepazone INN

Benicar film-coated tablets ℞ *antihypertensive; angiotensin II receptor antagonist* [olmesartan medoxomil] 5, 20, 40 mg

Benicar HCT film-coated tablets ℞ *antihypertensive; angiotensin II receptor antagonist; diuretic* [olmesartan medoxomil; hydrochlorothiazide] 20•12.5, 40•12.5, 40•25 mg

benidipine INN

benmoxin INN, DCF

benolizime INN

Benoquin cream ℞ *depigmenting agent for vitiligo* [monobenzone] 20%

benorilate INN, DCF [also: benorylate]

benorterone USAN, INN *antiandrogen*

benorylate BAN [also: benorilate]

benoxafos INN

benoxaprofen USAN, INN, BAN *anti-inflammatory; analgesic*

benoxinate HCl USP *topical ophthalmic anesthetic* [also: oxybuprocaine; oxybuprocaine HCl]

Benoxyl 5 lotion, mask (discontinued 2003) OTC *keratolytic for acne* [benzoyl peroxide] 5% ☒ PanOxyl

Benoxyl 10 lotion (discontinued 2003) OTC *topical keratolytic for acne* [benzoyl peroxide] 10%

benpenolisin INN

benperidol USAN, INN, BAN *antipsychotic*

benproperine INN [also: benproperine phosphate]

benproperine phosphate JAN [also: benproperine]

benrixate INN, DCF

Bensal HP ointment ℞ *antifungal; keratolytic* [benzoic acid; salicylic acid] 6%•3%

bensalan USAN, INN *disinfectant*

benserazide USAN, INN, BAN *decarboxylase inhibitor; antiparkinsonian adjunct* [also: benserazide HCl]

benserazide HCl JAN *decarboxylase inhibitor; antiparkinsonian adjunct* [also: benserazide]

bensuldazic acid INN, BAN

Bensulfoid cream OTC *topical acne treatment* [colloidal sulfur; resorcinol; alcohol] 8%•2%•12%

bensylyte HCl [see: phenoxybenzamine HCl]

Ben-Tann oral suspension ℞ *antihistamine* [diphenhydramine tannate] 25 mg/5 mL

bentazepam USAN, INN *sedative*

bentemazole INN

bentiamine INN

bentipimine INN

bentiromide USAN, INN, BAN, JAN *diagnostic aid for pancreas function*

bentonite NF, JAN *suspending agent*

bentoquatam USAN *topical skin protectant for allergic contact dermatitis and poison ivy exposure*

Bentyl capsules, tablets, IM injection, syrup ℞ *GI antispasmodic* [dicyclomine HCl] 10 mg; 20 mg; 10 mg/mL; 10 mg/5 mL ☑ Aventyl; Benadryl; Bontril

benurestat USAN, INN *urease enzyme inhibitor*

Benuryl ⒸⒶⓃ tablets ℞ *uricosuric for gout* [probenecid] 500 mg

Benylin Adult oral liquid OTC *antitussive* [dextromethorphan hydrobromide] 15 mg/5 mL ☑ Benadryl

Benylin DM syrup (discontinued 2002) OTC *antitussive* [dextromethorphan hydrobromide] 10 mg/5 mL ☑ Benadryl

Benylin DM 12-Hour; Benylin DM for Children 12-Hour ⒸⒶⓃ controlled-release syrup OTC *antitussive* [dextromethorphan polistirex] 30 mg/5 mL; 15 mg/5 mL ☑ Benadryl

Benylin DM-D; Children's Benylin DM-D ⒸⒶⓃ syrup OTC *antitussive; decongestant* [dextromethorphan hydrobromide; pseudoephedrine HCl] 15•30 mg/5 mL; 7.5•15 mg/5 mL ☑ Benadryl

Benylin DM-D-E ⒸⒶⓃ syrup OTC *antitussive; decongestant; expectorant* [dextromethorphan hydrobromide; pseudoephedrine HCl; guaifenesin; alcohol 5%] 15•30•100, 15•30•200 mg/5 mL ☑ Benadryl

Benylin DM-E ⒸⒶⓃ syrup OTC *antitussive; expectorant* [dextromethorphan hydrobromide; guaifenesin; alcohol 5%] 15•100 mg/5 mL ☑ Benadryl

Benylin Expectorant oral liquid OTC *antitussive; expectorant* [dextromethorphan hydrobromide; guaifenesin] 20•400 mg/20 mL ☑ Benadryl

Benylin First Defense ⒸⒶⓃ lozenges, syrup OTC *herbal remedy for coughs, nasal congestion, and sore throat due to cough or cold* [echinacea; menthol] 65•8 mg; 100•12.5 mg/10 mL

Benylin Multi-Symptom oral liquid (discontinued 2002) OTC *antitussive; decongestant; expectorant* [dextromethorphan hydrobromide; pseudoephedrine HCl; guaifenesin] 5•15•100 mg/5 mL ☑ Benadryl

Benylin Pediatric oral liquid OTC *antitussive* [dextromethorphan hydrobromide] 7.5 mg/5 mL ☑ Benadryl

Benz 42 *hydrophilic contact lens material* [hefilcon A]

Benza solution OTC *topical antiseptic* [benzalkonium chloride] 1:750

Benzac 5; Benzac 10 gel ℞ *keratolytic and antiseptic for acne* [benzoyl peroxide; alcohol] 5%•12%; 10%•12%

Benzac AC 2½; Benzac W 2½; Benzac AC 5; Benzac W 5; Benzac AC 10; Benzac W 10 gel ℞ *keratolytic for acne* [benzoyl peroxide] 2.5%; 2.5%; 5%; 5%; 10%; 10%

Benzac AC Wash 2½; Benzac AC Wash 5; Benzac W Wash 5; Benzac AC Wash 10; Benzac W Wash 10 topical liquid ℞ *keratolytic for acne* [benzoyl peroxide] 2.5%; 5%; 5%; 10%; 10%

BenzaClin gel ℞ *antibiotic and keratolytic for acne* [clindamycin phosphate; benzoyl peroxide] 1%•5%

5 Benzagel; 10 Benzagel gel (discontinued 2003) ℞ *keratolytic for acne* [benzoyl peroxide] 5%; 10%

Benzagel Wash gel ℞ *keratolytic and antiseptic for acne* [benzoyl peroxide; alcohol] 10%•14%

benzaldehyde NF *flavoring agent*

benzalkonium chloride (BAC) NF, INN, BAN, JAN *preservative; bacterio-*

static antiseptic; surfactant/wetting agent 17% topical

Benzamycin gel ℞ *antibiotic and keratolytic for acne* [erythromycin; benzoyl peroxide; alcohol 20%] 3%•5%

benzaprinoxide INN

benzarone INN, DCF

Benzashave shaving cream (discontinued 2003) ℞ *keratolytic for acne* [benzoyl peroxide] 5%, 10%

benzathine benzylpenicillin INN *natural penicillin antibiotic* [also: penicillin G benzathine; benzathine penicillin; benzylpenicillin benzathine]

benzathine penicillin BAN *natural penicillin antibiotic* [also: penicillin G benzathine; benzathine benzylpenicillin; benzylpenicillin benzathine]

benzathine penicillin G [see: penicillin G benzathine]

benzatropine INN *antiparkinsonian; anticholinergic* [also: benztropine mesylate; benztropine]

benzazoline HCl [see: tolazoline HCl]

benzbromaron JAN *uricosuric* [also: benzbromarone]

benzbromarone USAN, INN, BAN *uricosuric* [also: benzbromaron]

benzchinamide [see: benzquinamide]

benzchlorpropamide [see: beclamide]

Benzedrex inhaler ℞ *nasal decongestant* [propylhexedrine] 250 mg

benzene ethanol [see: phenylethyl alcohol]

benzene hexachloride, gamma [now: lindane]

benzeneacetic acid, sodium salt [see: sodium phenylacetate]

benzenebutanoic acid, sodium salt [see: sodium phenylbutyrate]

1,3-benzenediol [see: resorcinol]

benzenemethanol [see: benzyl alcohol]

benzestrofol [see: estradiol benzoate]

benzestrol USP, INN, BAN

benzethacil [see: penicillin G benzathine]

benzethidine INN, BAN, DCF

benzethonium chloride USP, INN, BAN, JAN *topical anti-infective; preservative*

benzetimide INN *anticholinergic* [also: benzetimide HCl]

benzetimide HCl USAN *anticholinergic* [also: benzetimide]

benzfetamine INN *anorexiant; CNS stimulant* [also: benzphetamine HCl; benzphetamine]

benzhexol BAN *anticholinergic; antiparkinsonian* [also: trihexyphenidyl HCl; trihexyphenidyl]

N-benzhydryl-N-methylpiperazine [see: cyclizine HCl]

benzilone bromide [see: benzilonium bromide]

benzilonium bromide USAN, INN, BAN *anticholinergic*

benzimidavir *investigational (Phase II) DNA inhibitor for AIDS-related cytomegalovirus infection*

2-benzimidazolepropionic acid [see: procodazole]

benzimidazoles, substituted *a class of gastric antisecretory agents that inhibit the ATPase "proton pump" within the cell* [also called: proton pump inhibitors; ATPase inhibitors]

benzin, petroleum JAN

benzindamine HCl [see: benzydamine HCl]

benzindopyrine INN *antipsychotic* [also: benzindopyrine HCl]

benzindopyrine HCl USAN *antipsychotic* [also: benzindopyrine]

benzinoform [see: carbon tetrachloride]

benziodarone INN, BAN, DCF

benzisoxazoles *a class of novel (atypical) antipsychotic agents*

benzmalecene INN

benzmethoxazone [see: chlorthenoxazine]

benznidazole INN

benzoaric acid [see: ellagic acid]

benzoate & phenylacetate [see: sodium benzoate & sodium phenylacetate]

benzobarbital INN

benzocaine USP, INN, BAN *topical anesthetic; nonprescription diet aid* [also: ethyl aminobenzoate] 5% topical

benzoclidine INN

benzoctamine INN, BAN *sedative; muscle relaxant* [also: benzoctamine HCl]

benzoctamine HCl USAN, INN *sedative; muscle relaxant* [also: benzoctamine]

Benzodent ointment OTC *topical oral anesthetic* [benzocaine] 20%

benzodepa USAN, INN *antineoplastic*

benzodiazepine HCl [see: medazepam HCl]

benzodiazepines *a class of nonbarbiturate sedative/hypnotics and anticonvulsants*

benzododecinium chloride INN

benzogynestryl [see: estradiol benzoate]

benzoic acid USP, JAN *antifungal; urinary acidifier*

benzoic acid, phenylmethyl ester [see: benzyl benzoate]

benzoic acid, potassium salt [see: potassium benzoate]

benzoic acid, sodium salt [see: sodium benzoate]

benzoin USP, JAN *topical protectant*

Benzoin Compound tincture OTC *skin protectant* [benzoin; aloe; alcohol 74–80%]

benzol [see: benzene ...]

benzonatate USP, INN, BAN *antitussive* 100 mg oral

benzophenone

benzopyrrolate [see: benzopyrronium]

benzopyrronium bromide INN

benzoquinone amidoinohydrazone thiosemicarbazone hydrate [see: ambazone]

benzoquinonium chloride

benzorphanol [see: levophenacylmorphan]

benzosulfinide [see: saccharin]

benzosulphinide sodium [see: saccharin sodium]

benzothiazepines *a class of calcium channel blockers*

benzothiozon [see: thioacetazone; thiacetazone]

benzotript INN

Benzox-10 gel (discontinued 2003) ℞ *keratolytic for acne* [benzoyl peroxide] 10%

benzoxiquine USAN, INN *antiseptic/disinfectant*

benzoxonium chloride INN

benzoyl *p*-aminosalicylate (B-PAS) [see: benzoylpas calcium]

benzoyl peroxide USAN, USP *keratolytic* 2.5%, 5%, 10% topical

benzoyl peroxide & erythromycin *keratolytic and antibiotic for acne* 5% • 3% topical

m-benzoylhydratropic acid [see: ketoprofen]

benzoylmethylecgonine [see: cocaine]

benzoylpas calcium USAN, USP *antibacterial; tuberculostatic* [also: calcium benzamidosalicylate]

benzoylsulfanilamide [see: sulfabenzamide]

benzoylthiamindisulfide [see: bisbentiamine]

benzoylthiaminmonophosphate [see: benfotiamine]

benzphetamine BAN *anorexiant; CNS stimulant* [also: benzphetamine HCl; benzfetamine]

benzphetamine chloride [see: benzphetamine HCl]

benzphetamine HCl NF *anorexiant; CNS stimulant* [also: benzfetamine; benzphetamine]

benzpiperylon [see: benzpiperylone]

benzpiperylone INN

benzpyrinium bromide NF, INN

benzquercin INN

benzquinamide USAN, INN, BAN *postanesthesia antinauseant and antiemetic*

benzthiazide USP, INN, BAN *diuretic; antihypertensive*

benztropine BAN *anticholinergic; antiparkinsonian* [also: benztropine mesylate; benzatropine]

benztropine mesylate USP *anticholinergic; antiparkinsonian* [also: benzatropine; benztropine] 0.5, 1, 2 mg oral

benztropine methanesulfonate [see: benztropine mesylate]

benzydamine INN, BAN *analgesic; antipyretic; anti-inflammatory* [also: benzydamine HCl]

benzydamine HCl USAN, JAN *analgesic; antipyretic; anti-inflammatory; investigational (orphan) radioprotectant for oral mucosa following radiation therapy for head and neck cancer* [also: benzydamine]

benzydroflumethiazide [see: bendroflumethiazide]

benzyl alcohol NF, INN, JAN *antimicrobial agent; antiseptic; local anesthetic*

benzyl analogue of serotonin (BAS) [see: benanserin HCl]

benzyl antiserotonin [see: benanserin HCl]

benzyl benzoate USP, JAN

benzyl carbinol [see: phenylethyl alcohol]

S-benzyl thiobenzoate [see: tibenzate]

benzylamide [see: beclamide]

benzylamines *a class of antifungals structurally related to the allylamines*

N-benzylanilinoacetamidoxime [see: cetoxime]

2-benzylbenzimidazole [see: bendazol]

benzyldimethyltetradecylammonium chloride [see: miristalkonium chloride]

benzyldodecyldimethylammonium chloride [see: benzododecinium chloride]

0-6-benzylguanine [see: alkylade]

benzylhexadecyldimethylammonium [see: cetalkonium]

benzylhexadecyldimethylammonium chloride [see: cetalkonium chloride]

benzylhydrochlorothiazide JAN

p-benzyloxyphenol [see: monobenzone]

benzylpenicillin INN, BAN *natural penicillin antibiotic; investigational (orphan) for penicillin hypersensitivity assessment*

benzylpenicillin benzathine JAN *natural penicillin antibiotic* [also: penicillin G benzathine; benzathine benzylpenicillin; benzathine penicillin]

benzylpenicillin potassium BAN, JAN *natural penicillin antibiotic* [also: penicillin G potassium]

benzylpenicillin procaine *natural penicillin antibiotic* [see: penicillin G procaine]

benzylpenicillin sodium BAN *natural penicillin antibiotic* [also: penicillin G sodium]

benzylpenicilloic acid [see: benzylpenicillin]

benzylpenicilloyl polylysine USP *diagnostic aid for penicillin sensitivity*

benzylpenilloic acid [see: benzylpenicillin]

benzylsulfamide INN, DCF

benzylsulfanilamide [see: benzylsulfamide]

BEP (bleomycin, etoposide, Platinol) *chemotherapy protocol for testicular cancer and germ cell tumors*

bepafant INN

bepanthen [see: panthenol]

beperidium iodide INN

bephene oxinaphthoate [see: bephenium hydroxynaphthoate]

bephenium embonate [see: bephenium hydroxynaphthoate]

bephenium hydroxynaphthoate USP, INN, BAN

bepiastine INN, DCF

bepridil INN, BAN *vasodilator; antianginal; calcium channel blocker* [also: bepridil HCl]

bepridil HCl USAN *vasodilator; antianginal; calcium channel blocker* [also: bepridil]

beractant USAN *pulmonary surfactant for neonatal respiratory distress syndrome or respiratory failure (orphan)*

beraprost USAN, INN *platelet aggregation inhibitor; peripheral vasodilator; investigational (Phase III) prostacyclin analogue for peripheral vascular disease (PVD); investigational (orphan) for pulmonary arterial hypertension (PAH)*

beraprost sodium USAN *platelet aggregation inhibitor*

berberine chloride JAN

berberine sulfate JAN

berberine tannate JAN

Berberis vulgaris *medicinal herb* [see: barberry]

berculon A [see: thioacetazone; thiacetazone]

berefrine USAN, INN *mydriatic*

bergamot, scarlet *medicinal herb* [see: Oswego tea]

bergamot, wild *medicinal herb* [see: wild bergamot]

bergamot oil (*Citrus aurantium; C. bergamia*) fruit peel *medicinal herb used in conjunction with long-wave UV light therapy for psoriasis and vitiligo; not generally regarded as safe and effective because of its photosensitizing properties*

bergenin JAN

Berinert-P ℞ *investigational (orphan) agent to prevent or treat acute attacks of angioedema* [C1-esterase-inhibitor, human]

berkelium *element (Bk)*

berlafenone INN

bermastine [see: barmastine]

bermoprofen INN

Berocca tablets ℞ *vitamin supplement* [multiple B vitamins; vitamin C; folic acid] ≛•500•0.5 mg

Berocca Plus tablets ℞ *vitamin/mineral/iron supplement* [multiple vitamins & minerals; ferrous fumarate; folic acid; biotin] ≛•27•0.8•0.15 mg

Berotec (widely available outside the U.S.) ℞ *investigational (NDA filed) bronchodilator; antiasthmatic; β-blocker* [fenoterol hydrobromide]

bertosamil INN

beryllium *element (Be)*

berythromycin USAN, INN *antiamebic; antibacterial*

besigomsin INN

besilate INN *combining name for radicals or groups* [also: besylate]

besipiridine INN *cognition enhancer for Alzheimer disease* [also: besipiridine HCl]

besipiridine HCl USAN *cognition enhancer for Alzheimer disease* [also: besipiridine]

besulpamide INN

besunide INN

besylate USAN *combining name for radicals or groups* [also: besilate]

beta alethine *investigational (Phase I/II, orphan) antineoplastic and immunostimulant for B-cell lymphoma, multiple myeloma, and metastatic melanoma*

beta blockers (β-blockers) *a class of cardiac agents characterized by their antihypertensive, antiarrhythmic, and antianginal actions; a class of topical antiglaucoma agents* [also called: beta-adrenergic antagonists]

beta carotene USAN, USP *vitamin A precursor* [also: betacarotene] 15 mg (25 000 IU) oral

beta cyclodextrin (β-cyclodextrin) *(previously used NF name)* [now: betadex]

betacarotene INN *vitamin A precursor* [also: beta carotene]

betacetylmethadol INN, BAN

Betachron E-R extended-release capsules (discontinued 2001) ℞ *antiarrhythmic; antihypertensive; antianginal; antiadrenergic (β-blocker); migraine prophylaxis* [propranolol HCl] 60, 80, 120, 160 mg

betadex USAN, INN *sequestering agent* [previous NF name: beta cyclodextrin]

beta-D-galactosidase *digestive enzyme* [see: tilactase]

Betadine aerosol, gauze pads, lubricating gel, cream, ointment, skin cleanser, foam, solution, swab, swabsticks OTC *broad-spectrum antimicrobial* [povidone-iodine] 5%; 10%; 5%; 5%; 10%; 7.5%; 7.5%; 10%; 10%; 10%

Betadine mouthwash, perineal wash, surgical scrub (discontinued 2003) OTC *broad-spectrum antimicrobial* [povidone-iodine] 0.5%; 10%; 7.5%

Betadine shampoo OTC *broad-spectrum antimicrobial for dandruff* [povidone-iodine] 7.5%

Betadine 5% Sterile Ophthalmic Prep solution ℞ *broad-spectrum antimicrobial for eye surgery* [povidone-iodine] 5%

Betadine First Aid Antibiotics Plus Moisturizer ointment OTC *antibiotic* [polymyxin B sulfate; bacitracin zinc] 10 000•500 IU/g

Betadine Medicated vaginal supposi-tories, vaginal gel OTC *antiseptic/ger-micidal; vaginal cleanser and deodorant* [povidone-iodine] 10%

Betadine Medicated Douche; Beta-dine Medicated Disposable Douche; Betadine Premixed Medicated Disposable Douche solution OTC *antiseptic/germicidal; vaginal cleanser and deodorant* [povi-done-iodine] 10%

Betadine Plus First Aid Antibiotics and Pain Reliever ointment OTC *topical antibiotic and anesthetic* [poly-myxin B sulfate; bacitracin zinc; pra-moxine HCl] 10 000 IU•500 IU•10 mg per g

Betadine PrepStick swab OTC *broad-spectrum antimicrobial* [povidone-iodine] 10%

Betadine PrepStick Plus swab OTC *broad-spectrum antimicrobial* [povi-done-iodine; alcohol] 10%• ?

beta-estradiol [see: estradiol]

beta-estradiol benzoate [see: estra-diol benzoate]

betaeucaine HCl [now: eucaine HCl]

Betagan Liquifilm eye drops ℞ *topical antiglaucoma agent (β-blocker)* [levo-bunolol HCl] 0.25%, 0.5% ② Betagen

Betagen ointment, solution, surgical scrub OTC *broad-spectrum antimicro-bial* [povidone-iodine] 1%; 10%; 7.5% ② Betagan

beta-glucocerebrosidase [see: alglu-cerase]

betahistine INN, BAN *vasodilator* [also: betahistine HCl; betahistine mesilate]

betahistine HCl USAN *vasodilator* [also: betahistine; betahistine mesilate]

betahistine mesilate JAN *vasodilator* [also: betahistine HCl; betahistine]

beta-hypophamine [see: vasopressin]

betaine HCl USP *electrolyte replenisher for homocystinuria* (orphan)

Betaject ⓒ injection ℞ *corticosteroidal anti-inflammatory* [betamethasone sodium phosphate; betamethasone acetate] 3•3 mg/mL

beta-lactams *a class of antibiotics*

beta-lactone [see: propiolactone]

betameprodine INN, BAN, DCF

betamethadol INN, BAN, DCF

betamethasone USAN, USP, INN, BAN, JAN *corticosteroidal anti-inflammatory*

betamethasone acetate USP, JAN *cor-ticosteroidal anti-inflammatory*

betamethasone acibutate INN, BAN *corticosteroidal anti-inflammatory*

betamethasone benzoate USAN, USP, BAN *topical corticosteroidal anti-inflammatory*

betamethasone dipropionate USAN, USP, BAN, JAN *topical corticosteroidal anti-inflammatory* 0.05% topical

betamethasone dipropionate, aug-mented *topical corticosteroidal anti-inflammatory* 0.05% topical

betamethasone dipropionate & clo-trimazole *corticosteroidal anti-inflam-matory; broad-spectrum antifungal* 0.05%•1% topical

betamethasone sodium phosphate USP, BAN, JAN *corticosteroidal anti-inflammatory*

betamethasone valerate USAN, USP, BAN, JAN *topical corticosteroidal anti-inflammatory; investigational (NDA filed) mousse for scalp psoriasis* 0.1% topical

betamicin INN *antibacterial* [also: beta-micin sulfate]

betamicin sulfate USAN *antibacterial* [also: betamicin]

betamipron INN

betanaphthol NF

betanidine INN *antihypertensive* [also: bethanidine sulfate; bethanidine; betanidine sulfate]

betanidine sulfate JAN *antihyperten-sive* [also: bethanidine sulfate; betan-idine; bethanidine]

Betapace tablets ℞ *antiarrhythmic (β-blocker) for life-threatening ventricular arrhythmias* (orphan) [sotalol HCl] 80, 120, 160, 240 mg

Betapace AF tablets ℞ *antiarrhythmic (β-blocker) for atrial fibrillation or atrial flutter* [sotalol HCl] 80, 120, 160 mg

betaprodine INN, BAN, DCF

beta-propiolactone [see: propiolactone]

beta-pyridylcarbinol [see: nicotinyl alcohol]

BetaRx *investigational (orphan) antidiabetic for type 1 patients on immunosuppression* [porcine islet preparation, encapsulated]

Betasept topical liquid OTC *broad-spectrum antimicrobial; germicidal* [chlorhexidine gluconate; alcohol 4%] 4%

Betaseron powder for subcu injection ℞ *immunomodulator for relapsing-remitting multiple sclerosis (orphan)* [interferon beta-1b] 0.25 mg (8 MIU)/dose

Betathine *investigational (orphan) antineoplastic and immunostimulant for multiple myeloma and metastatic melanoma* [beta alethine]

Betatrex cream, ointment, lotion (discontinued 2003) ℞ *corticosteroidal anti-inflammatory* [betamethasone valerate] 0.1%

Beta-Val cream, lotion ℞ *topical corticosteroidal anti-inflammatory* [betamethasone valerate] 0.1%

betaxolol INN, BAN *antianginal; antihypertensive; topical antiglaucoma agent (β-blocker)* [also: betaxolol HCl]

betaxolol HCl USAN, USP *antianginal; antihypertensive; topical antiglaucoma agent (β-blocker)* [also: betaxolol] 0.5% eye drops

Betaxon eye drops ℞ *topical antiglaucoma agent (β-blocker)* [levobetaxolol HCl] 0.5%

betazole INN [also: betazole HCl; ametazole]

betazole HCl USP [also: betazole; ametazole]

betazolium chloride [see: betazole HCl]

betel nut (*Areca catechu*) leaves and quids (a mixture of tobacco, powdered or sliced areca nut, and slaked lime wrapped in a *Piper betel* leaf) *medicinal herb used as a digestive aid and mild stimulant; not generally regarded as safe and effective as it causes leukoplakia and oral cancer*

beth root *medicinal herb* [see: birthroot]

bethanechol chloride USP, BAN, JAN *cholinergic urinary stimulant for postsurgical and postpartum urinary retention* 5, 10, 25, 50 mg oral

bethanidine BAN *antihypertensive* [also: bethanidine sulfate; betanidine; betanidine sulfate]

bethanidine sulfate USAN *antihypertensive; investigational (orphan) agent for the prevention and treatment of primary ventricular fibrillation* [also: betanidine; bethanidine; betanidine sulfate]

betiatide USAN, INN, BAN *pharmaceutic aid*

Betimol eye drops ℞ *antiglaucoma agent (β-blocker)* [timolol hemihydrate] 0.25%, 0.5%

Betonica officinalis *medicinal herb* [now: *Stachys officinalis*] [see: betony]

betony (*Stachys officinalis*) plant *medicinal herb for anxiety, delirium, diarrhea, fever, jaundice, liver and spleen sclerosis, migraine headache, mouth or throat irritation, nervousness, palpitations, and toothache; also used as a purgative and emetic agent*

Betoptic; Betoptic S Drop-Tainers (eye drops) ℞ *topical antiglaucoma agent (β-blocker)* [betaxolol HCl] 0.5%; 0.25%

betoxycaine INN

betoxycaine HCl [see: betoxycaine]

betula oil [see: methyl salicylate]

Betula spp. *medicinal herb* [see: birch]

Betuline lotion OTC *analgesic; counterirritant* [methyl salicylate; camphor; menthol; peppermint oil]

bevacizumab *antineoplastic; recombinant humanized monoclonal antibody (rhuMAb) to vascular endothelial growth factor (VEGF); angiogenesis inhibitor for metastatic colorectal cancer; investigational (Phase III) for breast, cervical, lung, and renal cancers*

bevantolol INN, BAN *antianginal; antihypertensive; antiarrhythmic* [also: bevantolol HCl]

bevantolol HCl USAN *antianginal; antihypertensive; antiarrhythmic* [also: bevantolol]

bevonium methylsulphate BAN [also: bevonium metilsulfate]

bevonium metilsulfate INN [also: bevonium methylsulphate]

bexarotene USAN, INN *synthetic retinoid analogue antineoplastic for cutaneous T-cell lymphoma (orphan); investigational (Phase III) for lung cancer*

bexlosteride USAN, INN *antineoplastic 5α-reductase inhibitor for prostate cancer*

Bextra film-coated caplets (discontinued 2005) ℞ *COX-2 inhibitor; nonsteroidal anti-inflammatory drug (NSAID) for osteoarthritis (OA), rheumatoid arthritis (RA), and primary dysmenorrhea; withdrawn from the market in 2005 for safety concerns* [valdecoxib] 10, 20 mg

Bexxar Dosimetric Package IV infusion ℞ *first of two steps in the radiotherapeutic treatment of non-Hodgkin lymphoma (NHL)* [tositumomab; iodine I 131 tositumomab] 450•35 mg (5 mCi of radiation)

Bexxar Therapeutic Package IV infusion ℞ *second of two steps in the radiotherapeutic treatment of non-Hodgkin lymphoma (NHL)* [tositumomab; iodine I 131 tositumomab] 450•35 mg (delivers 65–75 cGy of radiation)

bezafibrate USAN, INN, BAN, JAN *antihyperlipidemic*

bezitramide INN, BAN, DCF

bezomil INN *combining name for radicals or groups*

bFGF (basic fibroblast growth factor) [see: ersofermin]

B.F.I. Antiseptic powder OTC *topical antiseptic* [bismuth-formic-iodide] 16%

BHA (butylated hydroxyanisole) [q.v.]

BHAPs (bisheteroarylpiperazines) *a class of antiviral drugs*

BHD (BCNU, hydroxyurea, dacarbazine) *chemotherapy protocol*

BHDV; BHD-V (BCNU, hydroxyurea, dacarbazine, vincristine) *chemotherapy protocol*

BHT (butylated hydroxytoluene) [q.v.]

bialamicol INN, BAN *antiamebic* [also: bialamicol HCl]

bialamicol HCl USAN *antiamebic* [also: bialamicol]

biallylamicol [see: bialamicol]

biantrazole [now: losoxantrone HCl]

biapenem USAN, INN *antibacterial*

Biavax II powder for subcu injection ℞ *mumps and rubella vaccine* [mumps and rubella virus vaccine, live] 1000•20 000 U/0.5 mL

Biaxin Filmtabs (film-coated tablets), granules for oral suspension ℞ *macrolide antibiotic* [clarithromycin] 250, 500 mg; 125, 187.5, 250 mg/5 mL ⊡ Axid

Biaxin XL film-coated extended-release tablets ℞ *once-daily macrolide antibiotic* [clarithromycin] 500 mg

bibapcitide USAN *glycoprotein (GP) IIb/IIIa receptor antagonist; investigational (Phase III) diagnostic imaging aid for deep vein thrombosis*

bibenzonium bromide INN, BAN

bibrocathin [see: bibrocathol]

bibrocathol INN, DCF

bicalutamide USAN, INN, BAN *antiandrogen antineoplastic for prostatic cancer*

bicalutamide + LHRH-A (bicalutamide, goserelin acetate [Zoladex subcu implant]) *chemotherapy protocol for prostate cancer*

bicalutamide + LHRH-A (bicalutamide, leuprolide acetate [Lupron Depot injection]) *chemotherapy protocol for prostate cancer*

Bichloracetic Acid topical liquid ℞ *cauterant; keratolytic* [dichloroacetic acid] 10 mL ⊡ dichloroacetic acid

bicifadine INN *analgesic* [also: bicifadine HCl]

bicifadine HCl USAN *analgesic* [also: bicifadine]

Bicillin C-R; Bicillin C-R 900/300 Tubex (cartridge-needle unit) for deep IM injection ℞ *natural peni-*

cillin antibiotic [penicillin G benzathine; penicillin G procaine] 300 000•300 000, 600 000•600 000, 1 200 000•1 200 000 U; 900 000• 300 000 U 🔲 V-Cillin; Wycillin

Bicillin L-A Tubex (cartridge-needle unit) for deep IM injection ℞ *natural penicillin antibiotic* [penicillin G benzathine] 600 000, 1 200 000, 2 400 000 U

biciromab USAN, INN, BAN *antifibrin monoclonal antibody*

Bicitra oral solution ℞ *urinary alkalinizing agent* [sodium citrate; citric acid] 500•334 mg/5 mL

biclodil INN *antihypertensive; vasodilator* [also: biclodil HCl]

biclodil HCl USAN *antihypertensive; vasodilator* [also: biclodil]

biclofibrate INN, DCF

biclotymol INN, DCF

BiCNU powder for IV injection ℞ *nitrosourea-type alkylating antineoplastic for brain tumors, multiple myeloma, Hodgkin disease and non-Hodgkin lymphomas* [carmustine] 100 mg/dose

bicozamycin INN

Bicozene cream OTC *topical local anesthetic; antifungal* [benzocaine; resorcinol] 6%•1.67%

bicyclomycin [see: bicozamycin]

bidCAP (trademarked dosage form) *twice-daily capsule*

Bidhist extended-release tablets ℞ *antihistamine* [brompheniramine maleate] 6 mg

BiDil tablets ℞ *vasodilator for heart failure in black patients* [hydralazine HCl; isosorbide dinitrate] 37.5•20 mg

bidimazium iodide INN, BAN

bidisomide USAN, INN *antiarrhythmic*

Biebrich scarlet red [see: scarlet red]

Biebrich scarlet-picroaniline blue

bietamiverine INN

bietamiverine HCl [see: bietamiverine]

bietaserpine INN, DCF

bifemelane INN [also: bifemelane HCl]

bifemelane HCl JAN [also: bifemelane]

bifepramide INN

bifeprofen INN

bifeprunox *investigational (Phase III) dopamine agonist for schizophrenia*

Bifidobacterium longum infantis 35624 *investigational (orphan) agent for pediatric Crohn disease*

bifluranol INN, BAN

bifonazole USAN, INN, BAN, JAN *antifungal*

Big Shot B-12 tablets OTC *vitamin B_{12} supplement* [cyanocobalamin] 5000 μg

Bignonia sempervirens *medicinal herb* [see: gelsemium]

bilastine INN

bilberry (Myrtilli fructus; Vaccinium myrtillus) fruit *medicinal herb for cold hands and feet, diarrhea, edema, increasing microvascular blood flow, gastroenteritis, mucous membrane inflammation, night blindness, and varicose veins*

bile acid sequestrants *a class of antihyperlipidemic agents*

bile acids, conjugated *investigational (orphan) agent for steatorrhea in short bowel syndrome*

bile acids, oxidized [see: dehydrocholic acid]

bile salts BAN *digestive enzymes; laxative*

BiliCheck breath analyzer device *in vitro diagnostic aid for infant jaundice*

Bili-Labstix reagent strips *in vitro diagnostic aid for multiple urine products*

Bilopaque capsules (discontinued 2001) ℞ *radiopaque contrast medium for cholecystography* [tyropanoate sodium (57.4% iodine)] 750 mg (430.5 mg)

Biltricide film-coated tablets ℞ *anthelmintic for schistosomiasis (flukes)* [praziquantel] 600 mg

bimakalim INN

bimatoprost *topical prostamide analogue for glaucoma and ocular hypertension*

bimazol [see: carbimazole]

bimethadol [see: dimepheptanol]

bimethoxycaine lactate

bimosiamose disodium USAN *anti-inflammatory for asthma, psoriasis, and reperfusion injury following transplants or coronary revascularization*

bindarit USAN, INN *antirheumatic; investigational (orphan) for lupus nephritis*

bindazac [see: bendazac]

binedaline INN

binetrakin USAN, INN *immunomodulator for gastrointestinal carcinoma and rheumatoid arthritis*

binfloxacin USAN, INN *veterinary antibacterial*

binifibrate INN

biniramycin USAN, INN *antibacterial antibiotic*

binizolast INN

binodaline [see: binedaline]

binospirone INN *anxiolytic* [also: binospirone mesylate]

binospirone mesylate USAN *anxiolytic* [also: binospirone]

bioallethrin BAN *pediculicide*

Biobrane wound dressing *nylon fabric matrix bound to a silicon film*

Biobrane-L light adherence wound dressing *nylon fabric matrix bound to a silicon film*

Biocef capsules, powder for oral suspension ℞ *cephalosporin antibiotic* [cephalexin] 500 mg; 250 mg/5 mL

Bioclate powder for IV injection ℞ *antihemophilic to correct coagulation deficiency* [antihemophilic factor concentrate, recombinant] 250, 500, 1000 IU

BioCox intradermal injection (discontinued 2003) ℞ *diagnostic aid for coccidioidomycosis* [coccidioidin] 1:100, 1:10

Biocult-GC culture paddles for professional use *in vitro diagnostic aid for Neisseria gonorrhoeae*

Biodine Topical solution OTC *broad-spectrum antimicrobial* [povidone-iodine] 1%

Bio-E-Gel ℞ *investigational (Phase III) bioidentical human estrogen transdermal gel for postmenopausal symptoms* [estradiol]

bioflavonoids (vitamin P) *a group of more than 4000 natural substances with widespread biological activity, including anthelmintic, antimicrobial, antimalarial, antineoplastic, antioxidant, anti-inflammatory, and antiviral activity; historically named "vitamin P"*

biogastrone [see: carbenoxolone]

BioGlue ℞ *investigational (NDA filed) surgical adhesive for cardiovascular and pulmonary repair*

Biohist-LA sustained-release tablets ℞ *decongestant; antihistamine* [pseudoephedrine HCl; chlorpheniramine maleate] 120•12 mg

biological indicator for dry-heat sterilization USP *sterilization indicator*

biological indicator for ethylene oxide sterilization USP *sterilization indicator*

biological indicator for steam sterilization USP *sterilization indicator*

Bion Tears eye drops OTC *ophthalmic moisturizer/lubricant* [hydroxypropyl methylcellulose] 0.3%

bioral [see: carbenoxolone]

Bio-Rescue ℞ *investigational (orphan) chelating agent for acute iron poisoning* [dextran; deferoxamine]

bioresmethrin INN

bios I [see: inositol]

bios II [see: biotin]

Biosafe HbA1c (hemoglobin A1c) test kit for home use *in vitro diagnostic aid for glycemic control*

Biosafe PSA (prostate-specific antigen) test kit for home use *in vitro diagnostic aid for prostate function*

Biosafe Total Cholesterol (only) test kit for home use *in vitro diagnostic aid for hypercholesterolemia*

Biosafe Total Cholesterol Panel (includes HDL, LDL, and triglycerides) test kit for home use *in vitro diagnostic aid for hypercholesterolemia and hypertriglyceridemia*

Biosafe TSH (thyroid-stimulating hormone) test kit for home use *in vitro diagnostic aid for thyroid function*

biosynthetic human parathyroid hormone (1-34) [see: teriparatide]

Bio-Tab film-coated tablets (discontinued 2003) ℞ *tetracycline antibiotic* [doxycycline hyclate] 100 mg

Biotab tablets (discontinued 2002) OTC *decongestant; antihistamine; analgesic* [phenylpropanolamine HCl; phenyltoloxamine citrate; acetaminophen]

Biotel kidney reagent strips *in vitro diagnostic aid for urine hemoglobin, RBCs, and albumin (predictor of kidney diseases)*

biotexin [see: novobiocin]

Bio-Throid capsules ℞ *thyroid replacement therapy for hypothyroidism or thyroid cancer* [thyroid, desiccated (porcine)] 7.5, 15, 30, 60, 90, 120, 150, 180, 240 mg

biotin USP, INN, JAN *B complex vitamin; vitamin H*

Biotin Forte tablets OTC *vitamin supplement* [multiple B vitamins; vitamin C; folic acid; biotin] ±•200• 0.8•3 mg, ±•100•0.8•5 mg

BIP (bleomycin, ifosfamide [with mesna rescue], Platinol) *chemotherapy protocol for cervical cancer*

bipenamol INN *antidepressant* [also: bipenamol HCl]

bipenamol HCl USAN *antidepressant* [also: bipenamol]

biperiden USP, INN, BAN, JAN *anticholinergic; antiparkinsonian*

biperiden HCl USP, BAN, JAN *anticholinergic; antiparkinsonian*

biperiden lactate USP, BAN, JAN *anticholinergic; antiparkinsonian*

biphasic insulin [see: insulin, biphasic]

biphenamine HCl USAN *topical anesthetic; antibacterial; antifungal* [also: xenysalate]

biprofenide [see: bifepramide]

birch (Betula spp.) bark and leaves *medicinal herb for bladder problems, blood cleansing, and eczema*

birch oil, sweet [see: methyl salicylate]

bird lime *medicinal herb* [see: mistletoe]

bird pepper *medicinal herb* [see: cayenne]

bird's nest root *medicinal herb* [see: carrot]

biricodar dicitrate USAN *investigational (Phase II) multi-drug–resistance inhibitor for prostate and ovarian cancers*

biriperone INN

birthroot (Trillium erectum; T. grandiflorum; T. pendulum) plant *medicinal herb for insect and snake bites, stimulating menses and diaphoresis, and stopping bleeding after childbirth; also used as an antiseptic and astringent*

birthwort (Aristolochia clematitis) root and flowering plant *medicinal herb used as a diaphoretic, emmenagogue, febrifuge, oxytocic, and stimulant*

Bisac-Evac enteric-coated tablets, suppositories OTC *stimulant laxative* [bisacodyl] 5 mg; 10 mg

bisacodyl USP, INN, BAN, JAN *stimulant laxative* 5 mg oral; 10 mg suppositories

bisacodyl tannex USAN *stimulant laxative*

Bisa-Lax enteric-coated tablets, suppositories OTC *stimulant laxative* [bisacodyl] 5 mg; 10 mg

bisantrene INN *antineoplastic* [also: bisantrene HCl]

bisantrene HCl USAN *antineoplastic* [also: bisantrene]

bisaramil INN

bisatin [see: oxyphenisatin acetate]

bisbendazole INN

bisbentiamine INN, JAN

bisbutiamine [see: bisbutitiamine]

bisbutitiamine JAN

bis-chloroethyl-nitrosourea (BCNU) [see: carmustine]

bisdequalinium diacetate JAN

bisfenazone INN, DCF

bisfentidine INN

bisheteroarylpiperazines (BHAPs) *a class of antiviral drugs*

bishop's wort *medicinal herb* [see: nutmeg; betony]

bishydroxycoumarin [now: dicumarol]

bisibutiamine JAN [also: sulbutiamine]

Bismatrol chewable tablets, oral liquid OTC *antidiarrheal; antinauseant* [bismuth subsalicylate] 262 mg; 524 mg/5 mL

bismucatebrol [see: bibrocathol]

bismuth element (Bi)

bismuth, milk of USP *antacid; astringent*

bismuth aluminate USAN

bismuth betanaphthol USP
bismuth carbonate USAN
bismuth carbonate, basic [see: bismuth subcarbonate]
bismuth citrate USP
bismuth cream [see: bismuth, milk of]
bismuth gallate, basic [see: bismuth subgallate]
bismuth glycollylarsanilate BAN [also: glycobiarsol]
bismuth hydroxide [see: bismuth, milk of]
bismuth hydroxide nitrate oxide [see: bismuth subnitrate]
bismuth magma [now: bismuth, milk of]
bismuth magnesium aluminosilicate JAN
bismuth oxycarbonate [see: bismuth subcarbonate]
bismuth potassium tartrate NF
bismuth sodium triglycollamate USP
bismuth subcarbonate USAN, JAN *antacid; GI adsorbent*
bismuth subgallate USAN, USP *antacid; GI adsorbent*
bismuth subnitrate USP, JAN *skin protectant*
bismuth subsalicylate (BSS) USAN, JAN *antiperistaltic; antacid; GI adsorbent*
bisnafide dimesylate USAN *antineoplastic; DNA and RNA synthesis inhibitor*
bisobrin INN *fibrinolytic* [also: bisobrin lactate]
bisobrin lactate USAN *fibrinolytic* [also: bisobrin]
Bisolvon ℞ *investigational (orphan) agent for keratoconjunctivitis sicca of Sjögren syndrome* [bromhexine HCl]
bisoprolol USAN, INN, BAN *antihypertensive (β-blocker)*
bisoprolol fumarate USAN, JAN *antihypertensive (β-blocker)* 5, 10 mg oral
bisoprolol fumarate & hydrochlorothiazide *antihypertensive; β-blocker; diuretic* 2.5•6.5, 5•6.5, 10•6.5 mg oral
bisorcic INN

bisoxatin INN, BAN *laxative* [also: bisoxatin acetate]
bisoxatin acetate USAN *laxative* [also: bisoxatin]
Bispan ℞ *investigational agent for rheumatoid arthritis* [IPL-423 (code name —generic name not yet assigned)]
bispecific antibody 520C9x22 *investigational (orphan) for ovarian cancer*
bisphosphonates *a class of calcium-regulating agents that inhibit normal and abnormal bone resorption*
bispyrithione magsulfex USAN *antibacterial; antidandruff; antifungal*
bistort (Polygonum bistorta) *root medicinal herb for bleeding, cholera, cuts, diarrhea, dysentery, gum disease (mouthwash), and hemorrhoids*
bis-tropamide [now: tropicamide]
Bite Rx *solution* OTC *astringent wet dressing (Burow solution) for insect bites* [aluminum acetate] 0.5%
bithionol NF, INN, BAN, JAN *investigational anti-infective for paragonimiasis and fascioliasis*
bithionolate sodium USAN *topical anti-infective* [also: sodium bitionolate]
bithionoloxide INN
Bitin (available only from the Centers for Disease Control) ℞ *investigational anti-infective for paragonimiasis and fascioliasis* [bithionol]
bitipazone INN
bitolterol INN, BAN *sympathomimetic bronchodilator* [also: bitolterol mesylate; bitolterol mesilate]
bitolterol mesilate JAN *sympathomimetic bronchodilator* [also: bitolterol mesylate; bitolterol]
bitolterol mesylate USAN *sympathomimetic bronchodilator* [also: bitolterol; bitolterol mesilate]
bitoscanate INN
bitter ash *medicinal herb* [see: quassia; wahoo]
bitter ash; bitter quassia; bitter wood *medicinal herb* [see: quassia]
bitter buttons *medicinal herb* [see: tansy]
bitter cardamom (Alpinia fructus; A. oxyphylla) *medicinal herb for*

dementia, excessive water loss, and gastric lesions

bitter cucumber medicinal herb [see: bitter melon]

bitter dogbane medicinal herb [see: dogbane]

bitter grass medicinal herb [see: star grass]

bitter herb medicinal herb [see: centaury]

bitter melon (Momordica charantia) fruit, leaves, seeds, oil medicinal herb used as an antimicrobial and hypoglycemic; also used to reduce fertility in both males and females, and can act as an abortifacient

bitter quassia; bitter ash; bitter wood medicinal herb [see: quassia tree]

bitter tonics; bitters a class of agents that have a bitter taste, used as tonics, alteratives, or appetizers

bitter wintergreen medicinal herb [see: pipsissewa]

bitter wood; bitter ash; bitter quassia medicinal herb [see: quassia tree]

bitterroot; bitterwort medicinal herb [see: dogbane; gentian]

bitters; bitter tonics a class of agents that have a bitter taste, used as tonics, alteratives, or appetizers

bittersweet herb; bittersweet twigs medicinal herb [see: bittersweet nightshade]

bittersweet nightshade (Solanum dulcamara) medicinal herb for topical application on abrasions and felons; not generally regarded as safe and effective for internal use as it is highly toxic

bitterweed medicinal herb [see: fleabane; horseweed]

bitterwort; bitterroot medicinal herb [see: gentian]

bivalirudin USAN anticoagulant; thrombin inhibitor for DVT and unstable angina, and to prevent reocclusion in MI and angioplasty

bizelesin USAN, INN antineoplastic

B-Ject-100 injection ℞ parenteral vitamin therapy [multiple B vitamins]

black alder (Alnus glutinosa) bark and leaves medicinal herb used as an astringent, demulcent, emetic, hemostatic, and tonic

black alder dogwood medicinal herb [see: buckthorn; cascara sagrada]

black birch medicinal herb [see: birch]

black cherry; poison black cherry medicinal herb [see: belladonna]

black choke medicinal herb [see: wild black cherry]

black cohosh (Cimicifuga racemosa) root and rhizome medicinal herb for asthma, bronchitis, dysmenorrhea, dyspepsia, epilepsy, hypertension, hormone imbalance, lung disorders, menopause, rheumatism, snake bite, sore throat, St. Vitus dance, and tuberculosis

black currant (Ribes nigrum) medicinal herb [see: currant]

black dogwood medicinal herb [see: buckthorn; cascara sagrada]

black elder medicinal herb [see: elderberry]

black false hellebore (Veratrum niger) [see: hellebore]

black ginger medicinal herb [see: ginger]

black hellebore (Helleborus niger) [see: hellebore]

black mulberry (Morus nigra) medicinal herb [see: mulberry]

black oak (Quercus tinctoria) medicinal herb [see: white oak]

black poplar (Populus nigra; P. tremula) buds medicinal herb used as a diaphoretic, diuretic, expectorant, and vulnerary

black root medicinal herb [see: Culver root]

black sanicle medicinal herb [see: sanicle]

black snakeroot medicinal herb [see: black cohosh; sanicle]

black walnut (Juglans nigra) hulls and leaves medicinal herb for parasites, ringworm, skin rashes, and stopping lactation; also used as an external antiseptic

black widow spider antivenin [see: antivenin (Latrodectus mactans)]

black willow (Salix nigra) medicinal herb [see: willow]

blackberry (*Rubus fructicosus; R. villosus*) berries, leaves, and root bark *medicinal herb for bleeding, cholera, diarrhea in children, dysentery, sinus drainage, and vomiting*

Black-Draught syrup (discontinued 2003) OTC *stimulant laxative* [casanthranol; senna extract; alcohol 5%] 90•≙ mg/15 mL

Black-Draught tablets, chewable tablets, granules OTC *stimulant laxative* [sennosides] 6 mg; 10 mg; 20 mg/5 mL

blackwort *medicinal herb* [see: comfrey]

bladder fucus; bladderwrack *medicinal herb* [see: kelp (*Fucus*)]

bladderpod *medicinal herb* [see: lobelia]

Blairex Lens Lubricant solution OTC *rewetting solution for soft contact lenses*

Blairex Sterile Saline aerosol solution OTC *rinsing/storage solution for soft contact lenses* [sodium chloride (saline solution)]

blastomycin NF

blazing star *medicinal herb* [see: star grass]

blazing star (*Liatris scariosa; L. spicata; L. squarrosa*) root *medicinal herb used as a diuretic*

BlemErase lotion (discontinued 2003) OTC *keratolytic for acne* [benzoyl peroxide] 10%

Blenoxane powder for IM, IV, subcu, or intrapleural injection ℞ *glycopeptide antibiotic antineoplastic for Hodgkin and non-Hodgkin lymphomas, testicular and squamous cell carcinomas, and malignant pleural effusion (orphan)* [bleomycin sulfate] 15, 30 U

BLEO-COMF (bleomycin, cyclophosphamide, Oncovin, methotrexate, fluorouracil) *chemotherapy protocol*

bleomycin (BLM) INN, BAN *glycopeptide antibiotic antineoplastic* [also: bleomycin sulfate; bleomycin HCl] ② Cleocin

bleomycin HCl JAN *glycopeptide antibiotic antineoplastic* [also: bleomycin sulfate; bleomycin]

bleomycin sulfate USAN, USP, JAN *glycopeptide antibiotic antineoplastic for Hodgkin and non-Hodgkin lymphomas, testicular and squamous cell carcinomas, and malignant pleural effusion (orphan)* [also: bleomycin; bleomycin HCl] 15, 30 U injection

Bleph-10 eye drops, ophthalmic ointment ℞ *antibiotic* [sulfacetamide sodium] 10%

Blephamide eye drop suspension, ophthalmic ointment ℞ *corticosteroidal anti-inflammatory; antibiotic* [prednisolone acetate; sulfacetamide sodium] 0.2%•10%

blessed cardus; holy thistle *medicinal herb* [see: blessed thistle]

blessed thistle (*Cnicus benedictus*) plant *medicinal herb for blood cleansing, digestive disorders, headache, hormonal imbalance, lactation disorders, liver and gallbladder ailments, menstrual disorders, poor circulation, and strengthening heart and lungs*

Blighia sapida *medicinal herb* [see: ackee]

blind nettle (*Lamium album*) plant and flowers *medicinal herb used as an antispasmodic, astringent, expectorant, and styptic*

Blinx ophthalmic solution OTC *extraocular irrigating solution* [sterile isotonic solution]

BlisterGard topical liquid OTC *skin protectant*

Blistex ointment OTC *topical antipruritic/counterirritant; mild local anesthetic; vulnerary* [camphor; phenol; allantoin] 0.5%•0.5%•1%

Blistik lip balm OTC *antipruritic/counterirritant; mild local anesthetic; skin protectant; sunscreen (SPF 10)* [camphor; phenol; allantoin; dimethicone; padimate O; oxybenzone] 0.5%•0.5%•1%•2%•6.6%•2.5%

Blis-To-Sol topical liquid OTC *antifungal; keratolytic* [tolnaftate] 1%

Blis-To-Sol topical powder OTC *antifungal* [zinc undecylenate] 12%

BLM (bleomycin) [q.v.]

Blocadren tablets ℞ *antihypertensive; antianginal; migraine preventative; β-blocker* [timolol maleate] 5, 10, 20 mg

blocked ricin conjugated murine monoclonal antibodies (MAb) [see: ricin (blocked) conjugated murine MAb]

blood, whole USP *blood replenisher*

blood, whole human [now: blood, whole]

blood cells, human red [now: blood cells, red]

blood cells, red USP *blood replenisher*

blood group specific substances A, B & AB USP *blood neutralizer*

blood grouping serum, anti-A [see: anti-A blood grouping serum]

blood grouping serum, anti-B [see: anti-B blood grouping serum]

blood grouping serum, anti-C USP *for in vitro blood testing*

blood grouping serum, anti-c USP *for in vitro blood testing*

blood grouping serum, anti-D USP *for in vitro blood testing*

blood grouping serum, anti-E USP *for in vitro blood testing*

blood grouping serum, anti-e USP *for in vitro blood testing*

blood mononuclear cells, allogenic peripheral *investigational (orphan) agent for pancreatic cancer*

blood staunch *medicinal herb* [see: fleabane; horseweed]

blood volume expanders *a class of therapeutic blood modifiers used to increase the volume of circulating blood* [also called: plasma expanders]

bloodroot (Sanguinaria canadensis) root and rhizome *medicinal herb for diuresis, fever, inducing emesis, nasal polyps, rheumatism, sedation, skin cancer, stimulating menstrual flow, and warts; also used in toothpaste and mouthwash; not generally regarded as safe and effective for internal use*

Bluboro powder packets OTC *astringent wet dressing (modified Burow solution)* [aluminum sulfate; calcium acetate]

blue cohosh (Caulophyllum thalictroides) root *medicinal herb for cramps, epilepsy, induction of labor, menstrual flow stimulant, nerves, and chronic uterine problems*

blue curls *medicinal herb* [see: woundwort]

blue flag (Iris versicolor) root *medicinal herb used as a cathartic, diuretic, laxative, sialagogue, and vermifuge*

Blue Gel (discontinued 2003) OTC *pediculicide for lice* [pyrethrins; piperonyl butoxide; petroleum distillate] 0.3%•3%•1.2%

Blue Gel Muscular Pain Reliever gel OTC *topical analgesic; counterirritant* [menthol]

blue ginseng *medicinal herb* [see: blue cohosh]

blue gum tree *medicinal herb* [see: eucalyptus]

blue mountain tea *medicinal herb* [see: goldenrod]

blue pimpernel; blue skullcap *medicinal herb* [see: skullcap]

blue vervain (Verbena hastata) plant *medicinal herb for asthma, bladder and bowel disorders, bronchitis, colds, convulsions, cough, fever, insomnia, pulmonary tuberculosis, stomach upset, and worms*

blueberry *medicinal herb* [see: bilberry; blue cohosh]

bluebonnet; bluebottle *medicinal herb* [see: cornflower]

blue-green algae (Chloroplast membrane sulfolipids) *nutritional supplement for boosting the immune system*

bluensomycin INN *antibiotic*

BLyS (B lymphocyte stimulating) protein *investigational (orphan) natural immunostimulant for common variable immunodeficiency (CVI, CVID), autoimmune diseases, and B-cell tumors*

B-MOPP (bleomycin, nitrogen mustard, Oncovin, procarbazine, prednisone) *chemotherapy protocol*

BMP (BCNU, methotrexate, procarbazine) *chemotherapy protocol*

BMS 234475 *investigational (Phase II) second-generation protease inhibitor for HIV infection*

BMY-45622 *investigational (orphan) antineoplastic for ovarian cancer*

BOAP (bleomycin, Oncovin, Adriamycin, prednisone) *chemotherapy protocol*

Bo-Cal tablets OTC *dietary supplement* [calcium; vitamin D; magnesium] 250 mg•100 IU•125 mg

Body Fortress Natural Amino tablets OTC *protein supplement* [protein; lactalbumin hydrolysate] 1.67•1.5 g

boforsin [see: colforsin]

bofumustine INN

bogbean; bog myrtle *medicinal herb* [see: buckbean]

Boil-Ease ointment OTC *topical local anesthetic* [benzocaine] 20%

bolandiol INN *anabolic* [also: bolandiol dipropionate]

bolandiol dipropionate USAN, JAN *anabolic* [also: bolandiol]

bolasterone USAN, INN *anabolic steroid; also abused as a street drug*

bolazine INN

BOLD (bleomycin, Oncovin, lomustine, dacarbazine) *chemotherapy protocol*

Boldea fragrans medicinal herb [see: boldo]

boldenone INN, BAN *veterinary anabolic steroid; also abused as a street drug* [also: boldenone undecylenate]

boldenone undecylenate USAN *veterinary anabolic steroid; also abused as a street drug* [also: boldenone]

boldo (Peumus boldus) plant and leaves *medicinal herb for bile stimulation, colds, constipation, digestive disorders, earache, edema, gallstones, gonorrhea, gout, liver disease, rheumatism, syphilis, and worms*

Boldu boldus medicinal herb [see: boldo]

bolenol USAN, INN *anabolic*

bolmantalate USAN, INN, BAN *anabolic*

bolus alba [see: kaolin]

Bombay aloe *medicinal herb* [see: aloe]

bometolol INN

BOMP (bleomycin, Oncovin, Matulane, prednisone) *chemotherapy protocol*

BOMP; CLD-BOMP (bleomycin, Oncovin, mitomycin, Platinol) *chemotherapy protocol for cervical cancer*

Bonamil Infant Formula with Iron powder, oral liquid OTC *total or supplementary infant feeding* 453 g; 384, 946 mL

Bonamine Ⓒᴬᴺ chewable tablets OTC *anticholinergic; antihistamine; antivertigo agent; motion sickness preventative* [meclizine HCl] 25 mg ⃞ Bonine

bone ash [see: calcium phosphate, tribasic]

Bone Assure capsules OTC *vitamin/mineral/calcium supplement to maintain bone mineral density* [calcium (from bis-glycinate); magnesium (from oxide); zinc (from citrate); manganese (from citrate); trimethylglycine; multiple vitamins and minerals] 1000•320•12•3•100• ± per 6 capsules

Bone Meal tablets OTC *dietary supplement* [calcium; phosphorus] 236•118 mg

bone powder, purified [see: calcium phosphate, tribasic]

Bonefos Ⓒᴬᴺ capsules, IV infusion ℞ *bisphosphonate bone resorption inhibitor for hypercalcemia and osteolysis of malignancy (investigational (orphan) in the U.S.)* [clodronate disodium tetrahydrate] 400 mg; 60 mg/mL

boneset (Eupatorium perfoliatum) plant *medicinal herb for chills, colds, constipation, dengue fever, edema, fever, flu, pneumonia, and rheumatism*

Bone-Up capsules OTC *vitamin/mineral/calcium supplement to maintain bone mineral density* [calcium (hydroxyapatite); protein; magnesium (oxide); zinc (monomethionine); manganese; glucosamine HCl; multiple vitamins and minerals] 1000•1000•600•10•5•300• ± per 6 capsules

Bonine chewable tablets (discontinued 2004) OTC *anticholinergic; antihista-*

mine; *antivertigo agent; motion sickness preventative* [meclizine HCl] 25 mg

Boniva once-daily tablets, once-monthly tablets ℞ *bisphosphonate bone resorption inhibitor for postmenopausal osteoporosis; also used for metastatic bone disease* [ibandronate sodium] 2.5 mg; 150 mg

Boniva extended-release (3 month) tablets, IV depot ℞ *investigational (NDA filed) doseforms for postmenopausal osteoporosis* [ibandronate sodium]

Bontril slow-release capsules ℞ *anorexiant; CNS stimulant* [phendimetrazine tartrate] 105 mg ⏹ Bentyl; Vontrol

Bontril PDM tablets ℞ *anorexiant; CNS stimulant* [phendimetrazine tartrate] 35 mg

Bonviva (European name for U.S. product **Boniva**)

bookoo *medicinal herb* [see: buchu]

Boost oral liquid, pudding OTC *enteral nutritional therapy* [milk-based formula] 237 mL

Boostrix IM injection ℞ *active immunizing agent for tetanus, diphtheria, and pertussis; vaccine booster for adolescents (10–18 years)* [tetanus toxoid; diphtheria toxoid, reduced; acellular pertussis vaccine, adsorbed (TDaP; Tdap)] 5 LfU•2.5 LfU•8 μg per 0.5 mL dose

BOP (BCNU, Oncovin, prednisone) *chemotherapy protocol*

BOPAM (bleomycin, Oncovin, prednisone, Adriamycin, mechlorethamine, methotrexate) *chemotherapy protocol*

bopindolol INN

BOPP (BCNU, Oncovin, procarbazine, prednisone) *chemotherapy protocol*

boracic acid [see: boric acid]

borage (Borago officinalis) leaves *medicinal herb for bronchitis, colds, eye inflammation, hay fever, strengthening of heart, lactation stimulation, rashes, rheumatism, ringworm; not generally regarded as safe and effective*

borax [see: sodium borate]

Borbonia pinifolia *medicinal herb* [see: red bush tea]

boric acid NF, JAN *acidifying agent; ophthalmic emollient; antiseptic; astringent* 10% topical

2-bornanone [see: camphor]

bornaprine INN, BAN

bornaprolol INN

bornelone USAN, INN *ultraviolet screen*

bornyl acetate USAN

borocaptate sodium B 10 USAN *antineoplastic; radioactive agent* [also: sodium borocaptate (^{10}B)]

Borofair Otic ear drops ℞ *antibacterial; antifungal; astringent* [acetic acid; aluminum acetate] 2%• ²⁄

Borofax Skin Protectant ointment OTC *astringent* [zinc oxide] 15%

boroglycerin NF

boron *element (B); trace mineral for enhancing mental acuity and improving alertness; not generally regarded as safe and effective as it is highly toxic if taken internally or absorbed through broken skin*

Boropak powder packets OTC *astringent wet dressing (modified Burrow solution)* [aluminum sulfate; calcium acetate]

bortezomib *proteasome inhibitor; antineoplastic for multiple myeloma (orphan); investigational (Phase II) for mantle cell (non-Hodgkin) lymphoma*

bosentan USAN, INN *endothelin receptor antagonist (ERA) for pulmonary arterial hypertension (orphan)*

Boston Advance Cleaner; Boston Cleaner solution OTC *cleaning solution for rigid gas permeable contact lenses*

Boston Advance Comfort Formula solution OTC *disinfecting/wetting/soaking solution for rigid gas permeable contact lenses*

Boston Conditioning Solution OTC *disinfecting/wetting/soaking solution for rigid gas permeable contact lenses*

Boston Rewetting Drops OTC *rewetting solution for rigid gas permeable contact lenses*

Boston Simplicity Multi-Action solution OTC *disinfecting/wetting/soaking solution for rigid gas permeable contact lenses*

Boswellia serrata medicinal herb [see: frankincense]

Botanol ⓒ oral liquid OTC *dietary supplement* [potassium; magnesium; iron; iodine; herbal extracts] 779• 25.2•2.7•0.045•335 mg per 30 mL

botiacrine INN

Botox; Botox Cosmetic powder for injection ℞ *neurotoxin complex for blepharospasm and strabismus of dystonia (orphan), cervical dystonia (orphan), axillary hyperhidrosis, and cosmetic wrinkle treatments* [botulinum toxin, type A] 100 U/vial

BottomBetter ointment OTC *topical diaper rash treatment*

botulinum toxin, type A *neurotoxin complex derived from* Clostridium botulinum, *type A; treatment for blepharospasm and strabismus of dystonia (orphan), cervical dystonia (orphan), and cosmetic wrinkle treatments; investigational (orphan) for pediatric cerebral palsy*

botulinum toxin, type B *neurotoxin complex derived from* Clostridium botulinum, *type B; symptomatic treatment of cervical dystonia (orphan)*

botulinum toxin, type F *investigational (orphan) neurotoxin for cervical dystonia and essential blepharospasm*

botulism antitoxin USP *passive immunizing agent*

botulism equine antitoxin, trivalent *passive immunizing agent*

botulism immune globulin intravenous (BIG-IV) *treatment for infant botulism type A or B (orphan)*

Bounty Bears chewable tablets OTC *vitamin supplement* [multiple vitamins; folic acid] ±•0.3 mg

Bounty Bears Plus Iron chewable tablets OTC *vitamin/iron supplement* [multiple vitamins; iron; folic acid] ±•15•0.3 mg

bourbonal [see: ethyl vanillin]

bovactant BAN

bovine colostrum [see: *Cryptosporidium parvum* bovine colostrum IgG concentrate]

bovine fibrin BAN

bovine immunoglobulin concentrate [see: *Cryptosporidium parvum* bovine colostrum IgG concentrate]

bovine superoxide dismutase (bSOD) [see: orgotein]

bovine whey protein concentrate [see: *Cryptosporidium parvum* bovine colostrum IgG concentrate]

bower, virgin's *medicinal herb* [see: woodbine]

Bowman's root *medicinal herb* [see: Culver root]

box, mountain *medicinal herb* [see: uva ursi]

boxberry *medicinal herb* [see: wintergreen]

boxidine USAN, INN *antihyperlipoproteinemic*

Boyol salve OTC *topical anti-infective; anesthetic* [ichthammol; benzocaine] 10%• ± ⑨ boil

B-PAS (benzoyl para-aminosalicylate) [see: benzoylpas calcium]

BPD-MA (benzoporphyrin derivative) [see: verteporfin]

B-Plex tablets ℞ *vitamin supplement* [multiple B vitamins; vitamin C; folic acid] ± •500•0.5 mg

BrachySeed I-125 implants ℞ *radioactive brachytherapy* [iodine I 125 ceramic beads] 0.19–0.65 mCi (7–24.1 MBq)

BrachySeed Pd-103 implants ℞ *radioactive brachytherapy* [palladium Pd 103 ceramic beads] 1.0–1.8 mCi (37–66.6 MBq)

brallobarbital INN

bramble *medicinal herb* [see: blackberry]

BranchAmin 4% IV infusion ℞ *nutritional therapy for high metabolic stress* [multiple branched-chain essential amino acids]

branched-chain amino acids (BCAA) *investigational (orphan) for* amyotrophic lateral sclerosis [see: iso-leucine; leucine; valine]

brandy mint *medicinal herb* [see: peppermint]

Brasivol cream OTC *abrasive cleanser for acne* [aluminum oxide]

brasofensine maleate USAN *investigational dopamine reuptake inhibitor for Parkinson disease*

Brassica alba *medicinal herb* [see: mustard]

Bravelle powder for subcu or IM injection ℞ *follicle-stimulating hormone (FSH); ovulation stimulant for polycystic ovary disease and assisted reproductive technologies (ART)* [urofollitropin] 75 IU

brazergoline INN

Breathe Free nasal spray OTC *nasal moisturizer* [sodium chloride (saline solution)] 0.65%

Breezee Mist Aerosol powder OTC *antifungal; analgesic; anhidrotic* [undecylenic acid; menthol; aluminum chlorohydrate]

Breezee Mist Antifungal powder OTC *antifungal* [miconazole nitrate] [note: one of two different products with the same name] 2%

Breezee Mist Antifungal powder OTC *antifungal* [tolnaftate] [note: one of two different products with the same name] 1%

Breezee Mist Foot Powder OTC *anhidrotic* [talc; aluminum chlorohydrate]

brefonalol INN

bremazocine INN

Breonesin capsules (discontinued 2002) OTC *expectorant* [guaifenesin] 200 mg

brequinar INN *antineoplastic* [also: brequinar sodium]

brequinar sodium USAN *antineoplastic* [also: brequinar]

bretazenil USAN, INN *anxiolytic*

Brethaire oral inhalation aerosol (discontinued 2001) ℞ *sympathomimetic bronchodilator* [terbutaline sulfate] 0.2 mg/dose

Brethine tablets, IV or subcu injection ℞ *sympathomimetic bronchodila-*

tor [terbutaline sulfate] 2.5, 5 mg; 1 mg/mL ⓢ Banthine

bretylium tosilate INN *antiadrenergic; antiarrhythmic* [also: bretylium tosylate]

bretylium tosylate USAN, BAN *antiadrenergic; antiarrhythmic* [also: bretylium tosilate] 500, 1000 mg/vial injection

Brevibloc; Brevibloc Double Strength IV infusion ℞ *antiarrhythmic; β-blocker for supraventricular tachycardia* [esmolol HCl] 10, 250 mg/mL; 20 mg/mL

Brevicon tablets (in Wallettes of 28) ℞ *monophasic oral contraceptive* [norethindrone; ethinyl estradiol] 0.5 mg•35 μg

Brevital Sodium powder for IV injection ℞ *barbiturate general anesthetic* [methohexital sodium] 2.5 g ⓢ Bretylol

Brevoxyl Cleansing Lotion ℞ *keratolytic for acne* [benzoyl peroxide] 4%, 8%

Brevoxyl-4; Brevoxyl-8 gel ℞ *keratolytic for acne* [benzoyl peroxide] 4%; 8%

Brevoxyl-4 Creamy Wash; Brevoxyl-8 Creamy Wash topical liquid ℞ *keratolytic for acne* [benzoyl peroxide] 4%; 8%

brewer's yeast *natural source of protein and B-complex vitamins*

Brexidol 20 ⓒ tablets ℞ *analgesic; antirheumatic; nonsteroidal anti-inflammatory drug (NSAID)* [piroxicam betadex] 191.2 mg (=20 mg base)

Brexin-L.A. sustained-release capsules (discontinued 2003) ℞ *decongestant; antihistamine* [pseudoephedrine HCl; chlorpheniramine maleate] 120•8 mg

Bricanyl tablets, IV or subcu injection (discontinued 2001) ℞ *sympathomimetic bronchodilator* [terbutaline sulfate] 2.5, 5 mg; 1 mg/mL

Brietal Sodium ⓒ powder for IV injection (discontinued 2001) ℞ *barbiturate general anesthetic* [methohexital sodium] 10 mg/mL

brifentanil INN *narcotic analgesic* [also: brifentanil HCl]

brifentanil HCl USAN *narcotic analgesic* [also: brifentanil]

Brigham tea; Brigham Young weed *medicinal herb* [see: ephedra]

Brik-Paks (trademarked delivery form) *ready-to-use liquid containers*

brimonidine INN *ophthalmic α₂-adrenergic agonist for open-angle glaucoma and ocular hypertension* [also: brimonidine tartrate]

brimonidine tartrate USAN *selective α₂ agonist for open-angle glaucoma and ocular hypertension; investigational (orphan) for anterior ischemic optic neuropathy* [also: brimonidine] 0.2% eye drops

brinaldix [see: clopamide]

brinase INN [also: brinolase]

brinazarone INN

brindoxime INN

brineurin [now: abrineurin]

brinolase USAN *fibrinolytic enzyme* [also: brinase]

brinzolamide USAN, INN *topical carbonic anhydrase inhibitor for glaucoma*

Bristoject (trademarked delivery form) *prefilled disposable syringe*

Brite Eyes II eye drops OTC *moisturizer; lubricant; antioxidant and antiglycation agent to prevent free radical damage in the lens* [N-acetyl-L-carnitine; glycerin; carboxymethylcellulose sodium] 1%•1%•0.3%

British antilewisite (BAL) [now: dimercaprol]

British tobacco *medicinal herb* [see: coltsfoot]

brivudine INN

brobactam INN

brobenzoxaldine [see: broxaldine]

broclepride INN

brocresine USAN, INN, BAN *histidine decarboxylase inhibitor*

brocrinat USAN, INN *diuretic*

brodimoprim INN

brofaromine INN *investigational reversible/selective MAO inhibitor*

Brofed oral liquid ℞ *decongestant; antihistamine* [pseudoephedrine HCl; brompheniramine maleate] 60•8 mg/10 mL

brofezil INN, BAN

brofoxine USAN, INN *antipsychotic*

brolaconazole INN

brolamfetamine INN

bromacrylide INN

bromadel [see: carbromal]

Bromadine-DM syrup (discontinued 2002) ℞ *antitussive; decongestant; antihistamine* [dextromethorphan hydrobromide; pseudoephedrine HCl; brompheniramine maleate] 10•30•2 mg/5 mL

Bromadine-DX syrup ℞ *antitussive; decongestant; antihistamine* [dextromethorphan hydrobromide; pseudoephedrine HCl; brompheniramine maleate] 10•30•2 mg/5 mL

bromadoline INN *analgesic* [also: bromadoline maleate]

bromadoline maleate USAN *analgesic* [also: bromadoline]

Bromaline elixir (discontinued 2001) OTC *decongestant; antihistamine* [phenylpropanolamine HCl; brompheniramine maleate] 12.5•2 mg/5 mL

bromamid INN

Bromanate pediatric elixir OTC *decongestant; antihistamine* [pseudoephedrine HCl; brompheniramine maleate] 30•2 mg/10 mL

Bromanate DC Cough syrup (discontinued 2002) ℞ *narcotic antitussive; decongestant; antihistamine* [codeine phosphate; phenylpropanolamine HCl; brompheniramine maleate; alcohol] 10•12.5•2 mg/5 mL

Bromanate DM Cold & Cough pediatric elixir OTC *antitussive; decongestant; antihistamine* [dextromethorphan hydrobromide; pseudoephedrine HCl; brompheniramine maleate] 5•15•1 mg/5 mL

Bromanyl syrup (discontinued 2002) ℞ *narcotic antitussive; antihistamine* [codeine phosphate; bromodiphenhydramine HCl] 10•12.5 mg/5 mL

bromanylpromide [see: bromamid]

Bromarest DX Cough syrup (discontinued 2002) ℞ *antitussive; decongestant; antihistamine* [dextromethorphan hydrobromide; pseudoephedrine HCl; brompheniramine maleate; alcohol 0.95%] 10•30•2 mg/5 mL

Bromatane DX Cough syrup ℞ *antitussive; decongestant; antihistamine* [dextromethorphan hydrobromide; pseudoephedrine HCl; brompheniramine maleate; alcohol 1%] 20•60•4 mg/10 mL

Bromatapp extended-release tablets (discontinued 2001) OTC *decongestant; antihistamine* [phenylpropanolamine HCl; brompheniramine maleate] 75•12 mg

bromauric acid NF

bromazepam USAN, INN, BAN, JAN *benzodiazepine anxiolytic; minor tranquilizer*

bromazine INN, DCF *antihistamine* [also: bromodiphenhydramine HCl; bromodiphenhydramine]

bromazine HCl [see: bromodiphenhydramine HCl]

brombenzonium [see: bromhexine HCl]

bromchlorenone USAN, INN *topical anti-infective*

bromebric acid INN, BAN

bromelain JAN *anti-inflammatory; proteolytic enzymes* [also: bromelains]

bromelains USAN, INN, BAN *anti-inflammatory; proteolytic enzymes* [also: bromelain]

bromelin [see: bromelains]

bromerguride INN

brometenamine INN, DCF

bromethol [see: tribromoethanol]

Bromfed extended-release capsules ℞ *decongestant; antihistamine* [phenylephrine HCl; brompheniramine maleate] 15•12 mg

Bromfed syrup (discontinued 2003) OTC *decongestant; antihistamine* [pseudoephedrine HCl; brompheniramine maleate] 60•4 mg/10 mL ⑨ Bromphen

Bromfed tablets ℞ *decongestant; antihistamine* [pseudoephedrine HCl; brompheniramine maleate] 60•4 mg

Bromfed-DM Cough syrup ℞ *antitussive; decongestant; antihistamine* [dextromethorphan hydrobromide; pseudoephedrine HCl; brompheniramine maleate] 20•60•4 mg/10 mL

Bromfed-PD extended-release pediatric capsules ℞ *decongestant; antihistamine* [phenylephrine HCl; brompheniramine maleate] 7.5•6 mg

bromfenac INN *long-acting nonsteroidal anti-inflammatory drug (NSAID); analgesic; antipyretic* [also: bromfenac sodium]

bromfenac sodium USAN *long-acting nonsteroidal anti-inflammatory drug (NSAID); analgesic; antipyretic; topical treatment of ocular inflammation following cataract surgery* [also: bromfenac]

Bromfenex extended-release capsules ℞ *decongestant; antihistamine* [pseudoephedrine HCl; brompheniramine maleate] 120•12 mg

Bromfenex PD extended-release capsules ℞ *pediatric decongestant and antihistamine* [pseudoephedrine HCl; brompheniramine maleate] 60•6 mg

bromhexine INN, BAN *expectorant; mucolytic* [also: bromhexine HCl]

bromhexine HCl USAN, JAN *expectorant; mucolytic; investigational (orphan) for keratoconjunctivitis sicca of Sjögren syndrome* [also: bromhexine]

Bromhist-DM syrup ℞ *decongestant; antihistamine; antitussive; expectorant* [pseudoephedrine HCl; brompheniramine maleate; dextromethorphan hydrobromide; guaifenesin] 30•2•5•50 mg/5 mL

Bromhist-NR oral drops ℞ *pediatric decongestant and antihistamine* [pseudoephedrine HCl; brompheniramine maleate] 12.5•1 mg/mL

Bromhist-PDX oral drops ℞ *antitussive; decongestant; antihistamine* [dextromethorphan hydrobromide; pseudoephedrine HCl; brompheniramine maleate] 3•12.5•1 mg/mL

Bromhist-PDX syrup ℞ *decongestant; antihistamine; antitussive; expectorant* [phenylephrine HCl; brompheniramine maleate; dextromethorphan hydrobromide; guaifenesin] 5•2•5• 50 mg/5 mL

bromindione USAN, INN, BAN *anticoagulant*

bromine *element (Br)*

bromisoval INN [also: bromisovalum; bromvalerylurea; bromovaluree]

bromisovalum NF [also: bromisoval; bromvalerylurea; bromovaluree]

2-bromo-α-ergocryptine [see: bromocriptine]

bromocamphor [see: camphor, monobromated]

bromociclen INN [also: bromocyclen]

bromocriptine USAN, INN, BAN *dopamine agonist; prolactin enzyme inhibitor; antiparkinsonian*

bromocriptine mesilate JAN *dopamine agonist; prolactin enzyme inhibitor; antiparkinsonian* [also: bromocriptine mesylate]

bromocriptine mesylate USAN, USP *dopamine agonist; prolactin enzyme inhibitor; antiparkinsonian; investigational (NDA filed) agent for diabetic control of hypoglycemia* [also: bromocriptine mesilate] 2.5 mg oral

bromocyclen BAN [also: bromociclen]

bromodeoxyuridine [now: broxuridine]

bromodiethylacetylurea [see: carbromal]

bromodiphenhydramine BAN *antihistamine* [also: bromodiphenhydramine HCl; bromazine]

bromodiphenhydramine HCl USP *antihistamine* [also: bromazine; bromodiphenhydramine]

bromofenofos INN

bromoform USP

bromofos INN

1-bromoheptadecafluorooctane [see: perflubron]

bromoisovaleryl urea (BVU) [see: bromisovalum]

Bromophen T.D. sustained-release tablets (discontinued 2001) ℞

decongestant; antihistamine [phenylpropanolamine HCl; phenylephrine HCl; brompheniramine maleate] 15•15•12 mg ⑨ Bromphen

bromophenol blue

bromophin [see: apomorphine HCl]

bromophos [see: bromofos]

bromopride INN, DCF

Bromo-Seltzer effervescent granules OTC *antacid; analgesic; antipyretic* [sodium bicarbonate; citric acid; acetaminophen] 2781•2224•325 mg/dose

bromotheophyllinate aminoisobutanol [see: pamabrom]

bromotheophyllinate pyranisamine [see: pyrabrom]

bromotheophyllinate pyrilamine [see: pyrabrom]

8-bromotheophylline [see: pamabrom]

Bromotuss with Codeine syrup (discontinued 2002) ℞ *narcotic antitussive; antihistamine* [codeine phosphate; bromodiphenhydramine HCl] 10•12.5 mg/5 mL

bromovaluree DCF [also: bromisovalum; bromisoval; bromvalerylurea]

11-bromovincamine [see: brovincamine]

bromovinyl arabinosyluracil (BV-araU) [see: sorivudine]

bromoxanide USAN, INN *anthelmintic*

bromperidol USAN, INN, BAN, JAN *antipsychotic*

bromperidol decanoate USAN, BAN *antipsychotic*

Bromphen DC with Codeine Cough syrup (discontinued 2002) ℞ *narcotic antitussive; decongestant; antihistamine* [codeine phosphate; phenylpropanolamine HCl; brompheniramine maleate] 10•12.5•2 mg/5 mL

Bromphen DX Cough syrup (discontinued 2002) ℞ *antitussive; decongestant; antihistamine* [dextromethorphan hydrobromide; pseudoephedrine HCl; brompheniramine maleate; alcohol 0.95%] 10•30•2 mg/5 mL

brompheniramine INN, BAN *alkyl-amine antihistamine* [also: bromphen-iramine maleate]

Brompheniramine Cough syrup (discontinued 2002) OTC *antitussive; decongestant; antihistamine* [dextro-methorphan hydrobromide; pseudo-ephedrine HCl; brompheniramine maleate; alcohol 0.95%] 10•30•2 mg/5 mL

Brompheniramine DC Cough syrup (discontinued 2002) R *narcotic anti-tussive; decongestant; antihistamine* [codeine phosphate; phenylpropa-nolamine HCl; brompheniramine maleate; alcohol 1.15%] 10•12.5•2 mg/5 mL

brompheniramine maleate USP *alkylamine antihistamine* [also: brom-pheniramine] 10 mg/mL injection

brompheniramine maleate & pseu-doephedrine HCl *antihistamine; decongestant* 4•60 mg/5 mL oral

brompheniramine tannate *alkyl-amine antihistamine*

Brompton's Cocktail; Brompton's Mixture (refers to any oral narcotic/alcoholic solution containing mor-phine and either cocaine or a phe-nothiazine derivative) *prophylaxis for chronic, severe pain*

bromvalerylurea JAN [also: bromiso-valum; bromisoval; bromovaluree]

Bronchial capsules R *antiasthmatic; bronchodilator; expectorant* [theophyl-line; guaifenesin] 150•90 mg

Broncho Saline solution (discontin-ued 2002) OTC *diluent for inhalation bronchodilators; solution for tracheal lavage* [sodium chloride (saline solu-tion)] 0.9%

Broncholate softgels (discontinued 2002) R *bronchodilator; decongestant; expectorant* [ephedrine HCl; guaifen-esin] 12.5•200 mg ⊡ Brondelate

Broncholate syrup R *bronchodilator; decongestant; expectorant* [ephedrine HCl; guaifenesin] 12.5•200 mg/10 mL ⊡ Brondelate

Brondelate elixir R *antiasthmatic; bronchodilator; expectorant* [theophyl-line; guaifenesin] 192•150 mg/15 mL ⊡ Broncholate

Bronkaid Dual Action caplets OTC *bronchodilator; decongestant; expecto-rant* [ephedrine sulfate; guaifenesin] 25•400 mg

Bronkodyl capsules R *antiasthmatic; bronchodilator* [theophylline] 100, 200 mg

Bronkotuss Expectorant oral liquid (discontinued 2002) R *decongestant; antihistamine; expectorant* [ephedrine sulfate; chlorpheniramine maleate; guaifenesin; hydriodic acid; alcohol 5%] 8.2•4•100•1.67 mg/5 mL

bronopol INN, BAN, JAN

Brontex tablets, oral liquid (discontin-ued 2002) R *narcotic antitussive; expectorant* [codeine phosphate; guai-fenesin] 10•300 mg; 2.5•75 mg/5 mL

brook bean *medicinal herb* [see: buck-bean]

brooklime (Veronica beccabunga) plant *medicinal herb used as a diuretic, emmenagogue, and febrifuge*

broom (Cytisus scoparius) plant and bloom *medicinal herb for inducing bowel evacuation, diuresis, and emesis; also used as a homeopathic remedy for arrhythmias, diphtheria, and head and throat congestion*

broom, butcher's *medicinal herb* [see: butcher's broom]

broom, dyer's; green broom *medici-nal herb* [see: dyer's broom]

broparestrol INN, DCF

broperamole USAN, INN *anti-inflam-matory*

bropirimine USAN, INN *antineoplastic; antiviral*

broquinaldol INN

brosotamide INN, DCF

brosuximide INN

brotianide INN, BAN

brotizolam USAN, INN, BAN, JAN *hyp-notic*

brovanexine INN

brovavir [see: sorivudine]

BrōveX oral suspension ℞ *antihistamine* [brompheniramine tannate] 12 mg/5 mL

BrōveX CT chewable tablets ℞ *antihistamine* [brompheniramine tannate] 12 mg

brovincamine INN [also: brovincamine fumarate]

brovincamine fumarate JAN [also: brovincamine]

brown algae *medicinal herb* [see: kelp (*Laminaria*)]

brownwort *medicinal herb* [see: woundwort]

broxaldine INN, DCF

broxaterol INN

Broxine ℞ *investigational (NDA filed, orphan) radiosensitizer for primary brain tumors* [broxuridine]

broxitalamic acid INN

broxuridine INN *investigational (NDA filed, orphan) radiosensitizer for primary brain tumors*

broxyquinoline INN, DCF

brucine sulfate NF

bruisewort *medicinal herb* [see: comfrey; soapwort]

bryony (*Bryonia alba; B. dioica*) root *medicinal herb used as a pectoral and purgative; not generally regarded as safe and effective as root is poisonous in high doses (ingestion of as few as 40 berries can be fatal in adults, 15 in children)*

bryostatin-1 *investigational (orphan) agent for esophageal cancer; investigational (Phase I) for AIDS-related lymphomas*

B-Salt Forte ophthalmic solution (discontinued 2004) ℞ *intraocular irrigating solution* [sodium chloride (balanced saline solution)]

bSOD (bovine superoxide dismutase) [see: orgotein]

BSS (bismuth subsalicylate) [q.v.]

BSS; BSS Plus ophthalmic solution ℞ *intraocular irrigating solution* [sodium chloride (balanced saline solution)]

BTA Rapid Urine Test test kit for professional use *in vitro diagnostic aid for bladder tumor analytes in the urine*

BTA Stat Test test kit for home use *in vitro diagnostic aid for bladder tumor analytes in the urine* [rapid immunoassay (RIA)]

bucainide INN *antiarrhythmic* [also: bucainide maleate]

bucainide maleate USAN *antiarrhythmic* [also: bucainide]

bucco *medicinal herb* [see: buchu]

Bucet capsules ℞ *sedative; barbiturate analgesic* [butalbital; acetaminophen] 50•650 mg

bucetin INN, BAN, JAN

buchu (*Agathosma betulina; Barosma betulina; B. cenulata; B. serratifolia*) leaves *medicinal herb for edema, gas, gout, inflammation, kidney and urinary tract infections, and prostatitis; also used as a douche for leukorrhea and vaginal yeast infections*

buciclovir INN

bucillamine INN, JAN

bucindolol INN, BAN *antihypertensive* [also: bucindolol HCl]

bucindolol HCl USAN *antihypertensive* [also: bucindolol]

buckbean (*Menyanthes trifoliata*) leaves *medicinal herb used as a tonic, cathartic, diuretic, anthelmintic, and emetic*

buckeye; California buckeye; Ohio buckeye *medicinal herb* [see: horse chestnut]

buckhorn brake (*Osmunda cinnamomea; O. regalis*) root *medicinal herb used as a demulcent and tonic*

buckthorn (*Rhamnus cathartica; R. frangula*) bark and berries *medicinal herb for bleeding, bowel disorders, chronic constipation, fever, gallstones, lead poisoning, and liver disorders* [also see: cascara sagrada]

bucku *medicinal herb* [see: buchu]

bucladesine INN [also: bucladesine sodium]

bucladesine sodium JAN [also: bucladesine]

buclizine INN, BAN *antinauseant; antiemetic; anticholinergic; motion sickness relief* [also: buclizine HCl]

buclizine HCl USAN *antinauseant; antiemetic; anticholinergic; motion sickness relief* [also: buclizine]

buclosamide INN, BAN, DCF

bucloxic acid INN, DCF

bucolome INN, JAN

bucricaine INN

bucrilate INN *tissue adhesive* [also: bucrylate]

bucromarone USAN, INN *antiarrhythmic*

bucrylate USAN *tissue adhesive* [also: bucrilate]

bucumolol INN [also: bucumolol HCl]

bucumolol HCl JAN [also: bucumolol]

Budeprion SR sustained-release film-coated tablets ℞ *aminoketone antidepressant* [bupropion HCl] 100 mg

budesonide USAN, INN, BAN, JAN *corticosteroidal anti-inflammatory for chronic asthma, rhinitis, and inflammatory bowel disease*

budipine INN

budotitane INN

budralazine INN, JAN

bufenadine [see: bufenadrine]

bufenadrine INN

bufeniode INN, DCF

bufetolol INN [also: bufetolol HCl]

bufetolol HCl JAN [also: bufetolol]

bufexamac INN, BAN, JAN, DCF

bufezolac INN

buffered aspirin [see: aspirin, buffered]

Bufferin coated tablets, coated caplets OTC *analgesic; antipyretic; anti-inflammatory; antirheumatic* [aspirin (buffered with calcium carbonate, magnesium oxide, and magnesium carbonate)] 325, 500 mg

Bufferin AF Nite Time tablets OTC *antihistaminic sleep aid; analgesic* [diphenhydramine HCl; acetaminophen] 30•500 mg

Buffex tablets OTC *analgesic; antipyretic; anti-inflammatory; antirheumatic* [aspirin (buffered with aluminum glycinate and magnesium carbonate)] 325 mg

bufilcon A USAN *hydrophilic contact lens material*

buflomedil INN, BAN, DCF

bufogenin INN

buformin USAN, INN *antidiabetic*

bufrolin INN, BAN

bufuralol INN, BAN

bufylline BAN *diuretic; smooth muscle relaxant* [also: ambuphylline]

bugbane *medicinal herb* [see: hellebore; black cohosh]

bugleweed (*Lycopus virginicus*) plant *medicinal herb for cough, excessive menses, nervous indigestion, and other nervous disorders*

bugloss *medicinal herb* [see: borage]

Bugs Bunny Complete chewable tablets OTC *vitamin/mineral/calcium/iron supplement* [multiple vitamins & minerals; calcium; iron; folic acid; biotin] ±•100•18•0.4•0.04 mg

Bugs Bunny Plus Iron chewable tablets OTC *vitamin/iron supplement* [multiple vitamins; iron; folic acid] ±•15•0.3 mg

Bugs Bunny with Extra C Children's chewable tablets OTC *vitamin supplement* [multiple vitamins; folic acid] ±•0.3 mg

bugwort *medicinal herb* [see: black cohosh]

buku *medicinal herb* [see: buchu]

bulaquine INN

Bulk Forming Fiber Laxative film-coated tablets OTC *bulk laxative; antidiarrheal* [calcium polycarbophil] 625 mg

bulk-producing laxatives *a subclass of laxatives that work by increasing the hydration and volume of stool to stimulate peristalsis; also form an emollient gel to ease the movement of stool through the intestines* [see also: laxatives]

bull's foot *medicinal herb* [see: coltsfoot]

bumadizone INN, DCF

bumecaine INN

bumepidil INN

bumetanide USAN, USP, INN, BAN, JAN *loop diuretic* 0.25 mg/mL injection

bumetrizole USAN, INN *ultraviolet screen*

Bumex IV or IM injection (discontinued 2004) ℞ *loop diuretic* [bumetanide] 0.25 mg/mL

Bumex tablets ℞ *loop diuretic* [bumetanide] 0.5, 1, 2 mg

Buminate 5%; Buminate 25% IV infusion ℞ *blood volume expander for shock, burns, and hypoproteinemia* [human albumin] 5%; 25%

bunaftine INN

bunamidine INN, BAN *anthelmintic* [also: bunamidine HCl]

bunamidine HCl USAN *anthelmintic* [also: bunamidine]

bunamiodyl INN [also: buniodyl]

bunamiodyl sodium [see: bunamiodyl; buniodyl]

bunaprolast USAN, INN *antiasthmatic; 5-lipoxygenase inhibitor*

bunapsilate INN *combining name for radicals or groups*

bunazosin INN [also: bunazosin HCl]

bunazosin HCl JAN [also: bunazosin]

bundlin [now: sedecamycin]

buniodyl BAN [also: bunamiodyl]

bunitrolol INN [also: bunitrolol HCl]

bunitrolol HCl JAN [also: bunitrolol]

bunolol INN *antiadrenergic (β-receptor)* [also: bunolol HCl]

bunolol HCl USAN *antiadrenergic (β-receptor)* [also: bunolol]

Bupap caplets ℞ *analgesic; antipyretic; barbiturate sedative* [acetaminophen; butalbital] 650•50 mg

buparvaquone INN, BAN

buphenine INN, BAN *peripheral vasodilator* [also: nylidrin HCl]

Buphenyl tablets, powder for oral solution ℞ *antihyperammonemic for urea cycle disorders (orphan); investigational (orphan) for various sickling disorders* [sodium phenylbutyrate] 500 mg; 3 g/tsp., 8.6 g/tbsp.

bupicomide USAN, INN *antihypertensive*

bupivacaine INN, BAN *injectable local anesthetic* [also: bupivacaine HCl]

bupivacaine HCl USAN, USP, JAN *injectable local anesthetic* [also: bupivacaine] 0.25%, 0.5%, 0.75%

bupivacaine HCl & epinephrine *injectable local anesthetic; vasoconstrictor* 0.25%•1:200 000, 0.5%• 1:200 000, 0.75%•1:200 000

Bupivicaine Spinal injection ℞ *injectable local anesthetic for obstetrical use* [bupivacaine HCl; dextrose] 0.75%•8.25%

bupranol [see: bupranolol]

bupranolol INN, DCF [also: bupranolol HCl]

bupranolol HCl JAN [also: bupranolol]

Buprenex IV or IM injection ℞ *narcotic agonist-antagonist analgesic* [buprenorphine HCl] 0.3 mg/mL

buprenorphine INN, BAN *narcotic agonist-antagonist analgesic* [also: buprenorphine HCl]

buprenorphine HCl USAN, JAN *narcotic agonist-antagonist analgesic for inpatient treatment of opiate dependence (orphan)* [also: buprenorphine] 0.3 mg/mL injection

buprenorphine HCl & naloxone HCl *investigational (orphan) for opiate addictions*

bupropion BAN *aminoketone antidepressant; non-nicotine aid to smoking cessation* [also: bupropion HCl; amfebutamone]

bupropion HCl USAN *aminoketone antidepressant; non-nicotine aid to smoking cessation* [also: amfebutamone; bupropion] 75, 100, 150, 200 mg oral

buquineran INN, BAN

buquinolate USAN, INN *coccidiostat for poultry*

buquiterine INN

buramate USAN, INN *anticonvulsant; antipsychotic*

burdock (Arctium lappa; A. majus; A. minus) root *medicinal herb for arthritis, blood cleansing, dandruff, eczema, edema, fever, gout, kidney and lung disorders, rheumatism, skin diseases, and tumors; also used as an antimicrobial and diaphoretic*

burefrine [now: berefrine]

burnet (Pimpinella magna; P. saxifrage) root *medicinal herb used as an antispasmodic, astringent, carminative, diaphoretic, diuretic, stimulant, and stomachic*

burning bush *medicinal herb* [see: fraxinella; wahoo]

burodiline INN

Buro-Sol solution (discontinued 2004) OTC *astringent wet dressing (Burow solution)* [aluminum sulfate] 0.23%

Burow solution [see: aluminum acetate]

burr seed; turkey burr seed; clotbur; hareburr; hurr-burr; thorny burr *medicinal herb* [see: burdock]

burrage *medicinal herb* [see: borage]

buserelin INN, BAN *hormonal antineoplastic; gonad-stimulating principle; luteinizing hormone-releasing hormone analogue* [also: buserelin acetate]

buserelin acetate USAN, JAN *hormonal antineoplastic; gonad-stimulating principle; luteinizing hormone-releasing hormone analogue* [also: buserelin]

BuSpar tablets ℞ *nonsedating azaspirone anxiolytic* [buspirone HCl] 5, 10, 15, 30 mg

buspirone INN, BAN *nonsedating azaspirone anxiolytic* [also: buspirone HCl]

buspirone HCl USAN *nonsedating azaspirone anxiolytic* [also: buspirone] 5, 7.5, 10, 15, 30 mg oral

busulfan USP, INN, JAN *alkylating antineoplastic for chronic myelogenous leukemia (CML); pretreatment for bone marrow transplants (orphan); investigational (orphan) for neoplastic meningitis and primary brain malignancies* [also: busulphan]

Busulfex IV infusion ℞ *alkylating antineoplastic for chronic myelogenous leukemia (CML); pretreatment for bone marrow and stem cell transplants (orphan)* [busulfan] 6 mg/mL

busulphan BAN *alkylating antineoplastic* [also: busulfan]

butabarbital USP *sedative; hypnotic* [also: secbutobarbitone] ② butalbital

butabarbital sodium USP *sedative; hypnotic* [also: secbutabarbital sodium] 15, 30 mg oral; 30 mg/5 mL oral

butacaine INN, BAN [also: butacaine sulfate]

butacaine sulfate USP [also: butacaine]

butacetin USAN *analgesic; antidepressant*

butacetoluide [see: butanilicaine]

butaclamol INN *antipsychotic* [also: butaclamol HCl]

butaclamol HCl USAN *antipsychotic* [also: butaclamol]

butadiazamide INN

butafosfan INN, BAN

butalamine INN, BAN

butalbital USAN, USP, INN *barbiturate sedative* ② butabarbital; Butibel

butalbital & acetaminophen & caffeine *barbiturate sedative; analgesic* 50•325•40, 50•500•40 mg oral

butalbital & acetaminophen & caffeine & codeine phosphate *barbiturate sedative; analgesic; narcotic antitussive* 50•325•40•30 mg oral

butalbital & aspirin & caffeine *analgesic; barbiturate sedative* 50•325•40 mg oral

Butalbital Compound tablets, capsules ℞ *analgesic; barbiturate sedative* [aspirin; caffeine; butalbital] 325•40•50 mg

butalgin [see: methadone HCl]

butallylonal NF

butamben USAN, USP *topical anesthetic*

butamben picrate USAN *topical local anesthetic* 1% topical

butamirate INN *antitussive* [also: butamirate citrate; butamyrate]

butamirate citrate USAN *antitussive* [also: butamirate; butamyrate]

butamisole INN *veterinary anthelmintic* [also: butamisole HCl]

butamisole HCl USAN *veterinary anthelmintic* [also: butamisole]

butamiverine [see: butaverine]

butamoxane INN

butamyrate BAN *antitussive* [also: butamirate citrate; butamirate]

butane (n-butane) NF *aerosol propellant*

1,4-butanediol (1,4-B; BDO); butane-1,4-diol *precursor to gamma hydroxybutyrate (GHB); a formerly legal alternative to GHB, now also illegal (Schedule I)* [see: gamma hydroxybutyrate (GHB)]

butanilicaine INN, BAN

butanixin INN

butanserin INN

butantrone INN

butaperazine USAN, INN *antipsychotic*

butaperazine maleate USAN *antipsychotic*

butaprost USAN, INN, BAN *bronchodilator*

butaverine INN, DCF

butaxamine INN *antidiabetic; antihyperlipoproteinemic* [also: butoxamine HCl; butoxamine]

butcher's broom (*Ruscus aculeatus*) rhizomes *medicinal herb for atherosclerosis, circulatory disorders, hemorrhoids, thrombosis, varicose veins, and venous insufficiency; not generally regarded as safe and effective*

butedronate tetrasodium USAN *bone imaging aid*

butedronic acid INN

butelline [see: butacaine sulfate]

butenafine INN *antifungal*

butenafine HCl USAN *topical benzylamine antifungal*

butenemal [see: vinbarbital]

buteprate INN *former combining name for radicals or groups (name rescinded by the USAN)* [now: probutate]

buterizine USAN, INN *peripheral vasodilator*

Butesin Picrate ointment (discontinued 2004) OTC *local anesthetic* [butamben picrate] 1%

butetamate INN [also: butethamate]

butethal NF [also: butobarbitone]

butethamate BAN [also: butetamate]

butethamine HCl NF

butethanol [see: tetracaine]

Butex Forte capsules ℞ *analgesic; barbiturate sedative* [acetaminophen; butalbital] 650•50 mg

buthalital sodium INN [also: buthalitone sodium]

buthalitone sodium BAN [also: buthalital sodium]

buthiazide USAN *diuretic; antihypertensive* [also: butizide]

Butibel tablets, elixir ℞ *GI anticholinergic; sedative* [belladonna extract;

butabarbital sodium] 15•15 mg; 15•15 mg/5 mL ⊡ butalbital

butibufen INN

butidrine INN, DCF

butikacin USAN, INN, BAN *antibacterial*

butilfenin USAN, INN *hepatic function test*

butinazocine INN

butinoline INN

butirosin INN *antibacterial antibiotic* [also: butirosin sulfate; butirosin sulphate]

butirosin sulfate USAN *antibacterial antibiotic* [also: butirosin; butirosin sulphate]

butirosin sulphate BAN *antibacterial antibiotic* [also: butirosin sulfate; butirosin]

Butisol Sodium tablets, elixir ℞ *sedative; hypnotic* [butabarbital sodium] 15, 30, 50, 100 mg; 30 mg/5 mL ⊡ Butazolidin

butixirate USAN, INN *analgesic; antirheumatic*

butixocort INN

butizide INN *diuretic; antihypertensive* [also: buthiazide]

butobarbitone BAN [also: butethal]

butobendine INN

butoconazole INN, BAN *topical antifungal* [also: butoconazole nitrate]

butoconazole nitrate USAN, USP *topical antifungal* [also: butoconazole]

butocrolol INN

butoctamide INN [also: butoctamide semisuccinate]

butoctamide semisuccinate JAN [also: butoctamide]

butofilolol INN

butonate USAN, INN *anthelmintic*

butopamine USAN, INN *cardiotonic*

butopiprine INN, DCF

butoprozine INN *antiarrhythmic; antianginal* [also: butoprozine HCl]

butoprozine HCl USAN *antiarrhythmic; antianginal* [also: butoprozine]

butopyrammonium iodide INN

butopyronoxyl USP

butorphanol USAN, INN, BAN *analgesic; antitussive*

butorphanol tartrate USAN, USP, BAN, JAN *narcotic agonist-antagonist analge-*

sic; antitussive 10 mg nasal spray; 1, 2 mg/mL injection

butoxamine BAN *antidiabetic; antihyperlipoproteinemic* [also: butoxamine HCl; butaxamine]

butoxamine HCl USAN *antidiabetic; antihyperlipoproteinemic* [also: butaxamine; butoxamine]

2-butoxyethyl nicotinate [see: nicoboxil]

butoxylate INN

butoxyphenylacethydroxamic acid [see: bufexamac]

butriptyline INN, BAN *antidepressant* [also: butriptyline HCl]

butriptyline HCl USAN *antidepressant* [also: butriptyline]

butropium bromide INN, JAN

butterbur *(Petasites hybridus)* leaves and root *medicinal herb used as an analgesic for migraines and as an antispasmodic for asthma, cough, and gastrointestinal and urinary tract disorders; not generally regarded as safe and effective due to organ damage and carcinogenic properties*

buttercup *(Ranunculus acris; R. bulbosus; R. scleratus)* plant *medicinal herb used as an acrid, anodyne, antispasmodic, diaphoretic, and rubefacient*

butterfly weed *medicinal herb* [see: pleurisy root]

butternut *(Juglans cinerea)* bark, leaves, flowers *medicinal herb used as an anthelmintic, antiseptic, cathartic, cholagogue, and nervine*

butterweed *medicinal herb* [see: fleabane; horseweed]

butydrine [see: butidrine]

butyl alcohol NF *solvent*

butyl aminobenzoate (butyl *p*-aminobenzoate) [now: butamben]

butyl *p*-aminobenzoate picrate [see: butamben picrate]

butyl chloride NF

butyl 2-cyanoacrylate [see: enbucrilate]

butyl DNJ (deoxynojirimycin) [see: deoxynojirimycin]

butyl *p*-hydroxybenzoate [see: butylparaben]

butyl methoxydibenzoylmethane [see: avobenzone]

butyl nitrite; isobutyl nitrite *amyl nitrite substitutes, sold as euphoric street drugs, which produce a quick but short-lived "rush"* [see also: amyl nitrite; volatile nitrites]

butyl parahydroxybenzoate JAN *antifungal agent* [also: butylparaben]

***p*-butylaminobenzoyldiethylaminoethyl HCl** JAN

butylated hydroxyanisole (BHA) NF, BAN *antioxidant*

butylated hydroxytoluene (BHT) NF, BAN *antioxidant*

α-butylbenzyl alcohol [see: fenipentol]

1-butylbiguanide [see: buformin]

N-butyl-deoxynojirimycin [see: deoxynojirimycin]

1,4-butylene glycol (1,4-BG) *precursor to gamma hydroxybutyrate (GHB); a formerly legal alternative to GHB, now also illegal (Schedule I)* [see: gamma hydroxybutyrate (GHB)]

1,5-(butylimino)-1,5-dideoxy-D-glucitol *investigational (orphan) for Fabry disease and Gaucher disease*

butylmesityl oxide [see: butopyronoxyl]

butylparaben NF *antifungal agent* [also: butyl parahydroxybenzoate]

butylphenamide

butylphenylsalicylamide [see: butylphenamide]

butylscopolamine bromide JAN

butynamine INN

butyrate propionate [see: probutate; buteprate]

butyrophenones *a class of dopamine receptor antagonists with conventional (typical) antipsychotic activity* [also called: phenylbutylpiperadines]

butyrylcholesterinase *investigational (orphan) agent for reduction and clearance of serum cocaine levels and postsurgical apnea*

butyrylperazine [see: butaperazine]

O-butyrylthiamine disulfide [see: bisbutitiamine]

butyvinyl [see: vinylbital]

buzepide metiodide INN, DCF

BVAP (BCNU, vincristine, Adriamycin, prednisone) *chemotherapy protocol*

BV-araU (bromovinyl arabinosyluracil) [see: sorivudine]

BVCPP (BCNU, vinblastine, cyclophosphamide, procarbazine, prednisone) *chemotherapy protocol*

BVDS (bleomycin, Velban, doxorubicin, streptozocin) *chemotherapy protocol*

BVPP (BCNU, vincristine, procarbazine, prednisone) *chemotherapy protocol*

BVU (bromoisovaleryl urea) [see: bromisovalum]

BW 12C *investigational (orphan) agent for sickle cell disease*

Byclomine capsules, tablets ℞ *GI antispasmodic* [dicyclomine HCl] 10 mg; 20 mg ▣ Hycomine

Byetta subcu injection in prefilled pen injector ℞ *synthetic exendin-4 analogue to slow gastric emptying and improve glycemic control in type 2 diabetics* [exenatide] 5, 10 μg/dose

C (vitamin C) [see: ascorbic acid]

C & E softgels OTC *vitamin supplement* [vitamins C and E] 500•400 mg

C Factors "1000" Plus tablets OTC *vitamin C supplement with multiple bioflavonoids* [vitamin C; rose hips; citrus bioflavonoids; rutin; hesperidin] 1000•25•250•50•25 mg

C vitamin [see: ascorbic acid]

¹⁴C urea *diagnostic aid for H. pylori in the stomach* [also: carbon C 14 urea]

C1-esterase-inhibitor, human *investigational (orphan) agent to prevent or treat acute attacks of angioedema*

CA (cyclophosphamide, Adriamycin) *chemotherapy protocol*

CA (cytarabine, asparaginase) *chemotherapy protocol for acute myelocytic leukemia (AML)*

cA2 monoclonal antibodies (chimeric A2 MAb) [see: infliximab]

⁴⁵Ca [see: calcium chloride Ca 45]

⁴⁷Ca [see: calcium chloride Ca 47]

cabastine INN

cabbage, cow *medicinal herb* [see: masterwort; white pond lily]

cabbage, meadow; swamp cabbage *medicinal herb* [see: skunk cabbage]

cabbage, water *medicinal herb* [see: white pond lily]

cabergoline USAN, INN *dopamine agonist for hyperprolactinemia; investigational treatment for Parkinson disease and gynecologic disorders*

cabis bromatum [see: bibrocathol]

CABO (cisplatin, Abitrexate, bleomycin, Oncovin) *chemotherapy protocol for head and neck cancer*

CABOP; CA-BOP (Cytoxin, Adriamycin, bleomycin, Oncovin, prednisone) *chemotherapy protocol*

CABS (CCNU, Adriamycin bleomycin, streptozocin) *chemotherapy protocol*

cabufocon A USAN *hydrophobic contact lens material*

cabufocon B USAN *hydrophobic contact lens material*

CAC (cisplatin, ara-C, caffeine) *chemotherapy protocol*

cacao butter JAN

cactinomycin USAN, INN *antibiotic antineoplastic* [also: actinomycin C]

CAD (cyclophosphamide, Adriamycin, dacarbazine) *chemotherapy protocol*

CAD (cytarabine [and] daunorubi-cin) *chemotherapy protocol*

cade oil [see: juniper tar]

cadexomer INN

cadexomer iodine USAN, INN, BAN *antiseptic; antiulcerative wound dressing*

cadmium *element (Cd)*

cadralazine INN, BAN, JAN

Ca-DTPA (calcium pentetate) [see: pentetate calcium trisodium]

Caduet film-coated tablets Ŗ *calcium channel blocker and HMG-CoA reductase inhibitor for coronary artery disease (CAD)* [amlodipine besylate; atorvastatin] 2.5•10, 2.5•20, 2.5•30, 5•10, 5•20, 5•40, 5•80, 10•10, 10•20, 10•40, 10•80 mg

CAE (cyclophosphamide, Adria-mycin, etoposide) *chemotherapy protocol for small cell lung cancer (SCLC)* [also: ACE]

Caelyx ⓒ *injection Ŗ antineoplastic for ovarian carcinoma and AIDS-related Kaposi sarcoma* [doxorubicin HCl, liposome-encapsulated] 2 mg/mL

CAF (cyclophosphamide, Adria-mycin, fluorouracil) *chemotherapy protocol for breast cancer*

cafaminol INN

Cafatine suppositories Ŗ *migraine-specific vasoconstrictor* [ergotamine tartrate; caffeine] 2•200 mg

Cafatine-PB tablets Ŗ *migraine treatment; vasoconstrictor; anticholinergic; sedative* [ergotamine tartrate; caffeine; pentobarbital sodium; belladonna extract] 1•100•30•0.125 mg

Cafcit oral solution, injectable Ŗ *analeptic; CNS stimulant for apnea of prematurity (orphan)* [caffeine citrate] 20 mg/mL

cafedrine INN, BAN

Cafergot tablets, suppositories Ŗ *migraine treatment; vasoconstrictor* [ergotamine tartrate; caffeine] 1•100 mg; 2•100 mg

Caffedrine tablets OTC *CNS stimulant; analeptic* [caffeine] 200 mg

caffeic acid phenethyl ester (CAPE) *antimicrobial substance found in bee propolis*

caffeine USP, BAN, JAN *methylxanthine analeptic; CNS stimulant; diuretic; treatment for apnea of prematurity (orphan); potentiator of various NSAIDs*

caffeine citrate *methylxanthine analeptic; CNS stimulant for apnea of prematurity (orphan)*

caffeine monohydrate [see: caffeine, citrated]

caffeine nut *medicinal herb* [see: kola nut]

caffeine & sodium benzoate *analeptic for respiratory depression due to an overdose of CNS depressants* 250 mg/mL injection

CAFP (cyclophosphamide, Adria-mycin, fluorouracil, prednisone) *chemotherapy protocol*

CAFTH (cyclophosphamide, Adria-mycin, fluorouracil, tamoxifen, Halotestin) *chemotherapy protocol*

CAFVP (cyclophosphamide, Adria-mycin, fluorouracil, vincristine, prednisone) *chemotherapy protocol*

Cal Carb-HD powder for oral solution OTC *calcium supplement* [calcium carbonate] 2.5 g Ca/pkt.

Caladryl cream OTC *topical antihistamine; astringent; antipruritic/anesthetic* [diphenhydramine HCl; calamine] 1%•8% ② Benadryl

Caladryl lotion OTC *poison ivy treatment* [calamine; pramoxine HCl; alcohol 2.2%] 8%•1%

Caladryl Clear lotion OTC *poison ivy treatment* [pramoxine HCl; zinc acetate; alcohol 2%] 1%•0.1%

Caladryl for Kids cream (discontinued 2003) OTC *poison ivy treatment* [calamine; pramoxine HCl] 8%•1%

Calafol tablets Ŗ *vitamin/calcium supplement* [vitamins B_6 and B_{12}; folic acid; vitamin D_3; calcium] 25 mg•425 μg•1.6 mg•400 IU•400 mg

Cala-gen lotion (discontinued 2004) OTC *antipruritic; anesthetic; antihista-*

mine [diphenhydramine HCl; alcohol 2%] 1%

Calamatum spray (discontinued 2003) OTC *poison ivy treatment* [calamine; zinc oxide; menthol; camphor; benzocaine]

calamine USP, JAN *topical protectant; astringent; poison ivy treatment*

Calamine, Phenolated lotion OTC *poison ivy treatment* [calamine; zinc oxide; phenol] 8%•8%•1%

Calamine Lotion OTC *poison ivy treatment* [calamine; zinc oxide] 6.97%• 6.97%

calamint (*Calamintha officinalis*) *medicinal herb* [see: summer savory]

Calamintha hortensis medicinal herb [see: summer savory]

Calamintha montana medicinal herb [see: winter savory]

Calamox ointment (discontinued 2003) OTC *poison ivy treatment* [calamine] 17 g/100 g ② Camalox

calamus (*Acorus calamus*) rhizome *medicinal herb for anxiety, bad breath from smoking, colic, digestive disorders, fever, gas, irritated throat, and promoting wound healing; not generally regarded as safe and effective and is prohibited in the U.S. as a food additive or supplement*

Calamycin lotion OTC *antihistamine; astringent; anesthetic* [pyrilamine maleate; zinc oxide; calamine; benzocaine; chloroxylenol; alcohol 2%]

Calan film-coated tablets ℞ *antianginal; antiarrhythmic; antihypertensive; calcium channel blocker* [verapamil HCl] 40, 80, 120 mg ② kaolin; Kaon

Calan SR film-coated sustained-release tablets ℞ *antihypertensive; antianginal; antiarrhythmic; calcium channel blocker* [verapamil HCl] 120, 180, 240 mg ② kaolin; Kaon

calanolide A *investigational (Phase I/II) non-nucleoside reverse transcriptase inhibitor (NNRTI) for HIV infection*

Calcarb 600 with Vitamin D tablets OTC *calcium supplement* [calcium carbonate; vitamin D] 1.5 g (600 mg Ca)•125 IU

Cal-Carb Forte chewable tablets, caplets OTC *antacid; calcium supplement* [calcium carbonate] 1250 mg (500 mg Ca)

Calcet tablets OTC *dietary supplement* [calcium; vitamin D] 152.8 mg• 100 IU

Calcet Plus tablets OTC *vitamin/calcium/iron supplement* [multiple vitamins; calcium; iron; folic acid] ±• 152.8•18•0.8 mg

Calcibind powder for oral solution ℞ *antiurolithic to prevent stone formation in absorptive calciuria type I* [cellulose sodium phosphate] 300 g bulk pack

CalciCaps tablets OTC *dietary supplement* [dibasic calcium phosphate; calcium gluconate; calcium carbonate; vitamin D] 125 mg (Ca)•60 mg (P) •67 IU

CalciCaps with Iron tablets OTC *dietary supplement* [dibasic calcium phosphate; calcium gluconate; calcium carbonate; vitamin D; ferrous gluconate] 125 mg (Ca)•60 mg (P)•67 IU•7 mg

Calci-Chew chewable tablets OTC *calcium supplement* [calcium carbonate] 1250 mg (500 mg Ca)

Calciday-667 tablets (discontinued 2002) OTC *calcium supplement* [calcium carbonate] 667 mg (250 mg Ca)

calcidiol [see: calcifediol]

Calcidrine syrup (discontinued 2002) ℞ *narcotic antitussive; expectorant* [codeine phosphate; calcium iodide; alcohol 6%] 8.4•152 mg/5 mL

calcifediol (25-hydroxycholecalciferol; 25-hydroxyvitamin D₃) USAN, USP, INN *vitamin D precursor (converted to calcitriol in the body); calcium regulator for treatment of metastatic bone disease or hypocalcemia of chronic renal dialysis*

Calciferol IM injection ℞ *vitamin deficiency therapy for refractory rickets, familial hypophosphatemia, and hypo-*

parathyroidism [ergocalciferol (vitamin D₂)] 500 000 IU/mL

calciferol [now: ergocalciferol]

Calciferol Drops OTC *vitamin supplement* [ergocalciferol (vitamin D₂)] 8000 IU/mL

Calcijex injection ℞ *vitamin D therapy for hypoparathyroidism and hypocalcemia of chronic renal dialysis* [calcitriol] 1, 2 μg/mL

Calcimar subcu or IM injection ℞ *calcium regulator for hypercalcemia, Paget disease, and postmenopausal osteoporosis* [calcitonin (salmon)] 200 IU/mL

Calci-Mix capsules OTC *calcium supplement* [calcium carbonate] 1250 mg (500 mg Ca)

Calcionate syrup OTC *calcium supplement* [calcium glubionate] 1.8 g/5 mL

calcipotriene USAN *topical antipsoriatic* [also: calcipotriol]

calcipotriol INN, BAN *topical antipsoriatic* [also: calcipotriene]

Calciquid syrup OTC *calcium supplement* [calcium glubionate] 1.8 g/5 mL

calcitonin (human) USAN, INN, BAN, JAN *calcium regulator for symptomatic Paget disease (osteitis deformans) (orphan)* ☑ calcitriol

calcitonin (salmon) USAN, INN, BAN *calcium regulator for Paget disease (orphan), hypercalcemia, and postmenopausal osteoporosis*

calcitonin salmon (synthesis) JAN *synthetic analogue of calcitonin (salmon); calcium regulator* [also: salcatonin]

calcitonin salmon, recombinant *investigational (NDA filed) calcium regulator for hypercalcemia, postmenopausal osteoporosis, and Paget disease*

Cal-Citrate tablets, capsules OTC *calcium supplement* [calcium citrate] 250 mg Ca; 225 mg Ca

calcitriol (1,25-hydroxycholecalciferol; 1,25-hydroxyvitamin D₃) USAN, INN, BAN, JAN *physiologically active form of vitamin D; calcium regulator for hypoparathyroidism and hypocalcemia due to chronic renal dialysis; decreases the severity of psoriatic*

lesions 0.25, 0.5 μg oral; 1 μg/mL oral; 1, 2 μg injection ☑ calcitonin

calcium *element* (Ca)

calcium, oyster shell [see: calcium carbonate]

Calcium 600 tablets OTC *calcium supplement* [calcium carbonate] 1500 mg (600 mg Ca)

Calcium 600 + D tablets OTC *dietary supplement* [calcium; vitamin D] 600 mg•125 IU

Calcium 600 with Vitamin D tablets OTC *dietary supplement* [calcium; vitamin D] 600 mg•100 IU

calcium acetate USP, JAN *dietary calcium supplement (25% elemental calcium); buffering agent for hyperphosphatemia of end-stage renal disease (orphan)*

calcium alginate fiber *topical local hemostatic*

calcium aminacyl B-PAS (benzoyl para-aminosalicylate) [see: benzoylpas calcium]

calcium 4-aminosalicylate trihydrate [see: aminosalicylate calcium]

calcium amphomycin [see: amphomycin]

calcium antagonists *a class of coronary vasodilators that inhibit cardiac muscle contraction and slow cardiac electrical conduction velocity* [also called: calcium channel blockers; slow channel blockers]

calcium ascorbate (vitamin C) USP *water-soluble vitamin; antiscorbutic* 500 mg oral; 3256 mg/tsp. oral

calcium benzamidosalicylate INN, BAN *antibacterial; tuberculostatic* [also: benzoylpas calcium]

calcium benzoyl *p*-aminosalicylate (B-PAS) [see: benzoylpas calcium]

calcium benzoylpas [see: benzoylpas calcium]

calcium bis-dioctyl sulfosuccinate [see: docusate calcium]

calcium bis-glycinate *dietary calcium supplement*

calcium bromide JAN

calcium carbimide INN [also: cyanamide]

calcium carbonate USP *antacid; dietary calcium supplement (40% elemental calcium); investigational (orphan) for hyperphosphatemia of end-stage renal disease* [also: precipitated calcium carbonate] 500, 600, 650, 1250 mg oral; 1250 mg/5 mL oral

calcium carbonate, precipitated [now: calcium carbonate]

calcium carbophil *bulk laxative*

calcium caseinate *dietary calcium supplement; infant formula modifier*

calcium channel blockers *a class of coronary vasodilators that inhibit cardiac muscle contraction and slow cardiac electrical conduction velocity* [also called: calcium antagonists; slow channel blockers]

calcium chloride USP, JAN *calcium replenisher*

calcium chloride Ca 45 USAN *radioactive agent*

calcium chloride Ca 47 USAN *radioactive agent*

calcium chloride dihydrate [see: calcium chloride]

calcium citrate USP *dietary calcium supplement (21% elemental calcium)* 1.2, 4.5 g oral; 3.6 g/5 mL oral

calcium citrate tetrahydrate [see: calcium citrate]

calcium clofibrate INN

calcium cyanamide [see: calcium carbimide]

calcium D-glucarate tetrahydrate [see: calcium saccharate]

calcium D-gluconate lactobionate monohydrate [see: calcium glubionate]

calcium dioctyl sulfosuccinate [see: docusate calcium]

calcium disodium edathamil [see: edetate calcium disodium]

calcium disodium edetate JAN *heavy metal chelating agent* [also: edetate calcium disodium; sodium calcium edetate; sodium calciumedetate]

Calcium Disodium Versenate IM, IV, or subcu injection ℞ *chelating agent for acute or chronic lead poisoning and lead encephalopathy* [edetate calcium disodium] 200 mg/mL

calcium dobesilate INN

calcium doxybensylate [see: calcium dobesilate]

calcium edetate sodium [see: edetate calcium disodium]

calcium EDTA (ethylene diamine tetraacetic acid) [see: edetate calcium disodium]

calcium folinate INN, BAN, JAN *antianemic; folate replenisher; antidote to folic acid antagonist* [also: leucovorin calcium]

calcium glubionate USAN, INN *dietary calcium supplement*

calcium gluceptate USP *parenteral calcium replenisher* [also: calcium glucoheptonate] 1100 mg/5 mL injection

calcium glucoheptonate INN, DCF *parenteral calcium replenisher* [also: calcium gluceptate]

calcium gluconate (calcium D-gluconate) USP *dietary calcium supplement (9% elemental calcium); investigational (orphan) wash for hydrofluoric acid burns* 500, 650, 975, 1000 mg oral; 3.85 g/15 mL oral; 10% injection

calcium glycerinophosphate [see: calcium glycerophosphate]

calcium glycerophosphate NF, JAN

calcium hopantenate JAN

calcium hydroxide USP *astringent*

calcium hydroxide phosphate [see: calcium phosphate, tribasic]

calcium hypophosphite NF

calcium iodide *expectorant*

calcium iododocosanoate [see: iodobehenate calcium]

calcium lactate USP, JAN *dietary calcium supplement (13% elemental calcium)* 325, 650, 770 mg oral

calcium lactate hydrate [see: calcium lactate]

calcium lactate pentahydrate [see: calcium lactate]

calcium lactobionate USP *dietary calcium supplement*

calcium lactobionate dihydrate [see: calcium lactobionate]

calcium lactophosphate NF

calcium L-aspartate JAN

calcium levofolinate [see: levoleucovorin calcium]

calcium levulate [see: calcium levulinate]

calcium levulinate USP *dietary calcium supplement*

calcium levulinate dihydrate [see: calcium levulinate]

calcium mandelate USP

calcium oxide [see: lime]

calcium pantothenate (calcium D-pantothenate; vitamin B₅) USP, INN, JAN *water-soluble vitamin; enzyme cofactor* [also: pantothenic acid] 100, 218, 545 mg oral

calcium pantothenate, racemic (calcium DL-pantothenate) USP *water-soluble vitamin; enzyme cofactor*

calcium para-aminosalicylate JAN [also: aminosalicylate calcium]

calcium phosphate, dibasic USP, JAN *dietary calcium supplement; tablet base*

calcium phosphate, monocalcium [see: calcium phosphate, dibasic]

calcium phosphate, tribasic NF *dietary calcium supplement (39% elemental calcium)* [also: durapatite; hydroxyapatite]

Calcium + ⓒⓐⓝ oral liquid OTC *dietary supplement* [calcium; magnesium; vitamin D] 500 mg•200 mg•200 IU per 2 tsp. dose

calcium polycarbophil USAN, USP *bulk laxative; antidiarrheal*

calcium polystyrene sulfonate JAN *ion exchange resin for hyperkalemia*

calcium polysulfide & calcium thiosulfate [see: lime, sulfurated]

calcium saccharate USP, INN *stabilizer*

calcium silicate NF *tablet excipient*

calcium sodium ferriclate INN *hematinic* [also: ferriclate calcium sodium]

calcium stearate NF, JAN *tablet and capsule lubricant*

calcium sulfate NF *tablet and capsule diluent*

calcium tetracemine disodium [see: edetate calcium disodium]

calcium trisodium pentetate INN, BAN *plutonium chelating agent* [also: pentetate calcium trisodium]

calcium 10-undecenoate [see: calcium undecylenate]

calcium undecylenate USAN *antifungal*

calciumedetate sodium [see: edetate calcium disodium]

Calderol capsules Ŗ *vitamin D therapy for metastatic bone disease or hypocalcemia of chronic renal dialysis* [calcifediol] 20, 50 μg

Caldesene ointment OTC *moisturizer; emollient; astringent; antiseptic* [cod liver oil (vitamins A and D); zinc oxide; lanolin]

Caldesene topical powder OTC *antifungal* [calcium undecylenate] 10%

caldiamide INN *pharmaceutic aid* [also: caldiamide sodium]

caldiamide sodium USAN, BAN *pharmaceutic aid* [also: caldiamide]

Calel D tablets OTC *dietary supplement* [calcium carbonate; cholecalciferol] 500 mg•200 IU

Calendula officinalis *medicinal herb* [see: marigold]

CALF (cyclophosphamide, Adriamycin, leucovorin [rescue], fluorouracil) *chemotherapy protocol*

calfactant USAN *surface-active extract of saline lavage of calf lungs, used for prevention of respiratory distress syndrome (RDS) in premature infants* (orphan)

CALF-E (cyclophosphamide, Adriamycin, leucovorin [rescue], fluorouracil, ethinyl estradiol) *chemotherapy protocol*

CAL-G (cyclophosphamide, asparaginase, leurocristine, daunorubicin, prednisone) *chemotherapy protocol for acute lymphocytic leukemia (ALL)*

Cal-Gest chewable tablets OTC *calcium supplement* [calcium carbonate] 500 mg (200 mg Ca)

Calgonate wash ℞ *investigational (orphan) emergency treatment for hydrofluoric acid burns* [calcium gluconate]

Cal-Guard softgels (discontinued 2002) OTC *calcium supplement* [calcium carbonate] 125 mg (50 mg Ca)

California barberry *medicinal herb* [see: Oregon grape]

California buckthorn *medicinal herb* [see: buckthorn; cascara sagrada]

California false hellebore *(Veratrum californicum)* [see: hellebore]

californium *element (Cf)*

calioben [see: calcium iodobehenate]

Cal-Lac capsules OTC *calcium supplement* [calcium lactate] 500 mg

Calluna vulgaris *medicinal herb* [see: heather]

calmatives *a class of soothing agents that reduce excitement, nervousness, distress, or irritation* [also called: sedatives]

Calmol 4 rectal suppositories OTC *emollient; astringent* [cocoa butter; zinc oxide] 80%•10%

Calm-X tablets OTC *anticholinergic; antiemetic; antivertigo agent; motion sickness preventative* [dimenhydrinate] 50 mg

Calmylin ⓒ oral solution (discontinued 2001) OTC *antitussive; decongestant; expectorant* [dextromethorphan hydrobromide; pseudoephedrine HCl; guaifenesin] 3•6•20 mg/mL

Calmylin #1 ⓒ syrup (discontinued 2001) OTC *antihistamine* [dextromethorphan hydrobromide] 3 mg/mL

Calmylin #2 ⓒ oral solution (discontinued 2001) OTC *antitussive; decongestant* [dextromethorphan hydrobromide; pseudoephedrine HCl] 3•6 mg/mL

Calmylin #4 ⓒ oral solution (discontinued 2001) OTC *antitussive; antihistamine; expectorant* [dextromethorphan hydrobromide; diphenhydramine HCl; ammonium chloride] 2.5•3•25 mg/mL

Calmylin Cough & Cold ⓒ oral solution (discontinued 2001) OTC *antitussive; decongestant; expectorant; analgesic* [dextromethorphan hydrobromide; pseudoephedrine HCl; guaifenesin; acetaminophen] 1•2•6.67•21.67 mg/mL

Calmylin Expectorant ⓒ syrup (discontinued 2001) OTC *expectorant* [guaifenesin] 20 mg/mL

Calmylin Pediatric ⓒ syrup (discontinued 2001) OTC *pediatric antitussive and decongestant* [dextromethorphan hydrobromide; pseudoephedrine HCl] 1.5•3 mg/mL

Calmylin with Codeine ⓒ oral solution ℞ *narcotic antitussive; decongestant; expectorant* [codeine phosphate; pseudoephedrine HCl; guaifenesin] 0.66•6•20 mg/mL

Cal-Nate tablets ℞ *vitamin/mineral/calcium/iron supplement; stool softener* [multiple vitamins & minerals; calcium; iron; folic acid; docusate sodium] ±•125•27•1•50 mg

calomel NF

Calphosan IV injection ℞ *calcium replacement* [calcium glycerophosphate; calcium lactate] 50•50 mg/10 mL (0.08 mEq Ca/mL)

Calphron tablets (discontinued 2002) ℞ *calcium supplement; buffering agent for hyperphosphatemia in end-stage renal failure (orphan)* [calcium acetate] 667 mg

Cal-Plus tablets (discontinued 2002) OTC *calcium supplement* [calcium carbonate] 1500 mg (600 mg Ca)

calteridol INN *pharmaceutic aid* [also: calteridol calcium]

calteridol calcium USAN, BAN *pharmaceutic aid* [also: calteridol]

Caltha palustris *medicinal herb* [see: cowslip]

Caltrate 600 film-coated tablets OTC *calcium supplement* [calcium carbonate] 1500 mg (600 mg Ca)

Caltrate 600 + D tablets OTC *dietary supplement* [calcium carbonate; vitamin D] 600 mg•200 IU

Caltrate 600 + Iron/Vitamin D film-coated tablets OTC *dietary supplement* [calcium carbonate; ferrous fumarate; vitamin D] 600 mg•18 mg•125 IU

Caltrate Jr. chewable tablets (discontinued 2002) OTC *calcium supplement* [calcium carbonate] 750 mg (300 mg Ca)

Caltrate Plus tablets OTC *dietary supplement* [calcium carbonate; vitamin D; multiple minerals] 600 mg•200 IU• ≛

Caltro tablets OTC *dietary supplement* [calcium; vitamin D] 250 mg•125 IU

calumba; calumba root; calumbo *medicinal herb* [see: colombo]

calusterone USAN, INN *antineoplastic*

Calypte test kit for professional use *urine test for HIV-1 antibodies*

CAM (cyclophosphamide, Adriamycin, methotrexate) *chemotherapy protocol*

Cama Arthritis Pain Reliever tablets OTC *analgesic; antipyretic; antiinflammatory; antirheumatic* [aspirin (buffered with magnesium oxide and aluminum hydroxide)] 500 mg

camazepam INN

CAMB (Cytoxin, Adriamycin, methotrexate, bleomycin) *chemotherapy protocol*

cambendazole USAN, INN, BAN *anthelmintic*

CAMELEON (cytosine arabinoside, methotrexate, Leukovorin, Oncovin) *chemotherapy protocol*

camellia oil JAN

Camellia sinensis *medicinal herb* [see: green tea]

CAMEO (cyclophosphamide, Adriamycin, methotrexate, etoposide, Oncovin) *chemotherapy protocol*

Cameo Oil OTC *bath emollient*

CAMF (cyclophosphamide, Adriamycin, methotrexate, folinic acid) *chemotherapy protocol*

camiglibose USAN, INN *antidiabetic*

Camila tablets (in packs of 28) ℞ *oral contraceptive (progestin only)* [norethindrone] 0.35 mg

camiverine INN

camomile *medicinal herb* [see: chamomile]

camonagrel INN

camostat INN [also: camostat mesilate]

camostat mesilate JAN [also: camostat]

cAMP (cyclic adenosine monophosphate) [see: adenosine phosphate]

CAMP (cyclophosphamide, Adriamycin, methotrexate, procarbazine HCl) *chemotherapy protocol for non–small cell lung cancer (NSCLC)*

Campath IV infusion ℞ *immunosuppressant for B-cell chronic lymphocytic leukemia (orphan); investigational (Phase II) for non-Hodgkin lymphoma, organ transplants, and multiple sclerosis* [alemtuzumab] 30 mg/mL

camphetamide [see: camphotamide]

Campho-Phenique topical liquid, gel OTC *mild anesthetic; anti-infective; counterirritant* [camphor; phenol; eucalyptus oil] 10.8%•4.7%• ≛

Campho-Phenique Antibiotic Plus Pain Reliever ointment (discontinued 2001) OTC *topical antibiotic; local anesthetic* [polymyxin B sulfate; neomycin sulfate; bacitracin zinc; lidocaine] 5000 U•3.5 mg•500 U•40 mg per g

Campho-Phenique Cold Sore Treatment and Scab Relief cream OTC *anesthetic for cold sores and fever blisters* [pramoxine HCl; petrolatum] 1%•30

camphor (d-camphor; dl-camphor) USP, JAN *topical antipruritic; mild local anesthetic; counterirritant* [also: trans-π-oxocamphor]

camphor, monobromated USP

camphorated opium tincture [now: paregoric]

camphorated parachlorophenol [see: parachlorophenol, camphorated]

camphoric acid USP

camphotamide INN, DCF

Campral enteric-coated delayed-release tablets ℞ *GABA/taurine analogue for the treatment of alcoholism* [acamprosate calcium] 333 mg

Camptosar IV infusion ℞ *topoisomerase I inhibitor; antineoplastic for meta-*

static colorectal cancer [irinotecan HCl] 20 mg/mL

camptothecin-11 (CPT-11) [see: irinotecan]

camsilate INN *combining name for radicals or groups* [also: camsylate]

camsylate USAN, BAN *combining name for radicals or groups* [also: camsilate]

Camvirex ℞ *investigational (orphan) for pancreatic cancer and pediatric HIV/AIDS infections* [rubitecan]

camylofin INN, DCF

Canada fleabane *medicinal herb* [see: fleabane; horseweed]

Canada pitch tree *medicinal herb* [see: hemlock]

Canada root *medicinal herb* [see: pleurisy root]

Canada tea *medicinal herb* [see: wintergreen]

canaigre (*Rumex hymenosepalus*) *medicinal herb for a variety of disease states and used as a purported substitute for ginseng; not generally regarded as safe and effective because of high tannin content and possible mutagenic effect when used internally*

Canasa suppositories ℞ *anti-inflammatory for active ulcerative colitis, proctosigmoiditis, and proctitis* [mesalamine (5-aminosalicylic acid)] 500, 1000 mg

canbisol INN

Cancidas powder for IV infusion ℞ *antifungal for candidiasis, candidemia, invasive aspergillosis and other resistant fungal infections* [caspofungin acetate] 50, 70 mg/vial

candesartan USAN, INN *antihypertensive; angiotensin II receptor antagonist*

candesartan cilexetil USAN *antihypertensive; angiotensin II receptor antagonist; investigational (Phase II) for the prevention of diabetic retinopathy*

candicidin USAN, USP, INN, BAN *polyene antifungal*

Candida albicans skin test antigen *diagnostic aid for diminished cellular immunity; test for HIV patients to assess TB antigen response*

CandidaSure *reagent slides for professional use in vitro diagnostic aid for Candida albicans in the vagina*

Candin intradermal injection ℞ *diagnostic aid for diminished cellular immunity; test for HIV patients to assess TB antigen response* [Candida albicans skin test antigen] 0.1 mL

candleberry; candleberry myrtle *medicinal herb* [see: bayberry; tung seed]

candocuronium iodide INN

candoxatril USAN, INN, BAN *antihypertensive*

candoxatrilat USAN, INN, BAN *antihypertensive*

Canesten Topical ⒸⒶⓃ *cream* OTC *topical antifungal* [clotrimazole] 1%

Cankaid *oral solution* OTC *topical anti-inflammatory and anti-infective* [carbamide peroxide] 10%

cankerroot *medicinal herb* [see: gold thread]

canna; channa *medicinal herb* [see: kanna]

cannabinol INN, BAN *antiemetic; antinauseant; a nonpsychoactive derivative of the Cannabis sativa plant*

Cannabis sativa (marijuana; marihuana; hashish) *euphoric/hallucinogenic street drug made from the resin or dried leaves and flowering tops of the cannabis plant; medicinal herb for asthma, analgesia, leprosy, and loss of appetite; investigational (Phase II) for pain relief and sleep enhancement*

canrenoate potassium USAN *aldosterone antagonist* [also: canrenoic acid; potassium canrenoate]

canrenoic acid INN, BAN *aldosterone antagonist* [also: canrenoate potassium; potassium canrenoate]

canrenone USAN, INN *aldosterone antagonist*

cantharides JAN

cantharidin *topical keratolytic*

Cantil tablets ℞ *GI antispasmodic; anticholinergic; peptic ulcer adjunct* [mepenzolate bromide] 25 mg

Canvaxin ℞ *investigational (Phase III) theraccine for malignant melanoma*

CAO (cyclophosphamide, Adriamycin, Oncovin) *chemotherapy protocol*

CAP (cellulose acetate phthalate) [q.v.]

CAP (cyclophosphamide, Adriamycin, Platinol) *chemotherapy protocol for non–small cell lung cancer (NSCLC)*

CAP (cyclophosphamide, Adriamycin, prednisone) *chemotherapy protocol*

CAP; CAP-I (cyclophosphamide, Adriamycin, Platinol) *chemotherapy protocol*

CAP-II (cyclophosphamide, Adriamycin, high-dose Platinol) *chemotherapy protocol*

Capastat Sulfate powder for IM injection ℞ *tuberculostatic* [capreomycin sulfate] 1 g/vial ☒ Cepastat

CAP-BOP (cyclophosphamide, Adriamycin, procarbazine, bleomycin, Oncovin, prednisone) *chemotherapy protocol*

CAPE (caffeic acid phenethyl ester) *antimicrobial substance found in bee propolis*

Cape aloe *medicinal herb* [see: aloe]

cape gum *medicinal herb* [see: acacia]

capecitabine USAN, INN *oral fluoropyrimidine (a 5-FU prodrug) antineoplastic for metastatic breast and colorectal cancer; investigational (Phase III) for pancreatic cancer*

capers (Capparis spinosa) *flower buds and leaves medicinal herb for skin disorders and for reducing the effects of enlarged capillaries*

Capex shampoo ℞ *corticosteroidal antiinflammatory; antiseborrheic* [fluocinolone acetonide] 0.01%

capimorelin tartrate [see: capromorelin tartrate]

Capital with Codeine oral suspension ℞ *narcotic antitussive; analgesic* [codeine phosphate; acetaminophen] 12•120 mg/5 mL

Capitrol shampoo ℞ *antiseborrheic; antibacterial; antifungal* [chloroxine] 2% ☒ captopril

caplet (dosage form) *capsule-shaped tablet*

capmul 8210 [see: monoctanoin]

capobenate sodium USAN *antiarrhythmic*

capobenic acid USAN, INN *antiarrhythmic*

Capoten tablets ℞ *antihypertensive; angiotensin-converting enzyme (ACE) inhibitor; treatment for CHF and diabetic nephropathy* [captopril] 12.5, 25, 50, 100 mg

Capozide 25/15; Capozide 25/25; Capozide 50/15; Capozide 50/25 tablets ℞ *antihypertensive; angiotensin-converting enzyme (ACE) inhibitor; diuretic* [captopril; hydrochlorothiazide] 25•15 mg; 25•25 mg; 50•15 mg; 50•25 mg

Capparis spinosa *medicinal herb* [see: capers]

CAPPr (cyclophosphamide, Adriamycin, Platinol, prednisone) *chemotherapy protocol*

capreomycin INN, BAN *bactericidal antibiotic; tuberculostatic* [also: capreomycin sulfate]

capreomycin sulfate USAN, USP, JAN *bactericidal antibiotic; tuberculostatic* [also: capreomycin]

Caprogel ℞ *investigational (orphan) topical treatment for traumatic hyphema of the eye* [aminocaproic acid]

capromab INN *monoclonal antibody for diagnosis of prostate cancer* [also: capromab pendetide]

capromab pendetide USAN *monoclonal antibody for diagnosis of prostate cancer* [also: capromab]

capromorelin tartrate USAN *growth hormone secretagogue for anti-aging, congestive heart failure, and catabolic illness*

caproxamine INN, BAN

capsaicin *topical analgesic; counterirritant; investigational (orphan) for erythromelalgia and painful HIV-related neuropathy* 0.025%, 0.075% topical

Capsella bursa-pastoris *medicinal herb*
[see: shepherd's purse]

Capsicum frutescens; C. annuum
medicinal herb [see: cayenne]

capsicum oleoresin *topical analgesic;
counterirritant*

Capsin lotion OTC *topical analgesic*
[capsaicin] 0.025%, 0.075%

Capsulets (trademarked form) *sustained-release caplet*

captab (dosage form) *capsule-shaped
tablet*

captamine INN *depigmentor* [also: captamine HCl]

captamine HCl USAN *depigmentor*
[also: captamine]

captodiame INN, BAN

captodiame HCl [see: captodiame]

captodiamine HCl [see: captodiame]

captopril USAN, USP, INN, BAN, JAN
*antihypertensive; angiotensin-converting enzyme (ACE) inhibitor; treatment
for CHF and diabetic nephropathy*
12.5, 25, 50, 100 mg oral ⊡ Capitrol

captopril & hydrochlorothiazide
*antihypertensive; angiotensin-converting
enzyme (ACE) inhibitor; diuretic* 25•
15, 25•25, 50•15, 50•25 mg oral

capuride USAN, INN *hypnotic*

Capzasin-P cream OTC *topical analgesic*
[capsaicin] 0.025%

Carac cream ℞ *antineoplastic for actinic
keratoses and basal cell carcinomas*
[fluorouracil] 0.5%

caracemide USAN, INN *antineoplastic*

Carafate tablets, oral suspension ℞
treatment for duodenal ulcer [sucralfate] 1 g; 1 g/10 mL

caramel NF *coloring agent*

caramiphen INN, BAN *antitussive*

caramiphen edisylate *antitussive*

caramiphen HCl [see: caramiphen]

caraway (Carum carvi) NF *seeds
medicinal herb for acid indigestion,
appetite stimulation, colic, gas, gastrointestinal spasms, and uterine cramps*

caraway oil NF

carazolol INN, BAN

carbacephems *a class of bactericidal
antibiotics similar to second-generation
cephalosporins (q.v.)*

carbachol USP, INN, BAN, JAN *ophthalmic cholinergic; miotic for surgery;
antiglaucoma agent* [also: carbacholine chloride]

carbacholine chloride DCF *ophthalmic
cholinergic; miotic for surgery; antiglaucoma agent* [also: carbachol]

carbacrylamine resins

carbadipimidine HCl [see: carpipramine dihydrochloride]

carbadox USAN, INN, BAN *antibacterial*

carbaldrate INN

carbamate choline chloride [see:
carbachol]

carbamazepine USAN, USP, INN, BAN,
JAN *dibenzazepine anticonvulsant;
analgesic for trigeminal neuralgia; antipsychotic for manic episodes of a bipolar disorder* 100, 200 mg oral; 100
mg/5 mL oral

carbamide [see: urea]

carbamide peroxide USP *topical dental
anti-infective; cerumenolytic to emulsify and disperse ear wax*

N-carbamoylarsanilic acid [see: carbarsone]

carbamoylcholine chloride [see: carbachol]

O-carbamoylsalicylic acid lactam
[see: carsalam]

carbamylcholine chloride [see: carbachol]

carbamylglutamic acid *investigational
(orphan) treatment for N-acetylglutamate synthetase deficiency*

carbamylmethylcholine chloride
[see: bethanechol chloride]

carbantel INN *anthelmintic* [also: carbantel lauryl sulfate]

carbantel lauryl sulfate USAN *anthelmintic* [also: carbantel]

carbaril INN [also: carbaryl]

carbarsone USP, INN

carbaryl BAN [also: carbaril]

carbasalate calcium INN *analgesic*
[also: carbaspirin calcium]

carbaspirin calcium USAN *analgesic* [also: carbasalate calcium]

Carbastat solution Ɽ *direct-acting miotic for ophthalmic surgery* [carbachol] 0.01%

Carbatrol extended-release capsules Ɽ *anticonvulsant; analgesic for trigeminal neuralgia; antipsychotic* [carbamazepine] 100, 200, 300 mg

carbazeran USAN, INN *cardiotonic*

carbazochrome INN, JAN

carbazochrome salicylate INN

carbazochrome sodium sulfonate INN

carbazocine INN

carbenicillin INN, BAN *extended-spectrum penicillin antibiotic* [also: carbenicillin disodium; carbenicillin sodium]

carbenicillin disodium USAN, USP *extended-spectrum penicillin antibiotic* [also: carbenicillin; carbenicillin sodium]

carbenicillin indanyl sodium USAN, USP *extended-spectrum penicillin antibiotic* (base=76.4%) [also: carindacillin]

carbenicillin phenyl sodium USAN *antibacterial* [also: carfecillin]

carbenicillin potassium USAN *antibacterial*

carbenicillin sodium JAN *antibacterial* [also: carbenicillin disodium; carbenicillin]

carbenoxolone INN, BAN *corticosteroid; anti-inflammatory* [also: carbenoxolone sodium]

carbenoxolone sodium USAN *corticosteroid; anti-inflammatory* [also: carbenoxolone]

carbenzide INN

carbesilate INN *combining name for radicals or groups*

carbetapentane citrate NF *antitussive* [also: pentoxyverine]

carbetapentane tannate *antitussive*

carbetimer USAN, INN *antineoplastic*

carbetocin INN, BAN *uterotonic agent to prevent postpartum hemorrhage following cesarean section*

Carbex tablets Ɽ *dopaminergic antiparkinsonian (orphan)* [selegiline HCl] 5 mg

carbidopa USAN, USP, INN, BAN, JAN *decarboxylase inhibitor; antiparkinsonian adjunct*

carbidopa & levodopa *antiparkinsonian; dopamine precursor plus synergist* 10•100, 25•100, 25•250, 50•200 mg oral

carbifene INN *analgesic* [also: carbiphene HCl; carbiphene]

carbimazole INN, BAN

carbinoxamine INN, BAN *antihistamine for allergic rhinitis* [also: carbinoxamine maleate]

Carbinoxamine pediatric syrup, pediatric oral drops Ɽ *decongestant; antihistamine* [pseudoephedrine HCl; carbinoxamine maleate] 60•4 mg/5 mL; 25•2 mg/mL

Carbinoxamine Compound syrup, pediatric oral drops (discontinued 2004) Ɽ *antitussive; decongestant; antihistamine* [dextromethorphan hydrobromide; pseudoephedrine HCl; carbinoxamine maleate] 15•60•4 mg/5 mL; 4•25•2 mg/mL

carbinoxamine maleate USP *antihistamine for allergic rhinitis* [also: carbinoxamine]

carbinoxamine maleate & hydrocodone bitartrate & pseudoephedrine HCl *antihistamine; antitussive; decongestant* 2•5•30 mg/5 mL oral

carbinoxamine maleate & pseudoephedrine HCl *antihistamine; decongestant* 4•60 mg/5 mL oral; 2•25 mg/mL oral

carbinoxamine tannate *antihistamine for allergic rhinitis*

carbiphene BAN *analgesic* [also: carbiphene HCl; carbifene]

carbiphene HCl USAN *analgesic* [also: carbifene; carbiphene]

Carbiset tablets (discontinued 2002) Ɽ *decongestant; antihistamine* [pseudoephedrine HCl; carbinoxamine maleate] 60•4 mg

Carbiset-TR timed-release tablets (discontinued 2002) ℞ *decongestant; antihistamine* [pseudoephedrine HCl; carbinoxamine maleate] 120•8 mg

Carbocaine injection ℞ *injectable local anesthetic* [mepivacaine HCl] 1%, 1.5%, 2%, 3%

Carbocaine with Neo-Cobefrin injection ℞ *injectable local anesthetic; vasoconstrictor* [mepivacaine HCl; levonordefrin] 2%•1:20 000

carbocisteine INN, BAN *mucolytic* [also: carbocysteine]

carbocloral USAN, INN, BAN *hypnotic*

carbocromen INN *coronary vasodilator* [also: chromonar HCl]

carbocysteine USAN *mucolytic* [also: carbocisteine]

Carbodec tablets, syrup (discontinued 2002) ℞ *decongestant; antihistamine* [pseudoephedrine HCl; carbinoxamine maleate] 60•4 mg; 60•4 mg/5 mL

Carbodec DM syrup, pediatric drops (discontinued 2002) ℞ *antitussive; decongestant; antihistamine* [dextromethorphan hydrobromide; pseudoephedrine HCl; carbinoxamine maleate] 15•60•4 mg/5 mL; 4•25•2 mg/mL

Carbodec TR timed-release tablets (discontinued 2002) ℞ *decongestant; antihistamine* [pseudoephedrine HCl; carbinoxamine maleate] 120•8 mg

Carbodex DM pediatric oral drops ℞ *antitussive; decongestant; antihistamine* [dextromethorphan hydrobromide; pseudoephedrine HCl; carbinoxamine maleate] 4•15•2 mg/mL

Carbodex DM syrup ℞ *antitussive; decongestant; antihistamine* [dextromethorphan hydrobromide; pseudoephedrine HCl; brompheniramine maleate] 15•45•4 mg/5 mL

carbodimid calcium [see: calcium carbimide]

Carbofed DM pediatric oral drops ℞ *antitussive; decongestant; antihistamine* [dextromethorphan hydrobromide; pseudoephedrine HCl; carbinoxamine maleate] 4•15•1 mg/mL

Carbofed DM syrup ℞ *antitussive; decongestant; antihistamine* [dextromethorphan hydrobromide; pseudoephedrine HCl; brompheniramine maleate] 15•45•4 mg/5 mL

carbofenotion INN [also: carbophenothion]

carbol-fuchsin solution (or paint) USP *antifungal*

carbolic acid [see: phenol]

carbolin [see: carbachol]

Carbolith ⒸⒶⓃ capsules ℞ *antipsychotic for manic episodes* [lithium carbonate] 150, 300, 600 mg

carbolonium bromide BAN [also: hexcarbacholine bromide]

carbomer INN, BAN *emulsifying and suspending agent* [also: carbomer 910]

carbomer 1342 NF *emulsifying and suspending agent*

carbomer 910 USAN, NF *emulsifying and suspending agent* [also: carbomer]

carbomer 934 USAN, NF *emulsifying and suspending agent*

carbomer 934P USAN, NF *emulsifying and suspending agent*

carbomer 940 USAN, NF *emulsifying and suspending agent*

carbomer 941 USAN, NF *emulsifying and suspending agent*

carbomycin INN

carbon *element* (C)

carbon, activated

carbon C 13 urea *diagnostic aid for detection of H. pylori in the stomach*

carbon C 14 urea *diagnostic aid for H. pylori in the stomach* [also: ^{14}C urea]

carbon dioxide (CO_2) USP *respiratory stimulant*

carbon tetrachloride NF *solvent*

carbonic acid, calcium salt [see: calcium carbonate]

carbonic acid, dilithium salt [see: lithium carbonate]

carbonic acid, dipotassium salt [see: potassium carbonate]

carbonic acid, disodium salt [see: sodium carbonate]

carbonic acid, magnesium salt [see: magnesium carbonate]

carbonic acid, monoammonium salt [see: ammonium carbonate]

carbonic acid, monopotassium salt [see: potassium bicarbonate]

carbonic acid, monosodium salt [see: sodium bicarbonate]

carbonic anhydrase inhibitors *a class of diuretic agents that reduce the rate of aqueous humor formation, resulting in decreased intraocular pressure; available in both systemic (tablets) and topical (eye drops) forms*

carbonis detergens, liquor (LCD) [see: coal tar]

carbonyl iron *hematinic; iron supplement (100% elemental iron as microparticles)*

carbophenothion BAN [also: carbofenotion]

carboplatin USAN, INN, BAN *alkylating antineoplastic for ovarian and other cancers* 10 mg/mL, 50, 150, 450 mg/ dose injection

carboplatin & etoposide & paclitaxel *chemotherapy protocol for primary adenocarcinoma and small cell lung cancer (SCLC)*

carboplatin & gemcitabine *chemotherapy protocol for non–small cell lung cancer (NSCLC)*

carboprost USAN, INN, BAN *oxytocic*

carboprost methyl USAN *oxytocic*

carboprost trometanol BAN *oxytocic; prostaglandin-type abortifacient* [also: carboprost tromethamine]

carboprost tromethamine USAN, USP *oxytocic; prostaglandin-type abortifacient* [also: carboprost trometanol]

Carboptic Drop-Tainers (eye drops) ℞ *topical antiglaucoma agent; direct-acting miotic* [carbachol] 3%

carboquone INN

carbose D [see: carboxymethylcellulose sodium]

Carbo-Tax (carboplatin, Taxol) *chemotherapy protocol for ovarian cancer* [also: CaT]

carbovir *investigational (orphan) agent for AIDS and symptomatic HIV infections*

carboxyimamidate [see: carbetimer]

carboxymethylcellulose calcium NF *tablet disintegrant*

carboxymethylcellulose sodium USP *bulk laxative; suspending and viscosity-increasing agent; ophthalmic moisturizer; tablet excipient* [also: carmellose; carmellose sodium]

carboxymethylcellulose sodium 12 NF *suspending and viscosity-increasing agent*

carboxypeptidase G2 *investigational (orphan) agent for methotrexate toxicity*

carbromal NF, INN

carbubarb INN

carbubarbital [see: carbubarb]

carburazepam INN

carbutamide INN, BAN

carbuterol INN, BAN *bronchodilator* [also: carbuterol HCl]

carbuterol HCl USAN *bronchodilator* [also: carbuterol]

carcainium chloride INN

carcinoembryonic antigen (CEA)

cardamom seed NF

cardamom [see: bitter cardamom]

Cardec-DM pediatric syrup, pediatric drops (discontinued 2002) ℞ *antitussive; decongestant; antihistamine* [dextromethorphan hydrobromide; pseudoephedrine HCl; carbinoxamine maleate] 15•60•4 mg/5 mL; 4•25• 2 mg/mL

Cardec-DM syrup (discontinued 2004) ℞ *antitussive; decongestant; antihistamine* [dextromethorphan hydrobromide; pseudoephedrine HCl; carbinoxamine maleate] 15•60•4 mg/5 mL

Cardec-S oral liquid (discontinued 2004) ℞ *decongestant; antihistamine* [pseudoephedrine HCl; carbinoxamine maleate] 60•4 mg/5 mL

Cardene capsules ℞ *antianginal; antihypertensive; calcium channel blocker* [nicardipine HCl] 20, 30 mg ② Cardizem

Cardene I.V. injection ℞ *antihypertensive; calcium channel blocker* [nicardipine HCl] 2.5 mg/mL

Cardene SR sustained-release capsules R *antihypertensive; calcium channel blocker* [nicardipine HCl] 30, 45, 60 mg

cardiac glycosides *a class of cardiovascular drugs that increase the force of cardiac contractions* [also called: digitalis glycosides]

Cardiac T test *in vitro diagnostic aid for troponin T (indicator of cardiac damage) in whole blood*

cardiacs *a class of agents that stimulate or otherwise affect the heart (a term used in folk medicine)*

cardiamid [see: nikethamide]

cardin *medicinal herb* [see: blessed thistle]

Cardio-Green (CG) powder for IV injection (discontinued 2004) R *in vivo diagnostic aid for cardiac output, hepatic function, and ophthalmic angiography* [indocyanine green] 25, 50 mg

Cardiolite injection R *myocardial perfusion agent for cardiac SPECT imaging* [technetium Tc 99m sestamibi] 5 mL

Cardi-Omega 3 capsules OTC *dietary supplement* [omega-3 fatty acids; multiple vitamins & minerals] 1000• ≛ mg

cardioplegic solution (calcium chloride, magnesium chloride, potassium chloride, sodium chloride) [q.v.]

cardioprotective agents *a class of potent intracellular chelating agents which protect the heart from the effects of doxorubicin*

Cardioquin tablets (discontinued 2003) R *antiarrhythmic* [quinidine polygalacturonate] 275 mg

Cardiotek Rx coated tablets R *dietary supplement* [vitamins B_6 and B_{12}; folic acid; L-arginine HCl] 50•0.5•2• ≛ mg

Cardizem IV injection, Lyo-Ject (prefilled syringe) R *calcium channel blocker for atrial fibrillation or paroxysmal supraventricular tachycardia (PSVT)* [diltiazem HCl] 5 mg/mL; 25 mg ⊉ Cardene

Cardizem Monovial (single-use vial) (discontinued 2003) R *calcium channel blocker for atrial fibrillation or paroxysmal supraventricular tachycardia (PSVT)* [diltiazem HCl] 100 mg ⊉ Cardene

Cardizem tablets R *antianginal; antihypertensive; antiarrhythmic; calcium channel blocker* [diltiazem HCl] 30, 60, 90, 120 mg

Cardizem CD sustained-release capsules R *antihypertensive; antianginal; antiarrhythmic; calcium channel blocker* [diltiazem HCl] 120, 180, 240, 300, 360 mg

Cardizem LA extended-release caplets R *antihypertensive; antianginal; calcium channel blocker* [diltiazem HCl] 120, 180, 240, 300, 360, 420 mg

Cardizem SR sustained-release capsules (discontinued 2004) R *antihypertensive; antianginal; antiarrhythmic; calcium channel blocker* [diltiazem HCl] 60, 90, 120 mg

Cardizem XL R *investigational (NDA filed) h.s. dosing of Cardizem* [diltiazem HCl]

cardophyllin [see: aminophylline]

Cardura tablets R α_1-*adrenergic blocker for hypertension and benign prostatic hyperplasia (BPH)* [doxazosin mesylate] 1, 2, 4, 8 mg

Cardura XL R *investigational (NDA filed) sustained-release formulation* [doxazosin mesylate]

carebastine INN

carena [see: aminophylline]

carfecillin INN, BAN *antibacterial* [also: carbenicillin phenyl sodium]

carfenazine INN *antipsychotic* [also: carphenazine maleate; carphenazine]

carfentanil INN *narcotic analgesic* [also: carfentanil citrate]

carfentanil citrate USAN *narcotic analgesic* [also: carfentanil]

carfimate INN

cargentos [see: silver protein]

cargutocin INN

Carica papaya *medicinal herb* [see: papaya]

Carimune NF powder for IV infusion ℞ *passive immunizing agent for HIV and idiopathic thrombocytopenic purpura (ITP)* [immune globulin] 1, 3, 6, 12 g

carindacillin INN, BAN *extended-spectrum penicillin antibiotic* [also: carbenicillin indanyl sodium]

Cariporide ℞ *investigational (Phase III) for coronary artery bypass grafting*

Carisolv ⓒᴬᴺ gel ℞ *topical dissolution of dental caries* [sodium hypochlorite] 0.5%

carisoprodol USP, INN, BAN *skeletal muscle relaxant* 350 mg oral

carisoprodol & aspirin & codeine phosphate *skeletal muscle relaxant; narcotic analgesic* 200•325•16 mg oral

carline thistle (Carlina acaulis) root *medicinal herb used as a carminative, diaphoretic, digestive, diuretic, febrifuge, and, in large doses, an emetic and purgative*

carmantadine USAN, INN *antiparkinsonian*

carmellose INN *suspending agent; tablet excipient* [also: carboxymethylcellulose sodium; carmellose sodium]

carmellose sodium BAN *suspending agent; tablet excipient* [also: carboxymethylcellulose sodium; carmellose]

carmetizide INN

carminatives *a class of agents that relieve flatulence*

carminomycin HCl [now: carubicin HCl]

carmofur INN

Carmol 10 lotion OTC *moisturizer; emollient; keratolytic* [urea] 10%

Carmol 20 cream OTC *moisturizer; emollient; keratolytic* [urea] 20%

Carmol 40 cream, gel ℞ *moisturizer; emollient; keratolytic* [urea] 40%

Carmol HC cream ℞ *corticosteroidal anti-inflammatory; moisturizer; emollient* [hydrocortisone acetate; urea] 1%•10%

carmoxirole INN

carmustine USAN, INN, BAN *nitrosourea-type alkylating antineoplastic for brain tumors, multiple myeloma,* *Hodgkin disease, and non-Hodgkin lymphomas; polymer implant for recurrent malignant glioma (orphan)*

Carnation Follow-Up oral liquid, powder for oral liquid OTC *total or supplementary infant feeding*

Carnation Good Start [see: Good Start]

carnauba wax [see: wax, carnauba]

carnidazole USAN, INN, BAN *antiprotozoal*

carnitine INN *vitamin B$_t$*

L-carnitine [see: levocarnitine]

Carnitor tablets, oral solution, IV injection or infusion ℞ *dietary amino acid for primary and secondary genetic carnitine deficiency (orphan) and end-stage renal disease (orphan); investigational (orphan) for pediatric cardiomyopathy* [levocarnitine] 330 mg; 100 mg/mL; 500 mg/2.5 mL, 1 g/5 mL

carnosine *natural anti-carbonylation agent that prevents cross-linking of protein and collagen; antioxidant; dipeptide of β-alanine and L-histidine*

carocainide INN

Caroid enteric-coated tablets OTC *stimulant laxative* [bisacodyl] 5 mg

β-carotene [see: beta carotene]

caroverine INN

caroxazone USAN, INN *antidepressant*

carpenter's herb *medicinal herb* [see: woundwort]

carpenter's square *medicinal herb* [see: figwort]

carperidine INN, BAN

carperone INN

carphenazine BAN *antipsychotic* [also: carphenazine maleate; carfenazine]

carphenazine maleate USAN, USP *antipsychotic* [also: carfenazine; carphenazine]

carpindolol INN

carpipramine INN

carpipramine dihydrochloride [see: carpipramine]

carpolene [now: carbomer 934P]

carprazidil INN

carprofen USAN, INN, BAN *nonsteroidal anti-inflammatory drug (NSAID); analgesic; antipyretic*

carpronium chloride INN

Carpuject (trademarked delivery system) *prefilled syringe*

Carpuject Smartpak (trademarked delivery system) *prefilled cartridge-needle unit package*

CarraFoam; CarraWash topical liquid OTC *skin cleanser for incontinence care* [aloe vera; acemannan]

carrageenan NF *suspending and viscosity-increasing agent*

CarraKlenz topical liquid OTC *wound cleanser for intact skin* [aloe vera; acemannan]

CarraSmart gel OTC *hydrogel wound dressing* [acemannan]

Carrasyn; Carrasyn V gel OTC *hydrogel wound dressing* [acemannan]

carrot (*Daucus carota***)** oil from the dried seed and root *medicinal herb for edema, gas, and worms; also used as a nutritional and vitamin supplement and stimulant; may possibly protect the heart and liver*

carsalam INN, BAN

carsatrin INN *cardiotonic* [also: carsatrin succinate]

carsatrin succinate USAN *cardiotonic* [also: carsatrin]

cartazolate USAN, INN *antidepressant*

carteolol INN, BAN *topical antiglaucoma agent (β-blocker)* [also: carteolol HCl]

carteolol HCl USAN *topical antiglaucoma agent (β-blocker)* [also: carteolol] 1%

Carthamus tinctorius medicinal herb [see: safflower]

Cartia XT extended-release capsules ℞ *antihypertensive; antianginal; antiarrhythmic; calcium channel blocker* [diltiazem HCl] 120, 180, 240, 300 mg

carticaine BAN *amide local anesthetic for dentistry* [also: articaine]

Cartrix (delivery system) *prefilled syringes*

Cartrol Filmtabs (film-coated tablets) OTC *antihypertensive; β-blocker* [carteolol HCl] 2.5, 5 mg

carubicin INN *antineoplastic* [also: carubicin HCl]

carubicin HCl USAN *antineoplastic* [also: carubicin]

Carum carvi NF *medicinal herb* [see: caraway]

carumonam INN, BAN *antibacterial* [also: carumonam sodium]

carumonam sodium USAN *antibacterial* [also: carumonam]

carvedilol USAN, INN, BAN, JAN *antianginal; antihypertensive; α- and β-blocker for congestive heart failure*

carvotroline HCl USAN *antipsychotic*

Caryophyllus aromaticus medicinal herb [see: cloves]

carzelesin USAN *antineoplastic*

carzenide INN

casanthranol USAN, USP *stimulant laxative*

Cascara Aromatic oral liquid OTC *stimulant laxative* [cascara sagrada; alcohol 18%]

cascara fluidextract, aromatic USP *stimulant laxative; investigational (orphan) agent to speed the evacuation of an oral drug overdose* 2–6 mL oral

cascara sagrada USP *stimulant laxative* 325 mg oral

cascara sagrada (*Frangula purshiana; Rhamnus purshiana***)** bark *medicinal herb for constipation, cough, and gallbladder, intestinal, and liver disorders; chronic use can cause hypokalemia and melanosis coli* [also see: buckthorn]

cascarin [see: casanthranol]

Casec powder OTC *protein supplement* [calcium caseinate]

Casodex film-coated tablets ℞ *antiandrogen antineoplastic for prostatic cancer* [bicalutamide] 50 mg

caspofungin acetate USAN *systemic echinocandin antifungal for candidiasis, candidemia, invasive aspergillosis and other resistant fungal infections*

Cassia acutifolia; C. angustifolia; C. senna medicinal herb [see: senna]

CAST (Color Allergy Screening Test) reagent sticks for professional use *in vitro diagnostic aid for immunoglobulin E in serum*

Castaderm topical liquid OTC *antifungal; astringent; antiseptic* [resorcinol; boric acid; acetone; basic fuchsin; phenol; alcohol 9%]

Castel Minus; Castel Plus topical liquid OTC *antifungal* [resorcinol; acetone; basic fuchsin; alcohol 11.5%]

Castellani Paint Modified solution R *topical antifungal; antibacterial; keratolytic* [basic fuchsin; phenol; resorcinol]

Castellani's paint [see: carbol-fuchsin solution]

Castile soap

castor oil USP *stimulant laxative*

CaT (carboplatin, Taxol) *chemotherapy protocol for adenocarcinoma, non–small cell lung cancer (NSCLC), and ovarian cancer* [also: Carbo-Tax]

CAT (cytarabine, Adriamycin, thioguanine) *chemotherapy protocol*

Cataflam tablets R *analgesic; antiarthritic; nonsteroidal anti-inflammatory drug (NSAID) for ankylosing spondylitis* [diclofenac potassium] 50 mg

Catapres tablets R *antihypertensive* [clonidine HCl] 0.1, 0.2, 0.3 mg ⑨ Catarase; Combipres; Ser-Ap-Es

Catapres-TTS-1; Catapres-TTS-2; Catapres-TTS-3 7-day transdermal patch R *antihypertensive* [clonidine HCl] 0.1 mg/day (2.5 mg); 0.2 mg/day (5 mg); 0.3 mg/day (7.5 mg)

Catatrol R *investigational (NDA filed) bicyclic antidepressant; investigational (orphan) for cataplexy and narcolepsy* [viloxazine]

catchfly *medicinal herb* [see: dogbane]

catchweed *medicinal herb* [see: bedstraw]

catechol-O-methyltransferase (COMT) [see: COMT inhibitors]

catgut suture [see: absorbable surgical suture]

Catha edulis the plant from which cathinone, a naturally occurring stimulant, is derived [see also: cathinone; methcathinone]

Catharanthus roseus medicinal herb [see: periwinkle]

cathartics *a class of agents that cause vigorous evacuation of the bowels by increasing bulk, stimulating peristaltic action, etc.* [also called: purgatives]

Cathflo Activase powder for intra-catheter instillation R *tissue plasminogen activator (tPA) thrombolytic to keep open (TKO) central venous access devices (CVADs) (not therapeutic)* [alteplase] 2.2 mg/vial

cathine INN

cathinone INN *an extract of the* Catha edulis *plant, a naturally occurring stimulant* [see also: Catha edulis; methcathinone]

cathomycin sodium [see: novobiocin sodium]

catkins willow *medicinal herb* [see: willow]

catmint *medicinal herb* [see: catnip]

catnip (Nepeta cataria) plant *medicinal herb for colds, colic, convulsions, diarrhea, digestion, fever, flu, gas, hives, nervous conditions, and stimulating delayed menses*

Catrix Correction cream OTC *moisturizer; emollient*

catrup *medicinal herb* [see: catnip]

cat's claw (Uncaria guianensis; U. tomentosa) inner bark *medicinal herb for cancer, Candida infections, chronic fatigue, contraception, Crohn disease, diverticulitis, hypertension, irritable bowel, lupus, parasites, PMS, ulcers, and viral infections; also used as immune booster*

catswort *medicinal herb* [see: catnip]

Caucasian walnut *medicinal herb* [see: English walnut]

Caulophyllum thalictroides medicinal herb [see: blue cohosh]

caustics *a class of escharotic or corrosive agents that destroy living tissue* [also called: cauterants]

cauterants *a class of escharotic or corrosive agents that destroy living tissue* [also called: caustics]

CAV (cyclophosphamide, Adriamycin, vinblastine) *chemotherapy protocol*

CAV (cyclophosphamide, Adriamycin, vincristine) *chemotherapy protocol for small cell lung cancer (SCLC)* [also: VAC]

CAVe; CA·Ve (CCNU, Adriamycin, vinblastine) *chemotherapy protocol*

CAVE (cyclophosphamide, Adriamycin, vincristine, etoposide) *chemotherapy protocol for small cell lung cancer (SCLC)*

CAV/EP (cyclophosphamide, Adriamycin, vincristine, etoposide, Platinol) *chemotherapy protocol for small cell lung cancer (SCLC)*

Caverject intracavernosal injection, Luer-lock single-use autoinjector ℞ *vasodilator for erectile dysfunction* [alprostadil] 5, 10, 20, 40 μg/mL

Caverject Impulse powder for intracavernosal injection in prefilled syringe ℞ *vasodilator for erectile dysfunction* [alprostadil] 10, 20 μg/0.5 mL dose

CA·VP16; CAVP16 (cyclophosphamide, Adriamycin, VP·16) *chemotherapy protocol for small cell lung cancer (SCLC)*

cayenne (Capsicum annuum; C. frutescens) fruit *medicinal herb for arthritis, bleeding, cold feet, diabetes, high blood pressure, kidney disorders, rheumatism, poor circulation, strokes, topical neuritis syndromes, tumors, and ulcers*

CBV (cyclophosphamide, BCNU, VePesid) *chemotherapy protocol*

CBV (cyclophosphamide, BCNU, VP·16·213) *chemotherapy protocol*

CC (carboplatin, cyclophosphamide) *chemotherapy protocol for ovarian cancer*

CC·Galactosidase ℞ *investigational (orphan) enzyme replacement therapy for Fabry disease* [agalsidase alfa]

CCM (cyclophosphamide, CCNU, methotrexate) *chemotherapy protocol*

CCNU (chloroethyl-cyclohexylnitrosourea) [see: lomustine]

CCV·AV (CCNU, cyclophosphamide, vincristine [alternates with] Adriamycin, vincristine) *chemotherapy protocol*

CCVPP (CCNU, cyclophosphamide, Velban, procarbazine, prednisone) *chemotherapy protocol*

CD (cytarabine, daunorubicin) *chemotherapy protocol*

CD4 human truncated 369 AA polypeptide *investigational (orphan) treatment for AIDS*

CD4 immunoglobulin G, recombinant human *investigational (Phase I) antiviral for maternal/fetal transfer of HIV; investigational (orphan) for AIDS*

CD4 recombinant soluble human (rCD4) *investigational (Phase II, orphan) antiviral for AIDS*

CD5·T lymphocyte immunotoxin *investigational (orphan) agent for graft vs. host disease following bone marrow transplants*

CD20 *investigational for low-grade non-Hodgkin lymphoma*

CD·33 [see: ricin (blocked) conjugated murine MCA myeloid cells]

CdA (2·chloro·2′·deoxyadenosine) [see: cladribine]

CDB (cisplatin, dacarbazine, BCNU) *chemotherapy protocol for malignant melanoma*

CDC (carboplatin, doxorubicin, cyclophosphamide) *chemotherapy protocol*

CDDP; C·DDP (cis·diamminedichloroplatinum) [see: cisplatin]

CDDP/VP; CDDP/VP·16 (CDDP, VP·16) *chemotherapy protocol for pediatric brain tumors*

CDE (cyclophosphamide, doxorubicin, etoposide [filgrastim]) *chemotherapy protocol for HIV-related non-Hodgkin lymphoma*

CDP·571 *investigational (Phase III, orphan) anti-TNFα (tumor necrosis factor alpha) antibody CB-0010 for steroid-dependent Crohn disease; investigational for rheumatoid arthritis*

CDP·cholin [see: citicoline]

CEA (carcinoembryonic antigen)

CEA·Cide I·131 ℞ *investigational (orphan) antineoplastic for metastatic* *colorectal cancer* [iodine I 131–labeled labetuzumab]

CEA-Cide Y-90 ℞ *investigational (orphan) antineoplastic for colorectal, pancreatic, ovarian, and small cell lung cancer (SCLC)* [yttrium Y 90–labeled labetuzumab]

Ceanothus americanus medicinal herb [see: New Jersey tea]

CEA-Scan powder for injection ℞ *investigational (orphan) imaging agent for detection of recurrent or metastatic thyroid cancers; investigational (Phase III) for lung cancer* [arcitumomab] 1.25 mg

CEA-Vac ℞ *investigational (Phase III) vaccine for breast cancer*

CEB (carboplatin, etoposide, bleomycin) *chemotherapy protocol*

CECA (cisplatin, etoposide, cyclophosphamide, Adriamycin) *chemotherapy protocol*

Ceclor Pulvules (capsules), powder for oral suspension ℞ *cephalosporin antibiotic* [cefaclor] 250, 500 mg; 125, 187, 250, 375 mg/5 mL

Ceclor CD extended-release tablets (discontinued 2003) ℞ *cephalosporin antibiotic* [cefaclor] 375, 500 mg

Ceclor CDpak extended-release tablets (in compliance packs of 14) ℞ *cephalosporin antibiotic* [cefaclor] 500 mg

Cecon drops OTC *vitamin C supplement* [ascorbic acid] 100 mg/mL

Cedax capsules, powder for oral suspension ℞ *cephalosporin antibiotic* [ceftibuten] 400 mg; 90 mg/5 mL ⧉ Cidex

cedefingol USAN *antipsoriatic; antineoplastic adjunct*

cedelizumab USAN *monoclonal antibody; prophylaxis of rejection of solid organ allograft; immunomodulator for autoimmune diseases*

CEE (conjugated equine estrogen) [see: estrogens, conjugated]

CeeNu capsules, dose pack ℞ *nitrosourea-type alkylating antineoplastic for brain tumors and Hodgkin disease* [lomustine] 10, 40, 100 mg; 2 × 100 mg + 2 × 40 mg + 2 × 10 mg

CEF (cyclophosphamide, epirubicin, fluorouracil, [co-trimoxazole]) *chemotherapy protocol for breast cancer*

cefacetrile INN *antibacterial* [also: cephacetrile sodium]

cefacetrile sodium [see: cephacetrile sodium]

cefaclor USAN, USP, INN, BAN, JAN *second-generation cephalosporin antibiotic* 250, 500 mg oral; 125, 187, 250, 375 mg/5 mL oral

cefadroxil USAN, USP, INN, BAN *first-generation cephalosporin antibiotic* 500, 1000 mg oral

Cefadyl powder for IV or IM injection (discontinued 2004) ℞ *cephalosporin antibiotic* [cephapirin sodium] 1 g ⧉ Cefzil

cefalexin INN, JAN *first-generation cephalosporin antibiotic* [also: cephalexin]

cefaloglycin INN *antibacterial* [also: cephaloglycin]

cefalonium INN [also: cephalonium]

cefaloram INN [also: cephaloram]

cefaloridine INN *antibacterial* [also: cephaloridine]

cefalotin INN *first-generation cephalosporin antibiotic* [also: cephalothin sodium; cephalothin]

cefalotin sodium [see: cephalothin sodium]

cefamandole USAN, INN *second-generation cephalosporin antibiotic* [also: cephamandole]

cefamandole nafate USAN, USP *second-generation cephalosporin antibiotic* [also: cephamandole nafate]

cefamandole sodium USP *second-generation cephalosporin antibiotic*

cefaparole USAN, INN *antibacterial*

cefapirin INN, BAN *first-generation cephalosporin antibiotic* [also: cephapirin sodium]

cefapirin sodium [see: cephapirin sodium]

cefatrizine USAN, INN, BAN *antibacterial*

cefazaflur INN *antibacterial* [also: cefazaflur sodium]

cefazaflur sodium USAN *antibacterial* [also: cefazaflur]

cefazedone INN, BAN

cefazolin USP, INN *first-generation cephalosporin antibiotic* [also: cephazolin] 🔄 cephalothin; Zefazone

cefazolin sodium USAN, USP *first-generation cephalosporin antibiotic* [also: cephazolin sodium] 0.5, 1, 5, 10, 20 g injection 🔄 cephalothin; Zefazone

cefbuperazone USAN, INN *antibacterial*

cefcanel INN

cefcanel daloxate INN

cefdinir USAN, INN *third-generation cephalosporin antibiotic*

cefditoren pivoxil *broad-spectrum cephalosporin antibiotic*

cefedrolor INN

cefempidone INN, BAN

cefepime USAN, INN *third-generation cephalosporin antibiotic*

cefepime HCl USAN *third-generation cephalosporin antibiotic*

cefetamet USAN, INN *veterinary antibacterial*

cefetecol USAN, INN, BAN *antibacterial*

cefetrizole INN

cefivitril INN

cefixime USAN, USP, INN, BAN *third-generation cephalosporin antibiotic*

Cefizox powder or frozen premix for IV or IM injection ℞ *cephalosporin antibiotic* [ceftizoxime sodium] 0.5, 1, 2, 10 g

cefmenoxime INN *antibacterial* [also: cefmenoxime HCl]

cefmenoxime HCl USAN, USP *antibacterial* [also: cefmenoxime]

cefmepidium chloride INN

cefmetazole USAN, INN *second-generation cephalosporin antibiotic*

cefmetazole sodium USAN, USP, JAN *second-generation cephalosporin antibiotic*

cefminox INN

Cefobid powder or frozen premix for IV or IM injection ℞ *cephalosporin antibiotic* [cefoperazone sodium] 1, 2, 10 g

cefodizime INN *investigational cephalosporin antibiotic*

Cefol Filmtabs (film-coated tablets) ℞ *vitamin supplement* [multiple vitamins; folic acid] ± •0.5 mg

cefonicid INN, BAN *second-generation cephalosporin antibiotic* [also: cefonicid monosodium]

cefonicid monosodium USAN *second-generation cephalosporin antibiotic* [also: cefonicid]

cefonicid sodium USAN, USP *second-generation cephalosporin antibiotic*

cefoperazone INN, BAN *third-generation cephalosporin antibiotic* [also: cefoperazone sodium]

cefoperazone sodium USAN, USP *third-generation cephalosporin antibiotic* [also: cefoperazone]

ceforanide USAN, USP, INN, BAN *bactericidal antibiotic*

Cefotan powder or frozen premix for IV or IM injection ℞ *cephamycin antibiotic* [cefotetan disodium] 1, 2, 10 g

cefotaxime INN, BAN *third-generation cephalosporin antibiotic* [also: cefotaxime sodium] 🔄 cefoxitin

cefotaxime sodium USAN, USP *third-generation cephalosporin antibiotic* [also: cefotaxime] 0.5, 1, 2, 10, 20 g injection

cefotetan USAN, INN, BAN *cephamycin antibiotic*

cefotetan disodium USAN, USP *cephamycin antibiotic*

cefotiam INN, BAN *antibacterial* [also: cefotiam HCl]

cefotiam HCl USAN *antibacterial* [also: cefotiam]

cefoxazole INN [also: cephoxazole]

cefoxitin USAN, INN, BAN *cephamycin antibiotic* 🔄 cefotaxime

cefoxitin sodium USAN, USP, BAN *cephamycin antibiotic* 1, 2, 10 g/vial injection

cefpimizole USAN, INN *antibacterial*

cefpimizole sodium USAN, JAN *antibacterial*

cefpiramide USAN, USP, INN *antibacterial*

cefpiramide sodium USAN, JAN *antibacterial*

cefpirome INN, BAN *antibacterial* [also: cefpirome sulfate]

cefpirome sulfate USAN, JAN *antibacterial* [also: cefpirome]

cefpodoxime INN, BAN *broad-spectrum third-generation cephalosporin antibiotic* [also: cefpodoxime proxetil]

cefpodoxime proxetil USAN, JAN *broad-spectrum third-generation cephalosporin antibiotic* [also: cefpodoxime]

cefprozil USAN, INN *second-generation cephalosporin antibiotic*

cefprozil monohydrate

cefquinome INN, BAN *veterinary antibacterial*

cefquinome sulfate USAN *veterinary antibacterial*

cefradine INN *first-generation cephalosporin antibiotic* [also: cephradine]

cefrotil INN

cefroxadine USAN, INN *antibacterial*

cefsulodin INN, BAN *antibacterial* [also: cefsulodin sodium]

cefsulodin sodium USAN *antibacterial* [also: cefsulodin]

cefsumide INN

ceftazidime USAN, USP, INN, BAN, JAN *third-generation cephalosporin antibiotic*

cefteram INN

ceftezole INN

ceftibuten USAN, INN, BAN *third-generation cephalosporin antibiotic*

Ceftin film-coated tablets, oral suspension ℞ *cephalosporin antibiotic* [cefuroxime axetil] 125, 250, 500 mg; 125, 250 mg/5 mL

ceftiofur INN, BAN *veterinary antibacterial* [also: ceftiofur HCl]

ceftiofur HCl USAN *veterinary antibacterial* [also: ceftiofur]

ceftiofur sodium USAN *veterinary antibacterial*

ceftiolene INN

ceftioxide INN

ceftizoxime INN, BAN *third-generation cephalosporin antibiotic* [also: ceftizoxime sodium] ⊡ cefuroxime

ceftizoxime sodium USAN, USP *third-generation cephalosporin antibiotic* [also: ceftizoxime]

ceftriaxone INN, BAN *third-generation cephalosporin antibiotic* [also: ceftriaxone sodium]

ceftriaxone sodium USAN, USP *third-generation cephalosporin antibiotic* [also: ceftriaxone]

cefuracetime INN, BAN

cefuroxime USAN, INN, BAN *second-generation cephalosporin antibiotic* ⊡ ceftizoxime

cefuroxime axetil USAN, USP, BAN *second-generation cephalosporin antibiotic* 125, 250, 500 mg oral

cefuroxime pivoxetil USAN *second-generation cephalosporin antibiotic*

cefuroxime sodium USP, BAN *second-generation cephalosporin antibiotic* 0.75, 1.5, 7.5 g injection

cefuzonam INN

Cefzil film-coated tablets, powder for oral suspension ℞ *cephalosporin antibiotic* [cefprozil] 250, 500 mg; 125, 250 mg/5 mL ⊡ Cefadyl; Kefzol

Cefzon (foreign name for U.S. product Omnicef)

celandine (*Chelidonium majus*) root and plant *medicinal herb used as an analgesic, antispasmodic, caustic, diaphoretic, diuretic, narcotic, and purgative*

Celebrex capsules ℞ *antiarthritic; antipyretic; COX-2 inhibitor; nonsteroidal anti-inflammatory drug (NSAID); reduces polyp proliferation in familial adenomatous polyposis (FAP); investigational (Phase III) for bladder cancer* [celecoxib] 100, 200, 400 mg ⊡ Celexa; Cerebyx

celecoxib USAN *antiarthritic; antipyretic; COX-2 inhibitor; nonsteroidal anti-inflammatory drug (NSAID); reduces polyp proliferation in familial adenomatous polyposis (FAP)*

celery (*Apium graveolens*) root, stem, and seeds *medicinal herb for aiding digestion, arthritis, cancer, diuresis, gas, headache, hysteria, inducing menstruation, lumbago, nervousness, rheumatism, and terminating lactation*

Celestoderm-V; Celestoderm-V/2 ⓒᴬᴺ cream, ointment ℞ *corticosteroidal anti-inflammatory* [betamethasone valerate] 0.1%; 0.05%

Cellufresh eyedrops (handwritten)

Celestone syrup *corticosteroidal anti-inflammatory* [betamethasone] 0.6 mg/5 mL

Celestone tablets (discontinued 2005) *corticosteroidal anti-inflammatory* [betamethasone] 0.6 mg

Celestone Phosphate IV or IM injection ℞ *corticosteroidal anti-inflammatory* [betamethasone sodium phosphate] 4 mg/mL

Celestone Soluspan intrabursal, intra-articular, intralesional injection ℞ *corticosteroidal anti-inflammatory* [betamethasone sodium phosphate; betamethasone acetate] 3•3 mg/mL

Celexa film-coated tablets, oral solution ℞ *selective serotonin reuptake inhibitor (SSRI) for major depression* [citalopram hydrobromide] 10, 20, 40 mg; 10 mg/5 mL ▢ Celebrex

celgosivir HCl USAN *antiviral; α-glucosidase I inhibitor for HIV*

celiprolol INN, BAN *antihypertensive; antianginal; β-blocker* [also: celiprolol HCl]

celiprolol HCl USAN *investigational (NDA filed) antihypertensive; antianginal; β-blocker* [also: celiprolol]

cellacefate INN *tablet-coating agent* [also: cellulose acetate phthalate; cellacephate]

cellacephate BAN *tablet-coating agent* [also: cellulose acetate phthalate; cellacefate]

CellCept capsules, tablets, powder for oral suspension, powder for IV infusion ℞ *immunosuppressant for allogenic renal, hepatic, or cardiac transplants* [mycophenolate mofetil] 250 mg; 500 mg; 200 mg/mL; 500 mg/vial

cellulase USAN *digestive enzyme*

cellulolytic enzyme [see: cellulase]

cellulose *bulk laxative*

cellulose, absorbable [see: cellulose, oxidized]

cellulose, ethyl ester [see: ethylcellulose]

cellulose, hydroxypropyl methyl ether [see: hydroxypropyl methylcellulose]

cellulose, microcrystalline NF *tablet and capsule diluent* [also: dispersible cellulose]

cellulose, oxidized USP *topical local hemostatic*

cellulose, oxidized regenerated USP *local hemostatic*

cellulose, sodium carboxymethyl [see: carboxymethylcellulose sodium]

cellulose acetate NF *tablet-coating agent; insoluble polymer membrane*

cellulose acetate butyrate [see: cabufocon A; cabufocon B]

cellulose acetate dibutyrate [see: porofocon A; porofocon B]

cellulose acetate phthalate (CAP) NF *tablet-coating agent* [also: cellacefate; cellacephate]

cellulose carboxymethyl ether, sodium salt [see: carboxymethylcellulose sodium]

cellulose diacetate [see: cellulose acetate]

cellulose dihydrogen phosphate, disodium salt [see: cellulose sodium phosphate]

cellulose disodium phosphate [see: cellulose sodium phosphate]

cellulose ethyl ether [see: ethylcellulose]

cellulose gum, modified [now: croscarmellose sodium]

cellulose methyl ether [see: methylcellulose]

cellulose nitrate [see: pyroxylin]

cellulose sodium phosphate (CSP) USAN, USP *antiurolithic to prevent stone formation in absorptive hypercalciuria Type I*

cellulosic acid [see: cellulose, oxidized]

Celluvisc solution OTC *ophthalmic moisturizer/lubricant* [carboxymethylcellulose] 1%

celmoleukin INN *immunostimulant*

Celontin Kapseals (capsules) ℞ *succinimide anticonvulsant for absence (petit mal) seizures* [methsuximide] 150, 300 mg

celucloral INN, BAN

Cel·U·Jec IV, IM injection (discontinued 2002) R̥ *corticosteroid; antiinflammatory* [betamethasone sodium phosphate] 4 mg/mL

CEM (cytosine arabinoside, etoposide, methotrexate) *chemotherapy protocol*

Cenafed tablets, syrup OTC *nasal decongestant* [pseudoephedrine HCl] 60 mg; 30 mg/5 mL

Cenafed Plus tablets OTC *decongestant; antihistamine* [pseudoephedrine HCl; triprolidine HCl] 60•2.5 mg

Cena-K oral liquid R̥ *potassium supplement* [potassium chloride] 20, 40 mEq K/15 mL

Cenestin film-coated tablets R̥ *hormone replacement therapy for the treatment of postmenopausal symptoms* [synthetic conjugated estrogens, A] 0.3, 0.45, 0.625, 0.9, 1.25 mg

Cenogen Ultra capsules R̥ *vitamin/ mineral/iron supplement* [multiple vitamins & minerals; iron; folic acid] ≛•106•1 mg

Cenogen-OB capsules (discontinued 2004) R̥ *vitamin/mineral/iron supplement* [multiple vitamins & minerals; iron; folic acid] ≛•106•1 mg

Cenolate IV, IM, or subcu injection R̥ *vitamin C therapy; antiscorbutic* [sodium ascorbate] 562.5 mg/mL

Centany ointment R̥ *antibiotic for impetigo due to* S. aureus *or* S. pyogenes [mupirocin] 2%

Centaurea cyanus medicinal herb [see: cornflower]

centaury (Erythraea centaurium) plant *medicinal herb for aiding digestion, blood cleansing, fever, and promoting menstruation*

Centella asiatica medicinal herb [see: gotu kola]

Center-Al subcu or IM injection R̥ *allergenic sensitivity testing (subcu); allergenic desensitization therapy (IM)* [allergenic extracts, alum-precipitated]

centrazene [see: simtrazene]

centrophenoxine [see: meclofenoxate]

Centrum, Advanced Formula oral liquid OTC *vitamin/mineral/iron supplement* [multiple vitamins & minerals; ferrous fumarate; biotin; alcohol 6.7%] ≛•9•0.3 mg/15 mL

Centrum, Advanced Formula tablets OTC *vitamin/mineral/iron supplement* [multiple vitamins & minerals; ferrous fumarate; folic acid; biotin] ≛•18 mg•0.4 mg•30 µg

Centrum Jr. + Extra C; Centrum Jr. + Extra Calcium chewable tablets OTC *vitamin/mineral/calcium/iron supplement* [multiple vitamins & minerals; calcium; iron; folic acid; biotin] ≛•108•18•0.4•0.045 mg; ≛•160• 18•0.4•0.045 mg

Centrum Jr. with Iron tablets OTC *vitamin/mineral/iron supplement* [multiple vitamins & minerals; iron; folic acid; biotin] ≛•18 mg•0.4 mg•45 µg

Centrum Performance tablets OTC *vitamin/mineral/calcium/iron supplement* [multiple vitamins & minerals; calcium; iron; folic acid; biotin] ≛• 100•18 mg•0.4 mg•40 µg

Centrum Silver tablets OTC *geriatric vitamin/mineral supplement* [multiple vitamins & minerals; folic acid; biotin] ≛•400•30 µg

centruroides immune Fab 2 *investigational (orphan) antitoxin for scorpion stings*

Ceo-Two suppository OTC CO_2-*releasing laxative* [sodium bicarbonate; potassium bitartrate]

CEP (CCNU, etoposide, prednimustine) *chemotherapy protocol*

Cēpacol mouthwash/gargle OTC *oral antiseptic* [cetylpyridinium chloride] 0.05%

Cēpacol, Children's oral liquid (discontinued 2002) OTC *decongestant; analgesic* [pseudoephedrine HCl; acetaminophen] 15•160 mg/5 mL

Cēpacol Anesthetic troches OTC *topical oral anesthetic; antiseptic* [benzocaine; cetylpyridinium chloride] 10 mg•0.07%

Cēpacol Maximum Strength lozenges OTC *topical oral anesthetic* [benzocaine] 10 mg

Cēpacol Sore Throat oral liquid OTC *decongestant; analgesic* [pseudoephedrine HCl; acetaminophen] 60•640 mg/30 mL

Cēpacol Throat lozenges OTC *oral antiseptic* [cetylpyridinium chloride] 0.07%

Cēpacol Viractin cream, gel OTC *anesthetic for cold sores and fever blisters* [tetracaine HCl] 2%

Cēpastat Sore Throat lozenges OTC *topical antipruritic/counterirritant; mild local anesthetic* [phenol] 14.5, 29 mg ⊠ Capastat

cephacetrile sodium USAN, USP *antibacterial* [also: cefacetrile]

cephalexin USAN, USP, BAN *first-generation cephalosporin antibiotic* [also: cefalexin] 250, 500, 1000 mg oral; 125, 250 mg/5 mL oral ⊠ cefazolin; cephalothin

cephalexin HCl USAN, USP *first-generation cephalosporin antibiotic*

cephaloglycin USAN, USP, BAN *antibacterial* [also: cefaloglycin]

cephalonium BAN [also: cefalonium]

cephaloram BAN [also: cefaloram]

cephaloridine USAN, USP, BAN *antibacterial* [also: cefaloridine]

cephalosporin N [see: adicillin]

cephalosporins *a class of bactericidal antibiotics, divided into first-, second-, and third-generation; higher generations have increasing efficacy against gram-negative and decreasing efficacy against gram-positive bacteria*

cephalothin BAN *first-generation cephalosporin antibiotic* [also: cephalothin sodium; cefalotin] ⊠ cefazolin

cephalothin sodium USAN, USP *first-generation cephalosporin antibiotic* [also: cefalotin; cephalothin]

cephamandole BAN *second-generation cephalosporin antibiotic* [also: cefamandole]

cephamandole nafate BAN *second-generation cephalosporin antibiotic* [also: cefamandole nafate]

cephamycins *a class of bactericidal antibiotics similar to second-generation cephalosporins (q.v.)*

cephapirin sodium USAN, USP *first-generation cephalosporin antibiotic* [also: cefapirin] ⊠ cephradine

cephazolin BAN *first-generation cephalosporin antibiotic* [also: cefazolin]

cephazolin sodium BAN *first-generation cephalosporin antibiotic* [also: cefazolin sodium]

cephoxazole BAN [also: cefoxazole]

cephradine USAN, USP, BAN *first-generation cephalosporin antibiotic* [also: cefradine] 250, 500 mg oral; 125, 250 mg/5 mL oral ⊠ cephapirin

Cephulac oral/rectal solution ℞ *synthetic disaccharide used to prevent and treat portal-systemic encephalopathy* [lactulose] 10 g/15 mL

Ceplene ℞ *investigational (Phase III) histamine H₂ receptor agonist for malignant melanoma and acute myeloid leukemia (AML); investigational (Phase II) for hepatitis C and renal cell carcinoma* [histamine dihydrochloride]

Ceplene ℞ *investigational (Phase III) treatment for advanced metastatic melanoma* [histamine dihydrochloride]

CEPP (cyclophosphamide, etoposide, prednisone) *chemotherapy protocol for non-Hodgkin lymphoma*

CEPPB (cyclophosphamide, etoposide, prednisone, bleomycin) *chemotherapy protocol for non-Hodgkin lymphoma*

Ceptaz powder for IV or IM injection ℞ *cephalosporin antibiotic* [ceftazidime pentahydrate] 1, 2 g

CeraLyte powder for oral liquid, ready-to-use oral liquid OTC *supplementary feeding to maintain hydration and electrolyte balance in infants with diarrhea or vomiting* [rice-based formula]

ceramide trihexosidase (CTH) & agalsidase beta *investigational (orphan) enzyme replacement therapy for Fabry disease*

Cerebyx IV or IM injection ℞ *hydantoin anticonvulsant for grand mal sta-*

tus epilepticus (orphan) [fosphenytoin sodium (phenytoin sodium equivalent)] 75 (50) mg/mL ② Celebrex

Ceredase IV infusion ℞ glucocerebrosidase enzyme replacement in Gaucher disease type I (orphan); investigational (orphan) for types II and III [alglucerase] 10, 80 U/mL

Cerefolin tablets ℞ vitamin B supplement for hyperhomocystinemia [vitamins B_2, B_6, and B_{12}; L-methylfolate] 5•50•1•5.635 mg

cerelose [see: glucose]

Cereport ℞ investigational (Phase III) blood-brain barrier permeability-enhancing agent for carrying carboplatin to brain tumors [lobradimil]

Cerezyme powder for IV infusion ℞ enzyme replacement therapy for types I, II, and III Gaucher disease (orphan) [imiglucerase] 40 U/mL

cerium element (Ce)

cerium oxalate USP

cerivastatin sodium USAN HMG-CoA reductase inhibitor for hyperlipidemia and hypertriglyceridemia (discontinued 2001 due to safety concerns)

Cernevit-12 powder for IV injection ℞ parenteral vitamin therapy [multiple vitamins; folic acid; biotin] ±•414•60 µg

ceronapril USAN, INN antihypertensive

Cerose-DM oral liquid (discontinued 2002) OTC antitussive; decongestant; antihistamine [dextromethorphan hydrobromide; phenylephrine HCl; chlorpheniramine maleate; alcohol 2.4%] 15•10•4 mg/5 mL

Cerovite; Cerovite Advanced Formula tablets OTC vitamin/mineral/iron supplement [multiple vitamins & minerals; ferrous fumarate; folic acid; biotin] ±•18 mg•0.4 mg•30 µg

Cerovite Jr. tablets OTC vitamin/mineral/iron supplement [multiple vitamins & minerals; ferrous fumarate; folic acid; biotin] ±•18 mg•0.4 mg•45 µg

Cerovite Senior tablets OTC geriatric vitamin/mineral supplement [multiple vitamins & minerals; folic acid; biotin] ±•200•30 µg

Certagen film-coated tablets OTC vitamin/mineral/iron supplement [multiple vitamins & minerals; ferrous fumarate; folic acid; biotin] ±•18 mg•0.4 mg•30 µg

Certagen oral liquid OTC vitamin/mineral/iron supplement [multiple vitamins & minerals; iron; biotin; alcohol 6.6%] ±•9•0.3 mg

Certagen Senior tablets OTC geriatric vitamin/mineral supplement [multiple vitamins & minerals; folic acid; biotin] ±•200•30 µg

CertaVite tablets OTC vitamin/mineral/iron supplement [multiple vitamins & minerals; ferrous fumarate; folic acid; biotin] ±•18 mg•0.4 mg•30 µg

Certa-Vite Golden tablets OTC geriatric vitamin/mineral supplement [multiple vitamins & minerals; biotin] ±•30 µg

Certican (approved in Europe) ℞ investigational (NDA filed) agent for transplant rejection [everolimus]

Certiva IM injection (discontinued 2002) ℞ active immunizing agent for diphtheria, tetanus, and pertussis [diphtheria & tetanus toxoids & acellular pertussis (DTaP) vaccine] 15 Lf•6 Lf•40 µg per 0.5 mL

Cerubidine powder for IV injection ℞ antibiotic antineoplastic for multiple nonlymphocytic leukemias [daunorubicin HCl] 20 mg

ceruletide USAN, INN, BAN gastric secretory stimulant

ceruletide diethylamine USAN gastric secretory stimulant

Cerumenex ear drops ℞ cerumenolytic to emulsify and disperse ear wax [trolamine polypeptide oleate-condensate] 10%

Cervarix ℞ investigational human papilloma virus (HPV) vaccine to prevent cervical cancer

Cervidil vaginal insert ℞ prostaglandin for cervical ripening at term [dinoprostone] 10 mg

C.E.S. (CAN) sugar-coated tablets ℞ *estrogen replacement therapy for postmenopausal symptoms* [conjugated estrogens (from plants)] 0.4, 0.625, 0.9, 1.25 mg

Cesia tablets (in packs of 28) ℞ *triphasic oral contraceptive* [desogestrel; ethinyl estradiol]
Phase 1 (7 days): 100•25 μg;
Phase 2 (7 days): 125•25 μg;
Phase 3 (7 days): 150•25 μg

cesium *element* (Cs)

cesium (¹³¹Cs) **chloride** INN *radioactive agent* [also: cesium chloride Cs 131]

cesium chloride Cs 131 USAN *radioactive agent* [also: cesium (¹³¹Cs) chloride]

Ceta topical liquid OTC *soap-free therapeutic skin cleanser*

Ceta Plus capsules ℞ *narcotic analgesic* [hydrocodone bitartrate; acetaminophen] 5•500 mg

cetaben INN *antihyperlipoproteinemic* [also: cetaben sodium]

cetaben sodium USAN *antihyperlipoproteinemic* [also: cetaben]

Cetacaine topical liquid, gel, ointment, aerosol ℞ *local anesthetic; antiseptic* [benzocaine; tetracaine HCl; butamben] 14%•2%•2%

Cetacort lotion ℞ *topical corticosteroidal anti-inflammatory* [hydrocortisone] 0.25%, 0.5%

cetalkonium *antiseptic*

cetalkonium chloride USAN, INN, BAN *topical anti-infective*

Cetamide ophthalmic ointment ℞ *antibiotic* [sulfacetamide sodium] 10%

cetamolol INN *antiadrenergic (β-receptor)* [also: cetamolol HCl]

cetamolol HCl USAN *antiadrenergic (β-receptor)* [also: cetamolol]

Cetaphil cream, lotion, cleansing bar, cleansing solution OTC *soap-free therapeutic skin cleanser*

Cetapred ophthalmic ointment (discontinued 2003) ℞ *corticosteroidal anti-inflammatory; antibiotic* [prednisolone acetate; sulfacetamide sodium] 0.25%•10%

cethexonium chloride INN

cetiedil INN *peripheral vasodilator* [also: cetiedil citrate]

cetiedil citrate USAN *peripheral vasodilator; investigational (orphan) for sickle cell disease crisis* [also: cetiedil]

cetirizine INN, BAN *second-generation peripherally selective piperazine antihistamine for allergic rhinitis and chronic idiopathic urticaria* [also: cetirizine HCl]

cetirizine HCl USAN *second-generation peripherally selective piperazine antihistamine for allergic rhinitis and chronic idiopathic urticaria* [also: cetirizine]

cetobemidone [see: ketobemidone]

cetocycline INN *antibacterial* [also: cetocycline HCl]

cetocycline HCl USAN *antibacterial* [also: cetocycline]

cetofenicol INN *antibacterial* [also: cetophenicol]

cetohexazine INN

cetomacrogol 1000 INN, BAN

cetophenicol USAN *antibacterial* [also: cetofenicol]

cetophenylbutazone [see: kebuzone]

cetostearyl alcohol NF *emulsifying agent*

cetotetrine HCl [now: cetocycline HCl]

cetotiamine INN

cetoxime INN, BAN

cetoxime HCl [see: cetoxime]

Cetraria islandica *medicinal herb* [see: Iceland moss]

cetraxate INN *GI antiulcerative* [also: cetraxate HCl]

cetraxate HCl USAN *GI antiulcerative* [also: cetraxate]

cetrimide INN, BAN *topical antiseptic*

cetrimonium bromide INN *topical antiseptic* [also: cetrimonium chloride]

cetrimonium chloride BAN *topical antiseptic* [also: cetrimonium bromide]

cetrorelix acetate USAN *gonadotropin-releasing hormone (GnRH) antagonist for infertility*

Cetrotide subcu injection ℞ *gonadotropin-releasing hormone (GnRH) antagonist for infertility* [cetrorelix acetate] 0.25, 3 mg

cetuximab USAN *antineoplastic; epidermal growth factor receptor (EGFR)*

Cevalin   Chartix

blocker; treatment for metastatic colorectal cancer; investigational (orphan) for squamous cell carcinoma of the head and neck; investigational (Phase III) for pancreatic cancer

cetyl alcohol NF emulsifying and stiffening agent

cetyl esters wax NF stiffening agent

cetyldimethylbenzyl ammonium chloride [see: cetalkonium chloride]

cetylpyridinium chloride USP, INN, BAN topical antiseptic; preservative

cetyltrimethyl ammonium bromide

CEV (cyclophosphamide, etoposide, vincristine) chemotherapy protocol for small cell lung cancer (SCLC)

Cevi-Bid tablets OTC vitamin C supplement [ascorbic acid] 500 mg

Cevi-Fer timed-release capsules (discontinued 2005) ℞ hematinic; vitamin/iron supplement [ferrous fumarate (source of iron); ascorbic acid; folic acid] 63 (20)•300•1 mg

cevimeline HCl USAN cholinergic and muscarinic receptor agonist for dry mouth due to Sjögren syndrome

cevitamic acid [see: ascorbic acid]

cevitan [see: ascorbic acid]

ceylon gelatin [see: agar]

Cezin-S capsules ℞ geriatric vitamin/mineral supplement [multiple vitamins & minerals; folic acid] ±•0.5 mg

CF (carboplatin, fluorouracil) chemotherapy protocol for head and neck cancer

CF (cisplatin, fluorouracil) chemotherapy protocol for adenocarcinoma and head and neck cancer

CFC (chlorofluorocarbons) the type of propellant used in older aerosol and pressurized metered-dose inhaler (pMDI) delivery systems; these are being replaced with products that use HFA-134a propellant (q.v.)

CFL (cisplatin, fluorouracil, leucovorin [rescue]) chemotherapy protocol

CFM (cyclophosphamide, fluorouracil, mitoxantrone) chemotherapy protocol for breast cancer [also: CNF; FNC]

CFP (cyclophosphamide, fluorouracil, prednisone) chemotherapy protocol

CFPT (cyclophosphamide, fluorouracil, prednisone, tamoxifen) chemotherapy protocol

CFTR (cystic fibrosis transmembrane conductance regulator) [q.v.]

CG (Cardio-Green) [q.v.]

CG (chorionic gonadotropin) [see: gonadotropin, chorionic]

CGF (Chlorella growth factor) [q.v.]

CGF (Control Gel Formula) dressing [see: DuoDERM CGF]

CH1VPP; Ch1VPP (chlorambucil, vinblastine, procarbazine, prednisone) chemotherapy protocol

CHAD (cyclophosphamide, hexamethylmelamine, Adriamycin, DDP) chemotherapy protocol

chalk, precipitated [see: calcium carbonate, precipitated]

Chamaelirium luteum medicinal herb [see: false unicorn]

CHAMOCA (cyclophosphamide, hydroxyurea, actinomycin D, methotrexate, Oncovin, calcium folinate, Adriamycin) chemotherapy protocol for gestational trophoblastic neoplasm [also known as: modified Bagshawe protocol]

chamomile (Anthemis nobilis; Matricaria chamomilla) flowers medicinal herb for appetite stimulation, bronchitis, excessive menstruation with cramps, fever, gastrointestinal cramps, hysteria, inflammation, insomnia, nervousness, rheumatic disorders, and parasites

channa; canna medicinal herb [see: kanna]

CHAP (cyclophosphamide, Hexalen, Adriamycin, Platinol) chemotherapy protocol for ovarian cancer

CHAP (cyclophosphamide, hexamethylmelamine, Adriamycin, Platinol) chemotherapy protocol

Chap Stick Medicated Lip Balm stick, jar, squeezable tube OTC topical analgesic; counterirritant; moisturizer;

protectant; emollient [camphor; menthol; phenol] 1%•0.6%•0.5%

chaparral *(Larrea divaricata; L. glutinosa; L. tridentata)* leaves and stems *medicinal herb for arthritis, blood cleansing, bronchitis, cancer, chickenpox, colds, leukemia, rheumatic pain, stomach pain, and tumors; not generally regarded as safe and effective because of liver toxicity and stimulation of some tumors*

CharcoAid oral suspension OTC *adsorbent antidote for poisoning* [activated charcoal] 15 g/120 mL, 30 g/150 mL

CharcoAid 2000 oral liquid, granules OTC *adsorbent antidote for poisoning* [activated charcoal] 15 g/120 mL, 50 g/240 mL; 15 g

charcoal *gastric adsorbent/detoxicant; antiflatulent* 260 mg oral

charcoal, activated USP *general purpose antidote/adsorbent* 15, 30, 40, 120, 240 g, 208 mg/mL oral

Charcoal Plus enteric-coated tablets OTC *adsorbent; detoxicant* [activated charcoal] 250 mg

CharcoCaps capsules OTC *adsorbent; detoxicant; antiflatulent* [charcoal] 260 mg

Chardonna-2 tablets ℞ *GI anticholinergic; sedative* [belladonna extract; phenobarbital] 15•15 mg

chaste tree *(Vitex agnus-castus)* dried ripe fruit *medicinal herb for acne, balancing progesterone and estrogen production, increasing lactation, ovarian insufficiency, premenstrual breast pain, regulating menstrual cycle, and uterine bleeding*

chaulmosulfone INN

checkerberry *medicinal herb* [see: squaw vine; wintergreen]

cheese plant; cheeseflower *medicinal herb* [see: mallow]

cheese rennet *medicinal herb* [see: bedstraw]

Cheetah oral suspension ℞ *radiopaque contrast medium for gastrointestinal imaging* [barium sulfate] 2.2%

chelafrin [see: epinephrine]

Chelated Magnesium tablets (discontinued 2002) OTC *magnesium supplement* [magnesium amino acid chelate] 500 mg

Chelated Manganese tablets OTC *manganese supplement* [manganese] 20, 50 mg

chelating agents *a class of agents that prevent bodily absorption of and cause the excretion of substances such as heavy metals*

chelen [see: ethyl chloride]

Chelidonium majus *medicinal herb* [see: celandine]

Chelone glabra *medicinal herb* [see: turtlebloom]

Chemet capsules ℞ *heavy metal chelating agent for lead poisoning (orphan); investigational (orphan) for cystine kidney stones and mercury poisoning* [succimer] 100 mg

Chemo-Pin (trademarked form) *chemical-dispensing pin*

Chemstrip 2 GP; Chemstrip 2 LN; Chemstrip 4 the OB; Chemstrip 6; Chemstrip 7; Chemstrip 8; Chemstrip 9; Chemstrip 10 with SG; Chemstrip uGK reagent strips *in vitro diagnostic aid for multiple urine products*

Chemstrip bG reagent strips for home use *in vitro diagnostic aid for blood glucose*

Chemstrip K reagent strips for professional use *in vitro diagnostic aid for acetone (ketones) in the urine*

Chemstrip Micral reagent strips for professional use *in vitro diagnostic aid for albumin (protein) in the urine*

Chemstrip uG reagent strips for home use *in vitro diagnostic aid for urine glucose*

chenic acid [now: chenodiol]

Chenix tablets ℞ *anticholelithogenic for radiolucent gallstones (orphan)* [chenodiol] 250 mg

chenodeoxycholic acid INN, BAN *anticholelithogenic* [also: chenodiol]

chenodiol USAN *anticholelithogenic for radiolucent gallstones (orphan); investi-*

gational (orphan) for cerebrotendinous xanthomatosis [also: chenodeoxy-cholic acid]

Chenofalk ℞ *investigational (orphan) agent for cerebrotendinous xanthomatosis* [chenodiol]

Cheracol Cough syrup ℞ *narcotic antitussive; expectorant* [codeine phosphate; guaifenesin; alcohol 4.75%] 20•200 mg/10 mL

Cheracol D Cough Formula; Cheracol Plus syrup OTC *antitussive; expectorant* [dextromethorphan hydrobromide; guaifenesin; alcohol 4.75%] 20•200 mg/10 mL

Cheracol Nasal spray (discontinued 2001) OTC *nasal decongestant* [oxymetazoline HCl] 0.05%

Cheracol Sore Throat spray OTC *topical antipruritic/counterirritant; mild local anesthetic* [phenol] 1.4%

cherry, black; choke cherry; rum cherry *medicinal herb* [see: wild black cherry]

cherry, black; poison black cherry *medicinal herb* [see: belladonna]

cherry birch *medicinal herb* [see: birch]

cherry juice NF

chervil (Anthriscus cerefolium) flowering plant *medicinal herb used as a digestive, diuretic, expectorant, and stimulant*

chervil, sweet *medicinal herb* [see: sweet cicely]

chestnut *medicinal herb* [see: horse chestnut]

Chewable Multivitamins with Fluoride tablets ℞ *pediatric vitamin supplement and dental caries preventative* [multiple vitamins; fluoride; folic acid] ±•1•0.3 mg

Chewable Triple Vitamins with Fluoride tablets ℞ *pediatric vitamin supplement and dental caries preventative* [vitamins A, C, and D; fluoride] 2500 IU•60 mg•400 IU•1 mg

Chewable Vitamin C chewable tablets OTC *vitamin C supplement* [ascorbic acid and sodium ascorbate] 250, 500 mg

Chew-C chewable tablets OTC *vitamin supplement* [vitamin C (as ascorbic acid and sodium ascorbate)] 500 mg

ChexUP; Chex-Up; CHEX-UP (cyclophosphamide, hexamethylmelamine, fluorouracil, Platinol) *chemotherapy protocol*

CHF (cyclophosphamide, hexamethylmelamine, fluorouracil) *chemotherapy protocol*

Chibroxin Ocumeter (eye drops) (discontinued 2002) ℞ *topical fluoroquinolone antibiotic for bacterial conjunctivitis* [norfloxacin] 0.3%

chicken's toes *medicinal herb* [see: coral root]

chickweed (Stellaria media) plant *medicinal herb for appetite suppression, bleeding, blood cleansing, convulsions, obesity, skin rashes, and ulcers; also used as a homeopathic remedy for psoriasis and rheumatic pain*

chicory (Chicorium intybus) plant and root *medicinal herb for blood cleansing, cardiac disease, jaundice, liver disorders, promoting expectoration, and removal of calcium deposits*

Chiggerex ointment OTC *topical local anesthetic; analgesic; counterirritant* [benzocaine; camphor; menthol]

Chigger-Tox topical liquid OTC *local anesthetic* [benzocaine]

Chikusetsu ginseng (Panax pseudoginseng) *medicinal herb* [see: ginseng]

Children's Elixir DM Cough & Cold OTC *antitussive; decongestant; antihistamine* [dextromethorphan hydrobromide; pseudoephedrine HCl; brompheniramine maleate] 10•30•2 mg/10 mL

Children's Formula Cough syrup (discontinued 2002) OTC *antitussive; expectorant* [dextromethorphan hydrobromide; guaifenesin] 5•50 mg/5 mL

Children's Ibuprofen Cold oral suspension OTC *analgesic; antipyretic; nonsteroidal anti-inflammatory drug; nasal decongestant* [ibuprofen; pseudoephedrine] 100•15 mg/5 mL

Children's Loratadine syrup OTC
*nonsedating antihistamine for allergic
rhinitis* [loratadine] 5 mg/5 mL
chili pepper; chilies *medicinal herb*
[see: cayenne]
chillifolinum [see: quillifoline]
Chimaphila umbellata medicinal herb
[see: pipsissewa]
**chimeric (human-murine) G250
IgG monoclonal antibodies
(MAb)** *investigational (orphan) agent
for renal cell carcinoma*
**chimeric A2 (human-murine) IgG
monoclonal anti-TNF antibody
(cA2)** [see: infliximab]
**chimeric humanized monoclonal
antibodies (MAb) to** *Staphylococcus investigational (orphan) prophylaxis of* S. epidermidis *sepsis in low
birth weight infants*
**chimeric M-T412 (human-murine)
IgG monoclonal anti-CD4** [now:
priliximab]
chinchona *medicinal herb* [see: quinine]
Chinese cucumber *(Trichosanthes
kirilowii) gourd and root medicinal
herb for abscesses, amenorrhea, cough,
diabetes, edema, fever, inducing abortion, invasive moles, jaundice, poly-
uria, and tumors*
Chinese gelatin [see: agar]
Chinese isinglass [see: chiniofon]
Chinese rhubarb *medicinal herb* [see:
rhubarb]
chinethazone [see: quinethazone]
chiniofon NF, INN
Chionanthus virginica medicinal herb
[see: fringe tree]
Chirocaine local or epidural injection
℞ *long-acting local anesthetic* [levobu-
pivacaine HCl] 2.5, 5, 7.5 mg/mL
chitosamine [see: glucosamine]
chitosan *natural cellulose-like biopoly-
mer extracted from marine animal
exoskeletons and used as a treatment
for hypercholesterolemia, hyperlipidemia, and obesity; also used topically
as an antimicrobial and vulnerary*
chittem bark *medicinal herb* [see:
buckthorn; cascara sagrada]

**CHL + PRED (chlorambucil, pred-
nisone)** *chemotherapy protocol*
Chlamydiazyme reagent kit for professional use *in vitro diagnostic aid for
Chlamydia trachomatis* [solid phase
enzyme immunoassay]
Chlo-Amine chewable tablets OTC
antihistamine [chlorpheniramine mal-
eate] 2 mg
chlophedianol BAN *antitussive* [also:
chlophedianol HCl; clofedanol]
chlophedianol HCl USAN *antitussive*
[also: clofedanol; chlophedianol]
chlophenadione [see: clorindione]
chloquinate [see: cloquinate]
chloracyzine INN
Chlorafed oral liquid (discontinued
2002) OTC *decongestant; antihistamine*
[pseudoephedrine HCl; chlorpheniramine maleate] 30•2 mg/5 mL
Chlorafed; Chlorafed HS Timecelles
(sustained-release capsules) (discontinued 2002) ℞ *decongestant; antihistamine* [pseudoephedrine HCl; chlorpheniramine maleate] 120•8 mg;
60•4 mg
chloral betaine USAN, NF, BAN *sedative* [also: cloral betaine]
chloral hydrate USP, BAN *nonbarbiturate sedative and hypnotic; also abused
as a street drug* 500 mg oral; 250, 500
mg/5 mL oral
chloral hydrate betaine [see: chloral
betaine]
chloralformamide USP
chloralodol INN [also: chlorhexadol]
chloralose (α-chloralose) INN
chloralurethane [see: carbocloral]
chlorambucil USP, INN, BAN *nitrogen
mustard-type alkylating antineoplastic
for multiple leukemias and lymphomas*
chloramidobenzol [see: clofenamide]
chloramine [now: chloramine-T]
chloramine-T NF [also: tosylchloramide sodium]
chloramiphene [see: clomiphene cit-
rate]
chloramphenicol USP, INN, BAN, JAN
bacteriostatic antibiotic; antirickettsial 5
mg/mL eye drops; 10 mg/g topical

chloramphenicol palmitate USP, JAN *antibacterial; antirickettsial* 150 mg/5 mL oral

chloramphenicol pantothenate complex USAN *antibacterial; antirickettsial* [also: cloramfenicol pantotenate complex]

chloramphenicol sodium succinate USP, JAN *antibacterial; antirickettsial* 100 mg/mL injection

chloranautine [see: dimenhydrinate]

ChloraPrep One-Step swabs *topical antiseptic* [chlorhexidine gluconate; isopropyl alcohol] 2%•70%

chlorarsen [see: dichlorophenarsine HCl]

Chloraseptic mouthwash/gargle OTC *topical antipruritic/counterirritant; mild local anesthetic* [phenol] 1.4%

Chloraseptic, Children's lozenges OTC *topical oral anesthetic* [benzocaine] 5 mg

Chloraseptic, Children's throat spray OTC *topical antipruritic/counterirritant; mild local anesthetic* [phenol] 0.5%

Chloraseptic Sore Throat lozenges OTC *topical oral anesthetic; analgesic; counterirritant* [benzocaine; menthol] 6•10 mg

chlorazanil INN

chlorazanil HCl [see: chlorazanil]

chlorazodin INN [also: chloroazodin]

chlorazone [see: chloramine-T]

chlorbenzoxamine INN

chlorbenzoxamine HCl [see: chlorbenzoxamine]

chlorbetamide INN, BAN

chlorbutanol [see: chlorobutanol]

chlorbutin [see: chlorambucil]

chlorbutol BAN *antimicrobial agent* [also: chlorobutanol]

chlorcinnazine [see: clocinizine]

chlorcyclizine INN, BAN *topical antihistamine* [also: chlorcyclizine HCl]

chlorcyclizine HCl USP *topical antihistamine* [also: chlorcyclizine]

chlordantoin USAN, BAN *antifungal* [also: clodantoin]

chlordiazepoxide USP, INN, BAN, JAN *benzodiazepine anxiolytic; sedative; alcohol withdrawal aid*

chlordiazepoxide HCl USAN, USP, BAN, JAN *benzodiazepine anxiolytic; sedative; alcohol withdrawal aid; sometimes abused as a street drug* 5, 10, 25 mg oral

chlordiazepoxide HCl & clidinium bromide *anxiolytic; GI anticholinergic* 5•2.5 mg

chlordimorine INN

Chlordrine S.R. sustained-release capsules (discontinued 2002) ℞ *decongestant; antihistamine* [pseudoephedrine HCl; chlorpheniramine maleate] 120•8 mg

Chlorella *a genus of single-cell algae used as a source of multiple vitamins and minerals, protein, chlorellin, chlorophyll and Chlorella growth factor (q.v.); immune enhancer and chelator of heavy metals*

Chlorella **growth factor (CGF)** *natural extract of the nucleus of* Chlorella *algae (q.v.) that is widely used in wound healing and skin disorders*

Chloresium ointment, solution OTC *vulnerary and deodorant for wounds, burns, and ulcers* [chlorophyllin copper complex] 0.5%; 0.2%

Chloresium tablets OTC *systemic deodorant for ostomy, breath, and body odors* [chlorophyllin copper complex] 14 mg

chlorethate [see: clorethate]

chlorethyl [see: ethyl chloride]

chlorfenisate [see: clofibrate]

chlorfenvinphos BAN [also: clofenvinfos]

chlorguanide HCl [see: chloroguanide HCl]

chlorhexadol BAN [also: chloralodol]

chlorhexidine INN, BAN *antimicrobial* [also: chlorhexidine gluconate]

chlorhexidine gluconate USAN *antimicrobial; investigational (orphan) for oral mucositis in bone marrow transplant patients* [also: chlorhexidine]

chlorhexidine HCl USAN, BAN *topical anti-infective*

chlorhexidine phosphanilate USAN *antibacterial*

chlorimiphenin [see: imiclopazine]

chlorimpiphenine [see: imiclopazine]

chlorinated & iodized peanut oil [see: chloriodized oil]

chlorindanol USAN *spermaticide* [also: clorindanol]

chlorine *element (Cl)*

chloriodized oil USP

chlorisondamine chloride INN, BAN

chlorisondamone chloride [see: chlorisondamine chloride]

chlormadinone INN, BAN *progestin* [also: chlormadinone acetate]

chlormadinone acetate USAN, NF *progestin* [also: chlormadinone]

chlormerodrin NF, INN, BAN

chlormerodrin (^{197}Hg) INN *renal function test; radioactive agent* [also: chlormerodrin Hg 197]

chlormerodrin Hg 197 USAN, USP *renal function test; radioactive agent* [also: chlormerodrin (^{197}Hg)]

chlormerodrin Hg 203 USAN, USP *renal function test; radioactive agent*

chlormeroprin [see: chlormerodrin]

chlormethazanone [see: chlormezanone]

chlormethiazole BAN [also: clomethiazole]

chlormethine INN *nitrogen mustard-type alkylating antineoplastic* [also: mechlorethamine HCl; mustine; nitrogen mustard N-oxide HCl]

chlormethylencycline [see: clomocycline]

chlormezanone INN, BAN *mild anxiolytic*

chlormidazole INN, BAN

chlornaphazine INN

chloroacetic acid [see: monochloroacetic, dichloroacetic, or trichloroacetic acid]

8-chloroadenosine monophosphate, cyclic (8-Cl cAMP) [see: tocladesine]

chloroazodin USP [also: chlorazodin]

5-chlorobenzoxazolinone [see: chlorzoxazone]

chlorobutanol NF, INN *antimicrobial agent; preservative* [also: chlorbutol]

chlorochine [see: chloroquine]

chlorocresol USAN, NF, INN *antiseptic; disinfectant*

2-chloro-2′-deoxyadenosine (CdA) [now: cladribine]

chlorodeoxylincomycin [see: clindamycin]

chloroethane [see: ethyl chloride]

2-chloroethyl-3-sarcosinamide-1-nitrosourea *investigational (orphan) for malignant glioma*

chloroform NF *solvent*

chloroguanide HCl USP *antimalarial; dihydrofolate reductase inhibitor* [also: proguanil]

chloroguanide triazine pamoate [see: cycloguanil pamoate]

chloro-iodohydroxyquinoline [see: clioquinol]

chlorolincomycin [see: clindamycin]

chloromethapyrilene citrate [see: chlorothen citrate]

Chloromycetin powder for eye drops, ophthalmic ointment R *topical ophthalmic antibiotic* [chloramphenicol] 25 mg/15 mL; 10 mg/g

Chloromycetin Otic ear drops (discontinued 2003) R *broad-spectrum antibiotic* [chloramphenicol] 0.5%

Chloromycetin Sodium Succinate powder for IV injection R *broad-spectrum bacteriostatic antibiotic* [chloramphenicol sodium succinate] 100 mg/mL

p-chlorophenol [see: parachlorophenol]

chlorophenothane NF [also: clofenotane; dicophane]

chlorophenoxamide [see: clefamide]

chlorophenylmercury [see: phenylmercuric chloride]

chlorophyll, water soluble [see: chlorophyllin]

chlorophyllin *vulnerary; oral deodorant for ostomy, breath, and body odors; topical deodorant for wounds and ulcers* 20 mg oral

chlorophyllin copper complex USAN *oral deodorant for ostomy, breath, and* *body odors; topical deodorant for wounds and ulcers*

chloroprednisone INN

chloroprednisone acetate [see: chloroprednisone]

chloroprocaine INN *injectable local anesthetic* [also: chloroprocaine HCl]

chloroprocaine HCl USP *injectable local anesthetic; central or peripheral nerve block, including lumbar and epidural block* [also: chloroprocaine] 2%, 3% injection

Chloroptic eye drops (discontinued 2005) ℞ *topical ophthalmic antibiotic* [chloramphenicol] 5 mg/mL

Chloroptic S.O.P. ophthalmic ointment (discontinued 2005) ℞ *topical ophthalmic antibiotic* [chloramphenicol] 10 mg/g

chloropyramine INN [also: halopyramine]

chloropyrilene INN, BAN [also: chlorothen citrate]

chloroquine USP, INN, BAN *amebicide; antimalarial*

chloroquine diphosphate [see: chloroquine phosphate]

chloroquine HCl USP *amebicide; antimalarial* [also: chloroquine]

chloroquine phosphate USP, BAN *amebicide; antimalarial; lupus erythematosus suppressant* 250 mg oral

chloroserpidine INN

N-chlorosuccinimide [see: succinchlorimide]

chlorothen citrate NF [also: chloropyrilene]

chlorothenium citrate [see: chlorothen citrate]

chlorothenylpyramine [see: chlorothen]

chlorothiazide USP, INN, BAN *diuretic; antihypertensive* 250, 500 mg oral

chlorothiazide sodium USAN, USP *diuretic; antihypertensive*

chlorothymol NF

chlorotrianisene USP, INN, BAN *estrogen for hormone replacement therapy or inoperable prostatic cancer*

chloroxine USAN *antiseborrheic*

chloroxylenol USP, INN, BAN *bacteriostatic*

chlorozone [see: chloramine-T]

chlorpenthixol [see: clopenthixol]

Chlorphed-LA nasal spray (discontinued 2002) OTC *nasal decongestant* [oxymetazoline HCl] 0.05%

Chlorphedrine SR sustained-release capsules (discontinued 2002) ℞ *decongestant; antihistamine* [pseudoephedrine HCl; chlorpheniramine maleate] 120•8 mg

chlorphenamine INN *antihistamine* [also: chlorpheniramine maleate; chlorpheniramine]

chlorphenamine maleate [see: chlorpheniramine maleate]

chlorphenecyclane [see: clofenciclan]

chlorphenesin INN, BAN *skeletal muscle relaxant* [also: chlorphenesin carbamate]

chlorphenesin carbamate USAN, JAN *skeletal muscle relaxant* [also: chlorphenesin]

chlorphenindione [see: clorindione]

chlorpheniramine BAN *alkylamine antihistamine* [also: chlorpheniramine maleate; chlorphenamine] ⑨ chlorphentermine

chlorpheniramine maleate USP *alkylamine antihistamine* [also: chlorphenamine; chlorpheniramine] 4, 8, 12 mg oral

chlorpheniramine maleate & phenylpropanolamine HCl *antihistamine; decongestant* PPA was banned in all OTC products in 2001

chlorpheniramine maleate & pseudoephedrine HCl *antihistamine; decongestant* 8•120 mg oral

chlorpheniramine polistirex USAN *alkylamine antihistamine*

chlorpheniramine tannate & pseudoephedrine tannate *antihistamine; decongestant* 75•4.5 mg/5 mL oral

chlorpheniramine tannate & pyrilamine tannate & phenylephrine tannate *antihistamine; decongestant* 2•12.5•5 mg/5 mL oral

chlorphenoctium amsonate INN, BAN

chlorphenotane [see: chlorophenothane]

chlorphenoxamine INN, BAN [also: chlorphenoxamine HCl]

chlorphenoxamine HCl USP [also: chlorphenoxamine]

chlorphentermine INN, BAN *anorectic* [also: chlorphentermine HCl] ⑨ chlorpheniramine

chlorphentermine HCl USAN *anorectic* [also: chlorphentermine]

chlorphenylindandione [see: clorindione]

chlorphthalidone [see: chlorthalidone]

chlorprocaine chloride [see: chloroprocaine HCl]

chlorproethazine INN [also: chlorproethazine HCl]

chlorproethazine HCl [also: chlorproethazine]

chlorproguanil INN, BAN

chlorproguanil HCl [see: chlorproguanil]

chlorpromazine USP, INN, BAN *conventional (typical) phenothiazine antipsychotic for schizophrenia and manic episodes of a bipolar disorder; antiemetic for nausea and vomiting*

chlorpromazine HCl USP, BAN, JAN *phenothiazine antipsychotic for schizophrenia, manic episodes of a bipolar disorder, pediatric hyperactivity, and severe pediatric behavioral problems; treatment for acute intermittent porphyria, nausea/vomiting, and intractable hiccoughs* 10, 25, 50, 100, 200 mg oral; 100 mg/mL oral; 25 mg/mL injection

chlorpromazine hibenzate JAN *conventional (typical) phenothiazine antipsychotic for schizophrenia and manic episodes of a bipolar disorder; antiemetic for nausea and vomiting*

chlorpromazine phenolphthalinate JAN *conventional (typical) phenothiazine antipsychotic for schizophrenia and manic episodes of a bipolar disorder; antiemetic for nausea and vomiting*

chlorpromazine tannate USP, INN, BAN *conventional (typical) phenothiazine antipsychotic for schizophrenia and manic episodes of a bipolar disorder; antiemetic for nausea and vomiting*

chlorpropamide USP, INN, BAN, JAN *sulfonylurea antidiabetic* 100, 250 mg oral

chlorprophenpyridamine maleate [see: chlorpheniramine maleate]

chlorprothixene USAN, USP, INN, BAN *thioxanthene antipsychotic*

chlorpyrifos BAN

chlorquinaldol INN, BAN

Chlor-Rest tablets (discontinued 2001) OTC *decongestant; antihistamine* [phenylpropanolamine HCl; chlorpheniramine maleate] 18.7•2 mg

chlortalidone INN *antihypertensive; diuretic* [also: chlorthalidone]

chlortetracycline INN, BAN *antibiotic; antiprotozoal* [also: chlortetracycline bisulfate]

chlortetracycline bisulfate USP *antibiotic; antiprotozoal* [also: chlortetracycline]

chlortetracycline calcium *antibiotic; antiprotozoal*

chlortetracycline HCl USP, BAN *antibiotic; antiprotozoal*

chlorthalidone USAN, USP, BAN *antihypertensive; diuretic* [also: chlortalidone] 25, 50, 100 mg oral

chlorthenoxazin BAN [also: chlorthenoxazine]

chlorthenoxazine INN [also: chlorthenoxazin]

chlorthiazide [see: chlorothiazide]

chlortrianisestrol [see: chlorotrianisene]

Chlor-Trimeton Allergy 4 Hour syrup (discontinued 2001) OTC *antihistamine* [chlorpheniramine maleate] 2 mg/5 mL

Chlor-Trimeton Allergy 4 Hour tablets (discontinued 2002) OTC *antihistamine* [chlorpheniramine maleate] 4 mg

Chlor-Trimeton Allergy 8 Hour; Chlor-Trimeton Allergy 12 Hour timed-release tablets OTC *antihistamine* [chlorpheniramine maleate] 8 mg; 12 mg

Chlor-Trimeton Allergy-D 4 Hour tablets OTC *decongestant; antihista-*

mine [pseudoephedrine sulfate; chlorpheniramine maleate] 60•4 mg

Chlor-Trimeton Allergy-D 12 Hour sustained-release tablets OTC *decongestant; antihistamine* [pseudoephedrine sulfate; chlorpheniramine maleate] 120•8 mg

Chlor-Trimeton Allergy-Sinus caplets (discontinued 2001) OTC *decongestant; antihistamine; analgesic* [phenylpropanolamine HCl; chlorpheniramine maleate; acetaminophen] 12.5•2•500 mg

chlorzoxazone USP, INN, BAN, JAN *skeletal muscle relaxant* 250, 500 mg oral

chlosudimeprimylum [see: clopamide]

ChlVPP (chlorambucil, vinblastine, procarbazine, prednisone/prednisolone) *chemotherapy protocol for Hodgkin lymphoma* [note: prednisone is preferred in the U.S.; prednisolone is preferred in England]

ChlVPP/EVA (chlorambucil, vinblastine, procarbazine, prednisone/prednisolone, etoposide, vincristine, Adriamycin) *chemotherapy protocol for Hodgkin lymphoma* [note: prednisone is preferred in the U.S.; prednisolone is preferred in England]

CHO (cyclophosphamide, hydroxydaunomycin, Oncovin) *chemotherapy protocol*

CHO cells, recombinant [see: CD4, human truncated]

CHOB (cyclophosphamide, hydroxydaunomycin, Oncovin, bleomycin) *chemotherapy protocol*

CHOD (cyclophosphamide, hydroxydaunomycin, Oncovin, dexamethasone) *chemotherapy protocol*

choice dielytra *medicinal herb* [see: turkey corn]

Choice DM fingerstick test kit for home use OTC *in vitro diagnostic aid for glycosylated hemoglobin levels*

Choice dm oral liquid (discontinued 2005) OTC *enteral nutritional therapy*

for abnormal glucose tolerance [lactose-free formula] 240 mL

choke cherry; black choke *medicinal herb* [see: wild black cherry]

Cholac oral/rectal solution ℞ *synthetic disaccharide used to prevent and treat portal-systemic encephalopathy* [lactulose] 10 g/15 mL

cholagogues *a class of agents that stimulate the flow of bile into the duodenum*

cholalic acid [see: dehydrocholic acid]

cholecalciferol (vitamin D₃) USP, BAN, JAN *fat-soluble vitamin* [also: colecalciferol] 1000 IU oral

Choledyl SA sustained-action tablets (discontinued 2004) ℞ *antiasthmatic; bronchodilator* [oxtriphylline] 400, 600 mg

cholera vaccine USP *active bacterin for cholera (Vibrio cholerae)*

cholesterin [see: cholesterol]

cholesterol NF *emulsifying agent*

cholestrin [see: cholesterol]

cholestyramine BAN *bile salts ion-exchange resin; antihyperlipoproteinemic* [also: cholestyramine resin; colestyramine]

Cholestyramine Light powder for oral suspension ℞ *cholesterol-lowering antihyperlipidemic; also used for biliary obstruction* [cholestyramine resin] 4 g/dose

cholestyramine resin USP *bile salts ion-exchange resin; cholesterol-lowering antihyperlipidemic; also used for biliary obstruction* [also: colestyramine; cholestyramine] 4 g powder for oral solution

cholic acid [see: dehydrocholic acid]

Cholidase tablets OTC *dietary lipotropic with vitamin supplementation* [choline; inositol; vitamins B₆, B₁₂, and E] 185•150•2.5•0.005•7.5 mg

choline *dietary lipotropic supplement* 250, 300, 500, 650 mg oral

choline alfoscerate INN

choline bitartrate NF 250 mg oral

choline bromide hexamethylenedicarbamate [see: hexacarbacholine bromide]

choline chloride INN *investigational (orphan) for choline deficiency of long-term parenteral nutrition*

choline chloride acetate [see: acetyl-choline chloride]

choline chloride carbamate [see: carbachol]

choline chloride succinate [see: succinylcholine chloride]

choline dihydrogen citrate NF 650 mg oral

choline gluconate INN

choline glycerophosphate [see: choline alfoscerate]

choline perchlorate, nitrate ester [see: nitricholine perchlorate]

choline salicylate USAN, INN, BAN *analgesic; antipyretic; anti-inflammatory; antirheumatic*

choline theophyllinate INN, BAN *bronchodilator* [also: oxtriphylline]

cholinergic agonists *a class of agents that produce effects similar to those of the parasympathetic nervous system* [also called: parasympathomimetics]

cholinesterase inhibitors *a class of drugs which increase acetylcholine neurotransmitters, used as a cognition adjuvant in Alzheimer dementia* [also called: acetylcholinesterase (AChE) inhibitors]

Cholinoid capsules OTC *dietary lipotropic with vitamin supplementation* [choline; inositol; multiple B vitamins; vitamin C; lemon bioflavonoids] 111•111•≛•100•100 mg

Cholografin Meglumine injection ℞ *radiopaque contrast medium for cholecystography and cholangiography* [iodipamide meglumine (49.2% iodine)] 520 mg/mL (257 mg/mL)

chondodendron tomentosum [see: tubocurarine chloride]

chondrocyte-alginate *investigational (orphan) gel suspension for vesicoureteral reflux in children*

chondroitin 4-sulfate [see: danaparoid sodium]

chondroitin 6-sulfate [see: danaparoid sodium]

chondroitin sulfate *natural remedy for arthritis, blood clots, and extravasation from needle sticks after certain chemotherapy treatments*

chondroitin sulfate sodium JAN

chondroitin sulfuric acid *natural remedy* [see: chondroitin sulfate]

chondroitinase *investigational (orphan) agent for vitrectomy*

Chondrox capsules OTC *dietary supplement for osteoarthritis; protects and rebuilds cartilage in joints* [N-acetyl-D-glucosamine; glucosamine sulfate; chondroitin sulfate; manganese (from manganese aspartate)] 500•500•800•0.17 mg

Chondrus crispus medicinal herb [see: Irish moss]

chonsurid *natural remedy* [see: chondroitin sulfate]

Chooz chewable tablets OTC *antacid* [calcium carbonate] 500 mg

CHOP (cyclophosphamide, hydroxydaunomycin, Oncovin, prednisone) *chemotherapy protocol for non-Hodgkin lymphoma*

CHOP-BLEO (cyclophosphamide, hydroxydaunomycin, Oncovin, prednisone, bleomycin) *chemotherapy protocol for non-Hodgkin lymphoma*

CHOPE (cyclophosphamide, hydroxydaunomycin, Oncovin, prednisone, etoposide) *chemotherapy protocol*

CHOR (cyclophosphamide, hydroxydaunomycin, Oncovin, radiation therapy) *chemotherapy protocol*

Chorex-5 powder for IM injection ℞ *gonad-stimulating hormone for prepubertal cryptorchidism and hypogonadism; ovulation stimulant* [chorionic gonadotropin] 500 U/mL

Chorex-10 powder for IM injection (discontinued 2005) ℞ *gonad-stimulating hormone for prepubertal cryptorchidism and hypogonadism; ovulation stimulant* [chorionic gonadotropin] 1000 U/mL

choriogonadotropin alfa USAN, INN *recombinant human chorionic gonadotropin (rhCG); fertility stimulant for anovulatory women; adjuvant therapy for cryptorchidism*

chorionic gonadotrophin [see: gonadotropin, chorionic]

chorionic gonadotropin (CG) [see: gonadotropin, chorionic]

Choron-10 powder for IM injection ℞ *gonad-stimulating hormone for prepubertal cryptorchidism and hypogonadism; ovulation stimulant* [chorionic gonadotropin] 1000 U/mL

CHP (chlorhexidine phosphanilate) [q.v.]

Christmas factor [see: factor IX complex]

Chromagen capsules ℞ *hematinic* [ferrous fumarate; cyanocobalamin; ascorbic acid; intrinsic factor concentrate] 70•0.01•150•100 mg

Chromagen FA; Chromagen Forte capsules ℞ *vitamin/iron supplement* [vitamins B₁₂ & C; iron; folic acid] 0.01•150•70•1 mg; 0.01•60•151•1 mg

Chromagen OB capsules OTC *prenatal vitamin/mineral/iron supplement* [multiple vitamins & minerals; iron; folic acid] ±•28•1 mg

Chroma-Pak IV injection ℞ *chromium supplement* [chromic chloride hexahydrate (20% elemental chromium)] 20.5, 102.5 μg/mL (4, 20 μg Cr/mL)

chromargyre [see: merbromin]

chromated albumin [see: albumin, chromated Cr 51 serum]

Chromelin Complexion Blender topical suspension OTC *skin darkening agent for vitiligo and hypopigmented areas* [dihydroxyacetone] 5%

chromic acid, disodium salt [see: sodium chromate Cr 51]

chromic chloride USP *dietary chromium supplement (20% elemental chromium)* 20.5, 102.5 μg/mL (4, 20 μg Cr/mL) injection

chromic chloride Cr 51 USAN *radioactive agent*

chromic chloride hexahydrate [see: chromic chloride]

chromic phosphate Cr 51 USAN *radioactive agent*

chromic phosphate P 32 USAN, USP *antineoplastic; radioactive agent*

chromium *element (Cr); trace mineral important in glucose metabolism*

Chromium Chloride IV injection ℞ *intravenous nutritional therapy* [chromic chloride hexahydrate] 4 μg/mL

chromium chloride [see: chromic chloride Cr 51]

chromium chloride hexahydrate [see: chromic chloride]

chromium picolinate *dietary chromium supplement*

chromium polynicotinate *dietary chromium supplement*

chromocarb INN

chromonar HCl USAN *coronary vasodilator* [also: carbocromen]

Chronoforte capsules OTC *anti-aging supplement* [acetyl-L-carnitine; alpha lipoic acid; carnosine; nettle leaf; quercetin; biotin] 333.3•50•166.7•166.7•12.5•0.5 mg

Chronogesic ℞ *investigational (Phase III) narcotic analgesic for cancer-related pain* [sufentanil]

Chronosule (trademarked dosage form) *sustained-action capsule*

Chronotab (trademarked dosage form) *sustained-action tablet*

Chronovera Ⓒᴬᴺ delayed-onset, extended-release tablets ℞ *antihypertensive; calcium channel blocker* [verapamil HCl] 180, 240 mg

Chronulac oral/rectal solution ℞ *hyperosmotic laxative* [lactulose] 10 g/15 mL

Chrysanthemum parthenium *medicinal herb* [see: feverfew]

Chrysanthemum vulgare *medicinal herb* [see: tansy]

chrysazin *(withdrawn from market by FDA)* [see: danthron]

chrysin *natural aromatase inhibitor used to block the conversion of testosterone to estrogen*

CHVP (cyclophosphamide, hydroxydaunomycin, VM-26, prednisone) *chemotherapy protocol*

Chymodiactin powder for intradiscal injection (discontinued 2003) ℞ *proteolytic enzyme for herniated nucleus pulposus* [chymopapain] 4 nKat

chymopapain USAN, INN, BAN *proteolytic enzyme for herniated lumbar discs*

chymotrypsin USP, INN, BAN *proteolytic enzyme; zonulolytic for intracapsular lens extraction*

C.I. acid orange 24 monosodium salt (color index) [see: resorcin brown]

C.I. basic violet 3 (color index) [see: gentian violet]

C.I. basic violet 14 monohydrochloride (color index) [see: fuchsin, basic]

C.I. direct blue 53 tetrasodium salt (color index) [see: Evans blue]

C.I. mordant yellow 5, disodium salt (color index) [see: olsalazine sodium]

ciadox INN

Cialis film-coated tablets ℞ *phosphodiesterase type 5 (PDE5) inhibitor; selective vasodilator for erectile dysfunction (ED); investigational for female sexual dysfunction* [tadalafil] 5, 10, 20 mg

ciamexon INN, BAN

cianergoline INN

cianidanol INN

cianidol [see: cianidanol]

cianopramine INN

ciapilome INN

Ciba Vision Cleaner for Sensitive Eyes solution OTC *surfactant cleaning solution for soft contact lenses*

Ciba Vision Saline aerosol solution OTC *rinsing/storage solution for soft contact lenses* [sodium chloride (saline solution)]

Cibacalcin subcu or IM injection ℞ *calcium regulator for Paget disease (osteitis deformans) (orphan)* [calcitonin (human)] 0.5 mg/vial

cibenzoline INN, BAN *antiarrhythmic* [also: cifenline]

cibenzoline succinate JAN *antiarrhythmic* [also: cifenline succinate]

cicaprost INN *prostacyclin analogue*

cicarperone INN

cicely, sweet *medicinal herb* [see: sweet cicely]

Cichorium intybus *medicinal herb* [see: chicory]

ciclacillin INN, BAN *antibacterial* [also: cyclacillin]

ciclactate INN

ciclafrine INN *antihypotensive* [also: ciclafrine HCl]

ciclafrine HCl USAN *antihypotensive* [also: ciclafrine]

ciclazindol USAN, INN, BAN *antidepressant*

Ciclesonide ℞ *investigational (Phase III) for asthma*

ciclesonide *investigational (NDA filed) inhaled corticosteroid for persistent asthma*

cicletanine USAN, INN, BAN *antihypertensive*

ciclindole INN *antidepressant* [also: cyclindole]

cicliomenol INN

ciclobendazole INN, BAN *anthelmintic* [also: cyclobendazole]

ciclofenazine INN *antipsychotic* [also: cyclophenazine HCl]

ciclofenazine HCl [see: cyclophenazine HCl]

cicloheximide INN *antipsoriatic* [also: cycloheximide]

ciclonicate INN

ciclonium bromide INN

ciclopirox USAN, INN, BAN *topical antifungal for tinea pedis, tinea cruris, tinea corporis, tinea versicolor, candidiasis, seborrheic dermatitis, and onychomycosis* 0.77% topical

ciclopirox olamine USAN, USP, JAN *topical antifungal*

ciclopramine INN

cicloprofen USAN, INN, BAN *anti-inflammatory*

cicloprolol INN *antiadrenergic (β-receptor)* [also: cicloprolol HCl; cycloprolol]

cicloprolol HCl USAN *antiadrenergic (β-receptor)* [also: cicloprolol; cycloprolol]

ciclosidomine INN, BAN

ciclosporin INN *immunosuppressive* [also: cyclosporine; cyclosporin]

ciclotate INN *combining name for radicals or groups*

ciclotizolam INN, BAN

ciclotropium bromide INN

cicloxilic acid INN

cicloxolone INN, BAN

cicortonide INN

cicrotoic acid INN

Cidecin injection (name changed to Cubicin upon marketing release in 2003)

cideferron INN

Cidex; Cidex-7; Cidex Plus 28 solution OTC *broad-spectrum antimicrobial* [glutaral] 2%; 2%; 3.2% ⚕ Cedax

cidofovir USAN, INN *nucleoside antiviral for AIDS-related cytomegalovirus retinitis; investigational (Phase I/II) gel for AIDS-related genital herpes and Kaposi sarcoma*

cidoxepin INN *antidepressant* [also: cidoxepin HCl]

cidoxepin HCl USAN *antidepressant* [also: cidoxepin]

cifenline USAN *antiarrhythmic* [also: cibenzoline]

cifenline succinate USAN *antiarrhythmic* [also: cibenzoline succinate]

cifostodine INN

ciglitazone USAN, INN *antidiabetic*

cignolin [see: anthralin]

ciheptolane INN

ciladopa INN, BAN *antiparkinsonian; dopaminergic agent* [also: ciladopa HCl]

ciladopa HCl USAN *antiparkinsonian; dopaminergic agent* [also: ciladopa]

cilansetron INN *investigational treatment for irritable bowel syndrome*

cilastatin INN, BAN *enzyme inhibitor* [also: cilastatin sodium]

cilastatin sodium USAN, JAN *enzyme inhibitor* [also: cilastatin]

cilazapril USAN, INN, BAN, JAN *antihypertensive; ACE inhibitor*

cilazaprilat INN, BAN

cilexetil USAN *combining name for radicals or groups*

ciliary neurotrophic factor *investigational (orphan) agent for amyotrophic lateral sclerosis and other spinal muscular atrophies; investigational (Phase III) treatment for obesity in type 2 diabetics*

"cillins" *brief term for a class of antibiotics derived from various strains of the fungus Penicillium, or their semi-synthetic analogues, whose generic names end in "cillin," such as ampicillin* [properly called: penicillins]

cilmostim USAN *hematopoietic; macrophage colony-stimulating factor*

cilobamine INN *antidepressant* [also: cilobamine mesylate]

cilobamine mesylate USAN *antidepressant* [also: cilobamine]

cilofungin USAN, INN *antifungal*

cilomilast *phosphodiesterase type IV (PDE-IV) inhibitor; investigational (NDA filed) pulmonary anti-inflammatory for COPD*

ciloprost [see: iloprost]

cilostamide INN

cilostazol USAN, INN *vasodilator; antithrombotic; phosphodiesterase (PDE) III platelet aggregation inhibitor for intermittent claudication* 50, 100 mg oral

Ciloxan Drop-Tainers (eye drops), ointment ℞ *ophthalmic antibiotic* [ciprofloxacin HCl] 3.5 mg/mL; 0.3%

ciltoprazine INN

cilutazoline INN

cimaterol USAN, INN *repartitioning agent*

cimemoxin INN

cimepanol INN

cimetidine USAN, USP, INN, BAN, JAN *histamine H_2 antagonist for gastric ulcers* 200, 300, 400, 800 mg oral ⚕ dimethicone

cimetidine HCl USAN *histamine H_2 antagonist for gastric ulcers* 300 mg/5 mL oral; 300 mg/2 mL injection

cimetropium bromide INN

Cimicifuga racemosa *medicinal herb* [see: black cohosh]

cimoxatone INN

cinacalcet HCl *oral calcimimetic agent for hypercalcemia due to parathyroid carcinoma (orphan) and secondary hyperparathyroidism (SHPT) due to chronic kidney disease* (base=91%)

cinalukast USAN, INN *antiasthmatic*

cinametic acid INN

cinamolol INN

cinanserin INN *serotonin inhibitor* [also: cinanserin HCl]

cinanserin HCl USAN *serotonin inhibitor* [also: cinanserin]

cinaproxen INN

cincaine chloride [see: dibucaine HCl]

cinchocaine INN, BAN *local anesthetic* [also: dibucaine]

cinchocaine HCl BAN *local anesthetic* [also: dibucaine HCl]

Cinchona succirubra; C. ledgeriana; C. calisaya medicinal herb [see: quinine]

cinchonidine sulfate NF

cinchonine sulfate NF

cinchophen NF, INN, BAN

cinecromen INN

cinepaxadil INN

cinepazet INN, BAN *antianginal* [also: cinepazet maleate]

cinepazet maleate USAN *antianginal* [also: cinepazet]

cinepazic acid INN

cinepazide INN, BAN

cinfenine INN

cinfenoac INN, BAN

cinflumide USAN, INN *muscle relaxant*

cingestol USAN, INN *progestin*

cinitapride INN

cinmetacin INN

cinnamaldehyde NF

cinnamaverine INN

cinnamedrine USAN, INN *smooth muscle relaxant*

cinnamedrine HCl *smooth muscle relaxant*

cinnamic aldehyde [now: cinnamaldehyde]

cinnamon NF

cinnamon oil NF

cinnamon (*Cinnamonum zeylanicum*) bark and oil *medicinal herb for diarrhea, dysmenorrhea, gastrointestinal upset, microbial and fungal infections, and gas pain; also used as an aromatic, astringent, and stimulant*

cinnamon wood *medicinal herb* [see: sassafras]

cinnarizine USAN, INN, BAN *antihistamine*

cinnarizine clofibrate INN

cinnofuradione INN

cinnofuron [see: cinnofuradione]

cinnopentazone INN *anti-inflammatory* [also: cintazone]

cinnopropazone [see: apazone]

Cinobac capsules ℞ *urinary antibacterial* [cinoxacin] 250 mg

cinoctramide INN

cinodine HCl USAN *veterinary antibacterial*

cinolazepam INN

cinoquidox INN

cinoxacin USAN, USP, INN, BAN *urinary antibacterial*

cinoxate USAN, USP, INN *ultraviolet screen*

cinoxolone INN, BAN

cinoxopazide INN

cinperene USAN, INN *antipsychotic*

cinprazole INN

cinpropazide INN

cinquefoil (*Potentilla anserina; P. canadensis; P. reptans*) plant *medicinal herb used as an antispasmodic and astringent*

cinromide USAN, INN *anticonvulsant*

cintazone USAN *anti-inflammatory* [also: cinnopentazone]

cintramide INN *antipsychotic* [also: cintriamide]

cintredekin besudotox *investigational antineoplastic for brain tumors*

cintriamide USAN *antipsychotic* [also: cintramide]

cinuperone INN

cioteronel USAN, INN *antiandrogen*

cipamfylline USAN *antiviral agent; tumor necrosis factor alpha inhibitor*

cipemastat USAN, INN *matrix metalloproteinase inhibitor; investigational cartilage protective agent for rheumatoid arthritis*

cipionate INN *combining name for radicals or groups* [also: cypionate]

ciprafamide INN

Cipralan ℞ *investigational antiarrhythmic* [cifenline succinate]

Cipralex (name changed to Lexapro upon marketing release in 2002)

ciprazafone INN

ciprefadol INN *analgesic* [also: ciprefadol succinate]

ciprefadol succinate USAN *analgesic* [also: ciprefadol]

Cipro Cystitis Pack (6 film-coated tablets) ℞ *broad-spectrum fluoroquinolone antibiotic* [ciprofloxacin] 100 mg ⊡ Septa; Septra

Cipro film-coated tablets, powder for oral suspension ℞ *broad-spectrum fluoroquinolone antibiotic* [ciprofloxacin] 250, 500, 750 mg; 250, 500 mg/5 mL ⊡ Septa; Septra

Cipro HC Otic ear drop suspension ℞ *topical broad-spectrum fluoroquinolone antibiotic; corticosteroidal anti-inflammatory* [ciprofloxacin; hydrocortisone] 0.2%•1% (2•10 mg/mL)

Cipro I.V. ℞ *broad-spectrum fluoroquinolone antibiotic* [ciprofloxacin] 200, 400 mg/vial ⊡ Septa; Septra

Cipro XR film-coated extended-release tablets ℞ *broad-spectrum fluoroquinolone antibiotic* [ciprofloxacin] 500, 1000 mg

ciprocinonide USAN, INN *adrenocortical steroid*

Ciprodex ear drop suspension ℞ *broad-spectrum fluoroquinolone antibiotic; corticosteroidal anti-inflammatory* [ciprofloxacin HCl; dexamethasone] 0.3%•0.1%

ciprofibrate USAN, INN, BAN *antihyperlipoproteinemic*

ciprofloxacin USAN, INN, BAN *broad-spectrum fluoroquinolone antibiotic* 100, 250, 500, 750 mg oral; 250, 500 mg/5 mL oral; 0.3% eye drops

ciprofloxacin HCl USAN, USP, JAN *broad-spectrum bactericidal antibiotic*

cipropride INN

ciproquazone INN

ciproquinate INN *coccidiostat for poultry* [also: cyproquinate]

ciprostene INN *platelet antiaggregatory agent* [also: ciprostene calcium]

ciprostene calcium USAN *platelet antiaggregatory agent* [also: ciprostene]

ciproximide INN *antipsychotic; antidepressant* [also: cyproximide]

ciramadol USAN, INN *analgesic*

ciramadol HCl USAN *analgesic*

cirazoline INN

Circavite-T tablets OTC *vitamin/mineral/iron supplement* [multiple vitamins & minerals; iron] ≝•12 mg

cirolemycin USAN, INN *antineoplastic; antibacterial*

cisapride USAN, INN, BAN, JAN *peristaltic stimulant; treatment for nocturnal heartburn due to gastroesophageal reflux disease; (withdrawn from U.S. markets in 2000 due to increased cardiac arrhythmias)*

cisatracurium besylate USAN *nondepolarizing neuromuscular blocker*

CISCA; CisCA (cisplatin, cyclophosphamide, Adriamycin) *chemotherapy protocol for bladder cancer*

CISCA$_{II}$/VB$_{IV}$ (cisplatin, cyclophosphamide, Adriamycin, vinblastine, bleomycin) *chemotherapy protocol for germ cell tumors*

cisclomiphene [now: enclomiphene]

cisconazole USAN, INN *antifungal*

cis-DDP (diamminedichloroplatinum) [see: cisplatin]

cis-diamminedichloroplatinum (DDP) [see: cisplatin]

cismadinone INN

cisplatin USAN, USP, INN, BAN *alkylating antineoplastic for metastatic testicular tumors, metastatic ovarian tumors, and advanced bladder cancer* 1 mg/mL injection

cisplatin & docetaxel *chemotherapy protocol for bladder cancer and non–small cell lung cancer (NSCLC)*

cisplatin & fluorouracil *chemotherapy protocol for cervical cancer, used in conjunction with radiation therapy*

cisplatin & gemcitabine *chemotherapy protocol for metastatic bladder cancer*

cisplatin & vinorelbine *chemotherapy protocol for cervical cancer and non–small cell lung cancer (NSCLC)*

cis-**platinum** [now: cisplatin]

cis-**platinum II** [now: cisplatin]

9-*cis*-retinoic acid [see: alitretinoin]

13-*cis*-retinoic acid [see: isotretinoin]

cistinexine INN

citalopram INN, BAN *selective serotonin reuptake inhibitor (SSRI) for major depression*

citalopram hydrobromide USAN *selective serotonin reuptake inhibitor (SSRI) for major depression* 10, 20, 40 mg oral; 10 mg/5 mL oral

Citanest Forte injection Ŗ *injectable local anesthetic for dental procedures* [prilocaine HCl; epinephrine] 4%•1:200 000

Citanest Plain injection Ŗ *injectable local anesthetic for dental procedures* [prilocaine HCl] 4%

citatepine INN

citenamide USAN, INN *anticonvulsant*

citenazone INN

citicoline INN, JAN *investigational (Phase III) oral treatment for ischemic stroke and head trauma* [also: citicoline sodium]

citicoline & dizocilpine maleate *investigational (Phase III) neuroprotective treatment for stroke*

citicoline sodium USAN *investigational (Phase III) oral treatment for ischemic stroke and head trauma* [also: citicoline]

citiolone INN, DCF

Citra pH oral solution OTC *antacid* [sodium citrate] 450 mg/5 mL

Citracal tablets OTC *calcium supplement* [calcium citrate] 200 mg Ca ▨ Citrucel

Citracal Caplets + D OTC *dietary supplement* [calcium citrate; vitamin D] 315 mg•200 IU ▨ Citrucel

Citracal Liquitab effervescent tablets OTC *calcium supplement* [calcium citrate] 500 mg Ca ▨ Citrucel

Citracal Plus with Magnesium tablets OTC *dietary supplement* [calcium

citrate; vitamin D; multiple minerals] 250 mg Ca•125 IU•▵

Citracal Prenatal tablets Ŗ *calcium/iron supplement* [calcium citrate; iron; folic acid; docusate sodium] 125•1•27•50 mg

Citralax effervescent granules OTC *saline laxative* [magnesium citrate; magnesium sulfate]

citrate dextrose [see: ACD solution]

citrate of magnesia [see: magnesium citrate]

citrate phosphate dextrose [see: anticoagulant citrate phosphate dextrose solution]

citrate phosphate dextrose adenine [see: anticoagulant citrate phosphate dextrose adenine solution]

citrated caffeine NF [see: caffeine citrate]

citric acid USP *pH adjusting agent; urinary acidifier*

citric acid, magnesium oxide & sodium carbonate [see: Suby solution G]

citrin [see: bioflavonoids]

Citrocarbonate effervescent granules OTC *antacid* [sodium bicarbonate; sodium citrate] 780•1820 mg/dose

Citrolith tablets Ŗ *urinary alkalinizing agent* [potassium citrate; sodium citrate] 50•950 mg

citronella (Cymbopogon nardus; C. winterianus) oil *medicinal herb for gastrointestinal spasms, promoting diuresis, and worms; also used as an antibacterial; not generally regarded as safe and effective for internal use as it is highly toxic*

Citrotein oral liquid, powder for oral liquid OTC *enteral nutritional therapy* [lactose-free formula]

citrovorum factor [see: leucovorin calcium]

Citrucel powder, tablets OTC *bulk laxative* [methylcellulose] 2 g/tbsp. or scoop; 500 mg ▨ Citracal

Citrucel Sugar Free powder OTC *bulk laxative* [methylcellulose; phenylalanine] 2 g•52 mg per tbsp. ▨ Citracal

Citrus bergamia; C. aurantium medicinal herb [see: bergamot oil]

citrus bioflavonoids [see: bioflavonoids]

Citrus Calcium coated tablets OTC *calcium supplement* [calcium citrate] 200 mg Ca

Citrus limon medicinal herb [see: lemon]

Citrus paradisi medicinal herb [see: grapefruit]

civamide *investigational (orphan) agent for postherpetic neuralgia of the trigeminal nerve*

CIVPP (chlorambucil, vinblastine, procarbazine, prednisone) *chemotherapy protocol*

8-Cl cAMP (8-chloroadenosine monophosphate, cyclic) [see: tocladesine]

CLA (conjugated linoleic acid) [q.v.]

cladribine *antimetabolite antineoplastic for hairy-cell leukemia (orphan); investigational (orphan) for chronic lymphocytic leukemia, myeloid leukemia, multiple sclerosis, and non-Hodgkin lymphoma* 1 mg/mL injection

Claforan powder or frozen premix for IV or IM injection ℞ *cephalosporin antibiotic* [cefotaxime sodium] 0.5, 1, 2, 10 g

clamidoxic acid INN, BAN

clamoxyquin BAN *antiamebic* [also: clamoxyquin HCl; clamoxyquine]

clamoxyquin HCl USAN *antiamebic* [also: clamoxyquine; clamoxyquin]

clamoxyquine INN *antiamebic* [also: clamoxyquin HCl; clamoxyquin]

clanfenur INN

clanobutin INN

clantifen INN

clara cell 10kDa protein *investigational (orphan) for prevention of bronchopulmonary dysplasia in neonates with respiratory distress syndrome* ⚗ Clearasil

Claravis capsules ℞ *keratolytic for severe recalcitrant cystic acne* [isotretinoin] 10, 20, 40 mg

claretin-12 [see: cyanocobalamin] ⚗ Claritin; Clarityne

Clarinex film-coated tablets, syrup ℞ *nonsedating antihistamine for allergic rhinitis and chronic idiopathic urticaria* [desloratadine] 5 mg; 2.5 mg/5 mL

Clarinex RediTabs (rapidly disintegrating tablets) ℞ *nonsedating antihistamine for allergic rhinitis and chronic idiopathic urticaria* [desloratadine] 2.5, 5 mg

Clarinex-D 24 Hour extended-release tablets ℞ *nonsedating antihistamine plus decongestant for allergic rhinitis* [desloratadine; pseudoephedrine sulfate] 5•240 mg

Claripel cream ℞ *hyperpigmentation bleaching agent* [hydroquinone] 4%

clarithromycin USAN, INN, BAN, JAN *macrolide antibiotic* 250, 500, 1000 mg oral ⚗ dirithromycin; erythromycin

Claritin syrup OTC *nonsedating antihistamine for allergic rhinitis and chronic idiopathic urticaria* [loratadine] 1 mg/mL ⚗ claretin; Clarityne

Claritin 24-Hour Allergy tablets OTC *nonsedating antihistamine for allergic rhinitis and chronic idiopathic urticaria* [loratadine] 10 mg; 1 mg/mL ⚗ claretin; Clarityne

Claritin Hives Relief tablets OTC *nonsedating antihistamine for hives* [loratadine] 10 mg

Claritin Non-Drowsy Allergy tablets (name changed to **Claritin 24-Hour Allergy** in 2004)

Claritin RediTabs (rapidly disintegrating tablets) OTC *nonsedating antihistamine for allergic rhinitis and chronic idiopathic urticaria* [loratadine] 10 mg ⚗ claretin; Clarityne

Claritin-D 12 Hour; Claritin-D 24 Hour extended-release tablets OTC *decongestant; nonsedating antihistamine* [pseudoephedrine sulfate; loratadine] 120•5 mg; 240•10 mg

Clarityne (Mexican name for U.S. product Claritin) ⚗ claretin; Claritin

Claviceps purpurea medicinal herb [see: ergot]

clavulanate potassium USAN, USP *β-lactamase inhibitor; penicillin synergist*

clavulanic acid INN, BAN *β-lactamase inhibitor; penicillin synergist*

claw, scaly dragon's; turkey claw *medicinal herb* [see: coral root]

clay, kaolin *natural material* [see: kaolin]

clazolam USAN, INN *minor tranquilizer*

clazolimine USAN, INN *diuretic*

clazuril USAN, INN, BAN *coccidiostat for pigeons*

CLD-BOMP *chemotherapy protocol for cervical cancer* [see: BOMP]

Clean-N-Soak solution OTC *cleaning/ soaking solution for hard contact lenses*

Clear By Design gel (discontinued 2003) OTC *keratolytic for acne* [benzoyl peroxide] 2.5%

Clear Eyes eye drops OTC *topical ophthalmic decongestant and vasoconstrictor* [naphazoline HCl] 0.012%

Clear Eyes ACR eye drops OTC *topical ophthalmic decongestant and astringent* [naphazoline HCl; zinc sulfate] 0.012%•0.25%

Clear Total Lice Elimination System kit (shampoo + egg remover enzymes + nit comb) (discontinued 2003) OTC *pediculicide for lice* [pyrethrins; piperonyl butoxide] 0.3%•3%

Clear Tussin 30 oral liquid (discontinued 2002) OTC *antitussive; expectorant* [dextromethorphan hydrobromide; guaifenesin] 15•100 mg/5 mL

Clearasil lotion (discontinued 2003) OTC *keratolytic for acne* [benzoyl peroxide] 10% ⃞ clara cell

Clearasil Acne Treatment cream OTC *keratolytic for acne* [benzoyl peroxide] 10% ⃞ clara cell

Clearasil Acne-Fighting Pads OTC *keratolytic for acne* [salicylic acid; alcohol 2%] 2%

Clearasil Adult Care cream OTC *acne treatment* [sulfur; resorcinol; alcohol 10%]

Clearasil Antibacterial Soap bar OTC *medicated cleanser for acne* [triclosan]

Clearasil Clearstick topical liquid OTC *keratolytic for acne* [salicylic acid; alcohol 39%] 1.25%, 2%

Clearasil Daily Face Wash topical liquid OTC *medicated cleanser for acne* [triclosan] 0.3%

Clearasil Double Clear; Clearasil Double Textured medicated pads OTC *keratolytic for acne* [salicylic acid; alcohol 40%] 1.25%, 2%; 2%

Clearasil Medicated Deep Cleanser topical liquid OTC *keratolytic cleanser for acne* [salicylic acid; alcohol 42%] 0.5%

Clear-Atadine tablets OTC *nonsedating antihistamine for allergic rhinitis and chronic idiopathic urticaria* [loratadine] 10 mg

Clearblue Easy Digital Pregnancy Test test stick plus digital readout for home use *in vitro diagnostic aid; urine pregnancy test*

Clearblue Easy Ovulation Test test sticks for home use (7 sticks per package) OTC *in vitro diagnostic aid; urine ovulation test*

Clearblue Easy Pregnancy Test test stick for home use *in vitro diagnostic aid; urine pregnancy test*

Clearly Cala-gel OTC *topical antihistamine* [diphenhydramine HCl]

Clearplan Easy test kit for home use (discontinued 2004) *in vitro diagnostic aid to predict ovulation time*

Clearview Chlamydia test for professional use *in vitro diagnostic aid for Chlamydia trachomatis* [color-label immunoassay]

cleavers; cleaverwort *medicinal herb* [see: bedstraw]

clebopride USAN, INN *antiemetic*

clefamide INN, BAN

clemastine USAN, BAN *ethanolamine antihistamine*

clemastine fumarate USAN, USP, BAN *ethanolamine antihistamine* 1.34, 2.68 mg oral; 0.67 mg/5 mL

Clematis cirrhosa; C. virginiana *medicinal herb* [see: woodbine]

clemeprol INN, BAN

clemizole INN, BAN

clemizole penicillin INN, BAN

clenbuterol INN, BAN

Clenia cream, foaming wash ℞ *treatment for acne, rosacea, and seborrheic dermatitis* [sulfacetamide sodium; sulfur] 10%•5%

clenoliximab *investigational (Phase I/ II) anti-CD4 antibody for the treatment of rheumatoid arthritis*

clenpirin INN [also: clenpyrin]

clenpyrin BAN [also: clenpirin]

clentiazem INN *calcium channel antagonist* [also: clentiazem maleate]

clentiazem maleate USAN *calcium channel antagonist* [also: clentiazem]

Cleocin capsules ℞ *antibiotic; investigational (orphan) for AIDS-related* Pneumocystis carinii *pneumonia* [clindamycin HCl] 75, 150, 300 mg ▣ bleomycin; Lincocin

Cleocin vaginal cream in prefilled applicator, vaginal ovules (suppositories) ℞ *antibiotic for bacterial vaginosis* [clindamycin phosphate] 2%; 100 mg

Cleocin Pediatric granules for oral solution ℞ *antibiotic* [clindamycin palmitate HCl] 75 mg/5 mL

Cleocin Phosphate IV infusion, IM injection ℞ *antibiotic; investigational (orphan) for AIDS-related* Pneumocystis carinii *pneumonia* [clindamycin phosphate] 150 mg/mL

Cleocin T gel, lotion, topical suspension, pledgets ℞ *antibiotic for acne* [clindamycin phosphate] 1%

Clerz 2; Clerz Plus solution OTC *rewetting solution for hard or soft contact lenses*

cletoquine INN, BAN

Clexane (European name for U.S. product **Lovenox**)

clibucaine INN

click.easy (trademarked device) *reconstitution device for use with one.click prefilled auto-injector*

clidafidine INN

clidanac INN

clidinium bromide USAN, USP, INN, BAN *GI anticholinergic; peptic ulcer adjunct*

clidinium bromide & chlordiazepoxide HCl *GI anticholinergic; anxiolytic* 2.5•5 mg

Climara transdermal patch ℞ *estrogen replacement therapy for the treatment of postmenopausal symptoms and prevention of postmenopausal osteoporosis* [estradiol] 25, 37.5, 50, 60, 75, 100 μg/day

ClimaraPro transdermal patch ℞ *hormone replacement therapy for the treatment of postmenopausal symptoms and prevention of postmenopausal osteoporosis* [levonorgestrel; estradiol] 15• 45 μg/day

climazolam INN

climbazole INN, BAN

climiqualine INN

Clinac BPO gel ℞ *keratolytic for acne* [benzoyl peroxide] 7%

clinafloxacin HCl USAN *quinolone antibacterial*

Clinda-Derm topical solution (discontinued 2003) ℞ *antibiotic for acne* [clindamycin phosphate] 1%

Clindagel gel ℞ *antibiotic for acne* [clindamycin phosphate] 1%

ClindaMax gel, lotion, topical suspension ℞ *antibiotic for acne* [clindamycin phosphate] 1%

ClindaMax vaginal cream in prefilled applicators ℞ *antibiotic for bacterial vaginosis* [clindamycin phosphate] 2%

clindamycin USAN, INN, BAN *lincosamide antibiotic; investigational (orphan) for AIDS-related* Pneumocystis carinii *pneumonia*

clindamycin HCl USP, BAN *lincosamide antibiotic; investigational (orphan) for AIDS-related* Pneumocystis carinii *pneumonia* 75, 150, 300 mg oral

clindamycin HCl & primaquine phosphate *investigational (orphan) for AIDS-associated* Pneumocystis carinii *pneumonia*

clindamycin palmitate HCl USAN, USP *lincosamide antibiotic*

clindamycin phosphate USAN, USP *lincosamide antibiotic* 1% topical; 150 mg/mL injection

Clindesse vaginal cream in prefilled applicators ℞ *antibiotic for bacterial vaginosis* [clindamycin phosphate] 2%

Clindets topical suspension, pledgets ℞ *antibiotic for acne* [clindamycin; alcohol 52%] 1%

Clinipak (trademarked packaging form) *unit dose package*

Clinistix reagent strips for home use *in vitro diagnostic aid for urine glucose*

Clinitest reagent tablets for home use *in vitro diagnostic aid for urine glucose*

clinocaine HCl [see: procaine HCl]

clinofibrate INN

clinolamide INN

Clinoril tablets ℞ *antiarthritic; nonsteroidal anti-inflammatory drug (NSAID) for ankylosing spondylitis and acute bursitis/tendinitis* [sulindac] 150, 200 mg

clioquinol USP, INN, BAN *topical antibacterial and antifungal* 3% topical

clioxanide USAN, INN, BAN *anthelmintic* ⍰ Clinoxide

clipoxamine [see: cliropamine]

cliprofen USAN, INN *anti-inflammatory*

cliropamine INN

clobamine mesylate [now: cilobamine mesylate]

clobazam USAN, INN, BAN *minor benzodiazepine tranquilizer; anxiolytic*

clobedolum [see: clonitazene]

clobenoside INN

clobenzepam INN

clobenzorex INN

clobenztropine INN

clobetasol INN, BAN *topical corticosteroidal anti-inflammatory* [also: clobetasol propionate]

clobetasol propionate USAN *topical corticosteroidal anti-inflammatory for scalp dermatoses and plaque psoriasis* [also: clobetasol] 0.05% topical

clobetasone INN, BAN *topical corticosteroidal anti-inflammatory* [also: clobetasone butyrate]

clobetasone butyrate USAN *topical corticosteroidal anti-inflammatory* [also: clobetasone]

Clobex lotion, shampoo ℞ *corticosteroidal anti-inflammatory* [clobetasol propionate] 0.05%

clobutinol INN

clobuzarit INN, BAN

clocanfamide INN

clocapramine INN

clociguanil INN, BAN

clocinizine INN

clocortolone INN *topical corticosteroid* [also: clocortolone acetate]

clocortolone acetate USAN *topical corticosteroid* [also: clocortolone]

clocortolone pivalate USAN, USP *topical corticosteroid*

clocoumarol INN

Clocream cream OTC *moisturizer; emollient* [cod liver oil (vitamins A and E); cholecalciferol; vitamin A palmitate]

clodacaine INN

clodanolene USAN, INN *skeletal muscle relaxant*

clodantoin INN *antifungal* [also: chlordantoin]

clodazon INN *antidepressant* [also: clodazon HCl]

clodazon HCl USAN *antidepressant* [also: clodazon]

Cloderm cream ℞ *corticosteroidal anti-inflammatory* [clocortolone pivalate] 0.1%

clodoxopone INN

clodronate disodium *bisphosphonate bone resorption inhibitor for hypercalcemia of malignancy* [also: disodium clodronate]

clodronic acid USAN, INN, BAN *calcium regulator*

clofarabine *purine nucleoside antimetabolite antineoplastic for children with acute lymphoblastic leukemia (orphan); investigational (Phase III) for acute myelogenous leukemia*

Clofarex (name changed to **Clolar** upon marketing release in 2004)

clofazimine USAN, INN, BAN *bactericidal; tuberculostatic; leprostatic (orphan); available only to physicians enrolled in*

National Hansen Disease Programs through the FDA

clofedanol INN *antitussive* [also: chlophedianol HCl; chlophedianol]

clofedanol HCl [see: chlophedianol HCl]

clofenamic acid INN

clofenamide INN

clofenciclan INN

clofenetamine INN

clofenetamine HCl [see: clofenetamine]

clofenotane INN [also: chlorophenothane; dicophane]

clofenoxyde INN

clofenpyride [see: nicofibrate]

clofenvinfos INN [also: chlorfenvinphos]

clofeverine INN

clofexamide INN

clofezone INN

clofibrate USAN, USP, INN, BAN *triglyceride-lowering antihyperlipidemic for primary dysbetalipoproteinemia (type III hyperlipidemia) and hypertriglyceridemia (types IV and V hyperlipidemia)*

clofibric acid INN

clofibride INN

clofilium phosphate USAN, INN *antiarrhythmic*

clofinol [see: nicofibrate]

cloflucarban USAN *disinfectant* [also: halocarban]

clofluperol INN, BAN *antipsychotic* [also: seperidol HCl]

clofluperol HCl [see: seperidol HCl]

clofoctol INN

cloforex INN

clofurac INN

clogestone INN, BAN *progestin* [also: clogestone acetate]

clogestone acetate USAN *progestin* [also: clogestone]

cloguanamil INN, BAN [also: cloguanamile]

cloguanamile BAN [also: cloguanamil]

Clolar IV infusion ℞ *purine nucleoside antimetabolite antineoplastic for children with acute lymphoblastic leukemia (orphan); investigational (Phase III)*

for acute myelogenous leukemia [clofarabine] 1 mg/mL

clomacran INN, BAN *antipsychotic* [also: clomacran phosphate]

clomacran phosphate USAN *antipsychotic* [also: clomacran]

clomegestone INN *progestin* [also: clomegestone acetate]

clomegestone acetate USAN *progestin* [also: clomegestone]

clometacin INN

clometerone INN *antiestrogen* [also: clometherone]

clometherone USAN *antiestrogen* [also: clometerone]

clomethiazole INN [also: chlormethiazole]

clomethiazole edisylate USAN *GABA (A) receptor modulator for acute ischemic stroke*

clometocillin INN

Clomid tablets ℞ *ovulation stimulant* [clomiphene citrate] 50 mg

clomide [see: aklomide]

clomifene INN *gonad-stimulating principle; ovulation stimulant* [also: clomiphene citrate; clomiphene]

clomifenoxide INN

clominorex USAN, INN *anorectic*

clomiphene BAN *gonad-stimulating principle; ovulation stimulant* [also: clomiphene citrate; clomifene] ② clonidine

clomiphene citrate USAN, USP *gonad-stimulating principle; ovulation stimulant* [also: clomifene; clomiphene] 50 mg oral

clomipramine INN, BAN *tricyclic antidepressant for obsessive-compulsive disorders* [also: clomipramine HCl]

clomipramine HCl USAN *tricyclic antidepressant for obsessive-compulsive disorders* [also: clomipramine] 25, 50, 75 mg oral

clomocycline INN, BAN

clomoxir INN

Clomycin ointment (discontinued 2001) OTC *topical antibiotic; anesthetic* [polymyxin B sulfate; bacitracin;

neomycin sulfate; lidocaine] 5000
U•500 U•3.5 mg•40 mg per g

clonazepam USAN, USP, INN, BAN *anti-convulsant; anxiolytic for panic disorder; investigational (orphan) for hyperex-plexia (startle disease)* 0.5, 1, 2 mg oral

clonazoline INN

clonidine USAN, INN, BAN *centrally acting antiadrenergic antihypertensive; adjunct to epidural opioid analgesics for severe cancer pain (orphan)* ② clomi-phene; Klonopin; quinidine

clonidine HCl USAN, USP, BAN *centrally acting antiadrenergic antihyper-tensive; adjunct to epidural opioid anal-gesics for severe cancer pain (orphan)* 0.1, 0.2, 0.3 mg oral

clonitazene INN, BAN

clonitrate USAN, INN *coronary vasodilator*

clonixeril USAN, INN *analgesic*

clonixin USAN, INN *analgesic*

clopamide USAN, INN, BAN *antihyper-tensive; diuretic*

clopenthixol USAN, INN, BAN *antipsy-chotic*

cloperastine INN

cloperidone INN *sedative* [also: cloper-idone HCl]

cloperidone HCl USAN *sedative* [also: cloperidone]

clophenoxate [see: meclofenoxate]

clopidogrel INN, BAN *platelet aggrega-tion inhibitor for stroke, myocardial infarction, peripheral artery disease, and acute coronary syndrome*

clopidogrel bisulfate USAN *platelet aggregation inhibitor for stroke, myo-cardial infarction, peripheral artery dis-ease, and acute coronary syndrome*

clopidol USAN, INN, BAN *coccidiostat for poultry*

clopimozide USAN, INN *antipsychotic*

clopipazan INN *antipsychotic* [also: clo-pipazan mesylate]

clopipazan mesylate USAN *antipsy-chotic* [also: clopipazan]

clopirac USAN, INN, BAN *anti-inflam-matory*

cloponone INN, BAN

clopoxide [see: chlordiazepoxide]

clopoxide chloride [see: chlordiazep-oxide HCl]

Clopra tablets ℞ *antidopaminergic; antiemetic for chemotherapy; peristaltic* [metoclopramide HCl] 10 mg

cloprednol USAN, INN, BAN *corticoster-oid; anti-inflammatory*

cloprostenol INN, BAN *prostaglandin* [also: cloprostenol sodium]

cloprostenol sodium USAN *prostaglan-din* [also: cloprostenol]

cloprothiazole INN

cloquinate INN, BAN

cloquinozine INN

cloracetadol INN

cloral betaine INN *sedative* [also: chlo-ral betaine]

cloramfenicol pantotenate complex INN *antibacterial; antirickettsial* [also: chloramphenicol pantothenate com-plex]

cloranolol INN

clorarsen [see: dichlorophenarsine HCl]

clorazepate dipotassium USAN, USP *benzodiazepine anxiolytic; minor tran-quilizer; alcohol withdrawal aid; anti-convulsant adjunct* [also: dipotassium clorazepate] 3.75, 7.5, 15 mg oral

clorazepate monopotassium USAN *minor tranquilizer*

clorazepic acid BAN

cloretate INN *sedative; hypnotic* [also: clorethate]

clorethate USAN *sedative; hypnotic* [also: cloretate]

clorexolone USAN, INN, BAN *diuretic*

Clorfed extended-release tablets ℞ *decongestant; antihistamine* [pseudo-ephedrine HCl; chlorpheniramine maleate] 60•4 mg

clorgiline INN [also: clorgyline]

clorgyline BAN [also: clorgiline]

cloricromen INN

cloridarol INN

clorindanic acid INN

clorindanol INN *spermaticide* [also: chlorindanol]

clorindione INN, BAN

clormecaine INN

clorofene INN *disinfectant* [also: clorophene]

cloroperone INN *antipsychotic* [also: cloroperone HCl]

cloroperone HCl USAN *antipsychotic* [also: cloroperone]

clorophene USAN *disinfectant* [also: clorofene]

cloroqualone INN

clorotepine INN

Clorpactin WCS-90 powder for solution OTC *topical antimicrobial* [oxychlorosene sodium] 2 g

clorprenaline INN, BAN *adrenergic; bronchodilator* [also: clorprenaline HCl]

clorprenaline HCl USAN *adrenergic; bronchodilator* [also: clorprenaline]

Clorpres tablets ℞ *antihypertensive; diuretic* [clonidine HCl; chlorthalidone] 0.1•15 mg; 0.2•15 mg; 0.3•15 mg

clorquinaldol [see: chlorquinaldol]

clorsulon USAN, INN *antiparasitic; fasciolicide*

clortermine INN *anorectic* [also: clortermine HCl]

clortermine HCl USAN *anorectic* [also: clortermine]

closantel USAN, INN, BAN *anthelmintic*

closilate INN *combining name for radicals or groups* [also: closylate]

closiramine INN *antihistamine* [also: closiramine aceturate]

closiramine aceturate USAN *antihistamine* [also: closiramine]

clostebol INN [also: clostebol acetate]

clostebol acetate BAN [also: clostebol]

clostridial collagenase *investigational (Phase II, orphan) agent for advanced Dupuytren disease*

Clostridium botulinum toxin [see: botulinum toxin]

closylate USAN, BAN *combining name for radicals or groups* [also: closilate]

clotbur *medicinal herb* [see: burdock]

clothiapine USAN, BAN *antipsychotic* [also: clotiapine]

clothixamide maleate USAN *antipsychotic* [also: clotixamide]

clotiapine INN *antipsychotic* [also: clothiapine]

clotiazepam INN

cloticasone INN, BAN *anti-inflammatory* [also: cloticasone propionate]

cloticasone propionate USAN *anti-inflammatory* [also: cloticasone]

clotioxone INN

clotixamide INN *antipsychotic* [also: clothixamide maleate]

clotixamide maleate [see: clothixamide maleate]

Clotrimaderm ⓒ cream, topical solution, vaginal cream OTC *topical antifungal* [clotrimazole] 1%

clotrimazole (CLT) USAN, USP, INN, BAN, JAN *broad-spectrum antifungal; investigational (orphan) for sickle cell disease* 1% topical; 100 mg vaginal; 10 mg troches ⍰ co-trimoxazole

clotrimazole & betamethasone dipropionate *broad-spectrum antifungal; corticosteroidal anti-inflammatory* 1%•0.05% topical

clotrimidazole *investigational (orphan) for sickle cell disease*

cloudberry *medicinal herb* [see: blackberry]

clove oil NF

clover, king's; sweet clover *medicinal herb* [see: melilot]

clover, marsh *medicinal herb* [see: buckbean]

clover, purple; wild clover *medicinal herb* [see: red clover]

clover, winter *medicinal herb* [see: squaw vine]

cloves (*Caryophyllus aromaticus; Eugenia caryophyllata; Syzygium aromaticum*) seed and oil *medicinal herb for bad breath, bronchial secretions, dizziness, earache, fever, nausea, platelet aggregation inhibition, poor circulation, and thrombosis; also used topically as an analgesic and antiseptic*

clovoxamine INN

cloxacepride INN

cloxacillin INN, BAN *penicillinase-resistant penicillin antibiotic* [also: cloxacillin benzathine]

cloxacillin benzathine USP *penicillinase-resistant penicillin antibiotic* [also: cloxacillin]

cloxacillin sodium USAN, USP *penicillinase-resistant penicillin antibiotic*

Cloxapen capsules (discontinued 2002) ℞ *penicillinase-resistant penicillin antibiotic* [cloxacillin sodium] 250, 500 mg

cloxazolam INN

cloxestradiol INN

cloxifenol [see: triclosan]

cloximate INN

cloxiquine INN *antibacterial* [also: cloxyquin]

cloxotestosterone INN

cloxphendyl [see: cloxypendyl]

cloxypendyl INN

cloxyquin USAN *antibacterial* [also: cloxiquine]

clozapine USAN, INN, BAN *novel (atypical) dibenzapine antipsychotic for severe schizophrenia and recurrent suicidal behavior; sedative; also used for agitation and psychosis due to Alzheimer and other dementias* 12.5, 25, 100 mg oral

Clozaril tablets ℞ *novel (atypical) dibenzapine antipsychotic for severe schizophrenia and recurrent suicidal behavior; sedative; also used for agitation and psychosis due to Alzheimer and other dementias* [clozapine] 25, 100 mg

CLT (clotrimazole) [q.v.]

club, shepherd's *medicinal herb* [see: mullein]

club moss (*Lycopodium clavatum*) spores *medicinal herb used as a hemostatic and vulnerary*

cluster, wax *medicinal herb* [see: wintergreen]

C-Max gradual-release tablets OTC *vitamin/mineral supplement* [vitamin C; multiple minerals] 1 • ≝ g

CMC (carboxymethylcellulose) gum [see: carboxymethylcellulose sodium]

CMC (cyclophosphamide, methotrexate, CCNU) *chemotherapy protocol*

CMC-VAP (cyclophosphamide, methotrexate, CCNU, vincristine, Adriamycin, procarbazine) *chemotherapy protocol*

CMF; CMF-IV (cyclophosphamide, methotrexate, fluorouracil) *chemotherapy protocol for breast cancer*

CMF/AV (cyclophosphamide, methotrexate, fluorouracil, Adriamycin, Oncovin) *chemotherapy protocol*

CMFAVP (cyclophosphamide, methotrexate, fluorouracil, Adriamycin, vincristine, prednisone) *chemotherapy protocol*

CMFP; CMF-P (cyclophosphamide, methotrexate, fluorouracil, prednisone) *chemotherapy protocol for breast cancer*

CMFPT (cyclophosphamide, methotrexate, fluorouracil, prednisone, tamoxifen) *chemotherapy protocol*

CMFPTH (cyclophosphamide, methotrexate, fluorouracil, prednisone, tamoxifen, Halotestin) *chemotherapy protocol*

CMFT (cyclophosphamide, methotrexate, fluorouracil, tamoxifen) *chemotherapy protocol*

CMFVAT (cyclophosphamide, methotrexate, fluorouracil, vincristine, Adriamycin, testosterone) *chemotherapy protocol*

CMFVP (cyclophosphamide, methotrexate, fluorouracil, vincristine, prednisone) *chemotherapy protocol for breast cancer* [two dosing protocols: Cooper protocol and SWOG protocol]

CMH (cyclophosphamide, *m*-AMSA, hydroxyurea) *chemotherapy protocol*

C-MOPP (cyclophosphamide, mechlorethamine, Oncovin, procarbazine, prednisone) *chemotherapy protocol for Hodgkin or non-Hodgkin lymphoma*

CMV (cisplatin, methotrexate, vinblastine) *chemotherapy protocol for bladder cancer*

CMV-IGIV (cytomegalovirus immune globulin intravenous) [see: globulin, immune]

CN2 HCl [see: mechlorethamine HCl]

CNF (cyclophosphamide, Novantrone, fluorouracil) *chemotherapy protocol for breast cancer* [also: CFM; FNC]

Cnicus benedictus *medicinal herb* [see: blessed thistle]

CNOP (cyclophosphamide, Novantrone, Oncovin, prednisone) *chemotherapy protocol for non-Hodgkin lymphoma*

CO Fluoxetine ⒸⒶⓃ *capsules* ℞ *selective serotonin reuptake inhibitor (SSRI) for depression, obsessive-compulsive disorder (OCD), and bulimia nervosa* [fluoxetine HCl] 10, 20 mg

Co I (coenzyme I) [see: nadide]

CO_2 (carbon dioxide) [q.v.]

^{57}Co [see: cobaltous chloride Co 57]

^{57}Co [see: cyanocobalamin Co 57]

^{58}Co [see: cyanocobalamin (^{58}Co)]

^{60}Co [see: cobaltous chloride Co 60]

^{60}Co [see: cyanocobalamin Co 60]

coachweed *medicinal herb* [see: bedstraw]

coagulants *a class of agents that promote or accelerate clotting of the blood*

coagulation factor VIIa [see: factor VIIa, recombinant]

coagulation factor IX (human) [see: factor IX complex; nonacog alfa]

Coagulin-B ℞ *investigational (orphan) agent for moderate to severe hemophilia* [adeno-associated viral vector containing the gene for human coagulation Factor IX]

coakum *medicinal herb* [see: pokeweed]

coal tar USP *topical antieczematic; antiseborrheic*

co-amoxiclav (amoxicillin & potassium clavulanate) [q.v.]

COAP (cyclophosphamide, Oncovin, ara-C, prednisone) *chemotherapy protocol*

Co-Apap *tablets* (discontinued 2002) OTC *antitussive; decongestant; antihistamine; analgesic* [dextromethorphan hydrobromide; pseudoephedrine HCl; chlorpheniramine maleate; acetaminophen] 15•30•2•325 mg

COAP-BLEO (cyclophosphamide, Oncovin, ara-C, prednisone, bleomycin) *chemotherapy protocol*

Coated Aspirin; Coated Aspirin Extra Strength; Coated Aspirin Arthritis Pain Relief; Coated Aspirin Daily Low Dose ⒸⒶⓃ OTC *analgesic; antipyretic; anti-inflammatory; antirheumatic* [aspirin] 235 mg; 500 mg; 650 mg; 81 mg

COB (cisplatin, Oncovin, bleomycin) *chemotherapy protocol for head and neck cancer*

cobalamin concentrate USP *vitamin B_{12}; hematopoietic*

cobalt *element (Co)*

cobalt-labeled vitamin B_{12} [see: cyanocobalamin Co 57 & Co 60]

cobaltous chloride Co 57 USAN *radioactive agent*

cobaltous chloride Co 60 USAN *radioactive agent*

cobamamide INN

COBARTin ℞ *investigational (orphan) agent for steatorrhea in short bowel syndrome* [bile acids, conjugated]

cocaine USP, BAN *topical anesthetic for mucous membranes; widely abused as a street drug, derived from coca leaves* 4%, 10% *topical*

cocaine, crack *street drug made by converting cocaine HCl into a form that can be smoked, which causes a faster, more intense effect*

cocaine HCl USP *topical anesthetic for mucous membranes; widely abused as a street drug, derived from coca leaves* 135 mg oral; 4%, 10% *topical*

Cocaine Viscous *topical solution* ℞ *topical mucosal anesthesia* [cocaine] 4%, 10%

cocarboxylase INN [also: co-carboxylase]

co-carboxylase BAN [also: cocarboxylase]

cocashweed *medicinal herb* [see: life root]

coccidioidin USP *dermal coccidioidomycosis test*

cocculin [see: picrotoxin]

Cocculus lacunosus; C. suberosus *medicinal herb* [see: levant berry]

Cocculus palmatus medicinal herb [see: colombo]

Cochlearia armoracia medicinal herb [see: horseradish]

cocklebur *medicinal herb* [see: agrimony; burdock]

cockspur pepper *medicinal herb* [see: cayenne]

cockspur rye *medicinal herb* [see: ergot]

cocoa NF

cocoa *(Theobromo cacao)* bean *medicinal herb used as a cardiac stimulant, diuretic, and vasodilator*

cocoa butter NF *suppository base; emollient/protectant*

cocowort *medicinal herb* [see: shepherd's purse]

cod liver oil USP, BAN *vitamins A and D source; emollient/protectant*

cod liver oil, nondestearinated NF

codactide INN, BAN

Codal-DH syrup ℞ *narcotic antitussive; decongestant; antihistamine* [hydrocodone bitartrate; phenylephrine HCl; pyrilamine maleate] 1.66•5•8.33 mg/5 mL

Codal-DM syrup OTC *antitussive; decongestant; antihistamine* [dextromethorphan hydrobromide; phenylephrine HCl; pyrilamine maleate] 20•10•16.67 mg/10 mL

Codamine syrup, pediatric syrup (discontinued 2002) ℞ *narcotic antitussive; decongestant* [hydrocodone bitartrate; phenylpropanolamine HCl] 5•25 mg/5 mL; 2.5•12.5 mg/5 mL

CODE (cisplatin, Oncovin, doxorubicin, etoposide) *chemotherapy protocol for small cell lung cancer (SCLC)*

Codegest Expectorant oral liquid (discontinued 2002) ℞ *narcotic antitussive; decongestant; expectorant* [codeine phosphate; phenylpropanolamine HCl; guaifenesin] 10•12.5•100 mg/5 mL ② Codehist

Codehist DH elixir (discontinued 2002) ℞ *narcotic antitussive; decongestant; antihistamine* [codeine phosphate; pseudoephedrine HCl; chlorpheniramine maleate; alcohol 5.7%] 10•30•2 mg/5 mL ② Codegest

codehydrogenase I [see: nadide]

codeine USP, BAN *narcotic analgesic used as an antitussive; sometimes abused as a street drug* ② Kaodene

codeine & acetaminophen *narcotic analgesic* 15•300, 30•300, 60•300 mg oral; 12•30 mg/5 mL oral

codeine phosphate USP, BAN *narcotic analgesic used as an antitussive* 15 mg/5 mL oral; 15, 30 mg/mL injection

codeine phosphate & aspirin *narcotic antitussive; analgesic; antipyretic* 325•15 mg oral

codeine phosphate & aspirin & carisoprodol *narcotic analgesic; skeletal muscle relaxant* 16•325•200 mg oral

codeine phosphate & butalbital & acetaminophen & caffeine *narcotic antitussive; barbiturate sedative; analgesic* 30•50•325•40 mg oral

codeine phosphate & guaifenesin *antitussive; narcotic analgesic; expectorant* 10•300 mg oral; 10•100 mg/5 mL oral

codeine phosphate & promethazine HCl *narcotic antitussive; antihistamine* 10•6.25 mg/5 mL oral

codeine polistirex USAN *narcotic analgesic used as an antitussive*

codeine sulfate USP *narcotic analgesic used as an antitussive* 15, 30, 60 mg oral

codelcortone [see: prednisolone]

Codeprex extended-release oral suspension ℞ *narcotic antitussive; antihistamine* [codeine polistirex; chlorpheniramine polistirex] 20•4 mg/5 mL

co-dergocrine mesylate BAN *cognition adjuvant* [also: ergoloid mesylates]

Codiclear DH syrup ℞ *narcotic antitussive; expectorant* [hydrocodone bitartrate; guaifenesin] 5•100 mg/5 mL

Codimal capsules, film-coated tablets (discontinued 2002) OTC *decongestant;*

antihistamine; analgesic [pseudoephedrine HCl; chlorpheniramine maleate; acetaminophen] 30•2•325 mg

Codimal DH syrup ℞ *narcotic antitussive; decongestant; antihistamine* [hydrocodone bitartrate; phenylephrine HCl; pyrilamine maleate] 1.66•5•8.33 mg/5 mL

Codimal DM syrup OTC *antitussive; decongestant; antihistamine* [dextromethorphan hydrobromide; phenylephrine HCl; pyrilamine maleate] 20•10•16.67 mg/10 mL

Codimal PH syrup ℞ *narcotic antitussive; decongestant; antihistamine* [codeine phosphate; phenylephrine HCl; pyrilamine maleate] 20•10•16.66 mg/10 mL

Codimal-L.A.; Codimal-L.A. Half extended-release capsules (discontinued 2002) ℞ *decongestant; antihistamine* [pseudoephedrine HCl; chlorpheniramine maleate] 120•8 mg; 60•4 mg

codorphone [now: conorphone HCl]

codoxime USAN, INN *antitussive*

Coease intraocular injection ℞ *viscoelastic agent for ophthalmic surgery* [hyaluronate sodium] 12 mg/mL

coenzyme Q10 *natural enzyme cofactor used as a cardiac protectant, free radical scavenger, membrane stabilizer; investigational (orphan) for Huntington disease*

COF/COM (cyclophosphamide, Oncovin, fluorouracil + cyclophosphamide, Oncovin, methotrexate) *chemotherapy protocol*

coffeine [see: caffeine]

cofisatin INN

cofisatine [see: cofisatin]

cogazocine INN

Cogentin tablets, IV or IM injection ℞ *anticholinergic; antiparkinsonian* [benztropine mesylate] 0.5, 1, 2 mg; 1 mg/mL

Co-Gesic tablets ℞ *narcotic analgesic* [hydrocodone bitartrate; acetaminophen] 5•500 mg

Cognex capsules ℞ *reversible cholinesterase inhibitor; cognition adjuvant for*

Alzheimer dementia [tacrine HCl] 10, 20, 30, 40 mg

Cognitex; Cognitex with Pregnenolone softgels OTC *anti-aging supplement for improving mental function* [glyceryl phosphorylcholine; choline dihydrogen citrate; choline bitartrate; phosphatidylserine; vinpocetine; pantothenic acid; RNA/DNA; (pregnenolone)] 100•250•200•16.7•2.5•83.3•70.8•(8.3) mg

Co-Hist tablets (discontinued 2002) OTC *decongestant; antihistamine; analgesic* [pseudoephedrine HCl; chlorpheniramine maleate; acetaminophen] 30•2•325 mg

cohosh *medicinal herb* [see: black cohosh; blue cohosh; white cohosh]

Cola acuminata *medicinal herb* [see: kola nut]

Colace capsules, syrup, oral liquid OTC *laxative; stool softener* [docusate sodium] 50, 100 mg; 60 mg/15 mL; 150 mg/15 mL

Colace; Colace Infant/Child suppositories OTC *hyperosmolar laxative* [glycerin]

colaspase BAN *antineoplastic for acute lymphocytic leukemia (ALL)* [also: asparaginase]

Colazal capsules ℞ *gastrointestinal antiinflammatory for ulcerative colitis* [balsalazide disodium] 750 mg

Colazide (European name for U.S. product **Colazal**)

colchamine [see: demecolcine]

colchicine USP, JAN *gout suppressant; investigational (orphan) to stop the progression of multiple sclerosis* 0.6 mg oral; 1 mg injection

Colchicum autumnale; C. speciosum; C. vernum *medicinal herb* [see: autumn crocus]

Cold & Allergy elixir (discontinued 2001) OTC *decongestant; antihistamine* [phenylpropanolamine HCl; brompheniramine maleate] 12.5•2 mg/5 mL

cold cream USP

Cold Relief tablets (discontinued 2002) OTC *antitussive; decongestant; antihistamine; analgesic* [dextromethorphan hydrobromide; phenylpropanolamine HCl; chlorpheniramine maleate; acetaminophen] 10•12.5•2•325 mg

Cold Symptoms Relief tablets OTC *antitussive; decongestant; antihistamine; analgesic* [dextromethorphan hydrobromide; pseudoephedrine HCl; chlorpheniramine maleate; acetaminophen] 10•30•2•325 mg

Coldcough PD syrup ℞ *narcotic antitussive; decongestant; antihistamine* [dihydrocodeine bitartrate; phenylephrine HCl; chlorpheniramine maleate] 3•7.5•2 mg/5 mL

Coldec D extended-release caplets ℞ *decongestant; antihistamine* [pseudoephedrine HCl; carbinoxamine maleate] 80•8 mg

Coldec DM oral liquid ℞ *antitussive; decongestant; antihistamine* [dextromethorphan hydrobromide; pseudoephedrine HCl; brompheniramine maleate] 15•60•4 mg/5 mL

Cold-Gest sustained-release capsules (discontinued 2001) OTC *decongestant; antihistamine* [phenylpropanolamine HCl; chlorpheniramine maleate] 75•8 mg

Coldloc oral liquid (discontinued 2002) ℞ *decongestant; expectorant* [phenylpropanolamine HCl; phenylephrine HCl; guaifenesin] 20•5•100 mg/5 mL

Coldloc-LA sustained-release caplets (discontinued 2002) ℞ *decongestant; expectorant* [phenylpropanolamine HCl; guaifenesin] 75•600 mg

Coldmist JR sustained-release tablets ℞ *decongestant; expectorant* [pseudoephedrine HCl; guaifenesin] 48•595 mg

Coldmist LA extended-release caplets ℞ *decongestant; expectorant* [pseudoephedrine HCl; guaifenesin] 85•795 mg

Coldrine tablets (discontinued 2002) OTC *decongestant; analgesic* [pseudoephedrine HCl; acetaminophen] 30•325 mg

colecalciferol (vitamin D₃) INN *fat-soluble vitamin* [also: cholecalciferol]

colesevelam HCl USAN *bile acid sequestrant; nonabsorbable cholesterol-lowering polymer for hyperlipidemia*

Colestid tablets, granules ℞ *cholesterol-lowering antihyperlipidemic* [colestipol HCl] 1 g; 5 g/dose ⊠ colistin

colestipol INN, BAN *bile acid sequestrant; cholesterol-lowering antihyperlipidemic* [also: colestipol HCl] ⊠ colistin

colestipol HCl USAN, USP *bile acid sequestrant; cholesterol-lowering antihyperlipidemic* [also: colestipol] ⊠ colistin

colestolone USAN, INN *hypolipidemic*

colestyramine INN *bile salt ion-exchange resin; antihyperlipoproteinemic* [also: cholestyramine resin; cholestyramine]

colestyramine resin [see: cholestyramine]

colextran INN

Colfed-A sustained-release capsules ℞ *decongestant; antihistamine* [pseudoephedrine HCl; chlorpheniramine maleate] 120•8 mg

colfenamate INN

colforsin USAN, INN *antiglaucoma agent*

colfosceril palmitate USAN, INN, BAN *pulmonary surfactant for hyaline membrane disease and neonatal respiratory distress syndrome (orphan); investigational (orphan) for adult respiratory distress syndrome (ARDS)*

colic root *medicinal herb* [see: blazing star; star grass; wild yam]

colimecycline INN

colistimethate sodium USAN, USP, INN *bactericidal antibiotic* [also: colistin sulphomethate]

colistin INN, BAN *bactericidal antibiotic* [also: colistin sulfate] ⊠ Colestid; colestipol

colistin methanesulfonate [see: colistimethate sodium]

colistin sulfate USP *bactericidal antibiotic* [also: colistin]

colistin sulphomethate BAN *bactericidal antibiotic* [also: colistimethate sodium]

collagen *ophthalmic implant to block puncta and retain moisture; urethral injection for stress urinary incontinence*

collagen, purified bovine *injectable dermal filler for scars, wrinkles, and facial folds*

collagen, purified human *injectable dermal filler for scars, wrinkles, and facial folds*

collagen, purified type II *investigational (Phase III, orphan) oral treatment for juvenile rheumatoid arthritis*

collagen sponge, absorbable *topical local hemostat for surgery*

collagenase *topical proteolytic enzymes for necrotic tissue debridement; investigational (orphan) for Peyronie disease*

collagenase, clostridial [see: clostridial collagenase]

Collagenase Santyl ointment ℞ *proteolytic enzymes for debriding dermal ulcers and severely burned areas* [collagenase] 250 U/g

collard *medicinal herb* [see: skunk cabbage]

Collinsonia canadensis *medicinal herb* [see: stone root]

collodion USP *topical protectant*

colloidal aluminum hydroxide [see: aluminum hydroxide gel]

colloidal oatmeal *demulcent*

colloidal silicon dioxide [see: silicon dioxide, colloidal]

Collyrium for Fresh Eyes *ophthalmic solution* OTC *extraocular irrigating solution* [sterile isotonic solution]

Collyrium Fresh *eye drops* OTC *topical ophthalmic decongestant and vasoconstrictor* [tetrahydrozoline HCl] 0.05%

ColoCare *test kit for home use in vitro diagnostic aid for fecal occult blood*

colombo (Cocculus palmatus) *root medicinal herb used as an antiemetic and febrifuge*

colony-stimulating factors *a class of glycoproteins that stimulate the production of granulocytes and macrophages*

Color Allergy Screening Test (CAST) *reagent assay tubes in vitro diagnostic aid for immunoglobulin E in serum*

Color Ovulation Test *kit for home use* (discontinued 2004) *in vitro diagnostic aid to predict ovulation time*

ColoScreen *slide test for professional use in vitro diagnostic aid for fecal occult blood*

colterol INN *bronchodilator* [also: colterol mesylate]

colterol mesylate USAN *bronchodilator* [also: colterol]

colt's tail *medicinal herb* [see: fleabane; horseweed]

coltsfoot (Tussilago farfara) *buds, flowers, and leaves medicinal herb for asthma, bronchitis, dry cough, hay fever, lung disorders, excess mucus, and throat irritation*

Columbia Antiseptic *powder* OTC *astringent; antiseptic* [zinc oxide; talc; carbolic acid; boric acid]

columbine (Aquilegia vulgaris) *plant medicinal herb used as an astringent, diaphoretic, and diuretic*

Coly-Mycin M *powder for IV or IM injection* ℞ *bactericidal antibiotic* [colistimethate sodium] 150 mg

Coly-Mycin S Otic *suspension* ℞ *corticosteroidal anti-inflammatory; antibiotic* [hydrocortisone acetate; neomycin sulfate; colistin sulfate] 1%•4.71 mg•3 mg per mL

CoLyte *powder for oral solution* ℞ *pre-procedure bowel evacuant* [polyethylene glycol–electrolyte solution (PEG 3350)] 60 g/L

COM (cyclophosphamide, Oncovin, MeCCNU) *chemotherapy protocol*

COM (cyclophosphamide, Oncovin, methotrexate) *chemotherapy protocol*

COMA-A (cyclophosphamide, Oncovin, methotrexate/citrovo-

rum factor, Adriamycin, ara-C) *chemotherapy protocol*

COMB (cyclophosphamide, Oncovin, MeCCNU, bleomycin) *chemotherapy protocol*

COMB (Cytoxin, Oncovin, methotrexate, bleomycin) *chemotherapy protocol*

ComBgen tablets ℞ *vitamin B supplement* [vitamins B_6 and B_{12}; folic acid] 25•0.5•2.2 mg

CombiPatch transdermal patch ℞ *hormone replacement therapy for postmenopausal symptoms, hypogonadism, castration, and primary ovarian failure* [estradiol; norethindrone acetate] 5•14, 5•25 µg/day

Combipres 0.1; Combipres 0.2; Combipres 0.3 tablets ℞ *antihypertensive; diuretic* [clonidine HCl; chlorthalidone] 0.1•15 mg; 0.2•15 mg; 0.3•15 mg ⧉ Catapres

Combistix reagent strips *in vitro diagnostic aid for multiple urine products*

Combivent oral inhalation aerosol ℞ *anticholinergic bronchodilator for chronic bronchospasm with COPD* [ipratropium bromide; albuterol sulfate] 18•103 µg/dose

Combivir film-coated caplets ℞ *nucleoside reverse transcriptase inhibitor combination for HIV* [lamivudine; zidovudine] 150•300 mg

combretastatin A4 phosphate *investigational (orphan) agent for anaplastic, medullary, papillary, or follicular thyroid cancer*

Combunox film-coated caplets ℞ *narcotic analgesic* [oxycodone HCl; ibuprofen] 5•400 mg

COMe (Cytoxin, Oncovin, methotrexate) *chemotherapy protocol*

COMF (cyclophosphamide, Oncovin, methotrexate, fluorouracil) *chemotherapy protocol*

Comfort eye drops OTC *topical ophthalmic decongestant and vasoconstrictor* [naphazoline HCl] 0.03%

Comfort Tears eye drops OTC *ocular moisturizer/lubricant* [hydroxyethylcellulose]

ComfortCare GP Wetting & Soaking solution OTC *disinfecting/wetting/soaking solution for rigid gas permeable contact lenses*

Comfortine ointment (discontinued 2004) OTC *moisturizer; emollient; astringent; antiseptic* [vitamins A and D; lanolin; zinc oxide]

comfrey (*Symphytum officinale; S. tuberosum*) leaves and roots *medicinal herb for anemia, arthritis, blood cleansing, boils and sores, bruises, burns, edema, emphysema, fractures, gastric ulcers, hemorrhoids, and sprains; not generally regarded as safe and effective as it may be carcinogenic and hepatotoxic*

comfrey, spotted *medicinal herb* [see: lungwort]

Comhist tablets (discontinued 2002) ℞ *decongestant; antihistamine* [phenylephrine HCl; chlorpheniramine maleate; phenyltoloxamine citrate] 10•2•25 mg

Comhist LA long-acting capsules (discontinued 2002) ℞ *decongestant; antihistamine* [phenylephrine HCl; chlorpheniramine maleate; phenyltoloxamine citrate] 20•4•50 mg

COMLA (cyclophosphamide, Oncovin, methotrexate, leucovorin [rescue], ara-C) *chemotherapy protocol for non-Hodgkin lymphoma*

Commiphora abssynica; C. molmol; C. myrrha *medicinal herb* [see: myrrh]

Commiphora mukul *medicinal herb* [see: guggul]

Commit lozenges OTC *smoking deterrent; nicotine withdrawal aid* [nicotine polacrilex] 2, 4 mg

common bugloss *medicinal herb* [see: borage]

common elder *medicinal herb* [see: elderberry]

common flax *medicinal herb* [see: flaxseed]

comosain *investigational (orphan) proteolytic enzymes for debridement of severe burns*

COMP (CCNU, Oncovin, methotrexate, procarbazine) *chemotherapy protocol*

COMP (cyclophosphamide, Oncovin, methotrexate, prednisone) *chemotherapy protocol for pediatric Hodgkin lymphoma*

Compack (trademarked packaging form) *patient compliance package for oral contraceptives*

Compazine suppositories ℞ *conventional (typical) phenothiazine antipsychotic for schizophrenia; anxiolytic; antiemetic for nausea and vomiting; also used for acute treatment of migraine headaches* [prochlorperazine] 2.5, 5, 25 mg

Compazine syrup, IV or IM injection ℞ *conventional (typical) phenothiazine antipsychotic for schizophrenia; anxiolytic; antiemetic for nausea and vomiting; also used for acute treatment of migraine headaches* [prochlorperazine edisylate] 5 mg/5 mL; 5 mg/mL

Compazine tablets, Spansules (sustained-release capsules) ℞ *conventional (typical) phenothiazine antipsychotic for schizophrenia; anxiolytic; antiemetic for nausea and vomiting; also used for acute treatment of migraine headaches* [prochlorperazine maleate] 5, 10 mg; 10, 15 mg

Compete tablets OTC *vitamin/iron supplement* [multiple vitamins; ferrous gluconate; folic acid] ± •27•0.4 mg

Compleat Modified Formula closed system containers OTC *enteral nutritional therapy* [lactose-free formula]

Compleat Modified Formula ready-to-use oral liquid OTC *enteral nutritional therapy* [lactose-free formula]

Compleat Regular Formula ready-to-use oral liquid OTC *enteral nutritional therapy* [milk-based formula]

complement receptor type I, soluble recombinant human *investiga-tional (orphan) for adult respiratory distress syndrome*

Complete solution OTC *rewetting solution for soft contact lenses*

Complete All-in-One solution OTC *cleaning/disinfecting/rinsing/storage solution for soft contact lenses*

Complete Weekly Enzymatic Cleaner effervescent tablets OTC *enzymatic cleaner for soft contact lenses* [subtilisin A]

Complex 15 Face cream OTC *moisturizer; emollient*

Complex 15 Hand & Body cream, lotion OTC *moisturizer; emollient*

Comply oral liquid OTC *enteral nutritional therapy* [lactose-free formula]

component pertussis vaccine (alternate name for acellular pertussis vaccine) [see: diphtheria & tetanus toxoids & acellular pertussis (DTaP) vaccine, adsorbed]

Compound 347 liquid for vaporization ℞ *inhalation general anesthetic* [enflurane]

compound 42 [see: warfarin]

compound CB3025 [see: melphalan]

compound E [see: cortisone acetate]

compound F [see: hydrocortisone]

compound orange spirit [see: orange spirit, compound]

compound S [see: zidovudine]

compound solution of sodium chloride INN *fluid and electrolyte replenisher* [also: Ringer injection]

compound solution of sodium lactate INN *electrolyte and fluid replenisher; systemic alkalizer* [also: Ringer injection, lactated]

Compound W topical liquid, gel OTC *keratolytic* [salicylic acid in collodion] 17%

Compound W One Step Wart Remover for Kids pad OTC *keratolytic* [salicylic acid] 40%

Compoz gelcaps OTC *antihistaminic sleep aid* [diphenhydramine HCl] 25 mg

Compoz Nighttime Sleep Aid tablets OTC *antihistaminic sleep aid* [diphenhydramine HCl] 50 mg

compressible sugar [see: sugar, compressible]

Compro suppositories ℞ *conventional (typical) phenothiazine antipsychotic for schizophrenia; anxiolytic; antiemetic for nausea and vomiting; also used for acute treatment of migraine headaches* [prochlorperazine] 25 mg

Computer Eye Drops OTC *ophthalmic moisturizer and emollient* [glycerin] 1%

COMT (catechol-O-methyltransferase) inhibitors *a class of antiparkinson agents that stabilize serum levodopa levels by inhibiting an enzyme that breaks down the levodopa before it reaches the brain*

Comtan film-coated tablets ℞ *COMT inhibitor for Parkinson disease* [entacapone] 200 mg

Comtrex oral liquid (discontinued 2002) OTC *antitussive; decongestant; antihistamine; analgesic* [dextromethorphan hydrobromide; pseudoephedrine HCl; chlorpheniramine maleate; acetaminophen] 3.3•10•0.67•108.3 mg/5 mL

Comtrex, Cough Formula oral liquid (discontinued 2002) OTC *antitussive; decongestant; expectorant; analgesic* [dextromethorphan hydrobromide; pseudoephedrine HCl; guaifenesin; acetaminophen; alcohol 20%] 7.5•15•50•125 mg/5 mL

Comtrex Acute Head Cold caplets OTC *decongestant; antihistamine; analgesic* [pseudoephedrine HCl; brompheniramine maleate; acetaminophen] 30•2•500 mg

Comtrex Allergy-Sinus Treatment caplets, tablets OTC *decongestant; antihistamine; analgesic* [pseudoephedrine HCl; chlorpheniramine maleate; acetaminophen] 30•2•500 mg

Comtrex Cold & Cough Relief, Multi-Symptom; Multi-Symptom Comtrex Day & Night Cold & Cough Relief caplets OTC *antitussive; decongestant; antihistamine; analgesic* [dextromethorphan hydrobromide; pseudoephedrine HCl;

chlorpheniramine maleate; acetaminophen] 15•30•2•500 mg

Comtrex Day/Night Flu Therapy caplets OTC *decongestant; analgesic; antihistamine added PM* [pseudoephedrine HCl; acetaminophen; chlorpheniramine maleate added PM] 30•500 mg AM; 30•500•2 mg PM

Comtrex Flu Therapy & Fever Relief Day & Night, Multi-Symptom caplets (name changed to **Comtrex Day/Night Flu Therapy** in 2005)

Comtrex Liqui-Gels (liquid-filled capsules) (discontinued 2002) OTC *antitussive; decongestant; antihistamine; analgesic* [dextromethorphan hydrobromide; phenylpropanolamine HCl; chlorpheniramine maleate; acetaminophen] 10•12.5•2•325, 15•12.5•2•500 mg

Comtrex Multi-Symptom Cold & Flu Relief tablets, caplets (name changed to Comtrex Cough & Cold Relief, Multi-Symptom and/or Comtrex Day & Night Cold & Cough Relief, Multi-Symptom in 2002)

Comtrex Multi-Symptom Cold & Flu Relief Liqui-Gels (capsules) (discontinued 2002) OTC *antitussive; decongestant; antihistamine; analgesic* [dextromethorphan hydrobromide; phenylpropanolamine HCl; chlorpheniramine maleate; acetaminophen] 15•12.5•2•500 mg

Comtrex Multi-Symptom Deep Chest Cold softgels OTC *antitussive; decongestant; expectorant; analgesic* [dextromethorphan hydrobromide; pseudoephedrine HCl; guaifenesin; acetaminophen] 10•30•100•250 mg

Comtrex Multi-Symptom Non-Drowsy Cold & Cough Relief caplets OTC *antitussive; decongestant; analgesic* [dextromethorphan hydrobromide; pseudoephedrine HCl; acetaminophen] 15•30•500 mg

Comtrex Nighttime Cold & Cough oral liquid OTC *antitussive; decongestant; antihistamine; analgesic* [dextro-

methorphan hydrobromide; pseudoephedrine HCl; chlorpheniramine
maleate; acetaminophen] 5•10•
0.67•166.7 mg/5 mL

Comtrex Non-Drowsy caplets (name
changed to Comtrex Multi-Symptom Non-Drowsy Cold & Cough
Relief in 2002)

**Comtrex Sinus & Nasal Deconges-
tant** caplets OTC *decongestant; antihistamine; analgesic* [pseudoephedrine
HCl; brompheniramine maleate;
acetaminophen] 30•2•500 mg

Comtussin HC syrup ℞ *narcotic antitussive; decongestant; antihistamine*
[hydrocodone bitartrate; phenylephrine HCl; chlorpheniramine male-
ate] 5•10•4 mg/10 mL

Comvax IM injection ℞ *infant (1½–
15 months) vaccine for* H. influenzae
and hepatitis B [Hemophilus b purified capsular polysaccharide; Neisseria meningitidis OMPC; hepatitis B
virus vaccine] 7.5•125•5 μg/0.5 mL

Conceive Ovulation Predictor 5-
day test kit for professional use (discontinued 2004) *in vitro diagnostic
aid to predict ovulation time*

Conceive Pregnancy test kit for
home use *in vitro diagnostic aid; urine
pregnancy test*

Concentrated Cleaner solution OTC
*cleaning solution for rigid gas permeable
contact lenses*

Conceptrol Contraceptive Inserts
vaginal suppositories (discontinued
2002) OTC *spermicidal contraceptive*
[nonoxynol 9] 150 mg

**Conceptrol Disposable Contracep-
tive** vaginal gel OTC *spermicidal contraceptive* [nonoxynol 9] 4%

Concerta dual-release tablets ℞ *CNS
stimulant; once-daily treatment for
attention-deficit hyperactivity disorder
(ADHD)* [methylphenidate HCl]
18, 27, 36, 54, 72 mg (22% immediate release, 78% extended release)

Condylox solution, gel ℞ *topical
antimitotic for external genital and perianal warts* [podofilox] 0.5%

cone flower, purple *medicinal herb*
[see: echinacea]

conessine INN

conessine hydrobromide [see: cones-
sine]

Conex syrup (discontinued 2002) OTC
decongestant; expectorant [phenylpro-
panolamine HCl; guaifenesin] 12.5•
100 mg/5 mL

Conex with Codeine syrup (discontinued 2002) ℞ *narcotic antitussive;
decongestant; expectorant* [codeine
phosphate; phenylpropanolamine
HCl; guaifenesin] 10•12.5•100
mg/5 mL

confectioner's sugar [see: sugar, confectioner's]

Confide test kit for home use *in vitro
diagnostic aid for HIV in the blood*

congazone sodium [see: Congo red]

Congess JR capsules (discontinued
2002) ℞ *decongestant; expectorant*
[pseudoephedrine HCl; guaifenesin]
60•125 mg

Congess SR sustained-release capsules
(discontinued 2002) ℞ *decongestant;
expectorant* [pseudoephedrine HCl;
guaifenesin] 120•250 mg

Congestac caplets OTC *decongestant;
expectorant* [pseudoephedrine HCl;
guaifenesin] 60•400 mg

Congestaid tablets OTC *nasal decongestant* [pseudoephedrine HCl] 30 mg

Congestant D tablets (discontinued
2001) OTC *decongestant; antihistamine; analgesic* [phenylpropanol-
amine HCl; chlorpheniramine maleate; acetaminophen] 12.5•2•325 mg

Congestion Relief, Children's oral
liquid (discontinued 2002) OTC *nasal
decongestant* [pseudoephedrine HCl]
30 mg/5 mL

Congo red USP

conivaptan *investigational (NDA filed)
vasopressin antagonist for hyponatremia*

conjugated equine estrogen CEE)
[see: estrogens, conjugated]

conjugated estrogens [see: estrogens,
conjugated]

conjugated linoleic acid (CLA) *natural omega-6 essential fatty acid shown to be effective in weight management and cancer prevention*

conorphone INN *analgesic* [also: conorphone HCl]

conorfone HCl [see: conorphone HCl]

conorphone HCl USAN *analgesic* [also: conorfone]

CONPADRI; CONPADRI-I (cyclophosphamide, Oncovin, L-phenylalanine mustard, Adriamycin) *chemotherapy protocol*

Conray; Conray 30; Conray 43 injection (discontinued 2005) ℞ *radiopaque contrast medium* [iothalamate meglumine (47% iodine)] 600 mg/mL (282 mg/mL); 300 mg/mL (141 mg/mL); 430 mg/mL (202 mg/mL)

Conray 400 injection (discontinued 2001) ℞ *radiopaque contrast medium* [iothalamate sodium (59.9% iodine)] 668 mg/mL (400 mg/mL)

Consonar ℞ *investigational reversible/selective MAO inhibitor, type A* [brofaromine]

Constilac oral/rectal solution ℞ *hyperosmotic laxative* [lactulose] 10 g/15 mL

Constulose oral/rectal solution ℞ *hyperosmotic laxative* [lactulose] 10 g/15 mL

consumptive's weed *medicinal herb* [see: yerba santa]

Contac 12 Hour sustained-release capsules, sustained-release caplets (discontinued 2001) OTC *decongestant; antihistamine* [phenylpropanolamine HCl; chlorpheniramine maleate] 75•8 mg; 75•12 mg

Contac Cough & Chest Cold oral liquid (discontinued 2002) OTC *antitussive; decongestant; expectorant; analgesic* [dextromethorphan hydrobromide; pseudoephedrine HCl; guaifenesin; acetaminophen; alcohol 10%] 5•15•50•125 mg/5 mL

Contac Cough & Sore Throat oral liquid (discontinued 2002) OTC *antitussive; analgesic* [dextromethorphan hydrobromide; acetaminophen; alcohol 10%] 5•125 mg/5 mL

Contac Day & Night Allergy/Sinus Relief daytime caplets + nighttime caplets OTC *decongestant; analgesic; antihistamine/sleep aid added* PM [pseudoephedrine HCl; acetaminophen; diphenhydramine HCl added PM] 03/02 60•650 mg AM; 60•650•50 mg PM

Contac Day & Night Cold & Flu daytime caplets + nighttime caplets OTC *decongestant; analgesic; (antitussive added daytime; antihistamine/sleep aid added nighttime)* [pseudoephedrine HCl; acetaminophen; (dextromethorphan hydrobromide added daytime; diphenhydramine HCl added nighttime)] 60•650•30 mg daytime; 60•650•50 mg nighttime

Contac Severe Cold & Flu caplets OTC *antitussive; decongestant; antihistamine; analgesic* [dextromethorphan hydrobromide; pseudoephedrine HCl; chlorpheniramine maleate; acetaminophen] 15•30•2•500 mg

Contac Severe Cold & Flu Nighttime oral liquid (discontinued 2002) OTC *antitussive; decongestant; antihistamine; analgesic* [dextromethorphan hydrobromide; pseudoephedrine HCl; chlorpheniramine maleate; acetaminophen; alcohol 18.5%] 5•10•0.67•167 mg/5 mL

conteben [see: thioacetazone; thiacetazone]

ConTE-Pak-4 IV injection (discontinued 2003) ℞ *intravenous nutritional therapy* [multiple trace elements (metals)]

ContolRx toothpaste ℞ *dental caries preventative* [sodium fluoride] 1.1%

Contrin capsules ℞ *hematinic* [ferrous fumarate; cyanocobalamin; ascorbic acid; intrinsic factor concentrate; folic acid] 110 mg•15 μg•75 mg•240 mg•0.5 mg

Control timed-release capsules (discontinued 2001) OTC *diet aid* [phenylpropanolamine HCl] 75 mg

ControlPak (trademarked packaging form) *tamper-resistant unit-dose package*

Contuss oral liquid (discontinued 2002) ℞ *decongestant; expectorant* [phenylpropanolamine HCl; phenylephrine HCl; guaifenesin; alcohol 5%] 20•5•100 mg/5 mL

conval lily *medicinal herb* [see: lily of the valley]

Convallaria majalis *medicinal herb* [see: lily of the valley]

conventional (typical) antipsychotics *a class of dopamine receptor antagonists with a higher affinity to the D_2 than D_1 receptors and little affinity to the nondopaminergic receptors; high incidence of extrapyramidal side effects (EPS)* [compare to: novel (atypical) antipsychotics]

Convolvulus sepium *medicinal herb* [see: hedge bindweed]

convulsion root; convulsion weed *medicinal herb* [see: fit root]

Conyza canadensis *medicinal herb* [see: horseweed]

cool.click (trademarked device) *needle-free subcutaneous injector*

Cooper regimen *chemotherapy protocol for breast cancer* [see: CMFVP]

COP [see: creatinolfosfate]

COP (cyclophosphamide, Oncovin, prednisone) *chemotherapy protocol for non-Hodgkin lymphoma*

COP 1 (copolymer 1) [see: glatiramer acetate]

COPA (Cytoxin, Oncovin, prednisone, Adriamycin) *chemotherapy protocol*

COPA-BLEO (cyclophosphamide, Oncovin, prednisone, Adriamycin, bleomycin) *chemotherapy protocol*

COPAC (CCNU, Oncovin, prednisone, Adriamycin, cyclophosphamide) *chemotherapy protocol*

Copaxone subcu injection in Autoject2 (prefilled glass syringe) ℞ *immunomodulator for relapsing-remitting multiple sclerosis (orphan)* [glatiramer acetate] 20 mg

COPB (cyclophosphamide, Oncovin, prednisone, bleomycin) *chemotherapy protocol*

COP-BLAM (cyclophosphamide, Oncovin, prednisone, bleomycin, Adriamycin, Matulane) *chemotherapy protocol*

COP-BLEO (cyclophosphamide, Oncovin, prednisone, bleomycin) *chemotherapy protocol*

Cope tablets OTC *analgesic; antipyretic; anti-inflammatory; antacid* [aspirin; caffeine; magnesium hydroxide; aluminum hydroxide] 421•32•50•25 mg

COPE (cyclophosphamide, Oncovin, Platinol, etoposide) *chemotherapy protocol for small cell lung cancer (SCLC) and pediatric brain tumors*

Copegus film-coated tablets ℞ *nucleoside antiviral; combination therapy for chronic hepatitis C virus (HCV) infection* [ribavirin] 200 mg

Cophene No. 2 sustained-release capsules (discontinued 2002) ℞ *decongestant; antihistamine* [pseudoephedrine HCl; chlorpheniramine maleate] 120•12 mg

Cophene XP oral liquid (discontinued 2002) ℞ *narcotic antitussive; decongestant; expectorant* [hydrocodone bitartrate; pseudoephedrine HCl; guaifenesin; alcohol 12.5%] 5•60•200 mg/5 mL

Cophene-X capsules (discontinued 2002) ℞ *antitussive; decongestant; expectorant* [carbetapentane citrate; phenylephrine HCl; phenylpropanolamine HCl; potassium guaiacolsulfonate] 20•10•10•45 mg

copolymer 1 (COP 1) [see: glatiramer acetate]

copovithane BAN

COPP (CCNU, Oncovin, procarbazine, prednisone) *chemotherapy protocol*

COPP (cyclophosphamide, Oncovin, procarbazine, prednisone) *chemotherapy protocol for Hodgkin or non-Hodgkin lymphoma*

copper *element (Cu)*

copper chloride dihydrate [see: cupric chloride]

copper gluconate (copper D-gluconate) USP *dietary copper supplement*

copper sulfate pentahydrate [see: cupric sulfate]

copper 10-undecenoate [see: copper undecylenate]

copper undecylenate USAN

copperhead snake antivenin [see: antivenin (Crotalidae) polyvalent]

Coptis trifolia *medicinal herb* [see: gold thread]

Co-Pyronil 2 Pulvules (capsules) (discontinued 2002) OTC *decongestant; antihistamine* [pseudoephedrine HCl; chlorpheniramine maleate] 60•4 mg

CoQ10 [see: coenzyme Q10]

coral (*Goniopora* spp.; *Porite* spp.) *natural material used as a substrate for bone grafts and fractures and in reconstructive surgery*

coral root (*Corallorhiza odontorhiza*) *medicinal herb for diaphoresis, fever, insomnia, and sedation*

coral snake antivenin [see: antivenin (Micrurus fulvius)]

corbadrine INN *adrenergic; vasoconstrictor* [also: levonordefrin]

Cordarone tablets, IV infusion ℞ *antiarrhythmic for acute ventricular tachycardia and fibrillation (orphan)* [amiodarone HCl] 200 mg; 50 mg/mL

Cordox ℞ *investigational (Phase III) adjunct to coronary artery bypass graft (CABG) surgery; investigational (Phase III, orphan) cytoprotective agent for vaso-occlusive episodes of sickle cell disease* [fructose-1,6-diphosphate]

Cordran ointment, lotion, tape ℞ *corticosteroidal anti-inflammatory* [flurandrenolide] 0.05%; 0.05%; 4 μg/cm²

Cordran SP cream ℞ *corticosteroidal anti-inflammatory* [flurandrenolide] 0.05%

Coreg Tiltab (film-coated tablets) ℞ *antihypertensive; α- and β-blocker for congestive heart failure* [carvedilol] 3.125, 6.25, 12.5, 25 mg

Corgard tablets ℞ *antianginal; antihypertensive; antiadrenergic (β-blocker)* [nadolol] 20, 40, 80, 120, 160 mg

coriander (*Coriandrum sativum*) seed *medicinal herb used as antispasmodic, appetizer, carminative, and stomachic*

coriander oil NF

Coricidin D Cold, Flu, & Sinus tablets OTC *decongestant; antihistamine; analgesic* [pseudoephedrine HCl; chlorpheniramine maleate; acetaminophen] 30•2•325 mg

Coricidin HBP Chest Congestion & Cough softgels OTC *antitussive; expectorant* [dextromethorphan hydrobromide; guaifenesin] 10•200 mg

Coricidin HBP Cold & Flu tablets OTC *antihistamine; analgesic* [chlorpheniramine maleate; acetaminophen] 2•325 mg

Coricidin HBP Cough & Cold tablets OTC *antitussive; antihistamine* [dextromethorphan hydrobromide; chlorpheniramine maleate] 30•4 mg

Coricidin HBP Flu tablets OTC *antitussive; antihistamine; analgesic* [dextromethorphan hydrobromide; chlorpheniramine maleate; acetaminophen] 15•2•500 mg

Coricidin Sinus Headache tablets (discontinued 2001) OTC *decongestant; antihistamine; analgesic* [phenylpropanolamine HCl; chlorpheniramine maleate; acetaminophen] 12.5•2•500 mg

corkwood tree (*Duboisia myoporoides*) leaves *medicinal herb used as a central nervous system stimulant and in homeopathic therapy for eye disorders; not generally regarded as safe and effective as it contains scopolamine and related alkaloids, which may be fatal in high doses*

Corlopam IV infusion ℞ *rapid-acting vasodilator for in-hospital management of severe hypertension* [fenoldopam mesylate] 10 mg/mL

Corlux ℞ *investigational (Phase III) GR-II antagonist to reduce abnormal*

cortisol release in psychotic major depression [mifepristone]

Cormax ointment ℞ *corticosteroidal anti-inflammatory* [clobetasol propionate] 0.05%

cormed [see: nikethamide]

cormetasone INN *topical anti-inflammatory* [also: cormethasone acetate]

cormetasone acetate [see: cormethasone acetate]

cormethasone acetate USAN *topical anti-inflammatory* [also: cormetasone]

corn, turkey *medicinal herb* [see: turkey corn]

corn cockle (Agrostemma githago) seeds and root *medicinal herb for cancer, edema, exanthema, hemorrhoids, jaundice, and worms; also used as an emmenagogue and expectorant, and in homeopathic remedies for gastritis and paralysis; not generally regarded as safe and effective as it is extremely poisonous*

Corn Huskers lotion OTC *moisturizer; emollient*

corn oil NF *solvent; caloric replacement*

corn silk (stigmata maidis) *medicinal herb* [see: Indian corn]

cornflower (Centaurea cyanus) plant *medicinal herb for conjunctivitis, corneal ulcers and other eye disorders and for nervous disorders and poisonous bites and stings*

corpse plant *medicinal herb* [see: fit root]

corpus luteum extract [see: progesterone]

Corque cream ℞ *topical corticosteroidal anti-inflammatory; antifungal; antibacterial* [hydrocortisone; clioquinol] 1%•3%

Correctol enteric-coated tablets OTC *stimulant laxative* [bisacodyl] 5 mg

CortaGel OTC *corticosteroidal anti-inflammatory* [hydrocortisone] 1%

Cortaid cream, ointment OTC *corticosteroidal anti-inflammatory* [hydrocortisone acetate] 1%

Cortaid pump spray OTC *corticosteroidal anti-inflammatory* [hydrocortisone] 1%

Cortaid Faststick roll-on stick OTC *corticosteroidal anti-inflammatory* [hydrocortisone; alcohol 55%] 1%

Cortaid Intensive Therapy cream (discontinued 2004) OTC *corticosteroidal anti-inflammatory* [hydrocortisone] 1%

Cortaid with Aloe cream, ointment OTC *corticosteroidal anti-inflammatory* [hydrocortisone acetate] 0.5%

Cortane-B lotion ℞ *corticosteroidal anti-inflammatory; local anesthetic; antiseptic* [hydrocortisone acetate; pramoxine HCl; chloroxylenol] 1%•1%•0.1%

Cortane-B Aqueous; Cortane-B Otic ear drops ℞ *corticosteroidal anti-inflammatory; local anesthetic; bacteriostatic* [hydrocortisone; pramoxine HCl; chloroxylenol] 1%•1%•0.1%

Cortate ⓒᴬᴺ cream, ointment ℞ *corticosteroidal anti-inflammatory* [hydrocortisone acetate] 1%

Cortatrigen Modified ear drops, otic suspension ℞ *corticosteroidal anti-inflammatory; antibiotic* [hydrocortisone; neomycin sulfate; polymyxin B sulfate] 1%•5 mg•10 000 U per mL

Cort-Dome cream ℞ *corticosteroidal anti-inflammatory* [hydrocortisone] 0.5%, 1% ⑨ Cortone

Cort-Dome High Potency rectal suppositories ℞ *corticosteroidal anti-inflammatory* [hydrocortisone acetate] 25 mg

Cortef tablets, oral suspension ℞ *corticosteroid; anti-inflammatory* [hydrocortisone] 5, 10, 20 mg; 10 mg/5 mL

Cortef Feminine Itch cream OTC *corticosteroidal anti-inflammatory* [hydrocortisone acetate] 0.5%

Cortenema retention enema (discontinued 2004) ℞ *corticosteroidal anti-inflammatory for ulcerative colitis* [hydrocortisone] 100 mg/60 mL ⑨ quart enema

cortenil [see: desoxycorticosterone acetate]

cortexolone [see: cortodoxone]

Cortic-ND ear drops ℞ *corticosteroidal anti-inflammatory; local anesthetic; bacteriostatic* [hydrocortisone; pramoxine HCl; chloroxylenol] 1%•1%•0.1%

Corticaine cream OTC *corticosteroidal anti-inflammatory* [hydrocortisone acetate] 0.5%

corticorelin ovine triflutate USAN, INN *corticotropin-releasing hormone; diagnostic aid for Cushing syndrome and adrenocortical insufficiency* (orphan)

corticosteroids *a class of anti-inflammatory drugs*

corticotrophin INN, BAN *adrenocorticotropic hormone; corticosteroid; anti-inflammatory; diagnostic aid* [also: corticotropin]

corticotrophin-zinc hydroxide INN *adrenocorticotropic hormone; corticosteroid; anti-inflammatory; diagnostic aid* [also: corticotropin zinc hydroxide]

corticotropin USP *adrenocorticotropic hormone; corticosteroid; anti-inflammatory; diagnostic aid* [also: corticotrophin]

corticotropin, repository USP *adrenocorticotropic hormone; corticosteroid; anti-inflammatory; diagnostic aid*

corticotropin tetracosapeptide [see: cosyntropin]

corticotropin zinc hydroxide USP *adrenocorticotropic hormone; corticosteroid; anti-inflammatory; diagnostic aid* [also: corticotrophin-zinc hydroxide]

corticotropin-releasing factor *investigational (Phase I/II, orphan) agent for peritumoral brain edema*

Cortifoam intrarectal foam aerosol (discontinued 2004) ℞ *corticosteroidal anti-inflammatory for ulcerative proctitis* [hydrocortisone acetate] 90 mg/dose

cortisol [see: hydrocortisone]

cortisol 21-acetate [see: hydrocortisone acetate]

cortisol 21-butyrate [see: hydrocortisone butyrate]

cortisol 21-cyclopentanepropionate [see: hydrocortisone cypionate]

cortisol cyclopentylpropionate [see: hydrocortisone cypionate]

cortisol 21-valerate [see: hydrocortisone valerate]

cortisone INN, BAN *corticosteroid; anti-inflammatory* [also: cortisone acetate] ⑨ Cortizone

cortisone acetate USP *corticosteroid; anti-inflammatory* [also: cortisone] 25 mg oral

Cortisporin cream ℞ *corticosteroidal anti-inflammatory; antibiotic* [hydrocortisone acetate; neomycin sulfate; polymyxin B sulfate] 0.5%•0.5%•10 000 U per g

Cortisporin eye drop suspension ℞ *ophthalmic corticosteroidal anti-inflammatory; antibiotic* [hydrocortisone; neomycin sulfate; polymyxin B sulfate] 1%•0.35%•10 000 U per mL

Cortisporin ointment ℞ *corticosteroidal anti-inflammatory; antibiotic* [hydrocortisone; neomycin sulfate; bacitracin zinc; polymyxin B sulfate] 1%•0.5%•400 U•5000 U per g

Cortisporin ophthalmic ointment ℞ *ophthalmic corticosteroidal anti-inflammatory; antibiotic* [hydrocortisone; neomycin sulfate; bacitracin zinc; polymyxin B sulfate] 1%•0.35%•400 U/g•10 000 U/g

Cortisporin Otic ear drops, otic suspension ℞ *corticosteroidal anti-inflammatory; antibiotic* [hydrocortisone; neomycin sulfate; polymyxin B sulfate] 1%•5 mg•10 000 U per mL

Cortisporin-TC ear drop suspension ℞ *corticosteroidal anti-inflammatory; antibiotic; surface-active synergist* [hydrocortisone acetate; neomycin sulfate; colistin sulfate; thonzonium bromide] 10•3.3•3•0.5 mg/mL

cortisuzol INN

cortivazol USAN, INN *corticosteroid; anti-inflammatory*

Cortizone for Kids cream OTC *corticosteroidal anti-inflammatory* [hydrocortisone] 0.5%

Cortizone-5 cream (discontinued 2005) OTC *corticosteroidal anti-inflammatory* [hydrocortisone] 1% ꤺ cortisone

Cortizone-5 ointment OTC *corticosteroidal anti-inflammatory* [hydrocortisone] 0.5% ꤺ cortisone

Cortizone-10 ointment OTC *corticosteroidal anti-inflammatory* [hydrocortisone] 1%

Cortizone-10 Plus cream OTC *corticosteroidal anti-inflammatory* [hydrocortisone] 1%

Cortizone-10 Quickshot spray OTC *corticosteroidal anti-inflammatory* [hydrocortisone] 1%

cortodoxone USAN, INN, BAN *anti-inflammatory*

Cortone Acetate intra-articular or intralesional injection ℞ *corticosteroidal anti-inflammatory* [cortisone acetate] 50 mg/mL ꤺ Cort-Dome

Cortrosyn powder for IM or IV injection ℞ *multiple sclerosis; diagnostic aid for adrenal function; treatment for infantile spasms* [cosyntropin] 0.25 mg

Corvert IV infusion ℞ *antiarrhythmic for atrial fibrillation/flutter* [ibutilide fumarate] 0.1 mg/mL

corydalis (Corydalis cava) root *medicinal herb used as an antispasmodic, hypnotic, and antiparkinsonian*

Corydalis formosa *medicinal herb* [see: turkey corn]

Corynanthe johimbe *medicinal herb* [see: yohimbe]

Corzide 40/5; Corzide 80/5 tablets ℞ *antihypertensive; β-blocker; diuretic* [nadolol; bendroflumethiazide] 40•5 mg; 80•5 mg

Cosmederm-7 Ⓒᴬᴺ (trademarked ingredient) *topical anti-irritant* [strontium chloride]

Cosmegen powder for IV injection ℞ *antibiotic antineoplastic for various tumors, carcinomas, and sarcomas; potentiator for radiation therapy* [dactinomycin] 0.5 mg/vial

CosmoDerm gel for subcu injection ℞ *dermal filler for shallow scars and fine wrinkles* [collagen, purified human] 35 mg/mL

cosmoline [see: petrolatum]

CosmoPlast gel for subcu injection ℞ *dermal filler for scars, deep wrinkles, and facial folds* [collagen, purified human, cross-linked] 35 mg/mL

Cosopt eye drops ℞ *topical carbonic anhydrase inhibitor and beta-blocker for glaucoma* [dorzolamide HCl; timolol maleate] 2%•0.5%

cosyntropin USAN *adrenocorticotropic hormone; diagnostic aid for adrenal function* [also: tetracosactide; tetracosactrin]

Cotara ℞ *investigational (Phase III) agent for glioblastoma multiforme; investigational (Phase I/II) tumor necrosis therapy (TNT) for solid tumors; investigational (Phase I/II) for pancreatic, prostate, and liver cancers* [chimeric monoclonal antibody labeled with iodine-131]

cotarnine chloride NF

cotarnine HCl [see: cotarnine chloride]

Cotazym capsules (discontinued 2002) ℞ *digestive enzymes; antacid* [lipase; protease; amylase; calcium carbonate] 8000 U•30 000 U•30 000 U•25 mg

Cotazym-S capsules containing enteric-coated spheres (discontinued 2002) ℞ *digestive enzymes* [lipase; protease; amylase] 5000•20 000•20 000 USP units

cotinine INN *antidepressant* [also: cotinine fumarate]

cotinine fumarate USAN *antidepressant* [also: cotinine]

Cotridin Ⓒᴬᴺ syrup ℞ *narcotic antitussive; decongestant; antihistamine* [codeine phosphate; pseudoephedrine HCl; triprolidine HCl] 2•6•0.4 mg/mL

Cotridin Expectorant Ⓒᴬᴺ oral solution ℞ *narcotic antitussive; decongestant; antihistamine* [codeine phosphate; pseudoephedrine HCl; triprolidine HCl; guaifenesin] 2•6•0.4•20 mg/mL

Cotrim; Cotrim D.S. tablets ℞ *anti-infective; antibacterial* [trimethoprim; sulfamethoxazole] 80•400 mg; 160•800 mg ⊇ Cortin

Cotrim Pediatric oral suspension ℞ *anti-infective; antibacterial* [trimethoprim; sulfamethoxazole] 40•200 mg/5 mL

co-trimoxazole BAN [also: trimethoprim + sulfamethoxazole] ⊇ clotrimazole

cotriptyline INN

cotton, purified USP *surgical aid*

cottonseed oil NF *solvent*

cottonweed *medicinal herb* [see: milk-weed]

Co-Tuss V oral liquid (discontinued 2002) ℞ *narcotic antitussive; expectorant* [hydrocodone bitartrate; guaifenesin] 5•100 mg

couch grass (Agropyron repens) rhizomes, roots, and stems *medicinal herb for blood cleansing, cystitis, diabetes, jaundice, kidney problems, upper respiratory tract inflammation with mucous discharge, rheumatism, and urinary infections*

Cough syrup (discontinued 2002) OTC *antitussive; decongestant; expectorant* [dextromethorphan hydrobromide; phenylephrine HCl; guaifenesin] 10•5•100 mg/5 mL

Cough Formula oral liquid (discontinued 2002) OTC *antitussive; antihistamine* [dextromethorphan hydrobromide; chlorpheniramine maleate; alcohol 10%] 15•2 mg/5 mL

Cough Formula with Decongestant oral liquid (discontinued 2002) OTC *antitussive; decongestant* [dextromethorphan hydrobromide; pseudoephedrine HCl; alcohol 10%] 10•20 mg/5 mL

coughroot *medicinal herb* [see: birthroot]

coughweed *medicinal herb* [see: life root]

coughwort *medicinal herb* [see: coltsfoot]

Cough-X lozenges OTC *antitussive; topical oral anesthetic* [dextromethorphan hydrobromide; benzocaine] 5•2 mg

Coumadin tablets, powder for IV injection ℞ *coumarin-derivative anticoagulant* [warfarin sodium] 1, 2, 2.5, 3, 4, 5, 6, 7.5, 10 mg; 2 mg/mL ⊇ Kemadrin

coumafos INN [also: coumaphos]

coumamycin INN *antibacterial* [also: coumermycin]

coumaphos BAN [also: coumafos]

coumarin NF *anticoagulant; investigational (orphan) for renal cell carcinoma*

coumarins *a class of anticoagulants that interfere with vitamin K-dependent clotting factors*

coumazoline INN

coumermycin USAN *antibacterial* [also: coumamycin]

coumermycin sodium USAN *antibacterial*

coumetarol INN [also: cumetharol]

counterirritants *a class of agents that produce superficial irritation in one part of the body to relieve irritation in another part*

Covangesic tablets (discontinued 2001) OTC *decongestant; antihistamine; analgesic* [phenylpropanolamine HCl; phenylephrine HCl; chlorpheniramine maleate; pyrilamine maleate; acetaminophen] 12.5•7.5•2•12.5•275 mg

covatin HCl [see: captodiame HCl]

Covera-HS extended-release film-coated tablets ℞ *antihypertensive; antianginal; antiarrhythmic; calcium channel blocker* [verapamil HCl] 180, 240 mg ⊇ Provera

Coversyl ⓒⒶⓃ tablets ℞ *angiotensin-converting enzyme (ACE) inhibitor for essential hypertension; treatment for congestive heart failure (CHF)* [perindopril erbumine] 2, 4 mg

Coviracil (name changed to Emtriva upon marketing release in 2003) ℞

cow cabbage *medicinal herb* [see: masterwort; white pond lily]

cow parsnip *medicinal herb* [see: masterwort]

cowslip (Caltha palustris) plant *medicinal herb used as an analgesic, antispasmodic, diaphoretic, diuretic, expectorant, and rubefacient*

cowslip, Jerusalem *medicinal herb* [see: lungwort]

COX-2 (cyclooxygenase-2) inhibitors *a class of nonsteroidal anti-inflammatory drugs (NSAIDs) for osteoarthritis, rheumatoid arthritis, acute pain, and primary dysmenorrhea; these agents also have antipyretic activity*

Cozaar film-coated tablets ℞ *angiotensin II receptor antagonist for hypertension; treatment to delay the progression of diabetic nephropathy* [losartan potassium] 25, 50, 100 mg

CP (chlorambucil, prednisone) *chemotherapy protocol for chronic lymphocytic leukemia (CLL)*

CP (cyclophosphamide, Platinol) *chemotherapy protocol for ovarian cancer*

CP (cyclophosphamide, prednisone) *chemotherapy protocol*

CPB (cyclophosphamide, Platinol, BCNU) *chemotherapy protocol*

CPC (cyclophosphamide, Platinol, carboplatin) *chemotherapy protocol*

C.P.-DM pediatric oral drops ℞ *antitussive; decongestant; antihistamine* [dextromethorphan hydrobromide; pseudoephedrine HCl; carbinoxamine maleate] 4•15•1 mg/mL

C-Phed Tannate oral suspension ℞ *decongestant; antihistamine* [pseudoephedrine tannate; chlorpheniramine tannate] 150•9 mg/10 mL

CPM (CCNU, procarbazine, methotrexate) *chemotherapy protocol*

CPM 8/PSE 90/MSC 2.5 sustained-release tablets ℞ *antihistamine; decongestant; anticholinergic to dry mucosal secretions* [chorpheniramine maleate; pseudoephedrine HCl; methscopolamine nitrate] 8•90•2.5 mg

CPOB (cyclophosphamide, prednisone, Oncovin, bleomycin) *chemotherapy protocol*

CPT-11 (camptothecin-11) [see: irinotecan]

CP-Tannic oral suspension ℞ *decongestant; antihistamine* [pseudoephedrine tannate; chlorpheniramine tannate] 150•9 mg/10 mL

51Cr [see: albumin, chromated Cr 51 serum]

51Cr [see: chromic chloride Cr 51]

51Cr [see: chromic phosphate Cr 51]

51Cr [see: sodium chromate Cr 51]

cramp bark (Viburnum opulus) bark and berries *medicinal herb for asthma, convulsions, cramps, heart palpitations, hypertension, hysteria, leg cramps, nervousness, spasm, and urinary disorders*

crampweed *medicinal herb* [see: cinquefoil]

cranberry (Vaccinium edule; V. erythrocarpum; V. macrocarpon; V. oxycoccos; V. vitis) fruit *medicinal herb for bladder, kidney, and urinary tract infections; also used to decrease the rate of urine degradation and odor formation in incontinent patients*

cranesbill; spotted cranesbill *medicinal herb* [see: alum root]

Crantex ER extended-release capsules ℞ *decongestant; expectorant* [phenylephrine HCl; guaifenesin] 10•300 mg

Crataegus laevigata; C. monogyna; C. oxyacantha *medicinal herb* [see: hawthorn]

crawley; crawley root *medicinal herb* [see: coral root]

Creamy Tar shampoo OTC *antiseborrheic; antipsoriatic; antipruritic; antibacterial* [coal tar] 8.65%

Creapure ℞ *investigational (orphan) agent for amyotrophic lateral sclerosis (ALS)* [creatine]

creatine *investigational (orphan) agent for amyotrophic lateral sclerosis (ALS)*

creatinolfosfate INN

Creon delayed-release capsules containing enteric-coated microspheres (discontinued 2002) ℞ *porcine-derived digestive enzymes* [pancreatin (lipase; protease; amylase)] 300 mg (8000•13 000•30 000 USP units)

Creon 5; Creon 10: Creon 20 delayed-release capsules containing enteric-coated microspheres ℞ in the U.S, OTC in Canada *porcine-derived digestive enzymes* [lipase; protease; amylase] 5000•18 750•

16 600 USP units; 10 000•37 500•
33 200 USP units; 20 000•75 000•
66 400 USP units

Creon 25 Ⓒⓐⓝ delayed-release capsules containing enteric-coated microspheres OTC *porcine-derived digestive enzymes* [pancreatin (lipase; protease; amylase)] 300 mg (25 000•
62 500•74 700 USP units)

creosote carbonate USP

Creo-Terpin oral liquid OTC *antitussive* [dextromethorphan hydrobromide; alcohol 25%] 10 mg/15 mL

cresol NF *disinfectant*

cresotamide INN

cresoxydiol [see: mephenesin]

crestomycin sulfate [see: paromomycin sulfate]

Crestor tablets ℞ *HMG-CoA reductase inhibitor for hypercholesterolemia, mixed dyslipidemia, and hypertriglyceridemia* [rosuvastatin calcium] 5, 10, 20, 40 mg

Cresylate ear drops ℞ *antibacterial; antifungal* [m-cresyl acetate; chlorobutanol; alcohol] 25%•25%•1%

cresylic acid [see: cresol]

crilanomer INN

crilvastatin USAN, INN *antihyperlipidemic*

Crinone vaginal gel ℞ *natural progestin; hormone replacement or supplementation for assisted reproductive technology (ART) treatments* [progesterone] 4%, 8%

crisnatol INN *antineoplastic* [also: crisnatol mesylate]

crisnatol mesylate USAN *antineoplastic* [also: crisnatol]

Criticare HN ready-to-use oral liquid OTC *enteral nutritional therapy* [lactose-free formula]

Crixivan capsules ℞ *antiviral; HIV protease inhibitor* [indinavir sulfate] 100, 200, 333, 400 mg

crobefate INN *combining name for radicals or groups*

croconazole INN

crocus, autumn *medicinal herb* [see: autumn crocus]

Crocus sativus *medicinal herb* [see: saffron]

CroFab injection ℞ *treatment of pit viper (rattlesnake, copperhead, and cottonmouth moccasin) snake bites (orphan)* [antivenin (Crotalidae) polyvalent (ovine) Fab]

crofelemer USAN *investigational (Phase III) treatment for AIDS-related diarrhea; investigational (Phase II) antiviral for AIDS-related genital herpes*

crofilcon A USAN *hydrophilic contact lens material*

Crolom eye drops ℞ *mast cell stabilizer; ocular antiallergic and antiviral for vernal keratoconjunctivitis (orphan)* [cromolyn sodium] 4%

cromacate INN *combining name for radicals or groups*

cromakalim INN, BAN

Cro-Man-Zin tablets OTC *mineral supplement* [chromium; manganese; zinc] 0.2•5•25 mg

cromesilate INN *combining name for radicals or groups*

cromitrile INN *antiasthmatic* [also: cromitrile sodium]

cromitrile sodium USAN *antiasthmatic* [also: cromitrile]

cromoglicic acid INN *prophylactic antiasthmatic* [also: cromolyn sodium; cromoglycic acid]

cromoglycic acid BAN *prophylactic antiasthmatic* [also: cromolyn sodium; cromoglicic acid]

cromolyn sodium USAN, USP *anti-inflammatory; mast cell stabilizer for prophylactic treatment of allergy, asthma, and bronchospasm; treatment for mastocytosis and vernal keratoconjunctivitis (orphan)* [also: cromoglicic acid; cromoglycic acid] 20 mg/2 mL inhalation

Cronassial *investigational (orphan) agent for retinitis pigmentosa* [gangliosides, sodium salts]

cronetal [see: disulfiram]

cronidipine INN

cropropamide INN, BAN

croscarmellose INN *tablet disintegrant* [also: croscarmellose sodium]

croscarmellose sodium USAN, NF *tablet disintegrant* [also: croscarmellose]
crosfumaril [see: hemoglobin crosfumaril]
crospovidone NF *tablet excipient*
cross-linked carboxymethylcellulose sodium [now: croscarmellose sodium]
cross-linked carmellose sodium [see: croscarmellose sodium]
crotaline antivenin [see: antivenin (Crotalidae) polyvalent]
crotamiton USP, INN, BAN *scabicide; antipruritic*
crotetamide INN [also: crotethamide]
crotethamide BAN [also: crotetamide]
crotoniazide INN
crotonylidenisoniazid [see: crotoniazide]
crotoxyfos BAN
crowfoot *medicinal herb* [see: alum root; buttercup]
crowfoot buttercup; acrid crowfoot; cursed crowfoot; marsh crowfoot; meadow crowfoot; tall crowfoot; water crowfoot *medicinal herb* [see: buttercup]
crown, priest's *medicinal herb* [see: dandelion]
crude tuberculin [see: tuberculin, old]
Cruex cream OTC *antifungal* [clotrimazole] 1%
Cruex cream, aerosol powder OTC *antifungal* [undecylenic acid; zinc undecylenate] 20% total; 19% total
Cruex topical powder OTC *antifungal* [calcium undecylenate] 10%
crufomate USAN, INN, BAN *veterinary anthelmintic*
cryofluorane INN *aerosol propellant* [also: dichlorotetrafluoroethane]
cryptenamine acetates
Crypto-LA slide test for professional use *in vitro diagnostic aid for Cryptococcus neoformans antigens*
Cryptosporidium parvum bovine colostrum IgG concentrate *investigational (orphan) treatment of cryptosporidiosis-induced diarrhea in immunocompromised patients*

Cryselle tablets (in packs of 21 and 28) ℞ *monophasic oral contraceptive; emergency postcoital contraceptive* [norgestrel; ethinyl estradiol] 0.3 mg•30 μg
crystal violet [see: gentian violet]
crystallized trypsin [see: trypsin, crystallized]
Crystamine IM or subcu injection ℞ *hematinic; vitamin B_{12} supplement* [cyanocobalamin] 1000 μg/mL
Crysti 1000 IM or subcu injection ℞ *hematinic; vitamin B_{12} supplement* [cyanocobalamin] 1000 μg/mL
crystografin [see: meglumine diatriazole]
^{131}Cs [see: cesium chloride Cs 131]
CS-92 *investigational (Phase I/II) nucleoside reverse transcriptase inhibitor (NRTI) for HIV infection*
C-Solve OTC *lotion base*
CSP (cellulose sodium phosphate) [q.v.]
CT (cisplatin, Taxol) *chemotherapy protocol for ovarian cancer*
CT (cytarabine, thioguanine) *chemotherapy protocol*
CT-2584 mesylate *investigational (Phase II, orphan) antineoplastic for soft tissue sarcomas and malignant mesothelioma*
CT-3 *investigational anti-inflammatory*
CTAB (cetyltrimethyl ammonium bromide)
C-Tanna 12D tablets, oral suspension ℞ *pediatric antitussive, decongestant, and antihistamine* [carbetapentane tannate; phenylephrine tannate; pyrilamine tannate] 60•10•40 mg; 30•5•30 mg/5 mL
CTCb (cyclophosphamide, thiotepa, carboplatin) *chemotherapy protocol*
CTH (ceramide trihexosidase) [q.v.]
CTP-37 *investigational (Phase III) theraccine for cervical and pancreatic cancer; investigational (Phase II) for prostate and advanced colorectal cancers*

C/T/S topical solution (discontinued 2003) ℞ *antibiotic for acne* [clindamycin phosphate] 1%

CTX (cyclophosphamide) [q.v.]

Ctx-Plat (cyclophosphamide, Platinol) *chemotherapy protocol*

⁶⁴Cu [see: cupric acetate Cu 64]

cubeb (*Piper cubeba*) unripe berries *medicinal herb used as an antiseptic, antisyphilitic, carminative, diuretic, expectorant, stimulant, and stomachic*

Cubicin powder for IV infusion ℞ *cyclic lipopeptide antibiotic for skin and skin structure infections* [daptomycin] 250, 500 mg/vial

cucurbita (*Cucurbita maxima; C. moschata; C. pepa*) seeds *medicinal herb for prophylaxis, immobilizing, and aiding in the expulsion of intestinal worms and parasites; also used in prostate gland disorders*

Culturette 10 Minute Group A Strep ID slide test for professional use *in vitro diagnostic test for Group A streptococcal antigens in throat swabs* [latex agglutination test]

Culver physic *medicinal herb* [see: Culver root]

Culver root (*Varonicastrum virginicum*) *medicinal herb for blood cleansing, diarrhea, and liver and stomach disorders*

cumetharol BAN [also: coumetarol]

cumin (*Cuminum cyminum; C. odorum*) seeds and oil *medicinal herb for gastric cancer; also used as an antioxidant*

cupric acetate Cu 64 USAN *radioactive agent*

cupric chloride USP *dietary copper supplement*

cupric sulfate USP *antidote to phosphorus; dietary copper supplement* (40% elemental copper) 0.4, 2 mg/mL injection

Cuprimine capsules ℞ *metal chelating agent for rheumatoid arthritis, Wilson disease, and cystinuria* [penicillamine] 125, 250 mg

cuprimyxin USAN, INN *veterinary antibacterial; antifungal*

cuproxoline INN, BAN

Curaçao aloe *medicinal herb* [see: aloe]

curare [see: tubocurarine chloride]

Curcuma domestica; C. longa *medicinal herb* [see: turmeric]

cure-all *medicinal herb* [see: lemon balm]

curium *element* (Cm)

curled dock; curly dock *medicinal herb* [see: yellow dock]

curled mint *medicinal herb* [see: peppermint]

curls, blue *medicinal herb* [see: woundwort]

Curosurf intratracheal suspension ℞ *porcine lung extract for respiratory distress syndrome (RDS) in premature infants (orphan); also used for severe meconium aspiration in term infants* [poractant alfa] 1.5, 3 mL (120, 240 mg phospholipids)

curral [see: diallybarbituric acid]

currant (*Ribes nigrum; R. rubrum*) leaves and fruit *medicinal herb used as a diaphoretic and diuretic*

Curretab tablets (discontinued 2004) ℞ *synthetic progestin for secondary amenorrhea, abnormal uterine bleeding, and endometrial hyperplasia* [medroxyprogesterone acetate] 10 mg

custard apple *medicinal herb* [see: pawpaw]

Cūtar Bath Oil Emulsion OTC *antipsoriatic; antiseborrheic; antipruritic; emollient* [coal tar] 7.5%

Cūtemol cream OTC *moisturizer; emollient* [allantoin]

Cuticura Medicated Soap bar OTC *therapeutic skin cleanser* [triclocarban] 1%

Cutivate cream, ointment ℞ *corticosteroidal anti-inflammatory* [fluticasone propionate] 0.05%; 0.005%

CV (cisplatin, VePesid) *chemotherapy protocol*

CVA (cyclophosphamide, vincristine, Adriamycin) *chemotherapy protocol*

CVA-BMP; CVA + BMP (cyclophosphamide, vincristine, Adria-

mycin, BCNU, methotrexate, procarbazine) *chemotherapy protocol*

CVAD; C-VAD (cyclophosphamide, vincristine, Adriamycin, dexamethasone) *chemotherapy protocol*

CVB (CCNU, vinblastine, bleomycin) *chemotherapy protocol*

CVBD (CCNU, bleomycin, vinblastine, dexamethasone) *chemotherapy protocol*

CVD (cisplatin, vinblastine, dacarbazine) *chemotherapy protocol for malignant melanoma*

CVD+IL-2I (cisplatin, vinblastine, dacarbazine, interleukin-2, interferon alfa) *chemotherapy protocol for malignant melanoma*

CVEB (cisplatin, vinblastine, etoposide, bleomycin) *chemotherapy protocol*

CVI (carboplatin, VePesid, ifosfamide [with mesna rescue]) *chemotherapy protocol for non–small cell lung cancer (NSCLC)* [also: VIC]

CVM (cyclophosphamide, vincristine, methotrexate) *chemotherapy protocol*

CVP (cyclophosphamide, vincristine, prednisone) *chemotherapy protocol for non-Hodgkin lymphoma and chronic lymphocytic leukemia (CLL)*

CVPP (CCNU, vinblastine, procarbazine, prednisone) *chemotherapy protocol for Hodgkin lymphoma*

CVPP (cyclophosphamide, Velban, procarbazine, prednisone) *chemotherapy protocol*

CVPP-CCNU (cyclophosphamide, vinblastine, procarbazine, prednisone, CCNU) *chemotherapy protocol*

CY-1503 *investigational (Phase III, orphan) adjunct to surgery for congenital heart defects in newborns; investigational (orphan) for postischemic pulmonary reperfusion edema*

CY-1899 *investigational (orphan) agent for chronic active hepatitis B*

cyacetacide INN [also: cyacetazide]
cyacetazide BAN [also: cyacetacide]

CyADIC (cyclophosphamide, Adriamycin, DIC) *chemotherapy protocol*

cyamemazine INN
cyamepromazine [see: cyamemazine]
cyanamide JAN [also: calcium carbimide]
cyani *medicinal herb* [see: cornflower]
Cyanide Antidote Package ℞ *emergency treatment of cyanide poisoning* [sodium nitrite; sodium thiosulfate; amyl nitrite inhalant] 300 mg•12.5 g•0.3 mL

cyanoacetohydrazide [see: cyacetazide]
cyanoacrylate *topical skin adhesive for closing surgical incisions and traumatic lacerations; topical mucous membrane sealant and protectant for canker and mouth sores*

cyanocobalamin (vitamin B$_{12}$) USP, INN, BAN, JAN *water-soluble vitamin; hematopoietic* 50, 100, 250, 500, 1000 μg oral; 100, 1000 μg/mL injection

cyanocobalamin (^{57}Co) INN *pernicious anemia test; radioactive agent* [also: cyanocobalamin Co 57]

cyanocobalamin (^{58}Co) INN
cyanocobalamin (^{60}Co) INN *pernicious anemia test; radioactive agent* [also: cyanocobalamin Co 60]

cyanocobalamin Co 57 USAN, USP *pernicious anemia test; radioactive agent* [also: cyanocobalamin (^{57}Co)]

cyanocobalamin Co 60 USAN, USP *pernicious anemia test; radioactive agent* [also: cyanocobalamin (^{60}Co)]

Cyanoject IM or subcu injection ℞ *hematinic; vitamin B$_{12}$ supplement* [cyanocobalamin] 1000 μg/mL

cyclacillin USAN, USP *antibacterial* [also: ciclacillin]

cyclamate calcium NF
cyclamic acid USAN, BAN *non-nutritive sweetener (banned in the U.S.)*
cyclamide [see: glycyclamide]
cyclandelate INN, BAN, JAN *peripheral vasodilator; vascular smooth muscle relaxant*

cyclarbamate INN, BAN
cyclazocine USAN, INN *analgesic*
cyclazodone INN

Cyclessa tablets (in packs of 28) ℞ *triphasic oral contraceptive; emergency postcoital contraceptive* [desogestrel; ethinyl estradiol]
Phase 1 (7 days): 100•25 μg;
Phase 2 (7 days): 125•25 μg;
Phase 3 (7 days): 150•25 μg

cyclexanone INN

cyclic adenosine monophosphate (cAMP) [see: adenosine phosphate]

cyclic lipopeptides *a class of antibiotics that binds to bacterial membranes and causes a rapid depolarization of membrane potential, which inhibits RNA/DNA synthesis, leading to bacterial cell death*

cyclic propylene carbonate [see: propylene carbonate]

cyclindole USAN *antidepressant* [also: ciclindole]

Cyclinex-1 powder OTC *formula for infants with urea cycle disorders or gyrate atrophy*

Cyclinex-2 powder OTC *enteral nutritional therapy for urea cycle disorders or gyrate atrophy* [multiple essential amino acids]

cycliramine INN *antihistamine* [also: cycliramine maleate]

cycliramine maleate USAN *antihistamine* [also: cycliramine]

cyclizine USP, INN, BAN *antihistamine; antiemetic; anticholinergic; motion sickness relief*

cyclizine HCl USP, BAN *antiemetic*

cyclizine lactate USP, BAN *antinauseant*

cyclobarbital NF, INN [also: cyclobarbitone]

cyclobarbital calcium NF

cyclobarbitone BAN [also: cyclobarbital]

cyclobendazole USAN *anthelmintic* [also: ciclobendazole]

cyclobenzaprine INN *skeletal muscle relaxant* [also: cyclobenzaprine HCl]

cyclobenzaprine HCl USAN, USP *skeletal muscle relaxant* [also: cyclobenzaprine] 10 mg oral

cyclobutoic acid INN

cyclobutyrol INN

cyclocarbothiamine [see: cycotiamine]

Cyclocort ointment, cream, lotion ℞ *topical corticosteroidal anti-inflammatory* [amcinonide] 0.1%

cyclocoumarol BAN

cyclocumarol [see: cyclocoumarol]

α-cyclodextrin [see: alfadex]

Cyclofed Pediatric syrup ℞ *pediatric narcotic antitussive, decongestant, and expectorant* [codeine phosphate; pseudoephedrine HCl; guaifenesin; alcohol 6%] 10•30•100 mg/5 mL

cyclofenil INN, BAN

cyclofilcon A USAN *hydrophilic contact lens material*

cycloguanil embonate INN, BAN *antimalarial* [also: cycloguanil pamoate]

cycloguanil pamoate USAN *antimalarial* [also: cycloguanil embonate]

Cyclogyl Drop-Tainers (eye drops) ℞ *cycloplegic; mydriatic* [cyclopentolate HCl] 0.5%, 1%, 2%

cyclohexanehexol [see: inositol]

cyclohexanesulfamate dihydrate [see: sodium cyclamate]

cyclohexanesulfamic acid *(banned in the U.S.)* [see: cyclamic acid]

cycloheximide USAN *antipsoriatic* [also: cicloheximide]

p-**cyclohexylhydratropic acid** [see: hexaprofen]

N-cyclohexyllinoleamide [see: clinolamide]

4-cyclohexyloxybenzoate [see: cyclomethycaine]

1-cyclohexylpropyl carbamate [see: procymate]

N-cyclohexylsulfamic acid *(banned in the U.S.)* [see: cyclamic acid]

cyclomenol INN

cyclomethicone NF *wetting agent*

cyclomethycaine INN, BAN *local anesthetic* [also: cyclomethycaine sulfate]

cyclomethycaine sulfate USP *local anesthetic* [also: cyclomethycaine]

Cyclomydril Drop-Tainers (eye drops) ℞ *cycloplegic; mydriatic* [cyclopentolate HCl; phenylephrine HCl] 0.2%•1%

cyclonium iodide [see: oxapium iodide]

cyclooxygenase-2 (COX-2) inhibitors *a class of investigational anti-inflammatory drugs*

cyclopentamine INN, BAN [also: cyclopentamine HCl]

cyclopentamine HCl USP [also: cyclopentamine]

cyclopentaphene [see: cyclarbamate]

cyclopenthiazide USAN, INN, BAN *antihypertensive*

cyclopentolate INN, BAN *ophthalmic anticholinergic* [also: cyclopentolate HCl]

cyclopentolate HCl USP *ophthalmic anticholinergic; mydriatic; cycloplegic* [also: cyclopentolate] 1% eye drops

8-cyclopentyl 1,3-dipropylxanthine *investigational (orphan) for cystic fibrosis*

cyclophenazine HCl USAN *antipsychotic* [also: ciclofenazine]

cyclophosphamide USP, INN, BAN, JAN *nitrogen mustard–type alkylating antineoplastic; immunosuppressive* 25, 50 mg oral

cycloplegics *a class of drugs that paralyze the ciliary muscles of the eye*

cyclopolydimethylsiloxane [see: cyclomethicone]

cyclopregnol INN

cycloprolol BAN *antiadrenergic (β-receptor)* [also: cicloprolol HCl; cicloprolol]

cyclopropane USP, INN *inhalation general anesthetic*

Cycloprostin ℞ *investigational (orphan) heparin replacement for hemodialysis* [epoprostenol]

cyclopyrronium bromide INN

cycloserine (D-cycloserine) *investigational treatment for phobias and other severe anxiety disorders*

cycloserine (L-cycloserine) USP, INN, BAN, JAN *bacteriostatic; tuberculosis retreatment; investigational (orphan) for Gaucher disease*

cyclosporin BAN *immunosuppressant* [also: cyclosporine; ciclosporin]

cyclosporin A [now: cyclosporine]

cyclosporine USAN, USP *immunosuppressant for transplants (orphan), rheumatoid arthritis, and psoriasis; tear*

stimulant for Sjögren keratoconjunctivitis sicca (orphan); investigational (orphan) for corneal melting syndrome [also: ciclosporin; cyclosporin] 25, 100 mg oral; 100 mg/mL oral; 50 mg/mL injection

CycloTech (trademarked delivery device) *provides premeasured doses of oral liquids and records dosing times*

cyclothiazide USAN, USP, INN, BAN *diuretic; antihypertensive*

cyclovalone INN

cycobemin [see: cyanocobalamin]

Cycofed syrup ℞ *narcotic antitussive; decongestant* [codeine phosphate; pseudoephedrine HCl] 20•60 mg/5 mL

Cycofed Pediatric syrup (discontinued 2002) ℞ *narcotic antitussive; decongestant; expectorant* [codeine phosphate; pseudoephedrine HCl; guaifenesin; alcohol 6%] 10•30•100 mg

cycotiamine INN

cycrimine INN, BAN [also: cycrimine HCl]

cycrimine HCl USP [also: cycrimine]

Cycrin tablets (discontinued 2004) ℞ *synthetic progestin for secondary amenorrhea, abnormal uterine bleeding, and endometrial hyperplasia* [medroxyprogesterone acetate] 2.5, 5, 10 mg

Cydec pediatric oral drops ℞ *decongestant; antihistamine* [pseudoephedrine HCl; carbinoxamine maleate] 25•2 mg/mL

Cydec-DM syrup, pediatric oral drops ℞ *antitussive; decongestant; antihistamine* [dextromethorphan hydrobromide; pseudoephedrine HCl; carbinoxamine maleate] 15•60•4 mg/5 mL; 4•25•2 mg/mL

cyfluthrin BAN

cyhalothrin BAN

cyheptamide USAN, INN *anticonvulsant*

cyheptropine INN

CyHOP (cyclophosphamide, Halotestin, Oncovin, prednisone) *chemotherapy protocol*

Cyklokapron tablets, IV injection ℞ *systemic hemostatic* [tranexamic acid] 500 mg; 100 mg/mL

Cylert tablets, chewable tablets ℞ *CNS stimulant for attention-deficit hyperactivity disorder (ADHD)* [pemoline] 18.75, 37.5, 75 mg; 37.5 mg

Cylex; Cylex Sugar-Free throat lozenges OTC *topical oral anesthetic; antiseptic* [benzocaine; cetylpyridinium chloride] 15•5 mg

Cylexin ℞ *investigational (Phase III, orphan) adjunct to surgery for congenital heart defects in newborns; investigational (orphan) for postischemic pulmonary reperfusion edema* [CY-1503 (code name—generic name not yet assigned)]

Cymbalta enteric-coated pellets in capsules ℞ *selective serotonin and norepinephrine reuptake inhibitor (SSNRI) for major depressive disorder (MDD) and generalized anxiety disorder (GAD); analgesic for diabetic peripheral neuropathy (DPN); investigational (Phase II) for urinary incontinence* [duloxetine HCl] 20, 30, 60 mg

Cymbopogon citratus medicinal herb [see: lemongrass]

Cymbopogon nardus; C. winterianus medicinal herb [see: citronella]

cymemoxine [see: cimemoxin]

Cymevene (foreign name for U.S. product Cytovene)

Cynara scolymus medicinal herb [see: artichoke]

cynarine INN

Cyomin IM or subcu injection ℞ *hematinic; vitamin B_{12} supplement* [cyanocobalamin] 1000 μg/mL

cypenamine INN, BAN *antidepressant* [also: cypenamine HCl]

cypenamine HCl USAN *antidepressant* [also: cypenamine]

cypionate USAN, BAN *combining name for radicals or groups* [also: cipionate]

cypothrin USAN *veterinary insecticide*

cyprazepam USAN, INN *sedative*

cyprenorphine INN, BAN

cyprenorphine HCl [see: cyprenorphine]

Cypripedium pubescens medicinal herb [see: lady's slipper]

cyprodemanol [see: cyprodenate]

cyprodenate INN

cyproheptadine INN, BAN *nonselective piperidine antihistamine for hypersensitivity reactions; antipruritic* [also: cyproheptadine HCl]

cyproheptadine HCl USP, JAN *nonselective piperidine antihistamine for allergic rhinitis and type I hypersensitivity reactions; antipruritic; adjunctive anaphylactic therapy* [also: cyproheptadine] 4 mg oral; 2 mg/5 mL oral

cyprolidol INN *antidepressant* [also: cyprolidol HCl]

cyprolidol HCl USAN *antidepressant* [also: cyprolidol]

cyproquinate USAN *coccidiostat for poultry* [also: ciproquinate]

cyproterone INN, BAN *antiandrogen* [also: cyproterone acetate]

cyproterone acetate USAN *antiandrogen; investigational (orphan) for severe hirsutism* [also: cyproterone]

cyproximide USAN *antipsychotic; antidepressant* [also: ciproximide]

cyren A [see: diethylstilbestrol]

cyren B [see: diethylstilbestrol dipropionate]

cyromazine INN, BAN

Cystadane powder for oral solution ℞ *electrolyte replenisher for homocystinuria (orphan)* [betaine HCl] 1 g

Cystagon capsules ℞ *antiurolithic for nephropathic cystinosis (orphan)* [cysteamine bitartrate] 50, 150 mg

cystamin [see: methenamine]

cysteamine USAN, BAN *antiurolithic for nephropathic cystinosis (orphan)* [also: mercaptamine]

cysteamine bitartrate *antiurolithic for nephropathic cystinosis (orphan)*

cysteamine HCl USAN *antiurolithic; investigational (orphan) for corneal cystine crystal accumulation in cystinosis patients*

cysteine (L-cysteine) INN *nonessential amino acid; symbols: Cys, C; investigational (orphan) for erythropoietic protoporphyria photosensitivity* [also: cysteine HCl]

cysteine HCl (L-cysteine HCl) USP *nonessential amino acid* [also: cysteine] 50 mg/mL injection

L-cysteine HCl monohydrate [see: cysteine HCl]

Cystex tablets ℞ *urinary antibiotic; analgesic; acidifier* [methenamine; sodium salicylate; benzoic acid] 162•162.5•32 mg

cystic fibrosis gene therapy *investigational (orphan) agent for cystic fibrosis*

cystic fibrosis transmembrane conductance regulator (CFTR) *investigational (orphan) agent for cystic fibrosis*

cystic fibrosis transmembrane conductance regulator, recombinant adenovirus (AdGV-CFTR) *investigational (orphan) agent for cystic fibrosis*

cystine (L-cystine) USAN *amino acid*

Cysto-Conray; Cysto-Conray II intracavitary instillation (discontinued 2005) ℞ *radiopaque contrast medium for urological imaging* [iothalamate meglumine (47% iodine)] 430 mg/mL (202 mg/mL); 172 mg/mL (81 mg/mL)

cystogen [see: methenamine]

Cystografin; Cystografin Dilute intracavitary instillation ℞ *radiopaque contrast medium for urological imaging* [diatrizoate meglumine (46.67% iodine)] 300 mg/mL (141 mg/mL); 180 mg/mL (85 mg/mL)

Cystospaz tablets ℞ *GI/GU antispasmodic; antiparkinsonian; anticholinergic "drying agent" for allergic rhinitis and hyperhidrosis* [hyoscyamine sulfate] 0.15 mg

Cystospaz-M timed-release capsules (discontinued 2004) ℞ *GI/GU antispasmodic; antiparkinsonian; anticholinergic "drying agent" for allergic rhinitis and hyperhidrosis* [hyoscyamine sulfate] 0.375 mg

CYTABOM (cytarabine, bleomycin, Oncovin, mechlorethamine) *chemotherapy protocol*

Cytadren tablets ℞ *adrenal steroid inhibitor; antisteroidal antineoplastic for*

corticotropin-producing tumors [aminoglutethimide] 250 mg

cytarabine USAN, USP, INN, BAN *antimetabolite antineoplastic for various leukemias* 100, 500, 1000, 2000 mg injection ⑨ vidarabine

cytarabine, liposomal *antimetabolite antineoplastic for lymphomatous neoplastic meningitis (orphan)*

cytarabine HCl USAN *antiviral*

Cytisus scoparius *medicinal herb* [see: broom]

CytoGam IV infusion ℞ *prevention of primary cytomegalovirus in bone marrow and organ transplants from a CMV seropositive donor to an immunocompromised CMV seronegative recipient (orphan)* [cytomegalovirus immune globulin, solvent/detergent treated] 50 mg/mL

CytoImplant ℞ *investigational (orphan) agent for pancreatic cancer* [blood mononuclear cells, allogenic peripheral]

cytolin *investigational (Phase I/II) monoclonal antibody for AIDS*

cytomegalovirus immune globulin, human *prevention of primary cytomegalovirus in bone marrow and organ transplants from a CMV seropositive donor to an immunocompromised CMV seronegative recipient (orphan)*

cytomegalovirus immune globulin intravenous (CMV-IGIV) & ganciclovir sodium *investigational (orphan) for cytomegalovirus pneumonia in bone marrow transplant patients*

Cytomel tablets ℞ *synthetic thyroid hormone (T_3 fraction only)* [liothyronine sodium] 5, 25, 50 μg

cytoprotective agents *a class of drugs that provide prophylaxis against the side effects of antineoplastic agents*

Cytosar-U powder for subcu, intrathecal or IV injection (discontinued 2005) ℞ *antimetabolite antineoplastic for various leukemias* [cytarabine] 100, 500, 1000, 2000 mg/vial

cytosine arabinoside (ara-C) [see: cytarabine]

cytosine arabinoside HCl [now: cytarabine HCl]

Cytosol topical liquid ℞ *sterile irrigant* [physiological irrigating solution]

Cytotec tablets ℞ *prevents NSAID-induced gastric ulcers; has been used for cervical ripening and induction of labor; use by pregnant women can cause abortion, premature birth, or birth defects* [misoprostol] 100, 200 μg

cytotoxic lymphocyte maturation factor [see: edodekin alfa]

Cytovene capsules ℞ *antiviral for AIDS-related cytomegalovirus (CMV) infections (orphan) and CMV retinitis (orphan)* [ganciclovir] 250, 500 mg

Cytovene powder for IV infusion ℞ *antiviral for AIDS-related cytomegalovirus (CMV) infections (orphan)* [ganciclovir sodium] 500 mg/vial

Cytoxan tablets, powder for IV injection ℞ *nitrogen mustard-type alkylating antineoplastic for multiple leukemias, lymphomas, blastomas, sarcomas and organ cancers* [cyclophosphamide] 25, 50 mg; 100 mg

Cytra-2 solution ℞ *urinary alkalizing agent* [sodium citrate; citric acid] 500•334 mg/5 mL

Cytra-3 syrup ℞ *urinary alkalinizing agent* [potassium citrate; sodium citrate; citric acid] 550•500•334 mg/5 mL

Cytra-K oral solution ℞ *urinary alkalizing agent* [potassium citrate; citric acid] 1100•334 mg/5 mL

Cytra-LC solution ℞ *urinary alkalizing agent* [potassium citrate; sodium citrate; citric acid] 550•500•334 mg/5 mL

Cytuss HC oral liquid ℞ *narcotic antitussive; decongestant; antihistamine* [hydrocodone bitartrate; phenylephrine HCl; chlorpheniramine maleate] 5•10•4 mg/10 mL

CY-VA-DACT (Cytoxin, vincristine, Adriamycin, dactinomycin) *chemotherapy protocol*

CYVADIC; CY-VA-DIC; CyVADIC (cyclophosphamide, vincristine, Adriamycin, DIC) *chemotherapy protocol for bone and soft tissue sarcomas*

CYVMAD (cyclophosphamide, vincristine, methotrexate, Adriamycin, DTIC) *chemotherapy protocol*

D (vitamin D) [q.v.]

D-2.5-W; D-5-W; D-10-W; D-20-W; D-25-W; D-30-W; D-40-W; D-50-W; D-60-W; D-70-W ℞ *intravenous nutritional therapy* [dextrose]

D₂ (vitamin D₂) [see: ergocalciferol]

D₃ (vitamin D₃) [see: cholecalciferol]

d4T [see: stavudine]

D.A. chewable tablets ℞ *decongestant; antihistamine; anticholinergic to dry mucosal secretions* [phenylephrine HCl; chlorpheniramine maleate; methscopolamine nitrate] 10•2•1.25 mg

DA (daunorubicin, ara-C) *chemotherapy protocol for acute myelocytic leukemia (AML)*

D.A. II tablets ℞ *decongestant; antihistamine; anticholinergic to dry mucosal secretions* [phenylephrine HCl; chlorpheniramine maleate; methscopolamine nitrate] 10•4•1.25 mg

DAA (dihydroxyaluminum aminoacetate) [q.v.]

dacarbazine USAN, USP, INN, BAN *alkylating antineoplastic for metastatic malignant melanoma and Hodgkin disease* 100, 200 mg injection ⑨ Dicarbosil; procarbazine

dacemazine INN

dacisteine INN

dacliximab [now: daclizumab]

daclizumab USAN, INN, BAN *immuno-suppressant; monoclonal antibodies (MAb) to prevent acute rejection of organ and bone marrow transplants (orphan)*

Dacogen injection ℞ *antineoplastic; investigational (NDA filed, orphan) for myelodysplastic syndromes, chronic myelogenous leukemia, and sickle cell anemia; investigational (Phase III) for multiple myeloma* [decitabine]

Dacriose ophthalmic solution OTC *extraocular irrigating solution* [sterile isotonic solution]

dactinomycin USAN, USP, BAN *antibiotic antineoplastic for various tumors, carcinomas, and sarcomas; potentiator for radiation therapy* [also: actinomycin D]

dacuronium bromide INN, BAN

DADDS (diacetyl diaminodiphenyl-sulfone) [see: acedapsone]

dagapamil INN

daidzein *one of several soy isoflavones that provide cell-protective effects*

daidzin *isoform precursor to daidzein* [q.v.]

Daily Vitamins oral liquid OTC *vitamin supplement* [multiple vitamins]

Daily-Vite with Iron & Minerals tablets OTC *vitamin/mineral/iron supplement* [multiple vitamins & minerals; iron; folic acid; biotin] ≛•18•0.4• ≛ mg

Dairy Ease chewable tablets OTC *digestive aid for lactose intolerance* [lactase enzyme] 3000 U

daisy, wild *medicinal herb* [see: wild daisy]

Dakin solution [see: sodium hypochlorite]

Dalacin Ⓒᴬᴺ vaginal cream ℞ *lincosamide antibiotic for bacterial vaginosis* [clindamycin phosphate] 2% (100 mg/5 g dose)

Dalacin C Ⓒᴬᴺ capsules ℞ *lincosamide antibiotic* [clindamycin HCl] 150, 300 mg

Dalacin C Ⓒᴬᴺ granules for oral solution ℞ *lincosamide antibiotic* [clindamycin palmitate HCl] 75 mg/5 mL

Dalacin C Phosphate Ⓒᴬᴺ IV infusion, IM injection ℞ *lincosamide antibiotic; treatment for AIDS-related* Pneumocystis carinii *pneumonia* [clindamycin phosphate] 150 mg/mL

Dalacin T Ⓒᴬᴺ topical solution ℞ *topical antibiotic for acne* [clindamycin phosphate]

Dalalone intra-articular, intralesional, soft tissue, or IM injection ℞ *corticosteroid; anti-inflammatory* [dexamethasone sodium phosphate] 4 mg/mL

Dalalone D.P. intra-articular, soft tissue, or IM injection ℞ *corticosteroid; anti-inflammatory* [dexamethasone acetate] 16 mg/mL

Dalalone L.A. intralesional, intra-articular, soft tissue, or IM injection ℞ *corticosteroid; anti-inflammatory* [dexamethasone acetate] 8 mg/mL

dalanated insulin [see: insulin, dalanated]

dalbraminol INN

daledalin INN *antidepressant* [also: daledalin tosylate]

daledalin tosylate USAN *antidepressant* [also: daledalin]

dalfopristin USAN, INN *streptogramin antibacterial antibiotic for life-threatening infections*

dalfopristin & quinupristin *two streptogramin antibiotics that are synergistically bactericidal to gram-positive infections; investigational (NDA filed) for pneumonia*

Dallergy tablets, sustained-release caplets, syrup ℞ *decongestant; antihistamine; anticholinergic to dry mucosal secretions* [phenylephrine HCl; chlorpheniramine maleate; methscopolamine nitrate] 10•4•1.25 mg; 20•12•2.5 mg; 20•4•1.25 mg/10 mL

Dallergy-D syrup (discontinued 2002) OTC *decongestant; antihistamine* [phenylephrine HCl; chlorpheniramine maleate] 5•2 mg/5 mL

Dallergy-JR extended-release pediatric capsules, oral suspension ℞ *decongestant; antihistamine* [phenylephrine HCl; chlorpheniramine maleate] 20•4 mg; 20•4 mg/5 mL

Dalmane capsules ℞ *benzodiazepine sedative and hypnotic; anticonvulsant; muscle relaxant; also abused as a street drug* [flurazepam HCl] 15, 30 mg ⍰ Dialume

d′Alpha E 400; d′Alpha E 1000 softgels (discontinued 2004) OTC *vitamin supplement* [vitamin E (as *d*-alpha tocopherol)] 400 IU; 1000 IU

dalteparin sodium USAN, INN, BAN *a low molecular weight heparin–type anticoagulant and antithrombotic for prevention of deep vein thrombosis (DVT), unstable angina, and myocardial infarction*

daltroban USAN, INN *immunosuppressive*

Damason-P tablets ℞ *narcotic analgesic* [hydrocodone bitartrate; aspirin] 5•500 mg

dambose [see: inositol]

dametralast INN

damiana (Turnera aphrodisiaca; T. diffusa; T. microphylla) leaves *medicinal herb for bed-wetting, bronchitis, emphysema, headache, hormonal imbalance, hot flashes, menopause, and Parkinson disease; also used as an aphrodisiac*

damotepine INN

danaparoid sodium USAN, BAN *glycosaminoglycan anticoagulant and antithrombotic for prevention of deep vein thrombosis (DVT)*

danazol USAN, USP, INN, BAN *anterior pituitary suppressant; gonadotropin inhibitor for endometriosis, fibrocystic breast disease, and hereditary angioedema* 50, 100, 200 mg oral

dandelion (Leontodon taraxacum; Taraxacum officinale) leaves and root *medicinal herb for anemia, analgesia, blisters, blood cleansing, blood glucose regulation, constipation, diaphoresis, dyspepsia, edema, endurance, gallbladder disease, hypertension, and liver disorders*

daniplestim USAN *treatment for chemotherapy-induced bone marrow suppression*

daniquidone BAN

danitamon [see: menadione]

danitracen INN

Danocrine capsules (discontinued 2005) ℞ *gonadotropin inhibitor for endometriosis, fibrocystic breast disease, and hereditary angioedema* [danazol] 50, 100, 200 mg

danofloxacin INN *veterinary antibacterial* [also: danofloxacin mesylate]

danofloxacin mesylate USAN *veterinary antibacterial* [also: danofloxacin]

danosteine INN

danshen (Salvia miltiorrhiza) *medicinal herb for abdominal pain, bruises, circulatory problems, insomnia, menstrual irregularity, and stroke; also used as an aid in granulation of wounds*

danthron USP, BAN *(withdrawn from market by FDA)* [also: dantron] ⍰ Dantrium

Dantrium capsules, powder for IV injection ℞ *skeletal muscle relaxant; investigational (orphan) for neuroleptic malignant syndrome* [dantrolene sodium] 25, 50, 100 mg; 20 mg/vial (0.32 mg/mL) ⍰ danthron

dantrolene USAN, INN, BAN *skeletal muscle relaxant*

dantrolene sodium USAN, BAN *skeletal muscle relaxant; investigational (orphan) for neuroleptic malignant syndrome*

dantron INN *(withdrawn from market by FDA)* [also: danthron]

Dapacin Cold capsules (discontinued 2001) OTC *decongestant; antihistamine; analgesic* [phenylpropanolamine HCl; chlorpheniramine maleate; acetaminophen] 12.5•2•325 mg

Daphne mezereum medicinal herb [see: mezereon]

dapiprazole INN *α-adrenergic blocker; miotic; neuroleptic* [also: dapiprazole HCl]

dapoxetine *investigational (Phase III) agent for various urogenital indications, including premature ejaculation (PE)*

dapsone USAN, USP, BAN *bactericidal; leprostatic; herpetiform dermatitis suppressant; investigational (Phase III, orphan) for* Pneumocystis carinii *and toxoplasmosis* 25, 100 mg oral

dapsone & trimethoprim *investigational (Phase III) for* Pneumocystis carinii *pneumonia*

Daptacel IM injection R *active immunizing agent for diphtheria, tetanus, and pertussis* [diphtheria & tetanus toxoids & acellular pertussis (DTaP) vaccine, adsorbed] 15 Lf•5 Lf•10 μg per 0.5 mL dose

daptazole [see: amiphenazole]

daptomycin USAN, INN, BAN *cyclic lipopeptide antibiotic for skin and skin structure infections*

Daranide tablets (discontinued 2004) R *carbonic anhydrase inhibitor; diuretic* [dichlorphenamide] 50 mg ⍰ Daraprim

Daraprim tablets R *antimalarial; toxoplasmosis treatment adjunct* [pyrimethamine] 25 mg ⍰ Daranide

darbepoetin alfa USAN *hematopoietic; recombinant erythropoietin analogue for anemia associated with chronic renal failure*

darbufelone mesylate USAN *antiinflammatory; antiarthritic; cyclooxygenase inhibitor; 5-lipoxygenase inhibitor*

darenzepine INN

darglitazone sodium USAN *oral hypoglycemic*

darifenacin hydrobromide *selective muscarinic M_3 receptor antagonist for urinary frequency, urgency, and incontinence*

darodipine USAN, INN *antihypertensive; bronchodilator; vasodilator*

Darvocet A500 film-coated tablets R *narcotic analgesic* [propoxyphene napsylate; acetaminophen] 100•500 mg

Darvocet-N 50; Darvocet-N 100 tablets R *narcotic analgesic* [propoxyphene napsylate; acetaminophen] 50•325 mg; 100•650 mg ⍰ Darvon-N

Darvon Pulvules (capsules) R *narcotic analgesic* [propoxyphene HCl] 65 mg ⍰ Diovan

Darvon Compound 32; Darvon Compound 65 Pulvules (capsules) R *narcotic analgesic* [propoxyphene HCl; aspirin; caffeine] 32•389•32.4 mg; 65•389•32.4 mg ⍰ Diovan

Darvon-N film-coated tablets R *narcotic analgesic* [propoxyphene napsylate] 100 mg ⍰ Diovan

DAT (daunorubicin, ara-C, thioguanine) *chemotherapy protocol for acute myelocytic leukemia (AML)* [also: DCT; TAD]

datelliptium chloride INN

Datura stramonium medicinal herb [see: jimsonweed]

daturine hydrobromide [see: hyoscyamine hydrobromide]

DATVP (daunorubicin, ara-C, thioguanine, vincristine, prednisone) *chemotherapy protocol*

Daucus carota medicinal herb [see: carrot]

daunomycin [see: daunorubicin HCl]

daunorubicin (DNR) INN, BAN *anthracycline antibiotic antineoplastic for various leukemias* [also: daunorubicin HCl] ⍰ doxorubicin

daunorubicin citrate, liposomal *anthracycline antibiotic antineoplastic for advanced HIV-related Kaposi sarcoma (orphan)*

daunorubicin HCl USAN, USP, JAN *anthracycline antibiotic antineoplastic for various leukemias* [also: daunorubicin] 20, 50 mg injection ⍰ doxorubicin

DaunoXome IV infusion R *antibiotic antineoplastic for advanced AIDS-related Kaposi sarcoma (orphan)* [daunorubicin citrate, liposomal] 2 mg/mL (50 mg/dose)

DAV (daunorubicin, ara-C, VePesid) *chemotherapy protocol for acute myelocytic leukemia (AML)*

DAVA (desacetyl vinblastine amide) [see: vindesine]

DAVH (dibromodulcitol, Adriamycin, vincristine, Halotestin) *chemotherapy protocol*

davitamon [see: menadione]

Daxas ℞ *investigational (Phase III) agent for chronic obstructive pulmonary disease (COPD) and asthma* [roflumilast]

Dayalets Filmtabs (film-coated tablets) OTC *vitamin supplement* [multiple vitamins; folic acid] ±•0.4 mg

Dayalets + Iron Filmtabs (film-coated tablets) OTC *vitamin/iron supplement* [multiple vitamins; ferrous sulfate; folic acid] ±•18•0.4 mg

Dayhist-1 tablets OTC *antihistamine* [clemastine fumarate] 1.34 mg

Daypro film-coated caplets ℞ *antiarthritic; nonsteroidal anti-inflammatory drug (NSAID)* [oxaprozin] 600 mg

Daypro Alta film-coated caplets ℞ *antiarthritic; nonsteroidal anti-inflammatory drug (NSAID)* [oxaprozin potassium] 678 mg (=600 mg base)

DayQuil LiquiCaps (liquid-filled gelcaps), oral liquid (discontinued 2002) OTC *antitussive; decongestant; expectorant; analgesic* [dextromethorphan hydrobromide; pseudoephedrine HCl; guaifenesin; acetaminophen] 10•30•100•250 mg; 3.3•10•33.3•108.3 mg/5 mL

DayQuil Allergy Relief 4 Hour tablets (discontinued 2001) OTC *decongestant; antihistamine* [phenylpropanolamine HCl; brompheniramine maleate] 25•4 mg

DayQuil Allergy Relief 12 Hour extended-release tablets (discontinued 2001) OTC *decongestant; antihistamine* [phenylpropanolamine HCl; brompheniramine maleate] 75•12 mg

DayQuil Multi-Symptom Cold/Flu Relief LiquiCaps (liquid-filled gelcaps), oral liquid OTC *antitussive; decongestant; analgesic* [dextromethorphan hydrobromide; pseudoephedrine HCl; acetaminophen] 10•30•325 mg; 20•60•650 mg/30 mL

DayQuil Sinus Pressure & Pain Relief caplets (discontinued 2002) OTC *decongestant; analgesic; antipyretic* [pseudoephedrine HCl; acetaminophen] 30•500 mg

Dayto Himbin tablets (discontinued 2003) ℞ *alpha$_2$-adrenergic blocker for impotence; sympatholytic; mydriatic; may have aphrodisiac activity; no FDA-approved indications* [yohimbine HCl] 5.4 mg

Dayto Sulf vaginal cream (discontinued 2001) ℞ *broad-spectrum bacteriostatic* [sulfathiazole; sulfacetamide; sulfabenzamide] 3.42%•2.86%•3.7%

dazadrol INN *antidepressant* [also: dazadrol maleate]

dazadrol maleate USAN *antidepressant* [also: dazadrol]

Dazamide tablets (discontinued 2005) ℞ *carbonic anhydrase inhibitor diuretic; treatment for acute mountain sickness* [acetazolamide] 250 mg

dazepinil INN *antidepressant* [also: dazepinil HCl]

dazepinil HCl USAN *antidepressant* [also: dazepinil]

dazidamine INN

dazmegrel USAN, INN, BAN *thromboxane synthetase inhibitor*

dazolicine INN

dazopride INN *peristaltic stimulant* [also: dazopride fumarate]

dazopride fumarate USAN *peristaltic stimulant* [also: dazopride]

dazoquinast INN

dazoxiben INN, BAN *antithrombotic* [also: dazoxiben HCl]

dazoxiben HCl USAN *antithrombotic* [also: dazoxiben]

DBED (dibenzylethylenediamine dipenicillin G) [see: penicillin G benzathine]

DBM (dibromomannitol) [see: mitobronitol]

DC softgels OTC *laxative; stool softener* [docusate calcium] 240 mg

DC (daunorubicin, cytarabine) *chemotherapy protocol*

D&C Brown No. 1 (drugs & cosmetics) [see: resorcin brown]

DCA (desoxycorticosterone acetate) [q.v.]

DCA (dichloroacetate) [see: sodium dichloroacetate]

DCF (2′-deoxycoformycin) [see: pentostatin]

DCL (descarboethoxyloratadine) [q.v.]

DCMP (daunorubicin, cytarabine, mercaptopurine, prednisone) *chemotherapy protocol*

DCPM (daunorubicin, cytarabine, prednisone, mercaptopurine) *chemotherapy protocol*

DCT (daunorubicin, cytarabine, thioguanine) *chemotherapy protocol for acute myelocytic leukemia (AML)* [also: DAT; TAD]

DCV (DTIC, CCNU, vincristine) *chemotherapy protocol*

DCVax-Brain ℞ *investigational (Phase II, orphan) vaccine for glioblastoma multiforme* [dendritic cells pulsed with glioblastoma multiforme acid-eluted tumor antigens]

DCVax-Prostate ℞ *investigational (Phase II, orphan) vaccine for prostate cancer*

DDAVP tablets, nasal spray, rhinal tube, subcu or IV injection ℞ *posterior pituitary hormone for hemophilia A (orphan), von Willebrand disease (orphan), central diabetes insipidus, and nocturnal enuresis* [desmopressin acetate] 0.1, 0.2 mg; 10 μg/dose; 0.1 mg/mL; 15 μg/mL

DDAVP (1-deamino-8-D-arginine-vasopressin) [see: desmopressin acetate]

DDC; ddC (dideoxycytidine) [see: zalcitabine]

***o,p′*-DDD** [now: mitotane]

DDI; ddI (dideoxyinosine) [see: didanosine]

DDP; *cis*-DDP (diamminedichloroplatinum) [see: cisplatin]

DDS (diaminodiphenylsulfone) [now: dapsone]

DDT (dichlorodiphenyltrichloroethane) [see: chlorophenothane]

DDVP (dichlorovinyl dimethyl phosphate) [see: dichlorvos]

DEA (diethanolamine) [q.v.]

deacetyllanatoside C [see: deslanoside]

17-deacylnorgestimate [see: norelgestromin]

deadly nightshade *medicinal herb* [see: belladonna]

deadly nightshade leaf [see: belladonna extract]

deal pine *medicinal herb* [see: white pine]

1-deamino-8-D-arginine-vasopressin (DDAVP) [see: desmopressin acetate]

deanil INN *combining name for radicals or groups*

deanol BAN [also: deanol aceglumate]

deanol aceglumate INN [also: deanol]

deanol acetamidobenzoate

deba [see: barbital]

Debacterol oral solution with swab applicator ℞ *antiseptic and analgesic for ulcerating mouth and gum lesions such as aphthous ulcers (canker sores) and necrotizing ulcerative gingivitis (pyorrhea)* [sulfuric acid; sulfonated phenolics] 30%•50%

deboxamet INN

debrase *investigational (orphan) agent for debridement of acute, deep dermal burns*

Debridase ℞ *investigational (orphan) agent for debridement of acute, deep dermal burns* [debrase]

Debrisan beads, paste ℞ *debrider and cleanser for wet wounds* [dextranomer]

debrisoquin sulfate USAN *antihypertensive* [also: debrisoquine]

debrisoquine INN, BAN *antihypertensive* [also: debrisoquin sulfate]

Debrox ear drops OTC *agent to emulsify and disperse ear wax* [carbamide peroxide] 6.5%

Decadron tablets, elixir ℞ *corticosteroidal anti-inflammatory* [dexamethasone] 0.5, 0.75 mg ② Decaderm; Percodan

Decadron Phosphate intra-articular, intralesional, soft tissue or IM injection ℞ *corticosteroidal anti-inflammatory* [dexamethasone sodium phosphate] 4 mg/mL

Decadron Phosphate IV injection ℞ *corticosteroidal anti-inflammatory*

[dexamethasone sodium phosphate] 24 mg/mL

Decadron Phosphate Ocumeter (eye drops) ℞ *corticosteroidal anti-inflammatory* [dexamethasone sodium phosphate] 0.1%

Decadron with Xylocaine soft tissue injection ℞ *corticosteroidal anti-inflammatory* [dexamethasone sodium phosphate; lidocaine HCl] 4•10 mg/mL

Decadron-LA intralesional, intra-articular, soft tissue, or IM injection (discontinued 2004) ℞ *corticosteroidal anti-inflammatory* [dexamethasone acetate] 8 mg/mL

Deca-Durabolin IM injection (discontinued 2005) ℞ *anabolic steroid for anemia of renal insufficiency; sometimes abused as a street drug* [nandrolone decanoate (in oil)] 100, 200 mg/mL

Decagen tablets OTC *vitamin/mineral/iron supplement* [multiple vitamins & minerals; iron; folic acid; biotin] ±• 18 mg•0.4 mg•30 μg

Decaject intra-articular, intralesional, soft tissue, or IM injection ℞ *corticosteroidal anti-inflammatory* [dexamethasone sodium phosphate] 4 mg/mL

Decaject-L.A. intralesional, intra-articular, soft tissue, or IM injection ℞ *corticosteroidal anti-inflammatory* [dexamethasone acetate] 8 mg/mL

DECAL (dexamethasone, etoposide, cisplatin, ara-C, L-asparaginase) *chemotherapy protocol*

decamethonium bromide USP, INN [also: decamethonium iodide]

decamethonium iodide BAN [also: decamethonium bromide]

Decapinol oral rinse ℞ *gingivitis treatment*

decapinol [see: delmopinol]

Decavac IM injection ℞ *active immunizing agent for diphtheria and tetanus* [diphtheria & tetanus toxoids, adsorbed] 2•5 LfU per 0.5 mL dose

decavitamin USP

Decholin tablets OTC *laxative; hydrocholeretic* [dehydrocholic acid] 250 mg

decicain [see: tetracaine HCl]

decil INN *combining name for radicals or groups*

decimemide INN

decitabine USAN, INN, BAN *antineoplastic; investigational (NDA filed, orphan) for myelodysplastic syndromes, chronic myelogenous leukemia, and sickle cell anemia; investigational (Phase III) for multiple myeloma*

decitropine INN

declaben [now: lodelaben]

declenperone USAN, INN *veterinary sedative*

Declomycin capsules (discontinued 2003) ℞ *broad-spectrum antibiotic* [demeclocycline HCl] 150 mg

Declomycin film-coated tablets ℞ *broad-spectrum antibiotic* [demeclocycline HCl] 150, 300 mg

decloxizine INN

Decodult tablets OTC *decongestant; antihistamine; analgesic* [phenylephrine HCl; chlorpheniramine maleate; acetaminophen] 5•2•300 mg

Decofed syrup OTC *nasal decongestant* [pseudoephedrine HCl] 30 mg/5 mL

Decohistine DH oral liquid ℞ *narcotic antitussive; decongestant; antihistamine* [codeine phosphate; pseudoephedrine HCl; chlorpheniramine maleate; alcohol 5.8%] 10•30•2 mg/5 mL

Decolate tablets ℞ *decongestant; antihistamine; expectorant* [phenylephrine HCl; chlorpheniramine maleate; guaifenesin] 5•4•100 mg

decominol INN

Deconamine tablets, syrup ℞ *decongestant; antihistamine* [pseudoephedrine HCl; chlorpheniramine maleate] 60•4 mg; 30•2 mg/5 mL

Deconamine CX tablets, oral liquid (discontinued 2002) ℞ *narcotic antitussive; decongestant; expectorant* [hydrocodone bitartrate; pseudoephedrine HCl; guaifenesin] 5•30•300 mg; 5•60•200 mg/5 mL

Deconamine SR sustained-release capsules ℞ *decongestant; antihista-*

mine [pseudoephedrine HCl; chlorpheniramine maleate] 120•8 mg

Decongestabs sustained-release tablets (discontinued 2001) ℞ *decongestant; antihistamine* [phenylpropanolamine HCl; phenylephrine HCl; chlorpheniramine maleate; phenyltoloxamine citrate] 40•10•5•15 mg

Decongestant sustained-release tablets (discontinued 2001) ℞ *decongestant; antihistamine* [phenylpropanolamine HCl; phenylephrine HCl; chlorpheniramine maleate; phenyltoloxamine citrate] 40•10•5•15 mg

Decongestant tablets (discontinued 2002) OTC *decongestant; antihistamine; analgesic* [phenylephrine HCl; chlorpheniramine maleate; acetaminophen] 5•2•325 mg

Deconhist L.A. sustained-release tablets (discontinued 2001) ℞ *decongestant; antihistamine; anticholinergic* [phenylpropanolamine HCl; phenylephrine HCl; chlorpheniramine maleate; hyoscyamine sulfate; atropine sulfate; scopolamine hydrobromide] 50•25•8•0.19•0.04•0.01 mg

Deconomed SR sustained-release capsules ℞ *decongestant; antihistamine* [pseudoephedrine HCl; chlorpheniramine maleate] 120•8 mg

Deconsal II extended-release capsules ℞ *decongestant; expectorant* [phenylephrine HCl; guaifenesin] 20•375 mg

Deconsal II sustained-release tablets (discontinued 2004) ℞ *decongestant; expectorant* [pseudoephedrine HCl; guaifenesin] 60•600 mg ⑤ Deconal

Deconsal Sprinkle sustained-release capsules (discontinued 2002) ℞ *decongestant; expectorant* [phenylephrine HCl; guaifenesin] 10•300 mg ⑤ Deconal

decoquinate USAN, INN, BAN *coccidiostat for poultry*

dectaflur USAN, INN *dental caries prophylactic*

Decylenes ointment OTC *antifungal* [undecylenic acid; zinc undecylenate]

deditonium bromide INN

Deep-Down Rub OTC *analgesic; counterirritant* [methyl salicylate; menthol; camphor] 15%•5%•0.5%

deer musk *(Moschus moschiferus)* *natural remedy in ancient Chinese medicine; reported to have antianginal, antibacterial, antihistaminic, anti-inflammatory, CNS-depressant, and stimulant activity in clinical studies*

deerberry *medicinal herb* [see: holly; squaw vine; wintergreen]

DEET (diethyltoluamide) [q.v.]

DeFed-60 tablets (discontinued 2002) OTC *nasal decongestant* [pseudoephedrine HCl] 60 mg

Defen-LA sustained-release tablets (discontinued 2004) ℞ *decongestant; expectorant* [pseudoephedrine HCl; guaifenesin] 60•600 mg

deferasirox *investigational (NDA filed, orphan) once-daily oral iron chelator for chronic iron overload due to blood transfusions*

deferiprone *investigational (orphan) agent for chronic iron overload due to transfusion-dependent anemias*

deferoxamine USAN, INN *chelating agent for acute or chronic iron poisoning* [also: desferrioxamine]

deferoxamine HCl USAN *chelating agent for acute or chronic iron poisoning*

deferoxamine mesylate USAN, USP *chelating agent for acute or chronic iron poisoning* [also: desferrioxamine mesylate] 500, 2000 mg injection

defibrotide INN, BAN *investigational (orphan) agent for thrombotic thrombocytopenic purpura and hepatic veno-occlusive disease*

Definity injection ℞ *ultrasound contrast medium for cardiac imaging; investigational (NDA filed) for gynecologic imaging* [perflutren] 6.52 mg/mL

deflazacort USAN, INN, BAN *anti-inflammatory*

Deflux injectable gel ℞ *investigational treatment for pediatric vesicoureteral reflux (VUR)* [dextranomer microspheres in a NASHA carrier] 50 mg/mL

defosfamide INN

defungit sodium salt [see: bensul-dazic acid]

Defy eye drops ℞ topical ophthalmic antibiotic [tobramycin] 0.3%

Degas chewable tablets OTC antiflatu-lent [simethicone] 80 mg

Degest 2 eye drops OTC topical ophthalmic decongestant and vasoconstrictor [naphazoline HCl] 0.012%

Dehistine syrup ℞ decongestant; antihistamine; anticholinergic to dry mucosal secretions [phenylephrine HCl; chlorpheniramine maleate; methscopolamine nitrate] 20•4•2.5 mg/10 mL

dehydrated alcohol [see: alcohol, dehydrated]

dehydrex investigational (orphan) for recurrent corneal erosion

Dehydrex drops ℞ investigational (orphan) treatment for recurrent corneal erosion [dextran 70]

dehydroacetic acid NF preservative

dehydroandrosterone [see: prasterone]

dehydrocholate sodium USP [also: sodium dehydrocholate]

7-dehydrocholesterol, activated [now: cholecalciferol]

dehydrocholic acid USP, INN, BAN, JAN choleretic; laxative; investigational (orphan) agent for congenital errors of cholesterol and bile acid synthesis 250 mg oral

dehydrocholin [see: dehydrocholic acid]

dehydroemetine INN, BAN, DCF investigational anti-infective for amebiasis and amebic dysentery

dehydroepiandrosterone (DHEA) natural hormone precursor; investigational (NDA filed, orphan) for systemic lupus erythematosus (SLE); investigational (orphan) replacement therapy for adrenal insufficiency

dehydroepiandrosterone sulfate (DHEAS) investigational (Phase II) injectable antiasthmatic

dehydroepiandrosterone sulfate sodium investigational (orphan) agent

for re-epithelialization of serious burns and skin graft donor sites

Deka oral liquid ℞ decongestant; antihistamine; antitussive; expectorant [pseudoephedrine HCl; dexbrompheniramine maleate; dextromethorphan hydrobromide; guaifenesin] 15•0.5•15•100 mg/5 mL

Deka Pediatric oral drops ℞ decongestant; antihistamine; antitussive; expectorant [pseudoephedrine HCl; dexbrompheniramine maleate; dextromethorphan hydrobromide; guaifenesin] 12.5•0.5•4•40 mg/mL

Del Aqua-5; Del Aqua-10 gel (discontinued 2003) ℞ keratolytic for acne [benzoyl peroxide] 5%; 10%

delanterone INN

Delaprem (approved in several foreign countries) ℞ investigational (NDA filed) tocolytic and bronchodilator [hexoprenaline sulfate]

delapril INN antihypertensive; angiotensin-converting enzyme inhibitor [also: delapril HCl]

delapril HCl USAN antihypertensive; angiotensin-converting enzyme inhibitor [also: delapril]

Delatestryl IM injection ℞ androgen replacement for testosterone deficiency in men, delayed puberty in boys, and metastatic breast cancer in women; sometimes abused as a street drug [testosterone enanthate (in oil)] 200 mg/mL

delavirdine INN antiviral; non-nucleoside reverse transcriptase inhibitor (NNRTI) for HIV and AIDS [also: delavirdine mesylate]

delavirdine mesylate USAN antiviral; investigational (Phase III) non-nucleoside reverse transcriptase inhibitor (NNRTI) for HIV and AIDS [also: delavirdine]

delayed-release aspirin [see: aspirin]

Delcap (trademarked dosage form) unit dispensing cap

Delcort cream OTC topical corticosteroidal anti-inflammatory [hydrocortisone] 0.5%, 1% ▣ Dilacor

delequamine INN α_2 adrenoreceptor antagonist for sexual dysfunction [also: delequamine HCl]

delequamine HCl USAN α_2 adrenoreceptor antagonist for sexual dysfunction [also: delequamine]

delergotrile INN

Delestrogen IM injection ℞ estrogen replacement therapy for the treatment of postmenopausal symptoms and prevention of postmenopausal osteoporosis; hormonal antineoplastic for prostate and metastatic breast cancers [estradiol valerate in oil (synthetic estrogen)] 10, 20, 40 mg/mL

delfantrine INN

delfaprazine INN

Delfen Contraceptive vaginal foam OTC spermicidal contraceptive [nonoxynol 9] 12.5%

delmadinone INN, BAN progestin; antiandrogen; antiestrogen [also: delmadinone acetate]

delmadinone acetate USAN progestin; antiandrogen; antiestrogen [also: delmadinone]

delmetacin INN

delmopinol INN

Del-Mycin topical solution (discontinued 2003) ℞ antibiotic for acne [erythromycin] 2%

delnav [see: dioxathion]

delorazepam INN

deloxolone INN

m-delphene [see: diethyltoluamide]

delprostenate INN, BAN

Delsym extended-release oral suspension OTC antitussive [dextromethorphan polistirex] 30 mg/5 mL

Delta-Cortef tablets ℞ corticosteroid; anti-inflammatory [prednisolone] 5 mg

deltacortone [see: prednisone]

Delta-D tablets OTC vitamin supplement [cholecalciferol (vitamin D_3)] 400 IU

deltafilcon A USAN hydrophilic contact lens material

deltafilcon B USAN hydrophilic contact lens material

delta-1-hydrocortisone [see: prednisolone]

Deltasone tablets ℞ corticosteroid; anti-inflammatory [prednisone] 2.5, 5, 10, 20 mg

delta-9-tetrahydrocannabinol (THC) [see: dronabinol]

delta-9-THC (tetrahydrocannabinol) [see: dronabinol]

Delta-Tritex cream, ointment ℞ topical corticosteroidal anti-inflammatory [triamcinolone acetonide] 0.1%

Deltavac vaginal cream ℞ broad-spectrum antibiotic; antiseptic; vulnerary [sulfanilamide; aminacrine HCl; allantoin] 15%•0.2%•2%

deltibant USAN bradykinin antagonist for treatment of systemic inflammatory response syndrome

delta-stab [see: prednisolone]

delucemine HCl USAN NMDA receptor antagonist; neuroprotectant

Demadex tablets, IV injection ℞ antihypertensive; loop diuretic [torsemide] 5, 10, 20, 100 mg; 10 mg/mL

Demazin Repetabs (repeat-action tablets), syrup (discontinued 2001) OTC decongestant; antihistamine [phenylpropanolamine HCl; chlorpheniramine maleate] 25•4 mg; 12.5•2 mg/5 mL

dembrexine INN, BAN

dembroxol [see: dembrexine]

demecarium bromide USP, INN, BAN antiglaucoma agent; reversible cholinesterase inhibitor miotic

demeclocycline USP, BAN tetracycline antibiotic

demeclocycline HCl USP, BAN tetracycline antibiotic; antirickettsial 150, 300 mg oral

demecolcine INN, BAN

demecycline USAN, INN antibacterial

demegestone INN

demekastigmine bromide [see: demecarium bromide]

demelverine INN

Demerol tablets, syrup, IV or IM injection ℞ narcotic analgesic; also abused as a street drug [meperidine HCl] 50, 100 mg; 50 mg/5 mL; 25, 50, 75, 100 mg/mL

demetacin [see: delmetacin]

11-demethoxyreserpine [see: deserpidine]

demethylchlortetracycline (DMCT) [now: demeclocycline]

demethylchlortetracycline HCl [see: demeclocycline HCl]

N-demethylcodeine [see: norcodeine]

demexiptiline INN

Demi-Regroton tablets ℞ *antihypertensive; diuretic* [chlorthalidone; reserpine] 25•0.125 mg

democonazole INN

demoxepam USAN, INN *minor tranquilizer*

demoxytocin INN

Demser capsules ℞ *antihypertensive for pheochromocytoma* [metyrosine] 250 mg

demulcents *a class of agents that soothe irritated or abraded tissues, particularly mucous membranes*

Demulen 1/35; Demulen 1/50 tablets (in Compacks of 21 or 28) ℞ *monophasic oral contraceptive* [ethynodiol diacetate; ethinyl estradiol] 1 mg•35 μg; 1 mg•50 μg ⊠ Demerol; Demolin

denatonium benzoate USAN, NF, INN, BAN *alcohol denaturant; flavoring agent*

denaverine INN

Denavir cream ℞ *antiviral for recurrent herpes labialis* [penciclovir] 1%

denbufylline INN, BAN

dendritic cells pulsed with glioblastoma multiforme acid-eluted tumor antigens *investigational (orphan) agent for glioblastoma multiforme*

denileukin diftitox USAN, INN *antineoplastic for cutaneous T-cell lymphoma (orphan)*

denipride INN

denofungin USAN *antifungal; antibacterial*

denopamine INN

Denorex shampoo (discontinued 2003) OTC *antiseborrheic; antipsoriatic; antipruritic; antibacterial* [coal tar; menthol; alcohol] 9%•1.5•7.5%; 12.5%•1.5%•10.4%

Denorex Everyday Dandruff shampoo OTC *antiseborrheic; antibacterial; antifungal* [pyrithione zinc] 2%

denpidazone INN

Denquel toothpaste OTC *tooth desensitizer* [potassium nitrate] 5%

Denta 5000 Plus dental cream ℞ *topical caries preventative* [sodium fluoride] 1.1%

DentaGel ℞ *topical dental caries preventative* [sodium fluoride] 1.1%

dental antiformin [see: antiformin, dental]

dental-type silica [see: silica, dental-type]

Dentipatch transmucosal patch ℞ *mucous membrane anesthetic* [lidocaine HCl] 23, 46.1 mg

Dent's Lotion-Jel lotion/gel OTC *mucous membrane anesthetic* [benzocaine]

Dent's Toothache Gum; Dent's Toothache Drops OTC *topical oral anesthetic* [benzocaine]

denyl sodium [see: phenytoin sodium]

denzimol INN

deodorants *a class of agents that mask undesirable or offensive odors* [also called: antibromics]

2′-deoxycoformycin (DCF) [see: pentostatin]

deoxycorticosterone acetate [see: desoxycorticosterone acetate]

deoxycorticosterone pivalate [see: desoxycorticosterone pivalate]

deoxycortolone pivalate BAN *salt-regulating adrenocortical steroid* [also: desoxycorticosterone pivalate]

deoxycortone BAN *salt-regulating adrenocortical steroid* [also: desoxycorticosterone acetate; desoxycortone]

2′-deoxycytidine *investigational (orphan) host-protective agent in acute myelogenous leukemia*

deoxyephedrine HCl [see: methamphetamine HCl]

12-deoxyerythromycin [see: berythromycin]

deoxyribonuclease, recombinant human (rhDNase) [see: dornase alfa]

deoxyribonucleic acid (DNA)

15-deoxyspergualin trihydrochloride
[now: gusperimus trihydrochloride]

Depacin capsules OTC *analgesic; antipyretic* [acetaminophen] 325 mg

Depacon IV infusion ℞ *anticonvulsant* [valproate sodium] 500 mg/vial

Depade tablets (discontinued 2004) ℞ *narcotic antagonist for opiate dependence or overdose (orphan) and alcoholism* [naltrexone HCl] 50 mg

Depakene capsules ℞ *anticonvulsant* [valproic acid] 250 mg

Depakene syrup ℞ *anticonvulsant* [valproate sodium] 250 mg/5 mL

Depakote delayed-release enteric-coated tablets ℞ *anticonvulsant; antipsychotic for manic episodes of a bipolar disorder; migraine prophylaxis* [divalproex sodium] 125, 250, 500 mg

Depakote sprinkle capsules ℞ *anticonvulsant* [divalproex sodium] 125 mg

Depakote ER extended-release tablets ℞ *anticonvulsant; antipsychotic for manic episodes of a bipolar disorder; migraine headache preventative* [divalproex sodium] 250, 500 mg

depAndro 100; depAndro 200 IM injection (discontinued 2001) ℞ *androgen replacement for delayed puberty or breast cancer* [testosterone cypionate] 100 mg/mL; 200 mg/mL

Depen titratable tablets ℞ *metal chelating agent for rheumatoid arthritis, Wilson disease, and cystinuria* [penicillamine] 250 mg

depepsen [see: sodium amylosulfate]

depGynogen IM injection (discontinued 2003) ℞ *estrogen replacement therapy for the treatment of postmenopausal symptoms* [estradiol cypionate in oil] 5 mg/mL

depMedalone 40; depMedalone 80 intralesional, soft tissue, and IM injection ℞ *corticosteroid; anti-inflammatory; immunosuppressant* [methylprednisolone acetate] 40 mg/mL; 80 mg/mL

DepoCyt sustained-release intrathecal injection ℞ *antineoplastic for lymphomatous neoplastic meningitis (NM) arising from solid tumors or non-Hodgkin lymphoma (orphan)* [cytarabine, liposomal] 10 mg/mL

DepoDur extended-release liposomal suspension for epidural injection ℞ *narcotic analgesic* [morphine sulfate] 10 mg/mL

Depo-Estradiol IM injection ℞ *synthetic estrogen; hormone replacement therapy for the treatment of postmenopausal symptoms* [estradiol cypionate in oil] 5 mg/mL

DepoGen IM injection (discontinued 2003) ℞ *estrogen replacement therapy for the treatment of postmenopausal symptoms* [estradiol cypionate in oil] 5 mg/mL

Depoject intralesional, soft tissue, and IM injection ℞ *corticosteroid; anti-inflammatory; immunosuppressant* [methylprednisolone acetate] 40, 80 mg/mL

Depo-Medrol intralesional, soft tissue, and IM injection ℞ *corticosteroid; anti-inflammatory; immunosuppressant* [methylprednisolone acetate] 20, 40, 80 mg/mL

DepoMorphine ℞ *investigational (Phase II) sustained-release, encapsulated formulation to treat severe post-surgical pain* [morphine sulfate]

Deponit transdermal patch (discontinued 2005) ℞ *antianginal; vasodilator* [nitroglycerin] 16, 32 mg (0.2, 0.4 mg/hr.)

Depopred-40; Depopred-80 intralesional, soft tissue, and IM injection ℞ *corticosteroid; anti-inflammatory; immunosuppressant* [methylprednisolone acetate] 40 mg/mL; 80 mg/mL

Depo-Provera IM injection ℞ *hormonal antineoplastic adjunct for metastatic endometrial and renal carcinoma; long-term injectable contraceptive* [medroxyprogesterone acetate] 150, 400 mg/mL

Depo-Sub Q Provera 104 subcu injection in prefilled syringes ℞ *hormonal antineoplastic adjunct for meta-*

static endometrial and renal carcinoma; long-term injectable contraceptive [medroxyprogesterone acetate] 104 mg

Depotest 100; Depotest 200 IM injection (discontinued 2001) ℞ *androgen replacement for delayed puberty or breast cancer* [testosterone cypionate] 100 mg/mL; 200 mg/mL

Depo-Testadiol IM injection (discontinued 2004) ℞ *hormone replacement therapy for postmenopausal symptoms* [estradiol cypionate; testosterone cypionate] 2•50 mg/mL

Depotestogen IM injection (discontinued 2003) ℞ *hormone replacement therapy for postmenopausal symptoms* [estradiol cypionate; testosterone cypionate] 2•50 mg/mL

Depo-Testosterone IM injection ℞ *androgen replacement for testosterone deficiency in men; sometimes abused as a street drug* [testosterone cypionate (in oil)] 100, 200 mg/mL

depramine INN [also: balipramine]

deprenyl (L-deprenyl) [see: selegiline HCl]

depreotide USAN *radiopharmaceutical imaging agent for lung cancer; investigational (NDA filed) for malignant melanoma and neuroendocrine tumors*

depressants *a class of agents that reduce functional activity and vital energy in general by producing muscular relaxation and diaphoresis*

deprodone INN, BAN

Deproic Ⓒᴬᴺ capsules, syrup (discontinued 2001) ℞ *anticonvulsant* [valproic acid] 250, 500 mg; 250 mg/5 mL

Deproist Expectorant with Codeine oral liquid (discontinued 2002) ℞ *narcotic antitussive; decongestant; expectorant* [codeine phosphate; pseudoephedrine HCl; guaifenesin; alcohol 8.2%] 10•30•100 mg/5 mL

deprostil USAN, INN *gastric antisecretory*

deptropine INN, BAN

deptropine citrate [see: deptropine]

depurants; depuratives *a class of agents that purify or cleanse the sys-*

tem, particularly the blood [also called: pellants]

dequalinium chloride INN, BAN

Dequasine tablets OTC *dietary supplement* [multiple minerals & amino acids; vitamin C] ± •200 mg

deracoxib USAN *COX-2 inhibitor antiinflammatory and analgesic for osteoarthritis and rheumatoid arthritis*

deramciclane *serotonin 5-HT₂ receptor antagonist; investigational (Phase III) antidepressant and anxiolytic for general anxiety disorder (GAD)*

Derifil tablets OTC *systemic deodorant for ostomy, breath, and body odors* [chlorophyllin] 100 mg

Derma Viva lotion (discontinued 2004) OTC *moisturizer; emollient*

Dermabase OTC *cream base*

Dermabond topical liquid OTC *skin adhesive for closing surgical incisions and traumatic lacerations*

Dermacoat aerosol OTC *topical local anesthetic* [benzocaine] 4.5%

Dermacort cream, lotion ℞ *corticosteroidal anti-inflammatory* [hydrocortisone] 1% ⍰ DermiCort

Dermadrox ointment OTC *astringent; skin protectant; emollient* [aluminum hydroxide gel; zinc chloride; lanolin]

DermaFlex gel OTC *local anesthetic* [lidocaine] 2.5%

Dermal-Rub balm OTC *analgesic; counterirritant* [methyl salicylate; camphor; racemic manthol; cajuput oil]

Dermamycin cream, spray OTC *antihistamine* [diphenhydramine HCl] 2%

Derma-Pax lotion OTC *antihistamine; antiseptic; antipruritic* [pyrilamine maleate; chlorpheniramine maleate; alcohol 35%] 0.44%•0.06%

Dermarest gel OTC *antihistamine; antifungal* [diphenhydramine HCl; resorcinol] 2%•2%

Dermarest Dricort Creme OTC *corticosteroidal anti-inflammatory* [hydrocortisone acetate] 1%

Dermarest Plus gel, spray OTC *antihistamine; analgesic; counterirritant* [diphenhydramine HCl; menthol] 2%•1%

Dermasept Antifungal spray liquid OTC *antifungal; antiseptic; anesthetic; astringent* [tolnaftate; tannic acid; zinc chloride; benzocaine; methylbenzethonium HCl; undecylenic acid; alcohol 58.54%] 1.017%•6.098%• 5.081%•2.032%•3.049%•5.081%

Dermasil lotion OTC *bath emollient*

Derma-Smoothe/FS oil Ŗ *corticosteroidal anti-inflammatory; emollient* [fluocinolone acetonide] 0.01%

dermatan sulfate [see: danaparoid sodium]

dermatol [see: bismuth subgallate]

Dermatop E cream, ointment Ŗ *corticosteroidal anti-inflammatory* [prednicarbate] 0.1%

DermaVite tablets OTC *vitamin/mineral supplement* [multiple vitamins & minerals; folic acid; biotin] ±•400• 600 μg

Dermazinc shampoo OTC *antiseborrheic; antibacterial; antifungal* [pyrithione zinc] 0.25%

Derm-Cleanse topical liquid OTC *soap-free therapeutic skin cleanser*

Dermol HC anorectal cream, anorectal ointment Ŗ *corticosteroidal anti-inflammatory* [hydrocortisone] 1%, 2.5%; 1%

Dermolate Anti-Itch cream OTC *corticosteroidal anti-inflammatory* [hydrocortisone] 0.5%

Dermolin liniment OTC *analgesic; counterirritant; antiseptic* [methyl salicylate; camphor; racemic menthol; mustard oil; alcohol 8%]

Dermoplast aerosol spray, lotion OTC *local anesthetic; analgesic* [benzocaine; menthol] 20%•0.5%; 8%•0.5%

Dermovan OTC *cream base*

Dermprotective Factor (DPF) (trademarked ingredient) *aromatic syrup* [eriodictyon]

Dermtex HC with Aloe cream OTC *corticosteroidal anti-inflammatory* [hydrocortisone] 0.5%

Dermuspray aerosol spray Ŗ *enzyme for wound debridement* [trypsin; peruvian balsam] 0.1•72.5 mg/0.82 mL

derpanicate INN

DES (diethylstilbestrol) [q.v.]

desacetyl vinblastine amide (DAVA) [see: vindesine]

desacetyl-lanatoside C [see: deslanoside]

desaglybuzole [see: glybuzole]

desamino-oxytocin [see: demoxytocin]

desaspidin INN

descarboethoxyloratadine (DCL) *investigational antihistamine for allergy*

desciclovir USAN, INN *antiviral*

descinolone INN *corticosteroid; anti-inflammatory* [also: descinolone acetonide]

descinolone acetonide USAN *corticosteroid; anti-inflammatory* [also: descinolone]

Desenex cream OTC *antifungal* [clotrimazole] 1%

Desenex foam, soap OTC *antifungal* [undecylenic acid] 10%

Desenex powder, aerosol powder, ointment, cream OTC *antifungal* [undecylenic acid; zinc undecylenate] 25% total

Desenex, Prescription Strength spray liquid, spray powder OTC *antifungal* [miconazole nitrate] 2%

Desenex Antifungal cream OTC *antifungal* [miconazole nitrate] 2%

DesenexMax cream OTC *allylamine antifungal* [terbinafine HCl] 1%

deserpidine INN, BAN *antihypertensive; peripheral antiadrenergic; rauwolfia derivative* ⑨ desipramine

desert herb; desert tea *medicinal herb* [see: ephedra]

Desert Pure Calcium film-coated tablets OTC *calcium supplement* [calcium carbonate; vitamin D] 500 mg•125 IU

Desferal powder for IM, IV, or subcu injection Ŗ *chelating agent for acute or chronic iron poisoning* [deferoxamine mesylate] 500, 2000 mg ⑨ Disophrol

desferrioxamine BAN *chelating agent for acute or chronic iron poisoning* [also: deferoxamine]

desferrioxamine mesylate BAN *chelating agent for acute or chronic iron poisoning* [also: deferoxamine mesylate]

desflurane USAN, INN *inhalation general anesthetic*

desglugastrin INN

desipramine INN, BAN *tricyclic antidepressant* [also: desipramine HCl] ☑ deserpidine

desipramine HCl USAN, USP *tricyclic antidepressant* [also: desipramine] 10, 25, 50, 75, 100, 150 mg oral

desirudin USAN *anticoagulant; thrombin inhibitor for the prevention of deep vein thrombosis (DVT) in elective hip replacement surgery*

Desitin ointment OTC *moisturizer; emollient; astringent; antiseptic* [cod liver oil; zinc oxide]

Desitin Creamy ointment OTC *topical diaper rash treatment* [zinc oxide] 10%

Desitin with Zinc Oxide powder OTC *topical diaper rash treatment* [zinc oxide; corn starch] 10%•88.2%

deslanoside USP, INN, BAN *cardiotonic; cardiac glycoside*

desloratadine USAN *second-generation peripherally selective piperidine antihistamine for allergic rhinitis and chronic idiopathic urticaria; active metabolite of loratadine*

deslorelin USAN, INN *LHRH agonist; investigational (orphan) for central precocious puberty*

desmethylmoramide INN

desmophosphamide [see: defosfamide]

desmopressin INN, BAN *posterior pituitary antidiuretic hormone (ADH)* [also: desmopressin acetate]

desmopressin acetate USAN *antidiuretic; posterior pituitary antidiuretic hormone for hemophilia A (orphan), von Willebrand disease (orphan), and nocturnal enuresis* [also: desmopressin] 4 μg/mL injection; 10 μg nasal spray

desocriptine INN

Desogen tablets (in packs of 28) ℞ *monophasic oral contraceptive* [desogestrel; ethinyl estradiol] 0.15 mg•30 μg

desogestrel USAN, INN, BAN *progestin*

desolone [see: deprodone]

desomorphine INN, BAN

desonide USAN, INN, BAN *topical corticosteroidal anti-inflammatory* 0.05% topical

DesOwen ointment, cream, lotion ℞ *corticosteroidal anti-inflammatory* [desonide] 0.05%

Desoxi ⓒᴬᴺ cream, gel ℞ *corticosteroidal anti-inflammatory* [desoximetasone] 0.05%, 0.25%; 0.05%

desoximetasone USAN, USP, INN *topical corticosteroidal anti-inflammatory* [also: desoxymethasone] 0.05%, 0.25% topical ☑ dexamethasone

desoxycholic acid *increases secretion of bile acids*

desoxycorticosterone acetate (DCA; DOCA) USP *salt-regulating adrenocortical steroid* [also: desoxycortone; deoxycortone]

desoxycorticosterone pivalate USP *salt-regulating adrenocortical steroid* [also: deoxycortolone pivalate]

desoxycorticosterone trimethylacetate USP

desoxycortone INN *salt-regulating adrenocortical steroid* [also: desoxycorticosterone acetate; deoxycortone]

l-desoxyephedrine [see: levmetamfetamine]

desoxyephedrine HCl [see: methamphetamine HCl]

desoxymethasone BAN *topical corticosteroidal anti-inflammatory* [also: desoximetasone]

Desoxyn Gradumets (sustained-release tablets) (discontinued 2002) ℞ *CNS stimulant; sometimes abused as a street drug* [methamphetamine HCl] 5, 10, 15 mg ☑ digitoxin; digoxin

Desoxyn tablets ℞ *CNS stimulant; sometimes abused as a street drug* [methamphetamine HCl] 5 mg ☑ digitoxin; digoxin

desoxyribonuclease [see: fibrinolysin & desoxyribonuclease]

Despec oral liquid (discontinued 2002) ℞ *decongestant; expectorant* [phenylephrine HCl; phenylpropa-

nolamine HCl; guaifenesin] 20•5•
100 mg/5 mL

Desquam-E gel (discontinued 2003)
℞ *keratolytic for acne* [benzoyl peroxide] 2.5%

Desquam-E 5; Desquam-E 10 gel ℞ *keratolytic for acne* [benzoyl peroxide] 5%; 10%

Desquam-X cleansing bar ℞ *keratolytic for acne* [benzoyl peroxide] 10%

Desquam-X 5; Desquam-X 10 gel ℞ *keratolytic for acne* [benzoyl peroxide] 5%; 10%

Desquam-X 5 Wash; Desquam-X 10 Wash topical liquid (discontinued 2003) ℞ *keratolytic for acne* [benzoyl peroxide] 5%; 10%

de-Stat 3; de-Stat 4 solution OTC *cleaning/disinfecting/soaking solution for rigid gas permeable contact lenses*

destradiol [see: estradiol]

63-desulfohirudin [see: desirudin]

Desyrel film-coated tablets, Dividose (multiple-scored tablets) ℞ *antidepressant used for panic disorders, aggressive behavior, alcoholism, and cocaine withdrawal* [trazodone HCl] 50, 100 mg; 150, 300 mg

DET (diethyltryptamine) [q.v.]

Detachol topical liquid OTC *adhesive remover for the skin*

detajmium bitartrate INN

Detane gel OTC *topical local anesthetic* [benzocaine] 7.5%

detanosal INN

Detect-A-Strep slide tests for professional use *in vitro diagnostic aid for streptococcal antigens in throat swabs*

Detecto-Seal (trademarked packaging form) *tamper-resistant parenteral package*

deterenol INN *ophthalmic adrenergic* [also: deterenol HCl]

deterenol HCl USAN *ophthalmic adrenergic* [also: deterenol]

detergents *a class of agents that cleanse wounds and sores*

detigon HCl [see: chlophedianol HCl]

detirelix INN *luteinizing hormone-releasing hormone (LHRH) antagonist* [also: detirelix acetate]

detirelix acetate USAN *luteinizing hormone-releasing hormone (LHRH) antagonist* [also: detirelix]

detomidine INN, BAN *veterinary analgesic; sedative* [also: detomidine HCl]

detomidine HCl USAN *veterinary analgesic; sedative* [also: detomidine]

detorubicin INN

detralfate INN

Detrol film-coated tablets ℞ *muscarinic receptor antagonist for urinary frequency, urgency, and incontinence* [tolterodine tartrate] 1, 2 mg

Detrol LA extended-release capsules ℞ *muscarinic receptor antagonist for urinary frequency, urgency, and incontinence* [tolterodine tartrate] 2, 4 mg

detrothyronine INN

Detrusitol (European name for U.S. product Detrol)

Detussin oral liquid ℞ *narcotic antitussive; decongestant* [hydrocodone bitartrate; pseudoephedrine HCl; alcohol 5%] 5•60 mg/5 mL

Detussin Expectorant oral liquid (discontinued 2002) ℞ *narcotic antitussive; decongestant; expectorant* [hydrocodone bitartrate; pseudoephedrine HCl; guaifenesin; alcohol] 5•60•200 mg/5 mL

deuterium oxide USAN *radioactive agent*

devapamil INN

devazepide USAN *cholecystokinin antagonist*

devil's bones *medicinal herb* [see: wild yam]

devil's claw (Harpagophytum procumbens) root *medicinal herb for arrhythmias, arteriosclerosis, arthritis, blood cleansing, diabetes, hypertension, liver disease, lowering cholesterol, rheumatism, stomach disorders, and strengthening bladder and kidneys*

devil's club (Echinopanax horridum; Fatsia horrida; Oplopanax horridus; Panax horridum) cambium and stem *medicinal herb for arthritis, burns* *and cuts, colds, cough, fever, inducing vomiting and bowel evacuation, pneumonia, and tuberculosis*

devil's dung *medicinal herb* [see: asafetida]

devil's eye *medicinal herb* [see: henbane]

devil's fuge *medicinal herb* [see: mistletoe]

devil's shrub *medicinal herb* [see: Siberian ginseng]

Devrom chewable tablets OTC *systemic deodorizer for ostomy and incontinence odors* [bismuth subgallate] 200 mg

dewberry *medicinal herb* [see: blackberry]

Dex GG TR timed-release tablets ℞ *antitussive; expectorant* [dextromethorphan hydrobromide; guaifenesin] 60•1000 mg

Dex4 Glucose chewable tablets OTC *glucose elevating agent* [glucose]

dexa [see: dexamethasone]

Dexacidin eye drop suspension ℞ *ophthalmic corticosteroidal anti-inflammatory; antibiotic* [dexamethasone; neomycin sulfate; polymyxin B sulfate] 0.1%•0.35%•10 000 U/mL

Dexacidin ophthalmic ointment (name changed to Dexacine in 2002)

Dexacine ophthalmic ointment (discontinued 2004) ℞ *corticosteroidal anti-inflammatory; antibiotic* [dexamethasone; neomycin sulfate; polymyxin B sulfate] 0.1%•0.35%•10 000 U/g

Dexacort Phosphate Respihaler (oral inhalation aerosol) ℞ *corticosteroid for bronchial asthma* [dexamethasone sodium phosphate] 84 μg/dose

Dexacort Phosphate Turbinaire (nasal inhalation aerosol) ℞ *intranasal corticosteroidal anti-inflammatory* [dexamethasone sodium phosphate; alcohol 2%] 84 μg/dose

Dexafed Cough syrup (discontinued 2002) OTC *antitussive; decongestant; expectorant* [dextromethorphan hydrobromide; phenylephrine HCl; guaifenesin] 10•5•100 mg/5 mL

DexAlone liquid-filled gelcaps OTC *antitussive* [dextromethorphan hydrobromide] 30 mg

Dexameth tablets (discontinued 2004) ℞ *corticosteroidal anti-inflammatory* [dexamethasone] 0.5, 0.75, 1.5, 4 mg

dexamethasone USP, INN, BAN *corticosteroidal anti-inflammatory; investigational (orphan) for idiopathic intermediate uveitis* 0.25, 0.5, 0.75, 1, 1.5, 2, 4, 6 mg oral; 0.5 mg/5 mL oral ② desoximetasone

dexamethasone acefurate USAN, INN *corticosteroidal anti-inflammatory*

dexamethasone acetate USAN, USP, BAN *corticosteroidal anti-inflammatory* 8 mg/mL injection

dexamethasone dipropionate USAN *corticosteroidal anti-inflammatory*

Dexamethasone Intensol oral drops ℞ *corticosteroidal anti-inflammatory* [dexamethasone] 1 mg/mL

dexamethasone & neomycin sulfate & polymyxin B sulfate *topical ophthalmic corticosteroidal anti-inflammatory and antibiotic* 0.1%•0.35%•10 000 U/mL eye drops

dexamethasone sodium phosphate USP, BAN *corticosteroid; anti-inflammatory* 0.05%, 0.1% eye drops; 4, 10 mg/mL injection

dexamfetamine INN *CNS stimulant* [also: dextroamphetamine; dexamphetamine]

dexamisole USAN, INN *antidepressant*

dexamphetamine BAN *CNS stimulant* [also: dextroamphetamine; dexamfetamine]

Dexaphen S.A. sustained-release tablets (discontinued 2002) ℞ *decongestant; antihistamine* [pseudoephedrine sulfate; dexbrompheniramine maleate] 120•6 mg

Dexasone intra-articular, intralesional, soft tissue, or IM injection ℞ *corticosteroid; anti-inflammatory* [dexamethasone sodium phosphate] 4 mg/mL

Dexasone L.A. intralesional, intra-articular, soft tissue, or IM injection

Ŗ *corticosteroid; anti-inflammatory* [dexamethasone acetate] 8 mg/mL

Dexasporin ophthalmic ointment Ŗ *topical ophthalmic corticosteroidal anti-inflammatory; antibiotic* [dexamethasone; neomycin sulfate; polymyxin B sulfate] 0.1%•0.35%•10 000 U/g

Dexatrim extended-release tablets, timed-release capsules (discontinued 2001) OTC *diet aid* [phenylpropanolamine HCl] 75 mg

Dexatrim plus Vitamin C timed-release capsules (discontinued 2001) OTC *diet aid* [phenylpropanolamine HCl; vitamin C] 75•180 mg

Dexatrim Pre-Meal timed-release capsules (discontinued 2001) OTC *diet aid* [phenylpropanolamine HCl] 25 mg

dexbrompheniramine INN, BAN *alkylamine antihistamine* [also: dexbrompheniramine maleate]

dexbrompheniramine maleate USP *alkylamine antihistamine* [also: dexbrompheniramine]

dexchlorpheniramine INN *alkylamine antihistamine* [also: dexchlorpheniramine maleate]

dexchlorpheniramine maleate USP *alkylamine antihistamine* [also: dexchlorpheniramine] 4, 6 mg oral; 2 mg/5 mL oral

dexchlorpheniramine tannate *alkylamine antihistamine*

dexclamol INN *sedative* [also: dexclamol HCl]

dexclamol HCl USAN *sedative* [also: dexclamol]

Dexedrine Spansules (sustained-release capsules), tablets Ŗ *amphetamine; CNS stimulant; widely abused as a street drug* [dextroamphetamine sulfate] 5, 10, 15 mg; 5 mg ⑫ dextran

dexetimide USAN, INN, BAN *anticholinergic*

dexetozoline INN

dexfenfluramine INN, BAN *anorexiant; appetite suppressant; serotonin reuptake inhibitor* [also: dexfenfluramine HCl]

dexfenfluramine HCl USAN *anorexiant; appetite suppressant; serotonin reuptake inhibitor* [also: dexfenfluramine]

DexFerrum IV or IM injection Ŗ *hematinic* [iron dextran] 50, 100 mg/dose

DexFol tablets Ŗ *vitamin B supplement* [vitamins B_1, B_2, B_3, B_5, B_6, B_{12}, and C; folic acid; biotin] 1.5•1.5•20•10•50•1•60•5•0.3 mg

dexibuprofen USAN, INN *analgesic; cyclooxygenase inhibitor; anti-inflammatory*

dexibuprofen lysine USAN *analgesic; cyclooxygenase inhibitor; anti-inflammatory* [also: dexibuprofen]

deximafen USAN, INN *antidepressant*

dexindoprofen INN

Dexiron ⓒⓐⓃ IM injection Ŗ *hematinic* [iron dextran] 50 mg/mL

dexivacaine USAN, INN *anesthetic*

dexlofexidine INN

dexmedetomidine USAN, INN, BAN *sedative*

dexmedetomidine HCl *sedative for intubated and ventilated patients in an intensive care setting; premedication to anesthesia*

dexmethylphenidate HCl *CNS stimulant for attention-deficit hyperactivity disorder (ADHD) and narcolepsy; active isomer of methylphenidate HCl*

dexnorgestrel acetime [now: norgestimate]

Dexone intra-articular, intralesional, soft tissue, or IM injection (discontinued 2004) Ŗ *corticosteroidal anti-inflammatory* [dexamethasone sodium phosphate] 4 mg/mL

Dexone tablets (discontinued 2004) Ŗ *corticosteroidal anti-inflammatory* [dexamethasone] 0.5, 0.75, 1.5, 4 mg

Dexone LA intralesional, intra-articular, soft tissue, or IM injection Ŗ *corticosteroidal anti-inflammatory* [dexamethasone acetate] 8 mg/mL

dexormaplatin USAN, INN *antineoplastic*

dexoxadrol INN *CNS stimulant; analgesic* [also: dexoxadrol HCl]

dexoxadrol HCl USAN *CNS stimulant; analgesic* [also: dexoxadrol]

dexpanthenol USAN, USP, INN, BAN *cholinergic; antipruritic; postoperative prophylaxis for paralytic ileus* 250 mg/mL injection

dexpemedolac USAN *analgesic*

dexpropranolol HCl USAN *antiarrhythmic; antiadrenergic (β-receptor)* [also: dexpropranolol]

dexproxibutene INN

dexrazoxane USAN, INN, BAN *cardioprotectant for doxorubicin-induced cardiomyopathy (orphan); chelates intracellular iron* 250, 500 mg injection

dexsecoverine INN

dexsotalol HCl USAN *class III antiarrhythmic*

dextilidine INN

dextran INN, BAN *blood flow adjuvant; plasma volume extender* [also: dextran 40] ☒ Dexedrine; dextrin

dextran, high molecular weight [see: dextran 70]

dextran, low molecular weight [see: dextran 40]

dextran 1 *monovalent hapten for prevention of dextran-induced anaphylactic reactions; investigational (orphan) for cystic fibrosis*

dextran 40 USAN *blood flow adjuvant; plasma volume extender* [also: dextran] 10% injection

dextran 70 USAN *plasma volume extender; viscosity-increasing agent; investigational (orphan) for recurrent corneal erosion* 6% injection

dextran 75 USAN *plasma volume extender; viscosity-increasing agent* 6% injection

dextran sulfate *investigational (orphan) inhalant for cystic fibrosis*

dextran sulfate, sodium salt, aluminum complex [see: detralfate]

dextran sulfate sodium *investigational (orphan) agent for AIDS*

dextranomer INN, BAN *wound cleanser and debrider*

dextrates USAN, NF *tablet binder and diluent*

dextriferron NF, INN, BAN

dextrin NF, BAN *suspending agent; tablet binder and diluent* ☒ dextran

dextroamphetamine USAN *CNS stimulant; widely abused as a street drug, which causes strong psychic dependence* [also: dexamfetamine; dexamphetamine]

dextroamphetamine phosphate USP *CNS stimulant*

dextroamphetamine saccharate *CNS stimulant*

dextroamphetamine sulfate USP *CNS stimulant; widely abused as a street drug, which causes psychic dependence* 5, 10, 15 mg oral

dextrobrompheniramine maleate [see: dexbrompheniramine maleate]

dextrochlorpheniramine maleate [see: dexchlorpheniramine maleate]

dextrofemine INN

dextromethorphan USP, INN, BAN *antitussive*

dextromethorphan hydrobromide USP, BAN *antitussive*

dextromethorphan hydrobromide & guaifenesin *antitussive; expectorant* 30•500, 60•1000 mg oral

dextromethorphan polistirex USAN *antitussive*

dextromethorphan tannate *antitussive*

dextromoramide INN, BAN

dextromoramide tartrate [see: dextromoramide]

dextro-pantothenyl alcohol [see: dexpanthenol]

dextropropoxiphene chloride [see: propoxyphene HCl]

dextropropoxyphene INN, BAN *narcotic analgesic* [also: propoxyphene HCl]

dextropropoxyphene HCl BAN [also: propoxyphene HCl]

dextrorphan INN, BAN *adjunct to vasospastic therapy; investigational glutamate receptor antagonist for neurodegenerative disorders* [also: dextrorphan HCl]

dextrorphan HCl USAN *adjunct to vasospastic therapy; investigational glu-*

tamate receptor antagonist for neurodegenerative disorders [also: dextrorphan]

dextrose USP *fluid and nutrient replenisher; parenteral antihypoglycemic*

5% Dextrose and Electrolyte #48; 5% Dextrose and Electrolyte #75; 10% Dextrose and Electrolyte #48 IV infusion ℞ *intravenous nutritional/electrolyte therapy* [combined electrolyte solution; dextrose]

dextrose excipient NF *tablet excipient*

50% Dextrose with Electrolyte Pattern A (or N) IV infusion (discontinued 2001) ℞ *intravenous nutritional/electrolyte therapy* [combined electrolyte solution; dextrose]

Dextrostat tablets ℞ *amphetamine; CNS stimulant* [dextroamphetamine sulfate] 5, 10 mg

Dextrostix reagent strips for home use (discontinued 2004) *in vitro diagnostic aid for blood glucose*

dextrothyronine [see: detrothyronine]

dextrothyroxine BAN *antihyperlipidemic* [also: dextrothyroxine sodium]

dextrothyroxine sodium USAN, USP, INN *antihyperlipidemic* [also: dextrothyroxine]

dexverapamil INN *investigational adjunct to chemotherapy*

Dey-Dose (delivery system) *nebulizer*

Dey-Lute (delivery system) *nebulizer*

Dey-Pak Sodium Chloride 3% & 10% solution ℞ *for inducing sputum production for specimen collection* [sodium chloride] 3%; 10%

dezaguanine USAN, INN *antineoplastic*

dezaguanine mesylate USAN *antineoplastic*

dezinamide USAN, INN *anticonvulsant*

dezocine USAN, INN *narcotic analgesic*

DFMO (difluoromethylornithine) [see: eflornithine]

DFMO (difluoromethylornithine) HCl [see: eflornithine HCl]

DFMO-MGBG (eflornithine, mitoguazone) *chemotherapy protocol* [also see: DFMO; MGBG]

DFP (diisopropyl flurophosphate) [see: isoflurophate]

DFV (DDP, fluorouracil, VePesid) *chemotherapy protocol*

DHA (docosahexaenoic acid) [q.v.; also: doconexent]

DHAP (dexamethasone, high-dose ara-C, Platinol) *chemotherapy protocol for non-Hodgkin lymphoma*

DHC Plus capsules ℞ *narcotic analgesic* [dihydrocodeine bitartrate; acetaminophen; caffeine] 16•356.4•30 mg

DHE (dihydroergotamine) [see: dihydroergotamine mesylate]

D.H.E. 45 IV or IM injection ℞ *prophylaxis or treatment of migraine and cluster headaches* [dihydroergotamine mesylate] 1 mg/mL

DHEA (dehydroepiandrosterone) [q.v.]

DHPG (dihydroxy propoxymethyl guanine) [see: ganciclovir]

DHS Tar liquid shampoo, gel shampoo OTC *antiseborrheic; antipsoriatic; antipruritic; antibacterial* [coal tar] 0.5%

DHS Zinc shampoo OTC *antiseborrheic; antibacterial; antifungal* [pyrithione zinc] 2%

DHT tablets, Intensol (concentrated oral solution) ℞ *vitamin D therapy for tetany and hypoparathyroidism* [dihydrotachysterol] 0.125, 0.2, 0.4 mg; 0.2 mg/mL

DHT (dihydrotachysterol) [q.v.]

DHT (dihydrotestosterone) [see: androstanolone; stanolone]

DI (doxorubicin, ifosfamide [with mesna rescue]) *chemotherapy protocol for soft tissue sarcoma*

Diaβeta (or DiaBeta) tablets ℞ *sulfonylurea antidiabetic* [glyburide] 1.25, 2.5, 5 mg

Diabetic Tussin oral liquid OTC *expectorant* [guaifenesin] 100 mg/5 mL

Diabetic Tussin oral liquid (discontinued 2002) OTC *antitussive; decongestant; expectorant* [dextromethorphan hydrobromide; phenylephrine HCl; guaifenesin] 10•5•100 mg/5 mL

Diabetic Tussin DM oral liquid OTC *antitussive; expectorant* [dextrometh-

orphan hydrobromide; guaifenesin]
20•200, 20•400 mg/10 mL
Diabetic Tussin EX oral liquid (discontinued 2002) OTC *expectorant*
[guaifenesin] 100 mg/5 mL
Diabinese tablets R *sulfonylurea antidiabetic* [chlorpropamide] 100, 250 mg
diacerein INN
diacetamate INN, BAN
diacetolol INN, BAN *antiadrenergic (β-receptor)* [also: diacetolol HCl]
diacetolol HCl USAN *antiadrenergic (β-receptor)* [also: diacetolol]
diacetoxyphenylisatin [see: oxyphenisatin acetate]
diacetoxyphenyloxindol [see: oxyphenisatin acetate]
diacetrizoate sodium [see: diatrizoate sodium]
diacetyl diaminodiphenylsulfone (DADDS) [see: acedapsone]
diacetylated monoglycerides NF *plasticizer*
diacetylcholine chloride [see: succinylcholine chloride]
diacetyl-dihydroxydiphenylisatin [see: oxyphenisatin acetate]
diacetyldioxphenylisatin [see: oxyphenisatin acetate]
diacetylmorphine HCl USP *(heroin; banned in USA)* [also: diamorphine]
diacetylmorphine salts *(heroin; banned in USA)*
diacetylsalicylic acid [see: dipyrocetyl]
diacetyltannic acid [see: acetyltannic acid]
diacetylthiamine [see: acetiamine]
diagniol [see: sodium acetrizoate]
diallybarbituric acid [see: allobarbital]
diallylbarbituric acid [now: allobarbital]
diallylnortoxiferene dichloride [see: alcuronium chloride]
diallymal [see: allobarbital]
Dialpak (trademarked packaging form) *reusable patient compliance package for oral contraceptives*
Dialume capsules R *antacid* [aluminum hydroxide gel] 500 mg ⑨ Dalmane

Dialyte Pattern LM solution R *peritoneal dialysis solution* [multiple electrolytes; dextrose] 1.5%•*, 2.5%•*, 4.5%•*
Dialyvite 3000 tablets OTC *vitamin/ mineral supplement* [multiple vitamins & minerals; folic acid; biotin] *•3•0.3 mg
dia-mer-sulfonamides (sulfadiazine & sulfamerazine) [q.v.]
diamethine [see: dimethyltubocurarinium chloride; dimethyltubocurarine]
diamfenetide INN [also: diamphenethide]
diaminedipenicillin G [see: penicillin G benzathine]
diaminodiphenylsulfone (DDS) [now: dapsone]
3,4-diaminopyridine *investigational (orphan) for Lambert-Eaton myasthenic syndrome*
cis-diamminedichloroplatinum (DDP) [see: cisplatin]
diammonium phosphate [see: ammonium phosphate]
diamocaine INN, BAN *local anesthetic* [also: diamocaine cyclamate]
diamocaine cyclamate USAN *local anesthetic* [also: diamocaine]
diamorphine BAN *(heroin; banned in the U.S.)* [also: diacetylmorphine HCl]
Diamox powder for IV injection (discontinued 2005) R *carbonic anhydrase inhibitor diuretic; antiglaucoma; anticonvulsant; treatment for acute mountain sickness* [acetazolamide sodium] 500 mg
Diamox tablets, Sequels (sustained-release capsules) R *carbonic anhydrase inhibitor diuretic; antiglaucoma; anticonvulsant; treatment for acute mountain sickness* [acetazolamide] 125, 250 mg; 500 mg
diamphenethide BAN [also: diamfenetide]
diampromide INN, BAN
diampron [see: amicarbalide]
diamthazole BAN [also: dimazole]
diamthazole dihydrochloride [see: diamthazole]

Dianabol tablets (discontinued 1982) ℞ *steroid; discontinued for human use, but the veterinary product is still available and sometimes abused as a street drug* [methandrostenolone] 2.5, 5 mg

Diane-35 Ⓒᴬᴺ sugar-coated tablets ℞ *antiandrogen/estrogen for severe acne in women* [cyproterone acetate; ethinyl estradiol] 2•0.035 mg

diapamide USAN *diuretic; antihypertensive* [also: tiamizide]

Diaparene Baby cream OTC *topical diaper rash treatment*

Diaparene Cornstarch Baby powder OTC *topical diaper rash treatment* [corn starch; aloe]

Diaparene Diaper Rash ointment OTC *diaper rash treatment* [zinc oxide]

Diaper Guard ointment OTC *diaper rash treatment* [dimethicone; vitamins A, D, and E; zinc oxide] 1%• ± • ?

Diaper Rash ointment OTC *diaper rash treatment* [zinc oxide]

diaphene [see: dibromsalan]

diaphenylsulfone [see: dapsone]

diaphoretics *a class of agents that promote profuse perspiration* [also called: sudorifics]

Diapid nasal spray (discontinued 2001) ℞ *pituitary antidiuretic hormone for diabetes insipidus* [lypressin] 50 U/mL

Diar-Aid tablets OTC *antidiarrheal; GI adsorbent* [loperamide HCl] 2 mg

diarbarone INN

Diascan reagent strips for home use *in vitro diagnostic aid for blood glucose*

DiaScreen reagent strips for professional use *in vitro diagnostic aid for multiple disease markers in the urine*

Diasorb tablets, oral liquid OTC *antidiarrheal; GI adsorbent* [activated attapulgite] 750 mg; 750 mg/5 mL

Diastat rectal gel in a disposable applicator ("pediatric" and "adult" refer to the length of the applicator tip) ℞ *benzodiazepine anticonvulsant for acute repetitive seizures* (orphan) [diazepam] 2.5, 5, 10 mg (pediatric); 10, 15, 20 mg (adult)

Diastix reagent strips for home use *in vitro diagnostic aid for urine glucose*

diathymosulfone INN

diatrizoate meglumine USP *oral/parenteral radiopaque contrast medium (46.67% iodine)* [also: meglumine diatrizoate] 76% injection

diatrizoate methylglucamine [see: diatrizoate meglumine]

diatrizoate sodium USP *oral/rectal/parenteral radiopaque contrast medium (59.87% iodine)* [also: sodium amidotrizoate; sodium diatrizoate]

diatrizoate sodium I 125 USAN *radioactive agent*

diatrizoate sodium I 131 USAN *radioactive agent*

diatrizoic acid USAN, USP, BAN *radiopaque contrast medium* [also: amidotrizoic acid]

Diatx tablets ℞ *hematinic* [multiple B vitamins; folic acid; biotin] ± •5• 0.3 mg

Diatx Fe tablets ℞ *vitamin/mineral supplement for anemia* [multiple B vitamins; folic acid; biotin; ferrous fumarate] ± •5•0.3•100 mg

diaveridine USAN, INN, BAN *antibacterial*

diazacholesterol dihydrochloride [see: azacosterol HCl]

diazepam USAN, USP, INN, BAN, JAN *benzodiazepine anxiolytic; sedative; skeletal muscle relaxant; anticonvulsant for acute repetitive seizures* (orphan); *alcohol withdrawal aid; also abused as a street drug* 2, 5, 10 mg oral; 5 mg/5 mL oral; 5 mg/mL injection

Diazepam Intensol oral drops ℞ *benzodiazepine sedative; anxiolytic; skeletal muscle relaxant; anticonvulsant; also abused as a street drug* [diazepam; alcohol 19%] 5 mg/mL

diazinon BAN [also: dimpylate]

diaziquone USAN, INN *antineoplastic; investigational* (orphan) *for primary brain malignancies* (astrocytomas)

diazoxide USAN, USP, INN, BAN *emergency antihypertensive; vasodilator; glucose-elevating agent*

dibasic calcium phosphate [see: calcium phosphate, dibasic]

dibasic potassium phosphate [see: potassium phosphate, dibasic]

dibasic sodium phosphate [see: sodium phosphate, dibasic]

dibasol [see: bendazol]

dibazol [see: bendazol]

dibekacin INN, BAN

dibemethine INN

dibencil [see: penicillin G benzathine]

dibencozide [see: cobamamide]

Dibent IM injection ℞ GI antispasmodic [dicyclomine HCl] 10 mg/mL

dibenthiamine [see: bentiamine]

dibenzathione [see: sulbentine]

dibenzepin INN, BAN antidepressant [also: dibenzepin HCl]

dibenzepin HCl USAN antidepressant [also: dibenzepin]

dibenzodiazepines a class of novel (atypical) antipsychotic agents

dibenzothiazepines a class of novel (atypical) antipsychotic agents

dibenzothiazine [see: phenothiazine]

dibenzothiophene USAN keratolytic

dibenzoxazepines a class of dopamine receptor antagonists with antipsychotic, hypotensive, antiemetic, antispasmodic, and antihistaminic activity

dibenzoyl peroxide [see: benzoyl peroxide]

dibenzoylthiamin [see: bentiamine]

dibenzthion [see: sulbentine]

dibenzylethylenediamine dipenicillin G (DBED) [see: penicillin G benzathine]

Dibenzyline capsules ℞ antihypertensive for pheochromocytoma [phenoxybenzamine HCl] 10 mg

N,N-dibenzylmethylamine [see: dibemethine]

dibromodulcitol [see: mitolactol]

dibromohydroxyquinoline [see: broxyquinoline]

dibromomannitol (DBM) [see: mitobronitol]

dibromopropamidine BAN [also: dibrompropamidine]

4,5-dibromorhodamine 123 investigational (orphan) for chronic myelogenous leukemia

dibrompropamidine INN [also: dibromopropamidine]

dibromsalan USAN, INN disinfectant

dibrospidium chloride INN

dibucaine USP topical local anesthetic [also: cinchocaine] 1% topical

dibucaine HCl USP local anesthetic [also: cinchocaine HCl]

dibudinate INN combining name for radicals or groups

dibunate INN combining name for radicals or groups

dibuprol INN

dibupyrone INN, BAN

dibusadol INN

dibutoline sulfate

DIC (dimethyl imidazole carboxamide) [see: dacarbazine]

Dical CapTabs (capsule-shaped tablets) OTC dietary supplement [dibasic calcium phosphate; vitamin D] 117 mg (Ca)•90 mg (P)•133 IU

dicalcium phosphate [see: calcium phosphate, dibasic]

Dical-D chewable wafers (discontinued 2005) OTC dietary supplement [dibasic calcium phosphate; vitamin D] 232 mg (Ca)•180 mg (P)•200 IU

Dical-D tablets OTC dietary supplement [dibasic calcium phosphate; vitamin D] 105 mg (Ca)•81 mg (P)•120 IU

dicarbine INN

dicarfen INN

dichlofenthion BAN

dichloralantipyrine [see: dichloralphenazone]

dichloralphenazone (chloral hydrate & phenazone) BAN mild sedative

dichloralphenazone & acetaminophen & isometheptane mucate cerebral vasoconstrictor and analgesic for vascular and tension headaches; "possibly effective" for migraine headaches 100•325•65 mg oral

dichloralpyrine [see: dichloralphenazone]

dichloramine-T NF

dichloranilino imidazolin [see: clonidine HCl]

dichloren [see: mechlorethamine HCl]

dichlorisone INN

dichlorisone acetate [see: dichlorisone]

dichlormethazanone [see: dichlormezanone]

dichlormezanone INN

dichloroacetic acid *strong keratolytic/cauterant* ② Bichloracetic acid

dichlorodifluoromethane NF *aerosol propellant; topical refrigerant anesthetic*

dichlorodiphenyl trichloroethane (DDT) [see: chlorophenothane]

dichlorometaxylenol [see: dichloroxylenol]

dichloromethane [see: methylene chloride]

dichlorophen INN, BAN

dichlorophenarsine INN, BAN [also: dichlorophenarsine HCl]

dichlorophenarsine HCl USP [also: dichlorophenarsine]

dichlorotetrafluoroethane NF *aerosol propellant; topical refrigerant anesthetic* [also: cryofluorane]

dichlorovinyl dimethyl phosphate (DDVP) [see: dichlorvos]

dichloroxylenol INN, BAN

dichlorphenamide USP, BAN *carbonic anhydrase inhibitor; diuretic* [also: diclofenamide]

dichlorvos USAN, INN, BAN *anthelmintic*

dichysterol [see: dihydrotachysterol]

diciferron INN

dicirenone USAN, INN *hypotensive; aldosterone antagonist*

Dick test (scarlet fever streptococcus toxin)

diclazuril USAN, INN, BAN *coccidiostat for poultry; investigational for cryptosporidiosis in AIDS*

diclofenac INN, BAN *analgesic; antiarthritic; nonsteroidal anti-inflammatory drug (NSAID) for ankylosing spondylitis* [also: diclofenac potassium]

diclofenac potassium USAN *analgesic; antiarthritic; nonsteroidal anti-inflammatory drug (NSAID) for ankylosing*

spondylitis; topical treatment for actinic keratoses [also: diclofenac] 50 mg oral

diclofenac sodium USAN, JAN *analgesic; antiarthritic; nonsteroidal anti-inflammatory drug (NSAID) for ankylosing spondylitis; ocular treatment for cataract extraction and corneal refractive surgery; topical treatment for actinic keratoses (AK)* 25, 50, 75, 100 mg oral

diclofenamide INN *carbonic anhydrase inhibitor* [also: dichlorphenamide]

diclofensine INN

diclofibrate [see: simfibrate]

diclofurime INN

diclometide INN

diclonixin INN

dicloralurea USAN, INN *veterinary food additive*

Diclotec ⒸⒶⓃ *suppositories* ℞ *nonsteroidal anti-inflammatory drug (NSAID); antiarthritic; analgesic* [diclofenac sodium] 50, 100 mg

dicloxacillin USAN, INN, BAN *penicillinase-resistant penicillin antibiotic*

dicloxacillin sodium USAN, USP, BAN *penicillinase-resistant penicillin antibiotic* 250, 500 mg oral

dicobalt edetate INN, BAN

dicolinium iodide INN

Dicomal-DH *syrup* ℞ *narcotic antitussive; decongestant; antihistamine* [hydrocodone bitartrate; phenylephrine HCl; pyrilamine maleate] 1.66•5•8.33 mg/5 mL

Dicomal-DM *syrup* OTC *antitussive; decongestant; antihistamine* [dextromethorphan hydrobromide; phenylephrine HCl; pyrilamine maleate] 20•10•16.67 mg/10 mL

dicophane BAN [also: chlorophenothane; clofenotane]

dicoumarin [see: dicumarol]

dicoumarol INN *coumarin-derivative anticoagulant* [also: dicumarol]

dicresulene INN

Dictamnus albus *medicinal herb* [see: fraxinella]

dicumarol USAN, USP *coumarin-derivative anticoagulant* [also: dicoumarol] ② Demerol

dicyclomine BAN *anticholinergic* [also: dicyclomine HCl; dicycloverine]

dicyclomine HCl USP *GI antispasmodic; anticholinergic* [also: dicycloverine; dicyclomine] 10, 20 mg oral; 10 mg/5 mL oral; 10 mg/mL injection

dicycloverine INN *anticholinergic* [also: dicyclomine HCl; dicyclomine]

dicycloverine HCl [see: dicyclomine HCl]

dicysteine [see: cystine]

didanosine USAN, INN, BAN *antiviral nucleoside reverse transcriptase inhibitor for HIV-1 infections (orphan)* 200, 250, 400 mg oral

didehydrodideoxythymidine [see: stavudine]

Di-Delamine gel, spray OTC *topical antihistamine; bacteriostatic* [diphenhydramine HCl; tripelennamine HCl] 1%•0.5%•

2′,3′-dideoxyadenosine (ddA) *investigational (orphan) treatment for AIDS*

dideoxycytidine (DDC; ddC) [see: zalcitabine]

dideoxyinosine (DDI; ddI) [see: didanosine]

Didrex tablets ℞ *anorexiant* [benzphetamine HCl] 50 mg

Didrocal ⒸⒶ⒩ tablets (in a 90-day therapy pack) ℞ *bisphosphonate bone resorption inhibitor plus calcium supplement for established postmenopausal osteoporosis* [Phase 1 (14 days): etidronate disodium; Phase 2 (76 days): calcium carbonate] 400 mg; 1250 mg

Didro-Kit (Italian name for U.S. product Didronel)

Didronel tablets ℞ *bisphosphonate bone resorption inhibitor for Paget disease, heterotopic ossification, and hypercalcemia of malignancy (orphan)* [etidronate disodium] 200, 400 mg

Didronel IV infusion (discontinued 2004) ℞ *bisphosphonate bone resorption inhibitor for hypercalcemia of malignancy (orphan); investigational (orphan) for metabolic bone disease* [etidronate disodium] 300 mg/ampule

didrovaltrate INN

didroxane [see: dichlorophen]

dieldrin INN, BAN

dielytra; choice dielytra *medicinal herb* [see: turkey corn]

diemal [see: barbital]

dienestrol USP, INN *estrogen* [also: dienoestrol]

dienoestrol BAN *estrogen* [also: dienestrol]

dienogest INN

Diet Ayds candy (discontinued 2001) OTC *decrease taste perception of sweetness* [benzocaine] 6 mg

dietamiphylline [see: etamiphyllin]

dietamiverine HCl [see: bietamiverine HCl]

diethadione INN, BAN

diethanolamine NF *alkalizing agent*

diethazine INN, BAN

diethazine HCl [see: diethazine]

diethyl phthalate NF *plasticizer*

diethylamine *p*-aminobenzenestibonate [see: stibosamine]

3-diethylaminobutyranilide [see: octacaine]

diethylbarbiturate monosodium [see: barbital sodium]

diethylbarbituric acid [see: barbital]

diethylcarbamazine INN, BAN *anthelmintic for Bancroft filariasis, onchocerciasis, tropical eosinophilia, and loiasis* [also: diethylcarbamazine citrate]

diethylcarbamazine citrate USP *anthelmintic for Bancroft filariasis, onchocerciasis, tropical eosinophilia, and loiasis* [also: diethylcarbamazine]

diethylcarbamazine dihydrogen citrate [see: diethylcarbamazine citrate]

diethyldithiocarbamate *investigational (Phase II/III, orphan) immunomodulator for HIV and AIDS*

diethyldixanthogen [see: dixanthogen]

diethylenediamine citrate [see: piperazine citrate]

diethylenetriaminepentaacetic acid (DTPA) [see: pentetic acid]

N,N-diethyllysergamide [see: lysergide]

diethylmalonylurea [see: barbital]

diethylmalonylurea sodium [see: barbital sodium]

N,N-diethylnicotinamide [see: nikethamide]

diethylnorspermine *investigational (Phase I) anticancer agent*

diethylpropion BAN *anorexiant; CNS stimulant* [also: diethylpropion HCl; amfepramone] 75 mg oral

diethylpropion HCl USP *anorexiant; CNS stimulant* [also: amfepramone; diethylpropion] 25 mg oral

diethylstilbestrol (DES) USP, INN *hormonal antineoplastic for inoperable prostatic and breast cancer* [also: stilboestrol]

diethylstilbestrol diphosphate USP *hormonal antineoplastic* [also: fosfestrol]

diethylstilbestrol dipropionate NF

p-diethylsulfamoylbenzoic acid [see: etebenecid; ethebenecid]

diethylthiambutene INN, BAN

diethyltoluamide (DEET) USP, BAN *arthropod repellent*

diethyltryptamine (DET) *a hallucinogenic street drug closely related to dimethyltryptamine (DMT), but prepared synthetically*

N,N-diethylvanillamide [see: ethamivan]

dietifen INN

dietroxine [see: diethadione]

Dieutrim T.D. timed-release capsules (discontinued 2001) OTC *diet aid; decrease perception of sweetness* [phenylpropanolamine HCl; benzocaine] 75•9 mg

diexanthogen [see: dixanthogen]

difebarbamate INN

difemerine INN [also: difemerine HCl]

difemerine HCl [also: difemerine]

difemetorex INN

difenamizole INN

difencloxazine INN

difencloxazine HCl [see: difencloxazine]

difenidol INN *antiemetic; antivertigo* [also: diphenidol]

difenoximide INN *antiperistaltic* [also: difenoximide HCl]

difenoximide HCl USAN *antiperistaltic* [also: difenoximide]

difenoxin USAN, INN, BAN *antiperistaltic*

difenoxin HCl *antiperistaltic*

diferuloylmethane *investigational (orphan) agent for cystic fibrosis*

difetarsone INN, BAN

difeterol INN

Differin solution, gel, cream, single-use pledgets ℞ *synthetic retinoid analogue for acne* [adapalene] 0.1%

diflorasone INN, BAN *topical corticosteroidal anti-inflammatory* [also: diflorasone diacetate]

diflorasone diacetate USAN, USP *topical corticosteroidal anti-inflammatory* [also: diflorasone] 0.05% topical

difloxacin INN *anti-infective; DNA gyrase inhibitor* [also: difloxacin HCl]

difloxacin HCl USAN *anti-infective; DNA gyrase inhibitor* [also: difloxacin]

difluanazine INN *CNS stimulant* [also: difluanine HCl]

difluanazine HCl [see: difluanine HCl]

difluanine HCl USAN *CNS stimulant* [also: difluanazine]

Diflucan tablets, powder for oral suspension, IV infusion ℞ *systemic triazole antifungal* [fluconazole] 50, 100, 150, 200 mg; 10, 40 mg/mL; 2 mg/mL

diflucortolone USAN, INN, BAN *corticosteroid; anti-inflammatory*

diflucortolone pivalate USAN *corticosteroid; anti-inflammatory*

diflumidone INN, BAN *anti-inflammatory* [also: diflumidone sodium]

diflumidone sodium USAN *anti-inflammatory* [also: diflumidone]

diflunisal USAN, USP, INN, BAN *anti-inflammatory; analgesic; antipyretic; antiarthritic; antirheumatic* 250, 500 mg oral

difluoromethylornithine (DFMO) [see: eflornithine]

difluoromethylornithine HCl [see: eflornithine HCl]

difluprednate USAN, INN *anti-inflammatory*

difolliculin [see: estradiol benzoate]

diftalone USAN, INN *anti-inflammatory*

digalloyl trioleate USAN

Di-Gel oral liquid OTC *antacid; antiflatulent* [aluminum hydroxide; magnesium hydroxide; simethicone] 200•200•20 mg/5 mL

Di-Gel, Advanced Formula chewable tablets OTC *antacid; antiflatulent* [magnesium hydroxide; calcium carbonate; simethicone] 128•280•20 mg

Digepepsin dual-coated tablets (discontinued 2002) ℞ *digestive enzymes* [pancreatin; pepsin; bile salts] 300•250•150 mg

digestants; digestives *a class of agents that promote or aid in digestion*

Digestozyme tablets (discontinued 2002) ℞ *digestive enzymes; laxative; choleretic* [pancreatin; pepsin; dehydrocholic acid] 300•250•25 mg

Digibind powder for IV injection ℞ *antidote to digoxin/digitoxin overdose (orphan)* [digoxin immune Fab (ovine)] 38 mg/vial

Digidote ℞ *investigational (orphan) antidote to cardiac glycoside intoxication* [digoxin immune Fab (ovine)]

DigiFab powder for IV injection ℞ *antidote to digoxin/digitoxin overdose (orphan)* [digoxin immune Fab (ovine)] 40 mg/vial

digitalis USP *cardiotonic*

Digitalis ambigua; D. ferruginea; D. grandiflora; D. lanata; D. lutea; D. purpurea medicinal herb [see: foxglove]

digitalis glycosides *a class of cardiovascular drugs that increase the force of cardiac contractions* [also called: cardiac glycosides]

Digitek tablets ℞ *cardiac glycoside to increase cardiac output; antiarrhythmic* [digoxin] 0.125, 0.25 mg

digitoxin USP, INN, BAN *cardiotonic; cardiac glycoside; investigational (orphan) for soft tissue sarcomas and ovarian cancer* ☑ Desoxyn; digoxin

digitoxin, acetyl [see: acetyldigitoxin]

α-digitoxin monoacetate [see: acetyldigitoxin]

digitoxoside [see: digitoxin]

digolil INN *combining name for radicals or groups*

digoxin USP, INN, BAN *cardiotonic; cardiac glycoside antiarrhythmic* 0.125, 0.25 mg oral, 0.05 mg/mL oral, 0.1, 0.25 mg/mL injection ☑ Desoxyn; digitoxin

digoxin antibody [see: digoxin immune Fab]

digoxin immune Fab (ovine) *antidote to digoxin/digitoxin intoxication (orphan); investigational (orphan) for other cardiac glycoside intoxication*

Digoxin Injection C.S.D. ⒸⒶⓃ ℞ *cardiac glycoside to increase cardiac output; antiarrhythmic* [digoxin] 0.25 mg/mL

Digoxin Pediatric Injection C.S.D. ⒸⒶⓃ ℞ *cardiac glycoside to increase cardiac output; antiarrhythmic* [digoxin] 0.05 mg/mL

dihexyverine INN *anticholinergic* [also: dihexyverine HCl]

dihexyverine HCl USAN *anticholinergic* [also: dihexyverine]

Dihistine DH elixir ℞ *narcotic antitussive; decongestant; antihistamine* [codeine phosphate; pseudoephedrine HCl; chlorpheniramine maleate] 20•60•4 mg/10 mL

Dihistine Expectorant oral liquid (discontinued 2002) ℞ *narcotic antitussive; decongestant; expectorant* [codeine phosphate; pseudoephedrine HCl; guaifenesin; alcohol] 10•30•100 mg/5 mL

dihydan soluble [see: phenytoin sodium]

dihydralazine INN, BAN

dihydralazine sulfate [see: dihydralazine]

5,6-dihydro-5-azacytidine *investigational (orphan) for malignant mesothelioma*

dihydrobenzthiazide [see: hydrobentizide]

dihydrocodeine INN, BAN *narcotic analgesic* [also: dihydrocodeine bitartrate]

dihydrocodeine bitartrate USP *narcotic analgesic* [also: dihydrocodeine]

dihydrocodeinone bitartrate [see: hydrocodone bitartrate]

dihydroergocornine [see: ergoloid mesylates]

dihydroergocristine [see: ergoloid mesylates]

dihydroergocryptine [see: ergoloid mesylates]

dihydroergotamine (DHE) INN, BAN *antiadrenergic; anticoagulant; ergot alkaloid for rapid control of migraines* [also: dihydroergotamine mesylate; dihydroergotamine mesilate]

dihydroergotamine mesilate JAN *antiadrenergic; anticoagulant; ergot alkaloid for rapid control of migraines* [also: dihydroergotamine mesylate; dihydroergotamine]

dihydroergotamine mesylate USAN, USP *antiadrenergic; anticoagulant; ergot alkaloid for rapid control of migraines* [also: dihydroergotamine; dihydroergotamine mesilate] 1 mg/mL injection

dihydroergotamine methanesulfonate [see: dihydroergotamine mesylate]

dihydroergotoxine mesylate [now: ergoloid mesylates]

dihydroergotoxine methanesulfonate [now: ergoloid mesylates]

dihydroethaverine [see: drotaverine]

dihydrofollicular hormone [see: estradiol]

dihydrofolliculine [see: estradiol]

dihydrogenated ergot alkaloids [now: ergoloid mesylates]

dihydrohydroxycodeinone [see: oxycodone]

dihydrohydroxycodeinone HCl [see: oxycodone HCl]

6-dihydro-6-iminopurine [see: adenine]

dihydroindolones *a class of dopamine receptor antagonists with conventional (typical) antipsychotic activity* [also called: indolones]

dihydroisoperparine [see: drotaverine]

dihydromorphinone HCl [now: hydromorphone HCl]

dihydroneopine [see: dihydrocodeine bitartrate]

dihydropyridines *a class of calcium channel blockers*

dihydrostreptomycin (DST) INN *antibacterial* [also: dihydrostreptomycin sulfate]

dihydrostreptomycin sulfate USP *antibacterial* [also: dihydrostreptomycin]

dihydrostreptomycin-streptomycin [see: streptoduocin]

dihydrotachysterol (DHT) USP, INN, BAN, JAN *fat-soluble vitamin; synthetic reduction product of a vitamin D isomer; calcium regulator for tetany and hypoparathyroidism* 0.125, 0.2, 0.4 mg oral; 0.2 mg/mL oral

dihydrotestosterone (DHT) *investigational (Phase II, orphan) steroid for AIDS-wasting syndrome* [see: androstanolone; stanolone]

dihydrotheelin [see: estradiol]

dihydroxy(stearato)aluminum [see: aluminum monostearate]

dihydroxy propoxymethyl guanine (DHPG) [see: gancyclovir]

dihydroxyacetone *skin darkener for vitiligo and hypopigmented areas*

dihydroxyaluminum aminoacetate (DAA) USP *antacid*

dihydroxyaluminum sodium carbonate USP *antacid*

dihydroxyanthranol [see: anthralin]

dihydroxyanthraquinone *(withdrawn from market)* [see: danthron]

1,25-dihydroxycholecalciferol [see: calcitriol]

24,25-dihydroxycholecalciferol *investigational (orphan) for uremic osteodystrophy*

dihydroxyestrin [see: estradiol]

5,7-dihydroxyflavone [see: chrysin]

dihydroxyfluorane [see: fluorescein]

dihydroxyphenylalanine (DOPA) [see: levodopa]

dihydroxyphenylisatin [see: oxyphenisatin acetate]

dihydroxyphenyloxindol [see: oxyphenisatin acetate]

dihydroxyprogesterone acetophenide [see: algestone acetophenide]

dihydroxypropyl theophylline [see: dyphylline]

diiodobuphenine [see: bufeniode]

diiodohydroxyquin [now: iodoquinol]

diiodohydroxyquinoline INN, BAN *antiamebic* [also: iodoquinol]

diisopromine INN

diisopromine HCl [see: diisopromine]

diisopropanolamine NF *alkalizing agent*

diisopropyl flurophosphate (DFP) [see: isoflurophate]

diisopropyl flurophosphonate [see: isoflurophate]

diisopropyl phosphorofluoridate [see: isoflurophate]

2,6-diisopropylphenol [see: propofol]

Dilacor XR sustained-release capsules ℞ *antihypertensive; antianginal; antiarrhythmic; calcium channel blocker* [diltiazem HCl] 120, 180, 240 mg ⊇ Delcort

Dilantin Infatabs (chewable tablets) ℞ *hydantoin anticonvulsant* [phenytoin] 50 mg ⊇ Milontin; Mylanta; Xalatan

Dilantin Kapseals (capsules) ℞ *hydantoin anticonvulsant* [phenytoin sodium] 30, 100 mg ⊇ Milontin; Mylanta; Xalatan

Dilantin-125 oral suspension ℞ *hydantoin anticonvulsant* [phenytoin] 125 mg/5 mL ⊇ Milontin; Mylanta; Xalatan

Dilatrate-SR sustained-release capsules ℞ *antianginal; vasodilator* [isosorbide dinitrate] 40 mg

Dilatrend ℞ *antihypertensive; α- and β-blocker for congestive heart failure* [carvedilol]

Dilaudid tablets, oral liquid, subcu or IM injection, suppositories ℞ *narcotic analgesic; widely abused as a street drug* [hydromorphone HCl] 2, 4, 8 mg; 1 mg/mL; 1, 2, 4 mg/mL; 3 mg

Dilaudid Cough syrup ℞ *narcotic antitussive; expectorant* [hydromorphone HCl; guaifenesin; alcohol 5%] 1• 100 mg/5 mL

Dilaudid-HP subcu or IM injection; powder for subcu or IM injection ℞

narcotic analgesic [hydromorphone HCl] 10 mg/mL; 250 mg

dilazep INN

dilevalol INN, BAN *antihypertensive; antiadrenergic (β-receptor)* [also: dilevalol HCl]

dilevalol HCl USAN, JAN *antihypertensive; antiadrenergic (β-receptor)* [also: dilevalol]

dilithium carbonate [see: lithium carbonate]

dill (*Anethum graveolens*) fruit and seed *medicinal herb used as an aromatic, carminative, diaphoretic, stimulant, and stomachic*

dilmefone INN

Dilocaine injection (discontinued 2002) ℞ *injectable local anesthetic* [lidocaine HCl] 1%, 2%

Dilor elixir, IM injection (discontinued 2005) ℞ *antiasthmatic; bronchodilator* [dyphylline] 160 mg/15 mL; 250 mg/mL

Dilor tablets ℞ *antiasthmatic; bronchodilator* [dyphylline] 200 mg

Dilor 400 tablets ℞ *antiasthmatic; bronchodilator* [dyphylline] 400 mg

Dilor-G tablets, oral liquid (discontinued 2003) ℞ *antiasthmatic; bronchodilator; expectorant* [dyphylline; guaifenesin] 200•200 mg; 300•300 mg/15 mL

Dilotab tablets OTC *decongestant; analgesic; antipyretic* [pseudoephedrine HCl; acetaminophen] 30•500 mg

diloxanide INN, BAN, DCF

Diltia XT sustained-release capsules ℞ *antihypertensive; calcium channel blocker* [diltiazem HCl] 120, 180, 240 mg

diltiazem INN, BAN *coronary vasodilator; calcium channel blocker; antianginal; antihypertensive* [also: diltiazem HCl]

diltiazem HCl USAN, USP, JAN *coronary vasodilator; calcium channel blocker; antianginal; antihypertensive; antiarrhythmic* [also: diltiazem] 30, 60, 90, 120, 180, 240, 300, 360 mg oral; 5 mg/mL injection

diltiazem malate USAN *coronary vasodilator; calcium channel blocker; antianginal; antihypertensive; antiarrhythmic*

Dilt-XR extended-release capsules ℞ *antihypertensive; calcium channel blocker* [diltiazem HCl] 120, 180, 240 mg

Dilusol ⓐ OTC *topical solution base* [ethyl alcohol] 38.7%

Dilusol AHA ⓐ OTC *topical solution base* [ethyl alcohol with 8% glycolic acid (alpha hydroxy acid)]

diluted acetic acid [see: acetic acid, diluted]

diluted alcohol [see: alcohol, diluted]

diluted hydrochloric acid [see: hydrochloric acid, diluted]

diluted sodium hypochlorite [see: sodium hypochlorite, diluted]

dimabefylline INN

Dimacol caplets (discontinued 2002) OTC *antitussive; decongestant; expectorant* [dextromethorphan hydrobromide; pseudoephedrine HCl; guaifenesin] 10•30•100 mg ⊡ dimercaprol

dimantine INN *anthelmintic* [also: dymanthine HCl]

dimantine HCl INN [also: dymanthine HCl]

Dimaphen pediatric elixir OTC *decongestant; antihistamine* [pseudoephedrine HCl; brompheniramine maleate] 30•2 mg/10 mL

Dimaphen tablets, Release-Tabs (timed-release tablets) (discontinued 2001) OTC *decongestant; antihistamine* [phenylpropanolamine HCl; brompheniramine maleate] 25•4 mg; 75•12 mg

Dimaphen DM Cold & Cough pediatric elixir OTC *antitussive; decongestant; antihistamine* [dextromethorphan hydrobromide; pseudoephedrine HCl; brompheniramine maleate] 10•30•2 mg/10 mL

dimazole INN [also: diamthazole]

dimazole dihydrochloride [see: dimazole; diamthazole]

dimecamine INN

dimecolonium iodide INN

dimecrotic acid INN

dimedrol [see: diphenhydramine HCl]

dimefadane USAN, INN *analgesic*

dimefilcon A USAN *hydrophilic contact lens material*

dimefline INN, BAN *respiratory stimulant* [also: dimefline HCl]

dimefline HCl USAN *respiratory stimulant* [also: dimefline]

dimefocon A USAN *hydrophobic contact lens material*

dimekolin [see: dimecolonium iodide]

dimelazine INN

dimelin [see: dimecolonium iodide]

dimemorfan INN

dimenhydrinate USP, INN, BAN *antiemetic; anticholinergic; antivertigo; motion sickness prophylaxis* 50 mg oral; 12.5 mg/4 mL oral; 50 mg/mL injection ⊡ diphenhydramine

dimenoxadol INN [also: dimenoxadole]

dimenoxadole BAN [also: dimenoxadol]

dimepheptanol INN, BAN

dimepranol INN *immunomodulator* [also: dimepranol acedoben]

dimepranol acedoben USAN *immunomodulator* [also: dimepranol]

dimepregnen INN, BAN

dimepropion BAN [also: metamfepramone]

dimeprozan INN

dimeprozinum [see: dimeprozan]

dimercaprol USP, INN *chelating agent for arsenic, gold, and mercury poisoning; adjunct to lead poisoning* ⊡ Dimacol

dimercaptopropanol [see: dimercaprol]

2,3-dimercaptosuccinic acid (DMSA) [see: succimer]

dimesna INN

dimesone INN, BAN

Dimetabs tablets ℞ *anticholinergic; antiemetic; antivertigo agent; motion sickness preventative* [dimenhydrinate] 50 mg ⊡ Dimetane; Dimetapp

dimetacrine INN

dimetamfetamine INN

Dimetane Decongestant caplets, elixir (discontinued 2002) OTC *decongestant; antihistamine* [phenylephrine HCl; brompheniramine maleate] 10•4 mg; 5•2 mg/5 mL

Dimetane-DC Cough syrup (discontinued 2002) ℞ *narcotic antitussive; decongestant; antihistamine* [codeine phosphate; phenylpropanolamine

HCl; brompheniramine maleate; alcohol 0.95%] 10•12.5•2 mg/5 mL

Dimetane-DX Cough syrup (discontinued 2004) ℞ *antitussive; decongestant; antihistamine* [dextromethorphan hydrobromide; pseudoephedrine HCl; brompheniramine maleate; alcohol 1%] 20•60•4 mg/10 mL

Dimetapp tablets, Extentabs (long-acting tablets), elixir (discontinued 2001) OTC *decongestant; antihistamine* [phenylpropanolamine HCl; brompheniramine maleate] 25•4 mg; 75•12 mg; 12.5•2 mg/5 mL ⎙ Dimetabs

Dimetapp 4-Hour Liqui-Gels (liquid-filled capsules) (discontinued 2001) OTC *decongestant; antihistamine* [phenylpropanolamine HCl; brompheniramine maleate] 25•4 mg

Dimetapp 12-Hour Non-Drowsy Extentabs (extended-release tablets) OTC *decongestant* [pseudoephedrine HCl] 120 mg

Dimetapp Allergy liqui-gels (discontinued 2001) OTC *antihistamine* [brompheniramine maleate] 4 mg

Dimetapp Children's Cold & Fever oral suspension OTC *decongestant; analgesic* [pseudoephedrine HCl; ibuprofen] 15•100 mg

Dimetapp Children's Nighttime Flu syrup OTC *antitussive; decongestant; antihistamine; analgesic* [dextromethorphan hydrobromide; pseudoephedrine HCl; brompheniramine maleate; acetaminophen] 10•30•2•320 mg/10 mL

Dimetapp Children's Non-Drowsy Allergy orally disintegrating tablets, syrup OTC *nonsedating antihistamine for allergic rhinitis and chronic idiopathic urticaria* [loratadine] 10 mg; 5 mg/5 mL

Dimetapp Children's Non-Drowsy Flu syrup OTC *antitussive; decongestant; analgesic* [dextromethorphan hydrobromide; pseudoephedrine HCl; acetaminophen] 5•15•160 mg/5 mL

Dimetapp Cold & Allergy pediatric chewable tablets, quick-dissolve tablets (discontinued 2001) OTC *decongestant; antihistamine* [phenylpropanolamine HCl; brompheniramine maleate] 6.25•1 mg

Dimetapp Cold & Allergy pediatric elixir OTC *decongestant; antihistamine* [pseudoephedrine HCl; brompheniramine maleate] 30•2 mg/10 mL

Dimetapp Cold & Flu caplets (discontinued 2001) OTC *decongestant; antihistamine; analgesic* [phenylpropanolamine HCl; brompheniramine maleate; acetaminophen] 12.5•2•500 mg

Dimetapp Decongestant Pediatric oral drops OTC *nasal decongestant* [pseudoephedrine HCl] 7.5 mg/0.8 mL

Dimetapp Decongestant Plus Cough pediatric oral drops OTC *antitussive; decongestant* [dextromethorphan hydrobromide; pseudoephedrine HCl] 5•15 mg/1.6 mL

Dimetapp DM elixir (discontinued 2002) OTC *antitussive; decongestant; antihistamine* [dextromethorphan hydrobromide; phenylpropanolamine HCl; brompheniramine maleate] 10•12.5•2 mg/5 mL

Dimetapp DM Children's Cold & Cough elixir OTC *antitussive; decongestant; antihistamine* [dextromethorphan hydrobromide; pseudoephedrine HCl; brompheniramine maleate] 10•30•2 mg/10 mL

Dimetapp Long Acting Cough Plus Cold syrup OTC *antitussive; decongestant* [dextromethorphan hydrobromide; pseudoephedrine HCl] 7.5•15 mg/5 mL

Dimetapp Non-Drowsy Liqui-Gels (liquid-filled softgels) OTC *decongestant* [pseudoephedrine HCl] 30 mg

Dimetapp Sinus caplets OTC *decongestant; analgesic* [pseudoephedrine HCl; ibuprofen] 30•200 mg

dimethadione USAN, INN *anticonvulsant*

dimethazan

dimethazine [see: mebolazine]

dimethicone USAN, NF, BAN *lubricant and hydrophobing agent; soft tissue* *prosthetic aid* [also: dimeticone] 🔲 cimetidine

dimethicone 350 USAN *soft tissue prosthetic aid*

dimethindene BAN *antihistamine* [also: dimethindene maleate; dimetindene]

dimethindene maleate USP *antihistamine* [also: dimetindene; dimethindene]

dimethiodal sodium INN

dimethisoquin BAN [also: dimethisoquin HCl; quinisocaine]

dimethisoquin HCl USAN [also: quinisocaine; dimethisoquin]

dimethisterone USAN, NF, INN, BAN *progestin*

dimetholizine INN

dimethothiazine BAN *serotonin inhibitor* [also: fonazine mesylate; dimetotiazine]

dimethoxanate INN, BAN

dimethoxanate HCl [see: dimethoxanate]

2,5-dimethoxy-4-methylamphetamine (DOM) *a hallucinogenic street drug derived from amphetamine, popularly called STP*

dimethoxyphenyl penicillin sodium [see: methicillin sodium]

dimethpyridene maleate [see: dimethindene maleate]

dimethyl ketone [see: acetone]

dimethyl phthalate USP

dimethyl polysiloxane [see: dimethicone]

dimethyl sulfoxide (DMSO) USAN, USP, INN *solvent; anti-inflammatory for symptomatic relief of interstitial cystitis; investigational (orphan) for traumatic brain coma; investigational (orphan) topical treatment for scleroderma and extravasation of cytotoxic drugs* [also: dimethyl sulphoxide]

dimethyl sulphoxide BAN *topical anti-inflammatory; solvent* [also: dimethyl sulfoxide]

dimethyl triazeno imidazole carboxamide (DIC; DTIC) [see: dacarbazine]

3-(3,5-dimethyl-1H-methylene)-1,3-dihydro-indole-2-one *investigational (orphan) for Kaposi sarcoma and von Hippel-Lindau disease*

dimethylaminoethanol (DMAE) *natural precursor to the neurotransmitter acetylcholine; readily crosses the blood-brain barrier to enhance memory and cognitive function*

dimethylaminoethanol bitartrate *natural precursor to the neurotransmitter acetylcholine; readily crosses the blood-brain barrier to enhance memory and cognitive function* (base=37%)

dimethylaminophenazone [see: aminopyrine]

dimethylcysteine [see: penicillamine]

dimethylglycine HCl

dimethylhexestrol [see: methestrol]

1,5-dimethylhexylamine [see: octodrine]

5,5-dimethyl-2,4-oxazolidinedione (DMO) [see: dimethadione]

dimethyloxyquinazine [see: antipyrine]

o,α-dimethylphenethylamine [see: ortetamine]

dimethylsiloxane polymers [see: dimethicone]

dimethylthiambutene INN, BAN

dimethyltryptamine (DMT) *hallucinogenic street drug derived from a plant native to South America and the West Indies*

dimethyltubocurarine BAN [also: dimethyltubocurarinium chloride]

dimethyltubocurarine iodide [see: metocurine iodide]

dimethyltubocurarinium chloride INN [also: dimethyltubocurarine]

dimethylxanthine [see: theophylline]

dimeticone INN *lubricant and hydrophobing agent; soft tissue prosthetic aid* [also: dimethicone]

dimetindene INN *antihistamine* [also: dimethindene maleate; dimethindene]

dimetindene maleate [see: dimethindene maleate]

dimetipirium bromide INN

dimetofrine INN

dimetotiazine INN *serotonin inhibitor* [also: fonazine mesylate; dimethothiazine]

dimetridazole INN, BAN

dimevamide INN

dimevamide sulfate [see: dimevamide]

diminazene INN, BAN

dimoxamine HCl USAN *memory adjuvant*

dimoxaprost INN

dimoxyline INN

dimpylate INN [also: diazinon]

dinaline INN

Dinate IV or IM injection ℞ *anticholinergic; antiemetic; antivertigo agent; motion sickness preventative* [dimenhydrinate] 50 mg/mL

dinazafone INN

diniprofylline INN

dinitolmide INN, BAN

dinitrotoluamide [see: dinitolmide]

dinoprost USAN, INN, BAN *oxytocic; prostaglandin*

dinoprost trometamol BAN *oxytocic; prostaglandin* [also: dinoprost tromethamine]

dinoprost tromethamine USAN *oxytocic; prostaglandin-type abortifacient* [also: dinoprost trometamol]

dinoprostone USAN, INN, BAN *oxytocic for induction of labor; prostaglandin-type abortifacient; cervical ripening agent*

dinsed USAN, INN *coccidiostat for poultry*

Diocto oral liquid, syrup (discontinued 2004) OTC *laxative; stool softener* [docusate sodium] 150 mg/15 mL; 60 mg/15 mL

Diocto-C syrup (discontinued 2003) OTC *stimulant laxative; stool softener* [casanthranol; docusate sodium] 30•60 mg/15 mL

dioctyl calcium sulfosuccinate [now: docusate calcium]

dioctyl potassium sulfosuccinate [now: docusate potassium]

dioctyl sodium sulfosuccinate (DSS) [now: docusate sodium]

Diodex ⊛ eye drops ℞ *topical ophthalmic corticosteroidal anti-inflammatory* [dexamethasone sodium phosphate] 0.1%

diodone INN [also: iodopyracet]

diohippuric acid I 125 USAN *radioactive agent*

diohippuric acid I 131 USAN *radioactive agent*

diolamine USAN, INN *combining name for radicals or groups*

diolostene [see: methandriol]

dionin [see: ethylmorphine HCl]

diophyllin [see: aminophylline]

Dioscorea villosa *medicinal herb* [see: wild yam]

diosmin INN

Diostate D tablets OTC *dietary supplement* [calcium; phosphorus; vitamin D] 114 mg•88 mg•133 IU

diotyrosine I 125 USAN *radioactive agent*

diotyrosine I 131 USAN *radioactive agent*

Diovan capsules (discontinued 2002) ℞ *angiotensin II receptor antagonist; antihypertensive; treatment for congestive heart failure (CHF)* [valsartan] 80, 160 mg ⧖ Darvon

Diovan tablets ℞ *angiotensin II receptor antagonist; antihypertensive; treatment for congestive heart failure (CHF)* [valsartan] 40, 80, 160, 320 mg ⧖ Darvon

Diovan HCT tablets ℞ *antihypertensive; angiotensin II receptor antagonist; diuretic* [valsartan; hydrochlorothiazide] 80•12.5, 160•12.5, 160•25 mg ⧖ Darvon

dioxadilol INN

dioxadrol INN *antidepressant* [also: dioxadrol HCl]

dioxadrol HCl USAN *antidepressant* [also: dioxadrol]

***d*-dioxadrol HCl** [see: dexoxadrol HCl]

dioxamate INN, BAN

dioxaphetyl butyrate INN, BAN

dioxathion BAN [also: dioxation]

dioxation INN [also: dioxathion]

dioxethedrin INN

dioxethedrin HCl [see: dioxethedrin]

dioxifedrine INN

dioxindol [see: oxyphenisatin acetate]

dioxyanthranol [see: anthralin]

dioxyanthraquinone *(withdrawn from market)* [see: danthron]

dioxybenzone USAN, USP, INN *ultraviolet screen*

dipalmitoylphosphatidylcholine (DPPC) [see: colfosceril palmitate]

diparcol HCl [see: diethazine HCl]

dipegyl [see: niacinamide]

dipenicillin G [see: penicillin G benzathine]

dipenine bromide BAN [also: diponium bromide]

Dipentum capsules ℞ *anti-inflammatory for ulcerative colitis* [olsalazine sodium] 250 mg

diperodon USAN, INN, BAN *topical anesthetic*

diperodon HCl *topical anesthetic*

diphemanil methylsulfate USP *anticholinergic* [also: diphemanil metilsulfate; diphemanil methylsulphate]

diphemanil methylsulphate BAN *anticholinergic* [also: diphemanil methylsulfate; diphemanil metilsulfate]

diphemanil metilsulfate INN *anticholinergic* [also: diphemanil methylsulfate; diphemanil methylsulphate]

Diphen AF oral liquid OTC *antihistamine* [diphenhydramine HCl] 12.5 mg/5 mL

Diphen Cough syrup (discontinued 2002) OTC *antihistamine; antitussive* [diphenhydramine HCl; alcohol 5%] 12.5 mg/5 mL

diphenadione USP, INN, BAN

diphenan INN

diphenatil [see: diphemanil methylsulfate]

diphenchloxazine HCl [see: difencloxazine HCl]

diphenesenic acid [see: xenyhexenic acid]

Diphenhist caplets, oral liquid OTC *antihistamine* [diphenhydramine HCl] 25 mg; 12.5 mg/5 mL

Diphenhist softgels (discontinued 2002) OTC *antihistamine* [diphenhydramine HCl] 25 mg

diphenhydramine INN, BAN *ethanolamine antihistamine; anticholinergic; antiparkinsonian; motion sickness relief*

[also: diphenhydramine citrate] ⑨ dimenhydrinate

Diphenhydramine 50 capsules (discontinued 2001) OTC *antihistamine* [diphenhydramine HCl] 50 mg

diphenhydramine citrate USP *ethanolamine antihistamine; anticholinergic; antiparkinsonian; motion sickness relief* [also: diphenhydramine]

diphenhydramine HCl USP, BAN *ethanolamine antihistamine; antitussive; motion sickness preventative; sleep aid* 25, 50 mg oral; 50 mg/mL injection

diphenhydramine tannate *ethanolamine antihistamine; anticholinergic; antiparkinsonian; motion sickness relief*

diphenhydramine theoclate [see: dimenhydrinate]

diphenidol USAN, BAN *antiemetic; antivertigo* [also: difenidol]

diphenidol HCl USAN *antiemetic*

diphenidol pamoate USAN *antiemetic*

diphenmethanil methylsulfate [see: diphemanil methylsulfate]

diphenoxylate INN, BAN *antiperistaltic* [also: diphenoxylate HCl]

diphenoxylate HCl USP *antiperistaltic* [also: diphenoxylate]

diphenylacetylindandione [see: diphenadione]

diphenylalkylamines *a class of calcium channel blockers*

Diphenylan Sodium capsules ℞ *anticonvulsant* [phenytoin sodium] 30, 100 mg ⑨ Diphenylin

diphenylbutazone [see: phenylbutazone]

diphenylbutylpiperidines [see: phenylbutylpiperidines]

diphenylcyclopenone *investigational (orphan) agent for severe alopecia areata, alopecia totalis, and alopecia universalis*

diphenylhydantoin [now: phenytoin]

diphenylhydantoin sodium [now: phenytoin sodium]

diphenylisatin [see: oxyphenisatin]

diphenylpyraline INN, BAN *antihistamine* [also: diphenylpyraline HCl]

diphenylpyraline HCl USP *antihistamine* [also: diphenylpyraline]

diphetarsone [see: difetarsone]

diphexamide iodomethylate [see: buzepide metiodide]

diphosphonic acid [see: etidronic acid]

diphosphopyridine nucleotide (DPN) [now: nadide]

diphosphoric acid, tetrasodium salt [see: sodium pyrophosphate]

diphosphothiamin [see: co-carboxylase]

diphoxazide INN

diphtheria antitoxin USP *passive immunizing agent for diphtheria* [also: diphtheria toxoid] 500 U/mL injection

diphtheria CRM$_{197}$ conjugate *carrier protein for hemophilus b and pneumococcal vaccines*

diphtheria equine antitoxin *investigational passive immunizing agent (available only from the Centers for Disease Control and Prevention)*

diphtheria & tetanus toxoids, adsorbed (DT; Td) USP *active immunizing agent for diphtheria and tetanus* 2•2, 2•5, 2•10, 6.6•5, 7.5• 7.5, 10•5, 12.5•5, 15•10 LfU/0.5 mL injection

diphtheria & tetanus toxoids & acellular pertussis (DTaP) vaccine *active immunizing agent for diphtheria, tetanus, and pertussis*

diphtheria & tetanus toxoids & pertussis vaccine (DTP) USP *active immunizing agent for diphtheria, tetanus, and pertussis*

diphtheria & tetanus toxoids & whole-cell pertussis vaccine (DTwP) *active immunizing agent for diphtheria, tetanus, and pertussis* 6.5• 5•4, 10•5.5•4 LfU/0.5 mL injection

diphtheria toxin, diagnostic [now: diphtheria toxin for Schick test]

diphtheria toxin, inactivated diagnostic [now: Schick test control]

diphtheria toxin for Schick test USP *dermal diphtheria immunity test*

diphtheria toxoid USP *active immunizing agent for diphtheria* [also: diphtheria antitoxin]

diphtheria toxoid, adsorbed USP *active immunizing agent for diphtheria* 15 LfU/0.5 mL injection

dipipanone INN, BAN

dipipanone HCl [see: dipipanone]

dipiproverine INN

dipiproverine HCl [see: dipiproverine]

dipivalyl epinephrine (DPE) [now: dipivefrin]

dipivefrin USAN *ophthalmic adrenergic* [also: dipivefrine]

dipivefrin HCl USP *topical antiglaucoma agent* 0.1% eye drops

dipivefrine INN, BAN *ophthalmic adrenergic* [also: dipivefrin]

diponium bromide INN [also: dipenine bromide]

dipotassium carbonate [see: potassium carbonate]

dipotassium clorazepate INN *benzodiazepine anxiolytic; minor tranquilizer; anticonvulsant adjunct; alcohol withdrawal aid* [also: clorazepate dipotassium]

dipotassium hydrogen phosphate [see: potassium phosphate, dibasic]

dipotassium phosphate [see: potassium phosphate, dibasic]

dipotassium pyrosulfite [see: potassium metabisulfite]

diprafenone INN

diprenorphine INN, BAN

Diprivan *emulsion for IV* ℞ *general anesthetic* [propofol] 10 mg/mL

diprobutine INN, BAN

diprofene INN

diprogulic acid INN

diproleandomycin INN

Diprolene *ointment, gel, lotion* ℞ *topical corticosteroidal anti-inflammatory* [betamethasone dipropionate, augmented] 0.05%

Diprolene AF *cream* ℞ *topical corticosteroidal anti-inflammatory* [betamethasone dipropionate, augmented] 0.05%

diprophylline INN, BAN *bronchodilator* [also: dyphylline]

dipropylacetic acid [see: valproic acid]

2-dipropylaminoethyl diphenylthioacetate [see: diprofene]

1,1-dipropylbutylamine [see: diprobutine]

diproqualone INN

Diprosone ointment, cream, lotion, aerosol ℞ *corticosteroidal anti-inflammatory* [betamethasone dipropionate] 0.05%; 0.05%; 0.05%; 0.1%

diproteverine INN, BAN

diprothazine [see: dimelazine]

diprotrizoate sodium USP [also: sodium diprotrizoate]

diproxadol INN

Dipteryx odorata; D. oppositifolia medicinal herb [see: tonka bean]

dipyridamole USAN, USP, INN, BAN *coronary vasodilator; platelet aggregation inhibitor; diagnostic aid for coronary artery function* 25, 50, 75 mg oral

dipyrithione USAN, INN *antibacterial; antifungal*

dipyrocetyl INN

dipyrone USAN, BAN *analgesic; antipyretic* [also: metamizole sodium]

diquafosol tetrasodium *investigational (NDA filed) treatment for dry eye*

dirithromycin USAN, INN, BAN *macrolide antibiotic* ② clarithromycin; erythromycin

disaccharide tripeptide glycerol dipalmitoyl *investigational (orphan) immunostimulant for pulmonary and hepatic metastases of colorectal adenocarcinoma*

Disalcid film-coated tablets, capsules ℞ *analgesic; antipyretic; anti-inflammatory; antirheumatic* [salsalate] 500, 750 mg; 500 mg

disalicylic acid [see: salsalate]

Dis-Co Pack (trademarked packaging form) *unit-dose package*

discutients *a class of agents that cause a dispersal or disappearance of a pathological condition, such as a tumor*

disease-modifying antirheumatic drugs (DMARDs) *a class of agents that slow the progression of rheumatic arthritis (RA) by modifying immune system response; this is in contrast to NSAIDs, which treat only the symptoms of the disease*

disinfectants *a class of agents that inhibit the growth and development of microorganisms, usually on an inanimate surface, without necessarily killing them* [see also: antiseptics; germicides]

Disinfecting Solution OTC *chemical disinfecting solution for soft contact lenses*

Disipal ⒸⒶⓃ film-coated tablets (discontinued 2001) ℞ *anticholinergic; antiparkinsonian* [orphenadrine HCl] 50 mg

disiquonium chloride USAN, INN *antiseptic*

Disket (trademarked dosage form) *dispersible tablet*

Diskhaler (trademarked device) *inhalation powder dispenser* [used with a Rotadisk]

Diskus (trademarked device) *breath-activated inhalation powder dispenser*

Disobrom sustained-release tablets (discontinued 2002) ℞ *decongestant; antihistamine* [pseudoephedrine sulfate; dexbrompheniramine maleate] 120•6 mg

disobutamide USAN, INN *antiarrhythmic*

disodium carbenicillin [see: carbenicillin disodium]

disodium carbonate [see: sodium carbonate]

disodium cefotetan [see: cefotetan disodium]

disodium chromate [see: sodium chromate]

disodium clodronate tetrahydrate *bisphosphonate bone resorption inhibitor for hypercalcemia and osteolysis of malignancy* [approved in Canada; investigational (orphan) in the U.S.]

disodium cromoglycate (DSC; DSCG) [see: cromolyn sodium]

disodium dihydrogen methylenediphosphonate [see: medronate disodium]

disodium edathamil [see: edathamil disodium]

disodium edetate BAN *metal-chelating agent* [also: edetate disodium]

disodium ethylenediamine tetraacetate [see: edetate disodium]

disodium hydrogen phosphate [see: sodium phosphate]

disodium hydrogen phosphate heptahydrate [see: sodium phosphate, dibasic]

disodium hydrogen phosphate hydrate [see: sodium phosphate, dibasic]

(disodium) methylene diphosphonate (MDP) [now: medronate disodium]

disodium phosphate [see: sodium phosphate, dibasic]

disodium phosphate heptahydrate [see: sodium phosphate]

disodium phosphonoacetate monohydrate [see: fosfonet sodium]

disodium phosphorofluoridate [see: sodium monofluorophosphate]

disodium pyrosulfite [see: sodium metabisulfite]

disodium silibinin dihemisuccinate *investigational (orphan) antitoxin for* Amanita phalloides *(mushroom) intoxication*

disodium sulfate decahydrate [see: sodium sulfate]

disodium thiosulfate pentahydrate [see: sodium thiosulfate]

disofenin USAN, INN, BAN *carrier agent in diagnostic tests*

disogluside INN

Disophrol tablets, Chronotabs (sustained-action tablets) (discontinued 2002) OTC *decongestant; antihistamine* [pseudoephedrine sulfate; dexbrompheniramine maleate] 60•2 mg; 120•6 mg ② Desferal; disoprofol; Stilphostrol

disoprofol [see: propofol] ② Disophrol

disopromine HCl [see: diisopromine HCl]

disoproxil *combining name for radicals or groups* [also: soproxil]

disopyramide USAN, INN, BAN *antiarrhythmic for severe ventricular arrhythmias*

disopyramide phosphate USAN, USP, BAN *antiarrhythmic for severe ventricular arrhythmias* 100, 150 mg oral

disoxaril USAN, INN *antiviral*

Di-Spaz capsules, IM injection ℞ GI *antispasmodic* [dicyclomine HCl] 10 mg; 10 mg/mL

Dispenserpak (trademarked packaging form) *unit-of-use package*

DisperMox tablets for oral suspension ℞ *aminopenicillin antibiotic* [amoxicillin] 200, 400 mg

dispersible cellulose BAN *tablet and capsule diluent* [also: cellulose, microcrystalline]

Dispertab (trademarked dosage form) *delayed-release tablet*

Dispette (trademarked delivery system) *disposable pipette*

Dispos-a-Med (trademarked delivery form) *solution for inhalation*

distaquaine [see: penicillin V]

distigmine bromide INN, BAN

disulergine INN

disulfamide INN [also: disulphamide]

disulfiram USP, INN, BAN *deterrent to alcohol consumption*

disulfurous acid, dipotassium salt [see: potassium metabisulfite]

disulfurous acid, disodium salt [see: sodium metabisulfite]

disulphamide BAN [also: disulfamide]

disuprazole INN

** Dital** slow-release capsules (discontinued 2001) ℞ *anorexiant; CNS stimulant* [phendimetrazine tartrate] 105 mg

ditazole INN

ditekiren USAN *antihypertensive; renin inhibitor*

ditercalinium chloride INN

dithiazanine BAN [also: dithiazanine iodide]

dithiazanine iodide USP, INN [also: dithiazanine]

dithranol INN, BAN *topical antipsoriatic* [also: anthralin]

D.I.T.I.-2 vaginal cream ℞ *broad-spectrum antibiotic; antiseptic; vulnerary* [sulfanilamide; aminacrine HCl; allantoin] 15%•0.2%•2%

ditiocarb sodium INN

ditiomustine INN

ditolamide INN

ditophal INN, BAN

Ditropan tablets, syrup ℞ *urinary antispasmodic for urge urinary incontinence and frequency* [oxybutynin chloride] 5 mg; 5 mg/5 mL ⑤ Intropin

Ditropan XL extended-release tablets ℞ *urinary antispasmodic for urge urinary incontinence and frequency* [oxybutynin chloride] 5, 10, 15 mg

Diucardin tablets (discontinued 2003) ℞ *diuretic; antihypertensive* [hydroflumethiazide] 50 mg

Diurese tablets ℞ *diuretic; antihypertensive* [trichlormethiazide] 4 mg

diuretics *a class of agents that stimulate increased excretion of urine*

Diurigen tablets ℞ *diuretic* [chlorothiazide] 500 mg

Diuril tablets, oral suspension ℞ *diuretic* [chlorothiazide] 250, 500 mg; 250 mg/5 mL

Diutensen-R tablets ℞ *antihypertensive* [methyclothiazide; reserpine] 2.5•0.1 mg ⑤ Salutensin

divabuterol INN

divalproex sodium USAN *anticonvulsant; antipsychotic for manic episodes; migraine headache preventative; valproic acid derivative* [also: valproate semisodium; semisodium valproate]

divanilliden cyclohexanone [see: cyclovalone]

divaplon INN

Divide-Tab (trademarked dosage form) *scored tablet*

Dividose (trademarked dosage form) *multiple-scored tablets*

diviminol [see: viminol]

divinyl ether [see: vinyl ether]

divinyl oxide [see: vinyl ether]

dixamone bromide [see: methantheline bromide]

dixanthogen INN

dixarit [see: clonidine]

dizatrifone INN

dizocilpine INN *neuroprotective; NMDA (N-methyl-D-aspartate) antagonist* [also: dizocilpine maleate]

dizocilpine maleate USAN *neuroprotective; NMDA (N-methyl-D-aspartate) antagonist* [also: dizocilpine]

dizocilpine maleate & citicoline *investigational (Phase III) neuroprotective treatment for stroke*

D-Lay (trademarked dosage form) *timed-release tablet*

DMAE (dimethylaminoethanol) [q.v.]

DMARDs (disease-modifying antirheumatic drugs) *a class of agents that slow the progression of rheumatic arthritis (RA) by modifying immune system response; this is in contrast to NSAIDs, which treat only the symptoms of the disease*

DMax syrup ℞ *antitussive; decongestant; antihistamine* [dextromethorphan hydrobromide; phenylephrine HCl; carbinoxamine maleate] 15•8•4 mg/5 mL

DMax Pediatric oral drops ℞ *antitussive; decongestant; antihistamine* [dextromethorphan hydrobromide; phenylephrine HCl; carbinoxamine maleate] 4•2•1 mg/mL

DMC (dactinomycin, methotrexate, cyclophosphamide) *chemotherapy protocol*

DMCT (demethylchlortetracycline) [see: demeclocycline]

DML lotion OTC *moisturizer; emollient*

DML Forte cream OTC *moisturizer; emollient*

DMO (dimethyl oxazolidinedione) [see: dimethadione]

DMP 777 *investigational (orphan) agent for the management of cystic fibrosis lung disease*

d-MPH (d-methylphenidate HCl) [q.v.]

DMSA (dimercaptosuccinic acid) [see: succimer]

DMSO (dimethyl sulfoxide) [q.v.]

DMT (dimethyltryptamine) *street drug* [q.v.]

DNA (deoxyribonucleic acid)

DNA polymerase [see: reverse transcriptase inhibitors; non-nucleoside reverse transcriptase inhibitors]

DNase (recombinant human deoxyribonuclease I) [see: dornase alfa]

DNP-conjugated tumor vaccine *investigational (Phase III, orphan) theraccine for postsurgical stage III malignant melanoma*

DNR (daunorubicin) [q.v.]

Doak Tar bath oil, lotion (discontinued 2003) OTC *antiseborrheic; antipsoriatic; antipruritic; antibacterial* [coal tar] 0.8%; 2%

Doak Tar shampoo OTC *antiseborrheic; antipsoriatic; antipruritic; antibacterial* [coal tar] 1.2%

Doak Tar Distillate topical liquid (discontinued 2003) OTC *antiseborrheic; antipsoriatic; antipruritic; antibacterial* [coal tar] 40%

Doak Tar Oil topical liquid OTC *antiseborrheic; antipsoriatic; antipruritic; antibacterial* [coal tar] 0.8%, 2%

Doan's Pills caplets OTC *analgesic; antirheumatic* [magnesium salicylate] 325, 500 mg

Doan's P.M. caplets OTC *analgesic; antirheumatic; antihistaminic sleep aid* [magnesium salicylate; diphenhydramine HCl] 500•25 mg

DOAP (daunorubicin, Oncovin, ara-C, prednisone) *chemotherapy protocol*

dobupride INN

dobutamine USAN, INN, BAN *cardiotonic; vasopressor for shock* ⊡ *dopamine*

dobutamine HCl USAN, USP, BAN *cardiotonic; vasopressor for shock* 12.5 mg/mL injection

dobutamine lactobionate USAN *cardiotonic*

dobutamine tartrate USAN *cardiotonic*

Dobutrex IV infusion ℞ *vasopressor for cardiac shock* [dobutamine HCl] 12.5 mg/mL

DOCA (desoxycorticosterone acetate) [q.v.]

docarpamine INN

docebenone USAN, INN *5-lipoxygenase inhibitor*

docetaxel USAN, INN *antineoplastic for advanced or metastatic breast, prostate, and non–small cell lung cancer (NSCLC); analogue to paclitaxel; investigational (Phase III) for head and neck cancers*

docetaxel & cisplatin *chemotherapy protocol for bladder cancer and non–small cell lung cancer (NSCLC)*

dock, curled; curly dock; narrow dock; sour dock *medicinal herb* [see: yellow dock]

dock, patience; sweet dock *medicinal herb* [see: bistort]

doconazole USAN, INN *antifungal*

doconexent INN *omega-3 marine triglyceride* [also: docosahexaenoic acid (DHA)]

docosahexaenoic acid (DHA) *natural omega-3 fatty acid used to prevent a wide range of degenerative diseases; high concentrations are found in the brain, where supplementation may increase brain function; effective in treating depression and other brain disorders* [also: doconexent]

docosanol (n-docosanol) USAN *antiviral for herpes simplex labialis; topical treatment of oral herpes simplex type 1; investigational (Phase II) for HIV infection and AIDS-related Kaposi sarcoma*

docosil INN *combining name for radicals or groups*

Doctar shampoo (discontinued 2003) OTC *antiseborrheic; antipsoriatic; antipruritic; antibacterial* [coal tar] 0.5%

Docu oral liquid; syrup OTC *laxative; stool softener* [docusate sodium] 150 mg/15 mL; 20 mg/5 mL

docusate calcium USAN, USP *laxative; stool softener* 240 mg oral

docusate potassium USAN, USP *laxative; stool softener*

docusate sodium USAN, USP, BAN *stool softener; surfactant/wetting agent* [also: sodium dioctyl sulfosuccinate] 50, 100, 250 mg oral; 50 mg/15 mL oral

Docusate with Casanthranol capsules OTC *stool softener; stimulant laxative* [docusate sodium; casanthranol] 100•30 mg

dodecafluoropentane [see: perflenapent]

dodeclonium bromide INN

1-(11-dodecylamino-10-hydroxyundecyl)-3,7-dimethylxanthine hydrogen methanesulfonate *investigational (orphan) for hormone refractory prostate cancer*

2-dodecylisoquinolinium bromide [see: lauryl isoquinolinium bromide]

dofamium chloride INN, BAN

dofetilide USAN, INN, BAN *antiarrhythmic; potassium channel blocker*

dofosfate INN *combining name for radicals or groups*

dog grass *medicinal herb* [see: couch grass]

dog poison (*Aethusa cynapium*) plant *medicinal herb used as an antispasmodic and emetic in homeopathic remedies; not generally regarded as safe and effective as ingestion may be fatal*

dogbane (*Apocynum androsaemifolium*) root *medicinal herb used as a cathartic, diuretic, emetic, expectorant, stimulant, and sudorific*

dogwood, black; black alder dogwood *medicinal herb* [see: buckthorn; cascara sagrada]

DOK-Plus syrup OTC *stimulant laxative; stool softener* [casanthranol; docusate sodium; alcohol 10%] 30•60 mg/15 mL

Dolacet capsules R̸ *narcotic analgesic* [hydrocodone bitartrate; acetaminophen] 5•500 mg

dolantal [see: meperidine HCl]

dolantin [see: meperidine HCl]

dolasetron INN *serotonin 5-HT₃ receptor antagonist; antiemetic for nausea following chemotherapy, radiation, or surgery* [also: dolasetron mesylate]

dolasetron mesylate USAN *serotonin 5-HT₃ receptor antagonist; antiemetic for nausea following chemotherapy, radiation, or surgery* [also: dolasetron]

Dolgic caplets R̸ *analgesic; antipyretic; barbiturate sedative* [acetaminophen; butalbital] 650•50 mg

Dolgic LQ oral solution R̸ *analgesic; antipyretic; barbiturate sedative* [acetaminophen; butalbital; caffeine; alcohol 7.4%] 325•50•40 mg/15 mL

doliracetam INN

Dolobid film-coated tablets R̸ *analgesic; antiarthritic; antirheumatic; antiinflammatory; antipyretic* [diflunisal] 250, 500 mg

dolomite *nutritional supplement; source of calcium and magnesium*

Dolomite tablets OTC *mineral supplement* [calcium; magnesium] 130•78 mg

Dolono elixir OTC *analgesic; antipyretic* [acetaminophen] 160 mg/5 mL

Dolophine HCl subcu or IM injection (discontinued 2004) R̸ *narcotic analgesic; narcotic addiction detoxicant; often abused as a street drug* [methadone HCl] 10 mg/mL

Dolophine HCl tablets R̸ *narcotic analgesic; narcotic addiction detoxicant; often abused as a street drug* [methadone HCl] 5, 10 mg

Dolorac cream OTC *topical analgesic* [capsaicin] 0.025%

dolosal [see: meperidine HCl]

Dolsed sugar-coated tablets R̸ *urinary antibiotic; analgesic; antispasmodic; acidifier* [methenamine; phenyl salicylate; atropine sulfate; methylene blue; hyoscyamine sulfate; benzoic acid] 40.8•18.1•0.03•5.4•0.03•4.5 mg

dolvanol [see: meperidine HCl]

DOM (2,5-dimethoxy-4-methylamphetamine) *a hallucinogenic street drug derived from amphetamine, popularly called STP*

domazoline INN *anticholinergic* [also: domazoline fumarate]

domazoline fumarate USAN *anticholinergic* [also: domazoline]

Domeboro powder packets, effervescent tablets OTC *astringent wet dressing (modified Burow solution)* [aluminum sulfate; calcium acetate]

Domeboro Otic [see: Otic Domeboro]

Dome-Paste medicated gauze bandage OTC *protection and support of extremities* [zinc oxide; calamine; gelatin]

domestrol [see: diethylstilbestrol]

domibrom [see: domiphen bromide]

domiodol USAN, INN *mucolytic*

domiphen bromide USAN, BAN *topical anti-infective*

domipizone INN

Domol Bath and Shower Oil OTC *bath emollient*

domoprednate INN

domoxin INN

domperidone USAN, INN, BAN, JAN *antiemetic for diabetic gastroparesis and chronic gastritis*

Donatussin pediatric oral drops R̶ *decongestant; antihistamine; expectorant* [phenylephrine HCl; chlorpheniramine maleate; guaifenesin] 2•1•20 mg/mL

Donatussin syrup R̶ *antitussive; decongestant; antihistamine; expectorant* [dextromethorphan hydrobromide; phenylephrine HCl; chlorpheniramine maleate; guaifenesin] 15•10•2•100 mg/5 mL

Donatussin DC syrup R̶ *narcotic antitussive; decongestant; expectorant* [hydrocodone bitartrate; phenylephrine HCl; guaifenesin] 5•15•100 mg/10 mL

donepezil HCl USAN *reversible acetylcholinesterase (AChE) inhibitor; cognition adjuvant for Alzheimer dementia; also used for vascular dementia and memory improvement in multiple sclerosis patients*

donetidine USAN, INN, BAN *antagonist to histamine H_2 receptors*

dong quai (*Angelica polymorpha; A. sinensis; A. dahurica*) root *medicinal herb for allergies, anemia, blood cleansing, constipation, female hormonal problems, hypertension, internal bleeding, menopausal symptoms, nourishing brain, and ulcers; not generally regarded as safe and effective as it contains coumarins and safrole*

Donnagel chewable tablets, oral liquid (discontinued 2004) OTC *antidiarrheal; GI adsorbent* [attapulgite] 600 mg; 600 mg/15 mL ☒ Donnatal

Donnamar tablets (discontinued 2004) R̶ *GI/GU antispasmodic; antiparkinsonian; anticholinergic "drying agent" for allergic rhinitis and hyperhidrosis* [hyoscyamine sulfate] 0.125 mg

Donna-Sed elixir R̶ *GI antispasmodic; anticholinergic; sedative* [atropine sulfate; scopolamine hydrobromide; hyoscyamine hydrobromide; phenobarbital] 0.0194•0.0065•0.1037•16.2 mg/5 mL

Donnatal capsules (discontinued 2004) R̶ *GI antispasmodic; anticholinergic; sedative* [atropine sulfate; scopolamine hydrobromide; hyoscyamine sulfate; phenobarbital] 0.0194•0.0065•0.1037•16.2 mg ☒ Donnagel

Donnatal Extentabs (extended-release tablets), tablets, elixir R̶ *GI antispasmodic; anticholinergic; sedative* [atropine sulfate; scopolamine hydrobromide; hyoscyamine sulfate; phenobarbital] 0.0582•0.0195•0.3111•48.6 mg; 0.0194•0.0065•0.1037•16.2 mg; 0.0194•0.0065•0.1037•16.2 mg/5 mL ☒ Donnagel

Donnatal No. 2 tablets (discontinued 2004) R̶ *GI antispasmodic; anticholinergic; sedative* [atropine sulfate; scopolamine hydrobromide; hyoscyamine sulfate; phenobarbital] 0.0194•0.0065•0.1037•32.4 mg

Donnazyme tablets (discontinued 2002) R̶ *digestive enzymes* [pancreatin (lipase; protease; amylase)] 500 mg (1000•12 500•12 500 USP units) ☒ Entozyme

DOPA (dihydroxyphenylalanine) [see: levodopa]

L-dopa [see: levodopa]

dopamantine USAN, INN *antiparkinsonian*

dopamine INN, BAN *adrenergic; vasopressor for shock* [also: dopamine HCl] ☒ dobutamine; Dopram

dopamine HCl USAN, USP *adrenergic; vasopressor for shock* [also: dopamine] 40, 80, 160 mg/mL injection

dopamine HCl in 5% dextrose *adrenergic; vasopressor for shock* 80, 160, 320 mg/100 mL injection

dopaminergics *a class of antiparkinsonian agents that affect the dopamine neurotransmitters in the brain*

Dopar capsules ℞ *dopamine precursor; antiparkinsonian* [levodopa] 100, 250, 500 mg ☒ Dopram

dopexamine USAN, INN, BAN *cardiovascular agent*

dopexamine HCl USAN, BAN *cardiovascular agent*

Dopram IV injection or infusion ℞ *CNS stimulant; analeptic; adjunct to postanesthesia "stir-up"; respiratory stimulant for chronic obstructive pulmonary disease (COPD); also used for apnea of prematurity* [doxapram HCl] 20 mg/mL ☒ dopamine; Dopar

dopropidil INN

doqualast INN

Doral caplets ℞ *benzodiazepine sedative and hypnotic* [quazepam] 7.5, 15 mg

dorastine INN *antihistamine* [also: dorastine HCl]

dorastine HCl USAN *antihistamine* [also: dorastine]

Dorcol Children's Cold Formula oral liquid (discontinued 2002) OTC *pediatric decongestant and antihistamine* [pseudoephedrine HCl; chlorpheniramine maleate] 15•1 mg/5 mL

Dorcol Children's Cough syrup (discontinued 2002) OTC *pediatric antitussive, decongestant, and expectorant* [dextromethorphan hydrobromide; pseudoephedrine HCl; guaifenesin] 5•15•50 mg/5 mL

Dorcol Children's Decongestant oral liquid (discontinued 2002) OTC *nasal decongestant* [pseudoephedrine HCl] 15 mg/5 mL

doreptide INN

doretinel USAN, INN *antikeratinizing agent*

Dormarex 2 tablets OTC *antihistaminic sleep aid; motion sickness preventative* [diphenhydramine HCl] 50 mg

dormethan [see: dextromethorphan hydrobromide]

Dormin caplets, capsules OTC *antihistaminic sleep aid* [diphenhydramine HCl] 25 mg

dormiral [see: phenobarbital]

dormonal [see: barbital]

dornase alfa USAN, INN *reduces respiratory viscoelasticity of sputum in cystic fibrosis (orphan)*

Doryx coated pellets in capsules, delayed-release tablets ℞ *tetracycline antibiotic* [doxycycline hyclate] 75, 100 mg

dorzolamide HCl USAN *topical carbonic anhydrase inhibitor for glaucoma*

D.O.S. softgels OTC *laxative; stool softener* [docusate sodium] 100, 250 mg

Dosa-Trol Pack (trademarked dosage form) *unit-of-use package*

Dosepak (trademarked dosage form) *unit-of-use package*

dosergoside INN

Dosette (trademarked dosage form) *injectable unit-of-use system (vials, ampules, syringes, etc.)*

Dospan (trademarked form) *controlled-release tablets*

Dostinex tablets ℞ *dopamine agonist for hyperprolactinemia; investigational treatment for Parkinson disease and gynecologic disorders* [cabergoline] 0.5 mg

dosulepin INN *antidepressant* [also: dothiepin HCl; dothiepin; dosulepin HCl]

dosulepin HCl JAN *antidepressant* [also: dothiepin HCl; dosulepin; dothiepin]

dotarizine INN

dotefonium bromide INN

dothiepin BAN *antidepressant* [also: dothiepin HCl; dosulepin; dosulepin HCl]

dothiepin HCl USAN *antidepressant* [also: dosulepin; dothiepin; dosulepin HCl]

Double Antibiotic ointment OTC *antibiotic* [polymyxin B sulfate; bacitracin zinc] 10 000•500 U/g

Double Antibiotic Plus cream (discontinued 2003) OTC *antibiotic; local anesthetic* [polymyxin B sulfate; neomycin sulfate; pramoxine HCl] 5000 U•3.5 mg•10 mg per g

Double Ice ArthriCare [see: ArthriCare, Double Ice]

Double-Action Toothache Kit tablets + topical liquid OTC *analgesic; oral anesthetic* [(acetaminophen) + (benzocaine; alcohol 74%)] (325 mg) + (≚)

Dovobet (approved in 23 countries) ℞ *investigational (NDA filed) topical antipsoriatic and steroidal anti-inflammatory for plaque psoriasis* [calcipotriene; betamethasone dipropionate] 50 μg•0.5 mg

Dovonex cream, ointment, scalp solution ℞ *antipsoriatic* [calcipotriene] 0.005%

DOX → CMF, sequential (doxorubicin; cyclophosphamide, methotrexate, fluorouracil) *chemotherapy protocol for breast cancer*

doxacurium chloride USAN, INN, BAN *nondepolarizing neuromuscular blocker; muscle relaxant; adjunct to anesthesia*

doxaminol INN

doxapram INN, BAN *respiratory stimulant; analeptic* [also: doxapram HCl]

doxapram HCl USAN, USP *CNS stimulant; analeptic; adjunct to postanesthesia "stir-up"; respiratory stimulant for chronic obstructive pulmonary disease (COPD); also used for apnea of prematurity* [also: doxapram] 20 mg/mL injection

doxaprost USAN, INN *bronchodilator*

doxate [see: docusate sodium]

doxazosin INN, BAN *alpha₁-adrenergic blocker for hypertension and benign prostatic hyperplasia (BPH)* [also: doxazosin mesylate]

doxazosin mesylate USAN *alpha₁-adrenergic blocker for hypertension and benign prostatic hyperplasia (BPH)* [also: doxazosin] 1, 2, 4, 8 mg oral

doxefazepam INN

doxenitoin INN

doxepin INN, BAN *tricyclic antidepressant; anxiolytic; topical antihistamine* [also: doxepin HCl] ⬚ Doxidan; Loxitane

doxepin HCl USAN, USP *tricyclic antidepressant; anxiolytic; topical antihistamine* [also: doxepin] 10, 25, 50, 75, 100, 150 mg oral; 10 mg/mL oral

doxercalciferol USAN *synthetic vitamin D analogue; serum calcium regulator for hyperparathyroidism of chronic renal dialysis*

doxibetasol INN [also: doxybetasol]

Doxidan capsules (discontinued 2003) OTC *stimulant laxative; stool softener* [casanthranol; docusate sodium] 30• 100 mg

Doxidan delayed-release tablets OTC *stimulant laxative* [bisacodyl] 5 mg

doxifluridine INN, JAN *investigational antineoplastic*

Doxil IV injection ℞ *anthracycline antibiotic antineoplastic for ovarian cancer (orphan) and Kaposi sarcoma; investigational (NDA filed) for prostate cancer; investigational (Phase III) for breast cancer and multiple myeloma* [doxorubicin HCl, liposome-encapsulated] 20, 50 mg/vial

doxofylline USAN, INN *bronchodilator*

doxorubicin USAN, INN, BAN *anthracycline antibiotic antineoplastic* ⬚ daunorubicin

doxorubicin HCl USP *anthracycline antibiotic antineoplastic* 10, 20, 50 mg, 2 mg/mL injection

doxorubicin HCl, liposome-encapsulated (LED) *anthracycline antibiotic antineoplastic for ovarian cancer (orphan) and Kaposi sarcoma; investigational (NDA filed) for prostate cancer; investigational (Phase III) for breast cancer*

doxorubicin & vinorelbine *chemotherapy protocol for breast cancer*

doxpicodin HCl [now: doxpicomine HCl]

doxpicomine INN *analgesic* [also: doxpicomine HCl]

doxpicomine HCl USAN *analgesic* [also: doxpicomine]

Doxy 100; Doxy 200 powder for IV infusion ℞ *tetracycline antibiotic* [doxycycline hyclate] 100 mg/vial; 200 mg/vial

Doxy Caps capsules (discontinued 2003) ℞ *tetracycline antibiotic* [doxycycline hyclate] 100 mg

doxybetasol BAN [also: doxibetasol]

Doxychel Hyclate capsules, tablets, powder for IV injection (discontinued 2003) ℞ *tetracycline antibiotic* [doxycycline hyclate] 50, 100 mg; 50, 100 mg; 100, 200 mg

doxycycline USAN, USP, INN, BAN *tetracycline antibiotic; antirickettsial; malaria prophylaxis; investigational (Phase III) treatment for rosacea*

doxycycline calcium USP *tetracycline antibiotic; antiprotozoal*

doxycycline fosfatex USAN, BAN *tetracycline antibiotic*

doxycycline hyclate USP *tetracycline antibiotic; periodontitis treatment* 50, 100 mg oral; 100 mg/vial injection

doxycycline monohydrate *tetracycline antibiotic* 50, 100 mg oral

doxylamine INN, BAN *antihistamine; sleep aid* [also: doxylamine succinate]

doxylamine succinate USP *antihistamine; sleep aid* [also: doxylamine]

DPE (dipivalyl epinephrine) [now: dipivefrin]

DPF [see: Dermprotective Factor]

DPN (diphosphopyridine nucleotide) [now: nadide]

DPPC (dipalmitoylphosphatidylcholine) [see: colfosceril palmitate]

DPPE (diethyl-phenylmethyl-phenoxy ethenamine) HCl [see: tesmilifene HCl]

Dr. Brown's Home Drug Testing System *in vitro diagnostic aid for detection of multiple illicit drugs in the urine*

Dr. Dermi-Heal ointment OTC *vulnerary; antipruritic; astringent* [allantoin; zinc oxide; peruvian balsam] 1%•?•?

Dr. Edwards' Olive tablets OTC *stimulant laxative* [sennosides] 8.6 mg

Dr. Scholl's Advanced Pain Relief Corn Removers; Dr. Scholl's Callus Removers; Dr Scholl's Clear Away; Dr. Scholl's Corn Removers medicated discs OTC *keratolytic* [salicylic acid in a rubber-based vehicle] 40%

Dr. Scholl's Athlete's Foot powder, spray powder, spray liquid OTC *topical antifungal* [tolnaftate] 1%

Dr. Scholl's Clear Away OneStep; Dr. Scholl's OneStep Corn Removers medicated strips OTC *keratolytic* [salicylic acid in a rubber-based vehicle] 40%

Dr. Scholl's Corn/Callus Remover topical liquid OTC *keratolytic* [salicylic acid in flexible collodion] 17%

Dr. Scholl's Cracked Heel Relief cream OTC *topical local anesthetic; antiseptic* [lidocaine HCl; benzalkonium chloride] 2%•0.13%

Dr. Scholl's Moisturizing Corn Remover Kit medicated discs + cushions + moisturizing cream OTC *keratolytic* [salicylic acid in a rubber-based vehicle] 40%

Dr. Scholl's Tritin powder, spray powder OTC *topical antifungal* [tolnaftate] 1%

Dr. Scholl's Wart Remover Kit topical liquid + adhesive pads OTC *keratolytic* [salicylic acid in flexible collodion] 17%

Dr. Smith's Adult Care; Dr. Smith's Diaper ointment OTC *astringent; moisturizer; emollient* [zinc oxide] 10%

draflazine USAN *cardioprotectant*

dragée (French for "sugar plum") *a sugar-coated pill or medicated confection* [pronounced "drah zhá"]

dragon's claw, scaly *medicinal herb* [see: coral root]

dragonwort *medicinal herb* [see: bistort]

Dramamine oral liquid ℞ *antinauseant; antiemetic; antivertigo agent; motion sickness preventative* [dimenhydrinate] 15.62 mg/5 mL

Dramamine tablets, chewable tablets, oral liquid OTC *antinauseant; antiemetic; antivertigo agent; motion sickness preventative* [dimenhydrinate] 50 mg; 50 mg; 12.5 mg/4 mL

Dramamine, Children's oral liquid OTC *antinauseant; antiemetic; antivertigo agent; motion sickness preventative* [dimenhydrinate; alcohol 5%] 12.5 mg/5 mL

Dramamine II tablets (name changed to Dramamine Less Drowsy Formula in 2000)

Dramamine Less Drowsy Formula tablets OTC *anticholinergic; antihistamine; antivertigo agent; motion sickness preventative* [meclizine HCl] 25 mg

Dramanate IV or IM injection ℞ *antinauseant; antiemetic; antivertigo agent; motion sickness preventative* [dimenhydrinate] 50 mg/mL ⑨ Dommanate

dramarin [see: dimenhydrate]

dramedilol INN

Dramilin IV or IM injection ℞ *antinauseant; antiemetic; antivertigo agent; motion sickness preventative* [dimenhydrinate] 50 mg/mL

dramyl [see: dimenhydrate]

draquinolol INN

drazidox INN

dribendazole USAN, INN *anthelmintic*

dricol [see: amidephrine]

Dri/Ear ear drops OTC *antibacterial; antifungal* [boric acid] 2.75%

dried aluminum hydroxide gel [see: aluminum hydroxide gel, dried]

dried basic aluminum carbonate [see: aluminum carbonate, basic]

dried ferrous sulfate [see: ferrous sulfate, dried]

dried yeast [see: yeast, dried]

DriHist SR sustained-release caplets ℞ *decongestant; antihistamine; anticholinergic to dry mucosal secretions* [phenylephrine HCl; chlorphenir-

amine maleate; methscopolamine nitrate] 20•8•2.5 mg

drinidene USAN, INN *analgesic*

Drisdol capsules ℞ *vitamin deficiency therapy for refractory rickets, familial hypophosphatemia, and hypoparathyroidism* [ergocalciferol (vitamin D$_2$)] 50 000 IU

Drisdol Drops OTC *vitamin supplement* [ergocalciferol (vitamin D$_2$)] 8000 IU/mL

Dristan 12-Hr. nasal spray OTC *nasal decongestant* [oxymetazoline HCl] 0.05%

Dristan Cold, Maximum Strength caplets OTC *decongestant; antihistamine; analgesic* [pseudoephedrine HCl; brompheniramine maleate; acetaminophen] 30•2•500 mg

Dristan Cold Multi-Symptom Formula tablets OTC *decongestant; antihistamine; analgesic* [phenylephrine HCl; chlorpheniramine maleate; acetaminophen] 5•2•325 mg

Dristan Cold Non-Drowsy caplets OTC *decongestant; analgesic; antipyretic* [pseudoephedrine HCl; acetaminophen] 30•500 mg

Dristan Fast Acting Formula nasal spray OTC *nasal decongestant; antihistamine* [phenylephrine HCl; pheniramine maleate] 0.5%•0.2%

Dristan Saline Spray (discontinued 2002) OTC *nasal moisturizer* [sodium chloride (saline solution)]

Dristan Sinus caplets OTC *decongestant; analgesic* [pseudoephedrine HCl; ibuprofen] 30•200 mg

Drithocreme; Drithocreme HP 1%; Dritho-Scalp cream ℞ *topical antipsoriatic* [anthralin] 0.1%, 0.25%, 0.5%; 1%; 0.5%

Drixomed sustained-release tablets ℞ *decongestant; antihistamine* [pseudoephedrine sulfate; dexbrompheniramine maleate] 120•6 mg

Drixoral syrup (discontinued 2002) OTC *decongestant; antihistamine* [pseudoephedrine sulfate; brompheniramine maleate] 30•2 mg/5 mL

Drixoral 12 hour Non-Drowsy Formula extended-release tablets OTC *nasal decongestant* [pseudoephedrine sulfate] 120 mg

Drixoral Allergy Sinus extended-release tablets OTC *decongestant; antihistamine; analgesic* [pseudoephedrine sulfate; dexbrompheniramine maleate; acetaminophen] 60•3•500 mg

Drixoral Cold & Allergy sustained-action tablets OTC *decongestant; antihistamine* [pseudoephedrine sulfate; dexbrompheniramine maleate] 120•6 mg

Drixoral Cold & Flu; Drixoral Plus extended-release tablets (name changed to **Drixoral Allergy Sinus** in 2002)

Drixoral Cough & Congestion Liquid Caps (capsules) (discontinued 2002) OTC *antitussive; decongestant* [dextromethorphan hydrobromide; pseudoephedrine HCl] 30•60 mg

Drixoral Cough & Sore Throat Liquid Caps (liquid-filled capsules) (discontinued 2002) OTC *antitussive; analgesic* [dextromethorphan hydrobromide; acetaminophen] 15•325 mg

Drixoral Day; Drixoral N.D. (CAN) sustained-action tablets OTC *decongestant* [pseudoephedrine sulfate] 120 mg

Drixoral Night (CAN) tablets OTC *decongestant; antihistamine* [pseudoephedrine sulfate; dexbrompheniramine maleate] 60•2 mg

Drize sustained-release capsules (discontinued 2001) ℞ *decongestant; antihistamine* [phenylpropanolamine HCl; chlorpheniramine maleate] 75•12 mg

drobuline USAN, INN *antiarrhythmic*

drocarbil NF

drocinonide USAN, INN *anti-inflammatory*

droclidinium bromide INN

drocode [see: dihydrocodeine]

drofenine INN

droloxifene INN *investigational (Phase III) antineoplastic for breast cancer; investigational (Phase III) antiestrogen for postmenopausal osteoporosis*

droloxifene citrate USAN *antineoplastic; antiestrogen*

drometrizole USAN, INN *ultraviolet screen*

dromostanolone propionate USAN, USP *antineoplastic* [also: drostanolone]

dronabinol USAN, USP, INN *antiemetic for chemotherapy; appetite stimulant for AIDS patients (orphan); investigational (Phase II) for pain relief and sleep enhancement*

drop chalk [see: calcium carbonate]

dropberry *medicinal herb* [see: Solomon's seal]

Drop-Dose (trademarked delivery system) *prefilled eye drop dispenser*

dropempine INN

droperidol USAN, USP, INN, BAN *general anesthetic; antiemetic; antipsychotic*

Dropperettes (delivery system) *prefilled droppers*

droprenilamine USAN, INN *coronary vasodilator*

dropropizine INN, BAN

Drop-Tainers (trademarked packaging form) *prefilled eye drop dispenser*

drospirenone USAN *progestin; spironolactone analogue; aldosterone antagonist*

drostanolone INN, BAN *antineoplastic* [also: dromostanolone propionate]

drotaverine INN

drotebanol INN, BAN

Drotic ear drops ℞ *topical corticosteroidal anti-inflammatory; antibiotic* [hydrocortisone; neomycin sulfate; polymyxin B sulfate] 1%•5 mg•10 000 U per mL

drotrecogin alfa *antithrombotic; recombinant human activated protein C (rhAPC) for severe sepsis*

droxacin INN *antibacterial* [also: droxacin sodium]

droxacin sodium USAN *antibacterial* [also: droxacin]

Droxia capsules ℞ *sickle cell anemia treatment (orphan)* [hydroxyurea] 200, 300, 400 mg

droxicainide INN

droxicam INN

droxidopa INN

droxifilcon A USAN *hydrophilic contact lens material*

droxinavir HCl USAN *antiviral; HIV-1 protease inhibitor*

droxypropine INN, BAN

Dry E 400 tablets (discontinued 2004) OTC *vitamin supplement* [vitamin E (as d-alpha tocopheryl acid succinate)] 400 IU

Dry Eyes eye drops OTC *ophthalmic moisturizer/lubricant* [polyvinyl alcohol] 1.4%

Dry Eyes ophthalmic ointment OTC *ocular moisturizer/lubricant* [white petrolatum; mineral oil]

Dryopteris filix-mas medicinal herb [see: aspidium]

Dryox 2.5; Dryox 5; Dryox 10; Dryox 20 gel (discontinued 2003) OTC *keratolytic for acne* [benzoyl peroxide] 2.5%; 5%; 10%; 20%

Dryox 10S 5; Dryox 20S 10 gel (discontinued 2003) OTC *keratolytic for acne* [benzoyl peroxide; sulfur] 10%•5%; 20%•10%

Dryox Wash 5; Dryox Wash 10 topical liquid (discontinued 2003) OTC *keratolytic for acne* [benzoyl peroxide] 5%; 10%

Dryphen Multi-Symptom Formula tablets OTC *decongestant; antihistamine; analgesic* [phenylephrine HCl; chlorpheniramine maleate; acetaminophen] 5•2•325 mg

Drysol solution ℞ *astringent for hyperhidrosis* [aluminum chloride (hexahydrate)] 20%

Drytergent topical liquid OTC *soap-free therapeutic skin cleanser*

Drytex lotion OTC *keratolytic cleanser for acne* [salicylic acid; acetone; isopropyl alcohol] ±•10%•40%

Dryvax powder for reconstitution ℞ *active immunization against smallpox using the multiple-puncture technique (scarification); licensed for restricted use and available only from the CDC* [smallpox vaccine] 100 million infectious vaccinia viruses/mL

DSC; DSCG (disodium cromoglycate) [see: cromolyn sodium]

D-S-S capsules OTC *laxative; stool softener* [docusate sodium] 100 mg

DSS (dioctyl sodium sulfosuccinate) [now: docusate sodium]

DSS 100 Plus capsules (discontinued 2003) OTC *stimulant laxative; stool softener* [casanthranol; docusate sodium] 30•100 mg

DST (dihydrostreptomycin) [q.v.]

DT; Td (diphtheria & tetanus [toxoids]) *the designation DT (or TD) denotes the pediatric vaccine; Td denotes the adult vaccine* [see: diphtheria & tetanus toxoids, adsorbed]

DTaP (diphtheria & tetanus [toxoids] & acellular pertussis [vaccine]) [q.v.]

DTIC (dimethyl triazeno imidazole carboxamide) [see: dacarbazine]

DTIC & tamoxifen *chemotherapy protocol for malignant melanoma*

DTIC-ACTD; DTIC-ACT-D (DTIC, actinomycin D) *chemotherapy protocol*

DTIC-Dome IV injection ℞ *antineoplastic for metastatic malignant melanoma and Hodgkin disease* [dacarbazine] 100, 200 mg

DTP (diphtheria & tetanus [toxoids] & pertussis [vaccine]) [q.v.]

DTPA (diethylenetriaminepentaacetic acid) [see: pentetic acid]

DTPA (diethylenetriaminepentaacetic acid) technetium (^{99m}Tc), human serum albumin [see: technetium Tc 99m pentetate]

DTwP (diphtheria & tetanus [toxoids] & whole-cell pertussis [vaccine]) [q.v.]

Duac gel ℞ *antibiotic and keratolytic for acne* [clindamycin; benzoyl peroxide] 1%•5%

Duadacin capsules (discontinued 2001) OTC *decongestant; antihistamine; analgesic* [phenylpropanolamine HCl; chlorpheniramine maleate; acetaminophen] 12.5•2•325 mg

Duadacin Cold & Flu caplets (discontinued 2004) OTC *decongestant; antihistamine; analgesic* [pseudoephedrine HCl; chlorpheniramine maleate; acetaminophen] 30•2•500 mg

duazomycin USAN, INN *antineoplastic*

duazomycin A [see: duazomycin]

duazomycin B [see: azotomycin]

duazomycin C [see: ambomycin]

Duboisia myoporoides medicinal herb [see: corkwood]

duck's foot *medicinal herb* [see: mandrake]

ducodal [see: oxycodone]

Duet tablets ℞ *vitamin/mineral/calcium/ iron supplement* [multiple vitamins & minerals; calcium; iron] ≜•200• 29 mg

Dulcet (trademarked dosage form) *chewable tablet*

Dulcolax enteric-coated tablets, suppositories OTC *stimulant laxative* [bisacodyl] 5 mg; 10 mg

Dulcolax oral liquid OTC *saline laxative; antacid* [magnesium hydroxide] 400 mg/5 mL

Dulcolax Bowel Prep Kit 4 enteric-coated tablets + 1 suppository OTC *pre-procedure bowel evacuant* [bisacodyl] 5 mg; 10 mg

Dulcolax Stool Softener softgels OTC *laxative; stool softener* [docusate sodium] 100 mg

Dull-C powder OTC *vitamin C supplement* [ascorbic acid] 4.24 g/tsp.

dulofibrate INN

duloxetine INN *selective serotonin and norepinephrine reuptake inhibitor (SSNRI) for depression* [also: duloxetine HCl]

duloxetine HCl USAN *selective serotonin and norepinephrine reuptake inhibitor (SSNRI) for major depressive disorder (MDD) and generalized anxiety disorder (GAD); analgesic for diabetic peripheral neuropathy (DPN); investigational (Phase II) for urinary incontinence* [also: duloxetine]

dulozafone INN

dumorelin INN

duneryl [see: phenobarbital]

Duocaine injection ℞ *local anesthetic; peripheral nerve block for ophthalmologic surgery* [bupivacaine HCl; lidocaine HCl] 3.75•10 mg/mL

Duocet tablets ℞ *narcotic analgesic* [hydrocodone bitartrate; acetaminophen] 5•500 mg

Duo-Cyp IM injection (discontinued 2003) ℞ *hormone replacement therapy for postmenopausal symptoms* [estradiol cypionate; testosterone cypionate] 2•50 mg/mL

DuoDerm CGF; DuoDerm Extra Thin; DuoDerm Hydroactive adhesive dressings OTC *occlusive wound dressing* [hydrocolloid gel]

DuoDerm Hydroactive paste, granules OTC *wound dressing* [hydrocolloid gel] 30 g; 5 g

DuoFilm patch OTC *keratolytic* [salicylic acid in a rubber-based vehicle] 40%

DuoFilm topical liquid OTC *keratolytic* [salicylic acid in flexible collodion] 17%

DuoFilm Gel for Kids ⒸⒶⓃ OTC *topical keratolytic* [salicylic acid in flexible collodion] 11%

duometacin INN

duomycin [see: chlortetracycline HCl]

Duonate-12 pediatric oral suspension ℞ *decongestant; antihistamine* [phenylephrine tannate; pyrilamine tannate] 5•30 mg/5 mL

DuoNeb oral inhalation aerosol ℞ *anticholinergic bronchodilator for chronic obstructive pulmonary disease (COPD)* [ipratropium bromide; albuterol sulfate] 0.5•3 mg/dose

duoperone INN *neuroleptic* [also: duoperone fumarate]

duoperone fumarate USAN *neuroleptic* [also: duoperone]

DuoPlant gel ℞ *keratolytic* [salicylic acid in flexible collodion] 17%

duotal [see: guaiacol carbonate]

Duotan PD oral suspension ℞ *decongestant; antihistamine* [pseudoephedrine tannate; dexchlorpheniramine tannate] 75•2.5 mg/5 mL

Duo-Trach Kit pre-filled syringe with cannula (discontinued 2002) ℞ *injectable local anesthetic* [lidocaine HCl] 4%

DuoVisc prefilled syringes ℞ *dispersive/cohesive viscoelastic agent for ophthalmic surgery* [Viscoat (q.v.); ProVisc (q.v.)] 0.35•0.4, 0.5•0.55 mL

Duphalac oral/rectal solution ℞ *hyperosmotic laxative* [lactulose] 10 g/15 mL

Duplex topical liquid (discontinued 2004) OTC *soap-free therapeutic skin cleanser* [sodium lauryl sulfate] 15%

Duplex T shampoo (discontinued 2003) OTC *antiseborrheic; antipsoriatic; antipruritic; antibacterial* [coal tar] 10%

duponol [see: sodium lauryl sulfate]

dupracetam INN

Duracaps (dosage form) *sustained-release capsules*

DURAcare II solution OTC *surfactant cleaning solution for soft contact lenses*

Duraclon continuous epidural infusion ℞ *central analgesic; adjunct to opioid analgesics for severe cancer pain* (orphan) [clonidine HCl] 500 μg/mL

Duradrin capsules ℞ *cerebral vasoconstrictor and analgesic for vascular and tension headaches; "possibly effective" for migraine headaches* [isomethepene mucate; dichloralphenazone; acetaminophen] 65•100•325 mg

Duradryl syrup ℞ *decongestant; antihistamine; anticholinergic to dry mucosal secretions* [phenylephrine HCl; chlorpheniramine maleate; methscopolamine nitrate] 10•2•1.25 mg/5 mL

Duradryl JR pediatric capsules (discontinued 2004) ℞ *decongestant; antihistamine; anticholinergic to dry mucosal secretions* [phenylephrine HCl; chlorpheniramine maleate; methscopolamine nitrate] 10•4•1.25 mg

Duraflu tablets ℞ *antitussive; decongestant; expectorant; analgesic* [dextromethorphan hydrobromide; pseudoephedrine HCl; guaifenesin; acetaminophen] 20•60•200•500 mg

DuraGen ℞ *resorbable graft matrix to repair the dura mater following brain surgery or traumatic injury*

Duragesic-12; Duragesic-25; Duragesic-50; Duragesic-75; Duragesic-100 transdermal patch ℞ *narcotic analgesic* [fentanyl] 12.5 μg/hr.; 25 μg/hr.; 50 μg/hr.; 75 μg/hr.; 100 μg/hr.

Dura-Gest capsules (discontinued 2002) ℞ *decongestant; expectorant* [phenylephrine HCl; phenylpropanolamine HCl; guaifenesin] 45•5•200 mg

Durahist sustained-release tablets ℞ *decongestant; antihistamine; anticholinergic* [pseudoephedrine HCl; chlorpheniramine maleate; methscopolamine bromide] 60•8•1.25 mg

Duralex sustained-release capsules (discontinued 2002) ℞ *decongestant; antihistamine* [pseudoephedrine HCl; chlorpheniramine maleate] 120•8 mg

Duralith ⒸⒶⓃ sustained-release tablets ℞ *antipsychotic for manic episodes* [lithium carbonate] 300 mg

Duralone-40; Duralone-80 intralesional, soft tissue, and IM injection (discontinued 2004) ℞ *corticosteroid; anti-inflammatory; immunosuppressant* [methylprednisolone acetate] 40 mg/mL; 80 mg/mL

Duramist Plus 12-Hour Decongestant nasal spray OTC *nasal decongestant* [oxymetazoline HCl] 0.05%

Duramorph IV, IM, or subcu injection ℞ *narcotic analgesic* [morphine sulfate] 0.5, 1 mg/mL

duramycin *investigational (orphan) agent for cystic fibrosis*

Duranest; Duranest MPF injection (discontinued 2002) ℞ *injectable local anesthetic* [etidocaine HCl] [note: one of two different products with the same name] 1% ⓘ Duratest

Duranest; Duranest MPF injection (discontinued 2002) ℞ *injectable local anesthetic* [etidocaine; epinephrine] [note: one of two different products with the same name] 1%•1:200 000, 1.5%•1:200 000 ⓘ Duratest

durapatite USAN *prosthetic aid* [also: calcium phosphate, tribasic; hydroxyapatite]

Duraphen II extended-release tablets ℞ *decongestant; expectorant* [phenylephrine HCl; guaifenesin] 25•800 mg

DuraPrep Surgical Solution self-contained applicator OTC *broad-spectrum antimicrobial prep for surgical procedures* [iodine; isopropyl alcohol] 0.7%•74%

Durasal II sustained-release tablets ℞ *decongestant; expectorant* [pseudoephedrine HCl; guaifenesin] 60•600 mg

DuraSite (delivery system) *polymer-based eye drops*

DuraSolv (trademarked delivery system) *orally disintegrating tablets*

Durasphere injection ℞ *tissue-bulking agent for female stress urinary incontinence* [carbon-coated beads]

Dura-Tab (trademarked dosage form) *sustained-release tablet*

Dura-Tap/PD prolonged-action capsule (discontinued 2002) ℞ *pediatric decongestant and antihistamine* [pseudoephedrine HCl; chlorpheniramine maleate] 60•4 mg

Duratears Naturale ophthalmic ointment OTC *ocular moisturizer/lubricant* [white petrolatum; mineral oil; lanolin]

Duratest 100; Duratest 200 IM injection (discontinued 2001) ℞ *androgen replacement for delayed puberty or breast cancer* [testosterone cypionate] 100 mg/mL; 200 mg/mL ⊘ Duranest; Duratuss

Durathate-200 IM injection (discontinued 2001) ℞ *androgen replacement for delayed puberty or breast cancer* [testosterone enanthate] 200 mg/mL

Duration nasal spray OTC *nasal decongestant* [oxymetazoline HCl] 0.05%

Duratocin ⊛ IV injection ℞ *uterotonic agent to prevent postpartum hemorrhage following cesarean section* [carbetocin] 100 μg/mL

Duratuss tablets ℞ *decongestant; expectorant* [phenylephrine HCl; guaifenesin] 25•900 mg ⊘ Duratest

Duratuss DM elixir ℞ *antitussive; expectorant* [dextromethorphan hydrobromide; guaifenesin] 25•225 mg/5 mL

Duratuss G sustained-release film-coated caplets (discontinued 2003) ℞ *expectorant* [guaifenesin] 1200 mg

Duratuss GP extended-release tablets ℞ *decongestant; expectorant* [phenylephrine HCl; guaifenesin] 25•1200 mg ⊘ Duratest

Duratuss HD elixir ℞ *narcotic antitussive; decongestant; expectorant* [hydrocodone bitartrate; phenylephrine HCl; guaifenesin] 2.5•10•225 mg/5 mL

Dura-Vent long-acting tablets (discontinued 2002) ℞ *decongestant; expectorant* [phenylpropanolamine HCl; guaifenesin] 75•600 mg

Dura-Vent/A continuous-release capsule (discontinued 2001) ℞ *decongestant; antihistamine* [phenylpropanolamine HCl; chlorpheniramine maleate] 75•10 mg

Dura-Vent/DA sustained-release tablets ℞ *decongestant; antihistamine; anticholinergic to dry mucosal secretions* [phenylephrine HCl; chlorpheniramine maleate; methscopolamine nitrate] 20•8•2.5 mg

Duraxin capsules ℞ *antihistamine; analgesic* [phenyltoloxamine citrate; acetaminophen; salicylamide] 25•325•200 mg

Duricef capsules, tablets, powder for oral suspension ℞ *cephalosporin antibiotic* [cefadroxil] 500 mg; 1000 mg; 125, 250, 500 mg/5 mL

dusting powder, absorbable USP *surgical glove lubricant*

dutasteride USAN *5α-reductase blocker; inhibits the conversion of testosterone to dihydrotestosterone (DHT); treatment for benign prostatic hyperplasia (BPH); investigational (Phase III) for prostate cancer*

Dutonin (British name for U.S. product Serzone)

Duvoid tablets (discontinued 2001) ℞ *cholinergic urinary stimulant for postsurgical and postpartum urinary retention* [bethanechol chloride] 10, 25, 50 mg

DVB (DDP, vindesine, bleomycin) *chemotherapy protocol*

DVP (daunorubicin, vincristine, prednisone) *chemotherapy protocol for acute lymphocytic leukemia (ALL)*

DVPL-ASP (daunorubicin, vincristine, prednisone, L-asparaginase) *chemotherapy protocol*

dwarf ginseng *(Panax trifolius) medicinal herb* [see: ginseng]

dwarf palm; dwarf palmetto *medicinal herb* [see: saw palmetto]

dwarf sumach *medicinal herb* [see: sumach]

Dyazide capsules ℞ *antihypertensive; diuretic* [triamterene; hydrochlorothiazide] 37.5•25 mg ☒ thiazides; Tiazac

Dycill capsules (discontinued 2002) ℞ *penicillinase-resistant penicillin antibiotic* [dicloxacillin sodium] 250, 500 mg

dyclocaine BAN *topical anesthetic* [also: dyclonine HCl; dyclonine]

Dyclone solution (discontinued 2004) ℞ *anesthetic prior to upper GI and respiratory endoscopies* [dyclonine HCl] 0.5%, 1%

dyclonine INN *topical anesthetic* [also: dyclonine HCl; dyclocaine]

dyclonine HCl USP *topical anesthetic* [also: dyclonine; dyclocaine]

dydrogesterone USAN, USP, INN, BAN *progestin*

dyer's broom *(Genista tinctoria) flowering twigs medicinal herb used as an aperient, diuretic, stimulant, and vasoconstrictor*

dyer's bugloss *medicinal herb* [see: henna (Alkanna)]

dyer's saffron *medicinal herb* [see: safflower]

dyer's weed *medicinal herb* [see: goldenrod]

Dyflex-G tablets ℞ *antiasthmatic; bronchodilator; expectorant* [dyphylline; guaifenesin] 200•200 mg

dyflos BAN *antiglaucoma agent; irreversible cholinesterase inhibitor miotic* [also: isoflurophate]

Dy-G oral liquid ℞ *antiasthmatic; bronchodilator; expectorant* [dyphylline; guaifenesin] 100•100 mg/5 mL

dylate [see: clonitrate]

Dyline-GG tablets, oral liquid (discontinued 2005) ℞ *antiasthmatic; bronchodilator; expectorant* [dyphylline; guaifenesin] 200•200 mg; 300•300 mg/15 mL

Dylix elixir ℞ *antiasthmatic; bronchodilator* [dyphylline] 100 mg/15 mL

dymanthine HCl USAN *anthelmintic* [also: dimantine HCl]

Dymelor tablets ℞ *sulfonylurea antidiabetic* [acetohexamide] 250, 500 mg ☒ Demerol; Pamelor

Dymenate IV or IM injection ℞ *antinauseant; antiemetic; antivertigo; motion sickness preventative* [dimenhydrinate] 50 mg/mL

Dynabac enteric-coated delayed-release tablets ℞ *once-daily macrolide antibiotic for respiratory and dermatological infections* [dirithromycin] 250 mg

Dynacin capsules, film-coated tablets ℞ *tetracycline antibiotic* [minocycline HCl] 50, 75, 100 mg

DynaCirc capsules ℞ *antihypertensive; dihydropyridine calcium channel blocker* [isradipine] 2.5, 5 mg

DynaCirc CR controlled-release tablets ℞ *once-daily antihypertensive; dihydropyridine calcium channel blocker* [isradipine] 5, 10 mg

dynacoryl [see: nikethamide]

Dynafed; Dynafed Plus tablets (discontinued 2002) OTC *decongestant; analgesic; antipyretic* [pseudoephedrine HCl; acetaminophen] 30•500 mg

Dynafed Asthma Relief tablets OTC *bronchodilator; decongestant; expectorant* [ephedrine HCl; guaifenesin] 25•200 mg

Dynafed E.X. tablets OTC *analgesic; antipyretic* [acetaminophen] 500 mg

Dynafed Jr., Children's chewable tablets OTC *analgesic; antipyretic* [acetaminophen] 80 mg

Dyna-Hex Skin Cleanser; Dyna-Hex 2 Skin Cleanser topical liquid OTC *broad-spectrum antimicrobial; germicidal* [chlorhexidine gluconate; alcohol 4%] 4%; 2%

dynamine *investigational (orphan) agent for Lambert-Eaton myasthenic syndrome and Charcot-Marie-Tooth disease*

Dynapen capsules, powder for oral suspension (discontinued 2002) R̆ *penicillinase-resistant penicillin antibiotic* [dicloxacillin sodium] 125, 250, 500 mg; 62.5 mg/5 mL

dynarsan [see: acetarsone]

Dynepo (approved in Europe) R̆ *investigational (NDA filed) gene therapy for anemia of renal failure* [erythropoietin, gene-activated]

Dynex sustained-release caplets R̆ *decongestant; expectorant* [pseudoephedrine HCl; guaifenesin] 90•1200 mg

dyphylline USP *antiasthmatic; bronchodilator* [also: diprophylline] 200, 400 mg oral

dyphylline & guaifenesin *antiasthmatic; bronchodilator; expectorant* 200•200 mg oral

Dyphylline-GG elixir OTC *antiasthmatic; bronchodilator; expectorant* [dyphylline; guaifenesin] 100•100 mg/15 mL

Dyprotex pads OTC *topical diaper rash treatment* [zinc oxide; dimethicone] 40%•2.5%

Dyrenium capsules R̆ *antihypertensive; potassium-sparing diuretic* [triamterene] 50, 100 mg ② Pyridium

Dyrexan-OD sustained-release capsules (discontinued 2001) R̆ *anorexiant; CNS stimulant* [phendimetrazine tartrate] 105 mg

Dysport R̆ *investigational (orphan) agent for blepharospasm and strabismus of dystonia, pediatric cerebral palsy, and cervical dystonia* [botulinum toxin, type A]

dysprosium *element (Dy)*

Dytan chewable tablets, oral suspension R̆ *antihistamine* [diphenhydramine tannate] 25 mg; 25 mg/5 mL

Dytan-CS tablets R̆ *decongestant; antihistamine; antitussive* [phenylephrine tannate; diphenhydramine tannate; carbetapentane tannate] 10•25•30 mg

Dytan-D chewable tablets R̆ *decongestant; antihistamine* [phenylephrine tannate; diphenhydramine tannate] 10•25 mg

DZAPO (daunorubicin, azacitidine, ara-C, prednisone, Oncovin) *chemotherapy protocol*

E₂C (estradiol cypionate) [q.v.]

E5 monoclonal antibodies (MAb) [now: edobacomab]

EACA (epsilon-aminocaproic acid) [see: aminocaproic acid]

EAP (etoposide, Adriamycin, Platinol) *chemotherapy protocol for gastric and small bowel cancer*

ear, lion's *medicinal herb* [see: motherwort]

Ear-Dry ear drops OTC *antibacterial; antifungal* [boric acid] 2.75%

Ear-Eze ear drops R̆ *topical corticosteroidal anti-inflammatory; antibiotic* [hydrocortisone; neomycin sulfate; polymyxin B sulfate] 1%•5 mg•10 000 U per mL

EarSol ear drops (discontinued 2003) OTC *antiseptic* [alcohol] 44%

EarSol-HC ear drops OTC *topical corticosteroidal anti-inflammatory; antiseptic* [hydrocortisone; alcohol 44%] 1%

earthnut oil [see: peanut oil]

Easprin delayed-release enteric-coated tablets ℞ *analgesic; antipyretic; anti-inflammatory; antirheumatic* [aspirin] 975 mg

Easter giant *medicinal herb* [see: bistort]

Easy A1C fingerstick test kit for home use *in vitro diagnostic aid for glycosylated hemoglobin levels*

EasyInjector (trademarked device) *self-injector*

E-Base enteric-coated delayed-release caplets and tablets (discontinued 2005) ℞ *macrolide antibiotic* [erythromycin] 333, 500 mg

ebastine USAN, INN *antihistamine*

ebiratide INN

ebrotidine INN

ebselen INN

EC (etoposide, carboplatin) *chemotherapy protocol for lung cancer*

ecadotril USAN, INN *antihypertensive*

ecalcidene USAN *antipsoriatic*

ecamsule USAN *UVA sunscreen*

ecarazine [see: todralazine]

EC-ASA (enteric-coated aspirin) [see: aspirin]

ecastolol INN

Ecee Plus tablets OTC *vitamin/mineral supplement* [vitamins C and E; zinc sulfate; magnesium sulfate] 100•165•80•70 mg

echinacea (Echinacea angustifolia; E. purpurea; E. pallida) root *medicinal herb for anemia, blood diseases, blood poisoning, boils, dizziness, immune system stimulation, lymph disorders, promoting wound healing, prostate disorders, skin infections, and snake bites*

echinocandins *a class of antifungals* [also: glucan synthesis inhibitors]

Echinopanax horridum *medicinal herb* [see: devil's club]

ECHO (etoposide, cyclophosphamide, hydroxydaunomycin, Oncovin) *chemotherapy protocol*

EchoGen emulsion ℞ *investigational (NDA filed) ultrasound contrast agent for stress cardiography and transrectal prostate imaging* [perflenapent; perflisopent] 85%•15%

echothiophate iodide USP *antiglaucoma agent; irreversible cholinesterase inhibitor miotic* [also: ecothiopate iodide]

Echovist Ⓐ intrauterine suspension ℞ *ultrasound contrast medium for gynecological imaging* [galactose]

ecipramidil INN

eclanamine INN *antidepressant* [also: eclanamine maleate]

eclanamine maleate USAN *antidepressant* [also: eclanamine]

eclazolast USAN, INN *antiallergic; mediator release inhibitor*

EC-Naprosyn enteric-coated delayed-release tablets ℞ *antiarthritic; nonsteroidal anti-inflammatory drug (NSAID)* [naproxen] 375, 500 mg

ecogramostim BAN

ecomustine INN

econazole USAN, INN, BAN *topical antifungal*

econazole nitrate USAN, USP, BAN *topical antifungal* 1% topical

Econo B & C caplets OTC *vitamin supplement* [multiple B vitamins; vitamin C] ±•300 mg

Econopred; Econopred Plus Drop-Tainers (eye drop suspension) ℞ *topical ophthalmic corticosteroidal anti-inflammatory* [prednisolone acetate] 0.125%; 1%

ecopipam HCl USAN *selective dopamine receptor antagonist for addiction*

ecostigmine iodide [see: echothiophate iodide]

ecothiopate iodide INN, BAN *antiglaucoma agent; irreversible cholinesterase inhibitor miotic* [also: echothiophate iodide]

Ecotrin enteric-coated tablets, enteric-coated caplets OTC *analgesic; antipy-*

retic; anti-inflammatory; antiarthritic [aspirin] 325, 500 mg ℞ Edecrin

Ecotrin Adult Low Strength enteric-coated tablets OTC *analgesic; antipyretic; anti-inflammatory; antiarthritic* [aspirin] 81 mg

ecraprost USAN *treatment of peripheral occlusive disease*

ecteinascidin *investigational (Phase III) tetrahydroisoquinoline alkaloid for sarcoma*

ectylurea BAN

eculizumab *investigational (orphan) agent for idiopathic membranous glomerular nephropathy and paroxysmal nocturnal hemoglobinuria*

Ed A-Hist sustained-release tablets, oral liquid ℞ *decongestant; antihistamine* [phenylephrine HCl; chlorpheniramine maleate] 20•8 mg; 10•4 mg/5 mL

ED Tuss HC syrup ℞ *narcotic antitussive; decongestant; antihistamine* [hydrocodone bitartrate; phenylephrine HCl; chlorpheniramine maleate] 2.5•10•4 mg/5 mL

edamine [see: ethylenediamine]

EDAP (etoposide, dexamethasone, ara-C, Platinol) *chemotherapy protocol*

edathamil [now: edetate calcium disodium]

edathamil calcium disodium [now: edetate calcium disodium]

edathamil disodium [now: edetate disodium]

edatrexate USAN, INN *antineoplastic; methotrexate analogue*

Ed-Chlor-Tan caplets ℞ *antihistamine* [chlorpheniramine tannate] 8 mg

Edecrin tablets ℞ *antihypertensive; loop diuretic* [ethacrynic acid] 25, 50 mg ℞ Ecotrin; Ethaquin

Edecrin Sodium powder for IV injection ℞ *antihypertensive; loop diuretic* [ethacrynate sodium] 50 mg

edelfosine INN

edetate calcium disodium USAN, USP *heavy metal chelating agent for acute or chronic lead poisoning and lead encephalopathy* [also: sodium calcium edetate; sodium calciumedetate; calcium disodium edetate]

edetate dipotassium USAN *chelating agent*

edetate disodium USP *chelating agent; preservative; antioxidant* [also: disodium edetate] 150 mg/mL injection

edetate magnesium disodium *chelating agent for atherosclerosis*

edetate sodium USAN *chelating agent*

edetate trisodium USAN *chelating agent*

edetic acid NF, INN, BAN *chelating agent*

edetol USAN, INN *alkalizing agent*

Edex injection, pre-filled syringes ℞ *vasodilator for erectile dysfunction* [alprostadil] 10, 20, 40 μg/mL

Ed-Flex capsules ℞ *antihistamine; analgesic* [phenyltoloxamine citrate; acetaminophen; salicylamide] 20•300•200 mg

edifolone INN *antiarrhythmic* [also: edifolone acetate]

edifolone acetate USAN *antiarrhythmic* [also: edifolone]

Ed-In-Sol drops (discontinued 2005) OTC *hematinic; iron supplement* [ferrous sulfate (source of iron)] 75 mg/0.6 mL (15 mg/0.6 mL)

edisilate INN *combining name for radicals or groups* [also: edisylate]

edisylate USAN, BAN *combining name for radicals or groups* [also: edisilate]

edithamil [see: edetate ...]

edobacomab USAN *antiendotoxin monoclonal antibody for gram-negative sepsis; clinical trials discontinued 1997*

edodekin alfa USAN *antiasthmatic; investigational (Phase I/II) immunomodulator for AIDS-related Kaposi sarcoma; investigational (orphan) for renal cell carcinoma* [previously: interleukin 12 (IL-12)]

edogestrone INN, BAN

edonentan USAN *endothelin A (ETA) inhibitor for heart failure*

edoxudine USAN, INN *antiviral*

edrecolomab USAN *monoclonal antibody; antineoplastic adjuvant*

edrofuradene [see: nifurdazil]

edrophone chloride [see: edrophonium chloride]

edrophonium chloride USP, INN, BAN *cholinergic/anticholinesterase muscle stimulant; antidote to curare; myasthenia gravis diagnostic aid*

Ed-Spaz tablets ℞ *GI/GU antispasmodic; antiparkinsonian; anticholinergic "drying agent" for allergic rhinitis and hyperhidrosis* [hyoscyamine sulfate] 0.125 mg

EDTA (ethylenediaminetetraacetic acid) [see: edetate disodium]

EDTA calcium [see: edetate calcium disodium]

ED-TLC oral liquid ℞ *narcotic antitussive; decongestant; antihistamine* [hydrocodone bitartrate; phenylephrine HCl; chlorpheniramine maleate] 3.33•10•4 mg/10 mL

E.E.S. granules for oral suspension ℞ *macrolide antibiotic* [erythromycin ethylsuccinate] 200 mg/5 mL

EES (erythromycin ethylsuccinate) [q.v.]

E.E.S. 200 oral suspension ℞ *macrolide antibiotic* [erythromycin ethylsuccinate] 200 mg/5 mL

E.E.S. 400 film-coated tablets, oral suspension ℞ *macrolide antibiotic* [erythromycin ethylsuccinate] 400 mg; 400 mg/5 mL

efalizumab *recombinant humanized monoclonal antibody (rhuMAb) to leukocyte function–associated antigen-1 (LFA-1); immunosuppressant for moderate to severe plaque psoriasis*

efaproxiral *investigational (NDA filed) radiosensitizer for breast, lung, and brain tumors*

Efaproxyn ℞ *investigational (NDA filed) radiosensitizer for breast, lung, and brain tumors* [efaproxiral]

efaroxan INN, BAN

efavirenz *antiviral non-nucleoside reverse transcriptase inhibitor (NNRTI) for HIV infection*

efegatran sulfate USAN *antithrombotic*

efetozole INN

effector molecules *a class of cytotoxic or radioactive drugs delivered to specific tissue—usually a cancerous tumor—by targeted monoclonal antibody vehicles (T-MAVs; q.v.)*

Effer-K effervescent tablets ℞ *potassium supplement* [potassium bicarbonate; potassium citrate] 25 mEq K

Effervescent Potassium effervescent tablets ℞ *potassium supplement* [potassium bicarbonate; potassium citrate] 25 mEq K

Effervescent Potassium Chloride effervescent tablets for oral solution ℞ *potassium supplement* [potassium chloride] 25 mEq K

Effexor tablets ℞ *antidepressant for major depression* [venlafaxine HCl] 25, 37.5, 50, 75, 100 mg

Effexor XR extended-release capsules ℞ *antidepressant for major depression; anxiolytic for generalized anxiety disorder (GAD) and social anxiety disorder (SAD)* [venlafaxine HCl] 37.5, 75, 150 mg

Efidac 24 dual-release tablets OTC *antihistamine* [chlorpheniramine maleate] 16 mg (4 mg immediate release, 12 mg extended release)

Efidac 24 Pseudoephedrine dual-release tablets OTC *nasal decongestant* [pseudoephedrine HCl] 240 mg (60 mg immediate release, 180 mg extended release)

efletirizine *investigational second-generation peripherally selective piperazine antihistamine*

Eflone eye drop suspension ℞ *topical ophthalmic corticosteroidal anti-inflammatory* [fluorometholone acetate] 0.1%

eflornithine INN, BAN *antineoplastic; antiprotozoal; topical hair growth inhibitor* [also: eflornithine HCl]

eflornithine HCl USAN *antiprotozoal for Trypanosoma brucei gambiense (sleeping sickness) infection (orphan); topical hair growth inhibitor; investigational (Phase III) for bladder cancer; investigational (orphan) for AIDS-*

related Pneumocystis carinii *pneumonia (PCP)* [also: eflornithine]

efloxate INN

eflumast INN

Efodine ointment OTC *broad-spectrum antimicrobial* [povidone-iodine] 1%

eformoterol fumarate BAN *bronchodilator* [also: formoterol; formoterol fumarate]

EFP (etoposide, fluorouracil, Platinol) *chemotherapy protocol for gastric and small bowel cancer*

efrotomycin USAN, INN, BAN *veterinary growth stimulant*

Efudex cream, topical solution ℞ *antineoplastic for actinic keratoses and basal cell carcinomas* [fluorouracil] 5%; 2%, 5%

egtazic acid USAN, INN *pharmaceutic aid*

Egyptian privet *medicinal herb* [see: henna (*Lawsonia*)]

Egyptian thorn *medicinal herb* [see: acacia]

EHDP (ethane hydroxydiphosphonate) [see: etidronate disodium]

Ehrlich 594 [see: acetarsone]

Ehrlich 606 [see: arsphenamine]

eicosapentaenoic acid (EPA) *natural omega-3 fatty acid used to prevent a wide range of degenerative diseases; precursor to the anti-inflammatory and anticoagulant series 3 prostaglandins; effective in treating depression and other mental disorders* [also: icosapent]

8 in 1 (methylprednisolone, vincristine, lomustine, procarbazine, hydroxyurea, cisplatin, cytarabine, cyclophosphamide) *chemotherapy protocol*

8 in 1 (methylprednisolone, vincristine, lomustine, procarbazine, hydroxyurea, cisplatin, cytarabine, dacarbazine) *chemotherapy protocol for pediatric brain tumors*

8-MOP capsules ℞ *systemic psoralens for psoriasis, repigmentation of idiopathic vitiligo, and cutaneous T-cell lymphoma (CTCL); used to increase tolerance to sunlight and enhance pigmentation* [methoxsalen] 10 mg

einsteinium *element (Es)*

eIPV (enhanced, inactivated polio vaccine) [see: poliovirus vaccine, enhanced inactivated]

elacridar HCl USAN *chemotherapy potentiator; multi-drug-resistance inhibitor*

ELA-Max cream (name changed to L-M-X4 in 2003) OTC *local anesthetic* [lidocaine] 4%

elantrine USAN, INN *anticholinergic*

elanzepine INN

elastofilcon A USAN *hydrophilic contact lens material*

Elavil film-coated tablets (discontinued 2004) ℞ *tricyclic antidepressant* [amitriptyline HCl] 10, 25, 50, 75, 100, 150 mg ☒ Aldoril; Elidel; Eldepryl; Enovil; Equanil; Mellaril

Elavil IM injection (discontinued 2003) ℞ *tricyclic antidepressant* [amitriptyline HCl] 10 mg/mL ☒ Aldoril; Elidel; Eldepryl; Enovil; Equanil; Mellaril

elbanizine INN

elcatonin INN, JAN *investigational (orphan) intrathecal treatment of intractable pain*

eldacimibe USAN *antihyperlipidemic; antiatherosclerotic; AcylCoA transferase (ACAT) inhibitor*

Eldepryl capsules ℞ *dopaminergic antiparkinsonian (orphan)* [selegiline HCl] 5 mg ☒ Aldoril; Elavil; Enovil; Equanil; Mellaril

elder flower; elderberry (*Sambucus canadensis; S. ebulus; S. nigra; S. racemosa*) *berries and flowers medicinal herb for allergies, asthma, bronchitis, colds, constipation, edema, fever, hay fever, pneumonia, and sinus congestion; also used topically as an astringent*

Eldercaps capsules ℞ *vitamin/mineral supplement* [multiple vitamins & minerals; folic acid] ± • 1 mg

Eldertonic oral liquid OTC *vitamin/mineral supplement* [multiple B vitamins & minerals; alcohol 13.5%]

eldexomer INN

Eldisine ℞ *investigational (NDA filed) synthetic vinca alkaloid antineoplastic* *for leukemia, melanoma, breast and lung cancers* [vindesine sulfate]

Eldopaque; Eldopaque-Forte cream OTC *hyperpigmentation bleaching agent; sunscreen* [hydroquinone in a sunblock base] 2%; 4%

Eldoquin cream (discontinued 2003) OTC *hyperpigmentation bleaching agent* [hydroquinone] 2%

Eldoquin-Forte cream OTC *hyperpigmentation bleaching agent* [hydroquinone] 4%

elecampane (Inula helenium) root *medicinal herb for chronic bronchitis and cough*

electrocortin [see: aldosterone]

eledoisin INN

Elestat eye drops ℞ *selective H₁ antagonist; antihistamine; mast cell stabilizer* [epinastine HCl]

eletriptan hydrobromide USAN *vascular serotonin 5-HT₁ᵦ/₁ᴅ/₁ꜰ-receptor agonist for the acute treatment of migraine* (base=82.5%)

eleuthero (Eleutherococcus senticosus) root *medicinal herb for age spots, blood diseases, depression, hemorrhage, immune system stimulation, increasing endurance and longevity, normalizing blood pressure, platelet aggregation inhibition, sexual stimulation, and stress* [previously called: Siberian ginseng]

ELF (etoposide, leucovorin [rescue], fluorouracil) *chemotherapy protocol for gastric cancer*

elfazepam USAN, INN *veterinary appetite stimulant*

elfdock; elfwort *medicinal herb* [see: elecampane]

elgodipine INN

Elidel cream ℞ *nonsteroidal anti-inflammatory for atopic dermatitis* [pimecrolimus] 1% ② Elavil

Eligard sustained-release subcu injection ℞ *antihormonal antineoplastic for advanced prostate cancer* [leuprolide acetate] 7.5 mg (1-month depot), 22.5 mg (3-month depot), 30 mg (4-month depot), 45 mg (6-month depot)

Elimite cream ℞ *pediculicide for lice; scabicide* [permethrin] 5%

eliprodil INN *investigational treatment for ischemic stroke*

Elitek powder for IV infusion ℞ *antimetabolite antineoplastic for leukemia, lymphoma, and solid tumor malignancies* [rasburicase] 1.5 mg/vial

Elixomin elixir ℞ *antiasthmatic; bronchodilator* [theophylline] 80 mg/15 mL

Elixophyllin capsules, elixir ℞ *antiasthmatic; bronchodilator* [theophylline] 100, 200 mg; 80 mg/15 mL

Elixophyllin GG oral liquid ℞ *antiasthmatic; bronchodilator; expectorant* [theophylline; guaifenesin] 100•100 mg/15 mL

Elixophyllin-KI elixir ℞ *antiasthmatic; bronchodilator; expectorant* [theophylline; potassium iodide] 80•130 mg/ 15 mL

ElixSure Congestion; ElixSure Children's Congestion syrup OTC *decongestant* [pseudoephedrine HCl] 15 mg/5 mL

ElixSure Cough; ElixSure Children's Cough syrup OTC *antitussive* [dextromethorphan hydrobromide] 7.5 mg/ 5 mL

ElixSure Fever/Pain syrup OTC *analgesic; antipyretic* [acetaminophen] 160 mg/5 mL

ElixSure IB oral suspension OTC *analgesic; antipyretic* [ibuprofen] 100 mg/ 5 mL

ellagic acid INN

Ellence IV infusion ℞ *anthracycline antibiotic antineoplastic for breast cancer (orphan)* [epirubicin HCl] 2 mg/mL

Elliott's B solution *investigational (orphan) intrathecal chemotherapy diluent*

elliptinium acetate INN, BAN

elm, American; Indian elm; moose elm; red elm; rock elm; sweet elm; winged elm *medicinal herb* [see: slippery elm]

Elmiron capsules ℞ *urinary tract anti-inflammatory and analgesic for interstitial cystitis (orphan)* [pentosan polysulfate sodium] 100 mg

elmustine INN

elnadipine INN

Elocom Ⓒ ointment, cream, lotion ℞ *topical corticosteroidal anti-inflammatory* [mometasone furoate] 0.1%

Elocon ointment, cream, lotion ℞ *topical corticosteroidal anti-inflammatory* [mometasone furoate] 0.1%

Elon Barrier Protectant liquid OTC *skin protectant* [paraffin based]

Elon Dual Defense Antifungal Formula topical liquid OTC *antifungal* [undecylenic acid] 25%

Eloxatin IV infusion, powder for IV infusion ℞ *alkylating antineoplastic for metastatic ovarian and colorectal cancers (orphan); investigational (Phase III) for pancreatic cancer* [oxaliplatin] 50, 100 mg

elsamitrucin USAN, INN *antineoplastic*

Elspar powder for IV or IM injection ℞ *antineoplastic adjunct for acute lymphocytic leukemia* [asparaginase] 10 000 IU

eltanolone INN *investigational IV anesthetic*

eltenac INN

eltoprazine INN

Eltroxin tablets (discontinued 2003) ℞ *synthetic thyroid hormone (T_4 fraction only)* [levothyroxine sodium] 50, 75, 100, 125, 150, 200, 300 µg

elucaine USAN, INN *gastric anticholinergic*

Elymus repens medicinal herb [see: couch grass]

elziverine INN

EMA (estramustine L-alanine) [q.v.]

EMA 86 (etoposide, mitoxantrone, ara-C) *chemotherapy protocol for acute myelocytic leukemia (AML)*

EMACO (etoposide, methotrexate, actinomycin D, cyclophosphamide, Oncovin) *chemotherapy protocol*

Emadine eye drops ℞ *topical antihistamine for allergic conjunctivitis* [emedastine difumarate] 0.05%

Embeline ointment, gel, cream, scalp application ℞ *corticosteroidal anti-inflammatory* [clobetasol propionate] 0.05%

embinal [see: barbital sodium]

embonate INN, BAN *combining name for radicals or groups* [also: pamoate]

embramine INN, BAN

embramine HCl [see: embramine]

Embrex 600 chewable tablets ℞ *vitamin/mineral/calcium/iron supplement* [multiple vitamins & minerals; calcium; iron; folic acid] ≚•240•90•1 mg

embutramide USAN, INN, BAN *veterinary anesthetic; veterinary euthanasia*

Emcyt capsules ℞ *nitrogen mustard-type alkylating antineoplastic for metastatic or progressive prostatic carcinoma* [estramustine phosphate sodium] 140 mg

emedastine INN *ophthalmic antihistamine* [also: emedastine difumarate]

emedastine difumarate USAN, JAN *ophthalmic antihistamine* [also: emedastine]

Emend capsules ℞ *antiemetic for chemotherapy* [aprepitant] 80, 125 mg

emepronium bromide INN, BAN

emepronium carrageenate BAN

Emergent-Ez Kit (discontinued 2002) *carry-kit for medical personnel* [multiple drugs and devices for emergencies]

Emersal topical emulsion (discontinued 2004) ℞ *antipsoriatic; antiseborrheic* [ammoniated mercury; salicylic acid] 5%•2.5%

emetic herb; emetic weed *medicinal herb* [see: lobelia]

emetics *a class of agents that induce vomiting*

emetine BAN *antiamebic* [also: emetine HCl] ⓘ Emetrol

emetine bismuth iodide [see: emetine HCl]

emetine HCl USP *amebicide* [also: emetine]

Emetrol oral solution OTC *antiemetic for nausea associated with influenza, morning sickness, motion sickness, inhalation anesthesia, or food and drink indiscretions* [phosphorated carbohydrate solution (fructose, dextrose, and phosphoric acid)] 1.87 g•1.87 g•21.5 mg ② emetine

EMF oral liquid oTc *protein supplement* [multiple amino acids] 15 g protein

Emgel gel ℞ *antibiotic for acne* [erythromycin; alcohol 77%] 2%

emiglitate INN, BAN

emilium tosilate INN *antiarrhythmic* [also: emilium tosylate]

emilium tosylate USAN *antiarrhythmic* [also: emilium tosilate]

Eminase powder for IV injection (discontinued 2003) ℞ *thrombolytic enzyme for acute myocardial infarction* [anistreplase] 30 U/vial

emitefur USAN *antineoplastic for stomach, colorectal, breast, pancreatic, and non–small cell lung cancers (NSCLC)*

Emko; Emko Pre-Fil vaginal foam (discontinued 2002) oTc *spermicidal contraceptive* [nonoxynol 9] 8%

EMLA (eutectic mixture of local anesthetics) cream, adhesive disc ℞ *local anesthetic* [lidocaine; prilocaine] 2.5%•2.5%

emmenagogues *a class of agents that induce or increase menstruation*

Emollia lotion oTc *moisturizer; emollient*

emollient laxatives *a subclass of laxatives that work by retarding colonic absorption of fecal water to soften the stool and ease its movement through the intestines* [see also: laxatives]

emollients *a class of dermatological agents that soften and soothe the skin*

emonapride INN

emopamil INN

emorfazone INN

Empirin tablets oTc *analgesic; antipyretic; anti-inflammatory; antirheumatic* [aspirin] 325 mg

Empirin with Codeine No. 3 & No. 4 tablets ℞ *narcotic antitussive; analgesic; sometimes abused as a street drug* [codeine phosphate; aspirin] 30•325 mg; 60•325 mg

Emselex (European name for the U.S. product **Enablex**)

emtricitabine USAN *antiviral; nucleoside analogue reverse transcriptase*

inhibitor for HIV-1 infection; synthetic cytosine analogue

Emtriva capsules ℞ *antiviral for HIV-1 infection* [emtricitabine] 200 mg

emtryl [see: dimetridazole]

emu oil *natural remedy for arthritis pain, hair loss prevention, and chronic skin disorders*

emulsifying wax [see: wax, emulsifying]

Emulsoil oral emulsion oTc *stimulant laxative* [castor oil] 95%

E-Mycin enteric-coated tablets (discontinued 2005) ℞ *macrolide antibiotic* [erythromycin] 250, 333 mg

emylcamate INN, BAN

Enable ℞ *investigational (NDA filed) anti-inflammatory for rheumatoid arthritis and osteoarthritis* [tenidap]

Enablex extended-release tablets ℞ *selective muscarinic receptor antagonist for urinary frequency, urgency, and incontinence* [darifenacin hydrobromide] 7.5, 15 mg

enadoline INN *analgesic* [also: enadoline HCl]

enadoline HCl USAN *analgesic; investigational (orphan) for severe head injury* [also: enadoline]

enalapril INN, BAN *antihypertensive; angiotensin-converting enzyme (ACE) inhibitor* [also: enalapril maleate]

enalapril maleate USAN, USP *antihypertensive; angiotensin-converting enzyme (ACE) inhibitor; treatment for CHF* [also: enalapril] 2.5, 5, 10, 20 mg oral

enalapril maleate & hydrochlorothiazide *antihypertensive; angiotensin-converting enzyme (ACE) inhibitor; diuretic* 5•12.5, 10•25 mg oral

enalaprilat USAN, USP, INN, BAN *antihypertensive; angiotensin-converting enzyme (ACE) inhibitor* 1.25 mg/mL injection

enalkiren USAN, INN *antihypertensive; renin inhibitor*

enallynymal sodium [see: methohexital sodium]

enantate INN *combining name for radicals or groups* [also: enanthate]

[handwritten: Emsam]

enanthate USAN, USP, BAN *combining name for radicals or groups* [also: enantate]

enantiomer [def.] *One of a pair of chemical compounds having the same molecular formula, but with the atoms arranged in mirror image. Subdivided into (+) (formerly d- or dextro-) and (–) (formerly l- or levo-). [see also: isomer; racemic]*

Enbrel powder for subcu injection, pre-filled syringes ℞ *soluble tumor necrosis factor receptor (sTNFR) inhibitor for rheumatoid arthritis, juvenile rheumatoid arthritis (orphan), psoriatic arthritis, and ankylosing spondylitis; investigational (NDA filed) for congestive heart failure; investigational (orphan) for Wegener granulomatosis* [etanercept] 25 mg/vial; 50 mg 🄑 Incel

enbucrilate INN, BAN

encainide INN, BAN *antiarrhythmic* [also: encainide HCl]

encainide HCl USAN *antiarrhythmic* [also: encainide]

Encare vaginal suppositories OTC *spermicidal contraceptive* [nonoxynol 9] 2.27%

enciprazine INN, BAN *minor tranquilizer* [also: enciprazine HCl]

enciprazine HCl USAN *minor tranquilizer* [also: enciprazine]

enclomifene INN [also: enclomiphene]

enclomiphene USAN [also: enclomifene]

encyprate USAN, INN *antidepressant*

End Lice topical liquid (discontinued 2003) OTC *pediculicide for lice* [pyrethrins; piperonyl butoxide] 0.3%•3%

Endafed sustained-release capsules (discontinued 2002) ℞ *decongestant; antihistamine* [pseudoephedrine HCl; brompheniramine maleate] 120•12 mg

Endagen-HD oral liquid ℞ *narcotic antitussive; decongestant; antihistamine* [hydrocodone bitartrate; phenylephrine HCl; chlorpheniramine maleate] 3.33•10•4 mg/10 mL

Endal Expectorant syrup ℞ *narcotic antitussive; decongestant; expectorant* [codeine phosphate; phenylephrine HCl; guaifenesin; alcohol 5%] 12.5•4•125 mg/5 mL

Endal Nasal Decongestant timed-release caplets ℞ *decongestant; expectorant* [phenylephrine HCl; guaifenesin] 20•300 mg 🄑 Intal

Endal-HD syrup ℞ *narcotic antitussive; decongestant; antihistamine* [hydrocodone bitartrate; phenylephrine HCl; diphenhydramine HCl] 2•7.5•12.5 mg/5 mL

Endal-HD Plus syrup ℞ *narcotic antitussive; decongestant; antihistamine* [hydrocodone bitartrate; phenylephrine HCl; chlorpheniramine maleate] 3.5•7.5•2.5 mg/5 mL

endiemal [see: metharbital]

endive *medicinal herb* [see: chicory]

endive, white; wild endive *medicinal herb* [see: dandelion]

endixaprine INN

endobenzyline bromide

endocaine [see: pyrrocaine]

Endocet tablets ℞ *narcotic analgesic* [oxycodone HCl; acetaminophen] 5•325, 7.5•325, 7.5•500, 10•325, 10•650 mg

Endocodone tablets (discontinued 2005) ℞ *narcotic analgesic* [oxycodone HCl] 5 mg

endolate [see: meperidine HCl]

endomide INN

endomycin

Endospray ⒼⒶⒷ metered-dose spray OTC *topical anesthetic for oropharyngeal and endotracheal areas* [benzocaine; tetracaine] 18•2 mg/spray

endothelin-1 receptor antagonists *a class of vasodilator antihypertensives that block the action of endothelin-1 (ET-1), a vascular vasoconstrictor more potent than angiotensin II*

endothelin-A (EtA; ETA; ET$_A$) receptor antagonists *a class of antineoplastic agents that mediate the action of endothelin-1 (ET-1) to retard the proliferation of cancerous cells*

endralazine INN, BAN *antihypertensive* [also: endralazine mesylate]

endralazine mesylate USAN *antihypertensive* [also: endralazine]

Endrate IV infusion ℞ *chelating agent for hypercalcemia and ventricular arrhythmias due to digitalis toxicity* [edetate disodium] 150 mg/mL

endrisone INN *topical ophthalmic anti-inflammatory* [also: endrysone]

endrysone USAN *topical ophthalmic anti-inflammatory* [also: endrisone]

Enduret (trademarked dosage form) *prolonged-action tablet*

Enduron tablets ℞ *diuretic; antihypertensive* [methyclothiazide] 5 mg ⑨ Imuran; Inderal

Enduronyl; Enduronyl Forte tablets (discontinued 2003) ℞ *antihypertensive* [methyclothiazide; deserpidine] 5•0.25 mg; 5•0.5 mg ⑨ Inderal

Enecat CT concentrated rectal suspension ℞ *radiopaque contrast medium for gastrointestinal imaging* [barium sulfate] 5%

enefexine INN

Enerjets lozenges OTC *CNS stimulant; analeptic* [caffeine] 75 mg

enestebol INN

EnfaCare [see: Enfamil EnfaCare]

Enfalac AR ⒸⒶⓃ powder OTC *total or supplementary infant feeding; thickened formula* [cow's milk–based formula]

Enfalac Iron Fortified ⒸⒶⓃ oral liquid, powder for oral liquid OTC *total or supplementary infant feeding* [milk-based formula]

Enfalac ProSobee Soy ⒸⒶⓃ oral liquid, powder for oral liquid OTC *hypoallergenic infant food* [soy protein formula]

Enfalac Regular ⒸⒶⓃ oral liquid, powder for oral liquid OTC *total or supplementary infant feeding* [milk-based formula]

Enfalyte ready-to-use oral liquid OTC *supplementary feeding to maintain hydration and electrolyte balance in infants with diarrhea or vomiting* 33.8 oz bottles

Enfamil oral liquid, powder for oral liquid OTC *total or supplementary infant feeding*

Enfamil EnfaCare oral liquid, powder for oral liquid OTC *enriched formula for premature infants* [milk-based formula] 3 oz bottles; 14 oz cans

Enfamil Human Milk Fortifier powder OTC *supplement to breast milk*

Enfamil LactoFree oral liquid, concentrate for oral liquid, powder for oral liquid OTC *hypoallergenic infant formula* [milk-based formula, lactose free] 946 mL; 384 mL; 397 g

Enfamil LIPIL with Iron Nursette bottles, ready-to-use oral liquid, concentrate for oral liquid, powder for oral liquid OTC *infant formula fortified with omega-3 fatty acids* 3, 6 oz. bottles; 32 oz. cans; 13 oz. cans; 12.9, 25.9 oz. cans

Enfamil Low Iron oral liquid (discontinued 2003) OTC *total or supplementary infant feeding*

Enfamil Next Step oral liquid, powder for oral liquid OTC *total or supplementary infant feeding*

Enfamil Premature Formula oral liquid OTC *total or supplementary infant feeding*

Enfamil with Iron oral liquid, powder for oral liquid OTC *total or supplementary infant feeding*

enfenamic acid INN

enflurane USAN, USP, INN, BAN *inhalation general anesthetic* 125, 250 mL

enfuvirtide *fusion inhibitor that prevents HIV from binding to T-cells, thus preventing viral entry into healthy cells*

Engerix-B adult IM injection, pediatric IM injection ℞ *active immunizing agent for hepatitis B and D* [hepatitis B virus vaccine, recombinant] 20 μg/mL, 10 μg/0.5 mL

English elm (*Ulmus campestris*) *medicinal herb* [see: slippery elm]

English hawthorn *medicinal herb* [see: hawthorn]

English ivy (*Hedera helix*) leaves *medicinal herb used as an antispasmodic and antiexanthematous agent*

English oak (*Quercus robur*) *medicinal herb* [see: white oak]

English valerian *medicinal herb* [see: valerian]

English walnut (*Juglans regia*) leaves *medicinal herb used as an astringent*

englitazone INN *antidiabetic* [also: englitazone sodium]

englitazone sodium USAN *antidiabetic* [also: englitazone]

enhanced, inactivated polio vaccine (eIPV) [see: poliovirus vaccine, enhanced inactivated]

Enhancer oral suspension ℞ *radiopaque contrast medium for gastrointestinal imaging* [barium sulfate] 98%

enhexymal [see: hexobarbital]

eniclobrate

enilconazole USAN, INN, BAN *antifungal*

enilospirone INN

eniluracil USAN *antineoplastic potentiator for fluorouracil; uracil reductase inhibitor*

enisoprost USAN, INN *antiulcerative; investigational (orphan) to reduce cyclosporine nephrotoxicity following organ transplants*

Enisyl tablets OTC *dietary amino acid supplement* [L-lysine] 334, 500 mg

Enjuvia film-coated tablets ℞ *hormone replacement therapy for severe postmenopausal vasomotor symptoms* [synthetic conjugated estrogens, B] 0.3, 0.45, 0.625, 1.25 mg

Enlive! ready-to-use oral liquid OTC *enteral nutritional therapy* 240 mL

Enlon IV or IM injection ℞ *myasthenia gravis treatment; antidote to curare overdose* [edrophonium chloride] 10 mg/mL

Enlon Plus IV or IM injection ℞ *muscle stimulant; neuromuscular blocker antagonist* [edrophonium chloride; atropine sulfate] 10•0.14 mg

enloplatin USAN, INN *antineoplastic*

enocitabine INN

enofelast USAN, INN *antiasthmatic*

enolicam INN *anti-inflammatory; antirheumatic* [also: enolicam sodium]

enolicam sodium USAN *anti-inflammatory; antirheumatic* [also: enolicam]

Enomine capsules (discontinued 2002) ℞ *decongestant; expectorant* [phenylpropanolamine HCl; phenylephrine HCl; guaifenesin] 45•5•200 mg

enoxacin USAN, INN, BAN, JAN *broadspectrum fluoroquinolone antibiotic*

enoxamast INN

enoxaparin BAN *a low molecular weight heparin–type anticoagulant and antithrombotic for the prevention of deep vein thrombosis (DVT), unstable angina, and myocardial infarction* [also: enoxaparin sodium]

enoxaparin sodium USAN, INN *a low molecular weight heparin–type anticoagulant and antithrombotic for the prevention of deep vein thrombosis (DVT), unstable angina, and myocardial infarction* [also: enoxaparin]

enoximone USAN, INN, BAN *cardiotonic*

enoxolone INN, BAN

enphenemal [see: mephobarbital]

enpiprazole INN, BAN

enpiroline INN *antimalarial* [also: enpiroline phosphate]

enpiroline phosphate USAN *antimalarial* [also: enpiroline]

enprazepine INN

Enpresse tablets (in packs of 28) ℞ *triphasic oral contraceptive; emergency postcoital contraceptive* [levonorgestrel; ethinyl estradiol]
Phase 1 (6 days): 50•30 µg;
Phase 2 (5 days): 75•40 µg;
Phase 3 (10 days): 125•30 µg

enprofen [now: furaprofen]

enprofylline USAN, INN *bronchodilator*

enpromate USAN, INN *antineoplastic*

enprostil USAN, INN, BAN *investigational antisecretory and antiulcerative for acute peptic ulcers*

enramycin INN

enrofloxacin USAN, INN, BAN *veterinary antibacterial*

Enseal (trademarked dosage form) *enteric-coated tablet*

Ensure oral liquid, powder for oral liquid OTC *enteral nutritional therapy* [lactose-free formula]

Ensure pudding OTC *enteral nutritional therapy* [milk-based formula] 150 g

Ensure Glucerna beverage, bars OTC *diabetic nutritional supplements/snacks*

Ensure High Calcium ready-to-use oral liquid OTC *enteral nutritional therapy for postmenopausal women*

Ensure High Protein ready-to-use oral liquid OTC *enteral nutritional therapy* [lactose-free formula] 237 mL

Ensure HN; Ensure with Fiber ready-to-use oral liquid OTC *enteral nutritional therapy* [lactose-free formula]

Ensure Plus; Ensure Plus HN oral liquid OTC *enteral nutritional therapy* [lactose-free formula]

EN-tab (trademarked dosage form) *enteric-coated tablet*

entacapone USAN *catechol-O-methyltransferase (COMT) inhibitor for Parkinson disease*

entecavir USAN *nucleoside reverse transcriptase inhibitor (NRTI); antiviral for chronic hepatitis B virus (HBV) infection*

enteramine [see: serotonin]

Entero Vu oral liquid, powder for oral liquid Ŗ *radiopaque contrast agent for small bowel imaging* [barium sulfate] 600 mL; 100 g packets

Entero Vu 24% oral liquid Ŗ *radiopaque contrast agent for small bowel imaging* [barium sulfate] 600 mL

Entero-Test; Entero-Test Pediatric string capsules for professional use *in vitro diagnostic aid for GI disorders*

Entertainer's Secret oral spray OTC *saliva substitute*

Entex capsules (discontinued 2001) Ŗ *decongestant; expectorant* [phenylephrine HCl; phenylpropanolamine HCl; guaifenesin] 5•45•200 mg

Entex oral liquid Ŗ *decongestant; expectorant* [phenylephrine HCl; guaifenesin] 7.5•100 mg/5 mL

Entex ER extended-release capsules Ŗ *decongestant; expectorant* [phenylephrine HCl; guaifenesin] 10•300 mg

Entex HC oral liquid Ŗ *narcotic antitussive; decongestant; expectorant* [hydrocodone bitartrate; phenylephrine HCl; guaifenesin] 5•7.5•100 mg/5 mL

Entex LA dual-release capsules Ŗ *decongestant; expectorant* [phenylephrine HCl (extended release); guaifenesin (immediate release)] 30•400 mg

Entex LA long-acting tablets Ŗ *decongestant; expectorant* [phenylephrine HCl; guaifenesin] 30•600 mg

Entex PSE dual-release capsules Ŗ *decongestant; expectorant* [pseudoephedrine HCl (extended release); guaifenesin (immediate release)] 120•400 mg

Entex PSE sustained-release tablets Ŗ *decongestant; expectorant* [pseudoephedrine HCl; guaifenesin] 120•600 mg

Entocort ⒸⒶⓃ oral capsules for ileal release, retention enema Ŗ *steroidal anti-inflammatory for Crohn disease* [budesonide] 3 mg; 2 mg

Entocort EC oral capsules for ileal release Ŗ *corticosteroidal anti-inflammatory for Crohn disease* [budesonide (micronized)] 3 mg

Entri-Pak (dosage form) *liquid-filled pouch*

Entrition 0.5 oral liquid OTC *enteral nutritional therapy* [lactose-free formula]

Entrition HN Entri-Pak (liquid-filled pouch) OTC *enteral nutritional therapy* [lactose-free formula]

Entrobar oral suspension Ŗ *radiopaque contrast medium for gastrointestinal imaging* [barium sulfate] 50% (500 mL)

EntroEase oral suspension Ŗ *radiopaque contrast medium for gastrointestinal imaging* [barium sulfate] 13%

EntroEase Dry powder for oral suspension Ŗ *radiopaque contrast medium for gastrointestinal imaging* [barium sulfate] 92%

Entrophen Ⓒ enteric-coated tablets, enteric-coated caplets OTC *analgesic; antipyretic; anti-inflammatory; antirheumatic* [aspirin] 325, 500, 650 mg; 325, 650 mg

entsufon INN *detergent* [also: entsufon sodium]

entsufon sodium USAN *detergent* [also: entsufon]

Entuss Expectorant oral liquid (discontinued 2002) ℞ *narcotic antitussive; expectorant* [hydrocodone bitartrate; potassium guaiacolsulfonate] 5•300 mg/5 mL

Entuss Expectorant tablets (discontinued 2002) ℞ *narcotic antitussive; expectorant* [hydrocodone bitartrate; guaifenesin] 5•300 mg

Entuss-D oral liquid (discontinued 2002) ℞ *narcotic antitussive; decongestant* [hydrocodone bitartrate; pseudoephedrine HCl] 5•30 mg/5 mL

Entuss-D tablets (discontinued 2002) ℞ *narcotic antitussive; decongestant; expectorant* [hydrocodone bitartrate; pseudoephedrine HCl; guaifenesin] 5•30•300 mg

Entuss-D Jr. pediatric oral liquid (discontinued 2002) ℞ *narcotic antitussive; decongestant; expectorant* [hydrocodone bitartrate; pseudoephedrine HCl; guaifenesin; alcohol 5%] 2.5•30•100 mg/5 mL

Enuclene eye drops OTC *cleaning, wetting and lubricating agent for artificial eyes* [tyloxapol] 0.25%

Enulose oral/rectal solution ℞ *synthetic disaccharide used to prevent and treat portal-systemic encephalopathy* [lactulose] 10 g/15 mL

enviomycin INN

enviradene USAN, INN *antiviral*

Enviro-Stress slow-release tablets OTC *vitamin/mineral supplement* [multiple vitamins & minerals; folic acid] ±•0.4 mg

enviroxime USAN, INN *antiviral*

enzacamene USAN *ultraviolet sunscreen*

Enzone cream ℞ *topical corticosteroidal anti-inflammatory; local anesthetic*

[hydrocortisone acetate; pramoxine HCl] 1%•1%

Enzymatic Cleaner for Extended Wear tablets OTC *enzymatic cleaner for soft contact lenses* [pork pancreatin]

Enzyme chewable tablets (discontinued 2002) OTC *digestive enzymes* [amylase; protease; lipase; cellulase] 30•6•2•25 mg

EP (etoposide, Platinol) *chemotherapy protocol for adenocarcinoma, lung cancer, and testicular cancer*

EPA capsules OTC *dietary supplement* [omega-3 fatty acids] 1000 mg

EPA (eicosapentaenoic acid) [q.v.; also: icosapent]

epalrestat INN *investigational treatment for diabetic neuropathy*

epanolol USAN, INN, BAN

Epaxal Berna Ⓒ suspension for IM injection OTC *active immunizing agent for hepatitis A* [hepatitis A vaccine, inactivated] 0.5 mL

eperezolid USAN *antibacterial*

eperisone INN

epervudine INN

ephedra (Ephedra spp.) plant *medicinal herb for asthma, blood cleansing, bronchitis, bursitis, chills, colds, edema, fever, flu, headache, kidney disorders, nasal congestion, and venereal disease*

ephedrine USP, BAN *sympathomimetic bronchodilator; nasal decongestant; vasopressor for shock* ⯐ Appedrine; aprindine

ephedrine HCl USP, BAN *sympathomimetic bronchodilator; nasal decongestant; vasopressor for shock* ⯐ Appedrine; aprindine

ephedrine sulfate USP *sympathomimetic bronchodilator; nasal decongestant; vasopressor for acute hypotensive shock* [also: ephedrine sulphate] 25 mg oral; 50 mg/mL injection ⯐ Appedrine; aprindine

ephedrine sulphate BAN *sympathomimetic bronchodilator; nasal decongestant* [also: ephedrine sulfate] ⯐ Appedrine; aprindine

ephedrine tannate *sympathomimetic bronchodilator; nasal decongestant* ② Appedrine; aprindine

Epi-C concentrated oral suspension ℞ *radiopaque contrast medium for gastrointestinal imaging* [barium sulfate] 150%

epicainide INN

epicillin USAN, INN, BAN *antibacterial*

epicriptine INN

epidermal growth factor, human *investigational (orphan) for acceleration of corneal regeneration and the healing of severe burns*

epidermal growth factor receptor inhibitors *a class of antineoplastics*

epiestriol INN [also: epioestriol]

Epifoam aerosol foam ℞ *topical corticosteroidal anti-inflammatory; local anesthetic* [hydrocortisone acetate; pramoxine] 1%•1%

Epifrin eye drops (discontinued 2004) ℞ *antiglaucoma agent* [epinephrine HCl] 0.5%, 1%, 2% ② epinephrine; EpiPen

Epiject ⒸⒶⓃ IV infusion ℞ *anticonvulsant* [valproate sodium] 100 mg/mL

epilin [see: dietifen]

E-Pilo-1; E-Pilo-2; E-Pilo-4; E-Pilo-6 eye drops (discontinued 2004) ℞ *antiglaucoma agent* [pilocarpine HCl; epinephrine bitartrate] 1%•1%; 2%•1%; 4%•1%; 6%•1%

Epilyt lotion concentrate OTC *moisturizer; emollient*

epimestrol USAN, INN, BAN *anterior pituitary activator*

Epinal eye drops ℞ *topical antiglaucoma agent* [epinephryl borate] 0.5%, 1% ② Epitol

epinastine INN *ophthalmic antihistamine* [also: epinastine HCl]

epinastine HCl *ophthalmic antihistamine* [also: epinastine]

epinephran [see: epinephrine]

epinephrine USP, INN *vasoconstrictor; sympathomimetic bronchodilator; topical antiglaucoma agent; vasopressor for shock* [also: adrenaline] 1:1000, 1:10 000 (1, 0.1 mg/mL) injection ② Epifrin

epinephrine bitartrate USP *sympathomimetic bronchodilator; ophthalmic adrenergic; topical antiglaucoma agent*

epinephrine borate *topical antiglaucoma agent*

epinephrine HCl *sympathomimetic bronchodilator; nasal decongestant; topical antiglaucoma agent; vasopressor for shock* 0.1% eye drops

Epinephrine Mist inhalation aerosol OTC *sympathomimetic bronchodilator* [epinephrine] 0.22 mg/spray

epinephryl borate USAN, USP *adrenergic; topical antiglaucoma agent*

epioestriol BAN [also: epiestriol]

EpiPen; EpiPen Jr. auto-injector (automatic IM injection device) ℞ *emergency treatment of anaphylaxis; vasopressor for shock* [epinephrine] 1:1000 (1 mg/mL); 1:2000 (0.5 mg/mL) ② Epifrin

epipropidine USAN, INN *antineoplastic*

EpiQuin Micro cream ℞ *hyperpigmentation bleaching agent* [hydroquinone (in a base containing vitamins A, C, and E)] 4%

epirizole USAN, INN *analgesic; anti-inflammatory*

epiroprim INN

epirubicin INN, BAN *anthracycline antibiotic antineoplastic* [also: epirubicin HCl]

epirubicin HCl USAN, JAN *anthracycline antibiotic antineoplastic for breast cancer (orphan)* [also: epirubicin]

epirubicin & tamoxifen *chemotherapy protocol for breast cancer*

epitetracycline HCl USP *antibacterial*

epithiazide USAN, BAN *antihypertensive; diuretic* [also: epitizide]

epithioandrostanol [see: epitiostanol]

epitiostanol INN

epitizide INN *antihypertensive; diuretic* [also: epithiazide]

Epitol tablets ℞ *anticonvulsant; analgesic for trigeminal neuralgia; antipsychotic* [carbamazepine] 200 mg ② Epinal

Epival ⒸⒶⓃ enteric-coated tablets ℞ *anticonvulsant; antipsychotic for manic episodes of a bipolar disorder* [divalproex sodium] 125, 250, 500 mg

Epival ER ⒸⒶⓃ extended-release tablets ℞ *anticonvulsant* [divalproex sodium] 500 mg

Epivir film-coated tablets, oral solution ℞ *antiviral for HIV infection* [lamivudine] 150, 300 mg; 10 mg/mL

Epivir-HBV film-coated caplets, oral solution ℞ *antiviral for hepatitis B virus (HBV) infection* [lamivudine] 100 mg; 5 mg/mL

eplerenone USAN *aldosterone receptor antagonist for hypertension and congestive heart failure (CHF); improves survival after a cardiovascular event*

EPO (epoetin alfa) [q.v.]

EPO (evening primrose oil) [see: evening primrose]

EPOCH (etoposide, prednisone, Oncovin, cyclophosphamide, Halotestin) *chemotherapy protocol*

epoetin alfa (EPO) USAN, INN, BAN, JAN *hematopoietic to stimulate RBC production for anemia of chronic renal failure, HIV, and chemotherapy (orphan) and to reduce the need for blood transfusions in surgery; investigational (orphan) for myelodysplastic syndrome*

epoetin beta USAN, INN, BAN, JAN *investigational (orphan) hematinic for anemia of end-stage renal disease*

Epogen IV or subcu injection ℞ *hematopoietic to stimulate RBC production for anemia of chronic renal failure, HIV, and chemotherapy (orphan) and to reduce the need for blood transfusions in surgery* [epoetin alfa] 2000, 3000, 4000, 10 000, 20 000, 40 000 U/mL ⃞ "amp and gent" (ampicillin & gentamicin)

epoprostenol USAN, INN *platelet aggregation inhibitor and vasodilator for primary pulmonary hypertension (orphan); investigational (orphan) heparin replacement for hemodialysis*

epoprostenol sodium USAN, BAN *platelet aggregation inhibitor and vasodilator for hypertension*

epostane USAN, INN, BAN *interceptive*

epoxytropine tropate methylbromide [see: methscopolamine bromide]

epratuzumab *monoclonal antibody to CD22; investigational (Phase III, orphan) for AIDS-related non-Hodgkin lymphoma; investigational (Phase III) for systemic lupus erythematosus (SLE)*

eprazinone INN

eprinomectin USAN *veterinary antiparasitic*

episteride USAN, INN, BAN *alpha reductase inhibitor for benign prostatic hypertrophy*

eprosartan USAN *antihypertensive; angiotensin II receptor antagonist*

eprosartan mesylate USAN *antihypertensive; angiotensin II receptor antagonist*

eprovafen INN

eproxindine INN

eprozinol INN

epsikapron [see: aminocaproic acid]

epsilon-aminocaproic acid (EACA) [see: aminocaproic acid]

epsiprantel INN, BAN

Epsom salt granules OTC *saline laxative* [magnesium sulfate]

Epsom salt [see: magnesium sulfate]

e.p.t. Quick Stick test stick for home use *in vitro diagnostic aid; urine pregnancy test*

eptacog alfa (activated) *activated recombinant human blood coagulation Factor VII (rFVIIa) for hemophilia A and B*

eptaloprost INN

eptamestrol [see: etamestrol]

eptaprost [see: eptaloprost]

eptastatin sodium [see: pravastatin sodium]

eptastigmine INN *investigational treatment for Alzheimer disease*

eptazocine INN

eptifibatide *glycoprotein (GP) IIb/IIIa receptor antagonist; platelet aggregation inhibitor for acute coronary syndrome, unstable angina, myocardial infarction, and cardiac surgery*

Epulor oral liquid OTC *enteral nutritional therapy* [milk-based formula]

Epzicom film-coated tablets ℞ *once-daily nucleoside reverse transcriptase inhibitor (NRTI) antiviral combination* *for HIV infections* [abacavir sulfate; lamivudine] 600•300 mg

Equagesic tablets (discontinued 2004) ℞ *analgesic; antipyretic; anti-inflammatory; anxiolytic; sedative* [aspirin; meprobamate] 325•200 mg

Equalactin chewable tablets OTC *bulk laxative; antidiarrheal* [calcium polycarbophil] 625 mg

Equanil tablets (discontinued 2004) ℞ *anxiolytic* [meprobamate] 200, 400 mg ② Aldoril; Elavil; Eldepryl; Enovil; Mellaril

Equetro extended-release capsules ℞ *antipsychotic for manic episodes of a bipolar disorder* [carbamazepine] 100, 200, 300 mg

Equilet chewable tablets OTC *antacid* [calcium carbonate] 500 mg

equilin USP *estrogen*

Equipoise *brand name for boldenone undecylenate, a veterinary anabolic steroid abused as a street drug*

Equisetum arvens **medicinal herb** [see: horsetail]

Erbitux IV infusion ℞ *antineoplastic for metastatic colorectal cancer;investigational (orphan) for squamous cell carcinoma of the head and neck; investigational (Phase III) for pancreatic cancer* [cetuximab] 100 mg/vial

erbium *element (Er)*

erbulozole USAN, INN *antineoplastic adjunct*

erbumine USAN, INN, BAN *combining name for radicals or groups*

Ercaf tablets ℞ *migraine-specific vasoconstrictor* [ergotamine tartrate; caffeine] 1•100 mg

erdosteine INN

Erechtites hieracfolia **medicinal herb** [see: pilewort]

Ergamisol tablets ℞ *biological response modifier; antineoplastic adjunct for colon cancer* [levamisole HCl] 50 mg

ergocalciferol (vitamin D₂) USP, INN, BAN, JAN *fat-soluble vitamin for refractory rickets, familial hypophosphatemia, and hypoparathyroidism*

ergoloid mesylates USAN, USP *cognition adjuvant for age-related mental capacity decline* [also: co-dergocrine mesylate] 0.5, 1 mg oral

Ergomar sublingual tablets ℞ *prophylaxis or treatment of migraine and other vascular headaches* [ergotamine tartrate] 2 mg

ergometrine INN, BAN *oxytocic for induction of labor* [also: ergonovine maleate]

ergonovine maleate USP *oxytocic for the induction of labor and prevention of postpartum and postabortal hemorrhage* [also: ergometrine]

ergosterol, activated [see: ergocalciferol]

ergot (*Claviceps purpurea*) *dried sclerotia medicinal herb used as an abortifacient, emmenagogue, hemostatic, oxytocic, and vasoconstrictor; source of ergotamine and LSD*

ergot alkaloids [see: ergoloid mesylates]

ergotamine INN, BAN *migraine-specific analgesic* [also: ergotamine tartrate]

ergotamine tartrate USP *prophylaxis or treatment of migraine and other vascular headaches* [also: ergotamine]

ergotamine tartrate & caffeine *prophylaxis or treatment of migraine and other vascular headaches* 1•100 mg oral

Ergotrate Maleate IM or IV injection (discontinued 2004) ℞ *oxytocic for the induction of labor and prevention of postpartum and postabortal hemorrhage* [ergonovine maleate] 0.2 mg/mL

Ergotrate Maleate tablets ℞ *oxytocic for the induction of labor and prevention of postpartum and postabortal hemorrhage* [ergonovine maleate] 0.2 mg

ericolol INN

Erigeron canadensis **medicinal herb** [see: fleabane; horseweed]

eriodictyon NF

Eriodictyon californicum **medicinal herb** [see: yerba santa]

eritrityl tetranitrate INN *coronary vasodilator* [also: erythrityl tetranitrate]

erizepine INN

erlizumab USAN *monoclonal antibody to treat reperfusion injury following acute myocardial infarction*

erlotinib HCl *human epidermal growth factor receptor type 1 (HER-1; EGFR)/ tyrosine kinase inhibitor; antineoplastic for advanced or metastatic non–small cell lung and pancreatic cancer; investigational (Phase III) for breast cancer; investigational (orphan) for non-Hodgkin lymphoma*

E·R·O Ear Drops OTC *agent to emulsify and disperse ear wax* [carbamide peroxide] 6.5%

erocainide INN

errhines *a class of agents that promote nasal discharge or secretion*

Errin tablets (in packs of 28) ℞ *oral contraceptive (progestin only)* [norethindrone] 0.35 mg

ersofermin USAN, INN *wound healing agent; transglutaminase inhibitor for the treatment of scar tissue*

Ertaczo cream ℞ *antifungal* [sertaconazole nitrate] 2%

ertapenem sodium USAN *antibiotic* ⸺

Erwinase ℞ *investigational (orphan) antineoplastic for acute lymphocytic leukemia* [erwinia L-asparaginase]

erwinia L-asparaginase *investigational (orphan) antineoplastic for acute lymphocytic leukemia*

Ery Pads pledgets ℞ *antibiotic for acne* [erythromycin; alcohol 60.5%] 2%

ERYC delayed-release capsules containing enteric-coated pellets ℞ *macrolide antibiotic* [erythromycin] 250 mg ☒ ara-C

Erycette topical solution (discontinued 2003) ℞ *antibiotic for acne* [erythromycin] 2% ☒ Aricept

EryDerm 2% topical solution ℞ *antibiotic for acne* [erythromycin; alcohol 77%] 2%

Erygel gel (discontinued 2004) ℞ *antibiotic for acne* [erythromycin; alcohol 92%] 2%

Erymax topical solution (discontinued 2003) ℞ *antibiotic for acne* [erythromycin] 2%

Eryngium aquaticum *medicinal herb* [see: water eryngo]

EryPed chewable tablets (discontinued 2003) ℞ *macrolide antibiotic* [erythromycin ethylsuccinate] 200 mg

EryPed oral drops ℞ *macrolide antibiotic* [erythromycin ethylsuccinate] 100 mg/2.5 mL

EryPed 200; EryPed 400 oral suspension ℞ *macrolide antibiotic* [erythromycin ethylsuccinate] 200 mg/5 mL; 400 mg/5 mL

Ery-Tab enteric-coated delayed-release tablets ℞ *macrolide antibiotic* [erythromycin] 250, 333, 500 mg

erythorbic acid

Erythra-Derm topical solution (discontinued 2003) ℞ *antibiotic for acne* [erythromycin] 2%

Erythraea centaurium *medicinal herb* [see: centaury]

erythrityl tetranitrate USAN, USP *coronary vasodilator; antianginal* [also: eritrityl tetranitrate]

Erythrocin Lactobionate powder for IV injection ℞ *macrolide antibiotic* [erythromycin lactobionate] 500, 1000 mg/vial

Erythrocin Stearate Filmtabs (film-coated tablets) ℞ *macrolide antibiotic* [erythromycin stearate] 250, 500 mg

erythrol tetranitrate [now: erythrityl tetranitrate]

erythromycin USP, INN, BAN *macrolide antibiotic* 250, 500 mg oral; 2% topical; 0.5% ophthalmic ☒ clarithromycin; dirithromycin

erythromycin 2′-acetate octadecanoate [see: erythromycin acistrate]

erythromycin 2′-acetate stearate [see: erythromycin acistrate]

erythromycin acistrate USAN, INN *macrolide antibiotic*

erythromycin B [see: berythromycin]

erythromycin & benzoyl peroxide *antibiotic and keratolytic for acne* 3%• 5% topical

erythromycin estolate USAN, USP, BAN *macrolide antibiotic* 250, 500 mg/ 5 mL oral

erythromycin ethyl succinate BAN *macrolide antibiotic* [also: erythromycin ethylsuccinate]

erythromycin ethylcarbonate USP *macrolide antibiotic*

erythromycin ethylsuccinate (EES) USP *macrolide antibiotic* [also: erythromycin ethyl succinate] 400 mg oral; 200, 400 mg/5 mL oral

erythromycin gluceptate USP *macrolide antibiotic*

erythromycin glucoheptonate [see: erythromycin gluceptate]

erythromycin lactobionate USP *macrolide antibiotic*

erythromycin lauryl sulfate, propionyl [now: erythromycin estolate]

erythromycin monoglucoheptonate [see: erythromycin gluceptate]

erythromycin octadecanoate [see: erythromycin stearate]

erythromycin 2′-propanoate [see: erythromycin propionate]

erythromycin propionate USAN *macrolide antibiotic*

erythromycin 2′-propionate dodecyl sulfate [see: erythromycin estolate]

erythromycin propionate lauryl sulfate [now: erythromycin estolate]

erythromycin salnacedin USAN *macrolide antibiotic for acne vulgaris*

erythromycin stearate USP, BAN *macrolide antibiotic* 250, 500 mg oral

erythromycin stinoprate INN *macrolide antibiotic*

Erythronium americanum *medicinal herb* [see: adder's tongue]

erythropoietin, recombinant human (rEPO) [see: epoetin alfa; epoetin beta]

erythrosine sodium USP *dental disclosing agent*

Eryzole granules for oral suspension ℞ *antibiotic* [erythromycin ethylsuccinate; sulfisoxazole acetyl] 200•600 mg/5 mL

esafloxacin INN

esaprazole INN

escitalopram oxalate USAN *selective serotonin reuptake inhibitor (SSRI) for* *major depression and generalized anxiety disorder; isomer of citalopram*

Esclim transdermal patch ℞ *estrogen replacement therapy for the treatment of postmenopausal symptoms* [estradiol] 25, 37.5, 50, 75, 100 μg/day

esculamine INN

eseridine INN

eserine [see: physostigmine]

esflurbiprofen INN, BAN

Esgic caplets, capsules ℞ *analgesic; barbiturate sedative* [acetaminophen; caffeine; butalbital] 325•40•50 mg

Esgic-Plus caplets, capsules ℞ *analgesic; barbiturate sedative* [acetaminophen; caffeine; butalbital] 500•40•50 mg

ESHAP (etoposide, Solu-Medrol, high-dose ara-C, Platinol) *chemotherapy protocol for non-Hodgkin lymphoma*

ESHAP-MINE (alternating cycles of ESHAP and MINE) *chemotherapy protocol*

Esidrix tablets ℞ *antihypertensive; diuretic* [hydrochlorothiazide] 25, 50, 100 mg ⑨ Lasix

esilate INN *combining name for radicals or groups* [also: esylate]

Esimil tablets ℞ *antihypertensive; diuretic* [hydrochlorothiazide; guanethidine monosulfate] 25•10 mg ⑨ Estinyl; Isomil

Eskalith capsules ℞ *antipsychotic for manic episodes* [lithium carbonate] 300 mg

Eskalith tablets (discontinued 2005) ℞ *antipsychotic for manic episodes* [lithium carbonate] 300 mg

Eskalith CR controlled-release tablets ℞ *antipsychotic for manic episodes* [lithium carbonate] 450 mg

esmolol INN, BAN *antihypertensive; antiadrenergic (β-receptor)* [also: esmolol HCl]

esmolol HCl USAN *antihypertensive; antiarrhythmic; antiadrenergic (β-receptor)* [also: esmolol] 10 mg/mL injection

E-Solve OTC *lotion base*

esomeprazole magnesium USAN *proton pump inhibitor for gastric and duodenal ulcers, erosive esophagitis, GERD, and other gastroesophageal disorders; isomer of omeprazole*

esorubicin INN *antineoplastic* [also: esorubicin HCl]

esorubicin HCl USAN *antineoplastic* [also: esorubicin]

Esotérica Dry Skin Treatment lotion OTC *moisturizer; emollient*

Esotérica Facial; Esotérica Regular cream OTC *hyperpigmentation bleaching agent* [hydroquinone] 2%

Esotérica Fortified cream (discontinued 2003) OTC *hyperpigmentation bleaching agent; sunscreen* [hydroquinone; padimate O; oxybenzone] 2%•3.3%•2.5%

Esotérica Sensitive Skin Formula cream (discontinued 2003) OTC *hyperpigmentation bleaching agent* [hydroquinone] 1.5%

Esotérica Soap OTC *bath emollient*

Esotérica Sunscreen cream OTC *hyperpigmentation bleaching agent; sunscreen* [hydroquinone; padimate O; oxybenzone] 2%•3.3%•2.5%

esproquin HCl USAN *adrenergic* [also: esproquine]

esproquine INN *adrenergic* [also: esproquin HCl]

Essential ProPlus powder for oral solution OTC *oral protein supplement with vitamins and minerals* [soy protein; multiple vitamins and minerals]

Essential Protein powder OTC *oral protein supplement* [soy protein]

Estalis 140/50; Estalis 250/50 ⓒⒶⓃ transdermal patch ℞ *hormone replacement therapy for postmenopausal symptoms* [norethindrone acetate; estradiol-17β] 140•50 μg/day; 250•50 μg/day

Estar gel (discontinued 2004) OTC *antipsoriatic; antiseborrheic* [coal tar] 5%

estazolam USAN, INN *benzodiazepine sedative and hypnotic* 1, 2 mg oral

Ester-C Plus Multi-Mineral capsules OTC *vitamin C/mineral supplement*

with multiple bioflavonoids [vitamin C; acerola; rose hips; multiple minerals; citrus bioflavonoids; rutin] 425•12.5•12.5•±•50•5 mg

Ester-C Plus Vitamin C capsules OTC *vitamin C/calcium supplement with multiple bioflavonoids* [vitamin C; acerola; rose hips; calcium; citrus bioflavonoids; rutin] 500•10•10•62•25•5 mg; 1000•25•25•125•200•25 mg

esterified estrogens [see: estrogens, esterified]

esterifilcon A USAN *hydrophilic contact lens material*

estilben [see: diethylstilbestrol dipropionate]

Estinyl tablets (discontinued 2003) ℞ *estrogen replacement therapy for the treatment of postmenopausal symptoms; palliative therapy for breast and prostate cancers* [ethinyl estradiol] 0.02, 0.05, 0.5 mg ② Esimil

estolate INN *combining name for radicals or groups*

estomycin sulfate [see: paromomycin sulfate]

Estorra tablets (name changed to **Lunesta** in 2004)

Estrace tablets ℞ *estrogen replacement therapy for the treatment of postmenopausal symptoms and prevention of postmenopausal osteoporosis; palliative therapy for prostate and metastatic breast cancers* [estradiol, soy-derived] 0.5, 1, 2 mg

Estrace Vaginal cream ℞ *estrogen replacement for postmenopausal atrophic vaginitis* [estradiol] 0.1 mg/g

Estraderm transdermal patch ℞ *estrogen replacement therapy for the treatment of postmenopausal symptoms and prevention of postmenopausal osteoporosis* [estradiol] 50, 100 μg/day ② Estradurin

estradiol USP, INN *estrogen replacement therapy for the treatment of postmenopausal disorders and the prevention of postmenopausal osteoporosis; palliative therapy for breast and prostate cancers;*

may be naturally derived or a synthetic analogue [also: oestradiol] 0.5, 1, 2 mg oral

estradiol acetate *synthetic estrogen; hormone replacement therapy for the treatment of postmenopausal symptoms*

estradiol-17β *estrogen replacement therapy for postmenopausal disorders*

estradiol benzoate USP, INN, JAN [also: oestradiol benzoate]

estradiol 17-cyclopentanepropio-nate [see: estradiol cypionate]

estradiol cypionate USP *synthetic estrogen; hormone replacement therapy for the treatment of postmenopausal symptoms*

estradiol dipropionate NF, JAN

estradiol enanthate USAN *estrogen*

estradiol hemihydrate *synthetic estrogen; topical hormone therapy for atrophic vaginitis*

estradiol 17-heptanoate [see: estradiol enanthate]

estradiol monobenzoate [see: estradiol benzoate]

estradiol 17-nicotinate 3-propionate [see: estrapronicate]

estradiol phosphate polymer [see: polyestradiol phosphate]

Estradiol Transdermal System patch Rx *estrogen replacement therapy for the treatment of postmenopausal symptoms and prevention of postmenopausal osteoporosis* [estradiol] 50, 100 μg/day

estradiol 17-undecanoate [see: estradiol undecylate]

estradiol undecylate USAN, INN *estrogen*

estradiol valerate USP, INN, JAN *synthetic estrogen; hormone replacement therapy for the treatment of postmenopausal symptoms and the prevention of postmenopausal osteoporosis; hormonal antineoplastic for breast and prostate cancers* [also: oestradiol valerate]

Estra-L 40 IM injection Rx *estrogen replacement therapy for postmenopausal symptoms; antineoplastic for prostatic cancer* [estradiol valerate in oil] 40 mg/mL

estramustine USAN, INN, BAN *nitrogen mustard-type alkylating antineoplastic*

estramustine phosphate sodium USAN, BAN, JAN *nitrogen mustard-type alkylating antineoplastic for prostate cancer*

estramustine & vinblastine sulfate *chemotherapy protocol for prostate cancer*

estrapronicate INN

Estrasorb topical emulsion Rx *estrogen replacement therapy for postmenopausal symptoms* [estradiol hemihydrate] 2.5 mg/g (4.35 mg/pouch = 25 μg base/pouch)

Estratab tablets (discontinued 2003) Rx *estrogen replacement therapy for the treatment of postmenopausal symptoms; palliative therapy for breast and prostate cancers* [esterified estrogens] 0.3, 0.625, 2.5 mg ⧉ Ethatab

Estratest; Estratest H.S. sugar-coated tablets Rx *hormone replacement therapy for postmenopausal symptoms* [esterified estrogens; methyltestosterone] 1.25•2.5 mg; 0.625•1.25 mg

estrazinol INN *estrogen* [also: estrazinol hydrobromide]

estrazinol hydrobromide USAN *estrogen* [also: estrazinol]

Estring vaginal ring Rx *three-month estrogen replacement for postmenopausal atrophic vaginitis* [estradiol] 2 mg (7.5 μg/day)

estriol USP *estrogen* [also: estriol succinate; oestriol succinate]

estriol succinate INN *estrogen* [also: estriol; oestriol succinate]

estrobene [see: diethylstilbestrol]

estrobene DP [see: diethylstilbestrol dipropionate]

estrofurate USAN, INN *estrogen*

Estrogel transdermal gel Rx *estrogen replacement therapy for postmenopausal symptoms* [estradiol] 0.06%

Estrogel ⊛ transdermal gel Rx *estrogen replacement therapy for postmenopausal symptoms* [estrogen-17β] 0.06% (1.25 g/metered actuation)

estrogenic substances, conjugated [see: estrogens, conjugated] estrogenine [see: diethylstilbestrol]

estrogens *a class of sex hormones that includes estradiol, estrone, and estriol, also used as an antineoplastic*

estrogens, conjugated USP, JAN *a mixture of equine estrogens; hormone replacement therapy for the treatment of postmenopausal symptoms and prevention of postmenopausal osteoporosis; palliative therapy for breast and prostate cancers*

estrogens, esterified USP *a mixture of equine estrogens; hormone replacement therapy for the treatment of postmenopausal disorders; palliative therapy for breast and prostate cancers*

estrogens, synthetic conjugated, A *a mixture of 9 synthetic estrogenic substances; hormone replacement therapy for postmenopausal symptoms*

estrogens, synthetic conjugated, B *a mixture of 10 synthetic estrogenic substances; hormone replacement therapy for severe postmenopausal vasomotor symptoms*

estromenin [see: diethylstilbestrol]

estrone USP, INN *bioidentical human estrogen; natural hormone replacement therapy for postmenopausal disorders; palliative therapy for breast and prostate cancers* [also: oestrone]

Estrone Aqueous IM injection (discontinued 2003) ℞ *estrogen replacement therapy for postmenopausal symptoms; palliative therapy for breast and prostate cancers* [estrone] 5 mg/mL

estrone hydrogen sulfate [see: estrone sodium sulfate]

estrone sodium sulfate *synthetic estrogen*

Estrophasic (trademarked/patented dosing regimen) *gradual estrogen intake with steady progestin intake*

estropipate USP *natural estrogen replacement therapy for the treatment of postmenopausal symptoms and prevention of postmenopausal osteoporosis; a stabilized form of estrone, the bioidentical human estrogen* 0.75, 1.5, 3, 6 mg oral

Estrostep 21 tablets (in packs of 21) ℞ *triphasic oral contraceptive; treatment for acne vulgaris in females* [norethindrone acetate; ethinyl estradiol]
Phase 1 (5 days): 1000•20 μg;
Phase 2 (7 days): 1000•30 μg;
Phase 3 (9 days): 1000•35 μg

Estrostep Fe tablets (in packs of 28) ℞ *triphasic oral contraceptive; iron supplement* [norethindrone acetate; ethinyl estradiol; ferrous fumarate]
Phase 1 (5 days) 1•0.02•75 mg;
Phase 2 (7 days) 1•0.03•75 mg;
Phase 3 (9 days) 1•0.035•75 mg;
Counters (7 days) 0•0•75 mg

esuprone INN

esylate USAN, BAN *combining name for radicals or groups* [also: esilate]

eszopiclone *nonbarbiturate sedative and hypnotic for chronic insomnia*

etabenzarone INN

etabonate USAN, INN *combining name for radicals or groups*

etacepride INN

etacrynic acid INN, JAN *antihypertensive; loop diuretic* [also: ethacrynic acid]

etafedrine INN, BAN *adrenergic* [also: etafedrine HCl]

etafedrine HCl USAN *adrenergic* [also: etafedrine]

etafenone INN

etafilcon A USAN *hydrophilic contact lens material*

etamestrol INN

etaminile INN

etamiphyllin INN [also: etamiphylline]

etamiphyllin methesculetol [see: metescufylline]

etamiphylline BAN [also: etamiphyllin]

etamivan INN *central and respiratory stimulant* [also: ethamivan]

etamocycline INN

etamsylate INN *hemostatic* [also: ethamsylate]

etanercept USAN *soluble tumor necrosis factor receptor (sTNFR) inhibitor for rheumatoid arthritis, juvenile rheumatoid arthritis (orphan), psoriatic arthritis, and ankylosing spondylitis; investigational (NDA filed) for congestive heart failure; investigational (orphan) for Wegener granulomatosis*

etanidazole USAN, INN *antineoplastic; hypoxic cell radiosensitizer*

etanterol INN

etaperazine [see: perphenazine]

etaqualone INN

etarotene USAN, INN *keratolytic*

etasuline INN

etazepine INN

etazolate INN *antipsychotic* [also: etazolate HCl]

etazolate HCl USAN *antipsychotic* [also: etazolate]

etebenecid INN [also: ethebenecid]

etenzamide BAN [also: ethenzamide]

eterobarb USAN, INN, BAN *anticonvulsant*

etersalate INN

ethacridine INN [also: ethacridine lactate; acrinol] ⊡ ethacrynic

ethacridine lactate [also: ethacridine; acrinol]

ethacrynate sodium USAN, USP *antihypertensive; loop diuretic*

ethacrynic acid USAN, USP, BAN *antihypertensive; loop diuretic* [also: etacrynic acid] ⊡ ethacridine

ethambutol INN, BAN *bacteriostatic; primary tuberculostatic* [also: ethambutol HCl]

ethambutol HCl USAN, USP *bacteriostatic; primary tuberculostatic* [also: ethambutol] 400 mg oral

ethamivan USAN, USP, BAN *central and respiratory stimulant* [also: etamivan]

Ethamolin IV injection ℞ *sclerosing agent for bleeding esophageal varices (orphan)* [ethanolamine oleate] 5%

ethamsylate USAN, BAN *hemostatic* [also: etamsylate]

ethanol JAN *topical anti-infective/antiseptic; astringent; solvent; a widely abused "legal street drug" used to produce euphoria* [also: alcohol]

ethanol, dehydrated JAN *antidote* [also: alcohol, dehydrated]

ethanolamine oleate USAN *sclerosing agent for bleeding esophageal varices (orphan)* [also: monoethanolamine oleate]

ethanolamines *a class of antihistamines that includes diphenhydramine HCl and clemastine fumarate*

ethaverine INN *peripheral vasodilator*

ethaverine HCl *peripheral vasodilator* [see: ethaverine]

ethchlorvynol USP, INN, BAN *sedative; hypnotic*

ethebenecid BAN [also: etebenecid]

EtheDent chewable tablets ℞ *dental caries preventative* [sodium fluoride] 0.25, 0.5, 1 mg

EtheDent dental cream ℞ *topical caries preventative* [sodium fluoride] 1.1%

ethenzamide INN, JAN [also: etenzamide]

ether USP *inhalation anesthetic*

Ethezyme; Ethezyme 830 ointment ℞ *proteolytic enzyme for debridement of necrotic tissue; vulnerary* [papain; urea] 1 100 000 U•100 mg per gram; 830 000 IU•100 mg per gram

ethiazide INN, BAN

ethidium bromide [see: homidium bromide]

ethinamate USP, INN, BAN *sedative; hypnotic* ⊡ ethionamide

ethinyl estradiol USP *estrogen replacement therapy for the treatment of postmenopausal disorders; palliative therapy for prostate and breast cancers; investigational (orphan) for Turner syndrome* [also: ethinylestradiol; ethinyloestradiol]

ethinylestradiol INN *estrogen replacement therapy for the treatment of postmenopausal disorders; palliative therapy for prostate and breast cancers* [also: ethinyl estradiol; ethinyloestradiol]

ethinyloestradiol BAN *estrogen replacement therapy for the treatment of postmenopausal disorders; palliative therapy for prostate and breast cancers* [also: ethinyl estradiol; ethinylestradiol]

ethiodized oil USP *parenteral radiopaque contrast medium (37% iodine)*

ethiodized oil (¹³¹I) INN *antineoplastic; radioactive agent* [also: ethiodized oil I 131]

ethiodized oil I 131 USAN *antineoplastic; radioactive agent* [also: ethiodized oil (^{131}I)]

Ethiodol intracavitary instillation ℞ *radiopaque contrast medium for lymphography and gynecological imaging* [ethiodized oil (37% iodine)] 1284 mg/mL (475 mg/mL) ② ethynodiol

ethiofos [now: amifostine]

ethionamide USAN, USP, INN, BAN *bacteriostatic; tuberculosis retreatment* ② ethinamate

ethisterone NF, INN, BAN

Ethmozine film-coated tablets ℞ *antiarrhythmic for severe ventricular arrhythmias* [moricizine HCl] 200, 250, 300 mg

ethodryl [see: diethylcarbamazine citrate]

ethoglucid BAN [also: etoglucid]

ethoheptazine BAN [also: ethoheptazine citrate]

ethoheptazine citrate NF, INN [also: ethoheptazine]

ethohexadiol USP

ethomoxane INN, BAN

ethomoxane HCl [see: ethomoxane]

ethonam nitrate USAN *antifungal* [also: etonam]

ethopabate BAN

ethopropazine BAN *anticholinergic; antiparkinsonian* [also: ethopropazine HCl; profenamine]

ethopropazine HCl USP *anticholinergic; antiparkinsonian* [also: profenamine; ethopropazine]

ethosalamide BAN [also: etosalamide]

ethosuximide USAN, USP, INN, BAN *anticonvulsant* 250 mg oral; 250 mg/5 mL oral

ethotoin USP, INN, BAN *hydantoin anticonvulsant*

ethoxarutine [see: ethoxazorutoside]

ethoxazene HCl USAN *analgesic* [also: etoxazene]

ethoxazorutoside INN

ethoxyacetanilide (*withdrawn from market*) [see: phenacetin]

o-ethoxybenzamide [see: ethenzamide; etenzamide]

ethoxzolamide USP

Ethrane liquid for vaporization ℞ *inhalation general anesthetic* [enflurane]

ethybenztropine USAN, BAN *anticholinergic* [also: etybenzatropine]

ethyl acetate NF *solvent*

ethyl alcohol (EtOH; ETOH) [now: alcohol; ethanol]

ethyl aminobenzoate (ethyl p-aminobenzoate) JAN *topical anesthetic; nonprescription diet aid* [also: benzocaine]

ethyl 2-benzimidazolecarbamate [see: lobendazole]

ethyl N-benzylcyclopropanecarbamate [see: encyprate]

ethyl biscoumacetate NF, INN, BAN

ethyl biscumacetate [see: ethyl biscoumacetate]

ethyl carbamate [now: urethane]

ethyl carfluzepate INN

ethyl cartrizoate INN

ethyl chloride USP *topical local anesthetic; topical vapo-coolant*

ethyl dibunate USAN, INN, BAN *antitussive*

ethyl dirazepate INN

ethyl eicosapentaenoate *investigational (orphan) agent for Huntington disease*

ethyl ether [see: ether]

ethyl p-fluorophenyl sulfone [see: fluoresone]

ethyl p-hydroxybenzoate [see: ethylparaben]

ethyl loflazepate INN

ethyl nitrite NF

ethyl oleate NF *vehicle*

ethyl oxide [see: ether]

ethyl vanillin NF *flavoring agent*

ethylcellulose NF *tablet binder*

ethylchlordiphene [see: etofamide]

ethyldicoumarol [see: ethyl biscoumacetate]

ethylene NF *inhalation general anesthesia*

ethylene distearate [see: glycol distearate]

ethylenediamine USP, JAN

ethylenediaminetetraacetate [see: edetate disodium]

ethylenediaminetetraacetic acid (EDTA) [see: edetate disodium]

N,N-ethylenediarsanilic acid [see: difetarsone]

ethylenedinitrilotetraacetate disodium [see: edetate disodium]

ethylestrenol USAN, INN *anabolic steroid; also abused as a street drug* [also: ethyloestrenol; ethylnandrol]

ethylhexanediol [see: ethohexadiol]

2-ethylhexyl diphenyl phosphate [see: octicizer]

2-ethylhexyl p-methoxycinnamate [see: octinoxate]

2-ethylhexyl salicylate [see: octisalate]

ethylhydrocupreine HCl NF

ethylmethylthiambutene INN, BAN

ethylmorphine BAN [also: ethylmorphine HCl]

ethylmorphine HCl NF [also: ethylmorphine]

ethylnandrol JAN *anabolic steroid; also abused as a street drug* [also: ethylestrenol; ethyloestrenol]

ethylnorepinephrine HCl USP *sympathomimetic bronchodilator*

ethyloestradiol BAN *estrogen* [also: ethinyl estradiol]

ethyloestrenol BAN *anabolic steroid; also abused as a street drug* [also: ethylestrenol; ethylnandrol]

ethylpapaverine HCl [see: ethaverine HCl]

ethylparaben NF *antifungal agent*

ethylphenacemide [see: pheneturide]

ethylstibamine [see: stibosamine]

2-ethylthioisonicotinamide [see: ethionamide]

ethynerone USAN, INN *progestin*

ethynodiol BAN *progestin* [also: ethynodiol diacetate; etynodiol] ⊘ Ethiodol

ethynodiol diacetate USAN, USP *progestin* [also: etynodiol; ethynodiol]

(–)-5-ethynylnicotine [see: altinicline]

5-ethynyluracil [see: eniluracil]

Ethyol powder for IV infusion ℞ *chemoprotective agent for cisplatin and paclitaxel chemotherapy (orphan); investigational (orphan) for cyclophospha-* *mide; treatment for moderate to severe xerostomia following postoperative radiation therapy (orphan)* [amifostine] 500 mg/vial

ethypicone INN

ethypropymal sodium [see: probarbital sodium]

etibendazole USAN, INN *anthelmintic*

eticlopride INN

eticyclidine INN

etidocaine USAN, INN, BAN *injectable local anesthetic*

etidocaine HCl *injectable local anesthetic*

etidronate disodium USAN, USP *bisphosphonate bone resorption inhibitor for Paget disease, heterotopic ossification, and hypercalcemia of malignancy (orphan); investigational (orphan) for metabolic bone disease*

etidronate monosodium

etidronate sodium (*this term is used only when the form of sodium cannot be more accurately identified*)

etidronate tetrasodium

etidronate trisodium

etidronic acid USAN, INN, BAN *calcium regulator*

etifelmine INN

etifenin USAN, INN, BAN *diagnostic aid*

etifoxin BAN [also: etifoxine]

etifoxine INN [also: etifoxin]

etilamfetamine INN

etilefrine INN

etilefrine pivalate INN

etilevodopa *investigational (Phase III) antiparkinsonian agent*

etintidine INN *antagonist to histamine H_2 receptors* [also: etintidine HCl]

etintidine HCl USAN *antagonist to histamine H_2 receptors* [also: etintidine]

etiocholanedione *investigational (orphan) for aplastic anemia and Prader-Willi syndrome*

etipirium iodide INN

etiproston INN

etiracetam INN

etiroxate INN

etisazole INN, BAN

etisomicin INN, BAN

etisulergine INN

etizolam INN

etobedolum [see: etonitazene]

etocarlide INN

etocrilene INN *ultraviolet screen* [also: etocrylene]

etocrylene USAN *ultraviolet screen* [also: etocrilene]

etodolac USAN, INN, BAN *analgesic; antiarthritic; nonsteroidal anti-inflammatory drug (NSAID)* [also: etodolic acid] 200, 300, 400, 500, 600 mg oral

etodolic acid INN *analgesic; antiarthritic; nonsteroidal anti-inflammatory drug (NSAID)* [also: etodolac]

etodroxizine INN

etofamide INN

etofenamate USAN, INN, BAN *analgesic; anti-inflammatory*

etofenprox INN

etofibrate INN

etoformin INN *antidiabetic* [also: etoformin HCl]

etoformin HCl USAN *antidiabetic* [also: etoformin]

etofuradine INN

etofylline INN

etofylline clofibrate INN *antihyperlipoproteinemic* [also: theofibrate]

etoglucid INN [also: ethoglucid]

EtOH; ETOH (ethyl alcohol) [now: alcohol]

etolorex INN

etolotifen INN

etoloxamine INN

etomidate USAN, INN, BAN *rapid-acting nonbarbiturate general anesthetic; hypnotic*

etomidoline INN

etomoxir INN

etonam INN *antifungal* [also: ethonam nitrate]

etonam nitrate [see: ethonam nitrate]

etonitazene INN, BAN

etonogestrel USAN, INN *progestin*

etoperidone INN *antidepressant* [also: etoperidone HCl]

etoperidone HCl USAN *antidepressant* [also: etoperidone]

etophylate [see: acepifylline]

Etopophos powder for IV injection ℞ *antineoplastic for testicular and small cell lung cancers (SCLC)* [etoposide phosphate diethanolate] 119.3 mg/vial

etoposide USAN, INN, BAN *antineoplastic* 20, 30 mg/mL injection

etoposide & paclitaxel & carboplatin *chemotherapy protocol for primary adenocarcinoma and small cell lung cancer (SCLC)*

etoposide phosphate USAN *antineoplastic*

etoprindole INN

etoprine USAN *antineoplastic*

etoricoxib USAN *antiarthritic; antipyretic; COX-2 inhibitor; nonsteroidal anti-inflammatory drug (NSAID); investigational (NDA filed) for osteoarthritis, rheumatoid arthritis, musculoskeletal pain, and gout*

etorphine INN, BAN

etosalamide INN [also: ethosalamide]

etoxadrol INN *anesthetic* [also: etoxadrol HCl]

etoxadrol HCl USAN *anesthetic* [also: etoxadrol]

etoxazene INN *analgesic* [also: ethoxazene HCl]

etoxazene HCl [see: ethoxazene HCl]

etoxeridine INN, BAN

etozolin USAN, INN *diuretic*

etrabamine INN

Etrafon; Etrafon 2–10; Etrafon-A; Etrafon-Forte tablets ℞ *conventional (typical) phenothiazine antipsychotic for schizophrenia and psychotic disorders; antidepressant* [perphenazine; amitriptyline HCl] 2•25 mg; 2•10 mg; 4•10 mg; 4•25 mg

etretin [see: acitretin]

etretinate USAN, INN, BAN, JAN *systemic antipsoriatic; retinoic acid analogue*

etryptamine INN, BAN *CNS stimulant* [also: etryptamine acetate]

etryptamine acetate USAN *CNS stimulant* [also: etryptamine]

etybenzatropine INN *anticholinergic* [also: ethybenztropine]

etymemazine INN

etymemazine HCl [see: etymemazine]

etynodiol INN *progestin* [also: ethyno-diol diacetate; ethynodiol]

etyprenaline [see: isoetharine]

eucaine HCl NF

Eucalyptamint ointment, gel OTC *topical analgesic; counterirritant; antiseptic* [menthol; eucalyptus oil] 16%•
⚲; 8%• ⚲

eucalyptol USAN *topical bacteriostatic antiseptic/germicidal*

eucalyptus (Eucalyptus globulus) *oil medicinal herb for bronchitis, lung disorders, neuralgia, and skin sores; source of bioflavonoids*

eucalyptus oil NF *topical antiseptic*

eucatropine INN, BAN *ophthalmic anticholinergic* [also: eucatropine HCl]

eucatropine HCl USP *ophthalmic anticholinergic* [also: eucatropine]

Eucerin cream, lotion OTC *moisturizer; emollient*

Eucerin OTC *cream base*

Eucerin Itch-Relief Moisturizing spray OTC *counterirritant* [menthol] 0.15%

Eucerin Plus lotion OTC *moisturizer; emollient* [sodium lactate; urea] 5%•5%

eucodal [see: oxycodone]

Eudal-SR sustained-release tablets (discontinued 2002) ℞ *decongestant; expectorant* [pseudoephedrine HCl; guaifenesin] 120•400 mg

euflavine [see: acriflavine]

Euflex ⒸⒶⓃ tablets ℞ *antiandrogen antineoplastic adjunct to metastatic prostate cancer* [flutamide] 250 mg

Eugenia caryophyllata *medicinal herb* [see: cloves]

Eugenia pimenta *medicinal herb* [see: allspice]

eugenol USP *dental analgesic*

Euglucon ⒸⒶⓃ tablets ℞ *sulfonylurea antidiabetic* [glyburide] 2.5, 5 mg

eukadol [see: oxycodone]

Eulexin capsules ℞ *antiandrogen antineoplastic adjunct to metastatic prostate cancer* [flutamide] 125 mg

Euonymus atropurpureus *medicinal herb* [see: wahoo]

Eupatorium cannabinum *medicinal herb* [see: hemp agrimony]

Eupatorium perfoliatum *medicinal herb* [see: boneset]

Eupatorium purpureum *medicinal herb* [see: queen of the meadow]

Euphorbia poinsettia; E. pulcherrima *medicinal herb* [see: poinsettia]

euphoretics; euphoriants; euphora-gens *a class of agents that produce euphoria*

Euphrasia officinalis; E. rostkoviana; E. strica *medicinal herb* [see: eyebright]

euprocin INN *topical anesthetic* [also: euprocin HCl]

euprocin HCl USAN *topical anesthetic* [also: euprocin]

euquinine [see: quinine ethylcarbonate]

Eurax cream, lotion ℞ *scabicide; antipruritic* [crotamiton] 10% ⓈⒺ Serax; Urex

European alder; European black alder; European buckthorn *medicinal herb* [see: buckthorn]

European aspen *medicinal herb* [see: black poplar]

europium *element (Eu)*

EVA (etoposide, vinblastine, Adriamycin) *chemotherapy protocol for Hodgkin lymphoma*

Evac-Q-Kwik suppositories (discontinued 2003) OTC *stimulant laxative* [bisacodyl] 10 mg ⓈⒺ Evac-Q-Kit

Evac-Q-Kwik Kit oral solution + 2 tablets + 1 suppository (discontinued 2003) OTC *pre-procedure bowel evacuant* [Evac-Q-Mag (q.v.); Evac-Q-Tabs (q.v.); Evac-Q-Kwik suppository (q.v.)]

Evac-Q-Mag carbonated oral solution OTC *saline laxative* [magnesium citrate; citric acid; potassium citrate]

Evac-Q-Tabs tablets OTC *stimulant laxative* [bisacodyl] 5 mg

Evac-U-Gen chewable tablets OTC *stimulant laxative* [sennosides] 10 mg

evandamine INN

Evans blue USP *diagnostic aid for blood volume* [also: azovan blue] 5 mL injection

evening primrose *(Oenothera biennis)* bark, leaves, oil *medicinal herb for cardiovascular health, hypertension, mastalgia, multiple sclerosis, nerves, obesity, premenstrual syndrome, prostate disorders, rheumatoid arthritis, and skin disorders*

everlasting *(Anaphalis margaritacea; Gnaphalium polycephalum; G. uliginosum)* plant *medicinal herb used as an astringent, diaphoretic, febrifuge, pectoral, vermifuge, and vulnerary*

evernimicin USAN *investigational antibiotic*

Everone 200 IM injection (discontinued 2001) ℞ *androgen replacement for delayed puberty or breast cancer* [testosterone enanthate] 200 mg/mL

Evista film-coated tablets ℞ *selective estrogen receptor modulator (SERM) for the prevention and treatment of postmenopausal osteoporosis; investigational (Phase III) for breast cancer* [raloxifene HCl] 60 mg ☒ Avita

E-Vitamin ointment OTC *emollient* [vitamin E] 30 mg/g

E-VMAC (escalated methotrexate, vinblastine, Adriamycin, cisplatin) *chemotherapy protocol*

E-VMAC (escalated methotrexate, vinblastine, Adriamycin, cyclophosphamide) *chemotherapy protocol*

Evoclin topical foam ℞ *antibiotic for acne* [clindamycin phosphate] 1%

Evoxac capsules ℞ *cholinergic and muscarinic receptor agonist for treatment of dry mouth due to Sjögren syndrome* [cevimeline HCl] 30 mg

Evra [see: Ortho Evra]

Exact topical liquid (discontinued 2003) OTC *keratolytic cleanser for acne* [salicylic acid] 2%

Exact vanishing cream OTC *keratolytic for acne* [benzoyl peroxide] 5%

exalamide INN

exametazime USAN, INN, BAN *regional cerebral perfusion imaging aid*

Exanta tablets (approved in 14 European countries) ℞ *investigational (NDA filed) oral anticoagulant and direct thrombin inhibitor for the prevention of stroke due to atrial fibrillation and the prevention and treatment of a venous thromboembolic event (VTE)* [ximelagatran]

exaprolol INN *antiadrenergic (β-receptor)* [also: exaprolol HCl]

exaprolol HCl USAN *antiadrenergic (β-receptor)* [also: exaprolol]

exatecan mesylate USAN *antineoplastic; topoisomerase I inhibitor for skin cancer*

Excedrin Aspirin Free caplets, geltabs OTC *analgesic; antipyretic; anti-inflammatory* [acetaminophen; caffeine] 500•65 mg

Excedrin Extra Strength caplets, tablets, geltabs OTC *analgesic; antipyretic; anti-inflammatory* [acetaminophen; aspirin; caffeine] 250•250•65 mg

Excedrin Migraine tablets OTC *analgesic for relief of migraine headache syndrome, including prodrome, pain, and associated symptoms* [acetaminophen; aspirin; caffeine] 250•250•65 mg

Excedrin P.M. oral liquid, liquigels OTC *antihistaminic sleep aid; analgesic* [diphenhydramine HCl; acetaminophen] 50•1000 mg/30 mL; 25•500 mg

Excedrin P.M. tablets, caplets, geltabs OTC *antihistaminic sleep aid; analgesic* [diphenhydramine citrate; acetaminophen] 38•500 mg

Excedrin QuickTabs (orally dissolving tablets) OTC *analgesic; antipyretic; anti-inflammatory* [acetaminophen; caffeine] 500•65 mg

Excedrin Sinus tablets, caplets (discontinued 2002) OTC *decongestant; analgesic; antipyretic* [pseudoephedrine HCl; acetaminophen] 30•500 mg

Excedrin Tension Headache caplets, geltabs OTC *analgesic; antipyretic; anti-inflammatory* [acetaminophen; caffeine] 500•65 mg

Excita Extra premedicated condom OTC *spermicidal/barrier contraceptive* [nonoxynol 9] 8%

ExeFen-PD extended-release caplets ℞ *decongestant; expectorant* [phenylephrine HCl; guaifenesin] 10•600 mg

Exelderm solution ℞ *topical antifungal* [sulconazole nitrate] 1%

Exelon capsules, oral solution ℞ *acetylcholinesterase inhibitor to increase cognition in Alzheimer disease* [rivastigmine tartrate] 1.5, 3, 4.5, 6 mg; 2 mg/mL

exemestane INN *aromatase inhibitor; antihormonal antineoplastic for advanced breast cancer in postmenopausal women (orphan)*

exenatide *incretin memetic agent; synthetic exendin-4 analogue to slow gastric emptying and improve glycemic control in type 2 diabetics*

exepanol INN

Exgest LA long-acting tablets (discontinued 2002) ℞ *decongestant; expectorant* [phenylpropanolamine HCl; guaifenesin] 75•400 mg

Ex-Histine syrup ℞ *decongestant; antihistamine; anticholinergic to dry mucosal secretions* [phenylephrine HCl; chlorpheniramine maleate; methscopolamine bromide] 20•4•2.5 mg/10 mL

Exidine Skin Cleanser; Exidine-2 Scrub; Exidine-4 Scrub topical liquid OTC *broad-spectrum antimicrobial; germicidal* [chlorhexidine gluconate; alcohol 4%] 4%; 2%; 4%

exifone INN

exiproben INN

exisulind *investigational (NDA filed, orphan) antineoplastic for familial adenomatous polyposis (FAP; also known as adenomatous polyposis coli, or APC); investigational (Phase III) for lung cancer*

Exjade ℞ *investigational (NDA filed, orphan) once-daily oral iron chelator for chronic iron overload due to blood transfusions* [deferasirox]

Ex-Lax tablets, chocolated chewable tablets OTC *stimulant laxative* [sennosides] 15 mg

Ex-Lax Gentle Strength caplets OTC *stimulant laxative; stool softener* [sennosides; docusate sodium] 10•65 mg

Ex-Lax Maximum Relief tablets OTC *stimulant laxative* [sennosides] 25 mg

Ex-Lax Stool Softener caplets OTC *laxative; stool softener* [docusate sodium] 100 mg

Exna tablets (discontinued 2003) ℞ *diuretic; antihypertensive* [benzthiazide] 50 mg

EXO-226 *investigational (Phase III) albumin glycation inhibitor for the prevention and treatment of diabetes-related kidney disease*

Exocaine Medicated Rub; Exocaine Plus Rub OTC *analgesic; counterirritant* [methyl salicylate] 25%; 30%

Exosurf ℞ *investigational (orphan) pulmonary surfactant for adult respiratory distress syndrome (ARDS)* [colfosceril palmitate]

Exosurf Neonatal intratracheal suspension ℞ *pulmonary surfactant for hyaline membrane disease and respiratory distress syndrome (orphan)* [colfosceril palmitate] 108 mg

Exosurf Neonatal powder for injection (discontinued 2003) ℞ *pulmonary surfactant for hyaline membrane disease and respiratory distress syndrome (orphan)* [colfosceril palmitate] 108 mg

expectorants *a class of drugs that promote the ejection of mucus from the respiratory tract*

Expidet (trademarked dosage form) *fast-dissolving dose*

Exratuss oral suspension ℞ *antitussive; decongestant; antihistamine* [carbetapentane tannate; phenylephrine tannate; chlorpheniramine tannate] 30•12.5•4 mg

Exsel lotion/shampoo (discontinued 2004) ℞ *antiseborrheic; dandruff treatment* [selenium sulfide] 2.5%

exsiccated sodium arsenate [see: sodium arsenate, exsiccated]

Extencap (trademarked dosage form) *extended-release capsule*

extended insulin zinc [see: insulin zinc, extended]

Extendryl chewable tablets, syrup ℞ *decongestant; antihistamine; anticholin-*

ergic to dry mucosal secretions [phenylephrine HCl; chlorpheniramine maleate; methscopolamine nitrate] 10•2•1.25 mg; 20•4•2.5 mg/10 mL

Extendryl JR sustained-release pediatric capsules ℞ *decongestant; antihistamine; anticholinergic to dry mucosal secretions* [phenylephrine HCl; chlorpheniramine maleate; methscopolamine nitrate] 10•4•1.25 mg

Extendryl SR sustained-release capsules ℞ *decongestant; antihistamine; anticholinergic to dry mucosal secretions* [phenylephrine HCl; chlorpheniramine maleate; methscopolamine nitrate] 20•8•2.5 mg

Extentab (trademarked dosage form) *extended-release tablet*

Extina foam ℞ *investigational (Phase III) antifungal for seborrheic dermatitis* [ketoconazole]

Extra Action Cough syrup OTC *antitussive; expectorant* [dextromethorphan hydrobromide; guaifenesin] 20•200 mg/10 mL

"Extra Strength" products [see under product name]

Extraneal IV infusion (supplied in Ultrabag and Ambu-Flex) ℞ *peritoneal dialysis solution for end-stage renal disease (orphan)* [icodextrin] 75 g

Exubera ℞ *investigational (NDA filed) inhaled aerosol dry powder insulin*

eye balm; eye root *medicinal herb* [see: goldenseal]

Eye Drops OTC *topical ophthalmic decongestant and vasoconstrictor* [tetrahydrozoline HCl] 0.05%

Eye Irrigating Solution OTC *extraocular irrigating solution* [sterile isotonic solution]

Eye Irrigating Wash OTC *extraocular irrigating solution* [sterile isotonic solution]

Eye Scrub solution OTC *eyelid cleanser for blepharitis or contact lenses*

Eye Stream ophthalmic solution OTC *extraocular irrigating solution* [sterile isotonic solution]

Eye Wash ophthalmic solution OTC *extraocular irrigating solution* [sterile isotonic solution]

eyebright (*Euphrasia officinalis; E. rostkoviana; E. strica*) plant *medicinal herb for blood cleansing, cataracts, colds, conjunctivitis, eye disorders and infections, and stimulating liver function; not generally regarded as safe and effective for topical ophthalmic use*

Eye-Lube-A eye drops OTC *ophthalmic moisturizer/lubricant* [glycerin] 0.25%

Eye-Sed eye drops (discontinued 2001) OTC *ophthalmic astringent* [zinc sulfate] 0.25%

Eyesine eye drops (discontinued 2003) OTC *ophthalmic decongestant; vasoconstrictor* [tetrahydrozoline HCl] 0.05%

EZ Detect test kit for home use *in vitro diagnostic aid for fecal occult blood*

ezetimibe USAN *antihyperlipidemic; intestinal cholesterol absorption inhibitor*

Ezide tablets ℞ *antihypertensive; diuretic* [hydrochlorothiazide] 50 mg

ezlopitant USAN *substance P receptor antagonist for emesis, pain, and inflammation*

E-Z-Paque oral suspension ℞ *radiopaque contrast agent* [barium sulfate] 6.2, 10, 12 oz.

1+1-F Creme ℞ *topical corticosteroidal anti-inflammatory; antifungal; antibacterial; local anesthetic* [hydrocortisone; clioquinol; pramoxine] 1%•3%•1%

¹⁸F [see: fludeoxyglucose F 18]

¹⁸F [see: sodium fluoride F 18]

FABRase ℞ *investigational (orphan) enzyme replacement therapy for Fabry disease* [agalsidase alfa]

Fabrazyme powder for IV infusion ℞ *enzyme replacement therapy for Fabry disease (orphan)* [agalsidase beta] 5.5, 37 mg/dose

FAC (fluorouracil, Adriamycin, cyclophosphamide) *chemotherapy protocol for breast cancer*

FAC-LEV (fluorouracil, Adriamycin, Cytoxin, levamisole) *chemotherapy protocol*

FAC-M (fluorouracil, Adriamycin, cyclophosphamide, methotrexate) *chemotherapy protocol*

Fact Plus test kit for home use *in vitro diagnostic aid; urine pregnancy test*

Factive film-coated tablets ℞ *broad-spectrum fluoroquinolone antibiotic for respiratory tract infections* [gemifloxacin mesylate] 320 mg

factor II (prothrombin)

factor III [see: thromboplastin]

factor VIIa, recombinant *coagulant for hemophilia A and B (orphan)*

factor VIII [see: antihemophilic factor]

factor VIII (rDNA) BAN *blood coagulating factor*

factor VIII fraction BAN *blood coagulating factor*

factor VIII SQ, recombinant *investigational (orphan) for long-term hemophilia A treatment or for surgical procedures*

factor IX complex USP *systemic hemostatic; antihemophilic for hemophilia B (orphan)* [also: factor IX fraction; nonacog alfa]

factor IX fraction BAN *systemic hemostatic; antihemophilic* [also: factor IX complex; nonacog alfa]

factor XIII, plasma-derived *investigational (orphan) hemostatic for congenital factor XIII deficiency*

factor XIII, recombinant *investigational (orphan) hemostatic for congenital factor XIII deficiency*

Factrel powder for subcu or IV injection ℞ *gonadotropin releasing hormone* [gonadorelin HCl] 100, 500 µg

fadrozole INN *antineoplastic; aromatase inhibitor* [also: fadrozole HCl]

fadrozole HCl USAN *antineoplastic; aromatase inhibitor* [also: fadrozole]

falintolol INN

falipamil INN

Falkochol ℞ *investigational (orphan) agent for congenital errors of cholesterol and bile acid synthesis* [dehydrocholic acid]

false foxglove *medicinal herb* [see: feverweed]

false unicorn (Chamaelirium luteum) root *medicinal herb used for amenorrhea, morning sickness, and preventing miscarriages; also used for colic, cough, and digestive, kidney, and prostate problems; emetic in high doses*

false valerian *medicinal herb* [see: life root]

false vervain *medicinal herb* [see: blue vervain]

FAM (fluorouracil, Adriamycin, mitomycin) *chemotherapy protocol for adenocarcinoma and gastric cancer*

FAM-CF (fluorouracil, Adriamycin, mitomycin, citrovorum factor) *chemotherapy protocol*

famciclovir USAN, INN, BAN *oral antiviral for herpes simplex type 2 (HSV-2, genital herpes) and herpes zoster (shingles) infections; suppressive therapy for recurrent outbreaks*

FAME; FAMe (fluorouracil, Adriamycin, MeCCNU) *chemotherapy protocol*

famiraprinium chloride INN

FAMMe (fluorouracil, Adriamycin, mitomycin, MeCCNU) *chemotherapy protocol*

famotidine USAN, USP, INN, BAN *histamine H_2 antagonist for gastric ulcers* 10, 20, 40 mg oral; 10 mg/mL injection

famotine INN *antiviral* [also: famotine HCl]

famotine HCl USAN *antiviral* [also: famotine]

fampridine USAN, INN *investigational (orphan) agent for multiple sclerosis and spinal cord injury*

famprofazone INN, BAN

FAM-S (fluorouracil, Adriamycin, mitomycin, streptozocin) *chemotherapy protocol*

FAMTX (fluorouracil, Adriamycin, methotrexate [with leucovorin rescue]) *chemotherapy protocol for gastric cancer*

Famvir film-coated tablets ℞ *antiviral for herpes simplex virus type 2 (HSV-2, genital herpes) and herpes zoster (shingles) infections; suppressive therapy for recurrent outbreaks* [famciclovir] 125, 250, 500 mg

fananserin USAN *antipsychotic; antischizophrenic; dopamine D_2 and serotonin 5-HT_2 receptor antagonist*

fanetizole INN, BAN *immunoregulator* [also: fanetizole mesylate]

fanetizole mesylate USAN *immunoregulator* [also: fanetizole]

Fansidar tablets ℞ *antimalarial* [sulfadoxine; pyrimethamine] 500•25 mg

fanthridone BAN *antidepressant* [also: fantridone HCl; fantridone]

fantridone INN *antidepressant* [also: fantridone HCl; fanthridone]

fantridone HCl USAN *antidepressant* [also: fantridone; fanthridone]

FAP (fluorouracil, Adriamycin, Platinol) *chemotherapy protocol for gastric cancer*

Farbee with Vitamin C caplets OTC *vitamin supplement* [multiple B vitamins; vitamin C] ≜•300 mg

Fareston tablets ℞ *antiestrogen antineoplastic for metastatic breast cancer in postmenopausal women (orphan); investigational (orphan) for desmoid tumors* [toremifene citrate] 60 mg

farglitazar USAN *thiazolidinedione antidiabetic; increases cellular response to insulin without increasing insulin secretion*

farnesil INN *combining name for radicals or groups*

fasiplon INN

Faslodex prefilled syringe for IM injection (once monthly) ℞ *antiestrogen antineoplastic for metastatic breast cancer in postmenopausal women* [fulvestrant] 50 mg/mL

Faspak (trademarked form) *flexible plastic bag*

Fastic (Japanese name for U.S. product Starlix)

Fastin capsules (discontinued 2001) ℞ *anorexiant; CNS stimulant* [phentermine HCl] 30 mg

Fast-Trak (trademarked delivery system) *quick-loading syringe*

fat, hard NF *suppository base*

fat emulsion, intravenous *parenteral essential fatty acid replacement*

Father John's Medicine Plus oral liquid OTC *antitussive; decongestant; antihistamine* [dextromethorphan hydrobromide; phenylephrine HCl; chlorpheniramine maleate] 10•10•4 mg/30 mL

Fatsia horrida *medicinal herb* [see: devil's club]

FazaClo orally disintegrating tablets ℞ *novel (atypical) dibenzapine antipsychotic for severe schizophrenia and recurrent suicidal behavior; sedative; also used for agitation and psychosis due to Alzheimer disease* [clozapine] 25, 100 mg

fazadinium bromide INN, BAN

fazarabine USAN, INN *antineoplastic*

5-FC (5-fluorocytosine) [see: flucytosine]

FCAP (fluorouracil, cyclophosphamide, Adriamycin, Platinol) *chemotherapy protocol*

FCE (fluorouracil, cisplatin, etoposide) *chemotherapy protocol*

F-CL (fluorouracil, leucovorin calcium [rescue]) *chemotherapy protocol for colorectal cancer* [also: FU/LV]

FCP (fluorouracil, cyclophosphamide, prednisone) *chemotherapy protocol*

FD&C Red No. 2 (Food, Drug & Cosmetic Act) [see: amaranth]

FD&C Red No. 3 (Food, Drug & Cosmetic Act) [see: erythrosine sodium]

F-ddA (fluorodideoxyadenosine) [see: lodenosine]

FDDNP ([18F] fluoroethyl [methyl] amino-2-naphthyl ethylidene malononitrile) *PET scan contrast medium for detection of β-amyloid senile plaques and neurofibrillary tangles for early detection of Alzheimer disease*

18FDG (fludeoxyglucose) [see: fludeoxyglucose F 18]

FDh (2(3H) furanone di-hydro) *a precursor to gamma hydroxybutyrate (GHB); a formerly legal alternative to GHB, now also illegal (Schedule I); also known as gamma butyrolactone (GBL)* [see: gamma hydroxybutyrate (GHB)]

Fe50 (or Fe50) extended-release caplets (discontinued 2005) OTC *hematinic; iron supplement* [ferrous sulfate, dried (source of iron)] 160 mg (50 mg)

59Fe [see: ferric chloride Fe 59]

59Fe [see: ferric citrate (59Fe)]

59Fe [see: ferrous citrate Fe 59]

59Fe [see: ferrous sulfate Fe 59]

febantel USAN, INN, BAN *veterinary anthelmintic*

febarbamate INN

febricides *a class of agents that relieve or reduce fever* [also called: antifebriles; antipyretics; antithermics; febrifuges]

febrifuges *a class of agents that relieve or reduce fever* [also called: antifebriles; antipyretics; antithermics; febricides]

febuprol INN

febuverine INN

febuxostat *investigational (NDA filed) selective xanthine oxidase inhibitor for gout*

FEC (fluorouracil, epirubicin, cyclophosphamide) *chemotherapy protocol for breast cancer*

feclemine INN

feclobuzone INN

FED (fluorouracil, etoposide, DDP) *chemotherapy protocol for non–small cell lung cancer (NSCLC)*

Fedahist tablets (discontinued 2002) OTC *decongestant; antihistamine* [pseudoephedrine HCl; chlorpheniramine maleate] 60•4 mg

Fedahist Timecaps (timed-release capsules), Gyrocaps (extended-release capsules) (discontinued 2002) ℞ *decongestant; antihistamine* [pseudoephedrine HCl; chlorpheniramine maleate] 120•8 mg; 65•10 mg

fedotozine INN *investigational kappa selective opioid agonist for irritable bowel syndrome*

fedrilate INN

Feen-A-Mint enteric-coated tablets OTC *stimulant laxative* [bisacodyl] 5 mg

Feiba VH Immuno IV injection or drip ℞ *antihemophilic to correct factor VIII deficiency and coagulation deficiency* [anti-inhibitor coagulant complex, vapor heated and freeze-dried] (each bottle is labeled with dosage)

felbamate USAN, INN *anticonvulsant; adjunctive therapy for Lennox-Gastaut syndrome (orphan)*

Felbatol tablets, oral suspension (the FDA and the manufacturer strongly caution against its use due to adverse side effects) ℞ *anticonvulsant; adjunctive therapy for Lennox-Gastaut syndrome (orphan)* [felbamate] 400, 600 mg; 600 mg/5 mL

felbinac USAN, INN, BAN *anti-inflammatory*

Feldene capsules ℞ *antiarthritic; nonsteroidal anti-inflammatory drug (NSAID)* [piroxicam] 10, 20 mg

felipyrine INN

felodipine USAN, INN, BAN *vasodilator;
antihypertensive; calcium channel blocker*

felonwood; felonwort *medicinal herb*
[see: bittersweet nightshade]

felvizumab USAN *monoclonal antibody
for prophylaxis and treatment of respiratory syncytial virus (RSV)*

felypressin USAN, INN, BAN *vasoconstrictor*

Fem pH vaginal jelly OTC *antibacterial;
acidity modifier* [acetic acid, glacial;
oxyquinoline sulfate] 0.9%•0.025%

Fem-1 tablets OTC *analgesic; anti-inflammatory; diuretic* [acetaminophen;
pamabrom] 500•25 mg

female fern *(Polypodium vulgare)*
root *medicinal herb used as an anthelmintic, cholagogue, demulcent, and
purgative*

female regulator *medicinal herb* [see:
life root]

Femara film-coated tablets ℞ *aromatase inhibitor; estrogen antagonist; antineoplastic for early, advanced, or metastatic breast cancer in postmenopausal
women* [letrozole] 2.5 mg

FemBack caplets OTC *analgesic; antihistaminic sleep aid* [acetaminophen;
salicylamide; phenyltoloxamine cit-
rate] 150•150•44 mg

FemCal tablets (discontinued 2002)
OTC *dietary supplement* [calcium carbonate; vitamin D; multiple miner-
als] 250 mg•100 IU• ±

femhrt 1/5 tablets (in packs of 28) ℞
*synthetic/equine hormones; hormone
replacement therapy for postmenopausal symptoms* [norethindrone acetate;
ethinyl estradiol] 1 mg•5 μg

femhrtLo tablets (in packs of 28) ℞
*synthetic/equine hormones; hormone
replacement therapy for postmenopausal symptoms* [norethindrone acetate;
ethinyl estradiol] 0.5 mg•2.5 μg

Feminique Disposable Douche solution OTC *antiseptic; antifungal; vaginal
cleanser and deodorizer; acidity modifier* [sodium benzoate; sorbic acid;
lactic acid]

Feminique Disposable Douche solution OTC *vaginal cleanser and deodorizer; acidity modifier* [vinegar (acetic
acid)]

Femiron tablets (discontinued 2005)
OTC *hematinic; iron supplement* [fer-
rous fumarate (source of iron)] 63
mg (20 mg) ⚇ Remeron

Femiron Multi-Vitamins and Iron
tablets (discontinued 2005) OTC
vitamin/iron supplement [multiple
vitamins; ferrous fumarate; folic
acid] ± •20•0.4 mg

Femizol-M vaginal cream OTC *antifungal* [miconazole nitrate] 2%

femoxetine INN

FemPatch transdermal patch (discontinued 2003) ℞ *estrogen replacement
therapy for postmenopausal symptoms*
[estradiol] 25 μg/day

Femring vaginal ring ℞ *synthetic estrogen; three-month hormone replacement
for postmenopausal atrophic vaginitis*
[estradiol acetate] 12.4 mg (50 μg/
day), 24.8 mg (100 μg day)

FemSoft urethral insert *treatment for
stress urinary incontinence* [silicone
plug]

Femstat 3 vaginal cream in prefilled
applicator (discontinued 2004) OTC
antifungal [butoconazole nitrate] 2%

FemStat One vaginal cream (discontinued 2001) OTC *antifungal* [buto-
conazole nitrate] 2%

Femtrace tablets ℞ *synthetic estrogen;
hormone replacement for postmenopausal symptoms* [estradiol acetate] 0.45,
0.9, 1.8 mg

fenabutene INN

fenacetinol INN

fenaclon INN

fenadiazole INN

fenaftic acid INN

fenalamide USAN, INN *smooth muscle
relaxant*

fenalcomine INN

fenamifuril INN

fenamisal INN *antibacterial; tuberculostatic* [also: phenyl aminosalicylate]

fenamole USAN, INN *anti-inflammatory*

fenaperone INN

fenarsone [see: carbarsone]

fenasprate [see: benorilate]

fenbendazole USAN, INN, BAN *anthelmintic*

fenbenicillin INN [also: phenbenicillin]

fenbufen USAN, INN, BAN *anti-inflammatory*

fenbutrazate INN [also: phenbutrazate]

fencamfamin INN, BAN

fencamfamin HCl [see: fencamfamin]

fencarbamide INN *anticholinergic* [also: phencarbamide]

fenchlorphos BAN *systemic insecticide* [also: ronnel; fenclofos]

fencilbutirol USAN, INN *choleretic*

fenclexonium metilsulfate INN

fenclofenac USAN, INN, BAN *anti-inflammatory*

fenclofos INN *systemic insecticide* [also: ronnel; fenchlorphos]

fenclonine USAN, INN *serotonin inhibitor*

fenclorac USAN, INN *anti-inflammatory*

fenclozic acid INN, BAN

fendiline INN

fendizoate INN *combining name for radicals or groups*

fendosal USAN, INN, BAN *anti-inflammatory*

feneritrol INN

Fenesin sustained-release tablets (discontinued 2004) ℞ *expectorant* [guaifenesin] 600 mg

Fenesin DM tablets ℞ *antitussive; expectorant* [dextromethorphan hydrobromide; guaifenesin] 30•600 mg

fenestrel USAN, INN *estrogen*

fenethazine INN

fenethylline BAN *CNS stimulant* [also: fenethylline HCl; fenetylline]

fenethylline HCl USAN *CNS stimulant* [also: fenetylline; fenethylline]

fenetradil INN

fenetylline INN *CNS stimulant* [also: fenethylline HCl; fenethylline]

fenflumizole INN

fenfluramine INN, BAN *anorexiant; CNS depressant* [also: fenfluramine HCl]

fenfluramine HCl USAN *anorexiant; CNS depressant* [also: fenfluramine]

fenfluthrin INN, BAN

fengabine USAN, INN, BAN *mood regulator*

fenharmane INN

fenimide USAN, INN, BAN *antipsychotic*

feniodium chloride INN

fenipentol INN

fenirofibrate INN

fenisorex USAN, INN, BAN *anorectic*

fenleuton USAN *5-lipoxygenase inhibitor*

fenmetozole INN *antidepressant; narcotic antagonist* [also: fenmetozole HCl]

fenmetozole HCl USAN *antidepressant; narcotic antagonist* [also: fenmetozole]

fenmetramide USAN, INN, BAN *antidepressant*

fennel (Anethum foeniculum; Foeniculum officinale; F. vulgare) seeds *medicinal herb for colic, gas, intestinal problems, promoting expectoration, stimulating lactation and menses, and sedation in children*

fennel oil NF

fenobam USAN, INN *sedative*

fenocinol INN

fenoctimine INN *gastric antisecretory* [also: fenoctimine sulfate]

fenoctimine sulfate USAN *gastric antisecretory* [also: fenoctimine]

fenofibrate INN, BAN *antihyperlipidemic for primary hypercholesterolemia (types IIa and IIb hyperlipidemia), hypertriglyceridemia (types IV and V hyperlipidemia), and mixed dyslipidemia; also used for hyperuricemia* 67, 134, 200 mg oral

fenoldopam INN, BAN *vasodilator for hypertensive emergencies; dopamine agonist* [also: fenoldopam mesylate]

fenoldopam mesylate USAN *vasodilator for hypertensive emergencies; dopamine agonist* [also: fenoldopam] 10 mg/mL injection

fenoprofen USAN, INN, BAN *analgesic; antiarthritic; nonsteroidal anti-inflammatory drug (NSAID)*

fenoprofen calcium USAN, USP, BAN *analgesic; antiarthritic; nonsteroidal anti-inflammatory drug (NSAID)* 200, 300, 600 mg oral

fenoterol USAN, INN, BAN *bronchodilator; β-blocker* [also: fenoterol hydrobromide]

fenoterol hydrobromide JAN *investigational (NDA filed) bronchodilator; antiasthmatic; β-blocker* [also: fenoterol]

fenoverine INN

fenoxazol [see: pemoline]

fenoxazoline INN

fenoxazoline HCl [see: fenoxazoline]

fenoxedil INN

fenoxypropazine INN [also: phenoxypropazine]

fenozolone INN

fenpentadiol INN

fenperate INN

fenpipalone USAN, INN *anti-inflammatory*

fenpipramide INN, BAN

fenpiprane INN, BAN

fenpiprane HCl [see: fenpiprane]

fenpiverinium bromide INN

fenprinast INN *bronchodilator; antiallergic* [also: fenprinast HCl]

fenprinast HCl USAN *bronchodilator; antiallergic* [also: fenprinast]

fenproporex INN

fenprostalene USAN, INN, BAN *luteolysin*

fenquizone USAN, INN *diuretic*

fenretinide USAN, INN *synthetic retinoid; investigational (Phase III) chemopreventative for breast, bladder, oral, and skin cancers*

fenspiride INN *bronchodilator; antiadrenergic (α-receptor)* [also: fenspiride HCl]

fenspiride HCl USAN *bronchodilator; antiadrenergic (α-receptor)* [also: fenspiride]

fentanyl INN, BAN *narcotic analgesic; also abused as a street drug* [also: fentanyl citrate] 25, 50, 75, 100 μg/hr. transdermal ⧈ Sentinel

fentanyl citrate USAN, USP, JAN *narcotic analgesic; adjunct to anesthesia; also abused as a street drug* [also: fentanyl] 50 μg/mL injection

Fentanyl Oralet lozenges (discontinued 2005) ℞ *oral transmucosal narcotic analgesic for anesthesia premedication* [fentanyl citrate] 100, 200, 300, 400 μg

fenthion BAN

fentiazac USAN, INN, BAN *anti-inflammatory*

fenticlor USAN, INN, BAN *topical anti-infective*

fenticonazole INN, BAN *antifungal* [also: fenticonazole nitrate]

fenticonazole nitrate USAN *antifungal* [also: fenticonazole]

fentonium bromide INN

fenugreek (Trigonella foenum-graecum) seeds *medicinal herb for boils, bronchial secretions, cellulitis, diabetes, hypercholesterolemia, kidney stones, lung infections, promoting expectoration, stomach irritation, and tuberculosis*

fenyramidol INN *analgesic; skeletal muscle relaxant* [also: phenyramidol HCl]

fenyripol INN *skeletal muscle relaxant* [also: fenyripol HCl]

fenyripol HCl USAN *skeletal muscle relaxant* [also: fenyripol]

Feocyte prolonged-action tablets ℞ *hematinic* [iron (as ferrous fumarate, ferrous gluconate, and ferrous sulfate); desiccated liver; vitamins B_6, B_{12}, and C; folic acid] 110•15•2•0.05•100•0.8 mg

FeoGen capsules ℞ *hematinic* [ferrous fumarate; cyanocobalamin; ascorbic acid; intrinsic factor concentrate] 66•0.01•250•100 mg

FeoGen FA; FeoGen Forte gelcaps ℞ *hematinic; vitamin/iron supplement* [iron; vitamins B_{12} & C; folic acid] 66•0.01•250•1 mg; 151•0.01•60•1 mg

Feosol elixir (discontinued 2005) OTC *hematinic; iron supplement* [ferrous sulfate (source of iron)] 220 mg/5 mL (44 mg/5 mL) ⧈ Feostat; Fer-In-Sol; Festal

Feosol tablets OTC *hematinic; iron supplement* [carbonyl iron] [note: one of three different products with the same name] 45 mg

Feosol tablets OTC *hematinic; iron supplement* [ferrous sulfate (source of iron)] [note: one of three different products with the same name] 325 mg (65 mg)

Feosol tablets OTC *hematinic; iron supplement* [ferrous sulfate, dried (source of iron)] [note: one of three different products with the same name] 200 mg (65 mg)

Feostat chewable tablets OTC *hematinic; iron supplement* [ferrous fumarate (source of iron)] 100 mg (33 mg) ⊉ Feosol

Feostat suspension, drops (discontinued 2005) OTC *hematinic; iron supplement* [ferrous fumarate (source of iron)] 100 mg/5 mL (33 mg/5 mL); 45 mg/ 0.6 mL (15 mg/0.6 mL) ⊉ Feosol

fepentolic acid INN

fepitrizol INN

fepradinol INN

feprazone INN, BAN

fepromide INN

feprosidnine INN

Feratab tablets OTC *hematinic; iron supplement* [ferrous sulfate, dried (source of iron)] 187 mg (60 mg)

Fer-Gen-Sol drops OTC *hematinic; iron supplement* [ferrous sulfate (source of iron)] 75 mg/0.6 mL (15 mg/0.6 mL)

Fergon tablets OTC *hematinic; iron supplement* [ferrous gluconate (source of iron)] 225 mg (27 mg)

Feridex IV injection ℞ *contrast agent for MRI of the liver* [ferumoxides] (11.2 mg iron)

Fer-In-Sol drops OTC *hematinic; iron supplement* [ferrous sulfate (source of iron)] 75 mg/0.6 mL (15 mg/0.6 mL)

Fer-In-Sol syrup (discontinued 2005) OTC *hematinic* [ferrous sulfate (source of iron)] 90 mg/5 mL (18 mg/5 mL)

Fer-Iron drops (discontinued 2005) OTC *hematinic* [ferrous sulfate (source of iron)] 75 mg/0.6 mL (15 mg/0.6 mL)

fermium *element (Fm)*

fern; fern brake *medicinal herb* [see: buckhorn brake; female fern]

fern, flowering; king's fern; water fern *medicinal herb* [see: buckhorn brake]

fern-leaved foxglove *medicinal herb* [see: feverweed]

Fero-Folic-500 controlled-release Filmtabs (film-coated tablets) ℞ *hematinic* [ferrous sulfate; ascorbic acid; folic acid] 105•500•0.8 mg

Fero-Grad-500 controlled-release tablets OTC *hematinic; vitamin/iron supplement* [ferrous sulfate; sodium ascorbate] 105 mg Fe•500 mg

FeroSul tablets OTC *hematinic; iron supplement* [ferrous sulfate (source of iron)] 325 mg (65 mg)

Ferotrinsic capsules ℞ *hematinic* [ferrous fumarate; cyanocobalamin; ascorbic acid; intrinsic factor concentrate; folic acid] 110 mg•15 μg• 75 mg•240 mg•0.5 mg

Ferralet Plus tablets OTC *hematinic* [ferrous gluconate; cyanocobalamin; ascorbic acid; folic acid] 46 mg•25 μg•400 mg•0.8 mg

Ferretts film-coated caplets OTC *hematinic; iron supplement* [ferrous fumarate (source of iron)] 325 mg (106 mg)

Ferrex 150 capsules OTC *hematinic; iron supplement* [polysaccharide iron complex] 150 mg Fe

Ferrex 150 Forte capsules ℞ *hematinic* [polysaccharide iron complex; vitamin B_{12}; folic acid] 150 mg iron•25 μg•1 mg

Ferrex 150 Forte Plus capsules ℞ *hematinic* [polysaccharide iron complex; vitamins B_{12} and C; folic acid] 150•0.025•60•1 mg

Ferrex 150 Plus capsules OTC *hematinic; vitamin/iron supplement* [polysaccharide iron complex; vitamin C] 150 mg Fe•50 mg

Ferrex PC; Ferrex PC Forte film-coated tablets ℞ *vitamin/mineral/iron supplement for pregnancy and lactation* [multiple vitamins & minerals; polysaccharide iron complex; folic acid] ≟•60 mg Fe•1 mg

ferric ammonium citrate NF

ferric ammonium sulfate

ferric cacodylate NF

ferric chloride (FeCl₃)

ferric chloride Fe 59 (⁵⁹FeCl₃) USAN *radioactive agent*

ferric citrate (⁵⁹Fe) INN

ferric citrochloride NF

ferric fructose USAN, INN *hematinic*

ferric glycerophosphate NF

ferric hexacyanoferrate *investigational (orphan) agent for internal contamination with radioactive or nonradioactive cesium or thallium*

ferric hyaluronate *adhesion barrier for open gynecological and lower GI surgery*

ferric hydroxide sucrose complex [see: iron sucrose; saccharated ferric oxide]

ferric hypophosphite NF

ferric oxide NF *coloring agent*

ferric oxide, red NF

ferric oxide, yellow NF

ferric pyrophosphate, soluble NF

ferric subsulfate NF *hemostatic used in a solution or paste to control superficial bleeding from skin biopsies, cervical biopsies, colposcopy, etc.*

ferricholinate [see: ferrocholinate]

ferriclate calcium sodium USAN *hematinic* [also: calcium sodium ferriclate]

Ferriprox Ŗ *investigational (orphan) agent for chronic iron overload due to transfusion-dependent anemias* [deferiprone]

ferristene USAN *paramagnetic imaging agent for MRI*

Ferrlecit IV infusion Ŗ *hematinic for iron deficiency due to chronic hemodialysis with erythropoietin therapy* [sodium ferric gluconate (source of iron)] 62.5 mg Fe/5 mL

ferrocholate [see: ferrocholinate]

ferrocholinate INN

Ferromar sustained-release caplets OTC *hematinic* [ferrous fumarate; vitamin C] 201.5•200 mg

ferropolimaler INN

Ferro-Sequels timed-release tablets OTC *hematinic; iron supplement; stool softener* [ferrous fumarate (source of iron); docusate sodium] 150 (50)•100 mg

ferrotrenine INN

ferrous citrate Fe 59 USAN, USP *radioactive agent*

ferrous fumarate USP *hematinic; iron supplement (33% elemental iron)* 90, 324 mg oral

ferrous gluconate USP *hematinic; iron supplement (11.6% elemental iron)* 225, 300, 324, 325 mg oral

ferrous lactate NF

ferrous orotate JAN

ferrous sulfate (FeSO₄.7H₂O) USP, JAN *hematinic; iron supplement (20% elemental iron)* 325 mg oral; 220 mg/5 mL oral; 75 mg/0.6 mL oral

ferrous sulfate, dried (FeSO₄.xH₂O) USP *hematinic; iron supplement (30% elemental iron)* 160 mg oral

ferrous sulfate, exsiccated [see: ferrous sulfate, dried]

ferrous sulfate Fe 59 (⁵⁹FeSO₄) USAN *radioactive agent*

Fertinex subcu injection (discontinued 2003) Ŗ *follicle-stimulating hormone (FSH); ovulation stimulant for polycystic ovary disease (orphan) and assisted reproductive technologies (ART); investigational (orphan) for spermatogenesis in hormone-deficient males* [urofollitropin] 75, 150 IU

fertirelin INN, BAN *veterinary gonadotropin-releasing hormone* [also: fertirelin acetate]

fertirelin acetate USAN *veterinary gonadotropin-releasing hormone* [also: fertirelin]

ferucarbotran USAN *superparamagnetic diagnostic aid*

Ferula assafoetida; F. foetida; F. rubricaulis *medicinal herb* [see: asafetida; asafoetida]

ferumoxides USAN *diagnostic aid for magnetic resonance imaging of the liver*

ferumoxsil USAN *oral MRI contrast medium for upper GI tract imaging*

ferumoxtran-10 USAN *superparamagnetic diagnostic aid*

FeSO₄ (ferrous sulfate) [q.v.]

Fetal Fibronectin Test kit for professional use *in vitro diagnostic aid for fetal fibronectin in vaginal secretions at*

24–34 weeks, a predictor of preterm delivery

fetal neural cells [see: neural cells, porcine fetal]

fetid hellebore *(Helleborus foetidus)* [see: hellebore]

Fe-Tinic 150 capsules ℞ *hematinic* [polysaccharide-iron complex] 150 mg Fe

Fe-Tinic 150 Forte capsules ℞ *hematinic* [polysaccharide iron complex; vitamin B$_{12}$; folic acid] 150 mg Fe• 25 μg•1 mg

fetoxilate INN *smooth muscle relaxant* [also: fetoxylate HCl; fetoxylate]

fetoxylate BAN *smooth muscle relaxant* [also: fetoxylate HCl; fetoxilate]

fetoxylate HCl USAN *smooth muscle relaxant* [also: fetoxilate; fetoxylate]

fever root *medicinal herb* [see: coral root]

fever twig *medicinal herb* [see: bittersweet nightshade]

Feverall, Children's; Infant's Feverall; Junior Feverall suppositories OTC *analgesic; antipyretic* [acetaminophen] 120 mg; 80 mg; 325 mg

Feverall, Children's; Junior Feverall Sprinkle Caps (powder) OTC *analgesic; antipyretic* [acetaminophen] 80 mg; 160 mg ⊉ Fiberall

feverbush *medicinal herb* [see: winterberry]

feverfew *(Chrysanthemum parthenium; Leucanthemum parthenium; Pyrethrum parthenium; Tanacetum parthenium)* leaves and flowers *medicinal herb used as an aspirin substitute for chills, colds, fever, inflammation, and migraine and sinus headache*

feverweed *(Gerardia pedicularia)* plant *medicinal herb used as an antiseptic, diaphoretic, febrifuge, and sedative*

fexicaine INN, DCF

Fexicam ⒶⓊ suppositories ℞ *nonsteroidal anti-inflammatory drug (NSAID) for rheumatoid arthritis, osteoarthritis, ankylosing spondylitis, and primary dysmenorrhea* [piroxicam] 20 mg

fexinidazole INN

fexofenadine HCl USAN *second-generation peripherally selective piperidine anti-histamine for allergic rhinitis and chronic idiopathic urticaria* 30, 60, 180 mg oral

fezatione INN

fezolamine INN *antidepressant* [also: fezolamine fumarate]

fezolamine fumarate USAN *antidepressant* [also: fezolamine]

FGN-1 [now: exisulind]

fiacitabine (FIAC) USAN, INN *antiviral; investigational (Phase I/II) for HIV and AIDS*

fialuridine (FIAU) USAN, INN *antiviral; investigational (orphan) for chronic active hepatitis B*

Fiberall powder OTC *bulk laxative* [psyllium hydrophilic mucilloid] 3.5 g/tsp.

FiberCon tablets OTC *bulk laxative; antidiarrheal* [calcium polycarbophil] 500 mg

Fiberlan oral liquid OTC *enteral nutritional therapy* [lactose-free formula]

Fiber-Lax tablets OTC *bulk laxative; antidiarrheal* [calcium polycarbophil] 625 mg

FiberNorm tablets OTC *bulk laxative; antidiarrheal* [calcium polycarbophil] 625 mg

fibracillin INN

fibrin INN

fibrinase [see: factor XIII]

fibrinogen (^{125}I) INN [also: fibrinogen I 125]

fibrinogen, human USP *investigational (orphan)*

fibrinogen I 125 USAN *vascular patency test; radioactive agent* [also: fibrinogen (^{125}I)]

fibrinoligase [see: factor XIII]

fibrinolysin, human INN [also: plasmin]

fibrin-stabilizing factor (FSF) [see: factor XIII]

fibroblast growth factor, basic (bFGF) [see: ersofermin]

fibroblast interferon [now: interferon beta]

Fibrogammin P ℞ *investigational (orphan) hemostatic for congenital factor XIII deficiency* [factor XIII, plasma-derived]

fibronectin *investigational (orphan) for nonhealing corneal ulcers or epithelial defects*

Ficus carica medicinal herb [see: fig]

Fidelin ℞ *natural hormone precursor; investigational (NDA filed, orphan) for systemic lupus erythematosus (SLE); investigational (orphan) replacement therapy for adrenal insufficiency* [dehydroepiandrosterone (DHEA)]

fiduxosin HCl USAN α_{1a}-*adrenoceptor antagonist for benign prostatic hyperplasia (BPH)*

50% Dextrose with Electrolyte Pattern A (or N) IV *infusion* (discontinued 2001) ℞ *intravenous nutritional/electrolyte therapy* [combined electrolyte solution; dextrose]

fig (Ficus carica) *fruit medicinal herb used as a demulcent, emollient, and laxative*

figwort (Scrophularia nodosa) *leaves, stems, and roots medicinal herb for abrasions, athlete's foot, cradle cap, fever, impetigo, restlessness, skin diseases, and skin tumors*

filaminast USAN *selective phosphodiesterase IV inhibitor for asthma*

filenadol INN

filgrastim USAN, INN, BAN *hematopoietic stimulant for severe chronic neutropenia (orphan); investigational (Phase III, orphan) cytokine for AIDS-related cytomegalovirus retinitis; investigational (orphan) for myelodysplastic syndrome*

Filipendula ulmaria medicinal herb [see: meadowsweet]

filipin USAN, INN *antifungal*

Filmlok (trademarked dosage form) *film-coated tablet*

Filmseal (trademarked dosage form) *film-coated tablet*

Filmtabs (trademarked dosage form) *film-coated tablets*

FIME (fluorouracil, ICRF-159, MeCCNU) *chemotherapy protocol*

Finac lotion OTC *keratolytic for acne* [salicylic acid; isopropyl alcohol] 2%•22.5%

Finacea gel ℞ *antimicrobial and keratolytic for mild to moderate rosacea* [azelaic acid] 15%

Finajet; Finaplix *brand names for trenbolone acetate, a European veterinary anabolic steroid abused as a street drug*

finasteride USAN, INN, BAN α-*reductase inhibitor; androgen hormone inhibitor for benign prostatic hyperplasia (BPH) and androgenic alopecia in men*

Finevin cream ℞ *antimicrobial and keratolytic for inflammatory acne vulgaris* [azelaic acid] 20%

finger leaf *medicinal herb* [see: cinquefoil]

Fioricet tablets ℞ *analgesic; barbiturate sedative* [acetaminophen; caffeine; butalbital] 325•40•50 mg ⚠ Lorcet

Fioricet with Codeine capsules ℞ *narcotic antitussive; analgesic; barbiturate sedative* [codeine phosphate; acetaminophen; caffeine; butalbital] 30•325•40•50 mg

Fiorinal capsules ℞ *analgesic; barbiturate sedative* [aspirin; caffeine; butalbital] 325•40•50 mg ⚠ Florinef

Fiorinal with Codeine capsules ℞ *narcotic antitussive; analgesic; barbiturate sedative* [codeine phosphate; aspirin; caffeine; butalbital] 30•325•40•50 mg

Fiorinal-C ¼; Fiorinal-C ½ ⓒ capsules ℞ *narcotic antitussive; analgesic; barbiturate sedative* [codeine phosphate; aspirin; caffeine; butalbital] 15•330•40•50 mg; 30•330•40•50 mg

Fiortal capsules (discontinued 2004) ℞ *analgesic; barbiturate sedative* [aspirin; caffeine; butalbital] 325•40•50 mg

fipexide INN

fire ant venom allergenic extract *investigational (orphan) skin test and immunotherapy for fire ant reactions*

fireweed *medicinal herb* [see: pilewort]

First Choice reagent strips for home use *in vitro diagnostic aid for blood glucose*

First Response; First Response Early Result test stick for home use *in vitro diagnostic aid; urine pregnancy test*

First Response Ovulation Predictor test kit for home use *in vitro diagnostic aid to predict ovulation time*

fisalamine [see: mesalamine]

fit root (Monotropa uniflora) *medicinal herb used as an antispasmodic, febrifuge, nervine, and sedative*

FIV-ASA suppositories ℞ *anti-inflammatory for active ulcerative colitis, proctosigmoiditis, and proctitis* [mesalamine (5-aminosalicylic acid)] 500 mg

5 + 2 protocol (cytarabine, daunorubicin) *chemotherapy protocol for acute myelocytic leukemia (AML)*

5 + 2 protocol (cytarabine, mitoxantrone) *chemotherapy protocol for acute myelocytic leukemia (AML)*

5-ALA HCl; ALA [see: aminolevulinic acid HCl]

5% Alcohol and 5% Dextrose in Water; 10% Alcohol and 5% Dextrose in Water IV infusion ℞ *for caloric replacement and rehydration* [dextrose; alcohol] 5%•5%; 10%•5%

5 Benzagel; 10 Benzagel gel ℞ *topical keratolytic for acne* [benzoyl peroxide] 5%; 10%

5% Travert and Electrolyte No. 2; 10% Travert and Electrolyte No. 2 IV infusion ℞ *intravenous nutritional/electrolyte therapy* [combined electrolyte solution; invert sugar (50% dextrose + 50% fructose)]

506U78 *investigational (orphan) for chronic lymphocytic leukemia*

5-FC (5-fluorocytosine) [see: flucytosine]

five-finger grass; five fingers *medicinal herb* [see: cinquefoil]

five-fingers root *medicinal herb* [see: ginseng]

5-HT (5-hydroxytryptamine) [see: serotonin]

5-HT$_3$ (hydroxytryptamine) receptor antagonists *a class of antiemetic and antinauseant agents used primarily after emetogenic cancer chemotherapy* [also called: selective serotonin 5-HT$_3$ blockers]

5-HTP (5-hydroxytryptophan) [see: L-5 hydroxytryptophan]

FL (flutamide, leuprolide acetate) *chemotherapy protocol for prostate cancer*

FLAC (fluorouracil, leucovorin [rescue], Adriamycin, cyclophosphamide) *chemotherapy protocol*

flag, sweet; myrtle flag *medicinal herb* [see: calamus]

flag lily; poison flag; water flag *medicinal herb* [see: blue flag]

Flagyl film-coated tablets, capsules ℞ *antibiotic; antiprotozoal; amebicide* [metronidazole] 250, 500 mg; 375 mg

Flagyl ER film-coated extended-release tablets ℞ *once-daily antibiotic for bacterial vaginosis* [metronidazole] 750 mg

Flagyl IV powder for injection ℞ *antibiotic; antiprotozoal; amebicide* [metronidazole HCl] 500 mg

Flagyl IV RTU (ready-to-use) injection ℞ *antibiotic; antiprotozoal; amebicide* [metronidazole] 500 mg/100 mL

flamenol INN

Flanders Buttocks ointment OTC *topical diaper rash treatment* [zinc oxide; peruvian balsam]

flannel flower *medicinal herb* [see: mullein]

FLAP (fluorouracil, leucovorin [rescue], Adriamycin, Platinol) *chemotherapy protocol*

Flarex Drop-Tainers (eye drop suspension) ℞ *topical ophthalmic corticosteroidal anti-inflammatory* [fluorometholone acetate] 0.1%

FlashDose (trademarked delivery system) *orally disintegrating tablets*

Flatulex drops OTC *antiflatulent* [simethicone] 40 mg/0.6 mL

Flatulex tablets OTC *adsorbent; detoxicant; antiflatulent* [activated charcoal; simethicone] 250•80 mg

flavamine INN

flavine [see: acriflavine HCl]

flavocoxid *natural flavonoids and flavins; natural COX-2 inhibitor; analgesic and anti-inflammatory for the dietary management of osteoarthritis*

flavodic acid INN

flavodilol INN *antihypertensive* [also: flavodilol maleate]

flavodilol maleate USAN *antihypertensive* [also: flavodilol]

flavonoid [see: troxerutin]

Flavons tablets OTC *dietary supplement* [mixed bioflavonoids] 500 mg

Flavons-500 tablets OTC *dietary supplement* [citrus bioflavonoids] 500 mg

flavopiridol *investigational (Phase III) kinase inhibitor for lung cancer*

flavoxate INN, BAN *smooth muscle relaxant; urinary antispasmodic* [also: flavoxate HCl]

flavoxate HCl USAN *anticholinergic; smooth muscle relaxant; urinary antispasmodic* [also: flavoxate] 100 mg oral

flaxseed (Linum usitatissimum) *medicinal herb for arthritis, autoimmune diseases, colds, constipation, cough, heart disease, lowering cholesterol levels, skin disorders, and urinary tract infections*

flazalone USAN, INN, BAN *anti-inflammatory*

FLe (fluorouracil, levamisole) *chemotherapy protocol for colorectal cancer*

flea seed; fleawort *medicinal herb* [see: plantain]

fleabane; horseweed (Erigeron canadensis) *plant medicinal herb used as an astringent, diuretic, and hemostatic*

fleawort; flea seed *medicinal herb* [see: plantain]

Flebogamma 5% IV infusion R *passive immunizing agent for primary (inherited) immunodeficiency disorders* [immune globulin] 5% (50 mg/mL)

flecainide INN, BAN *antiarrhythmic* [also: flecainide acetate]

flecainide acetate USAN *antiarrhythmic* [also: flecainide] 50, 100, 150 mg oral

Fleet disposable enema OTC *saline laxative* [sodium phosphate, monobasic; sodium phosphate, dibasic] 7•19 g/118 mL dose

Fleet Babylax rectal liquid OTC *hyperosmolar laxative* [glycerin] 4 mL/dose

Fleet Bisacodyl disposable enema OTC *stimulant laxative* [bisacodyl] 10 mg/30 mL dose

Fleet Laxative enteric-coated tablets, suppositories OTC *stimulant laxative* [bisacodyl] 5 mg; 10 mg

Fleet Medicated Wipes cleansing pads OTC *moisturizer and cleanser for external rectal/vaginal areas; astringent; antiseptic; antifungal* [hamamelis water; glycerin; alcohol] 50%•10%•7%

Fleet Mineral Oil disposable enema OTC *emollient laxative* [mineral oil] 118 mL dose

Fleet Pain Relief anorectal wipes OTC *topical local anesthetic* [pramoxine HCl; glycerin] 1%•12%

Fleet Phospho-Soda oral solution OTC *saline laxative* [sodium phosphate, monobasic; sodium phosphate, dibasic] 2.4•0.9 g/5 mL

Fleet Prep Kits No. 1 to No. 3 OTC *pre-procedure bowel evacuant* [other Fleet products in combination kits]

FLEP (fluorouracil, leucovorin, etoposide, Platinol) *chemotherapy protocol*

flerobuterol INN

fleroxacin USAN, INN *antibacterial*

flesinoxan INN *investigational (Phase III) antidepressant and anxiolytic*

flestolol INN *antiadrenergic (β-receptor)* [also: flestolol sulfate]

flestolol sulfate USAN *antiadrenergic (β-receptor)* [also: flestolol]

fletazepam USAN, INN, BAN *skeletal muscle relaxant*

Fletcher's Castoria oral liquid OTC *stimulant laxative* [senna concentrate] 33.3 mg/mL

fleur-de-lis *medicinal herb* [see: blue flag]

Flex-all 454 gel OTC *analgesic; antipruritic; counterirritant; topical local anesthetic* [methyl salicylate; menthol] 2•16%

Flexaphen capsules R *skeletal muscle relaxant; analgesic* [chlorzoxazone; acetaminophen] 250•300 mg

Flex-Care Especially for Sensitive Eyes solution OTC *chemical disinfecting solution for soft contact lenses* [note: soft contact indication different from RGP contact indication for same product]

Flex-Care Especially for Sensitive Eyes solution OTC *disinfecting/wetting/soaking solution for rigid gas permeable contact lenses* [note: RGP contact indication different from soft contact indication for same product]

Flexderm sheets *absorbent wound dressing* [hydrogel polymer]

Flexeril film-coated tablets ℞ *skeletal muscle relaxant* [cyclobenzaprine HCl] 5, 10 mg ⊠ Flaxedil

FlexiGel Strands wound dressing OTC *absorbent dressing*

Flexoject IV or IM injection ℞ *skeletal muscle relaxant* [orphenadrine citrate] 30 mg/mL

Flexon IV or IM injection ℞ *skeletal muscle relaxant* [orphenadrine citrate] 30 mg/mL

FlexPack HP test for professional use *diagnostic aid for serum IgG antibodies to* H. pylori *(for peptic ulcers)*

FlexPen (trademarked form) *disposable prefilled self-injector for insulin*

Flex-Power Performance Sports cream OTC *analgesic* [trolamine salicylate] 10%

Flextra-DS tablets ℞ *analgesic; antipyretic; antihistaminic sleep aid* [acetaminophen; phenyltoloxamine citrate] 500•50 mg

Flexzan; Flexzan Extra adhesive sheets *absorbent, semi-occlusive wound dressing* [polyurethane foam]

flibanserin USAN *antidepressant*

Flintstones Children's; Flintstones Plus Calcium; Flintstones Plus Extra C Children's chewable tablets OTC *vitamin supplement* [multiple vitamins; folic acid] ≛•0.3 mg

Flintstones Complete chewable tablets OTC *vitamin/mineral/iron supplement* [multiple vitamins & minerals; iron; folic acid; biotin] ≛•18 mg•0.4 mg•40 μg

Flintstones Plus Iron chewable tablets OTC *vitamin/iron supplement*

[multiple vitamins; iron; folic acid] ≛•15•0.3 mg

Flo-Coat oral/rectal suspension ℞ *radiopaque contrast medium for gastrointestinal imaging* [barium sulfate] 100%

floctafenine USAN, INN, BAN *analgesic*

Flolan IV infusion ℞ *platelet aggregation inhibitor and vasodilator for primary pulmonary hypertension (orphan); investigational (orphan) heparin replacement for hemodialysis* [epoprostenol] 0.5, 1.5 mg

Flomax capsules ℞ *α₁-adrenergic blocker for benign prostatic hyperplasia (BPH)* [tamsulosin HCl] 0.4 mg ⊠ Slow-Mag; Zomig

flomoxef INN

Flonase nasal spray ℞ *corticosteroidal anti-inflammatory for seasonal or perennial rhinitis* [fluticasone propionate] 50 μg/dose

Flo-Pack (trademarked packaging form) *vial for IV drip*

flopropione INN

Floranex chewable tablets OTC *probiotic; dietary supplement* [Lactobacillus acidophilus; L. bulgaricus] 1 million CFU mixed culture

florantyrone INN, BAN

flordipine USAN, INN *antihypertensive*

floredil INN

Florentine iris *medicinal herb* [see: orris root]

floretione [see: fluoresone]

florfenicol USAN, INN, BAN *veterinary antibacterial*

Florical capsules, tablets OTC *calcium/fluoride supplement* [calcium carbonate; sodium fluoride] 364•8.3 mg

Florida Sunburn Relief lotion OTC *analgesic; antipruritic; counterirritant* [phenol; camphor; menthol; benzyl alcohol] 0.4%•0.2%•0.15%•3%

florifenine INN

Florinef Acetate tablets ℞ *replacement therapy for adrenocortical insufficiency in Addison disease* [fludrocortisone acetate] 0.1 mg ⊠ Fiorinal

Florone cream, ointment ℞ *corticosteroidal anti-inflammatory* [diflorasone diacetate] 0.05%

Florone E cream ℞ *corticosteroidal anti-inflammatory; emollient* [diflorasone diacetate] 0.05%

floropipamide [now: pipamperone]

floropipeton [see: propyperone]

Florvite drops ℞ *pediatric vitamin supplement and dental caries preventative* [multiple vitamins; sodium fluoride] ±•0.25, ±•0.5 mg/mL

Florvite; Florvite Half Strength chewable tablets ℞ *pediatric vitamin supplement and dental caries preventative* [multiple vitamins; sodium fluoride; folic acid] ±•1•0.3 mg; ±•0.5•0.3 mg

Florvite + Iron drops ℞ *pediatric vitamin/iron supplement and dental caries preventative* [multiple vitamins & minerals; sodium fluoride; ferrous sulfate] ±•0.25•10, ±•0.5•10 mg/mL

Florvite + Iron; Half Strength Florvite + Iron chewable tablets ℞ *pediatric vitamin/iron supplement and dental caries preventative* [multiple vitamins & minerals; sodium fluoride; ferrous sulfate; folic acid] ±•1•12•0.3 mg; ±•0.5•12•0.3 mg

flosequinan USAN, INN, BAN *antihypertensive; vasodilator*

flotrenizine INN

Flovent metered dose inhaler, Diskus (inhalation powder) ℞ *corticosteroidal antiasthmatic* [fluticasone propionate] 44, 110, 220 μg/dose; 50, 100, 250 μg/dose

Flovent Rotadisk (inhalation powder) (discontinued 2004) ℞ *corticosteroidal antiasthmatic* [fluticasone propionate] 50, 100, 250 μg/dose

Flovent HFA inhalation aerosol in a metered-dose inhaler ℞ *corticosteroidal antiasthmatic* [fluticasone propionate] 44, 110, 220 μg/dose

floverine INN

flower velure *medicinal herb* [see: coltsfoot]

flower-de-luce *medicinal herb* [see: blue flag]

floxacillin USAN *antibacterial* [also: flucloxacillin]

floxacrine INN

Floxin film-coated tablets, UroPak (3-day supply) ℞ *broad-spectrum fluoroquinolone antibiotic* [ofloxacin] 200, 300, 400 mg; 6 tablets × 200 mg

Floxin IV injection (discontinued 2004) ℞ *broad-spectrum fluoroquinolone antibiotic* [ofloxacin] 200, 400 mg/vial

Floxin Otic ear drops ℞ *broad-spectrum fluoroquinolone antibiotic* [ofloxacin] 0.3% (3 mg/mL)

Floxin Otic Singles (premeasured containers) ℞ *broad-spectrum fluoroquinolone antibiotic* [ofloxacin] 0.3% (0.75 mg per 0.25 mL container)

floxuridine USAN, USP, INN *antimetabolic antineoplastic for GI adenocarcinoma metastatic to the liver* 500 mg injection

Flu, Cold & Cough Medicine powder for oral solution (discontinued 2002) OTC *antitussive; decongestant; antihistamine; analgesic* [dextromethorphan hydrobromide; pseudoephedrine HCl; chlorpheniramine maleate; acetaminophen] 20•60•4•500 mg/pkt.

Flu OIA (Optical ImmunoAssay) test for professional use *rapid (less than 20 minutes) diagnostic aid for influenza A and B in sputum, nasal aspirate, or nasopharyngeal swab*

fluacizine INN

flualamide INN

fluanisone INN, BAN

Fluarix ℞ *investigational (NDA filed) vaccine for influenza virus types A and B* [influenza split-virus vaccine, inactivated]

fluazacort USAN, INN *anti-inflammatory*

flubanilate INN *CNS stimulant* [also: flubanilate HCl]

flubanilate HCl USAN *CNS stimulant* [also: flubanilate]

flubendazole USAN, INN, BAN *antiprotozoal*

flubenisolone [see: betamethasone]

flubepride INN

flubuperone [see: melperone]

flucarbril INN

flucetorex INN

flucindole USAN, INN *antipsychotic*

fluciprazine INN

fluclorolone acetonide INN, BAN *corticosteroid; anti-inflammatory* [also: flucloronide]

flucloronide USAN *corticosteroid; anti-inflammatory* [also: fluclorolone acetonide]

flucloxacillin INN, BAN *antibacterial* [also: floxacillin]

fluconazole USAN, INN, BAN *systemic triazole antifungal* 50, 100, 150, 200 mg oral; 2 mg/mL injection

flucrilate INN *tissue adhesive* [also: flucrylate]

flucrylate USAN *tissue adhesive* [also: flucrilate]

flucytosine USAN, USP, INN, BAN *systemic antifungal*

fludalanine USAN, INN *antibacterial*

Fludara powder for IV injection ℞ *antineoplastic for chronic lymphocytic leukemia (CLL) and non-Hodgkin lymphoma (orphan)* [fludarabine phosphate] 50 mg

fludarabine INN *antimetabolite antineoplastic* [also: fludarabine phosphate]

fludarabine phosphate USAN *antimetabolite antineoplastic for chronic lymphocytic leukemia (CLL) and non-Hodgkin lymphoma (orphan)* [also: fludarabine] 25 mg injection

fludazonium chloride USAN, INN *topical anti-infective*

fludeoxyglucose (^{18}F) INN *diagnostic aid; radioactive agent* [also: fludeoxyglucose F 18]

fludeoxyglucose F 18 USAN, USP *diagnostic aid; radioactive agent* [also: fludeoxyglucose (^{18}F)]

fludiazepam INN

fludorex USAN, INN *anorectic; antiemetic*

fludoxopone INN

fludrocortisone INN, BAN *salt-regulating adrenocortical steroid; mineralocorticoid* [also: fludrocortisone acetate]

fludrocortisone acetate USP *salt-regulating adrenocortical steroid; mineralocorticoid; for adrenocortical insufficiency in Addison disease* [also: fludrocortisone] 0.1 mg oral

fludroxicortide [see: flurandrenolide]

fludroxycortide INN *topical corticosteroid* [also: flurandrenolide; flurandrenolone]

flufenamic acid USAN, INN, BAN *anti-inflammatory*

flufenisal USAN, INN *analgesic*

flufosal INN

flufylline INN

flugestone INN, BAN *progestin* [also: flurogestone acetate]

flugestone acetate [see: flurogestone acetate]

fluindarol INN

fluindione INN

Flumadine film-coated tablets, syrup ℞ *antiviral; prophylaxis and treatment for influenza A virus* [rimantadine HCl] 100 mg; 50 mg/5 mL

flumazenil USAN, INN, BAN *benzodiazepine antagonist to reverse anesthesia or treat overdose* 0.1 mg/mL injection

flumazepil [see: flumazenil]

flumecinol INN *investigational (orphan) agent for neonatal hyperbilirubinemia*

flumedroxone INN, BAN

flumequine USAN, INN, BAN *antibacterial*

flumeridone USAN, INN, BAN *antiemetic*

flumetasone INN *corticosteroid; anti-inflammatory* [also: flumethasone]

flumethasone USAN, BAN *topical corticosteroidal anti-inflammatory* [also: flumetasone]

flumethasone pivalate USAN, USP, BAN *topical corticosteroidal anti-inflammatory*

flumethiazide INN, BAN

flumethrin BAN

flumetramide USAN, INN *skeletal muscle relaxant*

flumexadol INN

flumezapine USAN, INN, BAN *antipsychotic; neuroleptic*

fluminorex USAN, INN *anorectic*

FluMist prefilled single-use intranasal sprayers ℞ *flu vaccine* [influenza virus vaccine, live attenuated] 0.5 mL/dose

flumizole USAN, INN *anti-inflammatory*

flumoxonide USAN, INN *adrenocortical steroid*

flunamine INN

flunarizine INN, BAN *vasodilator* [also: flunarizine HCl]

flunarizine HCl USAN *vasodilator; investigational (orphan) for alternating hemiplegia* [also: flunarizine]

flunidazole USAN, INN *antiprotozoal*

flunisolide USAN, USP, INN, BAN *corticosteroidal anti-inflammatory for chronic asthma and rhinitis* 0.025% (25 μg/dose) nasal spray

flunisolide acetate USAN *anti-inflammatory*

flunitrazepam USAN, INN, BAN, JAN *benzodiazepine sedative and hypnotic; also abused as a "date rape" street drug*

flunixin USAN, INN, BAN *anti-inflammatory; analgesic*

flunixin meglumine USAN *anti-inflammatory; analgesic*

flunoprost INN

flunoxaprofen INN

fluocinolide [now: fluocinonide]

fluocinolone BAN *topical corticosteroidal anti-inflammatory* [also: fluocinolone acetonide]

fluocinolone acetonide USAN, USP, INN *topical corticosteroidal anti-inflammatory; ocular implant for uveitis (orphan)* [also: fluocinolone] 0.01%, 0.025% topical

fluocinonide USAN, USP, INN, BAN *topical corticosteroidal anti-inflammatory* 0.05% topical

fluocortin INN *anti-inflammatory* [also: fluocortin butyl]

fluocortin butyl USAN, BAN *anti-inflammatory* [also: fluocortin]

fluocortolone USAN, INN, BAN *corticosteroid; anti-inflammatory*

fluocortolone caproate USAN *corticosteroid; anti-inflammatory*

Fluogen IM injection, Steri-Vials, Steri-Dose (disposable syringes) (discontinued 2001) ℞ *flu vaccine* [influenza split-virus vaccine] 0.5 mL/dose

Fluonex cream ℞ *corticosteroidal anti-inflammatory* [fluocinonide] 0.05%

Fluonid topical solution ℞ *corticosteroidal anti-inflammatory* [fluocinolone acetonide] 0.01%

fluopromazine BAN *antipsychotic* [also: triflupromazine]

Fluoracaine eye drops ℞ *local anesthetic; corneal disclosing agent* [proparacaine HCl; fluorescein sodium] 0.5%•0.25%

fluoracizine [see: fluacizine]

fluorescein USP, BAN, JAN *ophthalmic diagnostic aid*

fluorescein, soluble [now: fluorescein sodium]

fluorescein sodium USP, BAN, JAN *ophthalmic diagnostic aid* 2% eye drops

fluorescein sodium & proparacaine HCl *corneal disclosing agent; topical ophthalmic anesthetic* 0.25%•0.5%

Fluorescite antecubital venous injection ℞ *ophthalmic diagnostic agent* [fluorescein sodium] 10%, 25%

Fluoresoft eye drops ℞ *diagnostic aid in fitting contact lenses* [fluorexon] 0.35%

fluoresone INN

Fluorets ophthalmic strips OTC *corneal disclosing agent* [fluorescein sodium] 1 mg

fluorexon *diagnosis and fitting aid for contact lenses*

fluorhydrocortisone acetate [see: fludrocortisone acetate]

Fluoride tablets OTC *dental caries preventative* [sodium fluoride] 2.21 mg

Fluoride Loz lozenges ℞ *topical dental caries preventative* [sodium fluoride] 2.21 mg

Fluorigard oral rinse OTC *topical dental caries preventative* [sodium fluoride; alcohol 6%] 0.05%

Fluori-Methane spray (discontinued 2005) ℞ *vapo-coolant anesthetic/analgesic* [trichloromonofluoromethane; dichlorodifluoromethane] 85%•15%

fluorine *element (F)*

fluorine F 18 fluorodeoxyglucose
[see: fludeoxyglucose F 18]

Fluorinse oral rinse ℞ *dental caries preventative* [sodium fluoride] 0.2%

Fluor-I-Strip; Fluor-I-Strip A.T. ophthalmic strips ℞ *corneal disclosing agent* [fluorescein sodium] 9 mg; 1 mg

Fluoritab chewable tablets, drops ℞ *dental caries preventative* [sodium fluoride] 1.1, 2.2 mg; 0.55 mg/drop

fluormethylprednisolone [see: dexamethasone]

5-fluorocytosine (5-FC) [see: flucytosine]

fluorodeoxyglucose F 18 [see: fludeoxyglucose F 18]

fluorodideoxyadenosine (F-ddA) [see: lodenosine]

fluorometholone USP, INN, BAN *topical ophthalmic corticosteroidal anti-inflammatory* 0.1% eye drops

fluorometholone acetate USAN *topical ophthalmic corticosteroidal anti-inflammatory*

fluoromethylene deoxycytidine (FMdC) [now: tezacitabine]

Fluor-Op eye drop suspension ℞ *corticosteroidal anti-inflammatory* [fluorometholone] 0.1%

Fluoroperm 32 ℞ *hydrophobic contact lens material* [paflufocon C]

Fluoroperm 62 ℞ *hydrophobic contact lens material* [paflufocon B]

Fluoroperm 92 ℞ *hydrophobic contact lens material* [paflufocon A]

Fluoroperm 151 ℞ *hydrophobic contact lens material* [paflufocon D]

Fluoroplex cream, topical solution ℞ *antineoplastic for actinic keratoses and basal cell carcinomas* [fluorouracil] 1%

fluoroquinolones *a class of synthetic, broad-spectrum, antimicrobial, bactericidal antibiotics*

fluorosalan USAN *disinfectant* [also: flusalan]

fluorouracil (5-FU) USAN, USP, INN, BAN *antimetabolite antineoplastic for colorectal (orphan), esophageal (orphan), breast, stomach, and pancreatic cancers; topical antineoplastic for actinic keratoses and basal cell carcinoma; investigational (orphan) for glioblastoma multiforme* 50 mg/mL injection; 2%, 5% topical

fluorouracil & cisplatin *chemotherapy protocol for cervical cancer, used in conjunction with radiation therapy*

fluorouracil & interferon alfa-2a *investigational (orphan) for esophageal and advanced colorectal carcinoma*

fluorouracil & leucovorin *antineoplastic for metastatic colorectal cancer (orphan)*

fluoruridine deoxyribose [see: floxuridine]

fluostigmine [see: isoflurophate]

Fluothane liquid for vaporization ℞ *inhalation general anesthetic* [halothane]

fluotracen INN *antipsychotic; antidepressant* [also: fluotracen HCl]

fluotracen HCl USAN *antipsychotic; antidepressant* [also: fluotracen]

fluoxetine USAN, INN, BAN *selective serotonin reuptake inhibitor (SSRI) for depression, obsessive-compulsive disorder, bulimia nervosa, premenstrual dysphoric disorder, and panic disorder*

fluoxetine HCl USAN *selective serotonin reuptake inhibitor (SSRI) for major depression, obsessive-compulsive disorder, bulimia nervosa, premenstrual dysphoric disorder, and panic disorder; investigational (orphan) for autism* 10, 20, 40 mg oral; 20 mg/5 mL oral

fluoximesterone [see: fluoxymesterone]

Flu-Oxinate eye drops ℞ *topical ophthalmic anesthetic; corneal disclosing agent* [benoxinate HCl; fluorescein sodium] 0.4%•0.25%

fluoxiprednisolone [see: triamcinolone]

fluoxymesterone USP, INN, BAN *oral androgen for hypogonadism or testosterone deficiency in men, delayed puberty in boys, and metastatic breast cancer in women* 10 mg oral

fluparoxan INN, BAN *antidepressant* [also: fluparoxan HCl]

fluparoxan HCl USAN *antidepressant* [also: fluparoxan]

flupenthixol BAN *thioxanthene antipsychotic* [also: flupentixol]

flupentixol INN *thioxanthene antipsychotic* [also: flupenthixol]

fluperamide USAN, INN *antiperistaltic*

fluperlapine INN

fluperolone INN, BAN *corticosteroid; anti-inflammatory* [also: fluperolone acetate]

fluperolone acetate USAN *corticosteroid; anti-inflammatory* [also: fluperolone]

fluphenazine INN, BAN *conventional (typical) phenothiazine antipsychotic for schizophrenia and psychotic disorders* [also: fluphenazine enanthate]

fluphenazine decanoate *conventional (typical) phenothiazine antipsychotic for schizophrenia and psychotic disorders; used for prolonged parenteral neuroleptic therapy* 25 mg/mL injection

fluphenazine enanthate USP *conventional (typical) phenothiazine antipsychotic for schizophrenia and psychotic disorders* [also: fluphenazine]

fluphenazine HCl USP, BAN *conventional (typical) phenothiazine antipsychotic for schizophrenia and psychotic disorders* 1, 2.5, 5, 10 mg oral; 2.5 mg/5 mL oral; 2.5 mg/L injection

flupimazine INN

flupirtine INN, BAN *non-narcotic analgesic* [also: flupirtine maleate]

flupirtine maleate USAN *non-narcotic analgesic* [also: flupirtine]

flupranone INN

fluprazine INN

fluprednidene INN, BAN

fluprednisolone USAN, NF, INN, BAN *corticosteroid; anti-inflammatory*

fluprednisolone valerate USAN *corticosteroid; anti-inflammatory*

fluprofen INN, BAN

fluprofylline INN

fluproquazone USAN, INN, BAN *analgesic*

fluprostenol INN, BAN *prostaglandin* [also: fluprostenol sodium]

fluprostenol sodium USAN *prostaglandin* [also: fluprostenol]

fluquazone USAN, INN *anti-inflammatory*

Flura tablets ℞ *dental caries preventative* [sodium fluoride] 2.2 mg

fluracil [see: fluorouracil]

fluradoline INN *analgesic* [also: fluradoline HCl]

fluradoline HCl USAN *analgesic* [also: fluradoline]

Flura-Drops ℞ *dental caries preventative* [sodium fluoride] 0.55 mg/drop

Flura-Loz lozenges ℞ *topical dental caries preventative* [sodium fluoride] 2.2 mg

flurandrenolide USAN, USP *topical corticosteroid* [also: fludroxycortide; flurandrenolone] 0.05% topical

flurandrenolone BAN *topical corticosteroid* [also: flurandrenolide; fludroxycortide]

flurantel INN

Flurate eye drops ℞ *topical ophthalmic anesthetic; corneal disclosing agent* [benoxinate HCl; fluorescein sodium] 0.4%•0.25%

flurazepam INN, BAN *benzodiazepine sedative and hypnotic; anticonvulsant; muscle relaxant; also abused as a street drug* [also: flurazepam HCl]

flurazepam HCl USAN, USP *benzodiazepine sedative and hypnotic; anticonvulsant; muscle relaxant; also abused as a street drug* [also: flurazepam] 15, 30 mg oral

flurbiprofen USAN, USP, INN, BAN *antiarthritic; nonsteroidal anti-inflammatory drug (NSAID)* 50, 100 mg oral

flurbiprofen sodium USP *prostaglandin synthesis inhibitor; antimiotic; ophthalmic nonsteroidal anti-inflammatory drug (NSAID)* 0.03% eye drops

Fluress eye drops ℞ *topical ophthalmic anesthetic; corneal disclosing agent* [benoxinate HCl; fluorescein sodium] 0.4%•0.25%

fluretofen USAN, INN *anti-inflammatory; antithrombotic*

flurfamide [now: flurofamide]

flurithromycin INN

flurocitabine USAN, INN *antineoplastic*

Fluro-Ethyl aerosol spray ℞ *topical refrigerant anesthetic* [ethyl chloride; dichlorotetrafluoroethane] 25%•75%

flurofamide USAN, INN *urease enzyme inhibitor*

flurogestone acetate USAN *progestin* [also: flugestone]

Flurosyn ointment, cream ℞ *topical corticosteroidal anti-inflammatory* [fluocinolone acetonide] 0.025%; 0.01, 0.025%

flurothyl USAN, USP, BAN *CNS stimulant* [also: flurotyl]

flurotyl INN *CNS stimulant* [also: flurothyl]

fluroxene USAN, NF, INN *inhalation anesthetic*

fluroxyspiramine [see: spiramide]

flusalan INN *disinfectant* [also: fluorosalan]

FluShield IM injection, Tubex (cartridge-needle unit) (discontinued 2002) ℞ *flu vaccine* [influenza purified split-virus vaccine] 0.5 mL/dose

flusoxolol INN, BAN

fluspiperone USAN, INN *antipsychotic*

fluspirilene USAN, INN, BAN *diphenylbutylpiperidine antipsychotic*

flutamide USAN, INN, BAN *antiandrogen antineoplastic for prostatic carcinoma* 125 mg oral

flutazolam INN

flutemazepam INN

Flutex ointment, cream ℞ *topical corticosteroidal anti-inflammatory* [triamcinolone acetonide] 0.025%, 0.1%, 0.5%

flutiazin USAN, INN *veterinary anti-inflammatory*

fluticasone INN, BAN *corticosteroidal anti-inflammatory for chronic asthma or rhinitis* [also: fluticasone propionate]

fluticasone propionate USAN *corticosteroidal anti-inflammatory for chronic asthma or rhinitis; topical treatment for dermatoses* [also: fluticasone] 0.005%, 0.05% topical

flutizenol INN

flutomidate INN

flutonidine INN

flutoprazepam INN

flutrimazole INN

flutroline USAN, INN *antipsychotic*

flutropium bromide INN

fluvastatin INN, BAN *HMG-CoA reductase inhibitor for hypercholesterolemia and atherosclerosis* [also: fluvastatin sodium]

fluvastatin sodium USAN *HMG-CoA reductase inhibitor for hypercholesterolemia, hypertriglyceridemia, and atherosclerosis* [also: fluvastatin]

Fluvirin IM injection, prefilled syringes ℞ *flu vaccine* [influenza split-virus vaccine] 0.5 mL/dose

fluvoxamine INN, BAN *selective serotonin reuptake inhibitor (SSRI) for obsessive-compulsive disorder* [also: fluvoxamine maleate]

fluvoxamine maleate USAN *selective serotonin reuptake inhibitor (SSRI) for obsessive-compulsive disorder; investigational (Phase III) for depression and panic disorder* [also: fluvoxamine] 25, 50, 100 mg oral

flux root *medicinal herb* [see: pleurisy root]

fluzinamide USAN, INN *anticonvulsant*

Fluzone IM injection, prefilled syringes ℞ *flu vaccine* [influenza split-virus vaccine] 0.5 mL/dose

Fluzone Preservative-Free: Pediatric Dose prefilled syringes for IM injection ℞ *flu vaccine* [influenza split-virus or whole-virus vaccine] 0.25 mL/dose

fluzoperine INN

flytrap *medicinal herb* [see: dogbane]

FMdC (fluoromethylene deoxycytidine) [now: tezacitabine]

FML; FML Forte eye drop suspension ℞ *ophthalmic corticosteroidal anti-inflammatory* [fluorometholone] 0.1%; 0.25%

FML S.O.P. ophthalmic ointment ℞ *topical ophthalmic corticosteroidal anti-inflammatory* [fluorometholone] 0.1%

FML-S eye drop suspension ℞ *corticosteroidal anti-inflammatory; antibiotic* [fluorometholone; sulfacetamide sodium] 0.1%•10%

FMS (fluorouracil, mitomycin, streptozocin) *chemotherapy protocol*

FMV (fluorouracil, MeCCNU, vincristine) *chemotherapy protocol*

FNC (fluorouracil, Novantrone, cyclophosphamide) *chemotherapy protocol for breast cancer* [also: CFN; CNF]

FNM (fluorouracil, Novantrone, methotrexate) *chemotherapy protocol*

foal's foot *medicinal herb* [see: coltsfoot]

FOAM (fluorouracil, Oncovin, Adriamycin, mitomycin) *chemotherapy protocol*

Foamicon chewable tablets OTC *antacid* [aluminum hydroxide; magnesium trisilicate] 80•20 mg

Focalin tablets ℞ *CNS stimulant for attention-deficit hyperactivity disorder (ADHD)* [dexmethylphenidate HCl] 2.5, 5, 10 mg

Focalin XR extended-release capsules ℞ *CNS stimulant for attention-deficit hyperactivity disorder (ADHD)* [dexmethylphenidate HCl] 5, 10, 20 mg

focofilcon A USAN *hydrophilic contact lens material*

fodipir USAN *excipient*

Foeniculum officinale; F. vulgare medicinal herb [see: fennel]

Foille spray OTC *local anesthetic; antiseptic* [benzocaine; chloroxylenol] 5%•0.63%

Foille Medicated First Aid ointment, aerosol spray OTC *local anesthetic; antiseptic* [benzocaine; chloroxylenol] 5%•0.1%; 5%•0.6%

Foille Plus aerosol spray OTC *local anesthetic; antiseptic* [benzocaine; chloroxylenol; alcohol 57.33%] 5%•0.6%

folacin [see: folic acid] ② Fulvicin

folate [see: folic acid]

folate sodium USP

Folergot-DF tablets ℞ *GI anticholinergic; sedative; analgesic* [belladonna alkaloids; phenobarbital; ergotamine tartrate] 0.2•40•0.6 mg

folescutol INN

Folgard tablets OTC *vitamin B supplement* [vitamins B_6 and B_{12}; folic acid] 10•0.115•0.8 mg

Folgard RX 2.2 film-coated tablets ℞ *vitamin B supplement* [vitamins B_6 and B_{12}; folic acid] 25•0.5•2.3 mg

folic acid USP, INN, BAN *vitamin B_c; vitamin M; hematopoietic; birth defect preventative* 0.4, 0.8, 1 mg oral; 5 mg/mL injection

folinate-SF calcium [see: leucovorin calcium]

folinic acid [see: leucovorin calcium]

follicle-stimulating hormone (FSH) BAN [also: menotropins]

follidrin [see: estradiol benzoate]

Follistim powder for subcu or IM injection ℞ *recombinant follicle-stimulating hormone (FSH) for the induction of ovulation in women and spermatogenesis in men* [follitropin beta] 75 IU

follitropin alfa INN *recombinant follicle-stimulating hormone (FSH) for the induction of ovulation or spermatogenesis (orphan); adjunct to assisted reproductive technologies (ART)*

follitropin beta INN *recombinant follicle-stimulating hormone (FSH) for the induction of ovulation in women and spermatogenesis in men*

follotropin [see: menotropins]

Follow-Up [see: Carnation Follow-Up]

Folpace tablets ℞ *vitamin/magnesium supplement* [vitamins B_6 and B_{12}; folic acid; vitamin E; magnesium] 25 mg• 425 μg•2.05 mg•100 IU•100 mg

Foltrin capsules ℞ *hematinic* [ferrous fumarate; cyanocobalamin; ascorbic acid; intrinsic factor concentrate; folic acid] 110 mg•15 μg•75 mg• 240 mg•0.5 mg

Foltx tablets ℞ *vitamin B therapy for arteriosclerosis, cardiovascular and peripheral vascular disease, and neurological disorders* [vitamins B_6 and B_{12}; folic acid] 25•2•2.5 mg

Folvite IM injection ℞ *hematinic* [folic acid] 5 mg/mL

fomepizole USAN, INN *antidote; alcohol dehydrogenase inhibitor for methanol or ethylene glycol poisoning (orphan)*

FOMI; FOMi (fluorouracil, Onco-vin, mitomycin) *chemotherapy protocol*

fomidacillin INN, BAN

fominoben INN [also: fominoben HCl]

fominoben HCl JAN [also: fominoben]

fomivirsen sodium *antisense drug for AIDS-related CMV retinitis*

fomocaine INN, BAN

fonatol [see: diethylstilbestrol]

fonazine mesylate USAN *serotonin inhibitor* [also: dimetotiazine; dimethothiazine]

fondaparinux sodium *selective factor Xa inhibitor; antithrombotic for prevention of deep vein thrombosis (DVT) and acute pulmonary embolism following orthopedic surgery*

fontarsol [see: dichlorophenarsine HCl]

fopirtoline INN

Foradil encapsulated powder for inhalation (used with an Aerolizer device) ℞ *β₂ agonist; twice-daily bronchodilator for asthma, COPD, and emphysema* [formoterol fumarate] 12 μg/dose

Forane liquid for vaporization ℞ *inhalation general anesthetic* [isoflurane]

forasartan USAN *antihypertensive; CHF treatment; angiotensin II receptor antagonist*

foreign colombo *medicinal herb* [see: colombo]

forfenimex INN

formaldehyde solution USP *disinfectant; anhidrotic for hyperhidrosis and bromhidrosis*

Formalyde-10 spray ℞ *anhidrotic for hyperhidrosis and bromhidrosis* [formaldehyde] 10%

formebolone INN, BAN

formetamide [see: formetorex]

formetorex INN

formidacillin [see: fomidacillin]

forminitrazole INN, BAN

formocortal USAN, INN, BAN *corticosteroid; anti-inflammatory*

formoterol INN *bronchodilator* [also: eformoterol; formoterol fumarate]

formoterol fumarate USAN, JAN *bronchodilator for asthma* [also: formoterol; eformoterol fumarate]

Formula 44 Cough Control Disks; Formula 44 Cough Silencers lozenges (discontinued 2002) OTC *antitussive; topical oral anesthetic* [dextromethorphan hydrobromide; benzocaine] 5•1.25 mg; 2.5•1 mg

Formula 405 cleansing bar OTC *therapeutic skin cleanser*

Formula B tablets ℞ *vitamin supplement* [multiple B vitamins; vitamin C; folic acid] ±•500•0.5 mg

Formula B Plus tablets ℞ *vitamin/mineral/iron supplement* [multiple vitamins & minerals; ferrous fumarate; folic acid; biotin] ±•27•0.8•0.15 mg

Formula EM oral solution OTC *antiemetic for nausea associated with influenza, morning sickness, motion sickness, inhalation anesthesia, or food and drink indiscretions* [phosphorated carbohydrate solution (fructose; dextrose; phosphoric acid)] 1.87 g•1.87 g•21.5 mg per 5 mL

Formula VM-2000 tablets OTC *dietary supplement* [multiple vitamins & minerals; multiple amino acids; iron; folic acid; biotin] ±•5 mg•0.2 mg•50 μg

Formulation R anorectal cream, anorectal ointment OTC *temporary relief of hemorrhoidal symptoms* [phenylephrine HCl] 0.25%

4'-formylacetanilide thiosemicarbazone [see: thioacetazone; thiacetazone]

foropafant INN

forskolin [see: colforsin]

Forta Drink powder OTC *enteral nutritional therapy* [lactose-free formula]

Forta Shake powder OTC *enteral nutritional therapy* [milk-based formula]

Fortamet extended-release film-coated tablets ℞ *biguanide antidiabetic* [metformin HCl] 500, 1000 mg

Fortaz powder or frozen premix for IV or IM injection ℞ *cephalosporin antibiotic* [ceftazidime] 0.5, 1, 2, 6 g

Fortel Midstream test stick for professional use *in vitro diagnostic aid; urine pregnancy test*

Fortel Plus test kit for home use *in vitro diagnostic aid; urine pregnancy test*

Fortéo subcu injection via prefilled self-injector ℞ *parathyroid hormone for postmenopausal osteoporosis in women and primary or hypogonadal osteoporosis in men* [teriparatide] 20 μg/day (750 μg/3 mL injector)

Fortical nasal delivery ℞ *investigational (NDA filed) calcium regulator for hypercalcemia, Paget disease, and post-menopausal osteoporosis* [calcitonin (salmon), recombinant]

fortimicin A [now: astromicin sulfate]

Fortovase softgels (discontinued 2005) ℞ *antiretroviral protease inhibitor for HIV* [saquinavir] 200 mg

40 winks capsules OTC *antihistaminic sleep aid* [diphenhydramine HCl] 50 mg

Forvade gel ℞ *investigational (Phase I/II) nucleoside antiviral for AIDS-related genital herpes* [cidofovir]

Forzest (Indian name for U.S. product Cialis)

Fosamax tablets, oral solution ℞ *bisphosphonate bone resorption inhibitor for Paget disease and corticosteroid-induced or age-related osteoporosis in men and women; investigational (orphan) for bone manifestations of Gaucher disease and pediatric osteogenesis imperfecta* [alendronate sodium] 5, 10, 35, 40, 70 mg; 70 mg/75 mL bottle

Fosamax Plus D tablets ℞ *bisphosphonate bone resorption inhibitor for Paget disease and corticosteroid-induced or age-related osteoporosis in men and women; vitamin D supplement* [alendronate sodium; cholecalciferol] 70 mg•2800 IU

fosamprenavir calcium USAN *antiretroviral; HIV-1 protease inhibitor; amprenavir prodrug*

fosamprenavir sodium USAN *antiretroviral; HIV-1 protease inhibitor; amprenavir prodrug*

fosarilate USAN, INN *antiviral*

fosazepam USAN, INN, BAN *hypnotic*

foscarnet sodium USAN, INN, BAN *antiviral for cytomegalovirus (CMV) and various herpes viruses (HSV-1, HSV-2)*

Foscavir IV injection ℞ *antiviral for cytomegalovirus (CMV) retinitis and herpes simplex virus (HSV) infections in immunocompromised patients* [foscarnet sodium] 24 mg/mL

foscolic acid INN

fosenazide INN

fosenopril sodium [see: fosinopril sodium]

fosfestrol INN, BAN *antineoplastic; estrogen* [also: diethylstilbestrol diphosphate]

fosfocreatinine INN

fosfomycin USAN, INN, BAN *antibacterial* [also: fosfomycin calcium; fosfomycin sodium]

fosfomycin calcium JAN *antibacterial* [also: fosfomycin; fosfomycin sodium]

fosfomycin sodium JAN *antibacterial* [also: fosfomycin; fosfomycin calcium]

fosfomycin tromethamine USAN *broad-spectrum bactericidal antibiotic for urinary tract infections*

fosfonet sodium USAN, INN *antiviral*

fosfosal INN

Fosfree tablets OTC *vitamin/iron supplement* [multiple vitamins; iron] ± •29 mg

fosfructose trisodium USAN *investigational (Phase III) cardioprotective agent used in coronary artery bypass graft surgery; investigational (Phase II) for pain during sickle cell crisis*

fosinopril INN, BAN *antihypertensive; angiotensin-converting enzyme (ACE) inhibitor* [also: fosinopril sodium]

fosinopril sodium USAN *antihypertensive; angiotensin-converting enzyme (ACE) inhibitor; adjunctive treatment for CHF* [also: fosinopril] 10, 20, 40 mg oral

fosinopril sodium & hydrochlorothiazide *antihypertensive; angiotensin-converting enzyme (ACE) inhibitor; diuretic* 10•12.5, 20•12.5 mg

fosinoprilat USAN, INN *antihypertensive*

fosmenic acid INN

fosmidomycin INN

fosphenytoin INN *hydantoin anticonvulsant* [also: fosphenytoin sodium]

fosphenytoin sodium USAN *hydantoin anticonvulsant for grand mal status epilepticus (orphan)* [also: fosphenytoin]

fospirate USAN, INN *veterinary anthelmintic*

fosquidone USAN, INN, BAN *antineoplastic*

Fosrenol chewable tablets ℞ *phosphate binder for hyperphosphatemia in endstage renal disease (ESRD)* [lanthanum carbonate] 250, 500 mg

fostedil USAN, INN *vasodilator; calcium channel blocker*

Fostex cleansing bar (discontinued 2003) OTC *keratolytic for acne* [benzoyl peroxide] 10% ⊡ pHisoHex

Fostex 10% BPO gel (discontinued 2003) OTC *keratolytic for acne* [benzoyl peroxide] 10%

Fostex 10% Wash topical liquid (discontinued 2003) OTC *keratolytic for acne* [benzoyl peroxide] 10%

Fostex Acne Cleansing cream OTC *keratolytic for acne* [salicylic acid] 2%

Fostex Acne Medication Cleansing bar OTC *medicated cleanser for acne* [salicylic acid] 2%

Fostex Medicated Cleansing Shampoo OTC *antiseborrheic; keratolytic* [sulfur; salicylic acid] 2%•2%

fostriecin INN *antineoplastic* [also: fostriecin sodium]

fostriecin sodium USAN *antineoplastic* [also: fostriecin]

Fostril lotion (discontinued 2004) OTC *acne treatment* [sulfur; zinc oxide]

fosveset USAN *ligant excipient*

fotemustine INN, BAN

fo-ti; ho-shou-wu (*Polygonum multiflorum*) root *medicinal herb for atherosclerosis, blood cleansing, constipation, improving liver and kidney function, insomnia, malaria, muscle aches, TB, and weak bones; also used to increase* *fertility, prevent aging, and promote longevity*

Fototar cream OTC *antipsoriatic; antiseborrheic* [coal tar] 2%

fotretamine INN

Fouchet reagent (solution)

4 Hair softgel capsules OTC *vitamin/mineral/iron supplement* [multiple vitamins & minerals; iron; folic acid; biotin] ±•2.5•33.3•0.25 mg

4 Nails softgel capsules OTC *vitamin/mineral/calcium/iron supplement* [multiple vitamins & minerals; calcium; iron; folic acid; biotin] ±•167•3•0.333•0.0083 mg

4 Trace Elements IV injection ℞ *intravenous nutritional therapy* [multiple trace elements (metals)]

4•Way Fast Acting nasal spray OTC *nasal decongestant* [phenylephrine HCl] 1%

4•Way Long Lasting nasal spray (discontinued 2002) OTC *nasal decongestant* [oxymetazoline HCl] 0.05%

40DS02 *investigational (orphan) for chronic iron overload due to transfusional treatments*

480848 *lipoprotein-associated phospholipase A2 (Lp-PLA2) blocker; investigational (Phase III) gene-based antiatherosclerotic agent*

4B5 antibody *investigational (Phase I) fully human monoclonal antibody for immunotherapy in melanoma patients*

Fourneau 309 (available only from the Centers for Disease Control) ℞ *antiparasitic for African trypanosomiasis and onchocerciasis* [suramin sodium]

foxglove (*Digitalis ambigua; D. ferriginea; D. grandiflora; D. lanata; D. lutea; D. purpurea*) leaves *medicinal herb for asthma, burns, congestive heart failure, edema, promoting wound healing, and sedation; not generally regarded as safe and effective for children as ingestion can be fatal*

foxglove, American; false foxglove; fern-leaved foxglove *medicinal herb* [see: feverweed]

foxtail *medicinal herb* [see: club moss]

frabuprofen INN

Fractar (trademarked ingredient) OTC *antipsoriatic; antiseborrheic* [crude coal tar]

Fragaria vesca medicinal herb [see: strawberry]

Fragmin deep subcu injection, prefilled syringes ℞ *anticoagulant/antithrombotic for prevention of deep vein thrombosis (DVT) after abdominal or hip replacement surgery, unstable angina, and myocardial infarction* [dalteparin sodium] 10 000, 25 000 IU (64, 160 mg)/mL; 2500, 5000 IU (16, 32 mg)/0.2 mL, 7500 IU (48 mg)/0.3 mL

framycetin INN, BAN *anti-infective wound dressing*

francium *element (Fr)*

Frangula purshiana medicinal herb [see: cascara sagrada]

frankincense (*Boswellia serrata*) leaves and bark *medicinal herb for anaphylaxis, arthritis, asthma, blood cleansing, bronchial disorders, dysentery, rheumatism, skin ailments, ulcers, and wound healing*

fraxinella (*Dictamnus albus*) root, plant, and seed *medicinal herb used as an anthelmintic, diuretic, emmenagogue, expectorant, and febrifuge*

Fraxiparine ⒸⒶⓃ subcu injection, prefilled syringes ℞ *anticoagulant/antithrombotic for prevention of deep vein thrombosis (DVT) after surgery, clotting during hemodialysis, unstable angina, and myocardial infarction* [nadroparin calcium] 9500 IU/mL; 0.2, 0.3, 0.4, 0.6, 0.8, 1 mL

Fraxiparine Forte ⒸⒶⓃ subcu injection, prefilled syringes ℞ *anticoagulant/ antithrombotic for prevention of deep vein thrombosis (DVT) after surgery, clotting during hemodialysis, unstable angina, and myocardial infarction* [nadroparin calcium] 19 000 IU/mL; 0.6, 0.8, 1 mL

FreAmine III 3% (8.5%) with Electrolytes IV infusion ℞ *total parenteral nutrition (8.5% only); peripheral parenteral nutrition (both)* [multiple essential and nonessential amino acids; electrolytes]

FreAmine III 8.5%; FreAmine III 10% IV infusion ℞ *total parenteral nutrition; peripheral parenteral nutrition* [multiple essential and nonessential amino acids]

FreAmine HBC 6.9% IV infusion ℞ *nutritional therapy for high metabolic stress* [multiple branched-chain essential and nonessential amino acids; electrolytes]

Free & Clear shampoo OTC *soap-free therapeutic cleanser*

Freedavite tablets OTC *vitamin/mineral/ iron supplement* [multiple vitamins & minerals; ferrous fumarate] ± • 10 mg

Freedox solution ℞ *investigational (NDA filed) lazaroid for subarachnoid hemorrhage (SAH), ischemic stroke, spinal cord and head injury* [tirilazad mesylate]

Freezone topical liquid OTC *keratolytic* [salicylic acid in a collodion-like vehicle] 13.6%

frentizole USAN, INN, BAN *immunoregulator*

fringe tree (*Chionanthus virginica*) bark *medicinal herb used as an aperient, diuretic, febrifuge, and tonic*

Frisium (available in Canada as Alti-Clobazam) ℞ *investigational benzodiazepine tranquilizer; anxiolytic* [clobazam]

fronepidil INN

frost plant; frost weed; frostwort *medicinal herb* [see: rock rose]

Frova film-coated tablets ℞ *vascular serotonin 5-HT$_{1B/1D}$ receptor agonist for the acute treatment of migraine* [frovatriptan succinate] 2.5 mg

frovatriptan succinate USAN *vascular serotonin 5-HT$_{1B/1D}$ receptor agonist for the acute treatment of migraine*

froxiprost INN

β-fructofuranosidase [see: sacrosidase]

fructose (D-fructose) USP *nutrient; caloric replacement* [also: levulose]

fructose-1,6-diphosphate (FDP) *investigational (Phase III) adjunct to* *coronary artery bypass graft (CABG) surgery; investigational (Phase III, orphan) cytoprotective agent for vaso-occlusive episodes of sickle cell disease*

Fruit C 100; Fruit C 200; Fruit C 500 chewable tablets OTC *vitamin C supplement* [ascorbic acid and calcium ascorbate] 100 mg; 200 mg; 500 mg

Fruity Chews chewable tablets OTC *vitamin supplement* [multiple vitamins; folic acid] ≚•0.3 mg

Fruity Chews with Iron chewable tablets OTC *vitamin/iron supplement* [multiple vitamins; iron; folic acid] ≚•12•0.3 mg

frusemide BAN *antihypertensive; loop diuretic* [also: furosemide]

FS Shampoo (name changed to Capex in 2003)

FSF (fibrin-stabilizing factor) [see: factor XIII]

FSH (follicle-stimulating hormone) [see: menotropins]

ftalofyne INN *veterinary anthelmintic* [also: phthalofyne]

ftaxilide INN

FTC [see: emtricitabine]

ftivazide INN

ftormetazine INN

ftorpropazine INN

5-FU (5-fluorouracil) [see: fluorouracil]

fubrogonium iodide INN

fuchsin, basic USP *topical antibacterial/ antifungal*

Fucidin Ⓒᴬᴺ cream, ointment ℞ *topical antibiotic* [fusidic acid] 2%

Fucidin H Ⓒᴬᴺ cream OTC *topical antibiotic and corticosteroidal anti-inflammatory* [fusidic acid; hydrocortisone] 2•1 mg/g

Fucus versiculosus medicinal herb [see: kelp]

FUDR powder for intra-arterial infusion ℞ *antimetabolic antineoplastic for GI adenocarcinoma metastatic to the liver* [floxuridine] 500 mg

FUDR; FUdR (5-fluorouracil deoxyribonucleoside) [see: floxuridine]

fuge, devil's *medicinal herb* [see: mistletoe]

Ful-Glo ophthalmic strips ℞ *corneal disclosing agent* [fluorescein sodium] 0.6 mg

Full Spectrum B tablets OTC *vitamin supplement* [multiple B vitamins]

fulmicoton [see: pyroxylin]

FU/LV (fluorouracil, leucovorin calcium [rescue]) *chemotherapy protocol for colorectal cancer* [also: F-CL]

FU/LV/CPT-11 (fluorouracil, leucovorin calcium [rescue], CPT-11) *chemotherapy protocol for metastatic colorectal cancer*

fulvestrant USAN *steroidal selective estrogen receptor down-regulator; antineoplastic for metastatic breast cancer in postmenopausal women*

Fulvicin P/G tablets (discontinued 2003) ℞ *systemic antifungal* [griseofulvin (ultramicrosize)] 125, 165, 250, 330 mg ◉ folacin; Furacin

Fulvicin U/F tablets (discontinued 2003) ℞ *systemic antifungal* [griseofulvin (microsize)] 250, 500 mg

FUM (fluorouracil, methotrexate) *chemotherapy protocol*

fumagillin INN, BAN

Fumaria officinalis medicinal herb [see: fumitory]

fumaric acid NF *acidifier*

Fumatinic sustained-release capsules ℞ *hematinic* [ferrous fumarate; cyanocobalamin; ascorbic acid] 200 mg (66 mg Fe)•5 μg•60 mg

fumitory (Fumaria officinalis) *plant medicinal herb for cardiovascular disorders, constipation, eczema, edema, and hepatobiliary disorders*

fumoxicillin USAN, INN *antibacterial*

Funduscein-10; Funduscein-25 antecubital venous injection ℞ *ophthalmic diagnostic agent* [fluorescein sodium] 10%; 25%

fungicidin [see: nystatin]

fungimycin USAN *antifungal*

Fungi-Nail topical liquid OTC *antifungal; keratolytic; anesthetic* [resorcinol; salicylic acid; chloroxylenol; benzocaine; alcohol 50%] 1%•2%•2%•0.5%

Fungizone cream, lotion (discontinued 2003) ℞ *polyene antifungal* [amphotericin B] 3%

Fungizone ointment (discontinued 2001) ℞ *polyene antifungal* [amphotericin B] 3%

Fungizone oral suspension (discontinued 2004) ℞ *systemic polyene antifungal; "swish and swallow" treatment for oral candidiasis* [amphotericin B] 100 mg/mL

Fungizone powder for IV infusion ℞ *systemic polyene antifungal* [amphotericin B deoxycholate] 50 mg/vial

Fung-O topical liquid OTC *keratolytic* [salicylic acid] 17%

Fungoid tincture OTC *antifungal* [miconazole nitrate] 2%

Fungoid-HC cream ℞ *corticosteroidal anti-inflammatory; antipruritic; antifungal; antibacterial* [miconazole nitrate; hydrocortisone] 2% ● 1%

FUP (fluorouracil, Platinol) *chemotherapy protocol for gastric cancer*

fuprazole INN

furacilin [see: nitrofurazone]

Furacin topical solution, cream ℞ *broad-spectrum antibacterial; adjunct to burn therapy and skin grafting* [nitrofurazone] 0.2% ② Fulvicin

Furacin Soluble Dressing ointment ℞ *broad-spectrum antibacterial; adjunct to burn therapy and skin grafting* [nitrofurazone] 0.2%

furacrinic acid INN, BAN

Furadantin oral suspension ℞ *urinary antibiotic* [nitrofurantoin] 25 mg/5 mL

furafylline INN

Furalan tablets ℞ *urinary antibiotic* [nitrofurantoin] 50, 100 mg

furalazine INN

furaltadone INN, BAN

Furamide (available only from the Centers for Disease Control) ℞ *investigational anti-infective for amebiasis* [diloxanide furoate]

2(3H) furanone di-hydro (FDh) *a precursor to gamma hydroxybutyrate (GHB); a formerly legal alternative to GHB, now also illegal (Schedule I); also*
known as gamma butyrolactone (GBL) [see: gamma hydroxybutyrate (GHB)]

furaprofen USAN, INN *anti-inflammatory*

furazabol INN

furazolidone USP, INN, BAN *bactericidal; antiprotozoal; treatment of diarrhea and enteritis due to bacterial or protozoal organisms*

furazolium chloride USAN, INN *antibacterial*

furazolium tartrate USAN *antibacterial*

furbucillin INN

furcloprofen INN

furegrelate INN *thromboxane synthetase inhibitor* [also: furegrelate sodium]

furegrelate sodium USAN *thromboxane synthetase inhibitor* [also: furegrelate]

furethidine INN, BAN

furfenorex INN

furfuryltrimethylammonium iodide [see: furtrethonium iodide]

furidarone INN

furmethoxadone INN

furobufen USAN, INN *anti-inflammatory*

furodazole USAN, INN *anthelmintic*

furofenac INN

furomazine INN

furomine USAN, INN, BAN *ligand*

furosemide USAN, USP, INN, JAN *antihypertensive; loop diuretic* [also: frusemide] 20, 40, 80 mg oral; 10 mg/mL oral; 40 mg/5 mL oral; 10 mg/mL injection ② torsemide

furostilbestrol INN

furoxicillin [see: fumoxicillin]

Furoxone oral liquid (discontinued 2005) ℞ *antibacterial* [furazolidone] 50 mg/15 mL

Furoxone tablets ℞ *bactericidal; antiprotozoal; treatment of diarrhea and enteritis due to bacterial or protozoal organisms* [furazolidone] 100 mg

fursalan USAN, INN *disinfectant*

fursultiamine INN

furterene INN

furtrethonium iodide INN

furtrimethonium iodide [see: furtrethonium iodide]

fusafungine INN, BAN

fusidate sodium USAN *antibacterial*

fusidic acid USAN, INN, BAN *topical antibacterial*

fusidic acid, sodium salt [see: fusidate sodium]

FUVAC (5-FU, vinblastine, Adriamycin, cyclophosphamide) *chemotherapy protocol*

Fuzeon powder for subcu injection ℞ *fusion inhibitor for HIV infection* [enfuvirtide] 90 mg/mL (108 mg/dose)

fuzlocillin INN, BAN

fytic acid INN

FZ (flutamide, Zoladex) *chemotherapy protocol for prostate cancer*

G17DT immunogen *investigational (orphan) agent for gastric cancer and adenocarcinoma of the pancreas*

G-3139 *investigational (Phase III) adjunct used with docetaxel for malignant melanoma, breast cancer, and other malignancies; investigational (Phase I/II) for AIDS-related non-Hodgkin lymphoma*

^{67}**Ga** [see: gallium citrate Ga 67]

GABA (gamma-aminobutyric acid) [see: γ-aminobutyric acid]

gabapentin USAN, INN *anticonvulsant; treatment for postherpetic neuralgia; investigational (orphan) for amyotrophic lateral sclerosis* 100, 300, 400, 600, 800 mg oral

Gabarone tablets ℞ *anticonvulsant for partial-onset seizures; treatment for postherpetic neuralgia* [gabapentin] 100, 300, 400 mg

Gabbromicina *investigational (orphan) agent for tuberculosis and Mycobacterium avium complex (MAC)* [aminosidine]

gabexate INN

Gabitril Filmtabs (film-coated tablets) ℞ *anticonvulsant adjunct for partial seizures* [tiagabine HCl] 2, 4, 12, 16, 20 mg ☒ Carbatrol

gaboxadol INN *investigational (Phase III) GABA$_A$ agonist for the treatment of insomnia*

gadobenate dimeglumine USAN *MRI diagnostic aid* [also: gadobenic acid]

gadobenic acid INN *MRI diagnostic aid* [also: gadobenate dimeglumine]

gadobutrol INN *investigational aid for MRI*

gadodiamide USAN, INN, BAN *parenteral MRI contrast medium*

gadofosveset trisodium USAN *contrast agent for vascular enhancement of MRI scans*

gadolinium *element (Gd)*

gadolinium texaphyrin (Gd-Tex) [now: motexafin gadolinium]

gadolinium-diethylenetriamine pentaacetic acid (Gd-DTPA) *investigational MRI contrast media for cardiac imaging*

gadopenamide INN

gadopentetate dimeglumine USAN *parenteral MRI contrast medium* [also: gadopentetic acid]

gadopentetic acid INN, BAN *parenteral MRI contrast medium* [also: gadopentetate dimeglumine]

gadoteric acid INN

gadoteridol USAN, INN, BAN *parenteral MRI contrast medium*

gadoversetamide USAN, INN *parenteral MRI contrast medium for imaging of the brain, head, and spine and liver structure and vascularity*

gadoxanum USAN *gadolinium-xanthan gum complex; diagnostic aid*

gadozelite USAN *gadolinium zeolite complex; diagnostic aid*

GA-EPO (gene-activated erythropoietin) [see: erythropoietin, gene-activated]

gaiactamine [see: guaiactamine]

gaietamine [see: guaiactamine]

galactagogues *a class of agents that promote or increase the flow of breast milk* [also called: lactogogues]

galactochitosan *investigational immune system stimulant and anticancer therapy*

α-D-galactopyranose [see: galactose]

galactose USAN *ultrasound contrast medium*

α-galactosidase [see: agalsidase alfa]

galamustine INN

galangal (*Alpinia galanga; A. officinarum*) *rhizomes medicinal herb for diuresis, fungal infections, gas, hypertension, tumors, ulcers, and worms; also used as an antiplatelet agent*

galantamine USAN, INN *acetylcholinesterase inhibitor to increase cognition in Alzheimer disease*

galantamine hydrobromide USAN *acetylcholinesterase inhibitor to increase cognition in Alzheimer disease*

galanthamine [see: galantamine]

galdansetron INN, BAN *antiemetic* [also: galdansetron HCl]

galdansetron HCl USAN *antiemetic* [also: galdansetron]

Galeopsis tetrahit medicinal herb [see: hemp nettle]

Galida ℞ *investigational (Phase III) peroxisome proliferator–activated receptor (PPAR) agonist for type 2 diabetes* [tesaglitazar]

Galium aparine; G. verum medicinal herb [see: bedstraw]

Galium odoratum medicinal herb [see: sweet woodruff]

gallamine BAN *neuromuscular blocker* [also: gallamine triethiodide]

gallamine triethiodide USP, INN *neuromuscular blocker; muscle relaxant* [also: gallamine]

gallamone triethiodide [see: gallamine triethiodide]

gallic acid NF

gallic acid, bismuth basic salt [see: bismuth subgallate]

gallium *element (Ga)*

gallium (⁶⁷Ga) citrate INN *radiopaque contrast medium; radioactive agent* [also: gallium citrate Ga 67]

gallium citrate Ga 67 USAN, USP *radiopaque contrast medium; radioactive agent* [also: gallium (⁶⁷Ga) citrate]

gallium nitrate USAN *bone resorption inhibitor for hypercalcemia of malignancy (orphan); investigational (Phase II) agent for AIDS-related non-Hodgkin lymphoma*

gallium nitrate nonahydrate [see: gallium nitrate]

gallopamil INN, BAN

gallotannic acid [see: tannic acid]

gallstone solubilizing agents *a class of drugs that dissolve gallstones*

galosemide INN

galsulfase *recombinant human enzyme N-acetylgalactosamine 4-sulfatase; treatment for mucopolysaccharidosis VI (MPS VI; Maroteaux-Lamy syndrome)*

galtifenin INN

Galzin *capsules* ℞ *copper blocking/complexing agent for Wilson disease (orphan)* [zinc acetate] 25, 50 mg

gamfexine USAN, INN *antidepressant*

Gamimune N *IV infusion (discontinued 2005)* ℞ *passive immunizing agent for HIV, ITP, and bone marrow transplantation; infection prophylaxis in pediatric HIV (orphan); investigational (orphan) for myocarditis and juvenile rheumatoid arthritis* [immune globulin, solvent/detergent treated] 5%, 10%

gamma benzene hexachloride [now: lindane]

gamma butyraldehyde (GHB-aldehyde) *a precursor to gamma hydroxybutyrate (GHB)* [see: gamma hydroxybutyrate (GHB)]

gamma butyrolactone (GBL) *precursor to gamma hydroxybutyrate (GHB); a formerly legal alternative to GHB, now also illegal (Schedule I); also known as 2(3H) furanone di-hydro (FDh)* [see: gamma hydroxybutyrate (GHB)]

gamma globulin [see: globulin, immune]

gamma hydroxybutyrate (GHB) *a CNS depressant used as an anesthetic in some countries; sometimes abused as a "date rape" street drug; illegal in the U.S. (Schedule I) as GHB, but available (Schedule III) as sodium oxybate to treat cataplexy due to narcolepsy* [also known as: sodium oxybate]

gamma oryzanol; gamma-oz *medicinal herb* [see: rice bran oil]

gamma-aminobutyric acid (GABA) [see: γ-aminobutyric acid]

Gammagard Liquid IV infusion ℞ *passive immunizing agent for HIV, idiopathic thrombocytopenic purpura (ITP), B-cell chronic lymphocytic leukemia, and Kawasaki syndrome* [immune globulin] 10%

Gammagard S/D freeze-dried powder for IV infusion (discontinued 2004) ℞ *passive immunizing agent for HIV, idiopathic thrombocytopenic purpura (ITP), B-cell chronic lymphocytic leukemia, and Kawasaki syndrome* [immune globulin, solvent/detergent treated] 50 mg/mL

gamma-hydroxybutyrate sodium [see: sodium oxybate]

gamma-linolenic acid (GLA) *natural omega-6 fatty acid; investigational (orphan) for juvenile rheumatoid arthritis*

Gamma-OH (banned in the U.S.; approved in Europe) ℞ *sedative; hypnotic; antidepressant* [gamma hydroxybutyrate (GHB)] 2.5 g

gammaphos [now: ethiofos]

Gammar-P I.V. (pasteurized) powder for IV infusion ℞ *passive immunizing agent and immunomodulator for HIV; pediatric treatment of primary immune deficiency (PID)* [immune globulin, heat treated; human albumin] 5%•3%

gamma-vinyl GABA (gamma-aminobutyric acid) [see: vigabatrin]

gamolenic acid INN, BAN

Gamulin Rh IM injection (discontinued 2001) ℞ *obstetric Rh factor immunity suppressant* [Rh$_O$(D) immune globulin] 300 μg

Gamunex IV infusion ℞ *passive immunizing agent for primary humoral immunodeficiency and idiopathic thrombocytopenic purpura* [immune globulin, chromatography purified] 10%

ganaxolone USAN *neuroactive steroid; investigational (orphan) for infantile spasms; investigational (Phase II) for migraine and adult epilepsy*

ganciclovir USAN, INN, BAN *antiviral for AIDS-related cytomegalovirus (CMV) infections (orphan) and CMV retinitis (orphan)* [also: ganciclovir sodium] 250, 500 mg oral

ganciclovir sodium USAN *antiviral for cytomegalovirus retinitis (orphan)* [also: ganciclovir]

ganciclovir sodium & cytomegalovirus immune globulin intravenous (CMV-IGIV) *investigational (orphan) for cytomegalovirus pneumonia in bone marrow transplant patients*

ganglefene INN

gangliosides, sodium salts *investigational (orphan) agent for retinitis pigmentosa*

Ganidin NR oral liquid ℞ *expectorant* [guaifenesin] 100 mg/5 mL

ganirelix INN *gonadotropin-releasing hormone (GnRH) antagonist for infertility* [also: ganirelix acetate]

ganirelix acetate USAN *gonadotropin-releasing hormone (GnRH) antagonist for infertility* [also: ganirelix] 250 μg/0.5 mL injection

Ganite IV infusion ℞ *bone resorption inhibitor for hypercalcemia of malignancy (orphan); investigational (Phase II) agent for AIDS-related non-Hodgkin lymphoma* [gallium nitrate] 25 mg/mL

Gani-Tuss NR oral liquid ℞ *narcotic antitussive; expectorant* [codeine phosphate; guaifenesin] 20•200 mg/10 mL

Gani-Tuss-DM NR oral liquid ℞ *antitussive; expectorant* [dextromethorphan hydrobromide; guaifenesin] 20•200 mg/10 mL

Gantanol tablets (discontinued 2001) ℞ *broad-spectrum sulfonamide bacteriostatic* [sulfamethoxazole] 500 mg

Gantrisin pediatric suspension ℞ *broad-spectrum sulfonamide antibiotic* [sulfisoxazole acetyl; alcohol 0.3%] 500 mg/5 mL

gapicomine INN

gapromidine INN

Garamicina (Mexican name for U.S. product Garamycin)

Garamycin cream, ointment (discontinued 2003) ℞ *antibiotic* [gentamicin sulfate] 0.1% ☑ Gamastan; kanamycin; Terramycin; Theramycin

Garamycin eye drops, ophthalmic ointment ℞ *ophthalmic antibiotic* [gentamicin sulfate] 3 mg/mL; 3 mg/g

Garamycin IV or IM injection ℞ *aminoglycoside antibiotic* [gentamicin sulfate] 40 mg/mL

garcinia (*Garcinia cambogia*) fruit *medicinal herb for appetite suppressant, thermogenesis, and weight control*

garden nightshade *medicinal herb* [see: bittersweet nightshade]

garden patience *medicinal herb* [see: yellow dock]

Garfield; Garfield Plus Extra C chewable tablets OTC *vitamin supplement* [multiple vitamins; folic acid] ± •0.3 mg

Garfield Complete with Minerals chewable tablets OTC *vitamin/mineral/iron supplement* [multiple vitamins & minerals; iron; folic acid; biotin] ± •18•0.4•0.04 mg

Garfield Plus Iron chewable tablets OTC *vitamin/iron supplement* [multiple vitamins; iron; folic acid] ± •15•0.3 mg

garget *medicinal herb* [see: pokeweed]

garlic (*Allium sativum*) bulb *medicinal herb for asthma, cancer immunity, diabetes, digestive disorders, ear infections, flatulence, hypercholesterolemia, hypertension, and infectious diseases*

Gas chewable tablets OTC *antiflatulent* [simethicone] 125 mg

gas gangrene antitoxin, pentavalent

gas gangrene antitoxin, polyvalent [see: gas gangrene antitoxin, pentavalent]

Gas Permeable Daily Cleaner solution OTC *cleaning solution for rigid gas permeable contact lenses*

Gas Relief chewable tablets, drops OTC *antiflatulent* [simethicone] 80, 125 mg; 40 mg/0.6 mL

Gas-Ban tablets OTC *antacid; antiflatulent* [calcium carbonate; simethicone] 300•40 mg

Gas-Ban DS oral liquid OTC *antacid; antiflatulent* [aluminum hydroxide; magnesium hydroxide; simethicone] 400•400•40 mg/5 mL

gastric acid inhibitors [see: proton pump inhibitors]

gastric mucin BAN

Gastroccult slide test for professional use *in vitro diagnostic aid for gastric occult blood*

Gastrocrom oral solution ℞ *mastocytosis treatment (orphan); investigational prophylactic treatment for food allergies* [cromolyn sodium] 100 mg/5 mL

Gastrografin oral solution ℞ *radiopaque contrast medium for gastrointestinal imaging* [diatrizoate meglumine; diatrizoate sodium (48.29% total iodine)] 660•100 mg/mL (367 mg/mL)

GastroMARK oral suspension (discontinued 2005) ℞ *MRI contrast medium for upper GI tract imaging* [ferumoxsil] 175 μg iron/mL

Gastrosed drops, tablets (discontinued 2004) ℞ *GI/GU antispasmodic; antiparkinsonian; anticholinergic "drying agent" for allergic rhinitis and hyperhidrosis* [hyoscyamine sulfate] 0.125 mg/mL; 0.125 mg

Gastro-Test string capsules for professional use *in vitro diagnostic aid for GI disorders*

Gastrozepine (approved in Europe) ℞ *investigational (NDA filed) treatment for peptic ulcers* [pirenzepine HCl]

Gas-X chewable tablets, softgels OTC *antiflatulent* [simethicone] 80, 125 mg; 125 mg

Gas-X with Maalox chewable tablets OTC *antiflatulent; antacid* [simethicone; calcium carbonate] 125•500 mg

gatifloxacin USAN *broad-spectrum fluoroquinolone antibiotic*

gaultheria oil [see: methyl salicylate]

Gaultheria procumbens medicinal herb [see: wintergreen]

gauze, absorbent USP *surgical aid*

gauze, petrolatum USP *surgical aid*

gauze bandage [see: bandage, gauze]

gavestinel USAN *N-methyl-D-aspartate (NMDA) receptor antagonist for stroke*

gavilimomab *investigational (orphan) agent for acute graft vs. host disease*

Gaviscon oral liquid OTC *antacid* [aluminum hydroxide; magnesium carbonate] 31.7•119.3 mg/5 mL

Gaviscon; Gaviscon-2 chewable tablets OTC *antacid* [aluminum hydroxide; magnesium trisilicate] 80•20 mg; 160•40 mg

Gaviscon Relief Formula chewable tablets, oral liquid OTC *antacid* [aluminum hydroxide; magnesium carbonate] 160•105 mg; 254•237.5 mg/5 mL

GBH *a mistaken acronym for gamma hydroxybutyrate (GHB)* [see: gamma hydroxybutyrate (GHB)]

GBL (gamma butyrolactone) *precursor to gamma hydroxybutyrate (GHB); a formerly legal alternative to GHB, now also illegal (Schedule I); also known as 2(3H) furanone di-hydro (FDh)* [see: gamma hydroxybutyrate (GHB)]

G-CSF (granulocyte colony-stimulating factor) [see: filgrastim]

Gd texaphyrin [see: motexafin gadolinum]

Gd-DTPA (gadolinium-diethylenetriamine pentaacetic acid) [q.v.]

Gebauer's Spray and Stretch spray Ŗ *vapo-coolant anesthetic/analgesic* [tetrafluoroethane; pentafluoropropane]

gedocarnil INN *investigational treatment of central nervous system disorders*

Gee-Gee tablets (discontinued 2002) OTC *expectorant* [guaifenesin] 200 mg

gefarnate INN, BAN

gefitinib *epidermal growth factor receptor-tyrosine kinase inhibitor (EGFR-TKI); antineoplastic for advanced or metastatic non–small cell lung cancer (NSCLC); investigational (Phase III) for head and neck cancers*

gelatin NF *encapsulating, suspending, binding and coating agent*

gelatin film, absorbable USP *topical local hemostat for surgery*

gelatin powder, absorbable *topical local hemostat for surgery*

gelatin solution, special intravenous [see: polygeline]

gelatin sponge, absorbable USP *topical local hemostat for surgery*

gelcaps (dosage form) *soft gelatin capsules*

Gelfilm; Gelfilm Ophthalmic Ŗ *topical local hemostat for surgery* [absorbable gelatin film]

Gelfoam powder Ŗ *topical local hemostat for surgery* [absorbable gelatin powder] ⑨ Ger-O-Foam

Gelfoam sponge, packs, dental packs, prostatectomy cones Ŗ *topical local hemostat for surgery* [absorbable gelatin sponge] ⑨ Ger-O-Foam

Gelhist pediatric oral suspension Ŗ *decongestant; antihistamine* [phenylephrine tannate; chlorpheniramine tannate; pyrilamine tannate] 5•2•12.5 mg/5 mL

Gel-Kam Rinse dental gel OTC *topical caries preventative* [stannous fluoride] 0.4%

Gelpirin-CCF tablets (discontinued 2001) OTC *decongestant; antihistamine; analgesic; expectorant* [phenylpropanolamine HCl; chlorpheniramine maleate; acetaminophen; guaifenesin] 12.5•1•325•25 mg

Gelseal (trademarked dosage form) *soft gelatin capsule*

gelsemium (*Bignonia sempervirens; Gelsemium nitidum; G. sempervirens*) *plant medicinal herb for asthma, neuralgia, and respiratory disorders; not* *generally regarded as safe and effective as it is highly toxic*

gelsolin, recombinant human *investigational (orphan) for respiratory symptoms of cystic fibrosis and bronchiectasis*

Gel-Tin gel OTC *topical dental caries preventative* [stannous fluoride] 0.4%

Gelusil chewable tablets OTC *antacid; antiflatulent* [aluminum hydroxide; magnesium hydroxide; simethicone] 200•200•25 mg

gemazocine INN

gemcadiol USAN, INN *antihyperlipoproteinemic*

gemcitabine USAN, INN, BAN *antimetabolite antineoplastic*

gemcitabine & carboplatin *chemotherapy protocol for non–small cell lung cancer (NSCLC)*

gemcitabine & cisplatin *chemotherapy protocol for metastatic bladder cancer*

gemcitabine HCl USAN *antimetabolite antineoplastic for advanced or metastatic breast, pancreatic, and non–small cell lung cancers (NSCLC); investigational (Phase III) for cervical cancer*

gemcitabine & vinorelbine *chemotherapy protocol for non–small cell lung cancer (NSCLC)*

gemcitabine-cis (gemcitabine, cisplatin) *chemotherapy protocol for non–small cell lung cancer (NSCLC)*

Gemcor film-coated tablets ℞ *antihyperlipidemic for hypercholesterolemia* [gemfibrozil] 600 mg

gemeprost USAN, INN, BAN *prostaglandin*

gemfibrozil USAN, USP, INN, BAN *triglyceride-lowering antihyperlipidemic for hypertriglyceridemia (types IV and V hyperlipidemia) and coronary heart disease* 600 mg oral

gemifloxacin mesylate USAN *broad-spectrum fluoroquinolone antibiotic for respiratory tract infections*

gemopatrilat USAN *vasopeptidase inhibitor (VPI); angiotensin-converting enzyme (ACE) inhibitor for hypertension and congestive heart failure*

gemtuzumab ozogamicin USAN *antibody-targeted chemotherapy agent for acute myeloid leukemia (orphan)*

Gemzar powder for IV infusion ℞ *antineoplastic for advanced or metastatic breast, pancreatic, and non–small cell lung cancers (NSCLC); investigational (Phase III) for cervical cancer* [gemcitabine HCl] 20 mg/mL

Genac tablets OTC *decongestant; antihistamine* [pseudoephedrine HCl; triprolidine HCl] 60•2.5 mg

Gen-Acebutolol ⓒAN film-coated tablets ℞ *antihypertensive; antianginal* [acebutolol HCl] 100, 200, 400 mg

Genacol tablets (discontinued 2001) OTC *antitussive; decongestant; antihistamine; analgesic* [dextromethorphan hydrobromide; phenylpropanolamine HCl; chlorpheniramine maleate; acetaminophen] 10•30•2•325 mg

Genacol Cold & Flu Relief tablets OTC *antitussive; decongestant; antihistamine; analgesic* [dextromethorphan hydrobromide; pseudoephedrine HCl; chlorpheniramine maleate; acetaminophen] 15•30•2•500 mg

Genahist tablets, capsules, oral liquid OTC *antihistamine* [diphenhydramine HCl] 25 mg; 25 mg; 12.5 mg/5 mL

Gen-Allerate tablets OTC *antihistamine* [chlorpheniramine maleate] 4 mg

Genamin Cold syrup (discontinued 2001) OTC *decongestant; antihistamine* [phenylpropanolamine HCl; chlorpheniramine maleate] 6.25•1 mg/5 mL

Gen-Amiodarone ⓒAN tablets ℞ *antiarrhythmic* [amiodarone HCl] 200 mg

Gen-Amoxicillin ⓒAN capsules ℞ *antibiotic* [amoxicillin trihydrate] 250, 500 mg

Genapap tablets, caplets OTC *analgesic; antipyretic* [acetaminophen] 325, 500 mg; 500 mg

Genapap, Children's chewable tablets, elixir OTC *analgesic; antipyretic* [acetaminophen] 80 mg; 160 mg/5 mL

Genapap, Infants' drops OTC *analgesic; antipyretic* [acetaminophen] 100 mg/mL

Genaphed tablets OTC *nasal decongestant* [pseudoephedrine HCl] 30 mg

Genasal nasal spray OTC *nasal decongestant* [oxymetazoline HCl] 0.05%

Genasense ℞ *investigational (NDA filed, orphan) antineoplastic for malignant melanoma; investigational (Phase III, orphan) for multiple myeloma and chronic lymphocytic leukemia (CLL)* [augmerosen]

Genasoft softgels OTC *laxative; stool softener* [docusate sodium] 100 mg

Genasoft Plus softgels (discontinued 2003) OTC *stimulant laxative; stool softener* [casanthranol; docusate sodium] 30•100 mg

Genaspor cream OTC *topical antifungal* [tolnaftate] 1%

Genatap elixir (discontinued 2001) OTC *decongestant; antihistamine* [phenylpropanolamine HCl; brompheniramine maleate] 12.5•2 mg/5 mL ⑨ Genapap

Genaton chewable tablets OTC *antacid* [aluminum hydroxide; magnesium trisilicate] 80•20 mg

Genaton oral liquid OTC *antacid* [aluminum hydroxide; magnesium carbonate] 31.7•137.3 mg/5 mL

Genaton, Extra Strength chewable tablets OTC *antacid* [aluminum hydroxide; magnesium carbonate] 160•105 mg

Genatuss syrup (discontinued 2002) OTC *expectorant* [guaifenesin; alcohol 3.5%] 100 mg/5 mL

Genatuss DM syrup OTC *antitussive; expectorant* [dextromethorphan hydrobromide; guaifenesin] 20•200 mg/10 mL

Gen-bee with C caplets OTC *vitamin supplement* [multiple B vitamins; vitamin C] ± •300 mg

Gencalc 600 film-coated tablets (discontinued 2002) OTC *calcium supplement* [calcium carbonate] 1500 mg (600 mg Ca)

Gen-Carbamazepine CR ⒸⒶⓃ filmcoated tablets ℞ *anticonvulsant; analgesic for trigeminal neuralgia; antimanic* [carbamazepine] 200, 400 mg

Gencold sustained-release capsules (discontinued 2001) OTC *decongestant; antihistamine* [phenylpropanolamine HCl; chlorpheniramine maleate] 75•8 mg

Gen-Cyproterone ⒸⒶⓃ tablets ℞ *antiandrogen* [cyproterone acetate] 50 mg

Gendecon tablets (discontinued 2002) OTC *decongestant; antihistamine; analgesic* [phenylephrine HCl; chlorpheniramine maleate; acetaminophen] 5•2•325 mg

Gendex 75 IV infusion ℞ *plasma volume expander for shock due to hemorrhage, burns, or surgery* [dextran 75] 6%

Gen-Doxazosin ⒸⒶⓃ tablets ℞ *antihypertensive (α-blocker); treatment for benign prostatic hyperplasia* [doxazosin mesylate] 1, 2, 4, 8 mg

Genebs tablets, caplets OTC *analgesic; antipyretic* [acetaminophen] 325, 500 mg; 500 mg

Generet-500 timed-release tablets OTC *hematinic* [ferrous sulfate; multiple B vitamins; sodium ascorbate] 105• ± •500 mg ⑨ Gentap

Generix-T tablets OTC *vitamin/mineral/iron supplement* [multiple vitamins & minerals; iron] ± •15 mg

GenESA computer-controlled IV infusion device ("GenESA System") ℞ *cardiac stressor for diagnosis of coronary artery disease* [arbutamine HCl] 0.05 mg/mL

Gen-Etodolac ⒸⒶⓃ capsules ℞ *analgesic; antiarthritic; nonsteroidal anti-inflammatory drug (NSAID)* [etodolac] 200, 300 mg

Genevax-HIV ℞ *investigational (Phase I/II) vaccine for HIV*

Geneye eye drops OTC *topical ophthalmic decongestant and vasoconstrictor* [tetrahydrozoline HCl] 0.05%

Geneye Extra eye drops OTC *topical ophthalmic decongestant, vasoconstric-*

tor, and lubricant [tetrahydrozoline HCl; polytheylene glycol 400] 0.05%•1%

Gen-Fenofibrate Micro ⓒ capsules ℞ antihyperlipidemic [fenofibrate, micronized] 200 mg

Genfiber powder OTC bulk laxative [psyllium hydrophilic mucilloid] 3.4 g/tsp.

Gen-Fluoxetine ⓒ capsules ℞ selective serotonin reuptake inhibitor (SSRI) for depression and obsessive-compulsive disorder (OCD) [fluoxetine HCl] 10, 20 mg

Gen-Fluvoxamine ⓒ film-coated tablets ℞ selective serotonin reuptake inhibitor (SSRI) depression and obsessive-compulsive disorder (OCD) [fluvoxamine maleate] 50, 100 mg

Gen-Gliclazide ⓒ tablets ℞ antidiabetic [gliclazide] 80 mg

Gen-Glybe ⓒ tablets ℞ sulfonylurea antidiabetic [glyburide] 2.5, 5 mg

Gengraf capsules, oral drops ℞ immunosuppressant for allogenic kidney, liver, and heart transplants (orphan), rheumatoid arthritis (RA), and psoriasis [cyclosporine] 25, 100 mg; 100 mg/mL

Gen-Ipratropium ⓒ inhalation solution ℞ bronchodilator for asthma [ipratropium bromide] 0.025%

Genista tinctoria medicinal herb [see: dyer's broom]

genistein one of several soy isoflavones that provide cell-protective effects

genistin isoform precursor to genistein [q.v.]

Genite oral liquid (discontinued 2002) OTC antitussive; decongestant; antihistamine; analgesic [dextromethorphan hydrobromide; pseudoephedrine HCl; doxylamine succinate; acetaminophen; alcohol 25%] 5•10• 1.25•167 mg/5 mL

Gen-K powder for oral solution ℞ potassium supplement [potassium chloride] 20 mEq K/pkt.

Gen-Metformin ⓒ film-coated tablets ℞ biguanide antidiabetic [metformin HCl] 500, 850 mg

Gen-Metoprolol ⓒ film-coated tablets ℞ antihypertensive; antianginal [metoprolol tartrate] 50, 100 mg

Gen-Naproxen EC ⓒ enteric-coated tablets ℞ antiarthritic; nonsteroidal anti-inflammatory drug (NSAID) [naproxen] 500 mg

genophyllin [see: aminophylline]

Genoptic eye drops ℞ topical ophthalmic antibiotic [gentamicin sulfate] 3 mg/mL

Genoptic S.O.P. ophthalmic ointment ℞ topical ophthalmic antibiotic [gentamicin sulfate] 3 mg/g

Genotropin MiniQuick (prefilled syringes in packs of 7) ℞ growth hormone for children or adults with congenital or endogenous growth hormone deficiency, children with Turner syndrome or renal-induced growth failure, or AIDS-wasting syndrome (orphan) [somatropin]

Genotropin powder for subcu injection ℞ growth hormone for children or adults with congenital or endogenous growth hormone deficiency, children with Turner syndrome or renal-induced growth failure, or AIDS-wasting syndrome (orphan) [somatropin] 1.5, 5.8 mg (4, 15 IU) per mL

Genpril film-coated tablets OTC analgesic; antiarthritic; antipyretic; nonsteroidal anti-inflammatory drug (NSAID) [ibuprofen] 200 mg

Genprin tablets OTC analgesic; antipyretic; anti-inflammatory; antirheumatic [aspirin] 325 mg

Gen-Ranitidine ⓒ film-coated tablets ℞ histamine H_2 antagonist for gastric and duodenal ulcers [ranitidine HCl] 150, 300 mg

Gentacidin eye drops ℞ ophthalmic antibiotic [gentamicin sulfate] 3 mg/mL

Gentacidin ophthalmic ointment (discontinued 2001) ℞ topical ophthalmic antibiotic [gentamicin sulfate] 3 mg/g

Gentak eye drops, ophthalmic ointment ℞ topical ophthalmic antibiotic [gentamicin sulfate] 3 mg/mL; 3 mg/g

gentamicin BAN *aminoglycoside antibiotic* [also: gentamicin sulfate] ☒ Jenamicin; kanamycin

gentamicin sulfate USAN, USP *aminoglycoside antibiotic* [also: gentamicin] 3 mg/mL eye drops; 3 mg/g ophthalmic; 0.1% topical; 10, 40 mg/mL injection

gentamicin sulfate, liposomal *investigational (orphan) agent for disseminated Mycobacterium avium-intracellulare infection*

gentamicin-impregnated polymethyl methacrylate (PMMA) beads *investigational (orphan) agent for chronic osteomyelitis*

GenTeal gel OTC *ophthalmic moisturizer/lubricant* [hydroxypropyl methylcellulose; carbopol 980]

GenTeal; GenTeal Mild eye drops OTC *ophthalmic moisturizer/lubricant* [hydroxypropyl methylcellulose]

gentian (*Gentiana lutea*) root *medicinal herb for aiding digestion, appetite stimulation, arthritis, hysteria, jaundice, liver disorders, and sore throat*

gentian violet USP *topical anti-infective/antifungal* [also: methylrosanilinium chloride] 1%, 2%

Gen-Ticlodipine ⒸⒶⓃ tablets ℞ *platelet aggregation inhibitor* [ticlodipine HCl] 250 mg

gentisic acid ethanolamide NF *complexing agent*

Gentlax tablets OTC *stimulant laxative* [bisacodyl] 5 mg

Gentle Cream OTC *moisturizer; emollient*

Gentran 40 IV injection ℞ *plasma volume expander for shock due to hemorrhage, burns, or surgery* [dextran 40] 10%

Gentran 70 IV infusion ℞ *plasma volume expander for shock due to hemorrhage, burns, or surgery* [dextran 70] 6%

Gen-Verapamil ⒸⒶⓃ film-coated tablets ℞ *antianginal; antiarrhythmic; antihypertensive* [verapamil HCl] 80, 120 mg

Genvir ℞ *investigational (Phase III) controlled-release form for acute genital herpes* [acyclovir]

Gen-Xene tablets (discontinued 2003) ℞ *benzodiazepine anxiolytic; minor tranquilizer; alcohol withdrawal aid; anticonvulsant adjunct* [chlorazepate dipotassium] 3.75, 7.5, 15 mg

Gen-Zopiclone ⒸⒶⓃ tablets ℞ *sedative; hypnotic* [zopiclone] 7.5 mg

Geocillin film-coated caplets ℞ *extended-spectrum penicillin antibiotic* [carbenicillin indanyl sodium] 500 mg (=382 mg base)

Geodon capsules ℞ *novel (atypical) dihydroindolone antipsychotic for schizophrenia and manic episodes of a bipolar disorder; also used for agitation or psychosis due to Alzheimer or other dementias* [ziprasidone HCl] 20, 40, 60, 80 mg

Geodon powder for IM injection ℞ *novel (atypical) antipsychotic for rapid control of acute agitation due to schizophrenia, Alzheimer disease, or other dementias* [ziprasidone mesylate] 20 mg/vial

gepefrine INN

gepirone INN *azapirone tranquilizer; anxiolytic; antidepressant* [also: gepirone HCl]

gepirone HCl USAN *investigational (NDA filed) azapirone tranquilizer; anxiolytic; antidepressant* [also: gepirone]

Geranium maculatum *medicinal herb* [see: alum root]

2-geranylhydroquinone [see: geroquinol]

Gerardia pedicularia *medicinal herb* [see: feverweed]

Geravim elixir OTC *vitamin/mineral supplement* [multiple B vitamins & minerals]

Geravite elixir OTC *geriatric vitamin supplement* [multiple B vitamins]

Gerber Baby Low Iron Formula oral liquid, powder for oral liquid OTC *total or supplementary infant feeding*

Gentle Ease (handwritten marginal note)

Gerber Soy Formula powder OTC *hypoallergenic infant formula* [soy protein formula]

Geref powder for IV injection ℞ *diagnostic aid for pituitary function; treatment for growth hormone deficiency (orphan), anovulation, and AIDS-related weight loss* [sermorelin acetate] 50 μg

Geri SS lotion OTC *moisturizer; emollient*

Geri-Hydrolac cream OTC *moisturizer; emollient* [ammonium lactate] 12%

Gerimal sublingual tablets, tablets ℞ *cognition adjuvant for age-related mental capacity decline* [ergoloid mesylates] 0.5, 1 mg; 1 mg

Gerimed film-coated tablets OTC *geriatric vitamin/mineral supplement* [multiple vitamins & minerals]

Geriot film-coated tablets OTC *hematinic; vitamin/mineral supplement* [carbonyl iron; multiple vitamins & minerals; folic acid; biotin] 50 mg•±•0.4 mg•45 μg

Geri-Soft lotion OTC *moisturizer; emollient*

Geritol Complete tablets OTC *vitamin/mineral/iron supplement* [multiple vitamins & minerals; ferrous fumarate; folic acid; biotin] ±•18 mg•0.4 mg•45 μg

Geritol Extend caplets OTC *vitamin/mineral/iron supplement* [multiple vitamins & minerals; ferrous fumarate; folic acid] ±•10•0.2 mg

Geritol Tonic oral liquid OTC *hematinic* [ferric pyrophosphate; multiple B vitamins; alcohol 12%] 18•± mg/15 mL

Geritonic oral liquid OTC *hematinic* [ferric ammonium citrate; liver fraction 1; multiple B vitamins & minerals; alcohol 20%] 105•375•± mg/15 mL

Gerivite oral liquid OTC *geriatric vitamin/mineral supplement* [multiple B vitamins & minerals; alcohol 18%]

Gerivites tablets (discontinued 2004) OTC *hematinic; vitamin/mineral supplement* [ferrous sulfate; multiple vitamins & minerals; folic acid] 50•±•0.4 mg

German valerian *medicinal herb* [see: valerian]

Germanin (available only from the Centers for Disease Control) ℞ *antiparasitic for African trypanosomiasis and onchocerciasis* [suramin sodium]

germanium *element* (Ge)

germicides *a class of agents that destroy micro-organisms* [see also: antiseptics; disinfectants]

geroquinol INN

Geroton Forte oral liquid OTC *geriatric vitamin/mineral supplement* [multiple B vitamins & minerals; alcohol 13.5%]

gesarol [see: chlorophenothane]

gestaclone USAN, INN *progestin*

gestadienol INN

gestanin [see: allyloestrenol]

gestodene USAN, INN, BAN *progestin*

gestonorone caproate USAN, INN *progestin* [also: gestronol]

gestrinone USAN, INN *progestin*

gestronol BAN *progestin* [also: gestonorone caproate]

Get Better Bear Sore Throat Pops OTC *throat emollient and protectant* [pectin] 19 mg

Gets-It topical liquid OTC *keratolytic* [salicylic acid; zinc chloride; alcohol 28%]

gevotroline INN *antipsychotic* [also: gevotroline HCl]

gevotroline HCl USAN *antipsychotic* [also: gevotroline]

Gevrabon oral liquid OTC *vitamin/mineral supplement* [multiple B vitamins & minerals; alcohol 18%]

Gevral tablets OTC *vitamin/mineral/iron supplement* [multiple vitamins & minerals; ferrous fumarate; folic acid] ±•18 mg•0.4 mg

Gevral Protein powder OTC *oral protein supplement* [calcium caseinate; sucrose]

G-F 20 [see: hylan G-F 20]

GFN (guaifenesin) [q.v.]

GFN 550/PSE 60/DM 30 sustained-release tablets ℞ *expectorant; decongestant; antitussive* [guaifenesin;

pseudoephedrine HCl; dextromethorphan hydrobromide] 550•60•30 mg

GFN 600/Phenylephrine 20 tablets ℞ *decongestant; expectorant* [phenylephrine HCl; guaifenesin] 20•600 mg

GFN 600/PSE 60/DM 30 sustained-release caplets ℞ *expectorant; decongestant; antitussive* [guaifenesin; pseudoephedrine HCl; dextromethorphan hydrobromide] 600•60•30 mg

GFN 1200/DM 60, GFN 1000/DM 50 sustained-release caplets ℞ *expectorant; antitussive* [guaifenesin; dextromethorphan hydrobromide] 1200•60 mg; 1000•50 mg

GFN 1200/DM 60/PSE 120 sustained-release caplets ℞ *expectorant; antitussive; decongestant* [guaifenesin; dextromethorphan hydrobromide; pseudoephedrine HCl] 1200•60•120 mg

GFN/PSE sustained-release tablets ℞ *expectorant; decongestant* [guaifenesin; pseudoephedrine HCl] 1200•120 mg

GHB (gamma hydroxybutyrate) *a CNS depressant used as an anesthetic in some countries, produced and abused as a "date rape" street drug in the U.S.; illegal in the U.S. (Schedule I)* [the sodium salt is medically known as sodium oxybate]

GHB-aldehyde (gamma butyraldehyde) *a precursor to gamma hydroxybutyrate (GHB)* [see: gamma hydroxybutyrate (GHB)]

GHRF; GH-RF (growth hormone-releasing factor) [q.v.]

Gilead, balm of *medicinal herb* [see: balm of Gilead]

ginger (Zingiber officinale) root *medicinal herb for childhood diseases, colds, colic, dizziness, fever, flu, gas pains, headache, indigestion, morning sickness, nausea, poor circulation, toothache, and vestibular disorders*

ginger, wild *medicinal herb* [see: wild ginger]

ginkgo (Ginkgo biloba) leaves *medicinal herb for Alzheimer disease, antioxidant, anxiety, asthma, attention-deficit disorder, chilblains, cerebral insufficiency, dementia, dizziness, memory loss, poor circulation, Raynaud disease, stroke, and tinnitus*

ginseng (Panax spp.) root *medicinal herb for age spots, blood diseases, depression, hemorrhage, increasing endurance and longevity, and stress; also used as an aphrodisiac* [also see: Siberian ginseng]

ginseng, blue; yellow ginseng *medicinal herb* [see: blue cohosh]

giparmen INN

giractide INN

girisopam INN

gitalin NF [also: gitalin amorphous]

gitalin amorphous INN [also: gitalin]

gitaloxin INN

gitoformate INN

gitoxin 16-formate [see: gitaloxin]

gitoxin pentaacetate [see: pengitoxin]

GLA (gamma-linolenic acid) [q.v.]

glacial acetic acid [see: acetic acid, glacial]

Gladase ointment ℞ *proteolytic enzyme for debridement of necrotic tissue; vulnerary* [papain; urea] 830 000 U•100 mg per gram

Gladase-C ointment ℞ *proteolytic enzyme for debridement of necrotic tissue; vulnerary; topical wound deodorant* [papain; urea; chlorophyllin copper complex] 521 700 U/g•10%•0.5%

glafenine INN, DCF, JAN

glaphenine [see: glafenine]

glatiramer acetate USAN *immunomodulator for relapsing-remitting multiple sclerosis (orphan)*

Glauber salt [see: sodium sulfate]

glaucarubin

Glaucon Drop-Tainers (eye drops) (discontinued 2004) ℞ *antiglaucoma agent* [epinephrine HCl] 1%, 2%

GlaucTabs tablets (discontinued 2003) ℞ *carbonic anhydrase inhibitor for glaucoma* [methazolamide] 25, 50 mg

glaze, pharmaceutical NF *tablet-coating agent*

glaziovine INN

Gleevec film-coated tablets ℞ *antineoplastic for chronic myeloid leukemia (CML) (orphan) and gastrointestinal stromal tumors (GIST)* [imatinib mesylate] 100, 400 mg

glemanserin USAN, INN *anxiolytic*

gleptoferron USAN, INN, BAN *veterinary hematinic*

Gliadel wafers ℞ *nitrosourea-type alkylating antineoplastic cerebral implants for excised brain tumors (orphan)* [carmustine] 7.7 mg

gliamilide USAN, INN *antidiabetic*

glibenclamide INN, BAN *sulfonylurea antidiabetic* [also: glyburide]

glibornuride USAN, INN, BAN *antidiabetic*

glibutimine INN

glicaramide INN

glicetanile INN *antidiabetic* [also: glicetanile sodium]

glicetanile sodium USAN *antidiabetic* [also: glicetanile]

gliclazide INN, BAN *sulfonylurea antidiabetic*

glicondamide INN

glidazamide INN

gliflumide USAN, INN *antidiabetic*

glimepiride USAN, INN, BAN *sulfonylurea antidiabetic*

glipentide [see: glisentide]

glipizide USAN, INN, BAN *sulfonylurea antidiabetic* 5, 10 mg oral

Glipizide ER extended-release tablets ℞ *sulfonylurea antidiabetic* [glipizide] 2.5, 5, 10 mg

gliquidone INN, BAN

glisamuride INN

glisentide INN

glisindamide INN

glisolamide INN

glisoxepide INN, BAN

Glivec (foreign name for U.S. product Gleevec)

globin zinc insulin INN [also: insulin, globin zinc]

globulin, aerosolized pooled immune *investigational (orphan) agent for respiratory syncytial virus lower respiratory tract disease*

globulin, immune USP *passive immunizing agent for HIV, ITP, B-cell CLL, and bone marrow transplantation; infection prophylaxis in pediatric HIV (orphan); investigational (orphan) for myocarditis and juvenile rheumatoid arthritis*

globulin, immune human serum [now: globulin, immune]

Glofil-125 injection ℞ *radiopaque contrast medium* [iothalamate sodium I 125 (59.9% iodine)] 1 mg/mL

Glossets (trademarked form) *sublingual or rectal administration*

gloxazone USAN, INN, BAN *veterinary anaplasmodastat*

gloximonam USAN, INN *antibacterial*

GlucaGen Diagnostic Kit IV injection ℞ *agent to inhibit movement of the gastrointestinal tract during radiographic procedures* [glucagon, recombinant] 1 mg

GlucaGen Emergency Kit; GlucaGen HypoKit subcu, IV, or IM injection ℞ *emergency treatment of hypoglycemic crisis* [glucagon, recombinant] 1 mg

glucagon USP, INN, BAN *antidiabetic; glucose elevating agent; diagnostic aid for GI imaging*

Glucagon Diagnostic Kit IM or IV injection ℞ *to inhibit GI tract movement during radiographic procedures* [glucagon, recombinant] 1 mg (1 U)

Glucagon Emergency Kit subcu, IM, or IV injection ℞ *emergency treatment for hypoglycemic crisis* [glucagon, recombinant] 1 mg (1 U)

glucalox INN [also: glycalox]

glucametacin INN

glucan synthesis inhibitors *a class of antifungals* [also: echinocandins]

D-glucaric acid, calcium salt tetrahydrate [see: calcium saccharate]

gluceptate USAN, USP, INN, BAN *combining name for radicals or groups*

gluceptate sodium USAN *pharmaceutic aid*

Glucerna; Glucerna Select; Glucerna Weight Loss Shake ready-to-use oral liquid OTC *enteral nutritional therapy for abnormal glucose tolerance*

D-glucitol [see: sorbitol]

D-glucitol hexanicotinate [see: sorbinicate]

β-glucocerebrosidase, macrophage-targeted [see: alglucerase]

glucocerebrosidase, recombinant retroviral vector *investigational (orphan) enzyme replacement for types I, II, or III Gaucher disease*

glucocerebrosidase-β-glucosidase [see: alglucerase]

glucocorticoids *a class of adrenal cortical steroids that modify the body's immune response*

Glucofilm reagent strips for home use *in vitro diagnostic aid for blood glucose*

glucoheptonic acid, calcium salt [see: calcium gluceptate]

glucomannan (*Amorphophallus konjac*) root *medicinal herb for constipation, diverticular disease, hemorrhoids, hypercholesterolemia, and obesity; it may produce altered insulin requirements or hypoglycemia in diabetics*

Glucometer Encore; Glucometer Elite reagent strips for home use *in vitro diagnostic aid for blood glucose*

D-gluconic acid, calcium salt [see: calcium gluconate]

D-gluconic acid, magnesium salt [see: magnesium gluconate]

D-gluconic acid, monopotassium salt [see: potassium gluconate]

D-gluconic acid, monosodium salt [see: sodium gluconate]

GlucoNorm ⊛ tablets ℞ *oral antidiabetic agent that stimulates release of insulin from the pancreas for type 2 diabetes* [repaglinide] 0.5, 1, 2 mg

Glucophage film-coated tablets ℞ *biguanide antidiabetic* [metformin HCl] 500, 850, 1000 mg

Glucophage XR extended-release tablets ℞ *once-daily biguanide antidiabetic* [metformin HCl] 500, 750 mg

β-D-glucopyranuronamide [see: glucuronamide]

glucosamine USAN, INN *pharmaceutic aid*

glucosamine sulfate *natural remedy for osteoarthritis*

d-glucose [see: dextrose]

glucose, liquid NF *tablet binder and coating agent; antihypoglycemic; diagnostic aid for diabetes* ② Glutose

d-glucose monohydrate [see: dextrose]

glucose oxidase

glucose polymers *caloric replacement*

Glucostix reagent strips for home use *in vitro diagnostic aid for blood glucose*

glucosulfamide INN

glucosulfone INN

glucosylceramidase [see: alglucerase]

Glucotrol tablets ℞ *sulfonylurea antidiabetic* [glipizide] 5, 10 mg

Glucotrol XL extended-release tablets ℞ *sulfonylurea antidiabetic* [glipizide] 2.5, 5, 10 mg

Glucovance film-coated caplets ℞ *antidiabetic combination for type 2 diabetes* [glyburide; metformin HCl] 1.25•250, 2.5•500, 5•500 mg

glucurolactone INN

glucuronamide INN, BAN

Glumetza extended-release tablets ℞ *once-daily biguanide antidiabetic* [metformin HCl] 500, 1000 mg

glunicate INN

gluside [see: saccharin]

gluside, soluble [see: saccharin sodium]

glusoferron INN

glutamic acid (L-glutamic acid) USAN, INN *nonessential amino acid; symbols: Glu, E* 340, 500 mg oral

glutamic acid HCl *gastric acidifier*

glutamine (L-glutamine) USAN, USP, JAN *nonessential amino acid that supplies energy to the brain to reduce fatigue and increase exercise endurance, combat hypoglycemia, and strengthen the GI tract; growth hormone secretagogue; investigational (orphan) for short bowel syndrome; symbols: Gln, Q*

glutamine & somatropin *investigational (orphan) for GI malabsorption due to short bowel syndrome*

glutaral USAN, USP, INN *disinfectant*

glutaraldehyde [see: glutaral]

Glutarex-1 powder OTC *formula for infants with glutaric aciduria type I*

Glutarex-2 powder OTC *enteral nutritional therapy for glutaric aciduria type I*

glutasin [see: glutamic acid HCl]

glutathione *endogenous antioxidant produced in the liver; unstable as an oral supplement, so levels are increased by using transdermal preparations, by supplementing its precursors, MSM and NAC (q.v.), or by regenerating it with SAMe (q.v.)*

L-**glutathione, reduced** *investigational (orphan) for AIDS-related cachexia*

glutaurine INN

glutethimide USP, INN, BAN *sedative; sometimes abused as a street drug* 250, 500 mg oral

Glutofac tablets OTC *vitamin/mineral supplement* [multiple vitamins & minerals]

Glutofac-ZX caplets ℞ *vitamin/mineral supplement* [multiple vitamins & minerals; folic acid; biotin] ± ● 1 ● 0.2 mg

Glutose gel OTC *glucose elevating agent* [glucose] 40% 🄐 glucose

Glyate syrup (discontinued 2002) OTC *expectorant* [guaifenesin; alcohol 3.5%] 100 mg/5 mL

glyburide USAN *sulfonylurea antidiabetic* [also: glibenclamide] 1.25, 1.5, 2.5, 3, 4.5, 5, 6 mg oral

glyburide & metformin HCl *sulfonylurea/biguanide antidiabetic combination for type 2 diabetes* 1.25 ● 250, 2.5 ● 500, 5 ● 500 mg oral

glybutamide [see: carbutamide]

glybuthiazol INN

glybuthizol [see: glybuthiazol]

glybuzole INN

glycalox BAN [also: glucalox]

glyceol *investigational (orphan) agent for decreasing intracranial hypertension or cerebral edema*

glycerides oleiques polyoxyethylenes [see: peglicol 5 oleate]

glycerin USP *humectant; solvent; osmotic diuretic; hyperosmotic laxative; emollient/protectant; ophthalmic moisturizer* [also: glycerol]

glycerol INN *humectant; solvent; osmotic diuretic; hyperosmotic laxative; emollient/protectant; monoctanoin component D* [also: glycerin]

glycerol, iodinated USAN, BAN *(disapproved for use as an expectorant in 1991)*

glycerol 1-decanoate *monoctanoin component B* [see: monoctanoin]

glycerol 1,2-dioctanoate *monoctanoin component C* [see: monoctanoin]

glycerol 1-octanoate *monoctanoin component A* [see: monoctanoin]

glycerol phosphate, manganese salt [see: manganese glycerophosphate]

glyceryl behenate NF *tablet and capsule lubricant*

glyceryl borate [see: boroglycerin]

glyceryl guaiacolate [now: guaifenesin]

glyceryl monostearate NF *emulsifying agent*

glyceryl triacetate [now: triacetin]

glyceryl trierucate *investigational (orphan) agent for adrenoleukodystrophy* [also: glyceryl trioleate]

glyceryl trinitrate BAN *coronary vasodilator* [also: nitroglycerin]

glyceryl trioleate *investigational (orphan) agent for adrenoleukodystrophy* [also: glyceryl trierucate]

glycerylaminophenaquine [see: glafenine]

Glyceryl-T capsules, oral liquid ℞ *antiasthmatic; bronchodilator; expectorant* [theophylline; guaifenesin] 150 ● 90 mg; 150 ● 90 mg/15 mL

glycinato dihydroxyaluminum hydrate [see: dihydroxyaluminum aminoacetate]

glycine USP, INN *nonessential amino acid; urologic irrigant; symbols: Gly, G* [also: aminoacetic acid] 1.5%

glycine aluminum-zirconium complex [see: aluminum zirconium tetrachlorohydrex gly; aluminum zirconium trichlorohydrex gly]

Glycine max *medicinal herb* [see: soy]

glycitein *one of several soy isoflavones that provide cell-protective effects*

glycitin *isoform precursor to glycitein* [q.v.]

glyclopyramide INN

glycobiarsol USP, INN [also: bismuth glycollylarsanilate]

glycocholate sodium [see: sodium glycocholate]

glycocoll [see: glycine]

Glycofed tablets (discontinued 2002) OTC *decongestant; expectorant* [pseudoephedrine HCl; guaifenesin] 30•100 mg

glycol distearate USAN *thickening agent*

GlycoLax powder for oral solution ℞ *laxative* [polyethylene glycol–electrolyte solution (PEG 3350)] 17 g/dose

glycolic acid *mild exfoliant and keratolytic*

glycolipodipsipeptides *a class of broad-spectrum antibiotics that are bactericidal against gram-positive aerobic and anaerobic bacteria*

p-**glycolophenetidide** [see: fenacetinol]

glycopeptides *a class of antibiotic antineoplastics*

glycophenylate [see: mepenzolate bromide]

glycoprotein (GP) IIb/IIIa receptor antagonists *a class of platelet aggregation inhibitors for acute coronary syndrome, unstable angina, myocardial infarction, and cardiac surgery*

glycopyrrolate USAN, USP GI *antispasmodic; antisecretory; peptic ulcer adjunct* [also: glycopyrronium bromide] 1, 2 mg oral; 0.2 mg/mL injection

glycopyrrone bromide [see: glycopyrrolate]

glycopyrronium bromide INN, BAN GI *antispasmodic; antisecretory; peptic ulcer adjunct* [also: glycopyrrolate]

glycosaminoglycans *a class of anticoagulants used for the prophylaxis of postoperative deep vein thrombosis (DVT)*

glycosides, cardiac *a class of cardiovascular drugs that increase the force of cardiac contractions* [also called: digitalis glycosides]

Glycotuss tablets (discontinued 2002) OTC *expectorant* [guaifenesin] 100 mg ⧈ Glytuss

Glycotuss-DM tablets (discontinued 2002) OTC *antitussive; expectorant*

[dextromethorphan hydrobromide; guaifenesin] 10•100 mg

glycyclamide INN, BAN

glycylcyclines *a class of bacteriostatic, antimicrobial antibiotics; a derivative of tetracyclines that have greater efficacy against tetracycline-resistant infections*

glycyrrhetinic acid [see: enoxolone]

glycyrrhiza NF

Glycyrrhiza glabra; G. palidiflora; G. uralensis medicinal herb [see: licorice]

glydanile sodium [now: glicetanile sodium]

glyhexamide USAN, INN *antidiabetic*

glyhexylamide [see: metahexamide]

glymidine BAN *antidiabetic* [also: glymidine sodium]

glymidine sodium USAN, INN *antidiabetic* [also: glymidine]

glymol [see: mineral oil]

Glynase PresTabs (micronized tablets) ℞ *sulfonylurea antidiabetic* [glyburide] 1.5, 3, 6 mg

glyoctamide USAN, INN *antidiabetic*

Gly-Oxide oral solution OTC *topical anti-inflammatory and anti-infective* [carbamide peroxide] 10%

glyparamide USAN *antidiabetic*

glyphylline [see: dyphylline]

glypinamide INN

glyprothiazol INN

glyprothizol [see: glyprothiazol]

Glyquin cream ℞ *hyperpigmentation bleaching agent* [hydroquinone (in a sunscreen base)] 4%

Glyquin-XM cream ℞ *hyperpigmentation bleaching agent* [hydroquinone (in a sunscreen base with vitamin E)] 4%

Glyset tablets ℞ *antidiabetic agent for type 2 diabetes; alpha-glucosidase inhibitor that delays the digestion of dietary carbohydrates* [miglitol] 25, 50, 100 mg

glysobuzole INN [also: isobuzole]

Glytuss film-coated tablets (discontinued 2002) OTC *expectorant* [guaifenesin] 200 mg ⧈ Glycotuss

GM-CSF (granulocyte-macrophage colony-stimulating factor) [see: regramostim; sargramostim; molgramostim]

G-myticin cream, ointment (discontinued 2003) ℞ *antibiotic* [gentamicin sulfate] 1 mg

Gnaphalium polycephalum; G. uliginosum medicinal herb [see: everlasting]

Gn-RH, GnRH (gonadotropin-releasing hormone) *an endogenous hormone, produced in the hypothalamus, which stimulates the release of luteinizing hormone (LH) and follicle-stimulating hormone (FSH) from the pituitary* [also known as: luteinizing hormone–releasing hormone (LH-RH)]

goatweed *medicinal herb* [see: St. John wort]

gold *element (Au)*

gold Au 198 USAN, USP *antineoplastic; liver imaging aid; radioactive agent*

gold sodium thiomalate USP *antirheumatic (50% gold)* [also: sodium aurothiomalate] 50 mg/mL injection

gold sodium thiosulfate NF [also: sodium aurotiosulfate]

gold thioglucose [see: aurothioglucose]

gold thread (*Coptis trifolia*) root *medicinal herb used as an antiphlogistic, bitter tonic, and sedative*

golden senecio *medicinal herb* [see: life root]

goldenrod (*Solidago nemoralis; S. odora; S. virgaurea*) leaves and flowering tops *medicinal herb used as an astringent, carminative, diaphoretic, diuretic, and stimulant*

goldenseal (*Hydrastis canadensis*) rhizome and root *medicinal herb used as an antibiotic and antiseptic and for internal bleeding, colon inflammation, eye infections, liver disorders, menorrhagia, mouth sores, muscular pain, sciatic pain, and vaginitis*

GoLYTELY powder for oral solution ℞ *pre-procedure bowel evacuant* [polyethylene glycol–electrolyte solution (PEG 3350)] 60 g/L

gonacrine [see: acriflavine]

Gonadimmune *investigational anti-gonadotropin-releasing hormone for prostate, breast, and endometrial cancer and endometriosis*

gonadorelin INN, BAN *gonad-stimulating principle* [also: gonadorelin acetate]

gonadorelin acetate USAN *gonad-stimulating principle for hypothalamic amenorrhea (orphan); diagnostic aid for fertility* [also: gonadorelin]

gonadorelin HCl USAN *gonad-stimulating principle; synthetic luteinizing hormone–releasing hormone (LH-RH); in vivo diagnostic aid for anterior pituitary function*

gonadotrophin, chorionic INN, BAN *gonad-stimulating principle* [also: gonadotropin, chorionic]

gonadotrophin, serum INN

gonadotropin, chorionic USP *gonad-stimulating hormone for prepubertal cryptorchidism and hypogonadism; ovulation stimulant* [also: gonadotrophin, chorionic] 500, 1000, 2000 U/mL injection

gonadotropin, serum [see: gonadotrophin, serum]

gonadotropin-releasing hormone (Gn-RH) *an endogenous hormone, produced in the hypothalamus, which stimulates the release of luteinizing hormone (LH) and follicle-stimulating hormone (FSH) from the pituitary* [also known as: luteinizing hormone–releasing hormone (LH-RH)]

gonadotropin-releasing hormone analogs *a class of hormonal antineoplastics*

gonadotropins *a class of hormones that stimulate the ovaries, including follicle-stimulating hormone and luteinizing hormone*

Gonak ophthalmic solution OTC *gonioscopic examination aid* [hydroxypropyl methylcellulose] 2.5% ◨ Gonic

Gonal-f subcu injection ℞ *recombinant follicle-stimulating hormone (FSH) for induction of ovulation or spermatogenesis (orphan); adjunct to assisted reproductive technologies (ART)* [follitropin alfa] 75, 450, 1050 IU

Gonal-f RFF Pen (prefilled syringes) ℞ *recombinant follicle-stimulating hormone (FSH) for induction of ovula-*

tion; adjunct to assisted reproductive technologies (ART) [follitropin alfa] 300, 450, 900 IU

Gonic powder for IM injection ℞ *gonad-stimulating hormone for prepubertal cryptorchidism and hypogonadism; ovulation stimulant* [chorionic gonadotropin] 1000 U/mL ⊡ Gonak

Goniopora spp. *natural material* [see: coral]

Gonioscopic Prism Solution Drop-Tainers (eye drops) OTC *agent for bonding gonioscopic prisms to eye* [hydroxyethyl cellulose]

Goniosol ophthalmic solution OTC *gonioscopic examination aid* [hydroxypropyl methylcellulose] 2.5%

Gonozyme Diagnostic reagent kit for professional use *in vitro diagnostic aid for Neisseria gonorrhoeae*

Good Sense Pain Relief Allergy Sinus gelcaps OTC *decongestant; antihistamine; analgesic* [pseudoephedrine HCl; chlorpheniramine maleate; acetaminophen] 30•2•500 mg

Good Sense Sinus caplets OTC *decongestant; antihistamine; analgesic* [pseudoephedrine HCl; chlorpheniramine maleate; acetaminophen] 30•2•500 mg

Good Start; Good Start Essentials; Good Start Supreme oral liquid, powder for oral liquid OTC *total or supplementary infant feeding*

GoodStart [see: Carnation Good Start]

Goody's Body Pain powder OTC *analgesic; antipyretic; anti-inflammatory* [acetaminophen; aspirin] 325•500 mg/dose

Goody's Extra Strength Headache powder OTC *analgesic; antipyretic; anti-inflammatory* [acetaminophen; aspirin; caffeine] 250•520•32.5 mg/dose

Goody's PM powder OTC *antihistaminic sleep aid; analgesic* [diphenhydramine citrate; acetaminophen] 38•500 mg

goose grass *medicinal herb* [see: bedstraw; cinquefoil]

goose hair; gosling weed *medicinal herb* [see: bedstraw]

Gordobalm OTC *analgesic; counterirritant; antiseptic* [methyl salicylate; menthol; camphor; alcohol 16%]

Gordochom topical solution OTC *antifungal; antiseptic* [undecylenic acid; chloroxylenol] 25%•3%

Gordofilm topical liquid ℞ *keratolytic* [salicylic acid in flexible collodion] 16.7%

Gordogesic Creme OTC *analgesic; counterirritant* [methyl salicylate] 10%

Gordon's Urea 40% cream ℞ *for removal of dystrophic nails* [urea] 40%

Gormel Creme OTC *moisturizer; emollient; keratolytic* [urea] 20%

goserelin USAN, INN, BAN *hormonal antineoplastic for prostate and breast cancer; luteinizing hormone-releasing hormone (LHRH) agonist* [also: goserelin acetate]

goserelin acetate JAN *hormonal antineoplastic for prostatic carcinoma, breast cancer, and endometriosis; luteinizing hormone-releasing hormone (LHRH) agonist* [also: goserelin]

gosling weed; goose grass; goose hair *medicinal herb* [see: bedstraw]

gossypol (Gossypium spp.) seed oil *medicinal herb for male and female contraception; not generally regarded as safe and effective as male sterility may be irreversible; investigational for metastatic endometrial carcinoma; investigational antiviral/interferon inducer for AIDS; investigational (orphan) for adrenal cortex cancer*

gotu kola (Centella asiatica; Hydrocotyle asiatica) entire plant *medicinal herb for abscesses, hypertension, contraception, leprosy, nervous breakdown, physical and mental fatigue, promoting wound healing, and rheumatism*

goutberry *medicinal herb* [see: blackberry]

govafilcon A USAN *hydrophilic contact lens material*

G/P 1200/600 sustained-release tablets ℞ *decongestant; expectorant* [pseudoephedrine HCl; guaifenesin] 60•1200 mg

GP IIb/IIIa inhibitors [see: glycoprotein (GP) IIb/IIIa receptor antagonists]

gp100 adenoviral gene therapy *investigational (Phase III, orphan) theraccine for metastatic melanoma*

gp120 (glycoprotein 120) antigens *investigational (Phase III) vaccine for HIV* [also: AIDS vaccine]

gp160 (glycoprotein 160) antigens *investigational (orphan) antiviral (therapeutic, Phase II) and vaccine (preventative, Phase I) for HIV and AIDS*

GP-500 tablets ℞ *decongestant; expectorant* [pseudoephedrine HCl; guaifenesin] 120•500 mg

gp96 heat shock protein-peptide complex *investigational (Phase III, orphan) antineoplastic for renal cell carcinoma and metastatic melanoma*

grace, herb of *medicinal herb* [see: rue]

Gradumet (trademarked dosage form) *controlled-release tablet*

graftskin *a living, bilayered skin construct for diabetic foot ulcers and pressure sores (the epidermal layer is living human keratinocytes; the dermal layer is living human fibroblasts)*

gramicidin USP, INN *antibacterial antibiotic*

gramicidin & neomycin sulfate & polymyxin B sulfate *topical antibiotic* 0.025 mg•1.75 mg•10 000 U per mL eye drops

gramicidin S INN

Graminis rhizoma *medicinal herb* [see: couch grass]

granisetron USAN, INN, BAN *serotonin 5-HT₃ receptor antagonist; antiemetic for nausea following chemotherapy, radiation, or surgery*

granisetron HCl USAN *serotonin 5-HT₃ receptor antagonist; antiemetic for nausea following chemotherapy, radiation, or surgery*

Granul-Derm aerosol spray ℞ *proteolytic enzyme for debridement of necrotic tissue* [trypsin; peruvian balsam] 0.1•72.5 mg/0.82 mL

Granulex aerosol spray ℞ *proteolytic enzyme for debridement of necrotic tissue* [trypsin; peruvian balsam] 0.1•72.5 mg/0.82 mL

granulocyte colony-stimulating factor (G-CSF), recombinant [see: filgrastim]

granulocyte-macrophage colony-stimulating factor (GM-CSF) [see: regramostim; sargramostim; molgramostim]

GranuMed aerosol spray ℞ *topical enzyme for wound debridement* [trypsin; peruvian balsam] 0.1•72.5 mg/0.82 mL

grape, bear's *medicinal herb* [see: uva ursi]

grape, Rocky Mountain; wild Oregon grape *medicinal herb* [see: Oregon grape]

grape seed (Vitis coigetiae; V. vinifera) oil *medicinal herb for dental caries; also used as a dietary source of essential fatty acids and tocopherols*

grape seed extract *natural free radical scavenger for inflammatory collagen disease and peripheral vascular disease; contains 92%–95% procyanidolic oligomers (PCOs)*

grapefruit (Citrus paradisi) *medicinal herb for potassium replacement; the pectin is used to help reduce cholesterol and promote regression of atherosclerosis*

grass burdock *medicinal herb* [see: burdock]

grass myrtle *medicinal herb* [see: calamus]

Gratiola officinalis *medicinal herb* [see: hedge hyssop]

gravelroot *medicinal herb* [see: queen of the meadow]

graybeard tree *medicinal herb* [see: fringe tree]

great wild valerian *medicinal herb* [see: valerian]

greater celandine *medicinal herb* [see: celandine]

green broom; greenweed *medicinal herb* [see: dyer's broom]

green hellebore (Veratrum viride) *medicinal herb* [see: hellebore]

green soap [see: soap, green]

green tea (Camellia sinensis) leaves *medicinal herb used as an antihyperlipidemic, antimicrobial, antineoplastic, and antioxidant; also used to promote longevity by attenuating severe fatal diseases*

Green Throat Spray; Red Throat Spray OTC *topical antipruritic/counterirritant; mild local anesthetic* [phenol] 1.4%

greenweed; green broom *medicinal herb* [see: dyer's broom]

grepafloxacin INN *broad-spectrum fluoroquinolone antibiotic*

grepafloxacin HCl USAN *broad-spectrum fluoroquinolone antibiotic*

Grifola frondosa *medicinal herb* [see: maitake mushrooms]

Grifols [see: Human Albumin Grifols]

Grifulvin V tablets, oral suspension (discontinued 2003) ℞ *systemic antifungal* [griseofulvin (microsize)] 250, 500 mg; 125 mg/5 mL

Grindelia squarrosia *medicinal herb* [see: gum weed]

Grisactin 250 capsules (discontinued 2004) ℞ *systemic antifungal* [griseofulvin (microsize)] 250 mg

Grisactin 500 tablets (discontinued 2004) ℞ *systemic antifungal* [griseofulvin (microsize)] 500 mg

Grisactin Ultra tablets (discontinued 2004) ℞ *systemic antifungal* [griseofulvin (ultramicrosize)] 250 mg

griseofulvin USP, INN, BAN *systemic antifungal* 125 mg/5 mL oral

Gris-PEG film-coated tablets ℞ *systemic antifungal* [griseofulvin (ultramicrosize)] 125, 250 mg

ground apple *medicinal herb* [see: chamomile]

ground berry *medicinal herb* [see: wintergreen]

ground holly *medicinal herb* [see: pipsissewa]

ground lemon *medicinal herb* [see: mandrake]

ground lily *medicinal herb* [see: birthroot]

ground raspberry *medicinal herb* [see: goldenseal]

ground squirrel pea *medicinal herb* [see: twin leaf]

ground thistle *medicinal herb* [see: carline thistle]

growth hormone, human (hGH) [see: somatropin]

growth hormone-releasing factor (GHRF; GH-RF) *investigational (orphan) for inadequate endogenous growth hormone in children*

G-strophanthin [see: ouabain]

GTI-2040 [see: antisense 20-mer phosphorothiolate oligonucleotide]

guabenxan INN

guacetisal INN

guafecainol INN

guaiac

guaiacol NF

p-**guaiacol** [see: mequinol]

guaiacol carbonate NF

guaiacol glyceryl ether [see: guaifenesin]

guaiactamine INN

guaiapate USAN, INN *antitussive*

guaiazulene soluble [see: sodium guaialenate]

guaietolin INN

Guaifed sustained-release capsules ℞ *decongestant; expectorant* [phenylephrine HCl; guaifenesin] 15•400 mg

Guaifed syrup OTC *decongestant; expectorant* [pseudoephedrine HCl; guaifenesin] 60•400 mg/10 mL

Guaifed-PD sustained-release capsules ℞ *decongestant; expectorant* [phenylephrine HCl; guaifenesin] 7.5•200 mg

guaifenesin USAN, USP, INN *expectorant* [also: guaiphenesin] 200, 400 mg oral; 100 mg/5 mL oral ⧠ guanfacine

guaifenesin & codeine phosphate *expectorant; narcotic antitussive; narcotic analgesic* 300•10 mg oral; 100•10 mg/5 mL oral

Guaifenesin DAC oral liquid (discontinued 2002) OTC *narcotic antitussive; decongestant; expectorant* [codeine phosphate; pseudoephedrine HCl; guaifenesin; alcohol 1.9%] 10•30•100 mg

guaifenesin & dextromethorphan hydrobromide *expectorant; antitussive* 500•30, 1000•60 mg oral

guaifenesin & dyphylline *expectorant; antiasthmatic; bronchodilator* 200•200 mg oral

guaifenesin & hydrocodone bitartrate *expectorant; narcotic antitussive* 100•5 mg/5 mL oral

Guaifenesin NR oral liquid ℞ *expectorant* [guaifenesin] 100 mg/5 mL

guaifenesin & phenylephrine HCl & phenylpropanolamine HCl *expectorant; decongestant* PPA banned in all OTC products in 2001

guaifenesin & pseudoephedrine HCl *expectorant; decongestant* 595•48, 600•60, 795•85 mg oral

Guaifenesin-DM extended-release caplets ℞ *antitussive; expectorant* [dextromethorphan hydrobromide; guaifenesin] 30•600 mg

Guaifenesin-DM syrup OTC *antitussive; expectorant* [dextromethorphan hydrobromide; guaifenesin] 20•200 mg/10 mL

Guaifenesin-DM NR oral liquid ℞ *antitussive; expectorant* [dextromethorphan hydrobromide; guaifenesin] 20•200 mg/10 mL

Guaifenex oral liquid (discontinued 2002) ℞ *decongestant; expectorant* [phenylpropanolamine HCl; phenylephrine HCl; guaifenesin] 20•5•100 mg/5 mL

Guaifenex DM extended-release caplets ℞ *antitussive; expectorant* [dextromethorphan hydrobromide; guaifenesin] 30•600 mg

Guaifenex G; Guaifenex LA extended-release caplets (discontinued 2004) ℞ *expectorant* [guaifenesin] 1200 mg; 600 mg

Guaifenex GP extended-release film-coated tablets ℞ *decongestant; expectorant* [pseudoephedrine HCl; guaifenesin] 120•1200 mg

Guaifenex PPA 75 extended-release tablets (discontinued 2002) ℞ *decongestant; expectorant* [phenylpropanolamine HCl; guaifenesin] 75•600 mg

Guaifenex PSE 60; Guaifenex PSE 120 extended-release caplets ℞ *decongestant; expectorant* [pseudoephedrine HCl; guaifenesin] 60•600 mg; 120•600 mg

Guaifenex-Rx extended-release tablets (AM and PM) (discontinued 2004) ℞ *decongestant; expectorant* [pseudoephedrine HCl + guaifenesin (AM); guaifenesin (PM)] 60•600 mg; 600 mg

Guaifenex-Rx DM extended-release tablets (AM and PM) (discontinued 2004) ℞ *decongestant + expectorant* (AM); *antitussive + expectorant* (PM) [pseudoephedrine HCl + guaifenesin (AM); dextromethorphan hydrobromide + guaifenesin (PM)] 60•600 mg; 30•600 mg

guaifylline INN *bronchodilator; expectorant* [also: guaithylline]

GuaiMAX-D extended-release caplets ℞ *decongestant; expectorant* [pseudoephedrine HCl; guaifenesin] 120•600 mg

guaimesal INN

Guaipax sustained-release tablets (discontinued 2002) ℞ *decongestant; expectorant* [phenylpropanolamine HCl; guaifenesin] 75•400 mg

Guaipax PSE sustained-release tablets ℞ *decongestant; expectorant* [pseudoephedrine HCl; guaifenesin] 120•600 mg

guaiphenesin BAN *expectorant* [also: guaifenesin]

guaisteine INN

Guaitab tablets (discontinued 2002) OTC *decongestant; expectorant* [pseudoephedrine HCl; guaifenesin] 60•400 mg

Guaitex LA sustained-release tablets (discontinued 2002) ℞ *decongestant;*

expectorant [phenylpropanolamine HCl; guaifenesin] 75•400 mg

Guaitex PSE tablets ℞ *decongestant; expectorant* [pseudoephedrine HCl; guaifenesin] 120•500 mg

guaithylline USAN *bronchodilator; expectorant* [also: guaifylline]

Guai-Vent/PSE sustained-release tablets ℞ *decongestant; expectorant* [pseudoephedrine HCl; guaifenesin] 120•600 mg

guamecycline INN, BAN

guanabenz USAN, INN *centrally acting antiadrenergic antihypertensive*

guanabenz acetate USAN, USP, JAN *centrally acting antiadrenergic antihypertensive* 4, 8 mg oral

guanacline INN, BAN *antihypertensive* [also: guanacline sulfate]

guanacline sulfate USAN *antihypertensive* [also: guanacline]

guanadrel INN *antihypertensive* [also: guanadrel sulfate]

guanadrel sulfate USAN, USP *antihypertensive* [also: guanadrel]

guanatol HCl [see: chloroguanide HCl]

guanazodine INN

guancidine INN *antihypertensive* [also: guancydine]

guancydine USAN *antihypertensive* [also: guancidine]

guanethidine INN, BAN *antihypertensive* [also: guanethidine monosulfate] ☒ guanidine

guanethidine monosulfate USAN, USP *antihypertensive; investigational (orphan) for reflex sympathetic dystrophy and causalgia* [also: guanethidine]

guanethidine sulfate USAN, USP, JAN *antihypertensive*

guanfacine INN, BAN *antihypertensive; antiadrenergic* [also: guanfacine HCl] ☒ guaifenesin

guanfacine HCl USAN *antihypertensive; antiadrenergic* [also: guanfacine] 1, 2 mg oral

guanidine HCl *cholinergic muscle stimulant* 125 mg oral ☒ guanethidine

guanisoquin sulfate USAN *antihypertensive* [also: guanisoquine]

guanisoquine INN *antihypertensive* [also: guanisoquin sulfate]

guanoclor INN, BAN *antihypertensive* [also: guanoclor sulfate]

guanoclor sulfate USAN *antihypertensive* [also: guanoclor]

guanoctine INN *antihypertensive* [also: guanoctine HCl]

guanoctine HCl USAN *antihypertensive* [also: guanoctine]

guanoxabenz USAN, INN *antihypertensive*

guanoxan INN, BAN *antihypertensive* [also: guanoxan sulfate]

guanoxan sulfate USAN *antihypertensive* [also: guanoxan]

guanoxyfen INN *antihypertensive; antidepressant* [also: guanoxyfen sulfate]

guanoxyfen sulfate USAN *antihypertensive; antidepressant* [also: guanoxyfen]

guar gum NF *dietary fiber supplement; tablet binder and disintegrant*

guarana (Paullinia cupana; P. sorbilis) seed paste *medicinal herb for dysentery, malaria, and weight reduction*

guaranine [see: caffeine]

guggul (Commiphora mukul) plant *medicinal herb for hypercholesterolemia and for arthritis and weight reduction in Ayurvedic medicine*

Guiadrine DM sustained-release caplets ℞ *antitussive; expectorant* [dextromethorphan hydrobromide; guaifenesin] 30•600 mg

Guiatex capsules, oral liquid (discontinued 2002) ℞ *decongestant; expectorant* [phenylephrine HCl; phenylpropanolamine HCl; guaifenesin] 5•45•200 mg; 5•20•100 mg/5 mL

Guiatex LA tablets (discontinued 2002) ℞ *decongestant; expectorant* [phenylpropanolamine HCl; guaifenesin] 75•400 mg

Guiatex PSE tablets (discontinued 2002) ℞ *decongestant; expectorant* [pseudoephedrine HCl; guaifenesin] 120•500 mg

Guiatuss syrup OTC *expectorant* [guaifenesin] 100 mg/5 mL ☒ Guiatussin

Guiatuss AC syrup ℞ *narcotic antitussive; expectorant* [codeine phosphate;

guaifenesin; alcohol 3.5%] 20•200 mg/10 mL

Guiatuss CF oral liquid (discontinued 2002) OTC *antitussive; decongestant; expectorant* [dextromethorphan hydrobromide; phenylpropanolamine HCl; guaifenesin; alcohol 4.75%] 10•12.5•100 mg/5 mL

Guiatuss DAC oral liquid (discontinued 2002) ℞ *narcotic antitussive; decongestant; expectorant* [codeine phosphate; pseudoephedrine HCl; guaifenesin; alcohol] 10•30•100 mg/5 mL

Guiatuss DM oral liquid OTC *antitussive; expectorant* [dextromethorphan hydrobromide; guaifenesin] 20•200 mg/10 mL

Guiatuss PE oral liquid (discontinued 2005) OTC *decongestant; expectorant* [pseudoephedrine HCl; guaifenesin] 60•200 mg/10 mL

Guiatussin DAC syrup (discontinued 2002) ℞ *narcotic antitussive; decongestant; expectorant* [codeine phosphate; pseudoephedrine HCl; guaifenesin; alcohol 1.6%] 10•30•100 mg/5 mL ⊡ Guiatuss

Guiatussin with Codeine Expectorant oral liquid (discontinued 2002) ℞ *narcotic antitussive; expectorant* [codeine phosphate; guaifenesin; alcohol 3.5%] 10•100 mg/5 mL

Guiatussin with Dextromethorphan oral liquid (discontinued 2002) OTC *antitussive; expectorant* [dextromethorphan hydrobromide; guaifenesin; alcohol 1.4%] 15•100 mg/5 mL

Guiavent capsules (discontinued 2002) ℞ *decongestant; expectorant* [pseudoephedrine HCl; guaifenesin] 120•250 mg

Guiavent PD pediatric capsules (discontinued 2002) ℞ *decongestant; expectorant* [pseudoephedrine HCl; guaifenesin] 60•300 mg

gum Arabic *medicinal herb* [see: acacia]

gum arabic [see: acacia]

gum ivy *medicinal herb* [see: English ivy]

gum myrrh tree *medicinal herb* [see: myrrh]

gum plant *medicinal herb* [see: comfrey; yerba santa]

gum senegal [see: acacia]

gum tree, hemlock *medicinal herb* [see: hemlock]

gum weed (Grindelia squarrosia) flowering top and leaves *medicinal herb for asthma, bronchitis, bladder infection, poison ivy and oak, and psoriasis and other skin disorders*

guncotton, soluble [see: pyroxylin]

gusperimus INN *immunosuppressant; investigational (orphan) for acute renal graft rejection* [also: gusperimus trihydrochloride; gusperimus HCl]

gusperimus HCl JAN *immunosuppressant* [also: gusperimus trihydrochloride; gusperimus]

gusperimus trihydrochloride USAN *immunosuppressant* [also: gusperimus; gusperimus HCl]

Gustase tablets (discontinued 2002) OTC *digestive enzymes* [amylase; protease; cellulase] 30•6•2 mg

Gustase Plus tablet (discontinued 2002) ℞ *digestive enzymes; sedative* [amylase; protease; cellulase; homatropine methylbromide; phenobarbital] 30•6•2•2.5•8 mg

gutta percha USP *dental restoration agent*

G•Well lotion, shampoo (discontinued 2003) ℞ *pediculicide for lice; scabicide* [lindane] 1%

gymnema (Gymnema melicida; G. sylvestre) leaves and roots *medicinal herb for diabetes, hyperactivity, and hypoglycemia*

Gynazole-1 vaginal cream in prefilled applicator ℞ *antifungal* [butoconazole nitrate] 2%

Gynecort Female Creme cream OTC *topical corticosteroidal anti-inflammatory* [hydrocortisone acetate] 1%

Gyne-Lotrimin 3 vaginal inserts, vaginal cream, combination pack (inserts + cream) OTC *antifungal* [clotrimazole] 200 mg; 2%; 200 mg + 1%

Gyne-Lotrimin 7 vaginal cream OTC *antifungal* [clotrimazole] 1%

gynergon [see: estradiol]

Gyne-Sulf vaginal cream (discontinued 2001) ℞ *broad-spectrum bacteriostatic* [sulfathiazole; sulfacetamide; sulfabenzamide] 3.42%•2.86%•3.7%

Gynodiol tablets ℞ *estrogen replacement therapy for the treatment of postmenopausal symptoms and prevention of postmenopausal osteoporosis; palliative therapy for prostate and metastatic breast cancers* [estradiol] 0.5, 1, 1.5, 2 mg

gynoestryl [see: estradiol]

Gynogen L.A. 20 IM injection (discontinued 2003) ℞ *estrogen replacement therapy for the treatment of postmenopausal symptoms; hormonal antineoplastic for prostate cancer* [estradiol valerate in oil] 20 mg/mL

Gynol II Contraceptive vaginal gel, vaginal jelly OTC *spermicidal contraceptive (for use with a diaphragm)* [nonoxynol 9] 2%; 3%

Gynostemma pentaphyllum *medicinal herb* [see: jiaogulan]

Gynovite Plus tablets OTC *vitamin/mineral/calcium/iron supplement* [multiple vitamins & minerals; calcium; iron; folic acid; biotin] ≛•83•3•0.067• ≟ mg

Gy-Pak (trademarked packaging form) *unit-of-issue package*

gypsy weed *medicinal herb* [see: speedwell]

Gyrocap (trademarked dosage form) *timed-release capsule*

H 9600 SR sustained-release caplets ℞ *decongestant; expectorant* [pseudoephedrine HCl; guaifenesin] 90•600 mg

H₁ blockers *a class of antihistamines* [also called: histamine H_1 antagonists]

H₂ blockers *a class of gastrointestinal antisecretory agents* [also called: histamine H_2 antagonists]

²H (deuterium) [see: deuterium oxide]

H₂¹⁵O [see: water O 15]

³H (tritium) [see: tritiated water]

HAART (highly active antiretroviral therapy) *multi-drug therapy given to HIV-positive patients to prevent progression to AIDS; a generic term applied to several different anti-HIV protocols*

Habitrol transdermal patch (discontinued 2003) ℞ *smoking deterrent; nicotine withdrawal aid* [nicotine] 17.5, 35, 52.5 mg

hachimycin INN, BAN

HAD (hexamethylmelamine, Adriamycin, DDP) *chemotherapy protocol*

hafnium *element* (Hf)

Hair Booster Vitamin tablets OTC *vitamin/mineral/iron supplement* [multiple B vitamins & minerals; iron; folic acid] ≛•18•0.4 mg

halarsol [see: dichlorophenarsine HCl]

halazepam USAN, USP, INN, BAN *benzodiazepine anxiolytic; sedative*

halazone USP, INN *disinfectant; water purifier*

halcinonide USAN, USP, INN, BAN *topical corticosteroidal anti-inflammatory*

Halcion tablets ℞ *benzodiazepine sedative and hypnotic* [triazolam] 0.125, 0.25 mg

Haldol IM injection ℞ *conventional (typical) butyrophenone antipsychotic; antispasmodic/antidyskinetic for Tourette syndrome; treatment for severe pediatric behavioral disorders such as aggression, combativeness, hyperexcitability, and poor impulse control* [haloperidol lactate] 5 mg/mL ⊡ Halenol; Halog

Haldol oral concentrate (discontinued 2003) ℞ *conventional (typical) butyrophenone antipsychotic; antispas-*

modic/antidyskinetic for Tourette syndrome; treatment for severe pediatric behavioral disorders such as aggression, combativeness, hyperexcitability, and poor impulse control [haloperidol lactate] 2 mg/mL ② Halenol; Halog

Haldol tablets (discontinued 2003) ℞ conventional (typical) butyrophenone antipsychotic; antispasmodic/antidyskinetic for Tourette syndrome; treatment for severe pediatric behavioral disorders such as aggression, combativeness, hyperexcitability, and poor impulse control [haloperidol] 0.5, 1, 2, 5, 10, 20 mg

Haldol Decanoate 50; Haldol Decanoate 100 long-acting IM injection ℞ conventional (typical) butyrophenone antipsychotic; antispasmodic/antidyskinetic for Tourette syndrome; treatment for severe pediatric behavioral disorders such as aggression, combativeness, hyperexcitability, and poor impulse control [haloperidol decanoate] 50 mg/mL; 100 mg/mL

Halenol, Children's oral liquid OTC analgesic; antipyretic [acetaminophen] 160 mg/5 mL

haletazole INN [also: halethazole]

halethazole BAN [also: haletazole]

Haley's M·O oral liquid OTC saline/emollient laxative [magnesium hydroxide; mineral oil] 900 mg•3.75 mL per 15 mL

Halfan tablets (discontinued 2003) ℞ antimalarial (orphan) [halofantrine HCl] 250 mg

HalfLytely Bowel Prep Kit enteric-coated delayed-release tablets + powder for oral solution ℞ pre-procedure bowel evacuant [bisacodyl + polyethylene glycol–electrolyte solution (PEG 3350)] 5 mg + 2 L

Halfprin; Halfprin 81 enteric-coated tablets OTC analgesic; antipyretic; antiinflammatory; antirheumatic [aspirin] 165 mg; 81 mg

Hall's Plus lozenges OTC topical oral analgesic; counterirritant; mild local anesthetic; antiseptic [menthol] 10 mg

Hall's Sugar Free Mentho-Lyptus lozenges OTC topical oral analgesic; counterirritant; mild local anesthetic; antiseptic [menthol; eucalyptus oil] 5•2.8, 6•2.8 mg

Halls Zinc Defense lozenges OTC topical anti-infective to relieve sore throat [zinc acetate] 5 mg

hallucinogens a class of agents that induce hallucinations

halobetasol propionate USAN topical corticosteroidal anti-inflammatory [also: ulobetasol] 0.05% topical

halocarban INN disinfectant [also: cloflucarban]

halocortolone INN

halocrinic acid [see: brocrinat]

halofantrine INN, BAN antimalarial [also: halofantrine HCl]

halofantrine HCl USAN antimalarial (orphan) [also: halofantrine]

Halofed tablets OTC nasal decongestant [pseudoephedrine HCl] 30, 60 mg

halofenate USAN, INN, BAN antihyperlipoproteinemic; uricosuric

halofuginone INN, BAN antiprotozoal [also: halofuginone hydrobromide]

halofuginone hydrobromide USAN antiprotozoal; investigational (orphan) for scleroderma [also: halofuginone]

Halog ointment, cream, solution ℞ corticosteroidal anti-inflammatory [halcinonide] 0.1% ② Haldol

Halog-E cream ℞ topical corticosteroidal anti-inflammatory; emollient [halcinonide] 0.1%

halometasone INN

halonamine INN

halopemide USAN, INN antipsychotic

halopenium chloride INN, BAN

haloperidol USAN, USP, INN, BAN conventional (typical) butyrophenone antipsychotic; antispasmodic/antidyskinetic for Tourette syndrome; treatment for severe pediatric behavioral disorders such as aggression, combativeness, hyperexcitability, and poor impulse control 0.5, 1, 2, 5, 10, 20 mg oral

haloperidol decanoate USAN, BAN conventional (typical) butyrophenone *antipsychotic; antispasmodic/antidyskinetic for Tourette syndrome; treatment for severe pediatric behavioral disorders such as aggression, combativeness, hyperexcitability, and poor impulse control* 50, 100 mg/mL injection

haloperidol lactate *conventional (typical) butyrophenone antipsychotic; antispasmodic/antidyskinetic for Tourette syndrome; treatment for severe pediatric behavioral disorders such as aggression, combativeness, hyperexcitability, and poor impulse control* 2 mg/mL oral; 5 mg/mL injection

Haloperidol Long Acting ⓒⒶⓃ *long-acting IM injection* ℞ *conventional (typical) butyrophenone antipsychotic; antispasmodic/antidyskinetic for Tourette syndrome; treatment for severe pediatric behavioral disorders such as aggression, combativeness, hyperexcitability, and poor impulse control* [haloperidol decanoate] 50, 100 mg/mL

halopone chloride [see: halopenium chloride]

halopredone INN *topical anti-inflammatory* [also: halopredone acetate]

halopredone acetate USAN *topical anti-inflammatory* [also: halopredone]

haloprogesterone USAN, INN *progestin*

haloprogin USAN, USP, INN, JAN *antibacterial; antifungal*

halopyramine BAN [also: chloropyramine]

Halotestin tablets (discontinued 2003) ℞ *androgen for hypogonadism or testosterone deficiency in men, delayed puberty in boys, and metastatic breast cancer in women* [fluoxymesterone] 2, 5, 10 mg ⊉ Halotex; Halotussin

Halotex cream, solution (discontinued 2004) ℞ *antifungal* [haloprogin] 1% ⊉ Halotestin

halothane USP, INN, BAN *inhalation general anesthetic*

Halotussin syrup OTC *expectorant* [guaifenesin; alcohol 3.5%] 100 mg/5 mL ⊉ Halotestin

Halotussin AC oral liquid (discontinued 2005) ℞ *narcotic antitussive; expectorant* [codeine phosphate; guaifenesin] 20•200 mg/10 mL

Halotussin DM oral liquid, sugar-free oral liquid (discontinued 2002) OTC *antitussive; expectorant* [dextromethorphan hydrobromide; guaifenesin] 10•100 mg/5 mL

haloxazolam INN

haloxon INN, BAN

halquinol BAN *topical anti-infective* [also: halquinols]

halquinols USAN *topical anti-infective* [also: halquinol]

Haltran tablets (discontinued 2005) OTC *analgesic; antiarthritic; antipyretic; nonsteroidal anti-inflammatory drug (NSAID)* [ibuprofen] 200 mg

HAM (hexamethylmelamine, Adriamycin, melphalan) *chemotherapy protocol*

HAM (hexamethylmelamine, Adriamycin, methotrexate) *chemotherapy protocol*

Hamamelis virginiana *medicinal herb* [see: witch hazel]

hamamelis water *medicinal herb* [see: witch hazel]

hamycin USAN, INN *antifungal*

HandiHaler (trademarked device) *inhalation powder dispenser*

hard fat [see: fat, hard]

hardock *medicinal herb* [see: burdock]

hareburr *medicinal herb* [see: burdock]

Harpagophytum procumbens *medicinal herb* [see: devil's claw]

hashish (*Cannabis sativa*) *euphoric/ hallucinogenic street drug made from the resin of the flowering tops of the cannabis plant*

Havrix adult IM injection, pediatric IM injection ℞ *immunization against hepatitis A virus (HAV)* [hepatitis A vaccine, inactivated] 1440 ELISA units (EL.U./mL); 360, 720 EL.U./0.5 mL

haw *medicinal herb* [see: hawthorn]

Hawaiian Tropic Cool Aloe with I.C.E. gel OTC *topical local anesthetic; analgesic; counterirritant* [lidocaine; menthol] ≜ • ≜

hawthorn (Crataegus laevigata; C. monogyna; C. oxyacantha) flowers, leaves, and berries *medicinal herb for angina pectoris, arrhythmias, arteriosclerosis, enlarged heart, high or low blood pressure, hypoglycemia, palpitations, and tachycardia; also used as an antiseptic*

Hayfebrol oral liquid OTC *decongestant; antihistamine* [pseudoephedrine HCl; chlorpheniramine maleate] 60•4 mg/10 mL

hazel, snapping; hazelnut *medicinal herb* [see: witch hazel]

HBIG (hepatitis B immune globulin) [q.v.]

hBNP (human B-type natriuretic peptide) [see: nesiritide; nesiritide citrate]

1% HC ointment ℞ *topical corticosteroidal anti-inflammatory* [hydrocortisone] 1%

HC (hydrocortisone) [q.v.]

4-HC (4-hydroperoxycyclophosphamide) [q.v.]

HC Derma-Pax topical liquid OTC *corticosteroidal anti-inflammatory; antihistamine; antiseptic* [hydrocortisone; pyrilamine maleate; chlorpheniramine maleate; chlorobutanol] 0.5%•0.44%•0.06%•25%

HCA (hydrocortisone acetate) [q.v.]

H-CAP (hexamethylmelamine, cyclophosphamide, Adriamycin, Platinol) *chemotherapy protocol*

hCG (human chorionic gonadotropin) [see: gonadotropin, chorionic]

HCT (hydrochlorothiazide) [q.v.]

HCTZ (hydrochlorothiazide) [q.v.]

HD 85 oral/rectal suspension ℞ *radiopaque contrast medium for gastrointestinal imaging* [barium sulfate] 85%

HD 200 Plus powder for oral suspension ℞ *radiopaque contrast medium for gastrointestinal imaging* [barium sulfate] 98%

HDCV (human diploid cell vaccine) [see: rabies vaccine]

HDMTX (high-dose methotrexate [with leucovorin rescue]) *chemotherapy protocol for bone sarcoma*

HDMTX-CF (high-dose methotrexate, citrovorum factor) *chemotherapy protocol*

HDMTX/LV (high-dose methotrexate, leucovorin [rescue]) *chemotherapy protocol*

HDPEB (high-dose PEB protocol) *chemotherapy protocol* [see: PEB]

HD-VAC (high-dose [methotrexate], vinblastine, Adriamycin, cisplatin) *chemotherapy protocol*

HE-2000 *investigational (Phase II) cellular energy regulator for HIV and AIDS*

Head & Shoulders; Head & Shoulders Dry Scalp shampoo OTC *antiseborrheic; antibacterial; antifungal* [pyrithione zinc] 1%

Head & Shoulders Intensive Treatment lotion/shampoo OTC *antiseborrheic; dandruff treatment* [selenium sulfide] 1%

heal-all *medicinal herb* [see: figwort; stone root; woundwort]

healing herb *medicinal herb* [see: comfrey]

Healon; Healon GV intraocular injection ℞ *viscoelastic agent for ophthalmic surgery* [hyaluronate sodium] 10 mg/mL; 14 mg/mL

Healon Yellow intraocular injection ℞ *viscoelastic agent for ophthalmic surgery; diagnostic agent* [hyaluronate sodium; fluorescein sodium] 10•0.005 mg/mL

Healon5 Ⓒᴬᴺ intraocular injection in preloaded syringes ℞ *viscoelastic agent for ophthalmic surgery* [hyaluronate sodium 5000] 23 mg/0.6 mL

heart, mother's; shepherd's heart *medicinal herb* [see: shepherd's purse]

Heartline enteric-coated tablets OTC *analgesic; antipyretic; anti-inflammatory; antirheumatic* [aspirin] 81 mg

heather (Calluna vulgaris) flowering shoots *medicinal herb used as an antiseptic, cholagogue, diaphoretic, diuretic, expectorant, and vasoconstrictor*

heavy liquid petrolatum [see: mineral oil]

heavy water (D₂O) [see: deuterium oxide]

Hectorol softgels ℞ *synthetic vitamin D analogue; calcium regulator for hyperparathyroidism secondary to chronic renal dialysis* [doxercalciferol] 2.5, 5 µg

hedaquinium chloride INN, BAN

Hedeoma pulegeoides medicinal herb [see: pennyroyal]

Hedera helix medicinal herb [see: English ivy]

hedge bindweed (*Convolvulus sepium*) flowering plant and roots *medicinal herb used as a cholagogue, febrifuge, and purgative*

hedge garlic (*Sisymbrium alliaria*) *medicinal herb* [see: garlic]

hedge hyssop (*Gratiola officinalis*) plant *medicinal herb used as a cardiac, diuretic, purgative, and vermifuge*

hedge-burs *medicinal herb* [see: bedstraw]

"hedgehog" proteins *a class of novel human proteins that induce the formation of regenerative tissue*

Heet Liniment OTC *analgesic; counterirritant; antiseptic* [methyl salicylate; camphor; capsaicin; alcohol 70%] 15%•3.6%•0.025%

hefilcon A USAN *hydrophilic contact lens material*

hefilcon B USAN *hydrophilic contact lens material*

hefilcon C USAN *hydrophilic contact lens material*

helenien [see: xantofyl palmitate]

Helianthemum canadense medicinal herb [see: rock rose]

helicon [see: aspirin]

Helicosol powder for oral solution ℞ *diagnostic aid for detection of H. pylori in the stomach* [carbon C 13 urea]

Helidac 14-day dose-pack ℞ *combination treatment for active duodenal ulcer with H. pylori infection* [bismuth subsalicylate (chewable tablets); metronidazole (tablets); tetracycline HCl (capsules)] 262.4 mg; 250 mg; 500 mg

heliomycin INN

heliox *helium-oxygen mixture used for respiratory distress* (usually an 80%• 20% mix)

Helistat sponge ℞ *topical local hemostat for surgery* [absorbable collagen sponge]

helium USP *diluent for gases; element (He)*

Helixate FS powder for IV injection ℞ *antihemophilic* [antihemophilic factor concentrate, recombinant, solvent/detergent-treated] 250, 500, 1000 IU

hellebore (*Helleborus* spp.; *Veratrum* spp.) rhizome *medicinal herb used as an antihypertensive; not generally regarded as safe and effective for internal consumption due to toxicity*

Helleborus spp. medicinal herb [see: hellebore]

helmet flower *medicinal herb* [see: aconite; sandalwood; skullcap]

helmet pod *medicinal herb* [see: twin leaf]

HEMA (2-hydroxyethyl methacrylate) *contact lens material*

Hemabate IM injection ℞ *prostaglandin-type abortifacient; for postpartum uterine bleeding* [carboprost tromethamine] 250 µg/mL

Hema-Check slide tests for home use *in vitro diagnostic aid for fecal occult blood*

Hema-Combistix reagent strips *in vitro diagnostic aid for multiple urine products*

Hemaspan timed-release tablets (discontinued 2005) OTC *hematinic; vitamin/iron supplement; stool softener* [ferrous fumarate (source of iron); ascorbic acid; docusate sodium] 330 (110)•200•20 mg

Hemastix reagent strips for professional use *in vitro diagnostic aid for urine occult blood*

Hematest reagent tablets for professional use *in vitro diagnostic aid for fecal occult blood*

hematin [now: hemin]

Hematinic tablets ℞ *hematinic* [ferrous fumarate; folic acid] 106 mg Fe•1 mg

Hematinic Plus tablets ℞ *hematinic; vitamin/mineral supplement* [multiple vitamins & minerals; ferrous fumarate; folic acid] ± • 106 mg Fe • 1 mg

hematinics *a class of iron-containing agents for the prevention and treatment of iron-deficiency anemia*

hematopoietics *a class of antianemic agents that promote the formation of red blood cells*

heme arginate *investigational (orphan) for acute symptomatic porphyria and myelodysplastic syndrome*

HemeSelect Collection kit for home use *in vitro diagnostic aid for fecal occult blood* [for use with HemeSelect Reagent kit]

HemeSelect Reagent kit for professional use *in vitro diagnostic aid for fecal occult blood* [for use with HemeSelect Collection kit]

hemiacidrin [see: citric acid, glucono-delta-lactone & magnesium carbonate]

hemin *enzyme inhibitor for acute intermittent porphyria (AIP), porphyria variegata, and hereditary coproporphyria (orphan)*

hemin & zinc mesoporphyrin *investigational (orphan) for acute porphyric syndromes*

hemlock *(Tsuga canadensis)* bark *medicinal herb used as an astringent, diaphoretic, and diuretic*

Hemoccult slide tests for professional use, test tape for professional use *in vitro diagnostic aid for fecal occult blood*

Hemoccult II slide tests for professional use *in vitro diagnostic aid for fecal occult blood*

Hemoccult II Dispenserpak; Hemoccult II Dispenserpak Plus slide tests for home use *in vitro diagnostic aid for fecal occult blood*

Hemoccult SENSA; Hemoccult II SENSA slide tests for professional use *in vitro diagnostic aid for fecal occult blood*

Hemocyte tablets OTC *hematinic; iron supplement* [ferrous fumarate (source of iron)] 324 mg (106 mg)

Hemocyte Plus elixir ℞ *hematinic* [polysaccharide-iron complex; multiple B vitamins & minerals; folic acid] 12 • ± • 0.33 mg

Hemocyte Plus tablets ℞ *hematinic* [ferrous fumarate; multiple B vitamins & minerals; sodium ascorbate; folic acid] 106 • ± • 200 • 1 mg

Hemocyte-F elixir ℞ *hematinic* [polysaccharide-iron complex; cyanocobalamin; folic acid] 100 mg Fe • 25 µg • 1 mg per 5 mL

Hemocyte-F tablets ℞ *hematinic* [ferrous fumarate; folic acid] 106 • 1 mg

Hemofil M IV injection ℞ *antihemophilic to correct coagulation deficiency* [antihemophilic factor concentrate] 10, 20, 30 mL

hemoglobin, recombinant human (rHb1.1) *investigational agent for chronic anemia*

hemoglobin crosfumaril USAN, INN *investigational (Phase III) blood substitute for perfusion deficit disorders and blood loss due to severe trauma*

Hemokine *investigational progenitor cell stimulator for neutropenia and thrombocytopenia* [muplestim]

Hemonyne IV infusion (discontinued 2001) ℞ *antihemophilic to correct factor IX deficiency (Christmas disease)* [coagulation factors II, VII, IX, and X, heat treated] 20, 40 mL

Hemopad fiber ℞ *topical hemostatic aid in surgery* [microfibrillar collagen hemostat]

Hemophilus b conjugate vaccine *active bacterin for* Haemophilus influenzae *type b*

Hemorid for Women cream OTC *topical local anesthetic and vasoconstrictor for hemorrhoids* [pramoxine HCl; phenylephrine HCl] 1% • 0.25%

Hemorid for Women lotion OTC *topical emollient and protectant for hemorrhoids* [mineral oil; petrolatum; glycerin]

Hemorid for Women rectal suppositories OTC *vasoconstrictor and astringent for hemorrhoids* [zinc oxide;
phenylephrine HCl] 11%•0.25%

Hemorrhoidal HC rectal suppositories ℞ *corticosteroidal anti-inflammatory for hemorrhoids* [hydrocortisone
acetate] 25 mg

hemostatics *a class of therapeutic blood
modifiers that arrest the flow of blood*
[see also: astringents; styptics]

Hemotene fiber ℞ *topical hemostatic
aid in surgery* [microfibrillar collagen
hemostat] 1 g

Hemovit film-coated tablets ℞ *hematinic* [multiple B vitamins; vitamin C;
folic acid; biotin] ±•60•1•0.3 mg

hemp *medicinal herb* [see: marijuana]

**hemp agrimony (Eupatorium can-
nabinum)** plant *medicinal herb used
as a cholagogue, diaphoretic, diuretic,
emetic, expectorant, and purgative*

hemp nettle (Galeopsis tetrahit)
plant *medicinal herb used as an astringent, diuretic, and expectorant*

Hem-Prep anorectal ointment, rectal
suppositories OTC *temporary relief of
hemorrhoidal symptoms; topical vasoconstrictor; astringent* [phenylephrine
HCl; zinc oxide] 0.025%•11%;
0.25%•11%

Hemril Uniserts (rectal suppositories)
OTC *temporary relief of hemorrhoidal
symptoms* [bismuth subgallate; bismuth resorcin compound; benzyl benzoate; peruvian balsam; zinc oxide]
2.25%•1.75%•1.2%•1.8%•11%

Hemril-HC Uniserts (suppositories)
℞ *corticosteroidal anti-inflammatory
for hemorrhoids* [hydrocortisone ace-
tate] 25 mg

henbane (Hyoscyamus niger) plant
*medicinal herb used as an anodyne,
antispasmodic, calmative, and narcotic;
primarily used externally because of its
high toxicity*

heneicosafluorotripropylamine [see:
perfluamine]

henna (Alkanna tinctoria) root
medicinal herb used as an astringent,

*antibiotic, and cosmetic dye; not gener-
ally regarded as safe and effective*

henna (Lawsonia inermis) leaves
medicinal herb used as an astringent

**HEOD (hexachloro-epoxy-octahy-
dro-dimethanonaphthalene)** [see:
dieldrin]

heparin BAN *anticoagulant; antithrombotic* [also: heparin calcium]

heparin, 2-0-desulfated *investigational
(orphan) for cystic fibrosis*

heparin calcium USP *anticoagulant;
antithrombotic* [also: heparin]

Heparin I.V. Flush prefilled syringe ℞
*IV flush for catheter patency (not ther-
apeutic)* [heparin sodium] 1 U/mL

Heparin Lock Flush solution ℞ *IV
flush for catheter patency (not therapeutic)* [heparin sodium] 10, 100 U/mL

heparin sodium USP, INN, BAN *anticoagulant; antithrombotic* 1000, 2000,
2500, 5000, 7500, 10 000, 20 000,
40 000 U/mL injection

**heparin sodium & sodium chloride
0.45%** *anticoagulant; antithrombotic*
12 500 U•250 mL, 25 000 U•250
mL, 25 000 U•500 mL

**heparin sodium & sodium chloride
0.9%** *anticoagulant; antithrombotic*
1000 U•500 mL, 2000 U•1000 mL

heparin sulfate [see: danaparoid
sodium]

heparin whole blood [see: blood,
whole]

heparinase 1 *investigational (Phase III)
agent for the reversal of heparin-induced
anticoagulation*

heparinase III *investigational cardioprotective agent*

HepatAmine IV infusion ℞ *nutritional
therapy for hepatic failure and hepatic
encephalopathy* [multiple branched-
chain essential and nonessential
amino acids; electrolytes]

**hepatica (Hepatica acutiloba; H.
triloba)** leaves and flowers *medicinal
herb used as a diuretic and pectoral*

Hepatic-Aid II Instant Drink powder OTC *enteral nutritional treatment*

for chronic liver disease [multiple branched chain amino acids]

hepatics *a class of agents that affect the liver (a term used in folk medicine)*

hepatitis A vaccine, inactivated *active immunizing agent for the hepatitis A virus (HAV)*

hepatitis B immune globulin (HBIG) USP *passive immunizing agent; investigational (orphan) prophylaxis against hepatitis B reinfection in liver transplant patients*

hepatitis B surface antigen (HBsAg) [see: hepatitis B virus vaccine, inactivated]

hepatitis B virus vaccine, inactivated USP *active immunizing agent for hepatitis B and D*

Hepflush-10 solution ℞ *IV flush for catheter patency (not therapeutic)* [heparin sodium] 10 U/mL

Hep-Forte capsules OTC *geriatric dietary supplement* [multiple vitamins & food products; folic acid; biotin] ± • 60• ? μg

Hep-Lock; Hep-Lock U/P solution ℞ *IV flush for catheter patency (not therapeutic)* [heparin sodium] 10, 100 U/mL

HEPP (H-chain ε [IgE] pentapeptide) [see: pentigetide]

hepronicate INN

Hepsera tablets ℞ *nucleotide analogue reverse transcriptase inhibitor for chronic hepatitis B virus (HBV) infection* [adefovir dipivoxil] 10 mg

heptabarb INN [also: heptabarbitone]

heptabarbital [see: heptabarb; heptabarbitone]

heptabarbitone BAN [also: heptabarb]

heptaminol INN, BAN

heptaminol HCl [see: heptaminol]

2-heptanamine [see: tuaminoheptane]

2-heptanamine sulfate [see: tuaminoheptane sulfate]

heptaverine INN

heptolamide INN

Heptovir ⓒᴬᴺ tablets, oral solution ℞ *antiviral nucleoside reverse transcriptase inhibitor for hepatitis B virus (HBV)* [lamivudine] 100 mg; 5 mg/mL

hepzidine INN

HER2 MAb (human epidermal growth factor receptor 2 monoclonal antibodies) [see: trastuzumab]

Heracleum lanatum medicinal herb [see: masterwort]

herb of grace *medicinal herb* [see: rue]

HercepTest test kit *diagnostic aid for the HER2 protein, used to screen patients who may benefit from treatment with Herceptin*

Herceptin powder for IV infusion ℞ *anti-HER2 monoclonal antibody for metastatic breast cancer; investigational (NDA filed) for ovarian and female genital tract cancers* [trastuzumab] 440 mg

Hercules woundwort *medicinal herb* [see: woundwort]

heroin *potent narcotic analgesic street drug which is highly addictive; banned in the U.S.* [medically known as diamorphine and diacetylmorphine HCl]

heroin HCl *(banned in the U.S.)* [see: diacetylmorphine HCl]

Herpecin-L lip balm OTC *vulnerary; sunblock* [allantoin; padimate O]

herpes simplex virus gene *investigational (orphan) for primary and metastatic brain tumors*

Herpetrol tablets (discontinued 2001) OTC *dietary supplement; claimed to prevent and treat herpes simplex infections* [L-lysine; multiple vitamins; zinc]

Herrick Lacrimal Plug ℞ *blocks the puncta and canaliculus to eliminate tear loss in keratitis sicca* [silicone plug]

HES (hydroxyethyl starch) [see: hetastarch]

Hespan IV infusion ℞ *plasma volume expander for shock due to hemorrhage, burns, surgery* [hetastarch] 6 g/100 mL ② Histatan

hesperidin *a bioflavonoid (q.v.)*

hesperidin methyl chalcone [see: bioflavonoids]

hetacillin USAN, USP, INN, BAN *antibacterial*

hetacillin potassium USAN, USP *antibacterial*

hetaflur USAN, INN, BAN *dental caries prophylactic*

hetastarch USAN, BAN *plasma volume extender* [also: hydroxyethylstarch] 6% in normal saline

heteronium bromide USAN, INN, BAN *anticholinergic*

Hetrazan tablets (available for compassionate use only) ℞ *anthelmintic for Bancroft filariasis, onchocerciasis, tropical eosinophilia, and loiasis* [diethylcarbamazine citrate] 50 mg

hexaammonium molybdate tetrahydrate [see: ammonium molybdate]

Hexabrix injection ℞ *radiopaque contrast medium* [ioxaglate meglumine; ioxaglate sodium (54.3% total iodine)] 393•196 mg/mL (320 mg/mL)

HexaCAF; Hexa-CAF (hexamethylmelamine, cyclophosphamide, amethopterin, fluorouracil) *chemotherapy protocol for ovarian cancer*

hexacarbacholine bromide INN [also: carbolonium bromide]

hexachlorane [see: lindane]

hexachlorocyclohexane [see: lindane]

hexachlorophane BAN *topical anti-infective; detergent* [also: hexachlorophene]

hexachlorophene USP, INN *topical anti-infective; detergent* [also: hexachlorophane]

hexacyclonate sodium INN

hexacyprone INN

hexadecanoic acid [see: palmitic acid]

hexadecanoic acid, methylethyl ester [see: isopropyl palmitate]

hexadecanol [see: cetyl alcohol]

hexadecylamine hydrofluoride [see: hetaflur]

hexadecylpyridinium chloride [see: cetylpyridinium chloride]

hexadecyltrimethylammonium bromide [see: cetrimonium bromide]

hexadecyltrimethylammonium chloride [see: cetrimonium chloride]

2,4-hexadienoic acid, potassium salt [see: potassium sorbate]

hexadiline INN

hexadimethrine bromide INN, BAN

hexadiphane [see: prozapine]

Hexadrol tablets, elixir (discontinued 2004) ℞ *corticosteroidal anti-inflammatory* [dexamethasone] 1.5, 4 mg; 0.5 mg/5 mL ☐ Hexalol

Hexadrol Phosphate intra-articular, intralesional, soft tissue, or IM injection ℞ *corticosteroidal anti-inflammatory* [dexamethasone sodium phosphate] 4, 10, 20 mg/mL

hexadylamine [see: hexadiline]

hexafluorenium bromide USAN, USP *skeletal muscle relaxant; succinylcholine synergist* [also: hexafluronium bromide]

hexafluorodiethyl ether [see: flurothyl]

hexaflurone bromide [see: hexafluorenium bromide]

hexafluronium bromide INN *skeletal muscle relaxant; succinylcholine synergist* [also: hexafluorenium bromide]

Hexalen capsules ℞ *antineoplastic for advanced ovarian adenocarcinoma (orphan)* [altretamine] 50 mg ☐ Hexalol

hexamarium bromide [see: distigmine bromide]

hexametazime BAN

hexamethone bromide [see: hexamethonium bromide]

hexamethonium bromide INN, BAN

hexamethylenamine [now: methenamine]

hexamethylenamine mandelate [see: methenamine mandelate]

hexamethylenetetramine [see: methenamine]

hexamethylmelamine (HMM; HXM) [see: altretamine]

hexamidine INN

hexamine hippurate BAN *urinary antibacterial* [also: methenamine hippurate]

hexamine mandelate [see: methenamine mandelate]

hexapradol INN

hexaprofen INN, BAN

hexapropymate INN, BAN

hexasonium iodide INN

hexavitamin USP

Hexavitamin tablets OTC *vitamin supplement* [multiple vitamins]

hexcarbacholine bromide INN [also: carbolonium bromide]

hexedine USAN, INN *antibacterial*

hexemal [see: cyclobarbital]

hexestrol NF, INN

hexetidine BAN

hexicide [see: lindane]

hexinol [see: cyclomenol]

hexobarbital USP, INN

hexobarbital sodium NF

hexobendine USAN, INN, BAN *vasodilator*

hexocyclium methylsulfate *peptic ulcer adjunct* [also: hexocyclium metilsulfate; hexocyclium methylsulphate]

hexocyclium methylsulphate BAN [also: hexocyclium methylsulfate; hexocyclium metilsulfate]

hexocyclium metilsulfate INN [also: hexocyclium methylsulfate; hexocyclium methylsulphate]

hexoprenaline INN, BAN *tocolytic; bronchodilator* [also: hexoprenaline sulfate]

hexoprenaline sulfate USAN, JAN *investigational (NDA filed) tocolytic; bronchodilator* [also: hexoprenaline]

hexopyrimidine [see: hexetidine]

hexopyrrolate [see: hexopyrronium bromide]

hexopyrronium bromide INN

hexydaline [see: methenamine mandelate]

hexylcaine INN *local anesthetic* [also: hexylcaine HCl]

hexylcaine HCl USP *local anesthetic* [also: hexylcaine]

hexylene glycol NF *humectant; solvent*

hexylresorcinol USP *anthelmintic; topical antiseptic*

1-hexyltheobromine [see: pentifylline]

H-F Gel ℞ *investigational (orphan) emergency treatment for hydrofluoric acid burns* [calcium gluconate]

HFA-134a (hydrofluoroalkane) *propellant used in CFC-free aerosol delivery systems*

hFSH (human follicle-stimulating hormone) [now: menotropins]

HFZ (homofenazine) [q.v.]

197Hg [see: chlormerodrin Hg 197]

197Hg [see: merisoprol acetate Hg 197]

197Hg [see: merisoprol Hg 197]

203Hg [see: chlormerodrin Hg 203]

203Hg [see: merisoprol acetate Hg 203]

hGH (human growth hormone) [see: somatropin]

hibenzate INN *combining name for radicals or groups* [also: hybenzate]

Hibiclens sponge/brush OTC *broad-spectrum antimicrobial; germicidal* [chlorhexidine gluconate; alcohol 4%] 4%

Hibiclens Antiseptic/AntiMicrobial Skin Cleanser topical liquid OTC *broad-spectrum antimicrobial; germicidal* [chlorhexidine gluconate; alcohol 4%] 4%

hibiscus (Hibiscus sabdariffa and other species) flowers and leaves *medicinal herb for cancer, edema, heart problems and nervous disorders; also used topically as an emollient; not generally regarded as safe and effective*

Hibistat Germicidal Hand Rinse topical liquid OTC *broad-spectrum antimicrobial; germicidal* [chlorhexidine gluconate; alcohol 70%] 0.5%

Hibistat Towelette OTC *broad-spectrum antimicrobial; germicidal* [chlorhexidine gluconate; alcohol 70%] 0.5%

HibTITER IM injection ℞ *pediatric (2–71 months) vaccine for Haemophilus influenzae type b (HIB)* [Hemophilus b conjugate vaccine (with a diphtheria CRM$_{197}$ carrier)] 10● (25) μg/0.5 mL

Hi-C DAZE (high-dose cytarabine, daunorubicin, azacitidine, etoposide) *chemotherapy protocol for acute myelogenous leukemia (AML)*

Hi-Cal VM nutrition bar OTC *enteral nutritional therapy for HIV and AIDS*

Hi-Cor 1.0; Hi-Cor 2.5 cream ℞ *topical corticosteroidal anti-inflammatory* [hydrocortisone] 1%; 2.5%

HIDA (hepatoiminodiacetic acid) [see: lidofenin]

HiDAC (high-dose ara-C) *chemotherapy protocol*

Hieracium pilosella *medicinal herb* [see: mouse ear]

high angelica *medicinal herb* [see: angelica]

high molecular weight dextran [see: dextran 70]

high osmolar contrast media (HOCM) *a class of older radiopaque agents that have a high osmolar concentration of iodine (the contrast agent), which corresponds to a higher incidence of adverse reactions* [also called: ionic contrast media]

High Potency N-Vites tablets oTC *vitamin supplement* [multiple B vitamins; vitamin C] ± •500 mg

High Potency Tar gel shampoo (discontinued 2003) oTC *antiseborrheic; antipsoriatic; antipruritic; antibacterial* [coal tar] 25%

hilafilcon A USAN *hydrophilic contact lens material*

hilafilcon B USAN *hydrophilic contact lens material*

hillberry *medicinal herb* [see: wintergreen]

Himalayan ginseng (*Panax pseudoginseng*) *medicinal herb* [see: ginseng]

hindheel *medicinal herb* [see: tansy]

hini *medicinal herb* [see: Culver root]

hioxifilcon A USAN *hydrophilic contact lens material*

Hipotest tablets oTC *dietary supplement* [multiple vitamins & minerals; multiple food products; calcium; iron; biotin] ± •53.5•50•0.001 mg

Hi-Po-Vites tablets oTC *dietary supplement* [multiple vitamins & minerals; multiple food products; iron; folic acid; biotin] ± •6•0.4•1 mg

Hiprex tablets ℞ *urinary antibiotic* [methenamine hippurate] 1 g

Hirudo medicinalis *natural treatment* [see: leeches]

Histacol DM syrup ℞ *decongestant; antihistamine; antitussive; expectorant* [pseudoephedrine HCl; brompheniramine maleate; dextromethorphan

hydrobromide; guaifenesin] 30•2•5•50/5 mL

Histade sustained-release capsules ℞ *decongestant; antihistamine* [pseudoephedrine HCl; chlorpheniramine maleate] 120•12 mg

Histagesic Modified tablets (discontinued 2002) oTC *decongestant; antihistamine; analgesic* [phenylephrine HCl; chlorpheniramine maleate; acetaminophen] 10•4•324 mg

Histalet syrup (discontinued 2002) ℞ *decongestant; antihistamine* [pseudoephedrine HCl; chlorpheniramine maleate] 45•3 mg/5 mL

Histalet Forte tablets (discontinued 2001) ℞ *decongestant; antihistamine* [phenylpropanolamine HCl; phenylephrine HCl; chlorpheniramine maleate; pyrilamine maleate] 50•10•4•25 mg

Histalet X tablets, syrup (discontinued 2002) ℞ *decongestant; expectorant* [pseudoephedrine HCl; guaifenesin] 120•400 mg; 45•200 mg/5 mL

histamine dihydrochloride USAN *investigational (Phase III) histamine H_2 receptor agonist for malignant melanoma and acute myeloid leukemia (AML); investigational (Phase II) for hepatitis C and renal cell carcinoma*

histamine H_1 antagonists *a class of antihistamines* [also called: H_1 blockers]

histamine H_2 antagonists *a class of gastrointestinal antisecretory agents* [also called: H_2 blockers]

histamine phosphate USP *gastric secretory stimulant; diagnostic aid for pheochromocytoma*

histantin [see: chlorcyclizine HCl]

histapyrrodine INN

Histatab Plus tablets oTC *decongestant; antihistamine* [phenylephrine HCl; chlorpheniramine maleate] 5•2 mg

Hista-Vadrin tablets (discontinued 2001) ℞ *decongestant; antihistamine* [phenylpropanolamine HCl; phenylephrine HCl; chlorpheniramine maleate] 40•5•6 mg

Hista-Vent DA sustained-release caplets ℞ *decongestant; antihistamine; anticholinergic to dry mucosal secretions* [phenylephrine HCl; chlorpheniramine maleate; methscopolamine nitrate] 20•8•2.5 mg

Histenol-Forte tablets OTC *antitussive; decongestant; analgesic* [dextromethorphan hydrobromide; pseudoephedrine HCl; acetaminophen] 10•30•325 mg

Histerone 100 IM injection (discontinued 2001) ℞ *androgen replacement for delayed puberty or breast cancer* [testosterone] 100 mg/mL

Histex oral liquid ℞ *decongestant; antihistamine* [pseudoephedrine HCl; chlorpheniramine maleate] 60•4 mg/10 mL

Histex I/E extended-release capsules ℞ *antihistamine for allergic rhinitis* [carbinoxamine maleate] 10 mg

Histex CT film-coated timed-release tablets ℞ *antihistamine for allergic rhinitis* [carbinoxamine maleate] 8 mg

Histex HC oral liquid ℞ *narcotic antitussive; decongestant; antihistamine* [hydrocodone bitartrate; pseudoephedrine HCl; carbinoxamine maleate] 5•30•2 mg/5 mL

Histex Pd oral liquid ℞ *antihistamine for allergic rhinitis* [carbinoxamine maleate] 4 mg/5 mL

Histex SR extended-release capsules ℞ *decongestant; antihistamine* [pseudoephedrine HCl; brompheniramine maleate] 120•10 mg

Histex SR film-coated, sustained-release tablets ℞ *decongestant; antihistamine; analgesic* [phenylephrine HCl; chlorpheniramine maleate; acetaminophen] 40•8•500 mg

histidine (L-histidine) USAN, USP, INN *amino acid (essential in infants and in renal failure, nonessential otherwise); symbols: His, H*

histidine monohydrochloride NF

495-L-histidineglucosylceramidase [see: imiglucerase]

Histine DM; Histinex DM syrup (discontinued 2002) ℞ *antitussive;*

decongestant; antihistamine [dextromethorphan hydrobromide; phenylpropanolamine HCl; brompheniramine maleate] 10•12.5•2 mg/5 mL

Histinex HC syrup ℞ *narcotic antitussive; decongestant; antihistamine* [hydrocodone bitartrate; phenylephrine HCl; chlorpheniramine maleate] 5•10•4 mg/10 mL

Histinex PV syrup ℞ *narcotic antitussive; decongestant; antihistamine* [hydrocodone bitartrate; pseudoephedrine HCl; chlorpheniramine maleate] 5•60•4 mg/10 mL

Histolyn-CYL intradermal injection ℞ *diagnostic aid for histoplasmosis* [histoplasmin (mycelial derivative)] 1:100

histoplasmin USP *dermal histoplasmosis test; Histoplasma capsulatum cultures in mycelial or yeast lysate form* 1:100 injection (yeast lysate form)

Histor-D syrup (discontinued 2002) ℞ *decongestant; antihistamine* [phenylephrine HCl; chlorpheniramine maleate; alcohol 2%] 5•2 mg/5 mL

Histosal tablets (discontinued 2001) OTC *decongestant; antihistamine; analgesic* [phenylpropanolamine HCl; pyrilamine maleate; acetaminophen; caffeine] 20•12.5•324•30 mg

histrelin USAN, INN *LHRH agonist; investigational (orphan) for acute intermittent porphyria, hereditary coproporphyria, and variegate porphyria*

histrelin acetate *LHRH agonist for palliative treatment of advanced prostate cancer and central precocious puberty (orphan)*

Histussin D oral liquid ℞ *narcotic antitussive; decongestant* [hydrocodone bitartrate; pseudoephedrine HCl] 5•60 mg/5 mL

Histussin HC syrup ℞ *narcotic antitussive; decongestant; antihistamine* [hydrocodone bitartrate; phenylephrine HCl; chlorpheniramine maleate] 2.5•5•2 mg/5 mL

HIV immune globulin (HIVIG) *investigational (Phase III, orphan)*

immunomodulator for AIDS and maternal/fetal HIV transfer

HIV immunotherapeutic (HIV-IT); HIV therapeutic *investigational (Phase II) gene therapy for HIV; investigational (Phase I–III) antiviral for symptomatic HIV*

HIV protease inhibitors *a class of antivirals that block HIV replication*

HIV vaccine [see: AIDS vaccine]

HIV-1 LA test [see: Recombigen HIV-1 LA]

HIV-1 peptide vaccine *investigational (Phase I) vaccine for HIV*

HIVAB HIV-1 EIA; HIVAB HIV-1/ HIV-2 EIA; HIVAB HIV-2 EIA reagent kit for professional use *in vitro diagnostic aid for HIV antibodies* [enzyme immunoassay (EIA)]

HIVAG-1 reagent kit for professional use *in vitro diagnostic aid for HIV antibodies* [enzyme immunoassay (EIA)]

hive vine *medicinal herb* [see: squaw vine]

Hi-Vegi-Lip tablets (discontinued 2002) OTC *digestive enzymes* [pancreatin (lipase; protease; amylase)] 2400 mg (4800•60 000•60 000 USP units)

Hivenyl ℞ *investigational (Phase III) histamine H_1 antagonist for skin allergies*

Hivid film-coated tablets ℞ *antiviral for advanced HIV infection (orphan)* [zalcitabine] 0.375, 0.75 mg

HK-Cardiosol *investigational heart preservation solution*

HMB (β-hydroxy-β-methylbutyrate) [q.v.]

HMB (homatropine methylbromide) [q.v.]

HMDP (hydroxymethylene diphosphonate) [see: oxidronic acid]

hMG (human menopausal gonadotropin) [see: menotropins]

HMG-CoA (3-hydroxy-3-methylglutaryl-coenzyme A) reductase inhibitors *a class of antihyperlipidemics that reduce serum LDL, VLDL, and triglycerides, but increase HDL* [also called: "statins"]

HMM (hexamethylmelamine) [see: altretamine]

HMR1964 *investigational (Phase III) for type 1 and type 2 diabetes*

HMS eye drop suspension ℞ *steroidal anti-inflammatory* [medrysone] 1%

HN₂ (nitrogen mustard) [see: mechlorethamine HCl]

HOAP-BLEO (hydroxydaunomycin, Oncovin, ara-C, prednisone, bleomycin) *chemotherapy protocol*

hoarhound *medicinal herb* [see: horehound]

hock heal *medicinal herb* [see: woundwort]

hog apple *medicinal herb* [see: mandrake; noni]

hogweed *medicinal herb* [see: broom; masterwort]

Hold, Children's lozenges (discontinued 2002) OTC *antitussive* [dextromethorphan hydrobromide] 5 mg

Hold DM lozenges OTC *antitussive* [dextromethorphan hydrobromide] 5 mg

holly (*Ilex aquifolium; I. opaca; I. vomitoria*) leaves and berries *medicinal herb used as a CNS stimulant and emetic; not generally regarded as safe and effective*

holly, ground *medicinal herb* [see: pipsissewa]

holly bay *medicinal herb* [see: magnolia]

holly-leaved barberry; holly mahonia *medicinal herb* [see: Oregon grape]

holmium *element (Ho)*

holy thistle; blessed cardus *medicinal herb* [see: blessed thistle]

homarylamine INN

homatropine BAN *ophthalmic anticholinergic* [also: homatropine hydrobromide]

homatropine hydrobromide USP *ophthalmic anticholinergic; cycloplegic; mydriatic* [also: homatropine] 5% eye drops

homatropine methylbromide USP, INN, BAN *anticholinergic*

Home Access; Home Access Express test kit for home use *in vitro diagnostic aid for HIV in the blood*

Home Access Hepatitis C Check test kit for home use *in vitro diagnostic aid for hepatitis C in the blood*

homidium bromide INN, BAN

Hominex-1 powder OTC *formula for infants with homocystinuria or hypermethioninemia*

Hominex-2 powder OTC *enteral nutritional therapy for homocystinuria or hypermethioninemia*

homochlorcyclizine INN, BAN

homofenazine (HFZ) INN

homomenthyl salicylate [see: homosalate]

homopipramol INN

homosalate USAN, INN *ultraviolet sunscreen*

4-homosulfanilamide [see: mafenide]

homprenorphine INN, BAN

honey *natural remedy used as an antibacterial and wound healing agent and as a gargle to promote expectoration; not generally regarded as safe and effective for infants because of possible* Clostridium botulinum *contamination*

honeybee venom *natural remedy* [see: bee venom]

honeybloom *medicinal herb* [see: dogbane]

hoodwart *medicinal herb* [see: skullcap]

HOP (hydroxydaunomycin, Oncovin, prednisone) *chemotherapy protocol*

hopantenic acid INN

hops (Humulus lupulus) flower *medicinal herb for aiding digestion, appetite stimulation, bronchitis, cystitis, delirium, edema, headache, hyperactivity, insomnia, intestinal cramps, menstrual disorders, nervousness, pain, excessive sexual desire, and TB*

hoquizil INN *bronchodilator* [also: hoquizil HCl]

hoquizil HCl USAN *bronchodilator* [also: hoquizil]

Hordeum vulgare *medicinal herb* [see: barley]

horehound (Marrubium vulgare) plant *medicinal herb for asthma, colds and cough, croup, inducing diaphoresis*

and diuresis, intestinal parasites, lung disorders, promoting expectoration, and respiratory disorders

horse chestnut (Aesculus californica; A. glabra; A. hippocastanum) nuts and leaves *medicinal herb for arthritis, colds and congestion, hemorrhoids, rheumatism, and varicose veins; not generally regarded as safe and effective for internal use as it is highly toxic*

horse-elder; horseheal *medicinal herb* [see: elecampane]

horsefoot; horsehoof *medicinal herb* [see: coltsfoot]

horsemint (Monarda punctata) leaves and flowering tops *medicinal herb used as a cardiac, carminative, diaphoretic, diuretic, emmenagogue, stimulant, and sudorific*

horseradish (Armoracia lapathiofolia; A. rusticana) root *medicinal herb for appetite stimulation, colic, cough, edema, expelling afterbirth, hay fever, poor circulation, sciatic pain, sinus disorders, and skin and internal tumors; also used as a vermifuge*

horsetail (Equisetum arvens) plant *medicinal herb for bladder disorders, brittle nails, glandular disorders, internal bleeding, nosebleeds, poor circulation, tuberculosis, and urinary disorders*

horseweed; fleabane (Erigeron canadensis) plant *medicinal herb used as an astringent, diuretic, and hemostatic*

ho-shou-wu; fo-ti (Polygonum multiflorum) root *medicinal herb for atherosclerosis, blood cleansing, constipation, improving liver and kidney function, insomnia, malaria, muscle aches, TB, and weak bones; also used to increase fertility, prevent aging, and promote longevity*

H.P. Acthar Gel IM or subcu injectable gel ℞ *corticosteroid; anti-inflammatory* [corticotropin repository] 80 U/mL

HPMCP (hydroxypropyl methylcellulose phthalate) [q.v.]

HPMPC (3-hydroxy-2-phosphonomethoxypropyl cytosine [dihydrate]) [see: cidofovir]

Hp-PAC Ⓒ blister packs for daily administration ℞ *multiple products for the eradication of* H. pylori [lansoprazole (delayed-release capsules); clarithromycin (tablets); amoxicillin trihydrate (capsules)] 30•500•500 mg

H-R Lubricating vaginal jelly OTC *lubricant* [hydroxypropyl methylcellulose]

5-HT (5-hydroxytryptamine) [see: serotonin]

HT (human thrombin) [see: thrombin]

HT; 3-HT (3-hydroxytyramine) [see: dopamine]

5-HTP (5-hydroxytryptophan) [see: L-5 hydroxytryptophan]

H-Tuss-D oral liquid (discontinued 2002) ℞ *narcotic antitussive; decongestant* [hydrocodone bitartrate; pseudoephedrine HCl; alcohol 5%] 5•60 mg/5 mL

Hu23F2G [see: rovelizumab]

Hu5c8 [see: ruplizumab]

huckleberry *medicinal herb* [see: bilberry]

HuM291 (human-mouse monoclonal antibody) [now: visilizumab]

Humalog vials for subcu injection, prefilled syringe cartridges, disposable pen injectors ℞ *rapid-acting insulin analogue for diabetes* [insulin lispro, human (rDNA)] 100 U/mL; 150 U/1.5 mL, 300 U/3 mL; 300 U/3 mL

Humalog Mix 50/50 vials for subcu injection, prefilled syringe cartridges, disposable pen injectors (discontinued 2002) ℞ *rapid-acting insulin analogue for diabetes* [insulin lispro protamine; insulin lispro, human (rDNA)] 50%•50% (100 U/mL total)

Humalog Mix 75/25 vials for subcu injection, disposable pen injectors ℞ *rapid-acting insulin analogue for diabetes* [insulin lispro protamine; insulin lispro, human (rDNA)] 75%•25% (100 U/mL total)

Humalog Mix25 Ⓒ prefilled syringe cartridges, disposable pen injectors ℞ *rapid-acting insulin analogue for diabetes* [insulin lispro protamine;

insulin lispro, human (rDNA)] 75%•25% (100 U/mL total)

human acid alpha-glucosidase *investigational (orphan) for glycogen storage disease type II*

human albumin [see: albumin, human]

Human Albumin Grifols IV infusion ℞ *blood volume expander for shock, burns, and hypoproteinemia* [human albumin] 25%

human amniotic fluid-derived surfactant [see: surfactant, human amniotic fluid derived]

human antihemophilic factor [see: antihemophilic factor]

human B-type natriuretic peptide (hBNP) [see: nesiritide; nesiritide citrate]

human chorionic gonadotropin (hCG) [see: gonadotropin, chorionic]

human complement receptor [see: complement receptor type I, soluble recombinant human]

human cytomegalovirus immune globulin [see: cytomegalovirus immune globulin, human]

human diploid cell vaccine (HDCV) [see: rabies vaccine]

human epidermal growth factor [see: epidermal growth factor, human]

human fibrinogen [see: fibrinogen, human]

human fibrinolysin [see: fibrinolysin, human]

human follicle-stimulating hormone (hFSH) [now: menotropins]

human growth hormone (hGH) JAN *growth hormone* [also: somatropin]

human growth hormone, recombinant (rhGH) [see: somatropin]

human growth hormone releasing factor (hGH-RF) [see: growth hormone-releasing factor (GH-RF)]

human immunodeficiency virus (HIV) immune globulin (HIVIG) [see: HIV immune globulin]

human insulin [see: insulin, human; insulin aspart; insulin aspart protamine]

human menopausal gonadotropin (hMG) [see: menotropins]

human respiratory syncytial virus immune globulin [see: respiratory syncytial virus immune globulin, human]

human retinal pigmented epithelial (RPE) cells on spherical cell-coated microcarriers (CCM) *investigational (Phase II, orphan) dopamine-producing brain implants for stage 3 and 4 Parkinson disease*

human serum albumin diethylene-triaminepentaacetic acid (DTPA) technetium (⁹⁹ᵐTc) JAN *radioactive agent* [also: technetium Tc 99m pentetate]

human superoxide dismutase (SOD) [see: superoxide dismutase, human]

human T-cell inhibitor [see: muromonab-CD3]

human T-cell lymphotrophic virus type III (HTLV-III) [now: human immunodeficiency virus (HIV)]

Human T-Lymphotropic Virus Type I EIA reagent kit for professional use *in vitro diagnostic aid for HTLV I antibody in serum or plasma* [enzyme immunoassay (EIA)]

Humate-P IV injection ℞ *antihemophilic for von Willebrand disease (orphan)* [antihemophilic factor VIII; von Willebrand factor] 20–40 IU/mL

Humatin capsules ℞ *aminoglycoside antibiotic; amebicide for acute and chronic intestinal amebiasis* [paromomycin sulfate] 250 mg

Humatrope powder for subcu or IM injection; prefilled cartridges for HumatroPen (self-injection device) ℞ *growth hormone for adults or children with congenital or endogenous growth hormone deficiency, children with Turner syndrome or renal-induced growth failure, or AIDS-wasting syndrome (orphan)* [somatropin] 5 mg (15 IU) per vial; 6, 12, 24 mg

HumatroPen (trademarked device) *subcu self-injector for Humatrope*

Humegon powder for IM injection (discontinued 2002) ℞ *ovulation stimulant for women; spermatogenesis stimulant for men* [menotropins] 75, 150 IU

Humibid CS tablets OTC *antitussive; expectorant* [dextromethorphan hydrobromide; guaifenesin] 20•400 mg

Humibid DM extended-release capsules ℞ *antitussive; expectorant* [dextromethorphan hydrobromide; guaifenesin; potassium guaiacolsulfonate] 50•400•200 mg

Humibid DM sustained-release caplets (discontinued 2004) ℞ *antitussive; expectorant* [dextromethorphan hydrobromide; guaifenesin] 30•600 mg

Humibid DM Sprinkle sustained-release capsules (discontinued 2002) ℞ *antitussive; expectorant* [dextromethorphan hydrobromide; guaifenesin] 15•300 mg

Humibid E tablets OTC *expectorant* [guaifenesin] 400 mg

Humibid L.A. sustained-release caplets (discontinued 2004) ℞ *expectorant* [guaifenesin; potassium guaiacolsulfonate] 600•300 mg

Humibid Pediatric sustained-release capsules (discontinued 2004) ℞ *expectorant* [guaifenesin] 300 mg

Humibid Sprinkle (name changed to Humibid Pediatric in 2002)

Humira subcu injection in prefilled self-injectors ℞ *disease-modifying antirheumatic drug (DMARD) for moderate to severe rheumatoid arthritis (RA)* [adalimumab] 40 mg/0.8 mL dose

HuMist Moisturizing nasal mist OTC *nasal moisturizer* [sodium chloride (saline solution)] 0.65%

Humorsol Ocumeter (eye drops) (discontinued 2004) ℞ *antiglaucoma agent; reversible cholinesterase inhibitor miotic* [demecarium bromide] 0.125%, 0.25%

Humulin 30/70 ⒸⒶⓃ subcu injection, prefilled syringe cartridges OTC *antidiabetic* [insulin; isophane insulin] 100 U/mL; 1.5 mL

Humulin 50/50 vials for subcu injection OTC *antidiabetic* [isophane human insulin (rDNA); human insulin (rDNA)] 100 U/mL

Humulin 70/30 prefilled syringe cartridges (discontinued 2004) OTC *antidiabetic* [isophane human insulin (rDNA); human insulin (rDNA)] 150 U/1.5 mL

Humulin 70/30 vials for subcu injection, disposable pen injectors OTC *antidiabetic* [isophane human insulin (rDNA); human insulin (rDNA)] 100 U/mL; 300 U/3 mL

Humulin L vials for subcu injection (discontinued 2005) OTC *antidiabetic* [insulin zinc, human (rDNA)] 100 U/mL

Humulin N prefilled syringe cartridges (discontinued 2004) OTC *antidiabetic* [isophane human insulin (rDNA)] 100 U/1.5 mL

Humulin N vials for subcu injection, disposable pen injectors OTC *antidiabetic* [isophane human insulin (rDNA)] 100 U/mL; 300 U/3 mL

Humulin R vials for subcu injection OTC *antidiabetic* [human insulin (rDNA)] 100 U/mL

Humulin R Regular U-500 (concentrated) vials for subcu injection ℞ *antidiabetic* [human insulin (rDNA)] 500 U/mL

Humulin U vials for subcu injection (discontinued 2005) OTC *antidiabetic* [insulin zinc, extended human (rDNA)] 100 U/mL

Humulin-U ⓒⒶⓃ subcu injection OTC *antidiabetic* [extended insulin zinc] 100 U/mL

Humulus lupulus medicinal herb [see: hops]

huperzine A *natural extract from Chinese club moss that enhances memory, focus, and concentration; prevents the breakdown of the neurotransmitter acetylcholine*

hurr-burr *medicinal herb* [see: burdock]

Hurricaine spray liquid, topical liquid, gel OTC *mucous membrane anesthetic* [benzocaine] 20%

HXM (hexamethylmelamine) [see: altretamine]

Hyacne ℞ *investigational (Phase III) acne treatment*

Hyalgan intra-articular injection in vials and prefilled syringes ℞ *viscoelastic lubricant and "shock absorber" for osteoarthritis and temporomandibular joint syndrome* [hyaluronate sodium] 20 mg/2 mL

hyalosidase INN, BAN

hyaluronan *viscoelastic lubricant and "shock absorber" for osteoarthritis of the knee*

hyaluronate sodium USAN, JAN *ophthalmic surgical aid; treatment for osteoarthritis and TMJ syndrome; veterinary synovitis agent* [also: hyaluronic acid]

hyaluronic acid BAN *ophthalmic surgical aid; treatment for osteoarthritis and TMJ syndrome; dermal filler for deep wrinkles and facial folds; veterinary synovitis agent* [also: hyaluronate sodium]

hyaluronidase USP, INN, BAN *adjuvant to increase the absorption and dispersion of injected drugs, hypodermoclysis, and subcutaneous urography; investigational (NDA filed) agent to clear vitreous hemorrhage; also used for diabetic retinopathy*

hyaluronoglucosaminidase [see: hyalosidase]

hyamate [see: buramate]

Hyate:C (Porcine) powder for IV injection ℞ *antihemophilic for patients with antibodies to human factor VIII* [antihemophilic factor concentrate, porcine] 400–700 porcine units

hybenzate USAN *combining name for radicals or groups* [also: hibenzate]

Hybrid Capture II Chlamydia Test reagent kit for professional use *in vitro diagnostic aid for* Chlamydia trachomatis

Hycamtin powder for IV injection ℞ *topoisomerase I inhibitor; antineoplastic*

for ovarian and small cell lung cancers; investigational (Phase II) for AIDS-related progressive multifocal leukoencephalopathy (PML) [topotecan HCl] 4 mg/dose

hycanthone USAN, INN *antischistosomal*

hycanthone mesylate *antischistosomal*

Hycet oral liquid R *narcotic analgesic* [hydrocodone bitartrate; acetaminophen; alcohol 7%] 2.5•108 mg/5 mL

hyclate INN *combining name for radicals or groups*

HycoClear Tuss syrup (discontinued 2002) R *narcotic antitussive; expectorant* [hydrocodone bitartrate; guaifenesin] 5•100 mg/5 mL

Hycodan tablets, syrup R *narcotic antitussive; anticholinergic* [hydrocodone bitartrate; homatropine methylbromide] 5•1.5 mg; 5•1.5 mg/5 mL ⑨ Hycomine; Vicodin

Hycomine syrup, pediatric syrup (discontinued 2002) R *narcotic antitussive; decongestant* [hydrocodone bitartrate; phenylpropanolamine HCl] 5•25 mg/5 mL; 2.5•12.5 mg/5 mL ⑨ Byclomine; Hycodan; Vicodin

Hycomine Compound tablets (discontinued 2002) R *narcotic antitussive; decongestant; antihistamine; analgesic* [hydrocodone bitartrate; phenylephrine HCl; chlorpheniramine maleate; acetaminophen; caffeine] 5•10•2•250•30 mg

Hycort cream, ointment R *topical corticosteroidal anti-inflammatory* [hydrocortisone] 1%

Hycosin Expectorant syrup R *narcotic antitussive; expectorant* [hydrocodone bitartrate; guaifenesin; alcohol 10%] 5•100 mg/5 mL

Hycotuss Expectorant syrup R *narcotic antitussive; expectorant* [hydrocodone bitartrate; guaifenesin; alcohol 10%] 5•100 mg/5 mL

hydantoins *a class of anticonvulsants*

Hydeltrasol IV, IM injection R *corticosteroid; anti-inflammatory* [prednisolone sodium phosphate] 20 mg/mL

Hydergine sublingual tablets, tablets, oral liquid R *cognition adjuvant for age-related mental capacity decline* [ergoloid mesylates] 0.5, 1 mg; 1 mg; 1 mg/mL ⑨ Hydramine

Hydergine LC liquid-filled capsules (discontinued 2004) R *cognition adjuvant for age-related mental capacity decline* [ergoloid mesylates] 1 mg

hydracarbazine INN

hydragogues *a class of purgatives that produce abundant watery discharge from the bowels*

hydralazine INN, BAN *antihypertensive; peripheral vasodilator* [also: hydralazine HCl]

hydralazine HCl USP, JAN *antihypertensive; peripheral vasodilator* [also: hydralazine] 10, 25, 50, 100 mg oral; 20 mg/mL injection

hydralazine polistirex USAN *antihypertensive*

Hydramine syrup, elixir R *antihistamine; antitussive* [diphenhydramine HCl] 12.5 mg/5 mL ⑨ Bydramine; Hydergine; Hydramyn; Hytramyn

hydrangea *(Hydrangea arborescens)* leaves and root *medicinal herb for arthritis, bladder infections, gallstones, gonorrhea, gout, kidney stones, rheumatism, and urinary disorders*

Hydrap-ES tablets R *antihypertensive; vasodilator; diuretic* [hydrochlorothiazide; reserpine; hydralazine HCl] 15•0.1•25 mg

hydrargaphen INN, BAN

hydrastine USP

hydrastine HCl USP

hydrastinine HCl NF

Hydrastis canadensis *medicinal herb* [see: goldenseal]

Hydrate IV or IM injection R *antinauseant; antiemetic; antivertigo; motion sickness preventative* [dimenhydrinate] 50 mg/mL

hydrazinecarboximidamide monohydrochloride [see: pimagedine HCl]

hydrazinoxane [see: domoxin]

Hydrea capsules R *antineoplastic for melanoma, squamous cell carcinoma,* *myelocytic leukemia, and ovarian cancer; sickle cell anemia treatment (orphan)* [hydroxyurea] 500 mg

Hydrisea lotion OTC *moisturizer; emollient* [Dead Sea salts]

Hydrisinol cream, lotion OTC *moisturizer; emollient*

Hydro Cobex IM injection ℞ *hematinic; vitamin B₁₂ supplement* [hydroxocobalamin] 1000 μg/mL

hydrobentizide INN

hydrobutamine [see: butidrine]

Hydrocare Cleaning and Disinfecting solution OTC *chemical disinfecting solution for soft contact lenses*

Hydrocare Preserved Saline solution OTC *rinsing/storage solution for soft contact lenses* [sodium chloride (preserved saline solution)]

Hydrocerin cream base, lotion base OTC *nontherapeutic base for compounding various dermatological preparations*

Hydrocet capsules ℞ *narcotic analgesic* [hydrocodone bitartrate; acetaminophen] 5•500 mg

hydrochloric acid NF *acidifying agent*

hydrochloric acid, diluted NF *acidifying agent*

hydrochlorothiazide (HCT; HCTZ) USP, INN, BAN *antihypertensive; diuretic* 12.5, 25, 50, 100 mg oral; 50 mg/5 mL oral; 100 mg/mL oral

hydrochlorothiazide & benazepril HCl *antihypertensive; diuretic; angiotensin-converting enzyme (ACE) inhibitor* 6.25•5, 12.5•10, 12.5•20, 25•20 mg oral

hydrochlorothiazide & bisoprolol fumarate *antihypertensive; diuretic; β-blocker* 6.5•2.5, 6.5•5, 6.5•10 mg oral

hydrochlorothiazide & captopril *antihypertensive; diuretic; angiotensin-converting enzyme (ACE) inhibitor* 15•25, 25•25, 15•50, 25•50 mg oral

hydrochlorothiazide & enalapril maleate *antihypertensive; diuretic; angiotensin-converting enzyme (ACE) inhibitor* 12.5•5, 25•10 mg oral

hydrochlorothiazide & fosinopril sodium *antihypertensive; diuretic;*

angiotensin-converting enzyme (ACE) inhibitor 12.5•10, 12.5•20 mg

hydrochlorothiazide & lisinopril *antihypertensive; diuretic; angiotensin-converting enzyme (ACE) inhibitor* 12.5•10, 12.5•20, 25•20 mg oral

hydrochlorothiazide & metoprolol tartrate *antihypertensive; diuretic; β-blocker* 25•50, 25•100, 50•00 mg oral

hydrochlorothiazide & quinapril HCl *antihypertensive; diuretic; angiotensin-converting enzyme (ACE) inhibitor* 12.5•10, 12.5•20, 25•20 mg oral

hydrochlorothiazide & triamterene *antihypertensive; potassium-sparing diuretic* 25•37.5 mg oral

hydrocholeretics *a class of gastrointestinal drugs that exert laxative effects and increase volume and water content of bile actions*

Hydrocil Instant powder OTC *bulk laxative* [psyllium hydrophilic mucilloid] 3.5 g/scoop

hydrocodone INN, BAN *antitussive* [also: hydrocodone bitartrate]

hydrocodone bitartrate USAN, USP *narcotic antitussive* [also: hydrocodone]

hydrocodone bitartrate & acetaminophen *narcotic antitussive; analgesic* 2.5•500, 5•325, 7.5•650, 7.5• 750, 10•325, 10•500, 10•650, 10• 750 mg oral; 2.5•167 mg/5 mL oral

hydrocodone bitartrate & guaifenesin *narcotic antitussive; expectorant* 5•100 mg/5 mL oral

hydrocodone bitartrate & ibuprofen *narcotic antitussive; analgesic* 7.5•200 mg oral

hydrocodone bitartrate & pseudoephedrine HCl & carbinoxamine maleate *narcotic antitussive; decongestant; antihistamine* 5•30•2 mg/5 mL oral

Hydrocodone Compound syrup (discontinued 2002) ℞ *narcotic antitussive; anticholinergic* [hydrocodone bitartrate; homatropine hydrobromide] 5•1.5 mg/5 mL

Hydrocodone CP syrup ℞ *narcotic antitussive; decongestant; antihistamine*

[hydrocodone bitartrate; phenylephrine HCl; chlorpheniramine maleate] 2.5•5•2 mg/5 mL

Hydrocodone GF syrup ℞ *narcotic antitussive; expectorant* [hydrocodone bitartrate; guaifenesin] 5•100 mg/5 mL

Hydrocodone HD oral liquid ℞ *narcotic antitussive; decongestant; antihistamine* [hydrocodone bitartrate; phenylephrine HCl; chlorpheniramine maleate] 3.33•10•4 mg/10 mL

Hydrocodone PA syrup, pediatric syrup (discontinued 2002) ℞ *narcotic antitussive; decongestant* [hydrocodone bitartrate; phenylpropanolamine HCl] 5•25 mg/5 mL; 2.5• 12.5 mg/5 mL

hydrocodone polistirex USAN *narcotic antitussive*

Hydrocol adhesive dressings *occlusive wound dressing* [hydrocolloid gel]

hydrocolloid gel *dressings for wet wounds*

Hydrocort cream ℞ *topical corticosteroidal anti-inflammatory* [hydrocortisone] 2.5%

hydrocortamate INN

hydrocortamate HCl [see: hydrocortamate]

hydrocortisone (HC) USP, INN, BAN *corticosteroid; anti-inflammatory* 5, 10, 20 mg oral; 0.5%, 1%, 2.5% topical

hydrocortisone aceponate INN *corticosteroid; anti-inflammatory*

hydrocortisone acetate (HCA) USP, BAN *corticosteroid; anti-inflammatory* 1% topical; 25 mg suppositories; 25, 50 mg/mL injection

hydrocortisone acetate & lidocaine HCl *corticosteroidal anti-inflammatory; local anesthetic* 3%•0.5% topical

hydrocortisone & acetic acid *corticosteroid; anti-inflammatory; acidifying agent* 1%•2% otic solution

hydrocortisone buteprate USAN [now: hydrocortisone probutate]

hydrocortisone butyrate BAN *topical corticosteroidal anti-inflammatory* [also: hydrocortisone probutate] 0.1% topical

hydrocortisone cyclopentylpropionate *corticosteroid; anti-inflammatory* [see: hydrocortisone cypionate]

hydrocortisone cypionate USP *corticosteroid; anti-inflammatory*

hydrocortisone hemisuccinate USP *corticosteroid; anti-inflammatory*

hydrocortisone & iodoquinol *corticosteroidal anti-inflammatory; amebicide; antimicrobial* 1%•1% topical

hydrocortisone & neomycin sulfate & polymyxin B sulfate *topical ophthalmic corticosteroidal anti-inflammatory and antibiotic* 1%•0.35%• 10 000 U/mL eye drops

hydrocortisone probutate USAN, USP *topical corticosteroidal anti-inflammatory* [previously known as: hydrocortisone buteprate]

hydrocortisone sodium phosphate USP, BAN *corticosteroid; anti-inflammatory*

hydrocortisone sodium succinate USP, BAN *corticosteroid; anti-inflammatory*

hydrocortisone valerate USAN, USP *topical corticosteroidal anti-inflammatory* 0.2% topical

Hydrocortone tablets ℞ *corticosteroid; anti-inflammatory* [hydrocortisone] 10, 20 mg

Hydrocortone Acetate intralesional, intra-articular, or soft tissue injection ℞ *corticosteroid; anti-inflammatory* [hydrocortisone acetate] 25, 50 mg/mL

Hydrocortone Phosphate IV, subcu, or IM injection ℞ *corticosteroid; anti-inflammatory* [hydrocortisone sodium phosphate] 50 mg/mL

Hydrocotyle asiatica *medicinal herb* [see: gotu kola]

Hydrocream Base OTC *cream base*

Hydro-Crysti 12 IM injection ℞ *hematinic; vitamin B_{12} supplement* [hydroxocobalamin] 1000 μg/mL

HydroDIURIL tablets ℞ *antihypertensive; diuretic* [hydrochlorothiazide] 25, 50, 100 mg

Hydro-DP syrup ℞ *narcotic antitussive; decongestant; antihistamine* [hydrocodone bitartrate; phenylephrine HCl; diphenhydramine HCl] 2•7.5•12.5 mg/5 mL

hydrofilcon A USAN *hydrophilic contact lens material*

hydroflumethiazide USP, INN, BAN *antihypertensive; diuretic* 50 mg oral

hydrofluoric acid *dental caries prophylactic*

hydrofluoroalkane (HFA) *propellant used in CFC-free aerosol delivery systems* [usually HFA-134a]

hydrogen *element (H)*

hydrogen peroxide USP *topical anti-infective*

hydrogen tetrabromoaurate [see: bromauric acid]

hydrogenated ergot alkaloids [now: ergoloid mesylates]

hydrogenated vegetable oil [see: vegetable oil, hydrogenated]

Hydrogesic capsules ℞ *narcotic analgesic* [hydrocodone bitartrate; acetaminophen] 5•500 mg

hydromadinone INN

Hydromet syrup ℞ *narcotic antitussive; anticholinergic* [hydrocodone bitartrate; homatropine methylbromide] 5•1.5 mg/5 mL

Hydromide syrup ℞ *narcotic antitussive; anticholinergic* [hydrocodone bitartrate; homatropine methylbromide] 5•1.5 mg/5 mL

hydromorphinol INN, BAN

hydromorphone INN, BAN *narcotic analgesic; widely abused as a street drug* [also: hydromorphone HCl]

hydromorphone HCl USP *narcotic analgesic; widely abused as a street drug* [also: hydromorphone] 2, 4, 8 mg oral; 1 mg/mL oral; 3 mg rectal; 1, 2, 4, 10 mg/mL injection

hydromorphone sulfate

Hydromox tablets (discontinued 2001) ℞ *diuretic; antihypertensive* [quinethazone] 50 mg

Hydron CP oral liquid ℞ *narcotic antitussive; decongestant; antihistamine* [hydrocodone bitartrate; phenyleph-

rine HCl; chlorpheniramine maleate] 5•10•2 mg/5 mL

Hydron EX; Hydron KGS oral liquid ℞ *narcotic antitussive; expectorant* [hydrocodone bitartrate; potassium guaiacolsulfonate] 2.5•120 mg/5 mL; 5•300 mg/5 mL

Hydron PSC oral liquid ℞ *narcotic antitussive; decongestant; antihistamine* [hydrocodone bitartrate; pseudoephedrine HCl; chlorpheniramine maleate] 5•30•2 mg/5 mL

Hydropane syrup ℞ *narcotic antitussive; anticholinergic* [hydrocodone bitartrate; homatropine methylbromide] 5•1.5 mg/5 mL

Hydro-Par tablets ℞ *antihypertensive; diuretic* [hydrochlorothiazide] 25, 50 mg

Hydro-PC; Hydro-PC II oral liquid ℞ *narcotic antitussive; decongestant; antihistamine* [hydrocodone bitartrate; phenylephrine HCl; chlorpheniramine maleate] 4•10•4 mg/10 mL; 4•15•4 mg/10 mL

Hydropel ointment OTC *skin protectant* [silicone; hydrophobic starch derivative] 30%•10%

Hydrophed tablets ℞ *antiasthmatic; bronchodilator; decongestant; antihistamine* [theophylline; ephedrine sulfate; hydroxyzine HCl] 130•25•10 mg

Hydrophilic OTC *ointment base*

hydrophilic ointment [see: ointment, hydrophilic]

hydrophilic petrolatum [see: petrolatum, hydrophilic]

Hydropres-50 tablets ℞ *antihypertensive; diuretic* [hydrochlorothiazide; reserpine] 50•0.125 mg

hydroquinone USP *hyperpigmentation bleaching agent* 3%, 4% topical

hydroquinone methyl ether [see: mequinol]

Hydro-Serp tablets ℞ *antihypertensive; diuretic* [hydrochlorothiazide; reserpine] 50•0.125 mg

Hydroserpine #1; Hydroserpine #2 tablets ℞ *antihypertensive; diuretic*

[hydrochlorothiazide; reserpine] 25•
0.125 mg; 50•0.125 mg

HydroSkin cream, lotion, ointment OTC *corticosteroidal anti-inflammatory* [hydrocortisone] 1%

hydrotalcite INN, BAN

HydroTex cream (discontinued 2003) ℞ *corticosteroidal anti-inflammatory* [hydrocortisone] 0.5%

Hydro-Tussin DM oral liquid ℞ *antitussive; expectorant* [dextromethorphan hydrobromide; guaifenesin] 20•200 mg/5 mL

Hydro-Tussin HC syrup ℞ *narcotic antitussive; decongestant; antihistamine* [hydrocodone bitartrate; pseudoephedrine HCl; chlorpheniramine maleate] 3•15•2 mg/5 mL

Hydro-Tussin HD oral liquid ℞ *narcotic antitussive; decongestant; expectorant* [hydrocodone bitartrate; pseudoephedrine HCl; guaifenesin] 5•60•200 mg/10 mL

hydroxamethocaine BAN [also: hydroxytetracaine]

hydroxidione sodium succinate [see: hydroxydione sodium succinate]

hydroxindasate INN

hydroxindasol INN

hydroxizine chloride [see: hydroxyzine HCl]

hydroxocobalamin USAN, USP, INN, BAN, JAN *vitamin B_{12}; hematopoietic* [also: hydroxocobalamin acetate] 1 mg/mL injection

hydroxocobalamin acetate JAN *vitamin B_{12}; hematopoietic* [also: hydroxocobalamin]

hydroxocobalamin & sodium thiosulfate *investigational (orphan) for severe acute cyanide poisoning*

hydroxocobemine [see: hydroxocobalamin]

3-hydroxy-2-phosphonomethoxypropyl cytosine (HPMPC) dihydrate [see: cidofovir]

N-hydroxyacetamide [see: acetohydroxamic acid]

4′-hydroxyacetanilide [see: acetaminophen]

4′-hydroxyacetanilide salicylate [see: acetaminosalol]

hydroxyamfetamine INN *ophthalmic adrenergic; mydriatic* [also: hydroxyamphetamine hydrobromide; hydroxyamphetamine]

hydroxyamphetamine BAN *ophthalmic adrenergic; mydriatic* [also: hydroxyamphetamine hydrobromide; hydroxyamfetamine]

hydroxyamphetamine hydrobromide USP *ophthalmic adrenergic/vasoconstrictor; mydriatic* [also: hydroxyamfetamine; hydroxyamphetamine]

4-hydroxyanisole (4HA); *p*-hydroxyanisole [see: mequinol]

hydroxyapatite BAN *prosthetic aid* [also: durapatite; calcium phosphate, tribasic]

2-hydroxybenzamide [see: salicylamide]

2-hydroxybenzoic acid [see: salicylic acid]

***o*-hydroxybenzyl alcohol** [see: salicyl alcohol]

hydroxybutanedioic acid [see: malic acid]

4-hydroxybutanoic acid [see: gamma hydroxybutyrate (GHB)]

4-hydroxybutanoic acid, sodium salt [see: sodium oxybate]

hydroxybutyrate sodium, gamma [see: sodium oxybate]

hydroxycarbamide INN *antineoplastic* [also: hydroxyurea]

hydroxychloroquine INN, BAN *antimalarial; lupus erythematosus suppressant* [also: hydroxychloroquine sulfate]

hydroxychloroquine sulfate USP *antimalarial; antirheumatic; lupus erythematosus suppressant* (base=77.5%) [also: hydroxychloroquine] 200 mg oral

25-hydroxycholecalciferol [see: calcifediol]

hydroxycincophene [see: oxycinchophen]

hydroxydaunomycin [see: doxorubicin]

14-hydroxydihydromorphine [see: hydromorphinol]

hydroxydione sodium succinate
INN, BAN

1α-hydroxyergocalciferol [see: doxercalciferol]

hydroxyethyl cellulose NF *suspending and viscosity-increasing agent; ophthalmic aid*

2-hydroxyethyl methacrylate (HEMA) *contact lens material*

hydroxyethyl starch (HES) [see: hetastarch]

hydroxyethylstarch JAN *plasma volume extender* [also: hetastarch]

hydroxyhexamide

3-hydroxyisovalerate; β-hydroxyisovalerate [see: β-hydroxy-β-methylbutyrate (HMB)]

hydroxylapatite [see: durapatite; calcium phosphate, tribasic]

hydroxymagnesium aluminate [see: magaldrate]

hydroxymesterone [see: medrysone]

6-hydroxymethylacylfulvene *investigational (orphan) for advanced or metastatic pancreatic cancer, ovarian cancer, or renal carcinoma*

β-hydroxy-β-methylbutyrate (HMB) *an endogenous metabolite of the amino acid L-leucine; a natural supplement taken to prevent exercise-induced muscle breakdown (proteolysis), resulting in larger muscle gains from resistance training; may have immunomodulatory effects*

hydroxymethylene diphosphonate (HMDP) [see: oxidronic acid]

hydroxymethylgramicidin [see: methocidin]

N-hydroxynaphthalimide diethyl phosphate [see: naftalofos]

hydroxypethidine INN, BAN

hydroxyphenamate USAN *minor tranquilizer* [also: oxyfenamate]

N-4-hydroxyphenylretinamide [see: fenretinide]

hydroxyprocaine INN, BAN

hydroxyprogesterone INN, BAN *synthetic progestin for amenorrhea, metrorrhagia, and dysfunctional uterine bleeding* [also: hydroxyprogesterone caproate]

hydroxyprogesterone caproate USP, INN, JAN *synthetic progestin for amenorrhea, metrorrhagia, and dysfunctional uterine bleeding* [also: hydroxyprogesterone] 125, 250 mg/mL IM injection (in oil)

2-hydroxypropanoic acid, calcium salt, hydrate [see: calcium lactate]

hydroxypropyl cellulose NF *topical protectant; emulsifying and coating agent* [also: hydroxypropylcellulose]

hydroxypropyl methylcellulose USP *suspending and viscosity-increasing agent; ophthalmic moisturizer and surgical aid* [also: hypromellose; hydroxypropylmethylcellulose]

hydroxypropyl methylcellulose 1828 USP

hydroxypropyl methylcellulose phthalate (HPMCP) NF *tablet-coating agent* [also: hydroxypropylmethylcellulose phthalate]

hydroxypropyl methylcellulose phthalate 200731 NF *tablet-coating agent*

hydroxypropyl methylcellulose phthalate 220824 NF *tablet-coating agent*

hydroxypropylcellulose JAN *topical protectant; emulsifying and coating agent* [also: hydroxypropyl cellulose]

hydroxypropylmethylcellulose JAN *suspending and viscosity-increasing agent; ophthalmic surgical aid* [also: hydroxypropyl methylcellulose; hypromellose]

hydroxypropylmethylcellulose phthalate JAN *tablet-coating agent* [also: hydroxypropyl methylcellulose phthalate]

hydroxypyridine tartrate INN

hydroxyquinoline *topical antiseptic*

4'-hydroxysalicylanilide [see: osalmid]

hydroxystearin sulfate NF

hydroxystenozole INN

hydroxystilbamidine INN, BAN *antileishmanial* [also: hydroxystilbamidine isethionate]

hydroxystilbamidine isethionate USP *antileishmanial* [also: hydroxystilbamidine]

hydroxysuccinic acid [see: malic acid]

hydroxytetracaine INN [also: hydroxamethocaine]

hydroxytoluic acid INN, BAN

5-hydroxytryptamine₁ (5-HT₁) [see: serotonin]

5-hydroxytryptamine₃ (5-HT₃) receptor antagonists *a class of antinauseant and antiemetic agents used primarily after emetogenic cancer chemotherapy*

5-hydroxytryptophan (5-HTP) [see: L-5 hydroxytryptophan]

3-hydroxytyramine (HT; 3-HT) [see: dopamine]

hydroxyurea USAN, USP, BAN *antimetabolite antineoplastic for melanoma, squamous cell carcinoma, myelocytic leukemia, and ovarian cancer; sickle cell anemia treatment (orphan); investigational adjunctive therapy for HIV* [also: hydroxycarbamide] 250, 500 mg oral

1α-hydroxyvitamin D₂ [see: doxercalciferol]

hydroxyzine INN, BAN *anxiolytic; minor tranquilizer; antiemetic; piperazine antihistamine; antipruritic* [also: hydroxyzine HCl]

hydroxyzine HCl USP *anxiolytic; minor tranquilizer; antiemetic; piperazine antihistamine; antipruritic* [also: hydroxyzine] 10, 25, 50 mg oral; 10 mg/5 mL oral; 25, 50 mg/mL injection

hydroxyzine pamoate USP *anxiolytic; minor tranquilizer; antiemetic; piperazine antihistamine; antipruritic* 25, 50, 100 mg oral

Hyflex-650 tablets ℞ *analgesic; antihistaminic sleep aid* [acetaminophen; phenyltoloxamine citrate] 650•60 mg

Hygenic Cleansing anorectal pads OTC *moisturizer and cleanser for external rectal/vaginal areas; astringent* [witch hazel] 50%

Hygroton tablets ℞ *antihypertensive; diuretic* [chlorthalidone] 25, 50, 100 mg ⊇ Regroton

Hylaform gel for subcu injection in prefilled syringes ℞ *dermal filler for wrinkles and facial folds* [hylan B] 5.5 mg/mL

hylan B *hyaluronic acid gel–based dermal filler*

hylan G-F 20 *hyaluronic acid gel-fluid polymer mixture for osteoarthritis and TMJ syndrome*

Hylorel tablets ℞ *antihypertensive* [guanadrel sulfate] 10, 25 mg

Hylutin IM injection (discontinued 2004) ℞ *synthetic progestin for amenorrhea, metrorrhagia, and dysfunctional uterine bleeding* [hydroxyprogesterone caproate in oil] 125, 250 mg/mL

hymecromone USAN, INN *choleretic*

hyoscine hydrobromide BAN *GI antispasmodic; prevent motion sickness; cycloplegic; mydriatic* [also: scopolamine hydrobromide]

hyoscine methobromide BAN *anticholinergic* [also: methscopolamine bromide]

hyoscyamine (L-hyoscyamine) USP, BAN *anticholinergic; urinary antispasmodic*

hyoscyamine hydrobromide USP *GI antispasmodic; anticholinergic*

hyoscyamine sulfate USP *GI/GU antispasmodic; antiparkinsonian; anticholinergic "drying agent" for allergic rhinitis and hyperhidrosis* [also: hyoscyamine sulphate] 0.375 mg oral; 0.125 mg/mL oral

hyoscyamine sulphate BAN *GI/GU antispasmodic; antiparkinsonian; anticholinergic "drying agent" for allergic rhinitis and hyperhidrosis* [also: hyoscyamine sulfate]

Hyoscyamus niger *medicinal herb* [see: henbane]

Hyosophen tablets, elixir ℞ *GI antispasmodic; anticholinergic; sedative* [atropine sulfate; scopolamine hydrobromide; hyoscyamine hydrobromide; phenobarbital] 0.0194•

0.0065•0.1037•16.2 mg; 0.0194•
0.0065•0.1037•16.2 mg/5 mL

Hypaque Meglumine 30% injection (discontinued 2001) ℞ *radiopaque contrast medium* [diatrizoate meglumine (46.67% iodine)] 300 mg/mL (141 mg/mL)

Hypaque Meglumine 60% injection ℞ *radiopaque contrast medium* [diatrizoate meglumine (46.67% iodine)] 600 mg/mL (282 mg/mL)

Hypaque Sodium oral/rectal solution (discontinued 2001) ℞ *radiopaque contrast medium for gastrointestinal imaging* [diatrizoate sodium (59.87% iodine)] 416.7 mg (249 mg)

Hypaque Sodium powder for oral/rectal solution ℞ *radiopaque contrast medium for gastrointestinal imaging* [diatrizoate sodium (59.87% iodine)] 1002 mg (600 mg)

Hypaque Sodium 20% intracavitary instillation ℞ *radiopaque contrast medium for urological imaging* [diatrizoate sodium (59.87% iodine)] 200 mg/mL (120 mg/mL)

Hypaque Sodium 25% injection (discontinued 2001) ℞ *radiopaque contrast medium* [diatrizoate sodium (46.67% iodine)] 250 mg/mL (150 mg/mL)

Hypaque Sodium 50% injection ℞ *radiopaque contrast medium* [diatrizoate sodium (46.67% iodine)] 500 mg/mL (300 mg/mL)

Hypaque-76 injection ℞ *radiopaque contrast medium* [diatrizoate meglumine; diatrizoate sodium (48.7% total iodine)] 660•100 mg/mL (370 mg/mL)

Hypaque-Cysto intracavitary instillation ℞ *radiopaque contrast medium for urological imaging* [diatrizoate meglumine (46.67% iodine)] 300 mg/mL (141 mg/mL)

Hypericum perforatum medicinal herb [see: St. John wort]

Hyperlyte; Hyperlyte R IV admixture (discontinued 2001) ℞ *intravenous electrolyte therapy* [combined electrolyte solution]

Hyperlyte CR IV admixture ℞ *intravenous electrolyte therapy* [combined electrolyte solution]

hyperosmotic laxatives a subclass of laxatives that use the osmotic effect to retain water in the intestines, lowering colonic pH and increasing peristalsis [see also: laxatives]

Hyperstat IV injection ℞ *vasodilator for hypertensive emergency* [diazoxide] 15 mg/mL ② Hyper-Tet; HyperHep

Hyphed oral liquid ℞ *narcotic antitussive; decongestant; antihistamine* [hydrocodone bitartrate; pseudoephedrine HCl; chlorpheniramine maleate; alcohol 5%] 5•60•4 mg/10 mL

Hy-Phen tablets ℞ *narcotic analgesic* [hydrocodone bitartrate; acetaminophen] 5•500 mg

hyphylline [see: dyphylline]

hypnogene [see: barbital]

hypnotics a class of agents that induce sleep

hypochlorous acid, sodium salt [see: sodium hypochlorite]

β-hypophamine [see: vasopressin]

α-hypophamine [see: oxytocin]

hypophosphorous acid NF antioxidant

Hyporet (trademarked delivery system) prefilled disposable syringe

HypoTears ophthalmic ointment OTC *ocular moisturizer/lubricant* [white petrolatum; mineral oil]

HypoTears; HypoTears PF eye drops OTC *ophthalmic moisturizer/lubricant* [polyvinyl alcohol] 1%

hyprolose [see: hydroxypropyl cellulose]

hypromellose INN, BAN suspending and viscosity-increasing agent [also: hydroxypropyl methylcellulose; hydroxypropylmethylcellulose]

Hyrexin-50 injection (discontinued 2002) ℞ *antihistamine; motion sickness preventative; sleep aid; antiparkinsonian* [diphenhydramine HCl] 50 mg/mL

Hyskon uterine infusion ℞ *hysteroscopy aid* [dextran 70; dextrose] 32%•10%

Hysone cream OTC *topical corticosteroidal anti-inflammatory; antifungal;*

antibacterial [hydrocortisone; clioquinol] 10•30 mg/g

hyssop (Hyssopus officinalis) leaves *medicinal herb for chronic hay fever, congestion, cough, lung ailments, promoting expectoration, and sore throat*

hyssop, hedge *medicinal herb* [see: hedge hyssop]

hyssop, Indian; wild hyssop *medicinal herb* [see: blue vervain]

hyssop, prairie *medicinal herb* [see: wild hyssop]

Hytakerol capsules ℞ *vitamin D therapy for tetany and hypoparathyroidism* [dihydrotachysterol] 0.125 mg

Hytinic capsules OTC *hematinic; iron supplement* [polysaccharide-iron complex] 150 mg Fe

Hytinic IM injection (discontinued 2005) ℞ *hematinic* [ferrous gluconate; multiple B vitamins; procaine HCl] 3 mg/mL• ± •2%

Hytone cream, lotion, ointment ℞ *topical corticosteroidal anti-inflamma-*

tory [hydrocortisone] 1%, 2.5%; 1%, 2.5%; 2.5% ⊡ Vytone

Hytone 1% ointment, spray ℞ *topical corticosteroidal anti-inflammatory* [hydrocortisone] 1%

Hytrin soft capsules ℞ *α₁-adrenergic blocker for hypertension and benign prostatic hyperplasia (BPH)* [terazosin HCl] 1, 2, 5, 10 mg

Hytrin ⊛ tablets, starter pack (1 mg × 7 + 2 mg × 7 + 5 mg × 14) ℞ *α₁-adrenergic blocker for hypertension and benign prostatic hyperplasia (BPH)* [terazosin HCl] 1, 2, 5, 10 mg

Hytuss tablets OTC *expectorant* [guaifenesin] 100 mg

Hytuss 2X capsules OTC *expectorant* [guaifenesin] 200 mg

Hyzaar film-coated tablets ℞ *antihypertensive; angiotensin II receptor antagonist; diuretic* [losartan potassium; hydrochlorothiazide] 50•12.5, 100•25 mg

I

¹²³I [see: iodohippurate sodium I 123]
¹²³I [see: sodium iodide I 123]
¹²⁵I [see: albumin, iodinated I 125 serum]
¹²⁵I [see: diatrizoate sodium I 125]
¹²⁵I [see: diohippuric acid I 125]
¹²⁵I [see: diotyrosine I 125]
¹²⁵I [see: fibrinogen I 125]
¹²⁵I [see: insulin I 125]
¹²⁵I [see: iodohippurate sodium I 125]
¹²⁵I [see: iodopyracet I 125]
¹²⁵I [see: iomethin I 125]
¹²⁵I [see: iothalamate sodium I 125]
¹²⁵I [see: liothyronine I 125]
¹²⁵I [see: oleic acid I 125]
¹²⁵I [see: povidone I 125]
¹²⁵I [see: rose bengal sodium I 125]
¹²⁵I [see: sodium iodide I 125]
¹²⁵I [see: thyroxine I 125]
¹²⁵I [see: triolein I 125]

¹³¹I [see: albumin, aggregated iodinated I 131 serum]
¹³¹I [see: albumin, iodinated I 131 serum]
¹³¹I [see: diatrizoate sodium I 131]
¹³¹I [see: diohippuric acid I 131]
¹³¹I [see: diotyrosine I 131]
¹³¹I [see: ethiodized oil I 131]
¹³¹I [see: insulin I 131]
¹³¹I [see: iodipamide sodium I 131]
¹³¹I [see: iodoantipyrine I 131]
¹³¹I [see: iodocholesterol I 131]
¹³¹I [see: iodohippurate sodium I 131]
¹³¹I [see: iodopyracet I 131]
¹³¹I [see: iomethin I 131]
¹³¹I [see: iothalamate sodium I 131]
¹³¹I [see: iotyrosine I 131]
¹³¹I [see: liothyronine I 131]
¹³¹I [see: macrosalb (¹³¹I)]
¹³¹I [see: oleic acid I 131]

¹³¹I [see: povidone I 131]
¹³¹I [see: rose bengal sodium I 131]
¹³¹I [see: sodium iodide I 131]
¹³¹I [see: thyroxine I 131]
¹³¹I [see: tolpovidone I 131]
¹³¹I [see: triolein I 131]
ibacitabine INN
ibafloxacin USAN, INN, BAN *antibacterial*
ibandronate sodium USAN *bisphosphonate bone resorption inhibitor for postmenopausal osteoporosis; also used for metastatic bone disease*
ibazocine INN
IBC (isobutyl cyanoacrylate) [see: bucrylate]
Iberet; Iberet-500 controlled-release Filmtabs (film-coated tablets) OTC *hematinic* [multiple B vitamins; ferrous sulfate; sodium ascorbate] ≛• 105•150 mg; ≛•105•500 mg
Iberet; Iberet-500 oral liquid (discontinued 2003) OTC *hematinic* [multiple B vitamins; ferrous sulfate] ≛•78.75 mg/15 mL
Iberet-Folic-500 controlled-release Filmtabs (film-coated tablets) ℞ *hematinic* [ferrous sulfate; multiple B vitamins; sodium ascorbate; folic acid] 105•≛•500•0.8 mg
iboga *(Tabernanthe iboga) euphoric/hallucinogenic street drug, the root of which is chewed or chopped into a fine powder and mixed with other drugs; doses high enough to induce hallucinations are also likely to cause death*
ibopamine USAN, INN, BAN *peripheral dopaminergic agent; vasodilator*
ibritumomab tiuxetan USAN *radioimmunotherapy carrier; radiolabeled with indium In 111 and yttrium Y 90 in the treatment protocol for non-Hodgkin B-cell lymphoma*
ibrotal [see: ibrotamide]
ibrotamide INN
IB-Stat oral spray ℞ *pediatric anticholinergic "drying agent" for allergic rhinitis and hyperhidrosis* [hyoscyamine sulfate] 0.125 mg/mL
ibudilast INN

ibufenac USAN, INN, BAN *analgesic; anti-inflammatory*
ibuprofen USAN, USP, INN, BAN *analgesic; antiarthritic; antipyretic; nonsteroidal anti-inflammatory drug (NSAID); investigational (orphan) IV treatment for patent ductus arteriosus* 200, 400, 600, 800 mg oral; 100 mg/5 mL oral; 40 mg/mL oral
ibuprofen aluminum USAN *anti-inflammatory*
ibuprofen & hydrocodone bitartrate *analgesic; narcotic antitussive* 200•7.5 mg oral
ibuprofen piconol USAN *topical anti-inflammatory*
Ibuprohm tablets ℞ *nonsteroidal anti-inflammatory drug (NSAID); antiarthritic; analgesic* [ibuprofen] 400 mg
ibuproxam INN
Ibutab tablets OTC *nonsteroidal anti-inflammatory drug (NSAID); antiarthritic; analgesic* [ibuprofen] 200 mg
ibutamoren mesylate USAN *growth hormone for congenital growth hormone deficiency, musculoskeletal impairment, and hip fractures*
ibuterol INN
ibutilide INN *antiarrhythmic* [also: ibutilide fumarate]
ibutilide fumarate USAN *antiarrhythmic for atrial fibrillation/flutter* [also: ibutilide]
ibuverine INN
ibylcaine chloride [see: butethamine HCl]
IC-351 *investigational (NDA filed) PDE-5 (phosphodiesterase-5) inhibitor for erectile dysfunction*
ICaps timed-release tablets OTC *vitamin/mineral supplement* [multiple vitamins & minerals]
ICaps Plus tablets OTC *vitamin/mineral supplement* [multiple vitamins & minerals]
Icar chewable tablets, oral suspension OTC *hematinic; iron supplement* [carbonyl iron] 15 mg; 15 mg/1.25 mL
icatibant acetate USAN *antiasthmatic*

ICE (idarubicin, cytarabine, etoposide) *chemotherapy protocol for acute myelogenous leukemia (AML)*

ICE (ifosfamide [with mesna rescue], carboplatin, etoposide) *chemotherapy protocol for osteosarcoma and lung cancer* [also: MICE]

Iceland moss (Cetraria islandica) plant *medicinal herb for anemia, bronchitis, hay fever, congestion, cough, digestive disorders, and lung disorders*

ICE-T (ifosfamide [with mesna rescue], carboplatin, etoposide, Taxol) *chemotherapy protocol for sarcoma, breast cancer, and non–small cell lung cancer (NSCLC)*

IC-Green powder for IV injection ℞ *in vivo diagnostic aid for cardiac output, hepatic function, and ophthalmic angiography* [indocyanine green] 25 mg

ichthammol USP, BAN *topical anti-infective* 10%, 20%

iclazepam INN

icodextrin INN, BAN *peritoneal dialysis solution for end-stage renal disease (orphan)*

icopezil maleate USAN *acetylcholinesterase inhibitor; cognition adjuvant for Alzheimer disease*

icosapent INN *omega-3 marine triglyceride* [also: eicosapentaenoic acid (EPA)]

icospiramide INN

icotidine USAN *antagonist to histamine H_1 and H_2 receptors*

ictasol USAN *disinfectant*

Ictotest reagent tablets for professional use *in vitro diagnostic aid for bilirubin in the urine*

Icy Hot balm, cream, stick OTC *analgesic; counterirritant* [methyl salicylate; menthol] 29%•7.6%; 30%•10%; 30%•10%

IDA-based BF 12 (idarubicin, cytarabine, etoposide) *chemotherapy protocol for acute myelogenous leukemia (AML)*

Idamycin powder for IV injection (discontinued 2004) ℞ *anthracycline antibiotic antineoplastic for acute myeloid leukemia (AML) (orphan);* *investigational (orphan) for pediatric use* [idarubicin HCl] 5, 10, 20 mg

Idamycin PFS powder for IV injection ℞ *anthracycline antibiotic antineoplastic for acute myeloid leukemia (AML) (orphan); investigational (orphan) for pediatric use* [idarubicin HCl] 1 mg/mL

idarubicin (IDR) INN, BAN *anthracycline antibiotic antineoplastic* [also: idarubicin HCl]

idarubicin HCl USAN, INN *anthracycline antibiotic antineoplastic for acute myeloid leukemia (AML) (orphan); investigational (orphan) for pediatric use* [also: idarubicin] 1 mg/mL injection

idaverine INN

idazoxan INN, BAN

idebenone INN, JAN *investigational treatment for Alzheimer disease*

idenast INN

Identi-Dose (trademarked dosage form) *unit dose package*

idoxifene USAN *antihormone antineoplastic; osteoporosis treatment; estrogen receptor antagonist for hormone replacement therapy*

idoxuridine (IDU) USAN, USP, INN, BAN, JAN *ophthalmic antiviral; investigational (orphan) for nonparenchymatous sarcomas*

IDR (idarubicin) [q.v.]

idralfidine INN

idremcinal USAN, INN *motilin agonist to stimulate gastrointestinal motility*

idrobutamine [see: butidrine]

idrocilamide INN

idropranolol INN

IDU (idoxuridine) [q.v.]

iduronidase [now: laronidase]

IE (ifosfamide [with mesna rescue], etoposide) *chemotherapy protocol for soft tissue sarcoma*

ifenprodil INN

ifetroban USAN *antithrombotic; anti-ischemic; antivasospastic*

ifetroban sodium USAN *antithrombotic; anti-ischemic; antivasospastic*

Ifex powder for IV injection ℞ *nitrogen mustard-type alkylating antineo-*

*plastic for testicular cancer (orphan);
investigational (orphan) for bone and
soft tissue sarcomas* [ifosfamide] 1, 3 g

IFN (interferon) [q.v.]

IFN-alpha 2 (interferon alfa-2) [see:
interferon alfa-2b, recombinant]

ifosfamide USAN, USP, INN, BAN *nitrogen mustard-type alkylating antineoplastic for testicular cancer (orphan);
investigational (orphan) for bone and
soft tissue sarcomas* 1, 3 g injection

**IfoVP (ifosfamide [with mesna res-
cue], VePesid)** *chemotherapy protocol for osteosarcoma*

ifoxetine INN

IG (immune globulin) [see: globulin,
immune]

IgE pentapeptide [see: pentigetide]

Igel 56 *hydrophilic contact lens material*
[hefilcon C]

IGF-1 (insulin-like growth factor-1)
[now: mecasermin]

IgG1 [see: immunoglobulin G1]

**IGIM (immune globulin intramus-
cular)** [see: globulin, immune]

**IGIV (immune globulin intrave-
nous)** [see: globulin, immune]

igmesine HCl USAN *sigma receptor lig-
and antidepressant*

IL-1, IL-2, etc. [see: interleukin-1,
interleukin-2, etc.]

IL-2 (interleukin-2) [see: aldesleukin;
teceleukin; celmoleukin]

ilepcimide USAN, INN *anticonvulsant;
investigational (orphan) for drug-resis-
tant generalized tonic-clonic epilepsy*

Iletin (U.S. products) [see under: Regular, NPH, and Lente]

Iletin Ⓒᴬᴺ subcu injection (discontinued 2001) OTC *antidiabetic* [insulin
(beef-pork)] 100 U/mL

Iletin Ⓒᴬᴺ subcu injection (discontinued 2001) OTC *antidiabetic* [insulin
zinc (beef-pork)] 100 U/mL

Iletin NPH Ⓒᴬᴺ subcu injection (discontinued 2001) OTC *antidiabetic*
[insulin (beef-pork)] 100 U/mL

Iletin II NPH Ⓒᴬᴺ subcu injection OTC
antidiabetic [insulin (pork)] 100 U/mL

Iletin II Pork Lente Ⓒᴬᴺ subcu injection OTC *antidiabetic* [insulin zinc
(pork)] 100 U/mL

Iletin II Pork NPH Ⓒᴬᴺ subcu injection OTC *antidiabetic* [insulin (pork)]
100 U/mL

Iletin II Pork Regular Ⓒᴬᴺ subcu
injection OTC *antidiabetic* [insulin
(pork)] 100 U/mL

Ilex aquifolium; I. opaca; I. vomitoria
medicinal herb [see: holly]

Ilex paraguariensis *medicinal herb* [see:
yerba maté]

Ilex verticillata *medicinal herb* [see:
winterberry]

Illicium anisatum; I. verum *medicinal
herb* [see: star anise]

ilmofosine USAN, INN *antineoplastic*

ilodecakin USAN, INN *interleukin 10,
human clone; immunomodulator for
Crohn disease, ulcerative colitis, rheumatoid arthritis (RA), and psoriasis*

ilomastat USAN *matrix metalloproteinase
(MMP) inhibitor for corneal ulcers,
inflammation, and cancers*

ilonidap USAN, INN *anti-inflammatory*

Ilopan IM injection, IV infusion ℞
postoperative ileus prophylactic [dex-
panthenol] 250 mg/mL

Ilopan-Choline tablets (discontinued
2002) ℞ *antiflatulent for splenic flex-
ure syndrome* [dexpanthenol; choline
bitartrate] 50•25 mg

iloperidone USAN, INN *investigational
(Phase III) selective serotonin and
dopamine antagonist for schizophrenia*

iloprost INN, BAN *prostacyclin analogue;
inhalation treatment for pulmonary
arterial hypertension (PAH) (orphan);
also used intravenously for systemic
sclerosis with Raynaud phenomenon*

Ilosone tablets, Pulvules (capsules),
oral suspension (discontinued 2005)
℞ *macrolide antibiotic* [erythromycin
estolate] 500 mg; 250 mg; 125, 250
mg/5 mL ⚑ inosine

Ilotycin ophthalmic ointment ℞ *antibiotic* [erythromycin] 0.5%

Ilotycin Gluceptate IV injection ℞ *macrolide antibiotic* [erythromycin gluceptate] 1 g/vial

Ilozyme tablets (discontinued 2002) ℞ *digestive enzymes* [lipase; protease; amylase] 11 000•30 000•30 000 USP units

I-L-X elixir OTC *hematinic* [ferrous gluconate; liver concentrate 1:20; multiple B vitamins] 70•98• ± mg/15 mL

I-L-X B₁₂ caplets OTC *hematinic* [carbonyl iron; desiccated liver; multiple B vitamins; ascorbic acid] 37.5• 130• ± •120 mg

I-L-X B₁₂ elixir OTC *hematinic* [ferric ammonium citrate; liver fraction 1; multiple B vitamins] 102•98• ± mg/15 mL

imafen INN *antidepressant* [also: imafen HCl]

imafen HCl USAN *antidepressant* [also: imafen]

Imager ac rectal suspension ℞ *radiopaque contrast medium for gastrointestinal imaging* [barium sulfate] 100%

imanixil INN

imatinib mesylate USAN *antineoplastic for chronic myeloid leukemia (CML) (orphan) and gastrointestinal stromal tumors (GIST)*

imazodan INN *cardiotonic* [also: imazodan HCl]

imazodan HCl USAN *cardiotonic* [also: imazodan]

imcarbofos USAN, INN *veterinary anthelmintic*

imciromab INN *antimyosin monoclonal antibody* [also: imciromab pentetate]

imciromab pentetate USAN, BAN *antimyosin monoclonal antibody; investigational (orphan) diagnostic aid for myocarditis and cardiac transplant rejection* [also: imciromab]

Imdur extended-release tablets ℞ *antianginal; vasodilator* [isosorbide mononitrate] 30, 60, 120 mg

imexon INN *investigational (orphan) for multiple myeloma*

IMF (ifosfamide [with mesna rescue], methotrexate, fluorouracil) *chemotherapy protocol*

imiclopazine INN

imidapril INN, BAN

imidazole carboxamide [see: dacarbazine]

imidazole salicylate INN

imidecyl iodine USAN *topical anti-infective*

imidocarb INN, BAN *antiprotozoal (Babesia)* [also: imidocarb HCl]

imidocarb HCl USAN *antiprotozoal (Babesia)* [also: imidocarb]

imidoline INN *antipsychotic* [also: imidoline HCl]

imidoline HCl USAN *antipsychotic* [also: imidoline]

imidurea NF *antimicrobial*

imiglucerase USAN, INN *glucocerebrosidase enzyme replacement for types I, II, and III Gaucher disease (orphan)*

Imigran (foreign name for U.S. product Imitrex)

imiloxan INN *antidepressant* [also: imiloxan HCl]

imiloxan HCl USAN *antidepressant* [also: imiloxan]

iminophenimide INN

iminostilbene [see: carbamazepine]

imipemide [now: imipenem]

imipenem USAN, USP, INN, BAN, JAN *carbapenem antibiotic*

imipramine INN, BAN *tricyclic antidepressant* [also: imipramine HCl] ⑦ Imferon; Norpramin; trimipramine

imipramine HCl USP *tricyclic antidepressant; treatment for childhood enuresis* [also: imipramine] 10, 25, 50 mg oral ⑦ Imferon; Norpramin; trimipramine

imipramine pamoate *tricyclic antidepressant* ⑦ Imferon; Norpramin; trimipramine

imipraminoxide INN

imiquimod USAN, INN *topical immunomodulator for external genital and perianal warts (condylomata acuminata), actinic keratoses, and superficial basal cell carcinoma (sBCC)*

imirestat INN

Imitrex film-coated tablets ℞ *vascular serotonin 5-HT₁ receptor agonist for the acute treatment of migraine headaches* [sumatriptan succinate] 25, 50, 100 mg

Imitrex nasal spray ℞ *vascular serotonin 5-HT₁ receptor agonist for the acute treatment of migraine headaches* [sumatriptan] 5, 20 mg/dose

Imitrex subcu injection in vials, prefilled syringes, or STATdose self-injector kits (two prefilled syringes) ℞ *vascular serotonin 5-HT₁ receptor agonist for the acute treatment of migraine and cluster headaches* [sumatriptan succinate] 6 mg/0.5 mL dose

ImmTher ℞ *investigational (orphan) immunostimulant for pulmonary and hepatic metastases of colorectal adenocarcinoma* [disaccharide tripeptide glycerol dipalmitoyl]

ImmuCyst ⓒ powder for intravesical instillation ℞ *antineoplastic for urinary bladder cancer* [BCG vaccine, live] 81 mg

Immun-Aid powder OTC *enteral nutritional therapy for immunocompromised patients*

immune globulin (IG) [see: globulin, immune]

immune globulin intramuscular [see: globulin, immune]

immune globulin intravenous (IGIV) [see: globulin, immune]

immune globulin intravenous pentetate USAN *radiodiagnostic imaging agent for inflammation and infection* [also: indium In 111 IGIV pentetate]

immune serum globulin (ISG) [see: globulin, immune]

Immunex CRP test kit for professional use *in vitro diagnostic aid for C-reactive protein (CRP) in blood to diagnose inflammatory conditions* [latex agglutination test]

Immuno-C ℞ *investigational (Phase II, orphan) treatment of cryptosporidiosis-induced diarrhea in immunocompromised patients* [*Cryptosporidium parvum* bovine colostrum IgG concentrate]

Immunocal powder for oral solution OTC *enteral nutritional therapy* [milk-based formula] 10 g/pkt.

ImmunoCAP Specific IgE blood test kit for professional use *in vitro diagnostic aid for IgE detection* [316 different allergens]

immunoglobulin G1 (mouse monoclonal 7E11-C5.3 antihuman prostatic carcinoma cell) disulfide [see: capromab pendetide]

immunoglobulin G1 (mouse monoclonal ZCE025 antihuman antigen CEA) disulfide [see: indium In 111 altumomab pentetate; altumomab]

immunoglobulin G2 (human-mouse monoclonal HuM291 anti-CD3 antigen) disulfide [now: visilizumab]

immunosuppressants *a class of drugs used to suppress the immune response, used primarily after organ transplantation surgery*

Imodium capsules ℞ *antidiarrheal* [loperamide HCl] 2 mg

Imodium ⓒ quick-dissolving lingual tablets OTC *antidiarrheal* [loperamide HCl] 2 mg

Imodium A-D caplets, oral liquid OTC *antidiarrheal* [loperamide HCl] 1 mg; 1 mg/5 mL

Imodium Advanced ⓒ chewable tablets OTC *antidiarrheal; antiflatulent* [loperamide HCl; simethicone] 2 • 125 mg

Imogam IM injection (discontinued 2001; replaced by Imogam Rabies-HT) ℞ *passive immunizing agent for rabies prophylaxis and treatment* [rabies immune globulin] 150 IU/mL

Imogam Rabies-HT IM injection ℞ *passive immunizing agent for use after rabies exposure* [rabies immune globulin, heat treated] 150 IU/mL

imolamine INN, BAN

Imovane ⓒ tablets ℞ *sedative; hypnotic* [zopiclone] 7.5 mg

Imovax intradermal (ID) injection, IM injection ℞ *rabies prophylaxis*

[rabies vaccine (HDCV)] 0.25 IU/
0.1 mL; 2.5 IU/mL

imoxiterol INN

impacarzine INN

Impact ready-to-use oral liquid OTC
enteral nutritional therapy [lactose-free
formula]

Impact Rubella slide test for professional use *in vitro diagnostic aid for
detection of rubella virus antibodies in
serum* [latex agglutination test]

*Impatiens balsamina; I. biflora; I.
capensis medicinal herb* [see: jewel-
weed]

IMPE [see: etipirium iodide]

impromidine INN, BAN *gastric secretion
indicator* [also: impromidine HCl]

impromidine HCl USAN *gastric secretion indicator* [also: impromidine]

improsulfan INN

Improved Analgesic ointment OTC
analgesic; counterirritant [methyl salicylate; menthol] 18.3%•16%

Improved Congestant tablets (discontinued 2002) OTC *antihistamine;
analgesic* [chlorpheniramine maleate;
acetaminophen] 2•325 mg

imuracetam INN

Imuran IV injection ℞ *immunosuppressant for organ transplantation
(orphan) and rheumatoid arthritis* [aza-
thioprine sodium] 100 mg ⊅
Enduron; Imferon

Imuran tablets ℞ *immunosuppressant for
organ transplantation (orphan) and rheumatoid arthritis* [azathioprine] 50 mg

Imuthiol ℞ *investigational (Phase II/III,
orphan) immunomodulator for HIV
and AIDS* [diethyldithiocarbamate]

¹¹¹In [see: indium In 111 altumomab
pentetate]

¹¹¹In [see: indium In 111 imciromab
pentetate]

¹¹¹In [see: indium In 111 murine anti-
CEA monoclonal antibody]

¹¹¹In [see: indium In 111 murine monoclonal antibody]

¹¹¹In [see: indium In 111 oxyquinoline]

¹¹¹In [see: indium In 111 pentetate]

¹¹¹In [see: indium In 111 pentetreo-
tide]

¹¹¹In [see: indium In 111 satumomab
pendetide]

¹¹¹In [see: pentetate indium disodium
In 111]

¹¹³ᵐIn [see: indium chlorides In 113m]

inactivated mumps vaccine [see:
mumps virus vaccine, inactivated]

**inactivated poliomyelitis vaccine
(IPV)** [see: poliovirus vaccine, inac-
tivated]

inactivated poliovirus vaccine (IPV)
[see: poliovirus vaccine, inactivated]

inamrinone USAN *cardiotonic* [also:
amrinone]

inamrinone lactate *vasodilator for
congestive heart failure* [previously
known as amrinone lactate; name
changed 2000]

inaperisone INN

Inapsine IV or IM injection ℞ *general
anesthetic; antiemetic* [droperidol] 2.5
mg/mL

incretin mimetic agents *a class of
antidiabetic drugs that improve the
body's normal glucose-sensing mecha-
nisms by activating the glucagon-like
peptide-1 (GLP-1) receptors*

indacrinic acid [see: indacrinone]

indacrinone USAN, INN *antihypertensive; diuretic*

indalpine INN, BAN

indanazoline INN

indanediones *a class of anticoagulants
that interfere with vitamin K–depen-
dent clotting factors*

indanidine INN

indanorex INN

indapamide USAN, INN, BAN *antihypertensive; diuretic* 1.25, 2.5 mg oral

indatraline INN

indecainide INN *antiarrhythmic* [also:
indecainide HCl]

indecainide HCl USAN *antiarrhythmic*
[also: indecainide]

indeloxazine INN *antidepressant* [also:
indeloxazine HCl]

indeloxazine HCl USAN *antidepressant*
[also: indeloxazine]

indenolol INN, BAN

Inderal tablets, IV injection ℞ *antianginal; antiarrhythmic; antihypertensive; antiadrenergic (β-blocker); migraine preventative* [propranolol HCl] 10, 20, 40, 60, 80 mg; 1 mg/mL ⑨ Enduron; Enduronyl; Inderide

Inderal LA long-acting capsules ℞ *antianginal; antihypertensive; antiadrenergic (β-blocker); migraine preventative* [propranolol HCl] 60, 80, 120, 160 mg

Inderide 40/25; Inderide 80/25 tablets ℞ *antihypertensive; β-blocker; diuretic* [propranolol HCl; hydrochlorothiazide] 40•25 mg; 80•25 mg ⑨ Inderal

Inderide LA 80/50; Inderide LA 120/50; Inderide LA 160/50 long-acting capsules (discontinued 2004) ℞ *antihypertensive; β-blocker; diuretic* [propranolol HCl; hydrochlorothiazide] 80•50 mg; 120•50 mg; 160•50 mg

Indian apple *medicinal herb* [see: mandrake]

Indian arrow; Indian arrow wood *medicinal herb* [see: wahoo]

Indian bark *medicinal herb* [see: magnolia]

Indian bay *medicinal herb* [see: laurel]

Indian corn (Zea mays) styles (silk) *medicinal herb used as an analgesic, diuretic, demulcent, and litholytic*

Indian cress (Tropaeolum majus) flowers, leaves, and seeds *medicinal herb used as an antiseptic and expectorant*

Indian elm *medicinal herb* [see: slippery elm]

Indian frankincense *medicinal herb* [see: frankincense]

Indian hemp *medicinal herb* [see: marijuana]

Indian hyssop *medicinal herb* [see: blue vervain]

Indian paint, red *medicinal herb* [see: bloodroot]

Indian paint, yellow *medicinal herb* [see: goldenseal]

Indian pipe *medicinal herb* [see: fit root]

Indian plant *medicinal herb* [see: bloodroot; goldenseal]

Indian poke (Veratrum viride) *medicinal herb* [see: hellebore]

Indian root *medicinal herb* [see: spikenard; wahoo]

Indian shamrock *medicinal herb* [see: birthroot]

Indian tobacco *medicinal herb* [see: lobelia]

Indiana protocol *chemotherapy protocol for ovarian cancer* [see: PAC-I]

indigo (Indigofera spp.) plant *medicinal herb for fever, hemorrhoids, inducing emesis, inflammation, liver cleansing, ovarian and stomach cancer, pain, scorpion bites, and worms; not generally regarded as safe and effective*

indigo, wild *medicinal herb* [see: wild indigo]

indigo carmine BAN *cystoscopy aid* [also: indigotindisulfonate sodium]

indigotindisulfonate sodium USP *cystoscopy aid* [also: indigo carmine]

indinavir USAN *antiviral; HIV-1 protease inhibitor*

indinavir sulfate USAN *antiviral; HIV-1 protease inhibitor*

indium *element (In)*

indium (^{111}In) diethylenetriamine pentaacetate JAN *radionuclide cisternography aid; radioactive agent* [also: indium In 111 pentetate]

indium chlorides In 113m USAN, USP *radioactive agent*

indium In 111 altumomab pentetate USAN *radiodiagnostic monoclonal antibody for colorectal carcinoma; anticarcinoembryonic antigen* [also: altumomab]

indium In 111 antimelanoma antibody XMMME-0001-DTPA [see: antimelanoma antibody]

indium In 111 CYT-103 [now: indium In 111 satumomab pendetide]

indium In 111 ibritumomab tiuxetan *radioimmunotherapy for non-Hodgkin B-cell lymphoma*

indium In 111 IGIV pentetate *radiodiagnostic imaging agent for inflamma-*

tion and infection [also: immune globulin intravenous pentetate]

indium In 111 imciromab pentetate *radioactive diagnostic aid for cardiac imaging*

indium In 111 murine monoclonal antibodies (2B8-MXDTPA) & yttrium Y 90 murine MAb (2B8-MXDTPA) *investigational (orphan) for non-Hodgkin B-cell lymphoma*

indium In 111 murine monoclonal antibodies (MAb) Fab to myosin [now: imciromab pentetate]

indium In 111 oxyquinoline USAN, USP *radioactive agent; diagnostic aid*

indium In 111 pentetate USP *radionuclide cisternography aid; radioactive agent* [also: indium (^{111}In) diethylenetriamine pentaacetate]

indium In 111 pentetreotide USAN *radioactive imaging agent for SPECT scans of neuroendocrine tumors; investigational (orphan) radiotherapeutic agent for somatostatin receptor–positive neuroendocrine tumors*

indium In 111 satumomab pendetide USAN *radiodiagnostic imaging aid for ovarian (orphan) and colorectal carcinoma* [also: satumomab]

indobufen INN

indocate INN

Indocin capsules, oral suspension, suppositories ℞ *antiarthritic; nonsteroidal anti-inflammatory drug (NSAID) for ankylosing spondylitis and acute bursitis/tendinitis* [indomethacin] 25, 50 mg; 25 mg/5 mL; 50 mg �ⓔ Lincocin; Minocin

Indocin I.V. powder for IV injection ℞ *prostaglandin synthesis inhibitor for neonatal closure of patent ductus arteriosus* [indomethacin sodium trihydrate] 1 mg

Indocin SR sustained-release capsules ℞ *antiarthritic; nonsteroidal anti-inflammatory drug (NSAID) for ankylosing spondylitis and acute bursitis/tendinitis* [indomethacin] 75 mg

indocyanine green USP, JAN *in vivo diagnostic aid for cardiac output, hepatic function, and ophthalmic angiography*

indolapril INN *antihypertensive* [also: indolapril HCl]

indolapril HCl USAN *antihypertensive* [also: indolapril]

indole 3-carbinol *natural phytochemical found in cruciferous vegetables; antioxidant and estrogen blocker shown effective against hormone-related cancers of the prostate, the uterus, and especially the breast; restores the p21 tumor suppressor gene*

indolidan USAN, INN, BAN *cardiotonic*

indolones *a class of dopamine receptor antagonists with conventional (typical) antipsychotic activity* [also called: dihydroindolones]

indometacin INN, JAN *antiarthritic; nonsteroidal anti-inflammatory drug (NSAID)* [also: indomethacin]

indometacin farnecil JAN *antiarthritic; nonsteroidal anti-inflammatory drug (NSAID)* [also: indomethacin]

indomethacin USAN, USP, BAN *antiarthritic; nonsteroidal anti-inflammatory drug (NSAID) for ankylosing spondylitis and acute bursitis/tendinitis* [also: indometacin; indometacin farnecil] 25, 50, 75 mg oral

indomethacin sodium USAN *anti-inflammatory*

indomethacin sodium trihydrate *neonatal closure of patent ductus arteriosus*

indopanolol INN

indopine INN

indoprofen USAN, INN, BAN *analgesic; anti-inflammatory*

indoramin USAN, INN, BAN *antihypertensive*

indoramin HCl USAN, BAN *antihypertensive*

indorenate INN *antihypertensive* [also: indorenate HCl]

indorenate HCl USAN *antihypertensive* [also: indorenate]

indoxole USAN, INN *antipyretic; anti-inflammatory*

indriline INN *CNS stimulant* [also: indriline HCl]

indriline HCl USAN *CNS stimulant* [also: indriline]

inductin [see: diphoxazide]

Infalyte oral solution OTC *electrolyte replacement* [sodium, potassium, and chloride electrolytes]

Infanrix IM injection ℞ *active immunizing agent for diphtheria, tetanus, and pertussis* [diphtheria & tetanus toxoids & acellular pertussis (DTaP) vaccine, adsorbed] 25 Lf•10 Lf•25 μg per 0.5 mL dose

Infantaire oral drops OTC *analgesic; antipyretic* [acetaminophen] 80 mg/0.8 mL

Infasurf intratracheal suspension ℞ *agent for prophylaxis and treatment of respiratory distress syndrome (RDS) in premature infants (orphan)* [calfactant] 6 mL

Infatab (trademarked dosage form) *pediatric chewable tablet*

INFeD IV or IM injection ℞ *hematinic* [iron dextran] 100 mg Fe/dose ② NSAID

Infergen subcu injection ℞ *consensus interferon for the treatment of chronic hepatitis C virus (HCV) infections* [interferon alfacon-1] 9, 15 μg/0.3 mL dose

Inflamase Mild; Inflamase Forte eye drops ℞ *corticosteroidal anti-inflammatory* [prednisolone sodium phosphate] 0.125%; 1%

infliximab *anti-inflammatory; anti-TNFα (tumor necrosis factor alpha) monoclonal antibody for Crohn disease (orphan), rheumatoid and psoriatic arthritis, and ankylosing spondylitis; also used for psoriasis and juvenile arthritis*

influenza purified surface antigen [see: influenza split-virus vaccine]

influenza split-virus vaccine *subcategory of influenza virus vaccine*

influenza subvirion vaccine [see: influenza split-virus vaccine]

influenza virus vaccine USP *active immunizing agent for influenza* [see the Web update (spwb.com) for specific strains used in the 2005–2006 flu season]

influenza whole-virus vaccine *subcategory of influenza virus vaccine*

infraRUB cream (discontinued 2004) OTC *analgesic; counterirritant* [methyl salicylate; menthol] 35%•10%

Infumorph 200; Infumorph 500 concentrate for continuous microinfusion ℞ *narcotic analgesic; intraspinal microinfusion for intractable chronic pain (orphan)* [morphine sulfate] 10 mg/mL (200 mg/vial); 25 mg/mL (500 mg/vial)

Infurfer ⒸⒶⓃ IV or IM injection ℞ *hematinic* [iron dextran] 50 mg/mL

Infuvite Adult IV infusion ℞ *multivitamin adjunct for adults receiving parenteral nutrition* [multiple vitamins; folic acid; biotin] ±•600•60 μg

Infuvite Pediatric IV infusion ℞ *multivitamin adjunct for infants and children receiving parenteral nutrition* [multiple vitamins; folic acid; biotin] ±•140•20 μg

INGN-201 *investigational (Phase III) gene therapy for head and neck cancers* [also: adenoviral p53 gene; p53 adenoviral gene]

INH (isonicotinic acid hydrazide) [see: isoniazid]

Inhal-Aid (trademarked form) *portable inhalation device*

inhalants *a class of street drugs that include nitrous oxide, volatile nitrites, and petroleum distillates* [see: nitrous oxide; volatile nitrites; petroleum distillate inhalants]

InhibiZone surface treatment ℞ *prophylactic antibiotic treatment for penile prostheses before implantation* [minocycline; rifampin] 3–10•9–25 mg (depending on prosthesis size)

inicarone INN

Inject-all (trademarked delivery system) *prefilled disposable syringe*

Inlay-Tabs (trademarked dosage form) *tablets with contrasting inlay*

InnoGel Plus gel packs + comb (discontinued 2003) OTC *pediculicide for lice* [pyrethrins; piperonyl butoxide technical] 0.3%•3%

Innohep deep subcu injection ℞ *anticoagulant/antithrombotic for prevention of* deep vein thrombosis (DVT) [tinzaparin sodium] 20 000 IU anti–factor Xa/mL

InnoLet prefilled disposable syringe OTC *device for self-administration of insulin* (available prefilled with Novolin 70/30 or Novolin N) [insulin] 1–40 U/injection

InnoPran XL long-acting capsules ℞ *antihypertensive; antiadrenergic (β-blocker)* [propranolol HCl] 80, 100 mg

Innovar injection (discontinued 2001) ℞ *narcotic analgesic; major tranquilizer* [fentanyl citrate; droperidol] 0.05•2.5 mg/mL

inocoterone INN *anti-acne* [also: inocoterone acetate]

inocoterone acetate USAN *anti-acne* [also: inocoterone]

INOmax inhalation gas ℞ *for neonatal hypoxic respiratory failure due to persistent pulmonary hypertension (orphan); investigational (orphan) for acute adult respiratory distress syndrome (ARDS)* [nitric oxide] 100, 800 ppm

inosine INN, JAN 🔲 Ilosone

inosine pranobex BAN, JAN *investigational antiviral/immunomodulator for AIDS; investigational (orphan) for subacute sclerosing panencephalitis*

inosiplex [now: inosine pranobex]

Inositech capsules OTC *vitamin B supplement* [inositol] 324 mg

inositol NF *dietary lipotropic supplement* 250, 500, 650 mg oral

inositol niacinate USAN *peripheral vasodilator* [also: inositol nicotinate]

inositol nicotinate INN, BAN *peripheral vasodilator* [also: inositol niacinate]

inotropes *a class of drugs that affect the force or energy of muscle contractions*

inprochone [see: inproquone]

inproquone INN, BAN

INSH (isonicotinoyl-salicylidene-hydrazine) [see: salinazid]

InspirEase (trademarked form) *portable inhalation device*

Inspra film-coated tablets ℞ *aldosterone receptor antagonist for hypertension and congestive heart failure (CHF);*

improves survival after a cardiovascular event [eplerenone] 25, 50 mg

Insta-Glucose gel OTC *glucose elevating agent* [glucose] 40%

insulin USP, JAN *antidiabetic* 🔲 inulin

insulin, biphasic INN, BAN *antidiabetic*

insulin, biphasic isophane BAN *antidiabetic*

insulin, dalanated USAN, INN *antidiabetic*

insulin, globin zinc USP [also: globin zinc insulin]

insulin, isophane USP, BAN, INN, JAN *antidiabetic*

insulin, neutral USAN, JAN *antidiabetic* [also: neutral insulin]

insulin, NPH (neutral protamine Hagedorn) [see: insulin, isophane]

insulin, protamine zinc (PZI) USP *antidiabetic* [also: insulin zinc protamine; protamine zinc insulin]

insulin argine INN *antidiabetic*

insulin aspart USAN, INN *antidiabetic; rapid-acting insulin analogue*

insulin aspart protamine *antidiabetic; intermediate-acting insulin analogue*

insulin defalan INN *antidiabetic*

insulin detemir USAN *antidiabetic; long-acting insulin formulation intended to provide continuous basal insulin levels through once- or twice-daily subcu injections*

insulin glargine INN *antidiabetic; long-acting, once-daily basal insulin analogue*

insulin glulisine *antidiabetic; rapid-onset, short-acting insulin analogue*

insulin human USAN, USP, INN, BAN, JAN *antidiabetic*

insulin human, isophane USP *antidiabetic*

insulin human zinc USP *antidiabetic*

insulin human zinc, extended USP *antidiabetic*

insulin I 125 USAN *radioactive agent*

insulin I 131 USAN *radioactive agent*

insulin lispro USAN, INN, BAN *antidiabetic*

insulin lispro protamine *antidiabetic*

Insulin Reaction gel OTC *glucose elevating agent* [glucose] 40%

insulin zinc USP, INN, BAN, JAN *antidiabetic*

insulin zinc, extended USP *antidiabetic* [also: insulin zinc suspension (crystalline)]

insulin zinc, prompt USP *antidiabetic* [also: insulin zinc suspension (amorphous)]

insulin zinc protamine JAN *antidiabetic* [also: insulin, protamine zinc; protamine zinc insulin]

insulin zinc suspension (amorphous) INN, BAN, JAN *antidiabetic* [also: insulin zinc, prompt]

insulin zinc suspension (crystalline) INN, BAN, JAN *antidiabetic* [also: insulin zinc, extended]

insulin-like growth factor-1, recombinant human (rhIGF-1) [now: mecasermin]

Insuman subcu injection OTC *investigational (Phase III) antidiabetic* [human insulin (rDNA)]

Intal solution for nebulization, aerosol spray ℞ *anti-inflammatory; mast cell stabilizer for prophylactic treatment of allergy, asthma, and bronchospasm* [cromolyn sodium] 20 mg/2 mL ampule; 800 μg/dose ▣ Endal

Integrilin IV injection ℞ *GP IIb/IIIa platelet aggregation inhibitor for acute coronary syndrome, unstable angina, myocardial infarction, and cardiac surgery* [eptifibatide] 0.75, 2 mg/mL

Intensol (trademarked form) *concentrated oral solution*

α-2-interferon [see: interferon alfa-2b, recombinant]

interferon, fibroblast [now: interferon beta]

interferon, leukocyte [now: interferon alfa-n3]

interferon α2b [see: interferon alfa-2b]

interferon αA [see: interferon alfa-2a]

interferon alfa JAN *investigational (Phase III) oral treatment for Sjögren syndrome; investigational (Phase II) for AIDS-related xerostomia; investigational (orphan) for oral human papillo-* mavirus (HPV) warts in HIV-infected patients

interferon alfa (BALL-1) JAN

interferon alfa-2 & interleukin-2 (aldesleukin) *chemotherapy protocol for renal cell carcinoma*

interferon alfa-2a (IFN-αA; rIFN-A) USAN, INN, BAN, JAN *antineoplastic/antiviral for hairy cell leukemia, hepatitis C, Kaposi sarcoma (orphan), and chronic myelogenous leukemia (orphan); investigational (orphan) for renal cell carcinoma*

interferon alfa-2a & fluorouracil *investigational (orphan) for esophageal carcinoma and advanced colorectal cancer*

interferon alfa-2a & teceleukin *investigational (orphan) for metastatic renal cell carcinoma and metastatic malignant melanoma*

interferon alfa-2b (IFN-α2) USAN, INN, BAN *antineoplastic for hairy-cell leukemia, malignant melanoma, AIDS-related Kaposi sarcoma (orphan), and various other cancers; antiviral for condylomata acuminata and chronic hepatitis B and C; investigational (Phase I/II) cytokine for AIDS*

interferon alfacon-1 USAN *bioengineered consensus interferon for the treatment of chronic hepatitis C virus (HCV) infections*

interferon alfa-n1 USAN, INN, BAN *antineoplastic; biological response modifier for chronic hepatitis C (orphan); investigational (Phase III) cytokine for HIV; investigational (orphan) for human papillomavirus in severe respiratory papillomatosis*

interferon alfa-n3 USAN *immunomodulator and antiviral for condylomata acuminata; investigational (Phase III) cytokine for HIV, AIDS, ARC, and hepatitis C*

interferon beta (IFN-B) BAN, JAN *antineoplastic; antiviral; immunomodulator*

interferon beta-1a USAN *immunomodulator for relapsing multiple sclerosis (orphan); investigational (orphan) for* non-A, non-B hepatitis, Kaposi sarcoma, brain tumors, and various other cancers

interferon beta-1b USAN *immunomodulator for relapsing-remitting multiple sclerosis (orphan)*

interferon gamma-1a JAN

interferon gamma-1b USAN, INN, BAN *antineoplastic; antiviral; immunoregulator for chronic granulomatous disease (orphan) and severe congenital osteopetrosis (orphan); investigational (orphan) for renal cell carcinoma*

interferon gamma-2a [see: interferon gamma-1b]

α-interferons [see: interferon alfa-n1 and -n3]

Intergel irrigating solution ℞ *adhesion barrier for open gynecological and lower GI surgical procedures* [ferric hyaluronate] 0.5%

interleukin-1 beta *investigational antineoplastic for melanoma; investigational liposome-encapsulated formulation for influenza A*

interleukin-1 receptor antagonist, recombinant human [now: anakinra]

interleukin-2 (aldesleukin) & interferon alfa-2 *chemotherapy protocol for renal cell carcinoma*

interleukin-2, liposome-encapsulated recombinant *investigational (orphan) for brain, central nervous system, kidney, and pelvic cancers*

interleukin-2, recombinant (IL-2) [see: aldesleukin; teceleukin; celmoleukin]

interleukin-10 (IL-10) [see: ilodecakin]

interleukin-11, recombinant human (rhIL-11) *platelet growth factor for thrombocytopenia of chemotherapy or radiation (orphan)* [also: oprelvekin]

interleukin-12 (IL-12) [see: edodekin alfa]

intermedine INN

intoplicine INN *investigational (Phase I) antineoplastic and topoisomerase I and II inhibitor*

Intrachol ℞ *investigational (orphan) for choline deficiency of long-term parenteral nutrition* [choline chloride]

IntraDose injectable gel ℞ *investigational (NDA filed, orphan) alkylating antineoplastic for squamous cell carcinoma of the head and neck; investigational (orphan) for metastatic malignant melanoma* [cisplatin; epinephrine]

Intralipid 10%; Intralipid 20% IV infusion ℞ *nutritional therapy* [fat emulsion]

IntraSite gel OTC *wound dressing* [graft T starch copolymer] 2%

intravascular perfluorochemical emulsion *synthetic blood oxygen carrier for PTCA*

intravenous fat emulsion [see: fat emulsion, intravenous]

intravenous immunoglobulin (IVIG) *investigational IV solution of concentrated antibodies for AIDS*

intrazole USAN, INN *anti-inflammatory*

Intrinsa transdermal patch ℞ *investigational (Phase III) hormone replacement therapy for female sexual dysfunction (FSD) and hypoactive sexual desire disorder (HSDD) in women* [testosterone]

intrinsic factor concentrate *antianemic to enhance the body's utilization of vitamin B_{12}*

intriptyline INN *antidepressant* [also: intriptyline HCl]

intriptyline HCl USAN *antidepressant* [also: intriptyline]

Introlan Half-Strength oral liquid OTC *enteral nutritional therapy* [lactose-free formula]

Introlite oral liquid OTC *enteral nutritional therapy* [lactose-free formula]

Intron A subcu or IM injection ℞ *antineoplastic for hairy cell leukemia, malignant melanoma, Kaposi sarcoma (orphan), and various other cancers; antiviral for condylomata acuminata and chronic hepatitis B and C; investigational (Phase I/II) cytokine for AIDS* [interferon alfa-2b] 3, 5, 10, 18, 25, 50 million IU/vial

Intropaste oral paste ℞ *radiopaque contrast medium for esophageal imaging* [barium sulfate] 70%

Intropin IV injection (discontinued 2004) ℞ *vasopressor for cardiac, pulmonary, traumatic, septic, or renal shock* [dopamine HCl] 40, 80, 160 mg/mL ② Ditropan; Isoptin

Inula helenium *medicinal herb* [see: elecampane]

inulin USP *diagnostic aid for renal function* 100 mg/mL injection ② insulin

Invanz IV or IM injection ℞ *broad-spectrum carbapenem antibiotic* [ertapenem sodium] 1 g/vial

invenol [see: carbutamide]

Inversine tablets ℞ *antiadrenergic; ganglionic blocker for severe hypertension* [mecamylamine HCl] 2.5 mg

invert sugar [see: sugar, invert]

Invirase capsules ℞ *antiretroviral protease inhibitor for HIV* [saquinavir mesylate] 200 mg

Invirase tablets ℞ *antiretroviral protease inhibitor for HIV* [saquinavir mesylate] 500 mg

iobenguane (¹³¹I) INN *radioactive agent* [also: iobenguane I 131]

iobenguane I 123 USP *radioactive agent*

iobenguane I 131 USAN *radioactive agent* [also: iobenguane (¹³¹I)]

iobenguane sulfate I 123 USAN *radiopharmaceutical diagnostic aid for adrenomedullary disorders and neuroendocrine tumors*

iobenguane sulfate I 131 USAN *diagnostic aid for pheochromocytoma* (orphan)

iobenzamic acid USAN, INN, BAN *radiopaque contrast medium for cholecystography*

Iobid DM sustained-release tablets ℞ *antitussive; expectorant* [dextromethorphan hydrobromide; guaifenesin] 30•600 mg

iobutoic acid INN

iocanlidic acid I 123 USAN *cardiac diagnostic aid*

Iocare Balanced Salt ophthalmic solution OTC *intraocular irrigating solution* [sodium chloride (balanced saline solution)]

iocarmate meglumine USAN *radiopaque contrast medium* [also: meglumine iocarmate]

iocarmic acid USAN, INN, BAN *radiopaque contrast medium*

iocetamic acid USAN, USP, INN, BAN *oral radiopaque contrast medium for cholecystography* (62% iodine)

Iocon shampoo (discontinued 2003) OTC *antiseborrheic; antipsoriatic; antipruritic; antibacterial* [coal tar; alcohol]

Iodal HD oral liquid (discontinued 2002) ℞ *narcotic antitussive; decongestant; antihistamine* [hydrocodone bitartrate; phenylephrine HCl; chlorpheniramine maleate] 1.67•5•2 mg/5 mL

iodamide USAN, INN, BAN *radiopaque contrast medium*

iodamide meglumine USAN *radiopaque contrast medium*

iodecimol INN

iodecol [see: iodecimol]

iodetryl INN

Iodex; Iodex-P ointment OTC *broad-spectrum antimicrobial* [povidone-iodine] 4.7%; 10%

Iodex with Methyl Salicylate ointment OTC *analgesic; counterirritant; anti-infective* [methyl salicylate; iodine] 4.8%•4.7%

iodinated (¹²⁵I) human serum albumin INN *radioactive agent; blood volume test* [also: albumin, iodinated I 125 serum]

iodinated (¹³¹I) human serum albumin INN, JAN *radioactive agent; intrathecal imaging agent; blood volume test* [also: albumin, iodinated I 131 serum]

iodinated glycerol [see: glycerol, iodinated]

iodinated I 125 albumin [see: albumin, iodinated I 125]

iodinated I 131 aggregated albumin [see: albumin, iodinated I 131 aggregated]

iodinated I 131 albumin [see: albumin, iodinated I 131]

iodine USP *broad-spectrum topical anti-infective; element (I) 2% topical*

iodine I 123 murine monoclonal antibodies (MAb) to alpha-feto-protein (AFP) *investigational (orphan) diagnostic aid for AFP-producing tumors, hepatocellular carcinoma, and hepatoblastoma*

iodine I 123 murine monoclonal antibodies (MAb) to human chorionic gonadotropin (hCG) *investigational (orphan) diagnostic aid for hCG-producing tumors*

iodine I 131 6B-iodomethyl-19-norcholesterol *investigational (orphan) for adrenal cortical imaging*

iodine I 131 metaiodobenzylguanidine sulfate [now: iobenguane sulfate I 131]

iodine I 131 murine monoclonal antibodies (MAb) to alpha-feto-protein (AFP) *investigational (orphan) treatment for AFP-producing tumors, hepatocellular carcinoma, and hepatoblastoma*

iodine I 131 murine monoclonal antibodies (MAb) to human chorionic gonadotropin (hCG) *investigational (orphan) treatment for hCG-producing tumors*

iodine I 131 murine monoclonal antibodies (MAb) IgG$_2$a to B cell5 *investigational (orphan) for B-cell leukemia and lymphoma*

iodine I 131 radiolabeled B1 monoclonal antibodies (MAb) *investigational (orphan) for non-Hodgkin B-cell lymphoma*

iodine I 131 tositumomab *radiotherapy for non-Hodgkin lymphoma (NHL); radiotherapeutic agent bound to NHL monoclonal antibody for targeted delivery of radiation* [see also: tositumomab]

iodipamide USP, BAN *parenteral radiopaque contrast medium* [also: adipiodone]

iodipamide meglumine USP, BAN *parenteral radiopaque contrast medium*

(49.42% iodine) [also: adipiodone meglumine]

iodipamide methylglucamine [see: iodipamide meglumine]

iodipamide sodium USP *parenteral radiopaque contrast medium*

iodipamide sodium I 131 USAN *radioactive agent*

iodisan [see: prolonium iodide]

iodixanol USAN, INN, BAN *parenteral radiopaque contrast medium (49.1% iodine)*

iodized oil NF

iodoalphionic acid NF [also: pheniodol sodium]

iodoantipyrine I 131 USAN *radioactive agent*

iodobehenate calcium NF

m-iodobenzylguanidine sulfate I 123 [see: iobenguane sulfate I 123]

iodocetylic acid (^{123}I) INN *diagnostic aid* [also: iodocetylic acid I 123]

iodocetylic acid I 123 USAN *diagnostic aid* [also: iodocetylic acid (^{123}I)]

iodochlorhydroxyquin [now: clioquinol]

iodocholesterol (^{131}I) INN *radioactive agent* [also: iodocholesterol I 131]

iodocholesterol I 131 USAN *radioactive agent* [also: iodocholesterol (^{131}I)]

iodoform NF

iodohippurate sodium I 123 USAN, USP *renal function test; radioactive agent*

iodohippurate sodium I 125 USAN *radioactive agent*

iodohippurate sodium I 131 USAN, USP *renal function test; radioactive agent* [also: sodium iodohippurate (^{131}I)]

iodohydroxyquin [see: clioquinol]

iodol USP

iodomethamate sodium NF

iodopanoic acid [see: iopanoic acid]

Iodopen IV injection R iodine supplement [sodium iodide (85% elemental iodine)] 118 μg/mL (100 μg I/mL)

iodophthalein, soluble [now: iodophthalein sodium]

iodophthalein sodium NF, INN

iodopyracet NF [also: diodone]

Iodoral

iodopyracet I 125 USAN *radioactive agent*

iodopyracet I 131 USAN *radioactive agent*

iodoquinol USAN, USP *antimicrobial; amebicide for intestinal amebiasis* [also: diiodohydroxyquinoline]

iodoquinol & hydrocortisone *amebicide; antimicrobial; corticosteroidal anti-inflammatory* 1%•1% topical

Iodosorb Ⓒᴬᴺ paste, ointment OTC *antibacterial; antiulcerative wound dressing* [cadexomer iodine] 0.9%

iodothiouracil INN, BAN

iodothymol [see: thymol iodide]

Iodotope capsules, oral solution ℞ *radioactive agent for hyperthyroidism and thyroid carcinoma* [sodium iodide I 131] 1–50 mCi; 7.05 mCi/mL

iodoxamate meglumine USAN, BAN *radiopaque contrast medium*

iodoxamic acid USAN, INN, BAN *radiopaque contrast medium*

iodoxyl [see: iodomethamate sodium]

Iofed extended-release capsules (discontinued 2002) ℞ *decongestant; antihistamine* [pseudoephedrine HCl; brompheniramine maleate] 120•12 mg

Iofed PD extended-release capsules (discontinued 2002) ℞ *pediatric decongestant and antihistamine* [pseudoephedrine HCl; brompheniramine maleate] 60•6 mg

iofendylate INN *radiopaque contrast medium* [also: iophendylate]

iofetamine (^{123}I) INN *diagnostic aid; radioactive agent* [also: iofetamine HCl I 123]

iofetamine HCl I 123 USAN *diagnostic aid; radioactive agent* [also: iofetamine (^{123}I)]

Iofoam (trademarked form) *foaming skin cleanser*

ioglicic acid USAN, INN, BAN *radiopaque contrast medium*

ioglucol USAN, INN *radiopaque contrast medium*

ioglucomide USAN, INN *radiopaque contrast medium*

ioglunide INN

ioglycamic acid USAN, INN, BAN *radiopaque contrast medium for cholecystography*

iogulamide USAN *radiopaque contrast medium*

iohexol USAN, INN, BAN *parenteral radiopaque contrast medium* (46.36% iodine)

Iohist D elixir (discontinued 2002) ℞ *decongestant; antihistamine* [phenylpropanolamine HCl; phenyltoloxamine citrate; pyrilamine maleate; pheniramine maleate] 25•4•4•4 mg/5 mL

Iohist DM syrup (discontinued 2002) ℞ *antitussive; decongestant; antihistamine* [dextromethorphan hydrobromide; phenylpropanolamine HCl; brompheniramine maleate] 10•12.5•2 mg/5 mL

iolidonic acid INN

iolixanic acid INN

iomeglamic acid INN

iomeprol USAN, INN, BAN *radiopaque contrast medium*

iomethin I 125 USAN *neoplasm test; radioactive agent* [also: iometin (^{125}I)]

iomethin I 131 USAN *neoplasm test; radioactive agent* [also: iometin (^{131}I)]

iometin (^{125}I) INN *neoplasm test; radioactive agent* [also: iomethin I 125]

iometin (^{131}I) INN *neoplasm test; radioactive agent* [also: iomethin I 131]

iometopane I 123 USAN *diagnostic imaging aid for dopamine and serotonin transporter sites*

iomorinic acid INN

Ionamin capsules ℞ *anorexiant; CNS stimulant* [phentermine HCl resin complex] 15, 30 mg

Ionax foam OTC *medicated cleanser for acne* [benzalkonium chloride]

Ionax Astringent Skin Cleanser topical liquid OTC *keratolytic cleanser for acne* [salicylic acid; isopropyl alcohol]

Ionax Scrub OTC *abrasive medicated cleanser for acne* [benzalkonium chloride]

ionic contrast media *a class of older radiopaque agents that, in general, have* a high osmolar concentration of iodine (the contrast agent), which corresponds to a higher incidence of adverse reactions [also called: high osmolar contrast media (HOCM)]

Ionil shampoo OTC *antiseborrheic; keratolytic; antiseptic* [salicylic acid; benzalkonium chloride]

Ionil Plus shampoo OTC *antiseborrheic; keratolytic* [salicylic acid] 2%

Ionil T shampoo OTC *antiseborrheic; antipsoriatic; keratolytic; antiseptic* [coal tar; salicylic acid; benzalkonium chloride]

Ionil-T Plus shampoo OTC *antiseborrheic; antipsoriatic; antipruritic; antibacterial* [coal tar] 2%

ionphylline [see: aminophylline]

iopamidol USAN, USP, INN, BAN *parenteral radiopaque contrast medium (49% iodine)*

iopanoic acid USP, INN, BAN *oral radiopaque contrast medium for cholecystography (66.68% iodine)*

iopentol USAN, INN, BAN *radiopaque contrast medium*

Iophen tablets, elixir, drops ℞ *expectorant* [iodinated glycerol] 30 mg; 60 mg/5 mL; 50 mg/mL

Iophen-C oral liquid (discontinued 2002) ℞ *narcotic antitussive; expectorant* [codeine phosphate; iodinated glycerol] 10•30 mg/5 mL

Iophen-DM oral liquid (discontinued 2002) ℞ *antitussive; expectorant* [dextromethorphan hydrobromide; iodinated glycerol] 10•30 mg/5 mL

iophendylate USP, BAN *radiopaque contrast medium* [also: iofendylate]

iophenoic acid INN [also: iophenoxic acid]

iophenoxic acid USP [also: iophenoic acid]

Iophylline elixir ℞ *antiasthmatic; bronchodilator; expectorant* [theophylline; iodinated glycerol] 120•30 mg/15 mL

Iopidine Drop-Tainers (eye drops) ℞ *topical sympathomimetic antiglaucoma agent* [apraclonidine HCl] 0.5%, 1%

ioprocemic acid USAN, INN *radiopaque contrast medium*

iopromide USAN, INN, BAN *parenteral radiopaque contrast medium (39% iodine)*

iopronic acid USAN, INN, BAN *radiopaque contrast medium for cholecystography*

iopydol USAN, INN, BAN *radiopaque contrast medium for bronchography*

iopydone USAN, INN, BAN *radiopaque contrast medium for bronchography*

Iosal II sustained-release tablets ℞ *decongestant; expectorant* [pseudoephedrine HCl; guaifenesin] 60•600 mg

iosarcol INN

iosefamic acid USAN, INN *radiopaque contrast medium*

ioseric acid USAN, INN *radiopaque contrast medium*

iosimide INN

iosulamide INN *radiopaque contrast medium* [also: iosulamide meglumine]

iosulamide meglumine USAN *radiopaque contrast medium* [also: iosulamide]

iosulfan blue *parenteral radiopaque contrast medium for lymphography*

iosumetic acid USAN, INN *radiopaque contrast medium*

iotalamic acid INN *radiopaque contrast medium* [also: iothalamic acid]

iotasul USAN, INN *radiopaque contrast medium*

iotetric acid USAN, INN *radiopaque contrast medium*

iothalamate meglumine USP *parenteral radiopaque contrast medium (47% iodine)* [also: meglumine iothalamate]

iothalamate sodium USP *parenteral radiopaque contrast medium (59.9% iodine)* [also: sodium iothalamate]

iothalamate sodium I 125 USAN *radioactive agent* [also: sodium iotalamate (^{125}I)]

iothalamate sodium I 131 USAN *radioactive agent* [also: sodium iotalamate (^{131}I)]

iothalamic acid USP, BAN *radiopaque contrast medium* [also: iotalamic acid]
iothiouracil sodium
iotranic acid INN
iotriside INN
iotrizoic acid INN
iotrol [now: iotrolan]
iotrolan USAN, INN, BAN *parenteral radiopaque contrast medium*
iotroxic acid USAN, INN, BAN *radiopaque contrast medium*
Iotussin HC syrup (discontinued 2002) ℞ *narcotic antitussive; decongestant; antihistamine* [hydrocodone bitartrate; phenylephrine HCl; chlorpheniramine maleate] 2.5•5•2 mg/5 mL
iotyrosine I 131 USAN *radioactive agent*
ioversol USAN, INN, BAN *parenteral radiopaque contrast medium* (47.3% iodine)
ioxabrolic acid INN
ioxaglate meglumine USAN *parenteral radiopaque contrast medium* [also: meglumine ioxaglate]
ioxaglate sodium USAN *parenteral radiopaque contrast medium* [also: sodium ioxaglate]
ioxaglic acid USAN, INN, BAN *radiopaque contrast medium*
ioxilan USAN, INN *diagnostic aid*
ioxitalamic acid INN
ioxotrizoic acid USAN, INN *radiopaque contrast medium*
iozomic acid INN
IPA (ifosfamide, Platinol, Adriamycin) *chemotherapy protocol for pediatric hepatoblastoma*
ipazilide fumarate USAN *antiarrhythmic*
ipecac USP *emetic*
ipecac, milk *medicinal herb* [see: birthroot; dogbane]
ipecac, powdered USP
ipexidine INN *dental caries prophylactic* [also: ipexidine mesylate]
ipexidine mesylate USAN, INN *dental caries prophylactic* [also: ipexidine]
IPL-423 *investigational agent for rheumatoid arthritis*
ipodate calcium USP *oral radiopaque contrast medium for cholecystography* (61.7% iodine)

ipodate sodium USAN, USP *oral radiopaque contrast medium for cholecystography* (61.4% iodine) [also: sodium ipodate; sodium iopodate]
IPOL subcu injection ℞ *poliomyelitis vaccine* [poliovirus vaccine, inactivated] 0.5 mL
Ipomoea pandurata *medicinal herb* [see: wild jalap]
Ipomoea violacea (**morning glory**) seeds *contain lysergic acid amide, chemically similar to LSD, which produces hallucinations when ingested as a street drug* [see also: LSD]
ipragratine INN
ipramidil INN
ipratropium bromide USAN, INN, BAN *anticholinergic bronchodilator for bronchospasm; antisecretory for rhinorrhea* 0.02%, 0.03%, 0.06% inhalation; 0.03%, 0.06% nasal spray
Ipravent [see: Apo-Ipravent]
iprazochrome INN
iprazone [see: isoprazone]
ipriflavone INN
iprindole USAN, INN, BAN *antidepressant*
Iprivasc powder for subcu injection ℞ *anticoagulant; thrombin inhibitor for the prevention of deep vein thrombosis (DVT) in elective hip replacement surgery* [desirudin] 15 mg/dose
iprocinodine HCl USAN, BAN *veterinary antibacterial*
iproclozide INN, BAN
iprocrolol INN
iprofenin USAN *hepatic function test*
iproheptine INN
iproniazid INN, BAN
ipronidazole USAN, INN, BAN *antiprotozoal* (Histomonas)
ipropethidine [see: properidine]
iproplatin USAN, INN, BAN *antineoplastic*
iprotiazem INN
iproxamine INN *vasodilator* [also: iproxamine HCl]
iproxamine HCl USAN *vasodilator* [also: iproxamine]
iprozilamine INN
ipsalazide INN, BAN

ipsapirone INN, BAN *anxiolytic* [also: ipsapirone HCl]

ipsapirone HCl USAN *anxiolytic* [also: ipsapirone]

Ipsatol Cough Formula for Children; Ipsatol Cough Formula for Adults oral liquid (discontinued 2002) OTC *antitussive; decongestant; expectorant* [dextromethorphan hydrobromide; phenylpropanolamine HCl; guaifenesin] 10•9•100 mg/5 mL

IPTD (isopropyl-thiadiazol) [see: glyprothiazol]

IPV (inactivated poliomyelitis vaccine) [see: poliovirus vaccine, inactivated]

IPV (inactivated poliovaccine) [see: poliovirus vaccine, inactivated]

iquindamine INN

Iquix eye drops ℞ *fluoroquinolone antibiotic for corneal ulcers* [levofloxacin] 1.5%

¹⁹²Ir [see: iridium Ir 192]

irbesartan USAN *angiotensin II receptor antagonist for hypertension; treatment to delay the progression of diabetic nephropathy*

Ircon tablets OTC *hematinic; iron supplement* [carbonyl iron] 66 mg

Ircon-FA tablets OTC *hematinic* [carbonyl iron; folic acid] 82 mg Fe•0.8 mg

Iressa film-coated tablets ℞ *antineoplastic for advanced or metastatic non–small cell lung cancer (NSCLC); investigational (Phase III) for head and neck cancers* [gefitinib] 250 mg

irgasan [see: triclosan]

iridium *element (Ir)*

iridium Ir 192 USAN *radioactive agent*

irindalone INN

irinotecan INN *topoisomerase I inhibitor; antineoplastic for metastatic colon and rectal cancers* [also: irinotecan HCl]

irinotecan HCl USAN, JAN *topoisomerase I inhibitor; antineoplastic for metastatic colorectal cancer* [also: irinotecan]

Iris florentina medicinal herb [see: orris root]

Iris versicolor medicinal herb [see: blue flag]

Irish broom *medicinal herb* [see: broom]

Irish moss (Chondrus crispus) *plant medicinal herb used as a demulcent*

irloxacin INN

irofulven USAN, INN *antineoplastic; DNA synthesis inhibitor; apoptosis inducer*

irolapride INN

Iromin-G tablets OTC *vitamin/iron supplement* [multiple vitamins; ferrous gluconate; folic acid] ≛•30•0.8 mg

iron *element (Fe)*

iron carbohydrate complex [see: polyferose]

iron dextran USP *hematinic*

iron heptonate [see: gleptoferron]

iron hydroxide sucrose complex [see: iron sucrose; saccharated ferric oxide]

iron oxide, saccharated [see: iron sucrose; saccharated ferric oxide]

iron perchloride [see: ferric chloride]

iron polymalether [see: ferropolimaler]

Iron Protein Plus capsules OTC *hematinic; iron supplement* [iron protein succinylate] 300 mg (15 mg Fe)

iron protein succinylate *hematinic (5% elemental iron)*

iron saccharate [see: iron sucrose; saccharated ferric oxide]

iron sorbitex USAN, USP *hematinic*

iron sucrose USAN *hematinic for iron deficiency due to chronic hemodialysis with erythropoietin therapy; also used in peritoneal dialysis and autologous blood donation* [also: saccharated ferric oxide]

iron sugar [see: iron sucrose; saccharated ferric oxide]

Iron-Folic 500 timed-release tablets OTC *hematinic* [ferrous sulfate; multiple B vitamins; sodium ascorbate; folic acid] 105•≛•500•0.8 mg

Irrigate eye wash (discontinued 2004) OTC *extraocular irrigating solution* [sterile isotonic solution]

irritant laxatives *a subclass of laxatives that work by direct action on the intestinal mucosa and nerve plexus to increase peristaltic action* [more commonly called stimulant laxatives]

irsogladine INN
irtemazole USAN, INN, BAN *uricosuric*
IS 5-MN (isosorbide 5-mononitrate) [see: isorbide mononitrate]
isaglidole INN
isamfazone INN
isamoltan INN
isamoxole USAN, INN, BAN *antiasthmatic*
isatoribine USAN *immunomodulator; cell growth regulator*
isaxonine INN
isbogrel INN
iseganan *antimicrobial* [also: iseganan HCl]
iseganan HCl USAN, INN *investigational (Phase III) antimicrobial rinse for oral mucositis, ventilator-associated pneumonia, and cystic fibrosis* [also: iseganan]
isepamicin USAN, INN, BAN *aminoglycoside antibiotic*
isethionate USAN, BAN *combining name for radicals or groups* [also: isetionate]
isetionate INN *combining name for radicals or groups* [also: isethionate]
ISG (immune serum globulin) [see: globulin, immune]
ISIS 2503 *investigational (Phase II) Ha-ras selective antisense inhibitor for colon, breast, pancreatic, and non–small cell lung cancers (NSCLC)*
Ismelin tablets ℞ *antihypertensive; investigational (orphan) for reflex sympathetic dystrophy and causalgia* [guanethidine monosulfate] 25 mg ⚠ Ritalin
Ismo film-coated tablets ℞ *antianginal; vasodilator* [isosorbide mononitrate] 20 mg
Ismotic solution ℞ *osmotic diuretic* [isosorbide] 45%
iso-alcoholic elixir NF
isoaminile INN, BAN
isoamyl *p*-methoxycinnamate [see: amiloxate]
isoamyl nitrate [see: amyl nitrite]
Iso-B capsules OTC *vitamin supplement* [multiple B vitamins; folic acid; biotin] ≟•200•100 μg
isobromindione INN
isobucaine HCl USP

isobutamben USAN, INN *topical anesthetic*
isobutane NF *aerosol propellant*
isobutyl *p*-aminobenzoate [see: isobutamben]
isobutyl α-phenylcyclohexaneglycolate [see: ibuverine]
isobutyl 2-cyanoacrylate (IBC) [see: bucrylate]
isobutyl nitrite; butyl nitrite *amyl nitrite substitutes, sold as euphoric street drugs, which produce a quick but short-lived "rush"* [see also: amyl nitrite; volatile nitrites]
***p*-isobutylhydratropohydroxamic acid** [see: ibuproxam]
isobutylhydrochlorothiazide [see: buthiazide]
isobutyramide *investigational (orphan) for sickle cell disease, beta-thalassemia syndrome, and beta-hemoglobinopathies*
isobuzole BAN [also: glysobuzole]
Isocaine HCl injection (discontinued 2002) ℞ *injectable local anesthetic* [mepivacaine HCl] 3%
Isocaine HCl injection (discontinued 2002) ℞ *injectable local anesthetic* [mepivacaine HCl; levonordefrin] 2%•1:20 000
Isocal oral liquid OTC *enteral nutritional therapy* [lactose-free formula]
Isocal HCN ready-to-use oral liquid OTC *enteral nutritional therapy* [lactose-free formula]
Isocal HN oral liquid OTC *enteral nutritional therapy* [lactose-free formula]
isocarboxazid USP, INN, BAN *antidepressant; MAO inhibitor*
Isochron extended-release tablets ℞ *antianginal; vasodilator* [isosorbide dinitrate] 40 mg
Isoclor Expectorant oral liquid (discontinued 2002) ℞ *narcotic antitussive; decongestant; expectorant* [codeine phosphate; pseudoephedrine HCl; guaifenesin; alcohol 5%] 10•30•100 mg/5 mL
Isocom capsules (discontinued 2002) ℞ *cerebral vasoconstrictor and analgesic for vascular and tension headaches;*

"possibly effective" for migraine headaches [isometheptene mucate; dichloralphenazone; acetaminophen] 65•100•325 mg

isoconazole USAN, INN, BAN *antibacterial; antifungal*

isocromil INN

Isocult for Bacteriuria culture paddles for professional use *in vitro diagnostic aid for nitrate, uropathogens, or bacteria in the urine*

Isocult for Candida culture paddles for professional use *in vitro diagnostic aid for* Candida albicans *in the vagina*

Isocult for N. gonorrhoeae and Candida culture test for professional use *in vitro diagnostic aid for gonorrhea and* Candida *in various specimens*

Isocult for Neisseria gonorrhoeae culture paddles for professional use *in vitro diagnostic aid for gonorrhea*

Isocult for Staphylococcus aureus culture paddles for professional use *in vitro diagnostic aid for* Staphylococcus aureus *in exudate*

Isocult for Streptococcal pharyngitis culture paddles for professional use *in vitro diagnostic test for streptococcal pharyngitis in throat swabs*

Isocult for T. vaginalis and Candida culture test for professional use *in vitro diagnostic aid for* Trichomonas *and* Candida *in vaginal or urethral cultures*

isodapamide [see: zidapamide]

d-**isoephedrine HCl** [see: pseudoephedrine HCl]

isoetarine INN *sympathomimetic bronchodilator* [also: isoetharine]

isoethadione [see: paramethadione]

isoetharine USAN, BAN *sympathomimetic bronchodilator* [also: isoetarine]

isoetharine HCl USP, BAN *sympathomimetic bronchodilator* 1% inhalation

isoetharine mesylate USP, BAN *sympathomimetic bronchodilator*

isofezolac INN

isoflupredone INN, BAN *anti-inflammatory* [also: isoflupredone acetate]

isoflupredone acetate USAN *anti-inflammatory* [also: isoflupredone]

isoflurane USAN, USP, INN, BAN *inhalation general anesthetic*

isoflurophate USP *antiglaucoma agent; irreversible cholinesterase inhibitor miotic* [also: dyflos]

Isoject (trademarked delivery system) *prefilled disposable syringe*

Isolan oral liquid OTC *enteral nutritional therapy* [lactose-free formula]

isoleucine (L-isoleucine) USAN, USP, INN, JAN *essential amino acid; symbols: Ile, I*

isoleucine & leucine & valine *investigational (orphan) for hyperphenylalaninemia*

Isolyte E; Isolyte S; Isolyte S pH 7.4 IV infusion ℞ *intravenous electrolyte therapy* [combined electrolyte solution]

Isolyte E with 5% Dextrose IV infusion (discontinued 2001) ℞ *intravenous nutritional/electrolyte therapy* [combined electrolyte solution; dextrose]

Isolyte G (H; M; P; R; S) with 5% Dextrose IV infusion ℞ *intravenous nutritional/electrolyte therapy* [combined electrolyte solution; dextrose]

Isolyte S pH 7.4 IV infusion ℞ *intravenous electrolyte therapy* [combined electrolyte solution]

isomazole INN *cardiotonic* [also: isomazole HCl]

isomazole HCl USAN *cardiotonic* [also: isomazole]

isomeprobamate [see: carisoprodol]

isomer [def.] *One of a group of chemical compounds having the same molecular formula, but differing in either the arrangement of atoms or the bonds between atoms in the compound.* [see also: enantiomer]

isomerol USAN *antiseptic*

isometamidium BAN [also: isometamidium chloride]

isometamidium chloride INN [also: isometamidium]

isomethadone INN, BAN

isomethepdrine chloride [see: isometheptene]

isometheptene INN, BAN

isometheptene HCl [see: isometheptene]

isometheptene mucate USP *cerebral vasoconstrictor; "possibly effective" for migraine headaches*

isometheptene mucate & dichloralphenazone & acetaminophen *cerebral vasoconstrictor and analgesic for vascular and tension headaches; "possibly effective" for migraine headaches* 65•100•325 mg oral

Isomil oral liquid, powder for oral liquid OTC *hypoallergenic infant food* [soy protein formula] 🔄 Esimil

Isomil DF ready-to-use oral liquid OTC *hypoallergenic infant food for management of diarrhea* [soy protein formula]

Isomil SF oral liquid OTC *hypoallergenic infant food* [soy protein formula, sucrose free]

isomolpan INN *antipsychotic; dopamine autoreceptor antagonist* [also: isomolpan HCl]

isomolpan HCl USAN *antipsychotic; dopamine autoreceptor antagonist* [also: isomolpan]

isomylamine HCl USAN *smooth muscle relaxant*

isoniazid USP, INN, BAN *bactericidal; primary tuberculostatic* 50, 100, 300 mg oral; 50 mg/5 mL oral

isonicophen [see: aconiazide]

isonicotinic acid hydrazide (INH) [see: isoniazid]

isonicotinic acid vanillylidenehydrazide [see: ftivazide]

1-isonicotinoyl-2-salicylidenehydrazine (INSH) [see: salinazid]

isonicotinylhydrazine [see: isoniazid]

isonixin INN

isooctadecanol [see: isostearyl alcohol]

isooctadecyl alcohol [see: isostearyl alcohol]

Isopan oral liquid OTC *antacid* [magaldrate] 540 mg/5 mL

Isopan Plus oral liquid OTC *antacid; antiflatulent* [magaldrate; simethicone] 540•40 mg/5 mL

Isopap capsules (discontinued 2002) ℞ *cerebral vasoconstrictor and analgesic for vascular and tension headaches; "possibly effective" for migraine headaches* [isometheptene mucate; dichloralphenazone; acetaminophen] 65•100•325 mg

isopentyl *p*-methoxycinnamate [see: amiloxate]

isopentyl nitrite [see: amyl nitrite]

isophenethanol [see: nifenalol]

isoprazone INN, BAN

isoprednidene INN, BAN

isopregnenone [see: dydrogesterone]

isoprenaline INN, BAN *sympathomimetic bronchodilator; vasopressor for shock* [also: isoproterenol HCl]

L-isoprenaline [see: levisoprenaline]

isoprenaline HCl [see: isoproterenol HCl]

isoprofen INN

isopropamide iodide USP, INN, BAN *peptic ulcer adjunct*

isopropanol [see: isopropyl alcohol]

isopropicillin INN

isoproponum iodide [see: isopropamide iodide]

7-isopropoxyisoflavone [see: ipriflavone]

isopropyl alcohol USP *topical anti-infective/antiseptic; solvent*

isopropyl alcohol, rubbing USP *rubefacient*

N-isopropyl meprobamate [see: carisoprodol]

isopropyl myristate NF *emollient*

isopropyl palmitate NF *oleaginous vehicle*

isopropyl sebacate

isopropyl unoprostone [see: unoprostone isopropyl]

isopropylantipyrine [see: propyphenazone]

isopropylarterenol HCl [see: isoproterenol HCl]

isopropylarterenol sulfate [see: isoproterenol sulfate]

isoproterenol HCl USP *sympathomimetic bronchodilator; vasopressor for* *shock* [also: isoprenaline] 1:5000, 1:50 000 (0.2, 0.02 mg/mL) injection

isoproterenol sulfate USP *sympathomimetic bronchodilator*

Isoptin film-coated tablets (discontinued 2001) ℞ *antianginal; antiarrhythmic; antihypertensive; calcium channel blocker* [verapamil HCl] 40, 80, 120 mg ⃰ Intropin

Isoptin IV injection (discontinued 2002) ℞ *antitachyarrhythmic; calcium channel blocker* [verapamil HCl] 5 mg/2 mL

Isoptin SR film-coated sustained-release tablets ℞ *antihypertensive; antianginal; antiarrhythmic; calcium channel blocker* [verapamil HCl] 120, 180, 240 mg

Isopto Atropine Drop-Tainers (eye drops) ℞ *cycloplegic; mydriatic* [atropine sulfate] 0.5%, 1%

Isopto Carbachol Drop-Tainers (eye drops) ℞ *antiglaucoma agent; direct-acting miotic* [carbachol] 0.75%, 1.5%, 3%

Isopto Carpine Drop-Tainers (eye drops) ℞ *topical antiglaucoma agent; direct-acting miotic* [pilocarpine HCl] 0.25%, 0.5%, 1%, 2%, 3%, 4%, 5%, 6%, 8%, 10% ⃰ Isopto Eserine

Isopto Cetamide Drop-Tainers (eye drops) ℞ *antibiotic* [sulfacetamide sodium] 15%

Isopto Cetapred eye drop suspension (discontinued 2003) ℞ *corticosteroidal anti-inflammatory; antibiotic* [prednisolone acetate; sulfacetamide sodium] 0.25%•10%

Isopto Homatropine Drop-Tainers (eye drops) ℞ *cycloplegic; mydriatic* [homatropine hydrobromide] 2%, 5%

Isopto Hyoscine Drop-Tainers (eye drops) ℞ *cycloplegic; mydriatic* [scopolamine hydrobromide] 0.25%

Isopto Plain; Isopto Tears Drop-Tainers (eye drops) OTC *ophthalmic moisturizer/lubricant* [hydroxypropyl methylcellulose] 0.5%

Isordil Tembid (sustained-release capsules and tablets) (discontinued 2004) ℞ *antianginal; vasodilator* [isosorbide dinitrate] 40 mg ⃰ Isuprel

Isordil Titradose (tablets), sublingual ℞ *antianginal; vasodilator* [isosorbide dinitrate] 5, 10, 20, 30, 40 mg; 2.5, 5, 10 mg ⃰ Isuprel

isosorbide USAN, USP, INN, BAN *osmotic diuretic; investigational (orphan) agent for Fabry disease*

isosorbide dinitrate USAN, USP, INN, BAN *coronary vasodilator; antianginal* 2.5, 5, 10, 20, 30, 40 mg oral

isosorbide mononitrate USAN, INN, BAN *coronary vasodilator; antianginal* 10, 20, 30, 60, 120 mg oral

Isosource; Isosource HN oral liquid OTC *enteral nutritional therapy* [lactose-free formula]

isospaglumic acid INN

isospirilene [see: spirilene]

isostearyl alcohol USAN *emollient; solvent*

isosulfamerazine [see: sulfaperin]

isosulfan blue USAN *lymphangiography aid* [also: sulphan blue]

isosulpride INN

Isotein HN powder OTC *enteral nutritional therapy* [lactose-free formula]

3-isothiocyanato-1-propene [see: allyl isothiocyanate]

isothiocyanic acid, allyl ester [see: allyl isothiocyanate]

isothipendyl INN, BAN

isothipendyl HCl [see: isothipendyl]

isotiquimide USAN, INN, BAN *antiulcerative*

Isotrate ER extended-release tablets ℞ *antianginal; vasodilator* [isosorbide dinitrate] 60 mg

isotretinoin USAN, USP, INN, BAN *systemic keratolytic for severe recalcitrant cystic acne; investigational (Phase III) for neuroblastoma*

isotretinoin anisatil USAN *keratolytic for acne vulgaris*

Isovorin ℞ *chemotherapy "rescue" agent (orphan)* [L-leucovorin]

Isovue-128 injection (discontinued 2001) ℞ *radiopaque contrast medium* [iopamidol (49% iodine)] 261 mg/mL (128 mg/mL)

Isovue-200; Isovue-250; Isovue-300; Isovue-370 injection ℞ *radiopaque contrast medium* [iopamidol (49% iodine)] 408 mg/mL (200 mg/mL); 510 mg/mL (250 mg/mL); 612 mg/mL (300 mg/mL); 755 mg/mL (370 mg/mL)

Isovue-M 200; Isovue-M 300 intrathecal injection ℞ *radiopaque contrast medium for myelography* [iopamidol (49% iodine)] 408 mg/mL (200 mg/mL); 612 mg/mL (300 mg/mL)

isoxaprolol INN

isoxepac USAN, INN, BAN *anti-inflammatory*

isoxicam USAN, INN, BAN *nonsteroidal anti-inflammatory drug (NSAID); antiarthritic; analgesic; antipyretic*

isoxsuprine INN, BAN *peripheral vasodilator* [also: isoxsuprine HCl]

isoxsuprine HCl USP, JAN *peripheral vasodilator* [also: isoxsuprine] 10, 20 mg oral

I-Soyalac oral liquid OTC *hypoallergenic infant food* [soybean protein formula]

isradipine USAN, INN, BAN *antihypertensive; dihydropyridine calcium channel blocker*

isrodipine [see: isradipine]

Istalol eye drops ℞ *topical antiglaucoma agent (β-blocker)* [timolol maleate] 0.5%

Istin (European name for U.S. product Norvasc)

Isuprel intracardiac, IV, IM, or subcu injection ℞ *vasopressor for cardiac, hypovolemic, or septic shock; sympathomimetic bronchodilator* [isoproterenol HCl] 1:5000, 1:50 000 (0.2, 0.02 mg/mL) ⚕ Isordil

Isuprel Mistometer (metered-dose inhalation aerosol), solution for inhalation (discontinued 2001) ℞ *sympathomimetic bronchodilator* [isoproterenol HCl] 103 μg/dose; 0.5% (1:200), 1% (1:100)

itanoxone INN

itasetron USAN *anxiolytic; antidepressant; antiemetic; serotonin 5-HT₃ receptor antagonist*

itazigrel USAN, INN *platelet antiaggregatory agent*

itazogrel [see: itazigrel]

Itch Relief Gel Spritz spray OTC *poison ivy treatment* [camphor] 0.5%

itchweed *(Veratrum viride)* *medicinal herb* [see: hellebore]

Itch-X spray, gel OTC *local anesthetic* [pramoxine HCl] 1%

itobarbital [see: butalbital]

itraconazole USAN, INN, BAN *systemic triazole antifungal* 100 mg oral

itramin tosilate INN [also: itramin tosylate]

itramin tosylate BAN [also: itramin tosilate]

itrocainide INN

iturelix USAN, INN *gonadotropin releasing hormone antagonist; ovarian and testicular steroid suppressant*

I-Valex-1 powder OTC *formula for infants with leucine catabolism disorder*

I-Valex-2 powder OTC *enteral nutritional therapy for leucine catabolism disorder*

Ivanaz injection ℞ *investigational (NDA filed) broad-spectrum carbapenem antibiotic* [MK-826 (code name —generic name not yet assigned)]

Ivarest cream OTC *poison ivy treatment* [calamine; diphenhydramine HCl] 14%•2%

Ivarest lotion (discontinued 2001) OTC *poison ivy treatment* [calamine; benzocaine] 14%•5%

ivarimod INN

Iveegam freeze-dried powder for IV infusion (discontinued 2004) ℞ *passive immunizing agent for HIV and Kawasaki syndrome; investigational (orphan) for acute myocarditis and juvenile rheumatoid arthritis* [immune globulin] 50 mg/mL

ivermectin USAN, INN, BAN *antiparasitic; anthelmintic for strongyloidiasis and onchocerciasis*

ivermectin component B$_{1a}$
ivermectin component B$_{1b}$
IVIG (intravenous immunoglobulin) [q.v.]
ivoqualine INN
ivy *medicinal herb* [see: American ivy; English ivy; poison ivy]
Ivy Block lotion OTC *preventative for poison ivy, oak, or sumac; use before the risk of exposure* [bentoquatam] 5%
Ivy Cleanse medicated wipes OTC *to remove toxic oils from poison ivy, oak, or sumac* [isopropanol; cetyl alcohol]
Ivy Soothe cream OTC *poison ivy treatment; corticosteroidal anti-inflammatory* [hydrocortisone] 1%
Ivy Stat gel OTC *poison ivy treatment; corticosteroidal anti-inflammatory* [hydrocortisone] 1%

Ivy Super Dry topical liquid OTC *poison ivy treatment* [zinc acetate; isopropanol; benzyl alcohol] 2%•35%•10%
Ivy-Chex spray (discontinued 2003) OTC *poison ivy treatment* [polyvinyl-pyrrolidone-vinylacetate copolymers; methyl salicylate; benzalkonium chloride]
Ivy-Dry lotion OTC *poison ivy treatment* [zinc acetate; isopropanol] 2%•12.5%
Ivy-Rid spray (discontinued 2003) OTC *poison ivy treatment* [polyvinyl-pyrrolidone-vinylacetate copolymers; benzalkonium chloride]
Ixel ℞ *investigational (Phase III) serotonin and norepinephrine reuptake inhibitor for depression and fibromyalgia syndrome* [milnacipran]
izonsteride USAN *antineoplastic 5α-reductase inhibitor for prostate cancer*

Januvia

jalap (*Ipomoea jalapa*) *medicinal herb* [see: wild jalap]
Jamaica mignonette *medicinal herb* [see: henna (*Lawsonia*)]
Jamaica pepper *medicinal herb* [see: allspice]
Jamaica sarsaparilla *medicinal herb* [see: sarsaparilla]
Jamaica sorrel *medicinal herb* [see: hibiscus]
Jantoven tablets ℞ *coumarin-derivative anticoagulant* [warfarin sodium] 1, 2, 2.5, 3, 4, 5, 6, 7.5, 10 mg
Japanese encephalitis (JE) virus vaccine *active immunization vaccine*
jasmine (*Jasminum officinale*) flowers *medicinal herb used as a calmative*
jaundice berry *medicinal herb* [see: barberry]
jaundice root *medicinal herb* [see: goldenseal]
java pepper *medicinal herb* [see: cubeb]
Jeffersonia diphylla *medicinal herb* [see: twin leaf]

Jenest-28 tablets (in packs of 28) (discontinued 2003) ℞ *biphasic oral contraceptive* [norethindrone; ethinyl estradiol]
Phase 1 (7 days): 500•35 µg;
Phase 2 (14 days): 1000•35 µg
Jersey tea *medicinal herb* [see: New Jersey tea]
Jerusalem cowslip; Jerusalem sage *medicinal herb* [see: lungwort]
jessamine, yellow *medicinal herb* [see: gelsemium]
Jesuit's bark *medicinal herb* [see: quinine]
Jets chewable tablets OTC *dietary supplement* [lysine; multiple vitamins] 300•± mg
JE-VAX powder for subcu injection ℞ *active immunizing agent* [Japanese encephalitis virus vaccine] 0.5 mL
Jevity; Jevity 1.5 Cal ready-to-use oral liquid OTC *enteral nutritional therapy* [lactose-free formula] 237 mL cans

Jevity Plus Ⓐ ready-to-use oral liquid OTC *enteral nutritional therapy* [lactose-free formula] 235 mL

jewelweed (Impatiens balsamina; I. biflora; I. capensis) juice *medicinal herb for prophylaxis and treatment of poison ivy rash*

Jew's harp plant *medicinal herb* [see: birthroot]

jiaogulan (Gynostemma pentaphyllum) leaves *medicinal herb used to regulate blood pressure and strengthen the immune system, and for its adaptogenic, antihyperlipidemic, antineoplastic, antioxidant, and cardio- and cerebrovascular protective effects*

jimsonweed (Datura stramonium) leaves and flowering tops *medicinal herb used as an analgesic, antiasthmatic, antispasmodic, hypnotic, and narcotic; also abused as a street drug*

jodphthalein sodium [see: iodophthalein sodium]

joe-pye weed *medicinal herb* [see: queen of the meadow]

jofendylate [see: iophendylate]

Johnswort *medicinal herb* [see: St. John's wort]

Jolivette tablets (in packs of 28) ℞ *oral contraceptive (progestin only)* [norethindrone] 0.35 mg

jopanoic acid [see: iopanoic acid]

josamycin USAN, INN *antibacterial*

jotrizoic acid [see: iotrizoic acid]

Juglans cinerea *medicinal herb* [see: butternut]

Juglans nigra *medicinal herb* [see: black walnut]

Juglans regia *medicinal herb* [see: English walnut]

Junel Fe 1/20; Junel Fe 1.5/30 tablets (in packs of 28) ℞ *monophasic oral contraceptive; iron supplement* [norethindrone acetate; ethinyl estradiol; ferrous fumarate] 1 mg•20 μg•75 mg; 1.5 mg•30 μg•75 mg

"Junior Strength" products [see under product name]

juniper (Juniperus communis) berries *medicinal herb for arthritis, bleeding, bronchitis, colds, edema, infections, kidney infections, pancreatic disorders, uric acid build-up, urinary disorders, and water retention*

juniper, prickly (Juniperus oxycedrus) *medicinal herb* [see: juniper]

juniper tar USP *antieczematic*

Just Tears eye drops OTC *ophthalmic moisturizer/lubricant* [polyvinyl alcohol] 1.4%

K+ 8; K+ 10 film-coated extended-release tablets ℞ *potassium supplement* [potassium chloride] 600 mg (8 mEq K); 750 mg (10 mEq K)

K+ Care powder for oral solution ℞ *potassium supplement* [potassium chloride] 15, 20, 25 mEq K/pkt.

K+ Care ET effervescent tablets ℞ *potassium supplement* [potassium bicarbonate] 20, 25 mEq K

⁴²K [see: potassium chloride K 42]

k82 ImmunoCap test kit for professional use *in vitro diagnostic aid for specific latex allergies*

KAb201 [see: anti-CEA sheep-human chimeric monoclonal antibodies (MAb) radiolabeled with iodine I 131]

Kadian polymer-coated sustained-release pellets in capsules ℞ *narcotic analgesic* [morphine sulfate] 20, 30, 50, 60, 100, 200 mg

kainic acid INN

Kala tablets OTC *probiotic; dietary supplement; fever blister treatment; not generally regarded as safe and effective as an antidiarrheal* [Lactobacillus acidophilus (soy-based)] 200 million CFU

kalafungin USAN, INN *antifungal*

Kaletra gelcaps, oral solution ℞ *antiviral protease inhibitor for HIV infection* [lopinavir; ritonavir] 133.3•33.3 mg; 80•20 mg/mL

kallidinogenase INN, BAN

Kalmia latifolia medicinal herb [see: mountain laurel]

kalmopyrin [see: calcium acetylsalicylate]

kalsetal [see: calcium acetylsalicylate]

Kaltostat; Kaltostat Fortex pads OTC *wound dressing* [calcium alginate fiber]

kalumb *medicinal herb* [see: colombo]

kanamycin INN, BAN *aminoglycoside antibiotic; tuberculosis retreatment* [also: kanamycin sulfate] ℞ Garamycin; gentamicin

kanamycin B [see: bekanamycin]

kanamycin sulfate USP *aminoglycoside antibiotic; tuberculosis retreatment* [also: kanamycin] 75, 500, 1000 mg/vial injection

Kank-a topical liquid/film OTC *mucous membrane anesthetic* [benzocaine] 20%

kanna (Sceletium tortuosum) *plant medicinal herb used as a antidepressant, anxiolytic, relaxant, and euphoriant*

Kantrex capsules, IV or IM injection, pediatric injection ℞ *aminoglycoside antibiotic* [kanamycin sulfate] 500 mg; 500, 1000 mg; 75 mg

Kao Lectrolyte powder for oral solution OTC *pediatric electrolyte replenisher*

Kaochlor 10%; Kaochlor S-F oral liquid (discontinued 2003) ℞ *potassium supplement* [potassium chloride; alcohol 5%] 20 mEq K/15 mL ☒ K-Lor

Kaodene Non-Narcotic oral liquid OTC *antidiarrheal; GI adsorbent; antacid* [kaolin; pectin; bismuth subsalicylate] 130•6.48• ☒ mg/mL

kaolin USP *clay natural material used topically as an emollient and drying agent and ingested for binding gastrointestinal toxins and controlling diarrhea* ☒ Calan; Kaon

Kaon elixir ℞ *potassium supplement* [potassium gluconate] 20 mEq K/15 mL ☒ Calan; kaolin

Kaon-Cl; Kaon-Cl 10 extended-release tablets ℞ *potassium supplement* [potassium chloride] 500 mg (6.7 mEq K); 750 mg (10 mEq K) ☒ Calan; kaolin

Kaon-Cl 20% oral liquid ℞ *potassium supplement* [potassium chloride; alcohol 5%] 40 mEq K/15 mL ☒ Calan; kaolin

Kaopectate caplets, oral liquid OTC *antidiarrheal; antinauseant* [bismuth subsalicylate] 262 mg; 262, 575 mg/15 mL

Kaopectate, Children's oral liquid OTC *antidiarrheal; antinauseant* [bismuth subsalicylate] 261 mg/15 mL ☒ Kapectalin

Kaopectate II caplets (discontinued 2004) OTC *antidiarrheal* [loperamide HCl] 2 mg

Kaopectate Advanced Formula oral liquid (discontinued 2004) OTC *antidiarrheal; GI adsorbent* [attapulgite] 750 mg/15 mL

Kaopectate Maximum Strength caplets OTC *antidiarrheal; GI adsorbent* [attapulgite] 750 mg

Kao-Spen oral suspension OTC *GI adsorbent; antidiarrheal* [kaolin; pectin] 5.2 g•260 mg per 30 mL

Kao-Tin oral liquid OTC *antidiarrheal; antinauseant* [bismuth subsalicylate] 262 mg/15 mL

Kapectolin oral liquid, oral suspension OTC *GI adsorbent; antidiarrheal* [bismuth subsalicylate] 262 mg/15 mL ☒ Kaopectate

Kapseal (trademarked dosage form) *capsules sealed with a band*

karaya gum (Sterculia tragacantha; S. urens; S. villosa) *medicinal herb used as a topical astringent and bulk laxative*

Karidium tablets, chewable tablets, drops ℞ *dental caries preventative* [sodium fluoride] 2.2 mg; 2.2 mg; 0.275 mg/drop

Karigel; Karigel-N gel ℞ *dental caries preventative* [sodium fluoride] 1.1%

Kariva tablets (in packs of 28) ℞ *biphasic oral contraceptive* [desogestrel; ethinyl estradiol]
Phase 1 (21 days): 150•20 μg;
Phase 2 (5 days): 0•10 μg

karyocyte growth factor [see: pegylated megakaryocyte growth and development factor, recombinant human]

kasal USAN *food additive*

kaugoed; kougoed *medicinal herb* [see: kanna]

kava kava (*Piper methysticum*) root *medicinal herb for insomnia and nervousness*

Kay Ciel oral liquid, powder for oral solution ℞ *potassium supplement* [potassium chloride] 20 mEq K/15 mL; 20 mEq K/pkt. ⊡ KCl

Kayexalate powder for oral or rectal suspension ℞ *potassium-removing agent for hyperkalemia* [sodium polystyrene sulfonate]

Kaylixir oral liquid ℞ *potassium supplement* [potassium gluconate; alcohol 5%] 20 mEq K/15 mL

K-C oral suspension OTC *antidiarrheal; GI adsorbent; antacid* [kaolin; pectin; bismuth subcarbonate] 5 g•260 mg•260 mg per 30 mL

KCl (potassium chloride) [q.v.] ⊡ Kay Ciel

K-Dur 10; K-Dur 20 controlled-release tablets ℞ *potassium supplement* [potassium chloride] 750 mg (10 mEq K); 1500 mg (20 mEq K)

kebuzone INN

Keflex Pulvules (capsules), oral suspension ℞ *cephalosporin antibiotic* [cephalexin] 250, 500 mg; 125, 250 mg/5 mL ⊡ Keflet; Keflin

Keftab tablets (discontinued 2005) ℞ *cephalosporin antibiotic* [cephalexin HCl] 500 mg

Kefurox powder for IV or IM injection (discontinued 2003) ℞ *cephalo-*

sporin antibiotic [cefuroxime sodium] 0.75, 1.5, 7.5 g

Kefzol powder or frozen premix for IV or IM injection (discontinued 2003) ℞ *cephalosporin antibiotic* [cefazolin sodium] 0.5, 1, 10, 20 g ⊡ Cefzil

kellofylline [see: visnafylline]

kelp (*Fucus versiculosus*) plant *medicinal herb for brittle fingernails, cleaning arteries, colitis, eczema, goiter, obesity, and toning adrenal, pituitary, and thyroid glands*

kelp (*Laminaria digitata; L. japonica*) plant *medicinal herb for cervical dilation and cervical ripening*

Kemadrin tablets ℞ *anticholinergic; antiparkinsonian* [procyclidine HCl] 5 mg ⊡ Coumadin

Kemsol ⊕ solution for bladder instillation ℞ *anti-inflammatory for symptomatic relief of interstitial cystitis* [dimethyl sulfoxide (DMSO)] 70%

Kemstro orally disintegrating tablets ℞ *skeletal muscle relaxant* [baclofen] 10, 20 mg

Kenaject-40 IM, intra-articular, intrabursal, intradermal injection ℞ *corticosteroid; anti-inflammatory* [triamcinolone acetonide] 40 mg/mL

Kenalog ointment, cream, lotion, aerosol spray ℞ *topical corticosteroidal anti-inflammatory* [triamcinolone acetonide] 0.025%, 0.1%, 0.5%; 0.025%, 0.1%, 0.5%; 0.025%, 0.1%; ⊉ ⊡ Ketalar

Kenalog in Orabase oral paste ℞ *corticosteroidal anti-inflammatory* [triamcinolone acetonide] 0.1%

Kenalog-10; Kenalog-40 IM, intra-articular, intrabursal, intradermal injection ℞ *corticosteroid; anti-inflammatory* [triamcinolone acetonide] 10 mg/mL; 40 mg/mL

Kenalog-H cream ℞ *corticosteroidal anti-inflammatory* [triamcinolone acetonide] 0.1%

Kendall compound A [see: dehydrocorticosterone]

Kendall compound B [see: corticosterone]

Kendall compound E [see: cortisone acetate]

Kendall compound F [see: hydrocortisone]

Kendall desoxy compound B [see: desoxycorticosterone acetate]

Kenonel cream ℞ *corticosteroidal anti-inflammatory* [triamcinolone acetonide] 1%

Kenral-MPA Ⓒᴬᴺ [see: Alti-MPA]

Kenwood Therapeutic oral liquid OTC *vitamin/mineral supplement* [multiple vitamins & minerals]

keoxifene HCl [now: raloxifene HCl]

Kepivance powder for IV injection ℞ *keratinocyte growth factor (KGF) for radiation- and chemotherapy-induced oral mucositis* [palifermin] 6.25 mg/dose

Keppra film-coated tablets, oral solution ℞ *anticonvulsant for partial-onset seizures* [levetiracetam] 250, 500, 750 mg; 100 mg/mL

keracyanin INN

Keralac cream ℞ *moisturizer; emollient; keratolytic* [urea] 50%

Keralac lotion ℞ *moisturizer; emollient; keratolytic* [urea; lactic acid; vitamin E] 35%•²•²

Keralac Nail Gel ℞ *moisturizer; emollient; keratolytic* [urea] 50%

Kerasal ointment OTC *keratolytic for calloused feet* [salicylic acid; urea] 5%•10%

keratolytics *a class of agents that cause sloughing of the horny layer of the epidermis and softening of the skin*

Keri; Keri Light lotion (discontinued 2004) OTC *moisturizer; emollient*

Keri Age Defy & Protect lotion OTC *moisturizer; emollient; sunscreen (SPF 15)* [octinoxate; oxybenzone] 7.5%•2%

Keri Creme (discontinued 2004) OTC *moisturizer; emollient*

Keri Nourishing Shea Butter lotion OTC *moisturizer; emollient*

Keri Original; Keri Advanced; Keri Sensitive Skin; Keri Shave Minimizing lotion OTC *moisturizer; emollient*

KeriCort-10 cream OTC *topical corticosteroidal anti-inflammatory* [hydrocortisone] 1%

Kerlone tablets ℞ *antihypertensive; β-blocker* [betaxolol HCl] 10, 20 mg

kernelwort *medicinal herb* [see: figwort]

Kerodex #51 cream OTC *skin protectant for dry or oily work*

Kerodex #71 cream OTC *water repellant skin protectant for wet work*

Kestrone 5 IM injection (discontinued 2003) ℞ *estrogen replacement therapy for postmenopausal symptoms; palliative therapy for inoperable prostatic and breast cancer* [estrone] 5 mg/mL

Ketalar IV or IM injection ℞ *rapid-acting general anesthetic; sometimes abused as a street drug due to its "dissociative state" effects* [ketamine HCl] 10, 50, 100 mg/mL ⑨ Kenalog

ketamine INN, BAN *a rapid-acting general anesthetic; sometimes abused as a street drug due to its "dissociative state" effects* [also: ketamine HCl]

ketamine HCl USAN, USP, JAN *a rapid-acting general anesthetic; sometimes abused as a street drug due to its "dissociative state" effects* [also: ketamine]

ketanserin USAN, INN, BAN *serotonin antagonist*

ketazocine USAN, INN *analgesic*

ketazolam USAN, INN, BAN *minor tranquilizer*

Ketek film-coated tablets ℞ *broad-spectrum ketolide antibiotic for respiratory tract infections* [telithromycin] 300, 400 mg

kethoxal USAN *antiviral* [also: ketoxal]

ketimipramine INN *antidepressant* [also: ketipramine fumarate]

ketimipramine fumarate [see: ketipramine fumarate]

ketipramine fumarate USAN *antidepressant* [also: ketimipramine]

7-KETO DHEA *investigational dehydroepiandrosterone (DHEA) derivative for Alzheimer disease*

ketobemidone INN, BAN

ketocaine INN

ketocainol INN

ketocholanic acid [see: dehydrocholic acid]

ketoconazole USAN, USP, INN, BAN *broad-spectrum imidazole antifungal; investigational (Phase III) for seborrheic dermatitis* 200 mg oral; 2% topical

Ketoderm ⓒᴬᴺ cream ℞ *topical antifungal* [ketoconazole] 2%

Keto-Diastix reagent strips *in vitro diagnostic aid for multiple urine products*

ketohexazine [see: cetohexazine]

ketolides *a class of oral antibiotics*

Ketonex-1 powder OTC *formula for infants with maple syrup urine disease*

Ketonex-2 powder *enteral nutritional therapy for maple syrup urine disease (MSUD)*

ketoprofen USAN, INN, BAN, JAN *analgesic; antiarthritic; antipyretic; nonsteroidal anti-inflammatory drug (NSAID)* 50, 75, 100, 150, 200 mg oral

ketorfanol USAN, INN *analgesic*

ketorolac INN, BAN *analgesic; nonsteroidal anti-inflammatory drug (NSAID)* [also: ketorolac tromethamine]

ketorolac tromethamine USAN *analgesic; nonsteroidal anti-inflammatory drug (NSAID)* [also: ketorolac] 10 mg oral; 15, 30 mg/mL injection

Ketostix reagent strips for home use *in vitro diagnostic aid for acetone (ketones) in the urine*

ketotifen INN, BAN *antihistamine; mast cell stabilizer* [also: ketotifen fumarate]

ketotifen fumarate USAN, JAN *antihistamine; mast cell stabilizer* [also: ketotifen]

ketotrexate INN

ketoxal INN *antiviral* [also: kethoxal]

Key-Plex injection ℞ *parenteral vitamin therapy* [multiple B vitamins; vitamin C] ≜ • 50 mg/mL

Key-Pred 25; Key-Pred 50 IM injection ℞ *corticosteroid; anti-inflammatory* [prednisolone acetate] 25 mg/mL; 50 mg/mL

Key-Pred-SP IV or IM injection ℞ *corticosteroid; anti-inflammatory* [prednisolone sodium phosphate] 20 mg/mL

K-G Elixir ℞ *potassium supplement* [potassium gluconate] 20 mEq K/15 mL

KGHB (potassium gamma hydroxybutyrate) [see: gamma hydroxybutyrate (GHB)]

khellin INN

khelloside INN

Kid Kare Children's Cough/Cold oral liquid OTC *antitussive; decongestant; antihistamine* [dextromethorphan hydrobromide; pseudoephedrine HCl; chlorpheniramine maleate] 10 • 30 • 2 mg/10 mL

Kid Kare Nasal Decongestant oral drops OTC *nasal decongestant* [pseudoephedrine HCl] 7.5 mg/0.8 mL

kidney root *medicinal herb* [see: queen of the meadow]

KIE syrup ℞ *bronchodilator; decongestant; expectorant* [ephedrine HCl; potassium iodide] 16 • 300 mg/10 mL

Kindercal oral liquid OTC *enteral nutritional therapy* [lactose-free formula]

Kinerase cream, lotion OTC *moisturizer; emollient* [N^6-furfuryladenine] 0.1%

Kinerase Intensive Eye Cream OTC *moisturizer; emollient* [kinetin; safflower oil] 0.125% • ≜

Kineret prefilled syringe for subcu injection ℞ *interleukin-1 receptor antagonist (IL-1ra); nonsteroidal anti-inflammatory drug (NSAID) for rheumatoid arthritis (RA)* [anakinra] 100 mg

Kinevac powder for IV injection ℞ *diagnostic aid for gallbladder function* [sincalide] 1 μg/mL

king's clover *medicinal herb* [see: melilot]

king's cure *medicinal herb* [see: pipsissewa]

king's fern *medicinal herb* [see: buckhorn brake]

kininase II inhibitors [see: angiotensin-converting enzyme inhibitors]

kinnikinnik *medicinal herb* [see: uva ursi]

Kionex powder for oral suspension ℞ *potassium-removing agent for hyper-*

kalemia [sodium polystyrene sulfonate] 15 g/dose

kitasamycin USAN, INN, BAN, JAN *antibacterial* [also: acetylkitasamycin; kitasamycin tartrate]

kitasamycin tartrate JAN *antibacterial* [also: kitasamycin; acetylkitasamycin]

KL4 surfactant *investigational (Phase II/III, orphan) for respiratory distress syndrome in adults and premature infants and meconium aspiration in newborn infants* [also: lucinactant]

Klamath weed *medicinal herb* [see: St. John's wort]

Klaron lotion ℞ *antibiotic for acne* [sulfacetamide sodium] 10%

KLB6; Ultra KLB6 softgels OTC *dietary supplement* [vitamin B₆; multiple food supplements] 3.5•≛ mg; 16.7•≛ mg

K-Lease extended-release capsules (discontinued 2004) ℞ *potassium supplement* [potassium chloride] 750 mg (10 mEq K)

Kleen-Handz solution OTC *topical antiseptic* [ethyl alcohol] 62%

Klerist-D tablets, sustained-release capsules (discontinued 2002) ℞ *decongestant; antihistamine* [pseudoephedrine HCl; chlorpheniramine maleate] 60•4 mg; 120•8 mg

Klonopin tablets, Rx Pak (prescription package), Tel-E-Dose (unit dose package), Wafers (orally disintegrating tablets) ℞ *anticonvulsant; anxiolytic for panic disorder; investigational (orphan) for hyperexplexia (startle disease)* [clonazepam] 0.5, 1, 2 mg; 0.5, 1, 2 mg; 0.5, 1, 2 mg; 0.125, 0.25, 0.5, 1, 2 mg 🔟 clonidine

K-Lor powder for oral solution ℞ *potassium supplement* [potassium chloride] 15, 20 mEq K/pkt. 🔟 Kaochlor

Klor-Con; Klor-Con/25 powder for oral solution ℞ *potassium supplement* [potassium chloride] 20 mEq K/pkt.; 25 mEq K/pkt.

Klor-Con 8; Klor-Con 10 film-coated extended-release tablets ℞ *potassium supplement* [potassium chloride] 600 mg (8 mEq K); 750 mg (10 mEq K)

Klor-Con M10; Klor-Con M15; Klor-Con M20 extended-release tablets ℞ *potassium supplement* [potassium chloride] 750 mg (10 mEq K); 1125 mg (15 mEq K); 1500 mg (20 mEq K)

Klor-Con/EF effervescent tablets ℞ *potassium supplement* [potassium bicarbonate; potassium citrate] 25 mEq K

Klorvess oral liquid, effervescent granules, effervescent tablets ℞ *potassium supplement* [potassium chloride] 20 mEq K/15 mL; 20 mEq K/pkt.; 20 mEq K

Klotrix film-coated controlled-release tablets ℞ *potassium supplement* [potassium chloride] 750 mg (10 mEq K) 🔟 Liotrix

Klout topical liquid OTC *pesticide-free lice removal agent* [acetic acid; isopropanol; sodium laureth sulfate]

K-Lyte ㊝ effervescent tablets ℞ *urinary alkalizer for hypocitruria* [potassium citrate] 2.5 g

K-Lyte; K-Lyte DS effervescent tablets ℞ *potassium supplement* [potassium bicarbonate; potassium citrate] 25 mEq K; 50 mEq K

K-Lyte/Cl powder for oral solution ℞ *potassium supplement* [potassium chloride] 25 mEq K/dose

K-Lyte/Cl; K-Lyte/Cl 50 effervescent tablets ℞ *potassium supplement* [potassium chloride] 25 mEq K; 50 mEq K

knitback; knitbone *medicinal herb* [see: comfrey]

knob grass; knob root *medicinal herb* [see: stone root]

K-Norm controlled-release capsules (discontinued 2004) ℞ *potassium supplement* [potassium chloride] 750 mg (10 mEq K)

knotted marjoram *medicinal herb* [see: marjoram]

knotweed (*Polygonum aviculare; P. hydropiper; P. persicaria; P. punctatum*) plant *medicinal herb used as an antiseptic, astringent, diaphoretic,* *diuretic, emmenagogue, rubefacient, and stimulant*

Koāte-DVI (double viral inactivation) powder for IV injection ℞ *antihemophilic to correct coagulation deficiency* [antihemophilic factor concentrate, solvent/detergent and dry heat treated]

Koāte-HP powder for IV injection (discontinued 2001) ℞ *antihemophilic to correct coagulation deficiency* [antihemophilic factor VIII] 250, 500, 1000, 1500 IU

Kof-Eze lozenges OTC *topical analgesic; counterirritant; mild local anesthetic* [menthol] 6 mg

Kogenate powder for IV injection ℞ *antihemophilic for treatment of hemophilia A and presurgical prophylaxis of hemophiliacs (orphan)* [antihemophilic factor concentrate, recombinant]

Kogenate FS powder for IV injection ℞ *antihemophilic for treatment of hemophilia A* [antihemophilic factor concentrate, recombinant; sucrose] 500 IU•28 mg

KOH (potassium hydroxide) [q.v.]

kola nut *(Cola acuminata)* seed *medicinal herb used as a stimulant; natural source of caffeine*

Kolephrin caplets OTC *decongestant; antihistamine; analgesic* [pseudoephedrine HCl; chlorpheniramine maleate; acetaminophen] 30•2•325 mg

Kolephrin GG/DM oral liquid OTC *antitussive; expectorant* [dextromethorphan hydrobromide; guaifenesin] 20•300 mg/10 mL

Kolephrin/DM caplets OTC *antitussive; decongestant; antihistamine; analgesic* [dextromethorphan hydrobromide; pseudoephedrine HCl; chlorpheniramine maleate; acetaminophen] 10•30•2•325 mg

kolfocon A USAN *hydrophobic contact lens material*

kolfocon B USAN *hydrophobic contact lens material*

kolfocon C USAN *hydrophobic contact lens material*

kolfocon D USAN *hydrophobic contact lens material*

Kolyum oral liquid ℞ *potassium supplement* [potassium gluconate; potassium chloride] 20 mEq K/15 mL

kombucha (yeast/bacteria/fungus symbiont) fermented tea *natural treatment for aging, cancer, intestinal disorders, and rheumatism*

Kondon's Nasal jelly (discontinued 2002) OTC *nasal decongestant* [ephedrine] 1%

Kondremul Plain emulsion OTC *emollient laxative* [mineral oil]

Konsyl powder for oral solution OTC *bulk laxative* [psyllium] 6 g/tsp. or pkt.

Konsyl Easy Mix Formula powder for oral solution OTC *bulk laxative with electrolytes* [psyllium; electrolytes] 6•±• g/tsp. or pkt.

Konsyl Fiber tablets OTC *bulk laxative; antidiarrheal* [calcium polycarbophil] 625 mg

Konsyl Orange powder for oral solution OTC *bulk laxative* [psyllium] 3.4 g/tbsp. or pkt.

Konsyl-D powder OTC *bulk laxative* [psyllium] 3.4 g/tsp.

Konyne 80 IV infusion (discontinued 2001) ℞ *antihemophilic to correct factor VIII (hemophilia A) and factor IX (hemophilia B; Christmas disease) deficiencies* [coagulation factors II, VII, IX, and X, heat treated] 20, 40 mL

Kophane Cough & Cold Formula oral liquid (discontinued 2002) OTC *antitussive; decongestant; antihistamine* [dextromethorphan hydrobromide; phenylpropanolamine HCl; chlorpheniramine maleate] 10•12.5•2 mg/5 mL

Korean ginseng *(Panax ginseng; P. shin-seng)* medicinal herb [see: ginseng]

Koromex vaginal cream (discontinued 2002) OTC *spermicidal contraceptive (for use with a diaphragm)* [octoxynol 9] 3%

Koromex vaginal foam, vaginal jelly (discontinued 2002) OTC *spermicidal*

contraceptive [nonoxynol 9] 12.5%; 3% Ⓡ Komex

Koromex Crystal Clear vaginal gel (discontinued 2002) OTC *spermicidal contraceptive (for use with a diaphragm)* [nonoxynol 9] 2%

kougoed; kaugoed *medicinal herb* [see: kanna]

Kovitonic oral liquid OTC *hematinic* [ferric pyrophosphate; multiple B vitamins; lysine; folic acid] 42•±• 10•0.1 mg/15 mL

K-Pek oral suspension OTC *antidiarrheal* [bismuth subsalicylate] 262 mg/15 mL

K-Pek II caplets OTC *antidiarrheal* [loperamide HCl] 2 mg

K-Phos M.F. tablets ℞ *urinary acidifier* [potassium acid phosphate; sodium acid phosphate] 155•350 mg (1.1 mEq K, 2.9 mEq Na)

K-Phos Neutral film-coated caplets ℞ *urinary acidifier; phosphorus supplement* [sodium phosphate, dibasic; potassium phosphate, monobasic; sodium phosphate, monobasic] 250 mg P

K-Phos No. 2 tablets ℞ *urinary acidifier* [potassium acid phosphate; sodium acid phosphate] 305•700 mg (2.3 mEq K, 5.8 mEq Na)

K-Phos Original tablets ℞ *urinary acidifier* [potassium acid phosphate] 500 mg (3.7 mEq K)

K.P.N. tablets OTC *vitamin/mineral/calcium/iron supplement* [multiple vitamins & minerals; calcium; iron; folic acid] ±•333•11•0.27 mg

^{81m}Kr [see: krypton Kr 81m]

^{85}Kr [see: krypton clathrate Kr 85]

Kredex (European name for U.S. product Coreg)

Kristalose powder for oral solution ℞ *hyperosmotic laxative* [lactulose] 10, 20 g/pkt.

Kronocap (trademarked dosage form) *sustained-release capsule*

Kronofed-A sustained-release capsules ℞ *decongestant; antihistamine* [pseudoephedrine HCl; chlorpheniramine maleate] 120•8 mg

Kronofed-A Jr. sustained-release pediatric capsules ℞ *decongestant; antihistamine* [pseudoephedrine HCl; chlorpheniramine maleate] 60•4 mg

krypton *element (Kr)*

krypton clathrate Kr 85 USAN *radioactive agent*

krypton Kr 81m USAN, USP *radioactive agent*

K-Tab film-coated extended-release tablets ℞ *potassium supplement* [potassium chloride] 750 mg (10 mEq K)

Kudrox oral suspension (discontinued 2004) OTC *antacid* [aluminum hydroxide; magnesium hydroxide; simethicone] 500•450•40 mg/5 mL

kudzu (*Pueraria lobata; P. thunbergiana*) root *medicinal herb for the management of alcoholism*

Kutapressin subcu or IM injection (discontinued 2004) ℞ *claimed to be an anti-inflammatory for multiple dermatoses* [liver derivative complex] 25.5 mg/mL

Kutrase capsules ℞ *porcine-derived digestive enzymes* [lipase; protease; amylase] 2400•30 000•30 000 USP units

Ku-Zyme capsules ℞ *porcine-derived digestive enzymes* [lipase; protease; amylase] 1200•15 000•15 000 USP units

Ku-Zyme HP capsules ℞ *porcine-derived digestive enzymes* [lipase; protease; amylase] 8000•30 000•30 000 USP units

K-vescent effervescent powder ℞ *potassium supplement* [potassium chloride] 20 mEq K/pkt.

Kwelcof oral liquid ℞ *narcotic antitussive; expectorant* [hydrocodone bitartrate; guaifenesin] 5•100 mg/5 mL

Kwellada-P Ⓒᴬᴺ creme rinse OTC *pediculicide for lice; scabicide* [permethrin] 1%

Kwellada-P Ⓒᴬᴺ lotion OTC *pediculicide for lice; scabicide* [permethrin] 5%

K-Y vaginal jelly OTC *lubricant* [glycerin; hydroxyethyl cellulose]

K-Y Plus vaginal gel OTC *spermicidal contraceptive (for use with a diaphragm)* [nonoxynol 9] 2.2%

kyamepromazin [see: cyamemazine]

Kytril film-coated tablets, oral solution, IV infusion ℞ *serotonin 5-HT₃ receptor antagonist; antiemetic for nau-* sea following chemotherapy, radiation, or surgery [granisetron HCl] 1 mg; 1 mg/5 mL; 0.1, 1 mg/mL

L-5 hydroxytryptophan (L-5HTP) *natural precursor to serotonin; investigational (orphan) for postanoxic intention myoclonus; investigational for depression and prophylaxis of migraine headaches*

LA-12 IM injection ℞ *hematinic; vitamin B_{12} supplement* [hydroxocobalamin] 1000 μg/mL

LAAM (*l*-acetyl-α-methadol [or] *l*-alpha-acetyl-methadol) [see: levomethadyl acetate]

labetalol INN, BAN *antihypertensive; antiadrenergic (α- and β-blocker)* [also: labetalol HCl]

labetalol HCl USAN, USP *antihypertensive; antiadrenergic (α- and β-blocker)* [also: labetalol] 100, 200, 300 mg oral; 5 mg/mL injection

labetuzumab *monoclonal antibody to CEA; investigational (orphan) for colorectal, pancreatic, ovarian, and small cell lung cancer*

Labrador tea (*Ledum groenlandicum; L. latifolium; L. palustre*) leaves *medicinal herb for bronchial infections, cough, diarrhea, headache, kidney disorders, lung infections, malignancies, rheumatism, and sore throat*

Labstix reagent strips *in vitro diagnostic aid for multiple urine products*

Lac-Hydrin cream, lotion ℞ *moisturizer; emollient* [ammonium lactate] 12%

Lac-Hydrin Five lotion OTC *moisturizer; emollient* [lactic acid]

LACI (lipoprotein-associated coagulation inhibitor) [see: tifacogin]

lacidipine USAN, INN, BAN *investigational antihypertensive; calcium channel blocker*

Lacipil (approved in Europe) ℞ *investigational antihypertensive; calcium channel blocker* [lacidipine]

LAC-Lotion ℞ *moisturizer; emollient* [ammonium lactate] 12%

Lacril eye drops OTC *ophthalmic moisturizer/lubricant* [hydroxypropyl methylcellulose] 0.5%

Lacri-Lube NP; Lacri-Lube S.O.P. ophthalmic ointment OTC *ocular moisturizer/lubricant* [white petrolatum; mineral oil; lanolin]

Lacrisert ophthalmic insert OTC *ophthalmic moisturizer/lubricant* [hydroxypropyl cellulose] 5 mg

lactagogues *a class of agents that promote or increase the flow of breast milk* [also called: galactagogues]

LactAid oral liquid, tablets OTC *digestive aid for lactose intolerance* [lactase enzyme] 250 U/drop; 3000 U

lactalfate INN

lactase enzyme *digestive enzyme for lactose intolerance*

lactated potassic saline [see: potassic saline, lactated]

lactated Ringer (LR) injection [see: Ringer injection, lactated]

lactated Ringer (LR) solution [see: Ringer injection, lactated]

lactic acid USP *pH adjusting agent*

LactiCare lotion OTC *emollient; moisturizer* [lactic acid]

LactiCare-HC lotion ℞ *topical corticosteroidal anti-inflammatory* [hydrocortisone] 1%, 2.5%

Lactinex granules, chewable tablets OTC *probiotic; dietary supplement; fever blister treatment; not generally regarded as safe and effective as an* antidiarrheal [*Lactobacillus acidophilus; L. bulgaricus*]

Lactinol lotion ℞ *emollient; moisturizer* [lactic acid] 10%

Lactinol·E cream ℞ *emollient; moisturizer* [lactic acid; vitamin E] 10% • 116.67 IU/g

lactitol INN, BAN

Lactobacillus acidophilus natural bacteria; probiotic; dietary supplement; not generally regarded as safe and effective as an antidiarrheal [also: acidophilus]

Lactobacillus bulgaricus natural bacteria; probiotic; dietary supplement; not generally regarded as safe and effective as an antidiarrheal

lactobin *investigational (orphan) for AIDS-related diarrhea*

lactobionic acid, calcium salt, dihydrate [see: calcium lactobionate]

Lactocal·F film-coated tablets ℞ *vitamin/mineral/calcium/iron supplement* [multiple vitamins & minerals; calcium; iron; folic acid] ± • 200 • 65 • 1 mg

lactoflavin [see: riboflavin]

LactoFree oral liquid, powder for oral liquid OTC *hypoallergenic infant formula* [milk-based formula, lactose free]

LactoFree LIPIL oral liquid, powder for oral liquid OTC *hypoallergenic infant formula fortified with omega-3 fatty acids* [milk-based formula, lactose free]

β-lactone [see: propiolactone]

γ-lactone D-glucofuranuronic acid [see: glucurolactone]

lactose NF *tablet and capsule diluent; dietary supplement*

Lactrase capsules OTC *digestive aid for lactose intolerance* [lactase enzyme] 250 mg

Lactrex 12% cream ℞ *emollient; moisturizer* [lactic acid] 12%

Lactuca sativa medicinal herb [see: lettuce]

Lactuca virosa medicinal herb [see: wild lettuce]

lactulose USAN, USP, INN, BAN *hyperosmotic laxative; synthetic disaccharide* used to prevent and treat portal-systemic encephalopathy 10 g/15 mL oral or rectal

ladakamycin [now: azacitidine]

Lady Esther cream OTC *moisturizer; emollient* [mineral oil]

lady's mantle (*Alchemilla xanthochlora; A. vulgaris*) plant *medicinal herb for diarrhea and other digestive disorders; also used as an astringent, anti-inflammatory agent, menstrual cycle regulator, and muscle relaxant*

lady's slipper (*Cypripedium pubescens*) root *medicinal herb for chorea, hysteria, insomnia, nervousness, and restlessness*

laidlomycin INN *veterinary growth stimulant* [also: laidlomycin propionate potassium]

laidlomycin propionate potassium USAN *veterinary growth stimulant* [also: laidlomycin]

Laki-Lorand factor [see: factor XIII]

lamb mint *medicinal herb* [see: peppermint; spearmint]

Lambda (name changed to **Fosrenol** upon marketing release in 2004)

lamb's quarter *medicinal herb* [see: birthroot]

Lamictal tablets, chewable/dispersible tablets ℞ *phenyltriazine anticonvulsant; adjunctive treatment for Lennox-Gastaut syndrome (orphan) and bipolar disorder* [lamotrigine] 25, 100, 150, 200 mg; 2, 5, 25 mg

lamifiban USAN, INN *glycoprotein (GP) IIb/IIIa receptor inhibitor; antiplatelet/antithrombotic agent for unstable angina*

lamifiban HCl USAN *glycoprotein (GP) IIb/IIIa receptor inhibitor; antiplatelet/antithrombotic agent for unstable angina*

Laminaria digitata; L. japonica medicinal herb [see: kelp]

Lamisil tablets ℞ *systemic allylamine antifungal for onychomycosis* [terbinafine HCl] 250 mg

Lamisil AT cream, spray, drops OTC *allylamine antifungal* [terbinafine HCl] 1%

Lamisil DermGel gel (discontinued 2002) ℞ *topical allylamine antifungal* [terbinafine HCl] 1%

Lamium album *medicinal herb* [see: blind nettle]

lamivudine USAN, INN, BAN *nucleoside reverse transcriptase inhibitor; antiviral for HIV and chronic hepatitis B infections*

lamotrigine USAN, INN, BAN *phenyltriazine anticonvulsant; adjunctive treatment for Lennox-Gastaut syndrome (orphan) and bipolar disorder*

Lampit (available only from the Centers for Disease Control) ℞ *investigational anti-infective for Chagas disease* [nifurtimox]

Lamprene capsules ℞ *bactericidal; tuberculostatic; leprostatic (orphan); available only to physicians enrolled in National Hansen Disease Programs through the FDA* [clofazimine] 50 mg

lamtidine INN, BAN

Lanabiotic ointment OTC *antibiotic; local anesthetic* [polymyxin B sulfate; neomycin sulfate; bacitracin zinc; lidocaine] 10 000 U•3.5 mg•500 U•40 mg per g

Lanacane spray, cream OTC *topical local anesthetic; antiseptic* [benzocaine; benzethonium chloride] 20%•0.1%; 6%•0.1%

Lanacaps (dosage form) *timed-release capsules*

Lanacort 5 cream, ointment OTC *topical corticosteroidal anti-inflammatory* [hydrocortisone acetate] 0.5%

Lanacort 10 cream OTC *topical corticosteroidal anti-inflammatory* [hydrocortisone acetate] 1%

Lanaphilic cream OTC *moisturizer; emollient; keratolytic* [urea] 20%

Lanaphilic OTC *ointment base*

Lanaphilic with Urea OTC *ointment base* [urea] 10%

Lanatabs (dosage form) *sustained-release tablets*

lanatoside NF, INN, BAN

Laniazid tablets ℞ *tuberculostatic* [isoniazid] 50 mg

Laniazid C.T. tablets ℞ *tuberculostatic* [isoniazid] 300 mg

lanolin USP *ointment base; water-in-oil emulsion; emollient/protectant*

lanolin, anhydrous USP *absorbent ointment base*

lanolin alcohols *ointment base ingredient*

Lanolor cream OTC *moisturizer; emollient*

Lanophyllin elixir ℞ *antiasthmatic; bronchodilator* [theophylline] 80 mg/ 15 mL

lanoteplase USAN *investigational (Phase III) thrombolytic and tissue plasminogen activator (tPA)*

Lanoxicaps capsules ℞ *cardiac glycoside to increase cardiac output; antiarrhythmic* [digoxin] 0.05, 0.1, 0.2 mg

Lanoxin tablets, pediatric elixir, IV or IM injection ℞ *cardiac glycoside to increase cardiac output; antiarrhythmic* [digoxin] 0.125, 0.25 mg; 0.05 mg/mL; 0.1, 0.25 mg/mL

lanreotide acetate USAN *antineoplastic*

lansoprazole USAN, INN, BAN *proton pump inhibitor for gastric and duodenal ulcers, erosive esophagitis, GERD, and other gastroesophageal disorders*

lanthanum *element (La)*

lanthanum carbonate *phosphate binder for hyperphosphatemia in end-stage renal disease (ESRD)*

Lantus prefilled cartridges for OptiPen One device (discontinued 2003) ℞ *human insulin analogue; long-acting, once-daily antidiabetic* [insulin glargine (rDNA)] 300 IU/3 mL

Lantus vials for subcu injection ℞ *human insulin analogue; long-acting, once-daily antidiabetic* [insulin glargine (rDNA)] 100 IU/mL

Lapacho colorado; L. morado *medicinal herb* [see: pau d'arco]

lapatinib *investigational treatment for breast cancer*

lapirium chloride INN *surfactant* [also: lapyrium chloride]

LAPOCA (**L-asparaginase, Oncovin, cytarabine, Adriamycin**) *chemotherapy protocol*

laprafylline INN

lapyrium chloride USAN *surfactant* [also: lapirium chloride]

laramycin [see: zorbamycin]

larch *(Larix americana; L. europaea)* bark, resin, young shoots, and needles *medicinal herb used as an anthelmintic, diuretic, laxative, and vulnerary; powdered bark is 98% arabinogalactans* [see also: arabinogalactans]

Largon IV or IM injection (discontinued 2004) R *sedative; analgesic adjunct* [propiomazine HCl] 20 mg/mL

Lariam tablets R *antimalarial for acute chloroquine-resistant malaria* (orphan) [mefloquine HCl] 250 mg

Larix americana; L. europaea medicinal herb [see: larch]

Larodopa capsules R *dopamine precursor; antiparkinsonian* [levodopa] 100, 250, 500 mg

Larodopa tablets R *dopamine precursor; antiparkinsonian* [levodopa] 100, 250, 500 mg

laronidase *enzyme replacement therapy for mucopolysaccharidosis I (MPS I)* (orphan)

laroxyl [see: amitriptyline]

Larrea divaricata; L. glutinosa; L. tridentata medicinal herb [see: chaparral]

lasalocid USAN, INN, BAN *coccidiostat for poultry*

Lasan cream, ointment R *topical antipsoriatic* [anthralin] 0.1%, 0.2%, 0.4%; 0.4%

Lasan HP-1 cream R *topical antipsoriatic* [anthralin] 1%

Lasix tablets, oral solution, IM or IV injection R *antihypertensive; loop diuretic* [furosemide] 20, 40, 80 mg; 10 mg/mL; 10 mg/mL ⊡ Esidrix; Lidex

lasofoxifene tartrate USAN *second-generation selective estrogen receptor modulator (SERM); investigational (NDA filed) for osteoporosis and the reduction of LDL cholesterol; investigational (Phase III) for breast cancer*

Lassar paste [betanaphthol (q.v.) + zinc oxide (q.v.)]

latamoxef INN, BAN *anti-infective* [also: moxalactam disodium]

latamoxef disodium [see: moxalactam disodium]

latanoprost USAN, INN *topical prostaglandin agonist for glaucoma and ocular hypertension*

latex agglutination test *in vitro diagnostic aid*

laudexium methylsulfate [see: laudexium metilsulfate; laudexium methylsulphate]

laudexium methylsulphate BAN [also: laudexium metilsulfate]

laudexium metilsulfate INN [also: laudexium methylsulphate]

lauralkonium chloride INN

laurel *(Laurus nobilis)* leaves and fruit *medicinal herb used as an aromatic, astringent, carminative, and stomachic*

laurel, mountain; rose laurel; sheep laurel *medicinal herb* [see: mountain laurel]

laurel, red; swamp laurel *medicinal herb* [see: magnolia]

laurel, spurge; spurge olive *medicinal herb* [see: mezereon]

laureth 4 USAN *surfactant*

laureth 9 USAN *spermaticide; surfactant*

laureth 10S USAN *spermaticide*

lauril INN *combining name for radicals or groups*

laurilsulfate INN *combining name for radicals or groups* [also: sodium lauryl sulfate]

laurixamine INN

laurocapram USAN, INN *excipient*

laurocapram & methotrexate *investigational (orphan) for topical treatment of mycosis fungoides*

lauroguadine INN

laurolinium acetate INN, BAN

lauromacrogol 400 INN

Laurus nobilis medicinal herb [see: laurel]

Laurus persea medicinal herb [see: avocado]

lauryl isoquinolinium bromide USAN *anti-infective*

lavender *(Lavandula spp.)* flowers, leaves, and oil *medicinal herb for acne, bile flow stimulation, diabetes, edema,* *flatulence, hyperactivity, insomnia, intestinal spasms, migraine headache, and stimulating menstrual flow*

lavender oil NF

lavoltidine INN *antiulcerative; histamine H₂-receptor blocker* [also: lavoltidine succinate; loxtidine]

lavoltidine succinate USAN *antiulcerative; histamine H₂-receptor blocker* [also: lavoltidine; loxtidine]

lawrencium *element (Lr)*

Lawsonia inermis medicinal herb [see: henna]

Laxative & Stool Softener softgels OTC *stimulant laxative; stool softener* [casanthranol; docusate sodium] 30• 100 mg

laxatives *a class of agents that promote evacuation of the bowels or have a mild purgative effect; subclasses: saline, stimulant, bulk-producing, emollient, stool-softening, and hyperosmotic* [see also: cathartics; purgatives; various subclasses]

Lax-Pills tablets OTC *stimulant laxative* [sennosides] 15, 25 mg

lazabemide USAN, INN *antiparkinsonian*

lazabemide HCl USAN *investigational treatment for Alzheimer disease*

lazaroids *a class of potent antioxidants that can protect against oxygen radical–mediated lipid peroxidation and progressive neuronal degeneration following brain or spinal trauma, subarachnoid hemorrhage, or stroke* [also called: 21-aminosteroids]

Lazer Creme OTC *moisturizer; emollient* [vitamins A and E] 3333.3• 116.67 U/g

Lazer Formalyde solution ℞ *anhidrotic for hyperhidrosis and bromhidrosis* [formaldehyde] 10%

LazerSporin-C ear drops ℞ *topical corticosteroidal anti-inflammatory; antibiotic* [hydrocortisone; neomycin sulfate; polymyxin B sulfate] 1%•5 mg•10 000 U per mL

LC-65 solution OTC *cleaning solution for hard, soft, or rigid gas permeable contact lenses*

L-Carnitine tablets, capsules OTC *dietary amino acid* [levocarnitine] 500 mg; 250 mg

LCD (liquor carbonis detergens) [see: coal tar]

LCR (leurocristine) [see: vincristine]

LCx *Neisseria gonorrhoeae* Assay reagent kit for professional use *in vitro diagnostic aid for* Neisseria gonorrhoeae

lead *element (Pb)*

lecimibide USAN *hypocholesterolemic; antihyperlipidemic*

lecithin NF *emulsifier; surfactant; natural phospholipid mixture of various phosphatidylcholines used as an antihypercholesterolemic and cognition enhancer for Alzheimer and other dementias* 420, 1200 mg oral

lecithol *natural remedy* [see: lecithin]

LED (liposome-encapsulated doxorubicin) [see: doxorubicin HCl, liposome-encapsulated]

Lederject (trademarked delivery system) *prefilled disposable syringe*

ledoxantrone trihydrochloride USAN *antineoplastic; topoisomerase II inhibitor* [previously: sedoxantrone trihydrochloride]

Ledum groenlandicum; L. latifolium; L. palustre medicinal herb [see: Labrador tea]

leeches (*Hirudo medicinalis*) *natural adjunct to postsurgical wound management*

leek (*Allium porrum*) *bulb, lower stem, and leaves medicinal herb used as an appetite stimulant, decongestant, and diuretic*

Leena tablets (in packs of 28) ℞ *triphasic oral contraceptive* [norethindrone; ethinyl estradiol]
Phase 1 (7 days): 500•35 μg;
Phase 2 (9 days): 1000•35 μg;
Phase 3 (5 days): 500•35 μg

lefetamine INN

leflunomide USAN, INN *anti-inflammatory for rheumatoid arthritis; investigational (orphan) for malignant glioma, ovarian cancer, and prevention of rejection of organ transplants; investi-*

gational (Phase II) for prostate and non–small cell lung cancers; investigational (Phase III) for first relapse glioblastoma multiforme 10, 20 mg oral

Legalon investigational (orphan) antitoxin for Amanita phalloides (mushroom) intoxication [disodium silibinin dihemisuccinate]

Legatrin PM caplets OTC prevention and treatment of nocturnal leg cramps [diphenhydramine HCl; acetaminophen] 50•500 mg

legs, red medicinal herb [see: bistort]

leiopyrrole INN

lemidosul INN

lemon (Citrus limon) fruit and peel medicinal herb used as an astringent, refrigerant, and source of vitamin C

lemon, ground; wild lemon medicinal herb [see: mandrake]

lemon balm (Melissa officinalis) plant medicinal herb used as an antispasmodic and sedative; also used for Graves disease and cold sores

lemon oil NF

lemon verbena (Aloysiatriphylla spp.) leaves and flowers medicinal herb for fever, flatulence, gastrointestinal spasms and other disorders, and sedation

lemon walnut medicinal herb [see: butternut]

lemongrass (Andropogon citratus; Cymbopogon citratus) leaves medicinal herb for colds, cough, fever, gastrointestinal spasm and other disorders, nervousness, pain, and rheumatism; also used as an antiemetic

Lemotussin-DM oral liquid ℞ antitussive; decongestant; antihistamine; expectorant [dextromethorphan hydrobromide; pseudoephedrine HCl; chlorpheniramine maleate; guaifenesin; potassium giaiacolsulfonate] 7.5•10•2•50•50 mg

lenalidomide investigational (NDA filed) immunomodulator for blood transfusions in patients with myelodysplastic syndrome (MDS)

lenampicillin INN

lenercept USAN tumor necrosis factor (TNF) receptor antagonist for septic shock, multiple sclerosis, inflammatory bowel disease, and rheumatoid arthritis

leniquinsin USAN, INN antihypertensive

lenitzol [see: amitriptyline]

lenograstim USAN, INN, BAN immunomodulator; antineutropenic; hematopoietic stimulant

lenperone USAN, INN antipsychotic

Lens Drops solution OTC rewetting solution for hard or soft contact lenses

Lens Lubricant solution OTC rewetting solution for hard or soft contact lenses

Lens Plus Daily Cleaner solution OTC surfactant cleaning solution for soft contact lenses

Lens Plus Oxysept products [see: Oxysept]

Lens Plus Rewetting Drops OTC rewetting solution for soft contact lenses

Lens Plus Sterile Saline aerosol solution OTC rinsing/storage solution for soft contact lenses [sodium chloride (saline solution)]

Lente Iletin II vials for subcu injection OTC antidiabetic [insulin zinc (pork)] 100 U/mL

lentin [see: carbachol]

lentinan JAN investigational (Phase II/III) immunomodulator for HIV and AIDS

Lentinula edodes medicinal herb [see: shiitake mushrooms]

Leontodon taraxacum medicinal herb [see: dandelion]

Leonurus cardiaca medicinal herb [see: motherwort]

leopard's bane medicinal herb [see: arnica]

Lepidium meyenii medicinal herb [see: maca]

lepirudin anticoagulant for heparin-associated thrombocytopenia (HAT) (orphan)

leprostatics a class of drugs effective against leprosy

leptacline INN

leptandra; purple leptandra medicinal herb [see: Culver root]

lercanidipine *investigational calcium channel blocker*

lergotrile USAN, INN *prolactin enzyme inhibitor*

lergotrile mesylate USAN *prolactin enzyme inhibitor*

leridistim USAN *interleukin-3 and granulocyte colony-stimulating factor receptor agonist for chemotherapy-induced neutropenia and thrombocytopenia*

Lescol capsules R HMG-CoA reductase inhibitor for hypercholesterolemia, hypertriglyceridemia, and atherosclerosis [fluvastatin sodium] 20, 40 mg

Lescol XL film-coated extended-release tablets R HMG-CoA reductase inhibitor for hypercholesterolemia, hypertriglyceridemia, and atherosclerosis [fluvastatin sodium] 80 mg

lesopitron INN *investigational anxiolytic*

lesser centaury *medicinal herb* [see: centaury]

Lessina film-coated tablets (in packs of 21 or 28) R *monophasic oral contraceptive; emergency postcoital contraceptive* [levonorgestrel; ethinyl estradiol] 0.1 mg•20 μg

leteprinim potassium USAN *investigational (Phase II) nerve growth factor for Alzheimer disease, spinal cord injury, and stroke*

letimide INN *analgesic* [also: letimide HCl]

letimide HCl USAN *analgesic* [also: letimide]

letosteine INN

letrazuril INN *investigational (Phase II) treatment for AIDS-related cryptosporidial diarrhea*

letrozole USAN, INN *aromatase inhibitor; estrogen antagonist; antineoplastic for early, advanced, or metastatic breast cancer in postmenopausal women*

lettuce (Lactuca sativa) *juice and leaves medicinal herb used as an anodyne, antispasmodic, expectorant, and sedative (for herbal medical use, common garden lettuce is harvested after it has gone to seed, and a milky juice is extracted)*

Leucanthemum parthenium *medicinal herb* [see: feverfew]

leucarsone [see: carbarsone]

leucine (L-leucine) USAN, USP, INN, JAN *essential amino acid; symbols: Leu, L*

leucine & isoleucine & valine *investigational (orphan) for hyperphenylalaninemia*

leucinocaine INN

leucocianidol INN

leucomycin [see: kitasamycin; spiramycin]

L-leucovorin *chemotherapy "rescue" agent (orphan)*

leucovorin calcium USP *antianemic; folate replenisher; antidote to folic acid antagonist; chemotherapy "rescue" agent (orphan)* [also: calcium folinate] 5, 15, 25 mg oral; 3, 10 mg injection; 50, 100, 350 mg/vial injection

leucovorin & fluorouracil *antineoplastic for metastatic colorectal cancer (orphan)*

leucovorin & methotrexate *antineoplastic for osteosarcoma (orphan)*

Leukeran film-coated tablets R *nitrogen mustard-type alkylating antineoplastic for multiple leukemias, lymphomas, and neoplasms* [chlorambucil] 2 mg

Leukine IV infusion R *myeloid reconstitution after autologous bone marrow transplant (orphan); investigational (Phase III) cytokine for HIV infection* [sargramostim] 250, 500 μg

leukocyte interferon [now: interferon alfa-n3]

leukocyte typing serum USP *in vitro blood test*

leukopoietin [see: sargramostim]

LeukoScan *investigational (Phase III) diagnostic aid for osteomyelitis; investigational (NDA filed) diagnostic aid for infectious lesions* [technetium Tc 99m sulesomab]

leukotriene receptor antagonists (LTRAs); leukotriene receptor inhibitors *a class of antiasthmatics that inhibit bronchoconstriction when* *used prophylactically (will not reverse bronchospasm)*

leupeptin *investigational (orphan) aid to microsurgical peripheral nerve repair*

leuprolide acetate USAN *testosterone suppressant; antihormonal antineoplastic for various cancers; LHRH agonist for central precocious puberty (orphan)* [also: leuprorelin] 5 mg/mL injection

leuprorelin INN, BAN *testosterone suppressant; antihormonal antineoplastic for various cancers* [also: leuprolide acetate]

leurocristine (LCR) [see: vincristine]

leurocristine sulfate [see: vincristine sulfate]

Leustatin IV infusion ℞ *antineoplastic for hairy-cell leukemia (orphan); investigational (orphan) for chronic lymphocytic leukemia, myeloid leukemia, multiple sclerosis, and non-Hodgkin lymphoma* [cladribine] 1 mg/mL

Leuvectin ℞ *investigational (Phase I/II, orphan) gene-based therapy for advanced metastatic renal cell carcinoma*

Levacet caplets OTC *analgesic; antihistaminic sleep aid* [aspirin; acetaminophen; salicylamide; phenyltoloxamine citrate; caffeine] 400•400•150•50•40 mg

levacetylmethadol INN *narcotic analgesic* [also: levomethadyl acetate]

levalbuterol *sympathomimetic bronchodilator; single-isomer albuterol*

levalbuterol HCl USAN *sympathomimetic bronchodilator; single-isomer albuterol*

levalbuterol sulfate USAN *sympathomimetic bronchodilator; single-isomer albuterol*

Levall 5.0 oral liquid ℞ *narcotic antitussive; decongestant; expectorant* [hydrocodone bitartrate; phenylephrine HCl; guaifenesin] 5•15•100 mg/5 mL

levallorphan INN, BAN [also: levallorphan tartrate] ② levorphanol

levallorphan tartrate USP [also: levallorphan]

levamfetamine INN *anorectic* [also: levamfetamine succinate; levamphetamine]

levamfetamine succinate USAN *anorectic* [also: levamfetamine; levamphetamine]

levamisole INN, BAN *biological response modifier; antineoplastic; veterinary anthelmintic* [also: levamisole HCl]

levamisole HCl USAN, USP *biological response modifier; antineoplastic; veterinary anthelmintic* [also: levamisole]

levamphetamine BAN *anorectic* [also: levamfetamine succinate; levamfetamine]

levant berry (Anamirta cocculus; A. paniculata) leaves and berries *medicinal herb for epilepsy, lice, malaria, morphine poisoning, and worms; not generally regarded as safe and effective for ingestion or topical application on abraded skin*

Levaquin film-coated tablets, oral solution, IV infusion ℞ *broad-spectrum fluoroquinolone antibiotic* [levofloxacin] 250, 500, 750 mg; 25 mg/mL; 250, 500, 750 mg

levarterenol [see: norepinephrine bitartrate]

levarterenol bitartrate [now: norepinephrine bitartrate]

Levatol tablets ℞ *antihypertensive; β-blocker* [penbutolol sulfate] 20 mg

Levbid extended-release tablets ℞ *GI/GU antispasmodic; antiparkinsonian; anticholinergic "drying agent" for allergic rhinitis or hyperhidrosis* [hyoscyamine sulfate] 0.375 mg

levcromakalim USAN, INN, BAN *antiasthmatic; antihypertensive*

levcycloserine USAN, INN *enzyme inhibitor*

levdobutamine INN *cardiotonic* [also: levdobutamine lactobionate]

levdobutamine lactobionate USAN *cardiotonic* [also: levdobutamine]

levdropropizine INN

Levemir subcu injection ℞ *antidiabetic; long-acting insulin formulation intended to provide continuous basal* *insulin levels through once- or twice-daily dosing* [insulin detemir]

levemopamil INN *investigational treatment for stroke*

levetiracetam USAN, INN *anticonvulsant for partial-onset seizures*

levisoprenaline INN

Levisticum officinale *medicinal herb* [see: lovage]

Levitra film-coated tablets ℞ *phosphodiesterase type 5 (PDE5) inhibitor; selective vasodilator for erectile dysfunction (ED)* [vardenafil HCl] 2.5, 5, 10, 20 mg

Levlen tablets (in Slidecases of 28) ℞ *monophasic oral contraceptive; emergency postcoital contraceptive* [levonorgestrel; ethinyl estradiol] 0.15 mg•30 μg

Levlite tablets (in Slidecases of 28) ℞ *monophasic oral contraceptive* [levonorgestrel; ethinyl estradiol] 0.1 mg•20 μg

levlofexidine INN

levmetamfetamine USAN, USP *nasal decongestant*

levobetaxolol INN *topical antiglaucoma agent (β-blocker)* [also: levobetaxolol HCl]

levobetaxolol HCl USAN *topical antiglaucoma agent (β-blocker)* [also: levobetaxolol]

levobunolol INN, BAN *topical antiglaucoma agent (β-blocker)* [also: levobunolol HCl]

levobunolol HCl USAN, USP *topical antiglaucoma agent (β-blocker)* [also: levobunolol] 0.25%, 0.5% eye drops

levobupivacaine HCl USAN *long-acting local anesthetic*

levocabastine INN, BAN *antihistamine* [also: levocabastine HCl]

levocabastine HCl USAN *antihistamine* [also: levocabastine]

levocarbinoxamine tartrate [see: rotoxamine tartrate]

levocarnitine USAN, USP, INN *dietary amino acid for primary and secondary genetic carnitine deficiency (orphan) and end-stage renal disease (orphan);* *investigational (orphan) for pediatric cardiomyopathy* 100, 300 mg/mL oral; 200 mg/mL injection

levocetirizine *investigational second-generation piperazine antihistamine for allergic rhinitis; isomer of cetirizine*

levodopa USAN, USP, INN, BAN, JAN *antiparkinsonian; dopamine precursor* ② methyldopa

levodopa & carbidopa *antiparkinsonian; dopamine precursor plus synergist* 100•10, 100•25, 200•50, 250•25 mg oral

Levo-Dromoran tablets; IV, IM, or subcu injection ℞ *narcotic analgesic* [levorphanol tartrate] 2 mg; 2 mg/mL

levofacetoperane INN

levofenfluramine INN

levofloxacin USAN, INN, JAN *broad-spectrum fluoroquinolone antibiotic* 750 mg oral

levofuraltadone USAN, INN *antibacterial; antiprotozoal*

levoglutamide INN, DCF [now: glutamine]

Levolet tablets ℞ *synthetic thyroid hormone (T_4 fraction only)* [levothyroxine sodium]

levoleucovorin calcium USAN *antidote to folic acid antagonists*

levomenol INN

levomepate [see: atromepine]

levomepromazine INN *analgesic* [also: methotrimeprazine]

levomethadone INN

levomethadyl acetate USAN *narcotic analgesic* [also: levacetylmethadol]

levomethadyl acetate HCl USAN *narcotic analgesic for management of opiate addiction (orphan)*

levomethorphan INN, BAN

levometiomeprazine INN

levomoprolol INN

levomoramide INN, BAN

levonantradol INN, BAN *analgesic* [also: levonantradol HCl]

levonantradol HCl USAN *analgesic* [also: levonantradol]

levonordefrin USP *adrenergic; vasoconstrictor* [also: corbadrine]

levonorgestrel USAN, USP, INN, BAN *progestin; contraceptive implant; emergency "morning after" oral contraceptive*

Levophed IV infusion ℞ *vasopressor for acute hypotensive shock* [norepinephrine bitartrate] 1 mg/mL

levophenacylmorphan INN, BAN

Levoprome IM injection (discontinued 2003) ℞ *central analgesic; CNS depressant* [methotrimeprazine HCl] 20 mg/mL

levopropicillin INN *antibacterial* [also: levopropylcillin potassium]

levopropicillin potassium [see: levopropylcillin potassium]

levopropoxyphene INN, BAN *antitussive* [also: levopropoxyphene napsylate]

levopropoxyphene napsylate USAN *antitussive* [also: levopropoxyphene]

levopropylcillin potassium USAN *antibacterial* [also: levopropicillin]

levopropylhexedrine INN

levoprotiline INN

Levora tablets (packs of 28) ℞ *monophasic oral contraceptive* [levonorgestrel; ethinyl estradiol] 0.15 mg•30 µg

levorin INN

levorphanol INN, BAN *narcotic analgesic* [also: levorphanol tartrate] ⑨ levallorphan

levorphanol tartrate USP *narcotic analgesic* [also: levorphanol] 2 mg oral

levosimendan USAN *investigational (Phase III) calcium sensitizer and vasodilator for decompensated heart failure*

Levo-T tablets (discontinued 2003) ℞ *synthetic thyroid hormone (T₄ fraction only)* [levothyroxine sodium] 25, 50, 75, 100, 125, 150, 200, 300 µg

Levothroid ⒸⒶⓃ tablets ℞ *synthetic thyroid hormone (T₄ fraction only)* [levothyroxine sodium] 25, 50, 75, 100, 112, 125, 150, 175, 200, 300 µg

Levothroid caplets, powder for injection ℞ *synthetic thyroid hormone (T₄ fraction only)* [levothyroxine sodium] 25, 50, 75, 88, 100, 112, 125, 150, 175, 200, 300 µg; 200 µg

levothyroxine sodium USP, INN *synthetic thyroid hormone (T₄ fraction only)* [also: thyroxine] 25, 50, 75, 88, 100, 112, 125, 137, 150, 175, 200, 300 µg oral; 200, 500 µg injection ⑨ liothyronine

levothyroxine sodium & tiratricol *investigational (orphan) to suppress thyroid-stimulating hormone (TSH) in thyroid cancer*

Levovist ⒸⒶⓃ powder for IV injection ℞ *ultrasound contrast medium for echocardiography* [galactose; palmitic acid]

levoxadrol INN *local anesthetic; smooth muscle relaxant* [also: levoxadrol HCl]

levoxadrol HCl USAN *local anesthetic; smooth muscle relaxant* [also: levoxadrol]

Levoxyl tablets ℞ *synthetic thyroid hormone (T₄ fraction only)* [levothyroxine sodium] 25, 50, 75, 88, 100, 112, 125, 137, 150, 175, 200, 300 µg

Levsin IV, IM, or subcu injection ℞ *GI/GU antispasmodic to reduce motility during radiologic imaging; preoperative antimuscarinic to reduce salivary and gastric secretions* [hyoscyamine sulfate] 0.5 mg/mL

Levsin tablets, drops, elixir ℞ *GI/GU antispasmodic; antiparkinsonian; anticholinergic "drying agent" for allergic rhinitis and hyperhidrosis* [hyoscyamine sulfate] 0.125 mg; 0.125 mg/mL; 0.125 mg/5 mL

Levsin PB drops ℞ *GI/GU antispasmodic; anticholinergic; sedative* [hyoscyamine sulfate; phenobarbital; alcohol 5%] 0.125•15 mg/mL

Levsin with Phenobarbital tablets ℞ *GI/GU antispasmodic; anticholinergic; sedative* [hyoscyamine sulfate; phenobarbital] 0.125•15 mg

Levsinex Timecaps (timed-release capsules) ℞ *GI/GU antispasmodic; antiparkinsonian; anticholinergic "drying agent" for allergic rhinitis or hyperhidrosis* [hyoscyamine sulfate] 0.375 mg

Levsin/SL sublingual tablets (also may be chewed or swallowed) ℞ *GI/GU*

antispasmodic; anticholinergic [hyoscyamine sulfate] 0.125 mg

Levulan Kerastick topical solution Ɍ *photosensitizer for photodynamic therapy of precancerous actinic keratoses of the face and scalp (for use with the BLU-U Blue Light Photodynamic Therapy Illuminator)* [aminolevulinic acid HCl] 20%

levulose BAN *nutrient; caloric replacement* [also: fructose]

Lexapro film-coated tablets, oral solution Ɍ *selective serotonin reuptake inhibitor (SSRI) for major depression and generalized anxiety disorder* [escitalopram oxalate] 5, 10, 20 mg; 5 mg/5 mL

lexipafant USAN *platelet activating factor (PAF) antagonist; investigational (Phase III) treatment for acute pancreatitis*

lexithromycin USAN, INN *antibacterial*

Lexiva film-coated caplets Ɍ *antiretroviral; HIV-1 protease inhibitor* [fosamprenavir calcium] 700 mg (=600 mg base)

lexofenac INN

Lexxel film-coated dual-release tablets Ɍ *antihypertensive; angiotensin-converting enzyme (ACE) inhibitor; calcium channel blocker* [enalapril maleate (immediate release); felodipine (extended release)] 5•5, 5•2.5 mg

LH-RF (luteinizing hormone–releasing factor) acetate hydrate [see: gonadorelin acetate]

LH-RF diacetate tetrahydrate [now: gonadorelin acetate]

LH-RF dihydrochloride [now: gonadorelin HCl]

LH-RF HCl [see: gonadorelin HCl]

LH-RH (luteinizing hormone–releasing hormone) *an endogenous hormone, produced in the hypothalamus, which stimulates the release of luteinizing hormone (LH) and follicle-stimulating hormone (FSH) from the pituitary* [also known as: gonadotropin-releasing hormone (Gn-RH)]

liarozole INN, BAN *antipsoriatic; aromatase inhibitor* [also: liarozole fumarate]

liarozole fumarate USAN *antipsoriatic; aromatase inhibitor; investigational (orphan) for congenital ichthyosis* [also: liarozole]

liarozole HCl USAN *antineoplastic for prostate cancer; aromatase inhibitor*

liatermin USAN *dopaminergic neuronal growth stimulator for Parkinson disease*

Liatris scariosa; L. spicata; L. squarrosa *medicinal herb* [see: blazing star]

libecillide INN

libenzapril USAN, INN *angiotensin-converting enzyme (ACE) inhibitor*

Librax capsules Ɍ *GI anticholinergic; anxiolytic* [methscopolamine nitrate; chlordiazepoxide HCl] 2.5•5 mg

Librel tablets Ɍ *investigational (Phase III) continuous-use oral contraceptive* [levonorgestrel; ethinyl estradiol]

Libritabs film-coated tablets (discontinued 2003) Ɍ *benzodiazepine anxiolytic; sedative* [chlordiazepoxide] 10, 25 mg

Librium capsules, powder for injection Ɍ *benzodiazepine anxiolytic; sedative; alcohol withdrawal aid; sometimes abused as a street drug* [chlordiazepoxide HCl] 5, 10, 25 mg; 100 mg

Lice-Enz foam shampoo (discontinued 2003) OTC *pediculicide for lice* [pyrethrins; piperonyl butoxide] 0.3%•3%

licofelone *investigational (Phase III) analgesic/antiarthritic/nonsteroidal anti-inflammatory drug (NSAID) with low gastric side effects*

licorice (Glycyrrhiza glabra; G. pallidiflora; G. uralensis) *root medicinal herb for Addison disease, blood cleansing, colds, cough, drug withdrawal, female disorders, hoarseness, hypoglycemia, lung disorders, sore throat, and stomach ulcers; also used as an expectorant and to increase energy*

licostinel USAN *investigational (Phase I) NMDA receptor antagonist for stroke*

licryfilcon A USAN *hydrophilic contact lens material*

licryfilcon B USAN *hydrophilic contact lens material*

Lid Wipes-SPF solution, pads (discontinued 2003) OTC *eyelid cleansing wipes for blepharitis or contact lenses*

LidaMantle cream ℞ *local anesthetic* [lidocaine HCl] 3%

LidaMantle HC cream ℞ *corticosteroidal anti-inflammatory; local anesthetic* [hydrocortisone acetate; lidocaine] 0.5%•3%

lidamidine INN *antiperistaltic* [also: lidamidine HCl]

lidamidine HCl USAN *antiperistaltic* [also: lidamidine]

Lidex cream, ointment, topical solution ℞ *topical corticosteroidal anti-inflammatory* [fluocinonide] 0.05% 🔁 Lasix; Lidox; Wydase

Lidex-E cream ℞ *corticosteroidal anti-inflammatory; emollient* [fluocinonide] 0.05%

lidimycin INN *antifungal* [also: lydimycin]

lidocaine USP, INN *topical local anesthetic; investigational (orphan) transdermal delivery for post-herpetic neuralgia* [also: lignocaine]

lidocaine benzyl benzoate [see: denatonium benzoate]

lidocaine HCl USP *local anesthetic; antiarrhythmic for acute ventricular arrhythmias* [also: lignocaine HCl] 2%, 3%, 4%, 5% topical; 1%, 2% IV injection; 4%, 10%, 20% IV admixture

lidocaine HCl in dextrose *injectable local anesthetic for obstetric use; IV infusion for acute ventricular arrhythmias* 1.5%•7.5%, 5%•7.5% injection; 0.2%, 0.4%, 0.8% infusion

lidocaine HCl & epinephrine *injectable local anesthetic; vasoconstrictor* 0.5%•1:200 000, 1%•1:100 000, 1%•1:200 000, 1.5%•1:200 000, 2%•1:50 000, 2%•1:100 000, 2%•1:200 000 injection

lidocaine HCl & hydrocortisone acetate *local anesthetic; corticosteroidal anti-inflammatory* 0.5%•3% topical

lidocaine & prilocaine *local anesthetic* 2.5%•2.5% topical

Lidocaine/Hydrocortisone Rectal cream in prefilled applicator ℞ *corticosteroidal anti-inflammatory; local anesthetic* [hydrocortisone acetate; lidocaine HCl] 0.5%•3%

Lidoderm transdermal patch ℞ *local anesthetic for post-herpetic neuralgia (orphan)* [lidocaine] 5%

lidofenin USAN, INN *hepatic function test*

lidofilcon A USAN *hydrophilic contact lens material*

lidofilcon B USAN *hydrophilic contact lens material*

lidoflazine USAN, INN, BAN *coronary vasodilator*

Lidoject-1; Lidoject-2 injection (discontinued 2002) ℞ *injectable local anesthetic* [lidocaine HCl] 1%; 2%

LidoPen auto-injector (automatic IM injection device) ℞ *emergency injection for cardiac arrhythmias* [lidocaine HCl] 300 mg/3 mL dose

Lidosense 4 cream OTC *local anesthetic* [lidocaine] 4%

Lidosite Topical System transdermal patch ℞ *local anesthetic* [lidocaine HCl; epinephrine] 10%•0.1%

LID-Pack ⓒⒶⓃ ophthalmic ointment + towelettes OTC *antibiotic* [polymyxin B sulfate; bacitracin zinc] 10 000• 500 U/g

lifarizine USAN, INN, BAN *platelet aggregation inhibitor*

life everlasting *medicinal herb* [see: everlasting]

Life Extension Booster; Life Extension Super Booster softgels OTC *vitamin/mineral supplement* [multiple vitamins & minerals]

Life Extension Herbal Mix powder for oral solution OTC *dietary supplement*

Life Extension Mix; Life Extension Mix with Niacin; Life Extension Mix without Copper caplets, capsules, powder for oral solution OTC *vitamin/mineral supplement* [multiple vitamins & minerals]

Life Extension Two-Per-Day tablets OTC *vitamin/mineral supplement* [multiple vitamins & minerals]

life root (Senecio aureus; S. jacoboea; S. vulgaris) *medicinal herb for childbirth pain, diaphoresis, edema, fever, and stimulation of labor and menses; not generally regarded as safe and effective for ingestion because of hepatotoxicity*

LifeCare bags (packaging form) *premixed IV infusion bags*

life-of-man *medicinal herb* [see: spikenard]

lifibrate USAN, INN *antihyperlipoproteinemic*

lifibrol USAN, INN *antihyperlipidemic*

LIG (lymphocyte immune globulin) [q.v.]

light mineral oil [see: mineral oil, light]

lignocaine BAN *topical local anesthetic* [also: lidocaine]

lignocaine HCl BAN *local anesthetic; antiarrhythmic* [also: lidocaine HCl]

lignosulfonic acid, sodium salt [see: polignate sodium]

lilopristone INN

lily, conval; May lily *medicinal herb* [see: lily of the valley]

lily, ground *medicinal herb* [see: birthroot]

lily, white pond; sweet water lily; sweet-scented pond lily; sweet-scented water lily; white water lily; toad lily *medicinal herb* [see: white pond lily]

lily of the valley (Convallaria majalis) *flower, leaves, and rhizome medicinal herb for arrhythmias, edema, epilepsy, and heart disorders*

limaprost INN

limarsol [see: acetarsone]

Limbitrol DS 10·25 tablets ℞ *antidepressant; anxiolytic* [chlordiazepoxide; amitriptyline HCl] 10•25 mg

Limbrel capsules ℞ *natural COX-2 inhibitor; analgesic and anti-inflammatory for the dietary management of osteoarthritis* [flavocoxid] 250 mg

lime USP *pharmaceutic necessity*

lime, sulfurated (calcium polysulfide, calcium thiosulfate) USP *wet dressing/soak for cystic acne and seborrhea*

lime tree *medicinal herb* [see: linden tree]

Lin-Amox ⓒ capsules, oral suspension ℞ *antibiotic* [amoxicillin trihydrate] 250, 500 mg; 125, 250 mg/5 mL

linarotene USAN, INN *antikeratinizing agent*

Lin-Buspirone ⓒ tablets ℞ *azaspirone anxiolytic* [buspirone HCl] 10 mg

Lincocin capsules, IV or IM injection ℞ *lincosamide antibiotic* [lincomycin HCl] 500 mg; 300 mg/mL ⚹ Cleocin; Indocin

lincomycin USAN, INN, BAN *lincosamide antibiotic*

lincomycin HCl USP *lincosamide antibiotic* 300 mg/mL injection

Lincorex IV or IM injection ℞ *lincosamide antibiotic* [lincomycin HCl] 300 mg/mL

lincosamides *a class of antimicrobial antibiotics with potentially serious side effects, to which bacterial resistance has been shown*

lindane USAN, USP, INN, BAN *pediculicide for lice; scabicide* 1% topical

linden tree (Tilia americana; T. cordata; T. europaea; T. platyphyllos) *flowers medicinal herb for diaphoresis, diarrhea, headache, hypertension, indigestion, nasal congestion, nervousness, skin moisturizer, stomach disorders, and throat irritation*

linezolid USAN *oxazolidinone antibiotic for gram-positive bacterial infections*

Linguets (trademarked form) *buccal tablets*

Linker protocol (daunorubicin, vincristine, prednisone, asparaginase, teniposide, cytarabine, methotrexate [with leucovorin rescue]) *chemotherapy protocol for acute lymphocytic leukemia (ALL)*

Lin-Megestrol ⓒ tablets ℞ *progestin; hormonal antineoplastic for advanced carcinoma of the breast or endometrium* [megestrol acetate] 40, 160 mg

linogliride USAN, INN *antidiabetic*

linogliride fumarate USAN *antidiabetic*

linolexamide [see: clinolamide]

linopiridine USAN, INN *cognition enhancer for Alzheimer disease*

Lin-Pravastatin Ⓒᴬᴺ *tablets* ℞ *HMG-CoA reductase inhibitor for hyperlipidemia and hypertriglyceridemia* [pravastatin sodium] 10, 20, 40 mg

linseed *medicinal herb* [see: flaxseed]

linsidomine INN

lint bells *medicinal herb* [see: flaxseed]

lintopride INN

Linum usitatissimum *medicinal herb* [see: flaxseed]

lion's ear; lion's tail *medicinal herb* [see: motherwort]

lion's tooth *medicinal herb* [see: dandelion]

Lioresal *caplets* ℞ *skeletal muscle relaxant* [baclofen] 10, 20 mg

Lioresal *intrathecal injection* ℞ *skeletal muscle relaxant for intractable spasticity due to spinal cord injury or disease (orphan); investigational (orphan) for dystonia* [baclofen] 0.05 mg/0.5 mL (50 μg/mL), 10 mg/20 mL (500 μg/mL), 10 mg/5 mL (2000 μg/mL)

liothyronine INN, BAN *radioactive agent* [also: liothyronine I 125] 🔁 levothyroxine

liothyronine I 125 USAN *radioactive agent* [also: liothyronine]

liothyronine I 131 USAN *radioactive agent*

liothyronine sodium USP, BAN *synthetic thyroid hormone (T₃ fraction only); treatment of myxedema coma or precoma (orphan)*

liotrix USAN, USP *synthetic thyroid hormone (a 4:1 mixture of T₄ and T₃)* 🔁 Klotrix

Lip Medex *ointment* OTC *topical antipruritic/counterirritant; mild local anesthetic* [camphor; phenol] 1%•0.54%

lipancreatin [see: pancrelipase]

lipase *digestive enzyme (digests fats)* [24 IU/mg in pancrelipase; 2 IU/mg in pancreatin]

lipase of pancreas [see: pancrelipase]

lipase triacylglycerol [see: pancrelipase]

Lipidil Supra Ⓒᴬᴺ *film-coated tables* ℞ *antihyperlipidemic for hypercholesterol-*

emia and hypertriglyceridemia [fenofibrate] 100, 160 mg

Lipil [see: Enfamil LIPIL; LactoFree LIPIL; ProSobee LIPIL]

Lipisorb *powder* OTC *enteral nutritional therapy* [lactose-free formula]

Lipitor *film-coated tablets* ℞ *HMG-CoA reductase inhibitor for hypercholesterolemia, dysbetalipoproteinemia, and hypertriglyceridemia; prevention of cardiovascular disease in high-risk patients* [atorvastatin calcium] 10, 20, 40, 80 mg

Lipoflavonoid *capsules* OTC *dietary lipotropic with vitamin supplementation* [choline; inositol; multiple B vitamins; vitamin C; lemon bioflavonoids] 111.3•111.3•≛•100•100 mg

Lipogen *capsules, caplets* OTC *dietary lipotropic with vitamin supplementation* [choline; inositol; multiple vitamins] 111•111•≛ mg

α-lipoic acid; lipoicin *natural antioxidant* [see: alpha lipoic acid]

Lipomul *oral liquid* OTC *dietary fat supplement* [corn oil] 10 g/15 mL

Liponol *capsules* OTC *dietary lipotropic with vitamin supplementation* [choline; inositol; methionine; multiple B vitamins] 115•83•110•≛ mg

lipopeptides [see: cyclic lipopeptides]

lipoprotein OspA, recombinant *(discontinued 2002) active immunizing agent against Lyme disease*

lipoprotein-associated coagulation inhibitor (LACI) [see: tifacogin]

liposomal gentamicin [see: gentamicin liposome]

liposome-encapsulated doxorubicin HCl (LED) [see: doxorubicin HCl, liposome-encapsulated]

liposome-encapsulated recombinant interleukin-2 [see: interleukin-2, liposome-encapsulated recombinant]

liposome-encapsulated T4 endonuclease V [see: T4 endonuclease V, liposome encapsulated]

Liposyn II 10%; Liposyn II 20%; Liposyn III 10%; Liposyn III

20% IV infusion ℞ *nutritional therapy* [fat emulsion]

Lipotriad caplets OTC *dietary lipotropic with vitamin supplementation* [choline; inositol; multiple vitamins] 111•⁑• ⁑ mg

lipotropics *a class of oral nutritional supplements*

Lipram 4500 delayed-release capsules containing enteric-coated microspheres ℞ *porcine-derived digestive enzymes* [lipase; protease; amylase] 4500•25 000•20 000 USP units

Lipram-CR5; Lipram-CR10; Lipram-CR20 delayed-release capsules containing enteric-coated microspheres ℞ *porcine-derived digestive enzymes* [lipase; protease; amylase] 5000•18 750•16 600 USP units; 10 000•37 500•33 200 USP units; 20 000•75 000•66 400 USP units

Lipram-PN10; Lipram-PN16; Lipram-PN20 delayed-release capsules containing enteric-coated microspheres ℞ *porcine-derived digestive enzymes* [lipase; protease; amylase] 10 000•30 000•30 000 USP units; 16 000•48 000•48 000 USP units; 20 000•44 000•56 000 USP units

Lipram-UL12; Lipram-UL18; Lipram-UL20 delayed-release capsules containing enteric-coated microspheres ℞ *porcine-derived digestive enzymes* [lipase; protease; amylase] 12 000•39 000•39 000 USP units; 18 000•58 500•58 500 USP units; 20 000•65 000•65 000 USP units

liquefied phenol [see: phenol, liquefied]

Liquibid sustained-release tablet ℞ *expectorant* [guaifenesin] 400 mg

Liquibid 1200 sustained-release tablet (discontinued 2004) ℞ *expectorant* [guaifenesin] 1200 mg

Liquibid-D; Liquibid-D 1200 sustained-release tablets ℞ *decongestant; expectorant* [phenylephrine HCl; guaifenesin] 40•600 mg; 40•1200 mg

Liquibid-PD sustained-release tablets ℞ *decongestant; expectorant* [phenylephrine HCl; guaifenesin] 25•275 mg

LiquiCaps (dosage form) *soft liquid-filled gelcaps*

Liqui-Char oral liquid OTC *adsorbent antidote for poisoning* [activated charcoal] 12.5 g/60 mL, 15 g/75 mL, 25 g/120 mL, 30 g/120 mL, 50 g/240 mL

Liqui-Coat HD concentrated oral suspension ℞ *radiopaque contrast medium for gastrointestinal imaging* [barium sulfate] 210%

Liquid Caps (dosage form) *soft liquid-filled gelcaps*

liquid glucose [see: glucose, liquid]

liquid petrolatum [see: mineral oil]

Liquid Pred syrup ℞ *corticosteroid; anti-inflammatory* [prednisone; alcohol 5%] 5 mg/5 mL

Liquid Tabs (dosage form) *liquid-filled tablets*

Liquidambar orientalis; L. styraciflua *medicinal herb* [see: storax]

Liqui-Doss emulsion OTC *emollient laxative* [mineral oil]

Liquifilm Tears; Liquifilm Forte eye drops OTC *ophthalmic moisturizer/lubricant* [polyvinyl alcohol] 1.4%; 3%

Liquifilm Wetting solution OTC *wetting solution for hard contact lenses*

Liqui-Gels (trademarked dosage form) *soft liquid-filled gelcaps*

Liqui-Histine DM syrup (discontinued 2002) ℞ *antitussive; decongestant; antihistamine* [dextromethorphan hydrobromide; phenylpropanolamine HCl; brompheniramine maleate] 10•12.5•2 mg/5 mL

Liqui-Histine-D elixir (discontinued 2001) ℞ *decongestant; antihistamine* [phenylpropanolamine HCl; phenyltoloxamine citrate; pyrilamine maleate; pheniramine maleate] 12.5•4•4•4 mg/5 mL

Liquimat lotion OTC *antibacterial and exfoliant for acne* [sulfur] 4%

Liquiprin Drops for Children OTC *analgesic; antipyretic* [acetaminophen] 80 mg/1.66 mL

Liquitab (trademarked dosage form) *chewable tablet*

liquor carbonis detergens (LCD) [see: coal tar]

liroldine INN

lisadimate USAN, INN *sunscreen*

lisinopril USAN, INN, BAN *antihypertensive; angiotensin-converting enzyme (ACE) inhibitor; adjunctive treatment for CHF* 2.5, 5, 10, 20, 30, 40 mg oral

lisinopril & hydrochlorothiazide *antihypertensive; angiotensin-converting enzyme (ACE) inhibitor; diuretic* 10•12.5, 20•12.5, 20•25 mg oral

lisofylline (LSF) USAN *acetyltransferase inhibitor; investigational (Phase III) immunomodulator and cytokine inhibitor for acute myeloid leukemia and bone marrow transplants; investigational agent for prevention of GI tract damage during chemotherapy; investigational (Phase II/III) for ARDS and acute lung injury*

Listerine; Cool-Mint Listerine; FreshBurst Listerine; Natural Citrus Listerine; Tartar Control Listerine mouthwash/gargle OTC *topical oral antiseptic; analgesic* [thymol; eucalyptol; methyl salicylate; menthol; alcohol 22%–26%] 0.06%•0.09%•0.06%•0.04%

Listermint Arctic Mint mouthwash/gargle OTC

lisuride INN [also: lysuride]

Lithane ⓒᴬⁿ capsules ℞ *antipsychotic for manic episodes* [lithium carbonate] 150, 300 mg

lithium *element (Li)*

lithium benzoate NF

lithium carbonate USAN, USP *antimanic; immunity booster in chemotherapy and AIDS* 150, 300, 450, 600 mg oral

lithium citrate USP *antimanic; immunity booster in chemotherapy and AIDS* 300 mg/5 mL oral

lithium hydroxide USP *antimanic*

lithium hydroxide monohydrate [see: lithium hydroxide]

lithium salicylate NF

Lithobid slow-release tablets ℞ *antipsychotic for manic episodes* [lithium carbonate] 300 mg

litholytics *a class of agents that dissolve stones or calculi* [see also: antilithics]

Lithonate capsules ℞ *antipsychotic for manic episodes* [lithium carbonate] 300 mg

Lithostat tablets ℞ *adjunctive therapy in chronic urea-splitting urinary tract infections* [acetohydroxamic acid] 250 mg

Lithotabs film-coated tablets ℞ *antipsychotic for manic episodes* [lithium carbonate] 300 mg

litracen INN

Little Colds Cough Formula oral drops OTC *antitussive* [dextromethorphan hydrobromide] 7.5 mg/mL

Little Colds for Infants and Children oral drops OTC *nasal decongestant* [phenylephrine HCl] 0.25%

Little Noses Gentle Formula, Infants and Children nose drops OTC *nasal decongestant* [phenylephrine HCl] 0.125%

Little Tummys Laxative oral drops OTC *stimulant laxative* [sennosides] 8.8 mg/mL

liver, desiccated; liver extracts *source of vitamin B_{12}*

Liver Combo No. 5 IM injection (discontinued 2004) ℞ *hematinic; vitamin B supplement* [liver extracts; vitamin B_{12}; folic acid] 10 μg•100 μg•0.4 mg per mL

liver derivative complex *claimed to be an anti-inflammatory for various dermatological conditions*

liver lily *medicinal herb* [see: blue flag]

liverleaf; liverwort *medicinal herb* [see: hepatica]

Livial (approved in Europe, Asia, and South America) ℞ *investigational (NDA filed) synthetic steroid for osteoporosis and other postmenopausal symptoms* [tibolone]

lividomycin INN

Livitrinsic-f capsules ℞ *hematinic* [ferrous fumarate; cyanocobalamin; ascorbic acid; intrinsic factor con-

centrate; folic acid] 110 mg•15 μg•
75 mg•240 mg•0.5 mg

Livostin eye drop suspension (discontinued 2005) ℞ *antihistamine for allergic conjunctivitis* [levocabastine HCl] 0.05%

Livostin ⒸⒶⓃ nasal spray ℞ *antihistamine for seasonal allergic rhinitis* [levocabastine HCl] 0.05%

lixazinone sulfate USAN *cardiotonic; phosphodiesterase inhibitor*

lixivaptan USAN *selective V2-receptor antagonist for nonhypovolemic hyponatremia*

LKV Infant Drops powder + liquid OTC *vitamin supplement* [multiple vitamins; biotin] ≟•75 μg/0.6 mL

LLD factor [see: cyanocobalamin]

10% LMD IV injection ℞ *plasma volume expander for shock due to hemorrhage, burns, or surgery* [dextran 40] 10%

LMD (low molecular weight dextran) [see: dextran 40]

LMF (Leukeran, methotrexate, fluorouracil) *chemotherapy protocol*

LMWD (low molecular weight dextran) [see: dextran 40]

L·M·X4 cream OTC *local anesthetic* [lidocaine, liposome-encapsulated] 4%

L·M·X5 anorectal cream OTC *local anesthetic* [lidocaine, liposome-encapsulated] 5%

Lobac capsules ℞ *skeletal muscle relaxant; analgesic* [salicylamide; phenyltoloxamine; acetaminophen] 200•20•300 mg

Lobana Body lotion OTC *moisturizer; emollient*

Lobana Body Shampoo; Lobana Liquid Lather topical liquid OTC *soap-free therapeutic skin cleanser* [chloroxylenol]

Lobana Derm-Ade cream OTC *moisturizer; emollient* [vitamins A, D, and E]

Lobana Peri-Garde ointment OTC *moisturizer; emollient; antiseptic* [vitamins A, D, and E; chloroxylenol]

lobelia (Lobelia inflata) plant (tincture) *medicinal herb for arthritis,*

asthma, bronchitis, hay fever, colds, cough, ear infections, epilepsy, fever, food poisoning, lockjaw, nervousness, pain, pneumonia, preventing miscarriage, whooping cough, and worms

lobeline INN *nicotine withdrawal aid* [also: lobeline HCl]

lobeline HCl JAN *nicotine withdrawal aid* [also: lobeline]

lobendazole USAN, INN *veterinary anthelmintic*

lobenzarit INN *antirheumatic* [also: lobenzarit sodium]

lobenzarit sodium USAN *antirheumatic* [also: lobenzarit]

lobradimil USAN *receptor-mediated permeabilizer; investigational (Phase III) blood-brain barrier permeability-enhancing agent for carrying carboplatin to brain tumors*

lobucavir USAN, INN *antiviral; investigational (Phase III) for AIDS-related asymptomatic cytomegalovirus (clinical trials discontinued 1999)*

lobuprofen INN

LoCholest; LoCholest Light powder for oral suspension ℞ *cholesterol-lowering antihyperlipidemic; also used for biliary obstruction* [cholestyramine resin] 4 g/dose

locicortolone dicibate INN

locicortone [see: locicortolone dicibate]

Locoid cream, ointment, solution ℞ *corticosteroidal anti-inflammatory* [hydrocortisone butyrate] 0.1%

Locoid Lipocream ℞ *corticosteroidal anti-inflammatory* [hydrocortisone butyrate (in an oil-in-water emulsion)] 0.1% (70% oil•30% water)

locust plant *medicinal herb* [see: senna]

lodaxaprine INN

lodazecar INN

lodelaben USAN, INN *antiarthritic; emphysema therapy adjunct*

lodenosine USAN *investigational (Phase II) reverse transcriptase antiviral for HIV infection*

Lodine film-coated tablets, capsules ℞ *analgesic; antiarthritic; nonsteroidal* *anti-inflammatory drug (NSAID)* [etodolac] 400, 500 mg; 200, 300 mg

Lodine XL film-coated extended-release tablets ℞ *once-daily analgesic and antiarthritic; nonsteroidal anti-inflammatory drug (NSAID)* [etodolac] 400, 500, 600 mg

lodinixil INN

lodiperone INN

Lodosyn tablets ℞ *decarboxylase inhibitor; antiparkinsonian adjunct (used with levodopa; no effect when given alone)* [carbidopa] 25 mg

lodoxamide INN, BAN *antiallergic; antiasthmatic* [also: lodoxamide ethyl]

lodoxamide ethyl USAN *antiallergic; antiasthmatic* [also: lodoxamide]

lodoxamide trometamol BAN *antiallergic; antiasthmatic* [also: lodoxamide tromethamine]

lodoxamide tromethamine USAN *antiasthmatic; antiallergic for vernal keratoconjunctivitis (orphan)* [also: lodoxamide trometamol]

Lodrane oral liquid ℞ *decongestant; antihistamine* [pseudoephedrine HCl; brompheniramine maleate] 60•4 mg/5 mL

Lodrane 12 D sustained-release tablets ℞ *decongestant; antihistamine* [pseudoephedrine HCl; brompheniramine maleate] 45•6 mg

Lodrane 24 extended-release capsules ℞ *antihistamine* [brompheniramine maleate] 12 mg

Lodrane D oral suspension ℞ *decongestant; antihistamine* [pseudoephedrine tannate; brompheniramine tannate] 90•8 mg/5 mL

Lodrane LD sustained-release capsules ℞ *decongestant; antihistamine* [pseudoephedrine HCl; brompheniramine maleate] 60•6 mg

Lodrane XR oral suspension ℞ *antihistamine* [brompheniramine tannate] 8 mg/5 mL

Loestrin 21 1/20; Loestrin 21 1.5/30 tablets (in packs of 21) ℞ *monophasic oral contraceptive* [norethindrone

acetate; ethinyl estradiol] 1 mg•20 μg; 1.5 mg•30 μg

Loestrin Fe 1/20; Loestrin Fe 1.5/30 tablets (in packs of 28) ℞ *monophasic oral contraceptive; iron supplement* [norethindrone acetate; ethinyl estradiol; ferrous fumarate] 1 mg•20 μg•75 mg; 1.5 mg•30 μg•75 mg

lofemizole INN *anti-inflammatory; analgesic; antipyretic* [also: lofemizole HCl]

lofemizole HCl USAN *anti-inflammatory; analgesic; antipyretic* [also: lofemizole]

Lofenalac powder for oral solution (name changed to **Phenyl-Free** in 2003)

lofendazam INN, BAN

lofentanil INN, BAN *narcotic analgesic* [also: lofentanil oxalate]

lofentanil oxalate USAN *narcotic analgesic* [also: lofentanil]

lofepramine INN, BAN *antidepressant* [also: lofepramine HCl]

lofepramine HCl USAN *antidepressant* [also: lofepramine]

lofexidine INN, BAN *antihypertensive* [also: lofexidine HCl]

lofexidine HCl USAN *centrally acting antiadrenergic antihypertensive; investigational (Phase III) treatment for opiate withdrawal syndrome* [also: lofexidine]

Lofibra capsules ℞ *antihyperlipidemic for primary hypercholesterolemia (types IIa and IIb hyperlipidemia), hypertriglyceridemia (types IV and V hyperlipidemia), and mixed dyslipidemia; also used for hyperuricemia* [fenofibrate] 67, 134, 200 mg

loflucarban INN

Logen tablets ℞ *antidiarrheal* [diphenoxylate HCl; atropine sulfate] 2.5• 0.025 mg

LoHist 12 Hour extended-release tablets ℞ *antihistamine* [brompheniramine tannate] 6 mg

LoKara lotion ℞ *corticosteroidal anti-inflammatory* [desonide] 0.05%

LOMAC (leucovorin, Oncovin, methotrexate, Adriamycin, cyclophosphamide) *chemotherapy protocol*

Lomanate oral liquid ℞ *antidiarrheal* [diphenoxylate HCl; atropine sulfate] 2.5•0.025 mg/5 mL

lombazole USAN, BAN

lomefloxacin USAN, INN, BAN *broad-spectrum fluoroquinolone antibiotic*

lomefloxacin HCl USAN *broad-spectrum fluoroquinolone antibiotic*

lomefloxacin mesylate USAN *antibacterial*

lometraline INN *antipsychotic; antiparkinsonian* [also: lometraline HCl]

lometraline HCl USAN *antipsychotic; antiparkinsonian* [also: lometraline]

lometrexol INN *antineoplastic* [also: lometrexol sodium]

lometrexol sodium USAN *antineoplastic* [also: lometrexol]

lomevactone INN

lomifylline INN

lomofungin USAN *antifungal*

Lomotil tablets, oral liquid ℞ *antidiarrheal* [diphenoxylate HCl; atropine sulfate] 2.5•0.025 mg; 2.5•0.025 mg/5 mL

lomustine USAN, INN, BAN *nitrosourea-type alkylating antineoplastic for brain tumors and Hodgkin disease*

lonafarnib *investigational (Phase III) antineoplastic for lung cancer*

Lonalac powder OTC *enteral nutritional therapy* [milk-based formula]

lonapalene USAN *antipsoriatic*

lonaprofen INN

lonazolac INN

lonidamine INN *investigational (Phase II) indazole-3-carboxylic acid for benign prostatic hyperplasia (BPH)*

Loniten tablets ℞ *antihypertensive; vasodilator* [minoxidil] 2.5, 10 mg ② clonidine

Lonox tablets ℞ *antidiarrheal* [diphenoxylate HCl; atropine sulfate] 2.5•0.025 mg ② Lovenox

loop diuretics *a class of diuretic agents that inhibit the reabsorption of sodium and chloride*

Lo/Ovral tablets (in Pilpaks of 21 or 28) ℞ *monophasic oral contraceptive; emergency postcoital contraceptive* [norgestrel; ethinyl estradiol] 0.3 mg•30 µg

loperamide INN, BAN *antiperistaltic; antidiarrheal* [also: loperamide HCl]

loperamide HCl USAN, USP, JAN *antiperistaltic; antidiarrheal* [also: loperamide] 2 mg oral; 1 mg/5 mL oral

loperamide oxide INN, BAN *antiperistaltic; antidiarrheal*

Lophophora williamsii *a flowering Mexican cactus whose heads (mescal buttons) are used to produce mescaline, a hallucinogenic street drug*

Lopid film-coated tablets ℞ *triglyceride-lowering antihyperlipidemic for hypertriglyceridemia (types IV and V hyperlipidemia) and coronary heart disease* [gemfibrozil] 600 mg (300 mg capsules available in Canada)

lopinavir USAN *antiviral protease inhibitor for HIV infection*

lopirazepam INN

loprazolam INN, BAN

lopremone [now: protirelin]

Lopressor tablets, IV injection ℞ *antianginal; antihypertensive; β-blocker* [metoprolol tartrate] 50, 100 mg; 1 mg/mL

Lopressor HCT 50/25; Lopressor HCT 100/25; Lopressor HCT 100/50 tablets ℞ *antihypertensive; β-blocker; diuretic* [metoprolol tartrate; hydrochlorothiazide] 50•25 mg; 100•25 mg; 100•50 mg

loprodiol INN

Loprox cream, gel, topical suspension, shampoo ℞ *antifungal for tinea pedis, tinea cruris, tinea corporis, tinea versicolor, candidiasis, and seborrheic dermatitis* [ciclopirox olamine] 1%

Loprox lotion (discontinued 2003) ℞ *antifungal* [ciclopirox olamine] 1%

Lorabid Pulvules (capsules), powder for oral suspension ℞ *carbacephem antibiotic* [loracarbef] 200, 400 mg; 100, 200 mg/5 mL

loracarbef USAN, INN *carbacephem antibiotic*

lorajmine INN *antiarrhythmic* [also: lorajmine HCl]

lorajmine HCl USAN *antiarrhythmic*
[also: lorajmine]

lorapride INN

loratadine USAN, INN, BAN *second-generation peripherally selective piperidine antihistamine for allergic rhinitis and chronic idiopathic urticaria* 10 mg oral

lorazepam USAN, USP, INN, BAN *benzodiazepine anxiolytic; preanesthetic sedative; anticonvulsant* 0.5, 1, 2 mg oral; 2, 4 mg/mL injection

Lorazepam Intensol oral drops ℞ *benzodiazepine anxiolytic; sedative; anticonvulsant* [lorazepam] 2 mg/mL

lorbamate USAN, INN *muscle relaxant*

lorcainide INN, BAN *antiarrhythmic*
[also: lorcainide HCl]

lorcainide HCl USAN *antiarrhythmic*
[also: lorcainide]

Lorcet Plus; Lorcet 10/650 tablets ℞ *narcotic analgesic* [hydrocodone bitartrate; acetaminophen] 7.5•650 mg; 10•650 mg

Lorcet-HD capsules ℞ *narcotic analgesic* [hydrocodone bitartrate; acetaminophen] 5•500 mg ② Fioricet

lorcinadol USAN, INN, BAN *analgesic*

loreclezole USAN, INN, BAN *antiepileptic*

Lorenzo oil (erucic acid and oleic acid) *natural treatment for childhood adrenoleukodystrophy and adrenomyeloneuropathy in adults*

lorglumide INN

lormetazepam USAN, INN, BAN *sedative; hypnotic*

lornoxicam USAN, INN, BAN *analgesic; anti-inflammatory*

Lorothidol (available only from the Centers for Disease Control) ℞ *investigational anti-infective for paragonimiasis and fascioliasis* [bithionol]

Loroxide lotion (discontinued 2003) OTC *keratolytic for acne* [benzoyl peroxide] 5.5%

lorpiprazole INN

Lortab elixir ℞ *narcotic analgesic* [hydrocodone bitartrate; acetaminophen] 2.5•167 mg/5 mL

Lortab 2.5/500; Lortab 5/500; Lortab 7.5/500; Lortab 10/500 tablets ℞ *narcotic analgesic* [hydrocodone bitartrate; acetaminophen] 2.5•500 mg; 5•500 mg; 7.5•500 mg; 10•500 mg

Lortab ASA tablets ℞ *narcotic analgesic* [hydrocodone bitartrate; aspirin] 5•500 mg

lortalamine USAN, INN *antidepressant*

Lortuss DM oral liquid OTC *antitussive; decongestant; antihistamine* [dextromethorphan hydrobromide; phenylephrine HCl; brompheniramine maleate] 15•7.5•2 mg/5 mL

Lortuss HC oral liquid ℞ *narcotic antitussive; decongestant* [hydrocodone bitartrate; phenylephrine HCl] 3.5•7.5 mg/5 mL

lorzafone USAN, INN *minor tranquilizer*

losartan INN *angiotensin II receptor antagonist for hypertension; treatment to delay the progression of diabetic nephropathy* [also: losartan potassium]

losartan potassium USAN *angiotensin II receptor antagonist for hypertension; treatment to delay the progression of diabetic nephropathy* [also: losartan]

Losec Ⓒᴬᴺ delayed-release tablets ℞ *proton pump inhibitor for gastric and duodenal ulcers and other gastroesophageal disorders* [omeprazole] 10, 20 mg

Losec 1-2-3 A Ⓒᴬᴺ ℞ *7-day regimen for eradication of H. pylori–associated peptic ulcer disease* [Losec, 20 mg b.i.d; amoxicillin, 1000 mg b.i.d; clarithromycin, 500 mg b.i.d.]

Losec 1-2-3 M Ⓒᴬᴺ ℞ *7-day regimen for eradication of H. pylori–associated peptic ulcer disease* [Losec, 20 mg b.i.d; metronidazole, 500 mg b.i.d; clarithromycin, 250 mg b.i.d.]

losigamone INN

losindole INN

losmiprofen INN

losoxantrone INN *antineoplastic* [also: losoxantrone HCl]

losoxantrone HCl USAN *antineoplastic* [also: losoxantrone]

losulazine INN *antihypertensive* [also: losulazine HCl]

losulazine HCl USAN *antihypertensive* [also: losulazine]

Lotemax eye drop suspension ℞ *corticosteroidal anti-inflammatory* [loteprednol etabonate] 0.5%

Lotensin tablets ℞ *antihypertensive; angiotensin-converting enzyme (ACE) inhibitor; also used for nondiabetic neuropathy* [benazepril HCl] 5, 10, 20, 40 mg

Lotensin HCT 5/6.25; Lotensin HCT 10/12.5; Lotensin HCT 20/12.5; Lotensin HCT 20/25 tablets ℞ *antihypertensive; angiotensin-converting enzyme (ACE) inhibitor; diuretic* [benazepril HCl; hydrochlorothiazide] 5•6.25 mg; 10•12.5 mg; 20•12.5 mg; 20•25 mg

loteprednol INN *corticosteroidal anti-inflammatory* [also: loteprednol etabonate]

loteprednol etabonate USAN *ophthalmic corticosteroidal anti-inflammatory* [also: loteprednol]

lotifazole INN

lotrafiban HCl USAN *platelet aggregation inhibitor; GP IIb/IIIa receptor antagonist*

Lotrel capsules ℞ *antihypertensive; angiotensin-converting enzyme (ACE) inhibitor; calcium channel blocker* [amlodipine besylate; benazepril HCl] 2.5•10, 5•10, 5•20, 10•20 mg

lotrifen INN

Lotrimin cream, solution, lotion (discontinued 2003) ℞ *antifungal* [clotrimazole] 1% ⊡ Otrivin

Lotrimin AF cream, topical solution, lotion OTC *antifungal* [clotrimazole] 1%

Lotrimin AF powder, spray powder, spray liquid OTC *antifungal* [miconazole nitrate] 2%

Lotrimin Ultra cream OTC *antifungal* [butenafine HCl] 1%

Lotrisone cream, lotion ℞ *corticosteroidal anti-inflammatory; antifungal* [betamethasone dipropionate; clotrimazole] 0.05%•1%

Lotronex film-coated tablets ℞ *serotonin 5-HT₃ receptor antagonist for irritable bowel syndrome (IBS)* [alosetron HCl] 0.562, 1.124 mg (=0.5, 1 mg base)

lotucaine INN

lousewort *medicinal herb* [see: betony; feverweed]

lovage (*Angelica levisticum; Levisticum officinale*) *leaves and roots medicinal herb for bad breath, boils, edema, flatulence, and sore throat; also used topically as a skin emollient*

lovastatin USAN, INN, BAN *HMG-CoA reductase inhibitor for hypercholesterolemia, hyperlipidemia, and atherosclerosis; also for primary prevention of coronary heart disease* 10, 20, 40 mg oral

Lovenox deep subcu injection, prefilled syringes ℞ *anticoagulant/antithrombotic for prevention of deep vein thrombosis (DVT) following knee, hip, or abdominal surgery, unstable angina, and myocardial infarction* [enoxaparin sodium] 300 mg; 30 mg/0.3 mL, 40 mg/0.4 mL, 60 mg/0.6 mL, 80, 120 mg/0.8 mL, 100, 150 mg/mL ⊡ Lonox

loviride USAN, INN *investigational nonnucleoside reverse transcriptase inhibitor (NNRTI) antiviral for HIV*

low molecular weight dextran (LMD; LMWD) [see: dextran 40]

low molecular weight heparins *a class of anticoagulants used for the prophylaxis or treatment of thromboembolic complications of surgery and ischemic complications of unstable angina or myocardial infarction*

low osmolar contrast media (LOCM) *a class of newer radiopaque agents that have a low osmolar concentration of iodine (the contrast agent), which corresponds to a lower incidence of adverse reactions* [also called: nonionic contrast media]

Lowila Cake bar OTC *soap-free therapeutic skin cleanser*

Low-Ogestrel tablets (in packs of 28) ℞ *monophasic oral contraceptive; emergency postcoital contraceptive* [norgestrel; ethinyl estradiol] 0.3 mg•30 μg

Lowsium Plus oral suspension OTC *antacid; antiflatulent* [magaldrate; simethicone] 540•40 mg/5 mL

loxanast INN

Loxapac ⓒ oral concentrate, IM injection (discontinued 2001) ℞ conventional (typical) dibenzoxazepine antipsychotic for schizophrenia [loxapine HCl] 25 mg/mL; 50 mg/mL

Loxapac ⓒ tablets (discontinued 2001) ℞ conventional (typical) dibenzoxazepine antipsychotic for schizophrenia [loxapine] 5, 10, 25, 50 mg

loxapine USAN, INN, BAN minor tranquilizer; conventional (typical) dibenzoxazepine antipsychotic for schizophrenia

loxapine HCl minor tranquilizer; conventional (typical) dibenzoxazepine antipsychotic for schizophrenia

loxapine succinate USAN minor tranquilizer; conventional (typical) dibenzoxazepine antipsychotic for schizophrenia 5, 10, 25, 50 mg oral

loxiglumide INN

Loxitane capsules ℞ conventional (typical) dibenzoxazepine antipsychotic for schizophrenia [loxapine succinate] 5, 10, 25, 50 mg ② doxepin

Loxitane C oral concentrate (discontinued 2003) ℞ conventional (typical) dibenzoxazepine antipsychotic for schizophrenia [loxapine HCl] 25 mg/mL

Loxitane IM injection (discontinued 2002) ℞ conventional (typical) dibenzoxazepine antipsychotic for schizophrenia [loxapine HCl] 50 mg/mL

loxoprofen INN

loxoribine USAN, INN immunostimulant; vaccine adjuvant; orphan status withdrawn 1996

loxotidine [now: lavoltidine succinate]

loxtidine BAN antiulcerative; histamine H_2-receptor blocker [also: lavoltidine succinate; lavoltidine]

lozilurea INN

Lozi-Tabs (trademarked form) lozenges

Lozol film-coated tablets ℞ antihypertensive; diuretic [indapamide] 1.25, 2.5 mg

L-PAM (L-phenylalanine mustard) [see: melphalan]

LR (lactated Ringer) solution [see: Ringer injection, lactated]

LSD (lysergic acid diethylamide) hallucinogenic street drug associated with disorders of sensory and temporal perception, depersonalization, and ataxia [medically known as lysergide]

LSF (lisofylline) [q.v.]

LTRAs (leukotriene receptor antagonists) a class of antiasthmatics

Lu texaphyrin [see: motexafin lutetium]

lubeluzole USAN, INN investigational neural protective for ischemic stroke

lubiprostone investigational (NDA filed) oral agent to increase fluid secretion in the small intestine for the treatment of chronic idiopathic constipation in adults

LubraSol Bath Oil (discontinued 2003) OTC bath emollient

Lubricating Jelly OTC vaginal lubricant [glycerin; propylene glycol]

Lubricoat (trademarked ingredient) surgical aid [ferric hyaluronate]

Lubriderm cream, lotion (discontinued 2004) OTC moisturizer; emollient

Lubriderm Bath Oil (discontinued 2004) OTC bath emollient

Lubriderm Daily Moisture with SPF 15 lotion OTC moisturizer; emollient; sunscreen [octinoxate; octisalate; oxybenzone] 7.5%•4%•3%

Lubrin vaginal inserts OTC lubricant for sexual intercourse [glycerin; caprylic triglyceride]

Lubriskin lotion OTC moisturizer; emollient

LubriTears eye drops OTC ophthalmic moisturizer/lubricant [hydroxypropyl methylcellulose] 0.3%

LubriTears ophthalmic ointment OTC ocular moisturizer/lubricant [white petrolatum; mineral oil; lanolin]

lucanthone INN, BAN antischistosomal [also: lucanthone HCl]

lucanthone HCl USAN, USP antischistosomal [also: lucanthone]

lucartamide INN

lucensomycin [see: lucimycin]

Lucentis

Lucidex enteric-coated tablets OTC *CNS stimulant; analeptic* [caffeine] 100 mg

Lucilia caesar natural treatment [see: maggots]

lucimycin INN

Ludiomil coated tablets (discontinued 2001) ℞ *tetracyclic antidepressant* [maprotiline HCl] 25, 50, 75 mg

Luer-lock (trademarked delivery device) *prefilled self-injection syringe*

lufironil USAN, INN *collagen inhibitor*

lufuradom INN

Lufyllin elixir, IM injection (discontinued 2005) ℞ *antiasthmatic; bronchodilator* [dyphylline] 100 mg/15 mL; 250 mg/mL

Lufyllin tablets ℞ *antiasthmatic; bronchodilator* [dyphylline] 200 mg

Lufyllin 400 tablets ℞ *antiasthmatic; bronchodilator* [dyphylline] 400 mg

Lufyllin-EPG tablets, elixir ℞ *antiasthmatic; bronchodilator; decongestant; expectorant; sedative* [dyphylline; ephedrine HCl; guaifenesin; phenobarbital] 100•16•200•16 mg; 150•24•300•24 mg/15 mL

Lufyllin-GG tablets, elixir ℞ *antiasthmatic; bronchodilator; expectorant* [dyphylline; guaifenesin] 200•200 mg; 100•100 mg/15 mL

Lugol solution ℞ *thyroid-blocking therapy; topical antimicrobial* [iodine; potassium iodide] 5%•10%

Lumenax (name changed to **Xifaxan** upon marketing release in 2004)

Lumigan eye drops ℞ *synthetic prostamide analogue for glaucoma and ocular hypertension* [bimatoprost] 0.03%

Luminal Sodium IV or IM injection ℞ *long-acting barbiturate sedative, hypnotic, and anticonvulsant; also abused as a street drug* [phenobarbital sodium] 130 mg/mL ② Tuinal

lumiracoxib *investigational (Phase III) antiarthritic for osteoarthritis; analgesic for acute pain; COX-2 inhibitor; nonsteroidal anti-inflammatory drug (NSAID)*

Lunelle IM injection ℞ *once-monthly injectable contraceptive* [estradiol cypionate; medroxyprogesterone acetate] 5•25 mg/0.5 mL

Lunesta film-coated tablets ℞ *nonbarbiturate sedative and hypnotic for chronic insomnia* [eszopiclone] 1, 2, 3 mg

lung surfactant, synthetic [see: colfosceril palmitate]

lungwort (*Pulmonaria officinalis*) flowering plant *medicinal herb used as an astringent, demulcent, emollient, expectorant, and pectoral*

2,6-lupetidine [see: nanofin]

lupitidine INN *veterinary antagonist to histamine H_2 receptors* [also: lupitidine HCl]

lupitidine HCl USAN *veterinary antagonist to histamine H_2 receptors* [also: lupitidine]

Lupron; Lupron Pediatric subcu injection (daily) ℞ *hormonal antineoplastic for prostatic cancer and central precocious puberty (orphan)* [leuprolide acetate] 5 mg/mL ② Mepron; Napron

Lupron Depot microspheres for IM injection (monthly) ℞ *hormonal antineoplastic for prostatic cancer, endometriosis, and uterine fibroids* [leuprolide acetate] 3.75, 7.5 mg ② Mepron; Napron

Lupron Depot–3 month; Lupron Depot–4 month microspheres for IM injection ℞ *hormonal antineoplastic for prostatic cancer* [leuprolide acetate] 11.5, 22.5 mg; 30 mg ② Mepron; Napron

Lupron Depot-Ped microspheres for IM injection (monthly) ℞ *hormonal antineoplastic for central precocious puberty (orphan)* [leuprolide acetate] 7.5, 11.25, 15 mg ② Mepron; Napron

luprostiol INN, BAN

Luride Lozi-Tabs (chewable tablets), drops, gel ℞ *dental caries preventative* [sodium fluoride] 0.25, 1.1, 2.2 mg; 1.1 mg/mL; 1.2%

Luride SF Lozi-Tabs (lozenges) ℞ *topical dental caries preventative* [sodium fluoride] 2.2 mg

lurosetron mesylate USAN *antiemetic*

lurtotecan dihydrochloride USAN *antineoplastic; topoisomerase I inhibitor*

Lusonal *oral liquid* ℞ *nasal decongestant* [phenylephrine HCl] 7.5 mg/5 mL

Lustra; Lustra-AF *cream* ℞ *hyperpigmentation bleaching agent* [hydroquinone] 4%

lutein *natural carotenoid used to prevent and treat age-related macular degeneration (AMD), retinitis pigmentosa (RP), and other retinal dysfunction*

luteinizing hormone–releasing factor acetate hydrate [see: gonadorelin acetate]

luteinizing hormone–releasing factor diacetate tetrahydrate [now: gonadorelin acetate]

luteinizing hormone–releasing factor dihydrochloride [now: gonadorelin HCl]

luteinizing hormone–releasing factor HCl [see: gonadorelin HCl]

luteinizing hormone–releasing hormone (LH-RH) *an endogenous hormone, produced in the hypothalamus, which stimulates the release of luteinizing hormone (LH) and follicle-stimulating hormone (FSH) from the pituitary* [also known as: gonadotropin-releasing hormone (Gn-RH)]

Lutera *tablets (in packs of 28)* ℞ *monophasic oral contraceptive* [levonorgestrel; ethinyl estradiol] 100•20 μg

lutetium *element (Lu)*

lutetium texaphyrin [now: motexafin lutetium]

Lu-Tex ℞ *investigational antineoplastic for the photodynamic treatment of cancer; investigational (Phase I/II) photosensitizer for ophthalmologic indications including age-related macular degeneration* [motexafin lutetium]

lutrelin INN *luteinizing hormone-releasing hormone (LHRH) agonist* [also: lutrelin acetate]

lutrelin acetate USAN *luteinizing hormone-releasing hormone (LHRH) agonist* [also: lutrelin]

Lutrepulse *powder for continuous ambulatory infusion* ℞ *gonadotropin-releasing hormone for hypothalamic amenorrhea (orphan)* [gonadorelin acetate] 0.8, 3.2 mg

Lutrin ℞ *investigational photodynamic therapy for recurrent breast cancer* [motexafin lutetium]

lutropin alfa USAN *recombinant human luteinizing hormone (rhLH); gonadotropin; ovulation stimulant for infertility due to chronic anovulation in hypogonadal women*

Luveris *powder for subcu injection* ℞ *gonadotropin; ovulation stimulant for infertility due to chronic anovulation in hypogonadal women* [lutropin alfa] 75 IU/dose

Luvox *film-coated tablets (discontinued 2004)* ℞ *selective serotonin reuptake inhibitor (SSRI) for obsessive-compulsive disorder (OCD)* [fluvoxamine maleate] 25, 50, 100 mg

luxabendazole INN, BAN

Luxiq *foam* ℞ *topical corticosteroidal anti-inflammatory for scalp dermatoses* [betamethasone valerate] 0.12%

L-VAM (leuprolide acetate, vinblastine, Adriamycin, mitomycin) *chemotherapy protocol*

lyapolate sodium USAN *anticoagulant* [also: sodium apolate]

lycetamine USAN *topical antimicrobial*

lycine HCl [see: betaine HCl]

lycopene *natural substance found in high concentration in ripe tomatoes; a member of the carotene family; used as an antineoplastic and antioxidant*

Lycopodium clavatum *medicinal herb* [see: club moss]

Lycopus virginicus *medicinal herb* [see: bugleweed]

Lyderm ⒸⒶⓃ *cream, ointment, gel* ℞ *topical corticosteroidal anti-inflammatory* [fluocinonide] 0.05%

lydimycin USAN *antifungal* [also: lidimycin]

Lyme borreliosis vaccine [see: lipoprotein OspA, recombinant]

lymecycline INN, BAN

LYMErix *IM injection (discontinued 2002)* ℞ *active immunizing agent* *against Lyme disease* [lipoprotein OspA, recombinant] 30 μg/0.5 mL

Lymphazurin 1% subcu injection ℞ *radiopaque contrast medium for lymphography* [isosulfan blue] 10 mg/mL (1%)

LymphoCide ℞ *investigational (Phase III, orphan) monoclonal antibodies for AIDS-related non-Hodgkin lymphoma* [yttrium Y 90–labeled epratuzumab]

lymphocyte immune globulin (LIG) *passive immunizing agent to prevent allograft rejection of renal transplants; treatment for aplastic anemia; investigational (orphan) for organ and bone marrow transplants* [also: antithymocyte globulin (ATG)]

lymphogranuloma venereum antigen USAN

LymphoScan ℞ *investigational (Phase III, orphan) for diagnostic aid for non-Hodgkin B-cell lymphoma, AIDS-related lymphomas, and other acute and chronic B-cell leukemias* [technetium Tc 99m bectumomab]

lynestrenol USAN, INN *progestin* [also: lynoestrenol]

lynoestrenol BAN *progestin* [also: lynestrenol]

Lyo-Ject (trademarked delivery system) *prefilled dual-chambered syringe with lyophilized powder and diluent*

Lypholized Vitamin B Complex & Vitamin C with B₁₂ injection ℞ *parenteral vitamin therapy* [multiple B vitamins; vitamin C] ± • 50 mg/mL

Lypholyte; Lypholyte II IV admixture ℞ *intravenous electrolyte therapy* [combined electrolyte solution]

lypressin USAN, USP, INN, BAN *posterior pituitary hormone; antidiuretic; vasoconstrictor*

Lyrica capsules ℞ *gabamimetic anticonvulsant; agent for the management of neuropathic pain from diabetic peripheral neuropathy (DPN) and postherpetic neuralgia (PHN); investigational (Phase III) for generalized anxiety disorder (GAD)* [pregabalin]

lysergic acid diethylamide (LSD) *street drug* [see: LSD; lysergide]

lysergide INN, BAN, DCF

lysine (L-lysine) USAN, INN *essential amino acid; symbols: Lys, K; natural remedy for the prophylaxis and treatment of recurrent oral and genital herpes simplex outbreaks; inhibits HSV replication* 312, 500, 1000 mg oral

lysine acetate USP *amino acid*

DL-lysine acetylsalicylate [see: aspirin DL-lysine]

lysine HCl USAN, USP *amino acid*

L-lysine monoacetate [see: lysine acetate]

L-lysine monohydrochloride [see: lysine HCl]

8-L-lysine vasopressin [see: lypressin]

Lysodren tablets ℞ *antibiotic antineoplastic for inoperable adrenal cortical carcinoma and Cushing syndrome* [mitotane] 500 mg

lysostaphin USAN *antibacterial enzyme; investigational agent for methicillin-resistant* Staphylococcus aureus (MRSA) *endocarditis*

lysuride BAN [also: lisuride]

M-CSF (macrophage colony-stimulating factor) [now: cilmostim]

M-2 protocol (vincristine, carmustine, cyclophosphamide, prednisone, melphalan) *chemotherapy protocol for multiple myeloma*

MAA (macroaggregated albumin) [see: albumin, aggregated]

Maalox chewable tablets (discontinued 2001) OTC *antacid* [aluminum hydroxide; magnesium hydroxide] 200•200, 350•350 mg ⊘ Marax

Maalox oral suspension OTC *antacid* [aluminum hydroxide; magnesium hydroxide] 225•200 mg/5 mL ☑ Marax

Maalox Antacid caplets (discontinued 2001) OTC *antacid* [calcium carbonate] 1 g

Maalox Antacid/Calcium Supplement chewable tablets OTC *antacid; calcium supplement* [calcium carbonate] 600 mg

Maalox Anti-Diarrheal caplets (discontinued 2001) OTC *antidiarrheal* [loperamide HCl] 2 mg

Maalox Anti-Gas chewable tablets OTC *antiflatulent* [simethicone] 80 mg

Maalox Anti-Gas, Extra Strength oral suspension OTC *antacid; antiflatulent* [aluminum hydroxide; magnesium hydroxide; simethicone] 500•450•40 mg/5 mL

Maalox H2 Acid Controller ⓒⒶⓃ film-coated tablets OTC *histamine H₂ antagonist for heartburn and acid indigestion* [famotidine] 10 mg

Maalox HRF (Heartburn Relief Formula) oral liquid (discontinued 2001) OTC *antacid* [aluminum hydroxide; magnesium carbonate] 140•175 mg/5 mL

Maalox Plus chewable tablets, oral suspension (discontinued 2001) OTC *antacid; antiflatulent* [aluminum hydroxide; magnesium hydroxide; simethicone] 200•200•25 mg; 500•450•40 mg/5 mL

Maalox Quick Dissolve chewable tablets OTC *antacid; calcium supplement* [calcium carbonate] 600, 1000 mg

Maalox TC oral suspension OTC *antacid* [aluminum hydroxide; magnesium hydroxide] 600•300 mg/5 mL

Maalox Therapeutic Concentrate oral suspension (renamed Maalox TC in 2003)

MAb; MAB (monoclonal antibodies)

MABOP (Mustargen, Adriamycin, bleomycin, Oncovin, prednisone) *chemotherapy protocol*

mabuterol INN

MAC (methotrexate, actinomycin D, chlorambucil) *chemotherapy protocol*

MAC; MAC III (methotrexate, actinomycin D, cyclophosphamide) *chemotherapy protocol for gestational trophoblastic neoplasm*

MAC (mitomycin, Adriamycin, cyclophosphamide) *chemotherapy protocol*

maca (*Lepidium meyenii*) root *medicinal herb used as an adaptogen, aphrodisiac in males, fertility aid in females, and to relieve stress*

MACC (methotrexate, Adriamycin, cyclophosphamide, CCNU) *chemotherapy protocol for non–small cell lung cancer (NSCLC)*

mace (*Myristica fragrans*) dried nutmeg aril (the fleshy network surrounding the seed) *medicinal herb* [see: nutmeg]

MACHO (methotrexate, asparaginase, cyclophosphamide, hydroxydaunomycin, Oncovin) *chemotherapy protocol*

MACOP-B (methotrexate, Adriamycin, cyclophosphamide, Oncovin, prednisone, bleomycin) *chemotherapy protocol for non-Hodgkin lymphoma*

macroaggregated albumin (MAA) [see: albumin, aggregated]

macroaggregated iodinated (¹³¹I) human albumin [see: macrosalb (¹³¹I)]

Macrobid capsules ℞ *urinary antibiotic* [nitrofurantoin (macrocrystals); nitrofurantoin monohydrate] 25•75 mg

Macrodantin capsules ℞ *urinary antibiotic* [nitrofurantoin (macrocrystals)] 25, 50, 100 mg

Macrodex IV infusion ℞ *plasma volume expander for shock due to hemorrhage, burns, or surgery* [dextran 70] 6%

macrogol 4000 INN, BAN [also: polyethylene glycol 4000]

macrogol ester 2000 INN *surfactant* [also: polyoxyl 40 stearate]

macrogol ester 400 INN *surfactant* [also: polyoxyl 8 stearate]

macrolides *a class of antibiotics that are bacteriostatic or bactericidal, depending on drug concentration*

macrophage colony-stimulating factor (M-CSF) [now: cilmostim]

macrophage-targeted β-glucocerebrosidase [now: alglucerase]

macrosalb (¹³¹I) INN, BAN

macrosalb (⁹⁹ᵐTc) INN, BAN [also: technetium (⁹⁹ᵐTc) labeled macroaggregated human ...]

Macroscint ℞ *investigational inflammation and infection imaging aid* [indium In 111 IGIV pentetate]

Macrotys actaeoides *medicinal herb* [see: black cohosh]

Macrulin *investigational (Phase I) oral agent for type 2 diabetes* [insulin]

Macugen intravitreous injection in prefilled syringes ℞ *pegylated VEGF (vascular endothelial growth factor) antagonist for neovascular (wet) age-related macular degeneration (AMD); investigational (Phase II) for diabetic retinopathy* [pegaptanib sodium] 0.3 mg/dose

MAD (MeCCNU, Adriamycin) *chemotherapy protocol*

mad-dog weed; mad weed *medicinal herb* [see: skullcap]

MADDOC (mechlorethamine, Adriamycin, dacarbazine, DDP, Oncovin, cyclophosphamide) *chemotherapy protocol*

madnep; madness *medicinal herb* [see: masterwort]

maduramicin USAN, INN *anticoccidial*

mafenide USAN, INN, BAN *bacteriostatic; adjunct to burn therapy*

mafenide acetate USP *broad-spectrum bacteriostatic to prevent meshed autograft loss on second- and third-degree burns (orphan)*

mafenide HCl

mafilcon A USAN *hydrophilic contact lens material*

mafoprazine INN

mafosfamide INN

Mag-200 tablets OTC *magnesium supplement* [magnesium oxide] 200 mg Mg

magaldrate USAN, USP, INN *antacid* 540 mg/5 mL oral

Magaldrate Plus oral suspension OTC *antacid; antiflatulent* [magaldrate; simethicone] 540•40 mg/5 mL

Magalox Plus chewable tablets OTC *antacid; antiflatulent* [aluminum hydroxide; magnesium hydroxide; simethicone] 200•200•25 mg

Magan tablets ℞ *analgesic; antirheumatic* [magnesium salicylate] 545 mg

Mag-Cal tablets OTC *dietary supplement* [calcium carbonate; vitamin D; multiple minerals] 416.7 mg•66.7 IU• ±

Mag-Cal Mega tablets OTC *mineral supplement* [magnesium; calcium] 800•400 mg

Mag-Caps capsules OTC *magnesium supplement* [magnesium oxide] 140 mg (85 mg Mg)

Mag-G tablets OTC *magnesium supplement* [magnesium gluconate dihydrate] 500 mg (27 mg Mg)

maggots (Lucilia caesar; Phaenicia sericata; Pharmia regina) *natural treatment for debriding necrotic tissue in abscesses, burns, cellulitis, gangrene, osteomyelitis, and ulcers*

magic mouthwash *a slang term for a combination of a local anesthetic plus one or more of the following: an antihistamine, a corticosteroid, an antifungal, an antibiotic—with or without an antacid used as a carrier*

Maginex enteric-coated tablets (discontinued 2004) OTC *magnesium supplement* [magnesium-L-aspartate HCl] 615 mg (61 mg Mg)

Maginex DS powder for oral liquid (discontinued 2004) OTC *magnesium supplement* [magnesium-L-aspartate HCl] 1230 mg (122 mg Mg)/pkt.

Magnacal ready-to-use oral liquid OTC *enteral nutritional therapy* [lactose-free formula]

Magnaprin; Magnaprin Arthritis Strength Captabs film-coated tablets OTC *analgesic; antipyretic; anti-*

inflammatory; antirheumatic [aspirin (buffered with aluminum hydroxide, magnesium hydroxide, and calcium carbonate)] 325 mg

MagneBind 200; MagneBind 300 tablets OTC *calcium/magnesium supplement that binds dietary phosphate* [magnesium carbonate; calcium carbonate] 200•400 mg; 300•250 mg

MagneBind 400 Rx tablets ℞ *calcium/magnesium supplement that binds dietary phosphate* [magnesium carbonate; calcium carbonate; folic acid] 400•200•1 mg

magnesia, milk of USP *antacid; saline laxative* [also: magnesium hydroxide] 400 mg/5 mL oral

magnesia magma [now: magnesia, milk of]

magnesium *element (Mg)*

magnesium aluminosilicate hydrate [see: almasilate]

magnesium aluminum silicate NF *suspending agent*

magnesium amino acid chelate *dietary magnesium supplement*

magnesium aspartate [see: potassium aspartate & magnesium aspartate]

magnesium carbonate USP *antacid; dietary magnesium supplement*

magnesium carbonate hydrate [see: magnesium carbonate]

magnesium chloride USP *electrolyte replenisher* 1.97 mEq/mL (20%) injection

magnesium chloride hexahydrate [see: magnesium chloride]

magnesium citrate USP *dietary magnesium supplement; saline laxative* 100 mg Mg oral; 1.75 g/30 mL oral

magnesium clofibrate INN

magnesium D-gluconate dihydrate [see: magnesium gluconate]

magnesium D-gluconate hydrate [see: magnesium gluconate]

magnesium EDTA (ethylene diamine tetraacetic acid) [see: edetate magnesium disodium]

magnesium gluconate USP *dietary magnesium supplement* 12.7 mg Mg oral

magnesium glycinate USAN

magnesium hydroxide USP *antacid; saline laxative* [also: magnesia, milk of]

magnesium hydroxycarbonate *antiurolithic*

magnesium oxide USP *antacid; sorbent; magnesium supplement* 400 mg oral

magnesium phosphate USP *antacid*

magnesium phosphate pentahydrate [see: magnesium phosphate]

magnesium salicylate USP *analgesic; antipyretic; anti-inflammatory; antirheumatic*

magnesium salicylate tetrahydrate [see: magnesium salicylate]

magnesium silicate NF *tablet excipient*

magnesium silicate hydrate [see: magnesium trisilicate]

magnesium stearate NF *tablet and capsule lubricant*

magnesium sulfate USP, JAN *anticonvulsant; saline laxative; electrolyte replenisher* 4%, 8%, 12.5%, 50% (0.325, 0.65, 1, 4 mEq/mL) injection

magnesium sulfate heptahydrate [see: magnesium sulfate]

magnesium trisilicate USP *antacid*

magnesium-L-aspartate HCl *dietary magnesium supplement*

Magnevist IV injection, prefilled syringes ℞ *MRI contrast medium* [gadopentetate dimeglumine] 469 mg/mL

magnolia (*Magnolia glauca*) bark *medicinal herb used as an antiperiodic, aromatic, astringent, diaphoretic, febrifuge, stimulant, and tonic*

Magnox oral suspension OTC *antacid* [aluminum hydroxide; magnesium hydroxide] 225•200 mg/5 mL

Magonate tablets, oral liquid OTC *magnesium supplement* [magnesium gluconate dihydrate] 500 mg (27 mg Mg); 1 g (54 mg Mg)/5 mL

Magonate Natal oral drops OTC *pediatric magnesium supplement* [magnesium gluconate] 3.52 mg Mg/mL

Mag-Ox 400 tablets OTC *antacid; magnesium supplement* [magnesium oxide] 400 mg (241 mg Mg)

Magsal tablets ℞ *analgesic; antipyretic; anti-inflammatory; antihistaminic sleep aid* [magnesium salicylate; phenyltoloxamine citrate] 600•25 mg

Mag-Tab SR sustained-release caplets OTC *magnesium supplement* [magnesium lactate dihydrate] 84 mg Mg

Magtrate tablets OTC *magnesium supplement* [magnesium gluconate] 500 mg (29 mg Mg)

mahogany birch; mountain mahogany *medicinal herb* [see: birch]

Mahonia aquifolium *medicinal herb* [see: Oregon grape]

ma-huang *medicinal herb* [see: ephedra]

MAID (mesna [rescue], Adriamycin, ifosfamide, dacarbazine) *chemotherapy protocol for soft tissue and bone sarcomas*

maitake mushrooms (*Grifola frondosa*) cap and stem *medicinal herb for cancer, diabetes, hypercholesterolemia, hypertension, obesity, and stimulation of the immune system*

maitansine INN *antineoplastic* [also: maytansine]

Maitec injection ℞ *investigational (orphan) agent for disseminated* Mycobacterium avium-intracellulare *infection* [gentamicin sulfate, liposomal]

Majorana hortensis *medicinal herb* [see: marjoram]

Major-Con chewable tablets OTC *antiflatulent* [simethicone] 80 mg

Major-gesic tablets OTC *antihistamine; analgesic* [phenyltoloxamine citrate; acetaminophen] 30•325 mg

malaleuca *medicinal herb* [see: tea tree oil]

Malarone; Malarone Pediatric film-coated tablets ℞ *malaria prophylaxis and treatment* [atovaquone; proguanil HCl (chloroguanide HCl)] 250•100 mg; 62.5•25 mg

malathion USP, BAN *pediculicide for lice*

maletamer INN *antiperistaltic* [also: malethamer]

malethamer USAN *antiperistaltic* [also: maletamer]

maleylsulfathiazole INN

malic acid NF *acidifying agent*

malidone [see: aloxidone]

Mallamint chewable tablets OTC *antacid* [calcium carbonate] 420 mg

Mallazine eye drops OTC *topical ophthalmic decongestant and vasoconstrictor* [tetrahydrozoline HCl] 0.05%

mallow (*Malva rotundifolia; M. sylvestris*) plant *medicinal herb used as an astringent, demulcent, emollient, and expectorant*

mallow, marsh (*Althaea officinalis*) *medicinal herb* [see: marsh mallow]

malonal [see: barbital]

malotilate USAN, INN *liver disorder treatment*

Malpighia glabra; M. punicifolia *medicinal herb* [see: acerola]

Maltsupex coated tablets, powder, oral liquid OTC *bulk laxative* [barley malt soup extract] 750 mg; 8 g/scoop; 16 g/tbsp.

Malva rotundifolia; M. sylvestris *medicinal herb* [see: mallow]

Mammol ointment OTC *emollient for nipples of nursing mothers* [bismuth subnitrate] 40%

m-AMSA (acridinylamine methanesulphon anisidide) [see: amsacrine]

Mandameth enteric-coated tablets ℞ *urinary antibiotic* [methenamine mandelate] 0.5, 1 g

Mandelamine film-coated tablets ℞ *urinary antibiotic* [methenamine mandelate] 0.5, 1 g

mandelic acid NF

Mandol powder for IV or IM injection (discontinued 2003) ℞ *cephalosporin antibiotic* [cefamandole nafate] 1 g ② nadolol

mandrake (*Mandragora officinarum; Podophyllum peltatum*) root and resin *medicinal herb for cancer, condylomata, constipation, fever, indigestion, liver disorders, lower bowel disorders, warts, and worms; not generally regarded as safe and effective for children or pregnant women*

Manerex Ⓒᴬᴺ film-coated tablets ℞ *antidepressant; MAO inhibitor* [moclobemide] 100, 150 mg

mangafodipir trisodium USAN *paramagnetic contrast agent for MRI of the liver*

manganese *element (Mn)*

manganese chloride USP *dietary manganese supplement* 0.1 mg/mL injection

manganese chloride tetrahydrate [see: manganese chloride]

manganese citrate *dietary manganese supplement (30% elemental manganese)*

manganese gluconate (manganese D-gluconate) USP *dietary manganese supplement*

manganese glycerophosphate NF

manganese hypophosphite NF

manganese phosphinate [see: manganese hypophosphite]

manganese sulfate USP *dietary manganese supplement* 0.1 mg/mL injection

manganese sulfate monohydrate [see: manganese sulfate]

mangofodipir trisodium *MRI contrast medium for liver imaging*

manidipine 6300 INN

manna sugar [see: mannitol]

mannite [see: mannitol]

mannitol (D-mannitol) USP *renal function test aid; antihypertensive; osmotic diuretic; urologic irrigant* 10%, 15%, 20%, 25% injection

mannitol hexanitrate INN

mannityl nitrate [see: mannitol hexanitrate]

D-mannoheptulose *the active principle in avocado that suppresses excess insulin production by the pancreas; investigational treatment for obesity and type 2 diabetes* [also: avocado sugar extract]

mannomustine INN, BAN

mannosulfan INN

manozodil INN

Mantoux test [see: tuberculin]

MAO inhibitors (monoamine oxidase inhibitors) [q.v.]

Maolate tablets ℞ *skeletal muscle relaxant* [chlorphenesin carbamate] 400 mg

Maox 420 tablets OTC *antacid* [magnesium oxide] 420 mg

MAP (mitomycin, Adriamycin, Platinol) *chemotherapy protocol*

Mapap tablets OTC *analgesic; antipyretic* [acetaminophen] 325, 500 mg

Mapap, Children's oral liquid OTC *analgesic; antipyretic* [acetaminophen] 160 mg/5 mL

Mapap Cold Formula tablets OTC *antitussive; decongestant; antihistamine; analgesic* [dextromethorphan hydrobromide; pseudoephedrine HCl; chlorpheniramine maleate; acetaminophen] 15•30•2•325 mg

Mapap Infant Drops OTC *analgesic; antipyretic* [acetaminophen] 100 mg/mL

Mapap Sinus geltabs OTC *decongestant; analgesic; antipyretic* [pseudoephedrine HCl; acetaminophen] 30•500 mg

maple lungwort *medicinal herb* [see: lungwort]

maprotiline USAN, INN *tetracyclic antidepressant*

maprotiline HCl USP *tetracyclic antidepressant* 25, 50, 75 mg oral

Maranox tablets OTC *analgesic; antipyretic* [acetaminophen] 325 mg

Marax tablets ℞ *antiasthmatic; bronchodilator; decongestant* [theophylline; ephedrine sulfate] 130•25 mg ⚠ Atarax; Maalox

Marax-DF pediatric syrup ℞ *antiasthmatic; bronchodilator; decongestant; antihistamine* [theophylline; ephedrine sulfate; hydroxyzine HCl] 97.5•18.75•7.5 mg/15 mL

Marblen tablets, oral liquid OTC *antacid* [calcium carbonate; magnesium carbonate] 520•400 mg; 540•400 mg/5 mL

Marcaine HCl injection ℞ *injectable local anesthetic* [bupivacaine HCl] 0.25%, 0.5%, 0.75%

Marcaine HCl injection ℞ *injectable local anesthetic* [bupivacaine HCl; epinephrine bitartrate] 0.25%•

1:200 000, 0.5%•1:200 000, 0.75%•
1:200 000 ⑨ Narcan

Marcaine Spinal injection (discontinued 2002) ℞ *injectable local anesthetic* [bupivacaine HCl] 0.75%

Marcillin capsules (discontinued 2002) ℞ *aminopenicillin antibiotic* [ampicillin] 500 mg

Marcof Expectorant syrup ℞ *narcotic antitussive; expectorant* [hydrocodone bitartrate; potassium guaiacolsulfonate] 5•300 mg/5 mL

mare's tail *medicinal herb* [see: fleabane; horseweed]

Marezine tablets OTC *antiemetic; anticholinergic; antihistamine; motion sickness preventative* [cyclizine HCl] 50 mg

Margesic capsules ℞ *analgesic; barbiturate sedative* [acetaminophen; caffeine; butalbital] 325•40•50 mg

Margesic H capsules ℞ *narcotic analgesic* [hydrocodone bitartrate; acetaminophen] 5•500 mg

maribavir USAN *antiviral for cytomegalovirus infections*

maridomycin INN

marigold (Calendula officinalis) florets *medicinal herb for bruises, cuts, dysmenorrhea, eye infections, fever, and skin diseases; not generally regarded as safe and effective*

marijuana ㉑ *approved for compassionate use in terminally ill patients*

marijuana; marihuana (Cannabis sativa) *euphoric/hallucinogenic street drug made from the dried leaves and flowering tops of the cannabis plant; medicinal herb for asthma, analgesia, leprosy, and loss of appetite; investigational for HIV*

marimastat USAN *investigational (Phase III) antineoplastic; matrix metalloproteinase (MMP) inhibitor*

Marine Lipid Concentrate softgels OTC *dietary supplement* [omega-3 fatty acids] 1200 mg

Marinol oil-filled gelcaps ℞ *antiemetic for chemotherapy; appetite stimulant for AIDS patients (orphan)* [dronabinol] 2.5, 5, 10 mg

mariptiline INN

marjoram (Majorana hortensis; Origanum vulgare) plant *medicinal herb for abdominal cramps, colic, headache, indigestion, respiratory problems, and violent cough*

Marlin Salt System tablets OTC *rinsing/storage solution for soft contact lenses* [sodium chloride (normal saline solution)] 250 mg

Marlin Salt System II tablets OTC *rinsing/storage solution for soft contact lenses* [sodium chloride (normal saline solution)] 250 mg

Marmine IV or IM injection ℞ *antinauseant; antiemetic; antivertigo; motion sickness preventative* [dimenhydrinate] 50 mg/mL

Marmine tablets OTC *antinauseant; antiemetic; antivertigo; motion sickness preventative* [dimenhydrinate] 50 mg

Marnatal-F film-coated tablets ℞ *vitamin/mineral/calcium/iron supplement* [multiple vitamins & minerals; calcium; iron; folic acid] ±•250•60•1 mg

Marogen ℞ *investigational (orphan) hematinic for anemia of end-stage renal disease* [epoetin beta]

maroxepin INN

Marplan tablets ℞ *antidepressant; monoamine oxidase (MAO) inhibitor* [isocarboxazid] 10 mg

Marpres tablets ℞ *antihypertensive; vasodilator; diuretic* [hydrochlorothiazide; reserpine; hydralazine HCl] 15•0.1•25 mg

Marrubium vulgare *medicinal herb* [see: horehound]

marsh clover; marsh trefoil *medicinal herb* [see: buckbean]

marsh mallow (Althaea officinalis) root *medicinal herb for asthma, boils, bronchial infections, cough, emphysema, infected wounds, kidney disorders, lung congestion, sore throat, and urinary bleeding*

MARstem ℞ *investigational (orphan) agent for myelodysplastic syndrome and* neutropenia due to bone marrow transplantation [angiotensin 1-7]

MART-1 adenoviral gene therapy investigational (orphan) for metastatic malignant melanoma

Marten-Tab caplets ℞ analgesic; barbiturate sedative [acetaminophen; butalbital] 325•50 mg

Marthritic tablets ℞ analgesic; antipyretic; anti-inflammatory; antirheumatic [salsalate] 750 mg

Marvelon ⓒ tablets (in packs of 21 or 28) ℞ monophasic oral contraceptive [desogestrel; ethinyl estradiol] 0.15 mg•30 μg

masoprocol USAN, INN antineoplastic for actinic keratoses (AK)

Massé Breast cream OTC moisturizer and emollient for nipples of nursing women

Massengill Baking Soda Freshness solution OTC vaginal cleanser and deodorizer; acidity modifier [sodium bicarbonate]

Massengill Disposable Douche solution OTC antiseptic/germicidal; vaginal cleanser and deodorizer; acidity modifier [cetylpyridinium chloride; lactic acid; sodium lactate]

Massengill Disposable Douche; Massengill Vinegar & Water Extra Mild solution OTC vaginal cleanser and deodorizer; acidity modifier [vinegar (acetic acid)]

Massengill Douche powder OTC astringent; analgesic; counterirritant; vaginal cleanser and deodorizer [ammonium alum; phenol; methyl salicylate; menthol; thymol]

Massengill Douche solution concentrate OTC vaginal cleanser and deodorizer; acidity modifier [lactic acid; sodium lactate; sodium bicarbonate]

Massengill Feminine Cleansing Wash topical liquid OTC for external perivaginal cleansing

Massengill Medicated towelettes OTC topical corticosteroidal anti-inflammatory [hydrocortisone] 0.5%

Massengill Medicated Douche with Cepticin; Massengill Medicated

Disposable Douche with Cepticin solution OTC antiseptic/germicidal; vaginal cleanser and deodorizer [povidone-iodine] 12%; 10%

Massengill Vinegar & Water Extra Cleansing with Puraclean solution OTC antiseptic/germicidal; vaginal cleanser and deodorizer; acidity modifier [cetylpyridinium chloride; vinegar (acetic acid)]

mast cell stabilizers a class of topical agents that inhibit the antigen-induced release of inflammatory mediators (e.g., various histamines and leukotrienes) from human mast cells; used on nasal, ophthalmological, and gastrointestinal mucosa [also known as: mediator release inhibitors]

masterwort (Heracleum lanatum) root and seed medicinal herb used as an antispasmodic, carminative, and stimulant

Mastisol topical liquid OTC adhesive for securing dressings, IV lines, etc. on the skin

maté medicinal herb [see: yerba maté]

Matricaria chamomilla medicinal herb [see: chamomile]

matrix metalloproteinase (MMP) inhibitors a class of investigational (Phase III) antineoplastics and investigational (orphan) agents to treat corneal ulcers

Matulane capsules ℞ antineoplastic for Hodgkin disease; investigational for other lymphomas, melanoma, brain tumors, and lung cancer [procarbazine HCl] 50 mg

Mavik ⓒ capsules ℞ antihypertensive; angiotensin-converting enzyme (ACE) inhibitor [trandolapril] 0.5, 1, 2 mg

Mavik tablets ℞ antihypertensive; angiotensin-converting enzyme (ACE) inhibitor; treatment for CHF [trandolapril] 1, 2, 4 mg

maxacalcitol USAN investigational vitamin D₃ analogue for the topical treatment of psoriasis

Maxair Autohaler (breath-activated metered-dose inhaler) ℞ sympatho-

mimetic bronchodilator [pirbuterol acetate] 0.2 mg/dose

Maxalt caplets ℞ *vascular serotonin 5-HT$_{1B/1D}$ receptor agonist for the acute treatment of migraine* [rizatriptan benzoate] 5, 10 mg

Maxalt-MLT orally disintegrating tablets ℞ *vascular serotonin 5-HT$_{1B/1D}$ receptor agonist for the acute treatment of migraine* [rizatriptan benzoate] 5, 10 mg

Maxalt-RPD ⒸⒶⓃ orally disintegrating tablets ℞ *vascular serotonin 5-HT$_{1B/1D}$ receptor agonist for the acute treatment of migraine* [rizatriptan benzoate] 5, 10 mg

Maxaquin film-coated tablets ℞ *broad-spectrum fluoroquinolone antibiotic* [lomefloxacin HCl] 400 mg

MaxEPA soft capsules OTC *dietary supplement* [omega-3 fatty acids; multiple vitamins & minerals] 1000• ± mg

Maxibolin *an anabolic steroid abused as a street drug* [see: ethylestrenol]

Maxicam ℞ *investigational (NDA filed) nonsteroidal anti-inflammatory drug (NSAID); antiarthritic; analgesic; antipyretic* [isoxicam]

Maxidex Drop-Tainers (eye drop suspension) ℞ *topical ophthalmic corticosteroidal anti-inflammatory* [dexamethasone] 0.1%

Maxidone caplets ℞ *narcotic analgesic* [hydrocodone bitartrate; acetaminophen] 10•750 mg

Maxifed caplets ℞ *decongestant; expectorant* [pseudoephedrine HCl; guaifenesin] 80•780 mg

Maxifed DM; Maxifed DMX sustained-release caplets OTC *antitussive; decongestant; expectorant* [dextromethorphan hydrobromide; pseudoephedrine HCl; guaifenesin] 30•60•580 mg; 40•80•780 mg

Maxifed-G sustained-release caplets OTC *decongestant; expectorant* [pseudoephedrine HCl; guaifenesin] 60•580 mg

Maxiflor cream, ointment ℞ *corticosteroidal anti-inflammatory* [diflorasone diacetate] 0.05%

Maxilube jelly OTC *vaginal lubricant*

Maximum Blue Label; Maximum Green Label tablets OTC *vitamin/mineral supplement* [multiple vitamins & minerals; folic acid; biotin] ± •130•50 µg

Maximum Red Label tablets OTC *vitamin/mineral/iron supplement* [multiple vitamins & minerals; iron; folic acid; biotin] ± •3.3 mg•0.13 mg•50 µg

"Maximum Strength" products [see under product name]

Maxiphen DM extended-release caplets ℞ *antitussive; decongestant; expectorant* [dextromethorphan hydrobromide; phenylephrine HCl; guaifenesin] 60•40•1000 mg

Maxipime powder for IV or IM injection ℞ *cephalosporin antibiotic* [cefepime HCl] 0.5, 1, 2 g

Maxitrol eye drop suspension, ophthalmic ointment ℞ *topical ophthalmic corticosteroidal anti-inflammatory; antibiotic* [dexamethasone; neomycin sulfate; polymyxin B sulfate] 0.1%• 0.35%•10 000 U/mL; 0.1%•0.35%• 10 000 U/g

Maxi-Tuss DM oral liquid ℞ *antitussive; expectorant* [dextromethorphan hydrobromide; guaifenesin] 20•200 mg/5 mL

Maxi-Tuss HC; Maxi-Tuss HCX oral liquid ℞ *narcotic antitussive; decongestant; antihistamine* [hydrocodone bitartrate; phenylephrine HCl; chlorpheniramine maleate] 2.5•10• 4 mg/5 mL; 6•12•2 mg/5 mL

Maxi-Tuss HCG oral liquid ℞ *narcotic antitussive; expectorant* [hydrocodone bitartrate; guaifenesin] 6•200 mg/5 mL

Maxivate lotion (discontinued 2004) ℞ *corticosteroidal anti-inflammatory* [betamethasone dipropionate] 0.05%

Maxivate ointment, cream ℞ *corticosteroidal anti-inflammatory* [betamethasone dipropionate] 0.05%

Maxi-Vite tablets OTC *vitamin/mineral/ calcium/iron supplement* [multiple vitamins & minerals; calcium; iron; folic acid; biotin] ± • 53.5 • 1.5 • 0.4 • 0.001 mg

Maxolon tablets ℞ *antidopaminergic; antiemetic for chemotherapy; peristaltic* [metoclopramide HCl] 10 mg

Maxovite sustained-release tablets OTC *vitamin/mineral supplement* [multiple vitamins & minerals; folic acid; biotin] ± • 330 • 11.7 µg

Maxzide tablets ℞ *antihypertensive; diuretic* [triamterene; hydrochlorothiazide] 37.5 • 25, 75 • 50 mg ⊡ Microzide

May apple *medicinal herb* [see: mandrake]

May bells; May lily *medicinal herb* [see: lily of the valley]

May bush; May tree *medicinal herb* [see: hawthorn]

May lily *medicinal herb* [see: lily of the valley]

maytansine USAN *antineoplastic* [also: maitansine]

May-Vita elixir (discontinued 2003) ℞ *vitamin supplement* [multiple B vitamins; folic acid] ± • 0.1 mg

Mazanor tablets (discontinued 2001) ℞ *anorexiant; CNS stimulant* [mazindol] 1 mg

mazapertine succinate USAN *antipsychotic; dopamine receptor antagonist*

mazaticol INN

MAZE (*m*-AMSA, azacitidine, etoposide) *chemotherapy protocol*

mazindol USAN, USP, INN, BAN *anorexiant; CNS stimulant; investigational (orphan) treatment for Duchenne muscular dystrophy* ⊡ mebendazole

mazipredone INN

MB (methylene blue) [q.v.]

m-BACOD; M-BACOD (methotrexate, bleomycin, Adriamycin, cyclophosphamide, Oncovin, dexamethasone) *chemotherapy protocol for non-Hodgkin lymphoma* ("m" is 200 mg/m^2; "M" is 3 g/m^2)

m-BACOD reduced dose (methotrexate, bleomycin, Adriamycin, cyclophosphamide, Oncovin, dexamethasone) *chemotherapy protocol for HIV-associated non-Hodgkin lymphoma*

M-BACOS (methotrexate, bleomycin, Adriamycin, cyclophosphamide, Oncovin, Solu-Medrol) *chemotherapy protocol*

MBC (methotrexate, bleomycin, cisplatin) *chemotherapy protocol for head and neck cancer*

MBD (methotrexate, bleomycin, DDP) *chemotherapy protocol*

MBR (methylene blue, reduced) [see: methylene blue]

MC (mitoxantrone, cytarabine) *chemotherapy protocol for acute myelocytic leukemia (AML)*

M-Caps capsules ℞ *urinary acidifier to control ammonia production* [racemethionine] 200 mg

MCBP (melphalan, cyclophosphamide, BCNU, prednisone) *chemotherapy protocol*

MCC (mycobacterial cell wall complex) [see: urocidin]

MCH (microfibrillar collagen hemostat) [q.v.]

MCK-442 investigational (Phase III) *non-nucleoside reverse transcriptase inhibitor (NNRTI) for AIDS*

MCP (melphalan, cyclophosphamide, prednisone) *chemotherapy protocol*

M-CSF (macrophage colony-stimulating factor) [now: cilmostim]

MCT oil OTC *dietary fat supplement* [medium chain triglycerides from coconut oil]

MCT (medium chain triglycerides) [q.v.]

MCV (methotrexate, cisplatin, vinblastine) *chemotherapy protocol*

MD-76 R injection ℞ *radiopaque contrast medium* [diatrizoate meglumine; diatrizoate sodium (48.7% total iodine)] 660 • 100 mg/mL (370 mg/mL)

MDA (methylenedioxyampheta-mine) [see: MDMA, MDEA]

MDEA (3,4-methylenedioxyetham-phetamine) *a hallucinogenic amphetamine derivative closely related to MDMA, abused as a street drug, which causes dependence* [also see: amphetamines; MDMA]

MD-Gastroview oral solution (discontinued 2005) ℞ *radiopaque contrast medium for gastrointestinal imaging* [diatrizoate meglumine; diatrizoate sodium (48.29% total iodine)] 660•100 mg/mL (367 mg/mL)

MDI (dosage form) *metered-dose inhaler*

MDMA (3,4-methylenedioxymeth-amphetamine) *widely abused hallucinogenic street drug that is chemically related to amphetamines and mescaline and causes dependence; investigational euphoric to counteract suicidal ideations and feelings of hopelessness in terminal cancer patients* [see also: amphetamines; mescaline; MDEA]

MDP (methylene diphosphonate) [now: medronate disodium]

MDX-240 *investigational (Phase II) virus-specific antibody for AIDS*

MEA (mercaptoethylamine) [see: mercaptamine]

meadow cabbage *medicinal herb* [see: skunk cabbage]

meadow sorrel *medicinal herb* [see: sorrel]

meadowsweet (Filipendula ulmaria) plant *medicinal herb used for ulcers and upper respiratory problems; also used as an astringent, diaphoretic, and diuretic*

mealberry *medicinal herb* [see: uva ursi]

mealy starwort *medicinal herb* [see: star grass]

measles, mumps & rubella virus vaccine, live USP *active immunizing agent for measles (rubeola), mumps, and rubella*

measles immune globulin USP

measles & rubella virus vaccine, live USP *active immunizing agent for measles (rubeola) and rubella*

measles virus vaccine, live USP *active immunizing agent for measles (rubeola)*

Mebadin (available only from the Centers for Disease Control) ℞ *investigational anti-infective for amebiasis and amebic dysentery* [dehydroemetine]

meballymal [see: secobarbital]

mebamoxine [see: benmoxin]

mebanazine INN, BAN

Mebaral tablets ℞ *long-acting barbiturate sedative, hypnotic, and anticonvulsant* [mephobarbital] 32, 50, 100 mg ⊉ Medrol

mebendazole USAN, USP, INN *anthelmintic for trichuriasis, enterobiasis, ascariasis, and uncinariasis* 100 mg oral ⊉ mazindol

mebenoside INN

mebeverine INN *smooth muscle relaxant* [also: mebeverine HCl]

mebeverine HCl USAN *smooth muscle relaxant* [also: mebeverine]

mebezonium iodide INN, BAN

mebhydrolin INN, BAN

mebiquine INN

mebolazine INN

mebrofenin USAN, INN *hepatobiliary function test*

mebrophenhydramine HCl [see: embramine HCl]

mebubarbital [see: pentobarbital]

mebumal [see: pentobarbital]

mebutamate USAN, INN *antihypertensive*

mebutizide INN

mecamylamine INN *antiadrenergic; ganglionic blocker for severe hypertension* [also: mecamylamine HCl]

mecamylamine HCl USP *antiadrenergic; ganglionic blocker for severe hypertension* [also: mecamylamine]

mecamylamine HCl & nicotine *investigational (Phase III) transdermal patch for smoking cessation*

mecarbinate INN

mecarbine [see: mecarbinate]

mecasermin USAN, INN, BAN *investigational (NDA filed, orphan) for amyotrophic lateral sclerosis, type 1 and type 2 diabetes, growth hormone insufficiency, and post-poliomyelitis syndrome* [previously known as insulin-like growth factor 1 (IGF-1)]

MeCCNU (methyl chloroethyl-cyclohexyl-nitrosourea) [see: semustine]

mecetronium ethylsulfate USAN *antiseptic* [also: mecetronium etilsulfate]

mecetronium etilsulfate INN *antiseptic* [also: mecetronium ethylsulfate]

mechlorethamine HCl USP *nitrogen mustard-type alkylating antineoplastic* [also: chlormethine; mustine; nitrogen mustard N-oxide HCl]

meciadanol INN

mecillinam INN, BAN *antibacterial* [also: amdinocillin]

mecinarone INN

Meclan cream (discontinued 2003) ℞ *antibiotic for acne* [meclocycline sulfosalicylate] 1% ⧄ Meclomen; Mezlin

meclizine HCl USP *antiemetic; antihistamine; anticholinergic; motion sickness relief* [also: meclozine] 12.5, 25, 50 mg oral ⧄ mescaline

meclocycline USAN, INN, BAN *topical antibiotic*

meclocycline sulfosalicylate USAN, USP *topical antibiotic*

meclofenamate sodium USAN, USP *analgesic; antiarthritic; nonsteroidal anti-inflammatory drug (NSAID)* 50, 100 mg oral

meclofenamic acid USAN, INN *nonsteroidal anti-inflammatory drug (NSAID)*

meclofenoxate INN, BAN

meclonazepam INN

mecloqualone USAN, INN *sedative; hypnotic*

mecloralurea INN

meclorisone INN, BAN *topical anti-inflammatory* [also: meclorisone dibutyrate]

meclorisone dibutyrate USAN *topical anti-inflammatory* [also: meclorisone]

mecloxamine INN

meclozine INN, BAN *antiemetic; antihistamine; anticholinergic; motion sickness relief* [also: meclizine HCl] ⧄ mescaline

mecobalamin USAN, INN *vitamin; hematopoietic*

mecrilate INN *tissue adhesive* [also: mecrylate]

mecrylate USAN *tissue adhesive* [also: mecrilate]

MECY (methotrexate, cyclophosphamide) *chemotherapy protocol*

mecysteine INN

Meda Cap capsules OTC *analgesic; antipyretic* [acetaminophen] 500 mg

Meda Tab tablets OTC *analgesic; antipyretic* [acetaminophen] 325 mg

Medacote lotion OTC *topical antihistamine; astringent; antipruritic* [pyrilamine maleate; zinc oxide] 1%• 2

Medalone 40; Medalone 80 [see: depMedalone 40; depMedalone 80]

medazepam INN *minor tranquilizer* [also: medazepam HCl]

medazepam HCl USAN *minor tranquilizer* [also: medazepam]

medazomide INN

medazonamide [see: medazomide]

Medebar Plus rectal suspension ℞ *radiopaque contrast medium for gastrointestinal imaging* [barium sulfate] 100%

Medent-DM sustained-release tablets ℞ *antitussive; decongestant; expectorant* [dextromethorphan hydrobromide; pseudoephedrine HCl; guaifenesin] 30•60•800 mg

Mederma gel OTC *moisturizer and emollient for scars* [PEG-4; onion extract; xanthan gum; allantoin]

Medescan oral suspension ℞ *radiopaque contrast medium for gastrointestinal imaging* [barium sulfate] 2.3%

medetomidine INN, BAN *veterinary analgesic; veterinary sedative* [also: medetomidine HCl]

medetomidine HCl USAN *veterinary analgesic; veterinary sedative* [also: medetomidine]

mediator release inhibitors *a class of topical agents that inhibit the antigen-induced release of inflammatory mediators (e.g., various histamines and leukotrienes) from human mast cells; used on nasal, ophthalmological, and gastro-*

intestinal mucosa [also known as: mast cell stabilizers]

medibazine INN

Medicago sativa medicinal herb [see: alfalfa]

medical air [see: air, medical]

Medicated Acne Cleanser OTC *topical acne treatment* [colloidal sulfur; resorcinol] 4%•2%

medicinal zinc peroxide [see: zinc peroxide, medicinal]

Medicone anorectal ointment OTC *topical local anesthetic* [benzocaine] 20%

Medicone rectal suppositories (discontinued 2004) OTC *topical vasoconstrictor for hemorrhoids* [phenylephrine HCl] 0.25%

Medi-First Sinus Decongestant tablets OTC *nasal decongestant* [pseudoephedrine HCl] 30 mg

medifoxamine INN

Medigesic capsules ℞ *analgesic; barbiturate sedative* [acetaminophen; caffeine; butalbital] 325•40•50 mg

Medihaler-Iso inhalation aerosol (discontinued 2001) ℞ *sympathomimetic bronchodilator* [isoproterenol sulfate] 80 μg/dose

medinal [see: barbital sodium]

Mediotic-HC ear drops ℞ *corticosteroidal anti-inflammatory; local anesthetic; bacteriostatic* [hydrocortisone; pramoxine HCl; chloroxylenol; benzalkonium chloride] 1%•1%•0.1%•0.01%

Mediplast plaster OTC *keratolytic* [salicylic acid] 40%

Mediplex Tabules (tablets) OTC *vitamin/mineral supplement* [multiple vitamins & minerals]

Mediplex Plus tablets OTC *vitamin/mineral supplement* [multiple vitamins & minerals; folic acid] ±•0.4 mg

Medi-Quik ointment (discontinued 2001) OTC *topical antibiotic* [polymyxin B sulfate; neomycin; bacitracin] 5000 U•3.5 mg•400 U per g

Medi-Quik spray OTC *topical local anesthetic; antiseptic* [lidocaine; benzalkonium chloride] 2%•0.13%

medium chain triglycerides (MCT) *dietary lipid supplement*

medorinone USAN, INN *cardiotonic*

medorubicin INN

Medotar ointment OTC *antipsoriatic; antiseborrheic; astringent; antiseptic* [coal tar; zinc oxide] 1%• ☲

Medralone 40; Medralone 80 intralesional, soft tissue, and IM injection (discontinued 2002) ℞ *corticosteroid; anti-inflammatory; immunosuppressant* [methylprednisolone acetate] 40 mg/mL; 80 mg/mL

medrogestone USAN, INN, BAN *progestin*

Medrol tablets, Dosepak (unit of use package) ℞ *corticosteroid; anti-inflammatory; immunosuppressant* [methylprednisolone] 2, 4, 8, 16, 24, 32 mg ⊘ Mebaral

medronate disodium USAN *pharmaceutic aid*

medronic acid USAN, INN, BAN *pharmaceutic aid*

medroxalol USAN, INN, BAN *antihypertensive*

medroxalol HCl USAN *antihypertensive*

medroxiprogesterone acetate [see: medroxyprogesterone acetate]

medroxyprogesterone INN, BAN *synthetic progestin for secondary amenorrhea or abnormal uterine bleeding; hormonal antineoplastic* [also: medroxyprogesterone acetate]

medroxyprogesterone acetate USP *synthetic progestin for secondary amenorrhea, abnormal uterine bleeding, and endometrial hyperplasia; hormonal antineoplastic* [also: medroxyprogesterone] 2.5, 5, 10 mg oral; 150 mg/mL depot injection

MED-Rx controlled-release tablets (14-day, 56-tablet regimen) (discontinued 2002) ℞ *decongestant; expectorant* [pseudoephedrine HCl + guaifenesin (blue tablets); guaifenesin (white tablets)] 60•600 mg; 600 mg

MED-Rx DM controlled-release tablets (14-day, 56-tablet regimen) ℞ *decongestant + expectorant (AM); antitussive + expectorant (PM)* [pseudoephedrine

HCl + guaifenesin (AM); dextromethorphan hydrobromide + guaifenesin (PM)] 60•600 mg; 30•600 mg

medrylamine INN

medrysone USAN, USP, INN *ophthalmic
corticosteroidal anti-inflammatory*

mefeclorazine INN

mefenamic acid USAN, USP, INN, BAN
*analgesic; nonsteroidal anti-inflamma-
tory drug (NSAID)*

mefenidil USAN, INN *cerebral vasodilator*

mefenidil fumarate USAN *cerebral
vasodilator*

mefenidramium metilsulfate INN

mefenorex INN *anorectic* [also: mefenorex HCl]

mefenorex HCl USAN *anorectic* [also:
mefenorex]

mefeserpine INN

mefexamide USAN, INN *CNS stimulant*

mefloquine USAN, INN, BAN *antimalarial*

mefloquine HCl USAN *antimalarial for
acute chloroquine-resistant malaria
(orphan)* 250 mg oral

Mefoxin powder or frozen premix for
IV or IM injection ℞ *cephamycin
antibiotic* [cefoxitin sodium] 1, 2, 10 g

mefruside USAN, INN *diuretic*

Mega AO 🅐🅝 tablets OTC *antioxidant/
vitamin supplement* [multiple vitamins; coenzyme Q10; folic acid; bio-
tin] ±•4•0.333•0.167 mg

Mega VM-80 tablets OTC *geriatric vita-
min/mineral supplement* [multiple
vitamins & minerals; folic acid; bio-
tin] ±•400•80 µg

Mega-B tablets OTC *vitamin supplement*
[multiple B vitamins; folic acid; bio-
tin] ±•100•100 µg

Megace tablets ℞ *progestin; hormonal
antineoplastic for advanced carcinoma
of the breast or endometrium* [mege-
strol acetate] 40 mg

Megace; Megace ES oral suspension
℞ *progestin; treatment for AIDS-related
anorexia and cachexia (orphan)* [mege-
strol acetate] 40 mg/mL; 125 mg/mL

**megakaryocyte growth and devel-
opment factor, pegylated, recombinant human** *investigational*

*(orphan) adjunct to hematopoietic stem
cell transplantation*

megallate INN *combining name for radicals or groups*

megalomicin INN *antibacterial* [also:
megalomicin potassium phosphate]

megalomicin potassium phosphate
USAN *antibacterial* [also: megalomicin]

Megaton elixir ℞ *vitamin/mineral supplement* [multiple B vitamins & minerals; folic acid] ±•0.1 mg

megestrol INN, BAN *progestin; hormonal antineoplastic for breast or endometrial cancer; investigational (Phase
III) for liver cancer* [also: megestrol
acetate]

megestrol acetate USAN, USP *progestin; hormonal antineoplastic for breast
or endometrial cancer; therapy for
AIDS-related anorexia and cachexia
(orphan)* [also: megestrol] 20, 40 mg
oral; 40 mg/mL oral

meglitinide INN

meglucycline INN

meglumine USP, INN *radiopaque contrast medium*

meglumine diatrizoate BAN *oral/
parenteral radiopaque contrast medium
(46.67% iodine)* [also: diatrizoate
meglumine]

meglumine iocarmate BAN *radiopaque contrast medium* [also: iocarmate meglumine]

meglumine iothalamate BAN *parenteral radiopaque contrast medium (47%
iodine)* [also: iothalamate meglumine]

meglumine ioxaglate BAN *radiopaque
contrast medium* [also: ioxaglate meg-
lumine]

meglutol USAN, INN *antihyperlipoproteinemic*

mel B [see: melarsoprol]

mel W [see: melarsonyl potassium]

meladrazine INN, BAN

melafocon A USAN *hydrophobic contact lens material*

melagatran *parenteral anticoagulant
and direct thrombin inhibitor*

Melaleuca alternifolia *medicinal herb*
[see: tea tree oil]

Melanex solution (discontinued 2003) ℞ *hyperpigmentation bleaching agent* [hydroquinone] 3%

melanoma vaccine *investigational (NDA filed, orphan) therapeutic vaccine for invasive stage III–IV melanoma; investigational (Phase III) for early-stage melanoma*

melarsonyl potassium INN, BAN

melarsoprol INN, BAN, DCF *investigational anti-infective for trypanosomiasis*

melatonin *natural sleep aid; investigational (orphan) for circadian rhythm sleep disorders in blind people with no light perception*

melengestrol INN *antineoplastic; progestin* [also: melengestrol acetate]

melengestrol acetate USAN *antineoplastic; progestin* [also: melengestrol]

meletimide INN

melfalan [see: melphalan]

Melfiat-105 Unicelles (sustained-release capsules) ℞ *anorexiant; CNS stimulant* [phendimetrazine tartrate] 105 mg

Melia azedarach medicinal herb [see: pride of China]

melilot *(Melilotus alba; M. officinalis)* flowering plant *medicinal herb used as an antispasmodic, diuretic, emollient, expectorant, and vulnerary*

melinamide INN

Melissa officinalis medicinal herb [see: lemon balm]

melitracen INN *antidepressant* [also: melitracen HCl]

melitracen HCl USAN *antidepressant* [also: melitracen]

melizame USAN, INN *sweetener*

Mellaril tablets, concentrate for oral solution (discontinued 2004) ℞ *conventional (typical) phenothiazine antipsychotic for schizophrenia; sedative; also used for agitation or psychosis due to Alzheimer or other dementias* [thioridazine HCl] 15, 100, 200 mg; 30 mg/mL ② Aldoril; Elavil; Eldepryl; Enovil; Equanil; Moderil

Mellaril-S oral suspension (discontinued 2003) ℞ *conventional (typical) phenothiazine antipsychotic for schizo-phrenia; sedative; also used for agitation or psychosis due to Alzheimer or other dementias* [thioridazine HCl] 25, 100 mg/5 mL

meloxicam USAN, INN, BAN *analgesic, antipyretic, and antiarthritic for osteoarthritis and rheumatoid arthritis; COX-2 inhibitor; nonsteroidal anti-inflammatory drug (NSAID)*

Melpaque HP cream ℞ *hyperpigmentation bleaching agent* [hydroquinone (in a sunscreen base)] 4%

melperone INN, BAN

melphalan (MPL) USAN, USP, INN, BAN, JAN *nitrogen mustard-type alkylating antineoplastic for multiple myeloma (orphan) and ovarian cancer; investigational (orphan) for metastatic melanoma*

Melquin HP cream ℞ *hyperpigmentation bleaching agent* [hydroquinone] 4%

memantine INN *NMDA (N-methyl-D-aspartate) antagonist; neuroprotective agent* [also: memantine HCl]

memantine HCl *NMDA (N-methyl-D-aspartate) antagonist for Alzheimer disease; investigational (Phase III) neuroprotective agent for diabetic neuropathy, vascular dementia, Parkinson disease, and AIDS dementia* [also: memantine]

Memorette (trademarked packaging form) *patient compliance package*

memotine INN *antiviral* [also: memotine HCl]

memotine HCl USAN *antiviral* [also: memotine]

menabitan INN *analgesic* [also: menabitan HCl]

menabitan HCl USAN *analgesic* [also: menabitan]

Menactra IM injection ℞ *meningitis vaccine for adolescents and adults (11–55 years)* [meningococcal polysaccharide vaccine, groups A, C, Y, and W-135, conjugated to diphtheria toxoid] 4•4•4•4•48 μg per 0.5 mL dose

menadiol BAN *vitamin K₄; prothrombogenic* [also: menadiol sodium diphosphate]

menadiol sodium diphosphate USP *vitamin K₄; prothrombogenic* [also: menadiol]

menadiol sodium sulfate INN

menadione USP *vitamin K₃; prothrombogenic*

menadione sodium bisulfite USP, INN

Menadol captabs OTC *analgesic; antiarthritic; antipyretic; nonsteroidal antiinflammatory drug (NSAID)* [ibuprofen] 200 mg

menaphthene [see: menadione]

menaphthone [see: menadione]

menaphthone sodium bisulfite [see: menadione sodium bisulfite]

menaquinone *vitamin K₂; prothrombogenic*

menatetrenone INN

menbutone INN, BAN

mendelevium *element (Md)*

Menest film-coated tablets ℞ *hormone replacement therapy for the treatment of postmenopausal symptoms; palliative therapy for prostate and breast cancers* [esterified estrogens (equine estrogen mixture)] 0.3, 0.625, 1.25, 2.5 mg

menfegol INN

menglytate INN

menichlopholan [see: niclofolan]

Meni-D capsules ℞ *anticholinergic; antivertigo agent; motion sickness preventative* [meclizine HCl] 25 mg

meningococcal polysaccharide vaccine, group A USP *active bacterin for meningitis (Neisseria meningitidis)*

meningococcal polysaccharide vaccine, group C USP *active bacterin for meningitis (Neisseria meningitidis)*

meningococcal polysaccharide vaccine, group W-135 *active bacterin for meningitis (Neisseria meningitidis)*

meningococcal polysaccharide vaccine, group Y *active bacterin for meningitis (Neisseria meningitidis)*

Menispermum cocculus; M. lacunosum *medicinal herb* [see: levant berry]

menitrazepam INN

menoctone USAN, INN *antimalarial*

menogaril USAN, INN *antibiotic antineoplastic*

Menomune-A/C/Y/W-135 powder for subcu injection ℞ *meningitis vaccine* [meningococcal polysaccharide vaccine, groups A, C, Y, and W-135] 50 μg of each group per 0.5 mL dose

Menopur powder for IM injection ℞ *ovulation stimulant for women; spermatogenesis stimulant for men* [menotropins] 150 IU

Menostar transdermal patch ℞ *estrogen replacement therapy for postmenopausal symptoms* [17β-estradiol] 14 μg/day

menotropins USAN, USP *gonadotropin; gonad-stimulating principle for the induction of ovulation in women and the stimulation of spermatogenesis in men*

Men-Phor lotion OTC *analgesic; counterirritant; moisturizer* [menthol; camphor] 0.5%•0.5%

Mentax cream ℞ *benzylamine antifungal* [butenafine HCl] 1%

Mentha piperita medicinal herb [see: peppermint]

Mentha pulegium medicinal herb [see: pennyroyal]

Mentha spicata medicinal herb [see: spearmint]

menthol USP *topical analgesic and antipruritic; counterirritant; mild local anesthetic*

Menthol Cough Drops lozenges OTC *topical oral analgesic; counterirritant; mild local anesthetic; antiseptic* [menthol] 6.5 mg

Mentholatum vaporizing ointment OTC *counterirritant; cough suppressant* [menthol; camphor] 9%•1.3%

Mentholatum Cherry Chest Rub for Kids vaporizing ointment OTC *counterirritant; cough suppressant* [menthol; camphor; eucalyptus oil] 4.7%•2.6%•1.2%

menthyl anthranilate [see: meradimate]

Menyanthes trifoliata medicinal herb [see: buckbean]

meobentine INN *antiarrhythmic* [also: meobentine sulfate]

meobentine sulfate USAN *antiarrhythmic* [also: meobentine]

mepacrine INN *anthelmintic; antimalarial* [also: quinacrine HCl]

mepacrine HCl [see: quinacrine HCl]

meparfynol [see: methylpentynol]

mepartricin USAN, INN *antifungal; antiprotozoal*

mepazine acetate [see: pecazine]

mepenzolate bromide USP, INN *GI antispasmodic; anticholinergic; peptic ulcer adjunct*

mepenzolate methylbromide [see: mepenzolate bromide]

mepenzolone bromide [see: mepenzolate bromide]

Mepergan injection (discontinued 2004) ℞ *narcotic analgesic; sedative* [meperidine HCl; promethazine HCl] 25•25 mg/mL

Mepergan Fortis capsules (discontinued 2004) ℞ *narcotic analgesic; sedative* [meperidine HCl; promethazine HCl] 50•25 mg

meperidine HCl USP *narcotic analgesic; also abused as a street drug* [also: pethidine] 50, 100 mg oral; 50 mg/5 mL oral; 25, 50, 75, 100 mg/mL injection ⊉ meprobamate

Mephaquin ℞ *antimalarial for acute chloroquine-resistant malaria (orphan)* [mefloquine HCl]

mephenesin NF, INN

mephenhydramine [see: moxastine]

mephenoxalone INN

mephentermine INN *adrenergic; vasoconstrictor; vasopressor for hypotensive shock* [also: mephentermine sulfate]

mephentermine sulfate USP *adrenergic; vasoconstrictor; vasopressor for hypotensive shock* [also: mephentermine]

mephenytoin USAN, USP, INN *hydantoin anticonvulsant* [also: methoin] ⊉ Mephyton

mephobarbital USP, JAN *anticonvulsant; sedative* [also: methylphenobarbital; methylphenobarbitone]

Mephyton tablets ℞ *coagulant to correct anticoagulant-induced prothrombin deficiency; vitamin K supplement* [phytonadione] 5 mg ⊉ mephenytoin; methadone

mepicycline [see: pipacycline]

MEPIG (mucoid exopolysaccharide *Pseudomonas* [hyper]immune globulin) [q.v.]

mepindolol INN, BAN

mepiperphenidol bromide

mepiprazole INN, BAN

mepirizole [see: epirizole]

mepiroxol INN

mepitiostane INN

mepivacaine INN *local anesthetic* [also: mepivacaine HCl]

mepivacaine HCl USP *local anesthetic* [also: mepivacaine] 3% injection

mepivacaine HCl & levonordefrin *injectable local anesthetic; vasoconstrictor* 2%•1:20 000 injection

mepixanox INN

mepolizumab USAN, INN *immunomodulator*

mepramidil INN

meprednisone USAN, USP, INN

meprobamate USP, INN, BAN, JAN *anxiolytic; sedative; hypnotic; minor tranquilizer; also abused as a street drug* 200, 400 mg oral ⊉ meperidine

Mepron oral suspension ℞ *antiprotozoal for AIDS-related Pneumocystis carinii pneumonia (orphan); investigational (orphan) for AIDS-related Toxoplasma gondii encephalitis* [atovaquone] 750 mg/5 mL ⊉ Lupron; Napron

meproscillarin INN, BAN

meprothixol BAN [also: meprotixol]

meprotixol INN [also: meprothixol]

meprylcaine INN *local anesthetic* [also: meprylcaine HCl]

meprylcaine HCl USP *local anesthetic* [also: meprylcaine]

meptazinol INN, BAN *analgesic* [also: meptazinol HCl]

meptazinol HCl USAN *analgesic* [also: meptazinol]

mepyramine INN, BAN *antihistamine* [also: pyrilamine maleate]

mepyramine maleate [see: pyrilamine maleate]

mepyrium [see: amprolium]

mepyrrotazine [see: dimelazine]

mequidox USAN, INN *antibacterial*

mequinol USAN, INN *hyperpigmentation bleaching agent*

mequitamium iodide INN

mequitazine INN, BAN

mequitazium iodide [see: mequitamium iodide]

meradimate USAN *ultraviolet A sunscreen*

meragidone sodium

meralein sodium USAN, INN *topical anti-infective*

meralluride NF, INN

merbaphen USP

merbromin NF, INN *general antiseptic*

mercaptamine INN *antiurolithic* [also: cysteamine]

mercaptoarsenical [see: arsthinol]

mercaptoarsenol [see: arsthinol]

mercaptoethylamine (MEA) [see: mercaptamine]

mercaptomerin (MT6) INN [also: mercaptomerin sodium]

mercaptomerin sodium USP [also: mercaptomerin]

mercaptopurine (6-MP) USP, INN *antimetabolite antineoplastic for acute lymphocytic, lymphoblastic, myelogenous, and myelomonocytic leukemias* 50 mg oral

mercuderamide INN

mercufenol chloride USAN *topical anti-infective*

mercumatilin sodium INN

mercuric oxide, yellow NF *ophthalmic antiseptic (FDA ruled it "not safe and effective" in 1992)*

mercuric salicylate NF

mercuric succinimide NF

mercurobutol INN

mercurophylline NF, INN

mercurous chloride [see: calomel]

mercury *element (Hg)*

mercury, ammoniated USP *topical anti-infective; antipsoriatic*

mercury amide chloride [see: mercury, ammoniated]

mercury oleate NF

merethoxylline procaine

mergocriptine INN

Meridia capsules ℞ *anorexiant for the treatment of obesity* [sibutramine HCl] 5, 10, 15 mg

merisoprol acetate Hg 197 USAN *radioactive agent*

merisoprol acetate Hg 203 USAN *radioactive agent*

merisoprol Hg 197 USAN *renal function test; radioactive agent*

Meritene powder OTC *enteral nutritional therapy* [milk-based formula]

meropenem USAN, INN, BAN *broad-spectrum carbapenem antibiotic for intra-abdominal and complicated skin structure infections, and bacterial meningitis*

Merrem powder for IV infusion ℞ *broad-spectrum carbapenem antibiotic for intra-abdominal and complicated skin structure infections, and bacterial meningitis* [meropenem] 500, 1000 mg

mersalyl INN

mersalyl sodium [see: mersalyl]

Mersol solution, tincture OTC *antiseptic; antibacterial; antifungal* [thimerosal] 1:1000

mertiatide INN

Meruvax II powder for subcu injection ℞ *rubella vaccine* [rubella virus vaccine, live] 0.5 mL

mesabolone INN

mesalamine USAN *anti-inflammatory; treatment of ulcerative colitis and proctitis* [also: mesalazine] 4 g/60 mL enema

mesalazine INN, BAN *anti-inflammatory; treatment of ulcerative colitis and proctitis* [also: mesalamine]

mescaline *hallucinogenic street drug derived from the flowering heads (mescal buttons) of a Mexican cactus* ⧉ meclizine

Mescolor sustained-release film-coated tablets (discontinued 2005) ℞ *decongestant; antihistamine; anticholinergic to dry mucosal secretions* [pseudoephedrine HCl; chlorpheniramine maleate; methscopolamine nitrate] 120•8•2.5 mg

meseclazone USAN, INN *anti-inflammatory*

mesembryanthemum *medicinal herb* [see: kanna]

mesifilcon A USAN *hydrophilic contact lens material*

mesilate INN *combining name for radicals or groups* [also: mesylate]

mesna USAN, INN, BAN *prophylaxis for ifosfamide-induced hemorrhagic cystitis (orphan); investigational (orphan) treatment for cyclophosphamide-induced hemorrhagic cystitis* 100 mg/mL injection, 400 mg oral

Mesnex film-coated caplets, IV injection ℞ *prophylaxis for ifosfamide-induced hemorrhagic cystitis (orphan); investigational (orphan) treatment for cyclophosphamide-induced hemorrhagic cystitis* [mesna] 400 mg; 100 mg/mL

mesocarb INN

meso-inositol [see: inositol]

meso-NDGA (nordihydroguaiaretic acid) [see: masoprocol]

meso-nordihydroguaiaretic acid (NDGA) [see: masoprocol]

mesoridazine USAN, INN *phenothiazine antipsychotic*

mesoridazine besylate USP *conventional (typical) phenothiazine antipsychotic for schizophrenia*

mespiperone C 11 USAN *radiopharmaceutical imaging aid for PET scans of the brain (produced at bedside for immediate administration)*

mespirenone INN

mestanolone INN, BAN

mestenediol [see: methandriol]

mesterolone USAN, INN, BAN *androgen; also abused as a street drug*

Mestinon tablets, Timespan (extended-release tablets), syrup, IM or IV injection ℞ *cholinergic/anticholinesterase muscle stimulant; muscle relaxant reversal; treatment for myasthenia gravis* [pyridostigmine bromide] 60 mg; 180 mg; 60 mg/5 mL; 5 mg/mL ☑ Mesantoin; Metatensin

mestranol USAN, USP, INN *estrogen*

mesudipine INN

mesulergine INN

mesulfamide INN

mesulfen INN [also: mesulphen]

mesulphen BAN [also: mesulfen]

mesuprine INN *vasodilator; smooth muscle relaxant* [also: mesuprine HCl]

mesuprine HCl USAN *vasodilator; smooth muscle relaxant* [also: mesuprine]

mesuximide INN *succinimide anticonvulsant* [also: methsuximide]

mesylate USAN, USP, BAN *combining name for radicals or groups* [also: mesilate]

metabromsalan USAN, INN *disinfectant*

metabutethamine HCl NF

metabutoxycaine HCl NF

metacetamol INN, BAN

metaclazepam INN

metacycline INN *antibacterial* [also: methacycline]

Metadate CD dual-release capsules, sprinkle caps ℞ *CNS stimulant; once-daily treatment for attention-deficit hyperactivity disorder (ADHD)* [methylphenidate HCl] 10, 20, 30 mg (30% immediate release; 70% extended release)

Metadate ER extended-release tablets ℞ *CNS stimulant for attention-deficit hyperactivity disorder (ADHD) and narcolepsy* [methylphenidate HCl] 10, 20 mg

Metadol ⊛ oral liquid ℞ *narcotic analgesic; treatment for opioid dependence* [methadone HCl] 10 mg/mL

Metaglip film-coated tablets ℞ *antidiabetic combination for type 2 diabetes* [glipizide; metformin HCl] 2.5•250, 2.5•500, 5•500 mg

metaglycodol INN

metahexamide INN

metahexanamide [see: metahexamide]

Metahydrin tablets ℞ *diuretic; antihypertensive* [trichlormethiazide] 4 mg ☑ Metandren

metalkonium chloride INN

metallibure INN *anterior pituitary activator for swine* [also: methallibure]

metalol HCl USAN *antiadrenergic (β-receptor)*

metamelfalan INN

metamfazone INN [also: methamphazone]

metamfepramone INN [also: dimepropion]

metamfetamine INN *CNS stimulant; widely abused as a street drug* [also: methamphetamine HCl]

metamizole sodium INN *analgesic; antipyretic* [also: dipyrone]

metampicillin INN

Metamucil capsules OTC *bulk laxative* [psyllium husk] 520 mg

Metamucil effervescent powder OTC *bulk laxative; antacid* [psyllium hydrophilic mucilloid; sodium bicarbonate; potassium bicarbonate] 3.4• ? • ? g/pkt.

Metamucil wafers OTC *bulk laxative* [psyllium husk] 3.4 g

Metamucil Original Texture; Metamucil Smooth Texture powder OTC *bulk laxative* [psyllium husk] 3.4 g/dose

metandienone INN [also: methandrostenolone; methandienone]

metanixin INN

metaoxedrine chloride [see: phenylephrine HCl]

metaphosphoric acid, potassium salt [see: potassium metaphosphate]

metaphosphoric acid, trisodium salt [see: sodium trimetaphosphate]

metaphyllin [see: aminophylline]

metapramine INN

metaproterenol polistirex USAN *sympathomimetic bronchodilator* [also: orciprenaline] ? metoprolol

metaproterenol sulfate USAN, USP *sympathomimetic bronchodilator* 10, 20 mg oral; 0.4%, 0.6%, 5% inhalation

metaradrine bitartrate [see: metaraminol bitartrate]

metaraminol INN *adrenergic; vasopressor for acute hypotensive shock, anaphylaxis, or traumatic shock* [also: metaraminol bitartrate]

metaraminol bitartrate USP *adrenergic; vasopressor for acute hypotensive shock, anaphylaxis, or traumatic shock* [also: metaraminol]

Metastat (name changed to Metadol upon marketing release in 2001)

Metastron IV injection ℞ *analgesic for metastatic bone pain* [strontium chloride Sr 89] 10.9–22.6 mg/mL (4 mCi)

Metatensin #2; Metatensin #4 tablets ℞ *antihypertensive* [trichlormethiazide; reserpine] 2•0.1 mg; 4•0.1 mg ? Mesantoin; Mestinon

metaterol INN

metaxalone USAN, INN, BAN *skeletal muscle relaxant* ? metolazone

metazamide INN

metazepium iodide [see: buzepide metiodide]

metazide INN

metazocine INN, BAN

metbufen INN

metcaraphen HCl

metembonate INN *combining name for radicals or groups*

meteneprost USAN, INN *oxytocic; prostaglandin*

metenolone INN *anabolic steroid; also abused as a street drug* [also: methenolone acetate; methenolone; metenolone acetate]

metenolone acetate JAN *anabolic steroid; also abused as a street drug* [also: methenolone acetate; metenolone; methenolone]

metenolone enanthate JAN *anabolic steroid; also abused as a street drug* [also: methenolone enanthate]

metergoline INN, BAN

metergotamine INN

metescufylline INN

metesculetol INN

metesind glucuronate USAN *specific thymidylate synthase (TS) inhibitor antineoplastic* ? medicine

metethoheptazine INN

metetoin INN *anticonvulsant* [also: methetoin]

metformin USAN, INN, BAN *biguanide antidiabetic* [also: metformin HCl]

Metformin ER extended-release caplets Ɽ *biguanide antidiabetic* [metformin HCl] 500 mg

metformin HCl USAN, JAN *biguanide antidiabetic* [also: metformin] 500, 850, 750, 1000 mg oral

metformin HCl & glyburide *biguanide/sulfonylurea antidiabetic combination for type 2 diabetes* 250•1.25, 500•2.5, 500•5 mg oral

methacholine bromide NF

methacholine chloride USP, INN *cholinergic; bronchoconstrictor for in vivo pulmonary challenge tests*

methacrylic acid copolymer NF *tablet-coating agent*

methacycline USAN *antibacterial* [also: metacycline]

methacycline HCl USP *gram-negative and gram-positive bacteriostatic; antirickettsial*

methadol [see: dimepheptanol]

methadone INN *narcotic analgesic; narcotic addiction detoxicant; often abused as a street drug* [also: methadone HCl] ☑ Mephyton

methadone HCl USP *narcotic analgesic; narcotic addiction detoxicant; often abused as a street drug* [also: methadone] 5, 10, 40 mg oral; 5, 10 mg/5 mL oral; 10 mg/mL oral; 10 mg/mL injection

methadonium chloride [see: methadone HCl]

Methadose tablets, dispersible tablets, oral concentrate Ɽ *narcotic analgesic; narcotic addiction detoxicant; often abused as a street drug* [methadone HCl] 5, 10 mg; 40 mg; 10 mg/mL

methadyl acetate USAN *narcotic analgesic* [also: acetylmethadol]

methafilcon B USAN *hydrophilic contact lens material*

Methagual OTC *analgesic; counterirritant* [methyl salicylate; guaiacol] 8%•2%

Methalgen cream OTC *analgesic; counterirritant* [methyl salicylate; menthol; camphor; mustard oil]

methallenestril INN

methallenestrol [see: methallenestril]

methallibure USAN *anterior pituitary activator for swine* [also: metallibure]

methalthiazide USAN *diuretic; antihypertensive*

methamoctol

methamphazone BAN [also: metamfazone]

methamphetamine HCl USP *CNS stimulant; widely abused as a street drug* [also: metamfetamine] 5 mg oral

methampyrone [now: dipyrone]

methanabol [see: methandriol]

methandienone BAN [also: methandrostenolone; metandienone]

methandriol

methandrostenolone USP *steroid; discontinued for human use, but the veterinary product is still available and sometimes abused as a street drug* [also: metandienone; methandienone]

methaniazide INN

methanol [see: methyl alcohol]

methantheline bromide USP *peptic ulcer adjunct* [also: methanthelinium bromide]

methanthelinium bromide INN, BAN *anticholinergic* [also: methantheline bromide]

methaphenilene INN, BAN [also: methaphenilene HCl]

methaphenilene HCl NF [also: methaphenilene]

methapyrilene INN [also: methapyrilene fumarate]

methapyrilene fumarate USP [also: methapyrilene]

methapyrilene HCl USP

methaqualone USAN, USP, INN, BAN *hypnotic; sedative; widely abused as a street drug, which leads to dependence*

methaqualone HCl USP

metharbital USP, INN, JAN *anticonvulsant* [also: metharbitone]

metharbitone BAN *anticonvulsant* [also: metharbital]

methastyridone INN

Methatropic capsules OTC *dietary lipotropic with vitamin supplementation* [choline; inositol; methionine; multiple B vitamins] 115•83•110• ± mg

methazolamide USP, INN *carbonic anhydrase inhibitor for glaucoma* 25, 50 mg oral

Methblue 65 tablets ℞ *urinary anti-infective and antiseptic; antidote to cyanide poisoning* [methylene blue] 65 mg

methcathinone *a highly addictive manufactured street drug similar to cathinone, with amphetamine-like effects* [see also: cathinone; *Catha edulis*]

methdilazine USP, INN *phenothiazine antihistamine; antipruritic*

methdilazine HCl USP *phenothiazine antihistamine; antipruritic*

methenamine USP, INN *urinary antibiotic* ⊡ methionine

methenamine hippurate USAN, USP *urinary antibiotic* [also: hexamine hippurate]

methenamine mandelate USP *urinary antibiotic* 0.5, 1 g oral; 0.5 g/5 mL oral

methenamine sulfosalicylate *topical antipsoriatic*

methenolone BAN *anabolic steroid; also abused as a street drug* [also: methenolone acetate; metenolone; metenolone acetate]

methenolone acetate USAN *anabolic steroid; also abused as a street drug* [also: metenolone; methenolone; metenolone acetate]

methenolone enanthate USAN *anabolic steroid; also abused as a street drug* [also: metenolone enanthate]

metheptazine INN

Methergine coated tablets, IV or IM injection ℞ *oxytocic for induction of labor, control of postpartum uterine atony, and postpartum hemorrhage* [methylergonovine maleate] 0.2 mg; 0.2 mg/mL

methestrol INN

methetharimide [see: bemegride]

methetoin USAN *anticonvulsant* [also: metetoin]

methicillin sodium USAN, USP *penicillinase-resistant penicillin antibiotic* [also: meticillin]

methimazole USP *thyroid inhibitor* [also: thiamazole] 5, 10 mg oral

methindizate BAN [also: metindizate]

methiodal sodium USP, INN

methiomeprazine INN

methiomeprazine HCl [see: methiomeprazine]

methionine (DL-methionine) NF, JAN *urinary acidifier* [also: racemethionine] 500 mg oral

methionine (L-methionine) USAN, USP, INN, JAN *essential amino acid; symbols: Met, M; investigational (orphan) for AIDS myelopathy* ⊡ methenamine

methionyl neurotropic factor, brain-derived, recombinant *investigational (orphan) for amyotrophic lateral sclerosis*

methionyl stem cell factor, recombinant human *investigational (orphan) for progressive bone marrow failure*

N-methionylleptin (human) [see: metreleptin]

methiothepin [see: metitepine]

methisazone USAN *antiviral* [also: metisazone]

methisoprinol [now: inosine pranobex]

Methitest tablets ℞ *androgen for hypogonadism or testosterone deficiency in men, delayed puberty in boys, and metastatic breast cancer in women; also abused as a street drug* [methyltestosterone] 10, 25 mg

methitural INN

methixene HCl USAN *smooth muscle relaxant* [also: metixene] ⊡ methoxsalen

methocamphone methylsulfate [see: trimethidinium methosulfate]

methocarbamol USP, INN, BAN, JAN *skeletal muscle relaxant* 500, 750 mg oral; 100 mg/mL injection

methocidin INN

methohexital USP, INN *barbiturate general anesthetic* [also: methohexitone]

methohexital sodium USP *barbiturate general anesthetic*

methohexitone BAN *barbiturate general anesthetic* [also: methohexital]

methoin BAN *anticonvulsant* [also: mephenytoin]

methonaphthone [see: menbutone]
methophedrine [see: methoxyphedrine]
methophenazine [see: metofenazate]
methopholine USAN *analgesic* [also: metofoline]
methoprene INN
methopromazine INN
methopromazine maleate [see: methopromazine]
methopyrimazole [see: epirizole]
d-**methorphan** [see: dextromethorphan]
d-**methorphan hydrobromide** [see: dextromethorphan hydrobromide]
methoserpidine INN, BAN
methotrexate (MTX) USAN, USP, INN, BAN, JAN *antimetabolite antineoplastic for leukemia, lymphoma, and various solid tumors; systemic antipsoriatic; antirheumatic for juvenile rheumatoid arthritis (orphan) 2.5 mg oral*
methotrexate & laurocapram *investigational (orphan) for topical treatment of mycosis fungoides*
methotrexate & leucovorin *antineoplastic for osteosarcoma (orphan)*
Methotrexate LPF Sodium *preservative-free injection* R *antimetabolite antineoplastic for leukemia, lymphoma, and various solid tumors; systemic antipsoriatic; antirheumatic* [methotrexate sodium] *2.5 mg/mL*
methotrexate sodium USP *antirheumatic; systemic antipsoriatic; antimetabolite antineoplastic for leukemia, lymphoma, various solid tumors, and osteogenic sarcoma (orphan) 20, 1000 mg/vial injection; 2.5 mg/mL injection*
methotrimeprazine USAN, USP *central analgesic; CNS depressant* [also: levomepromazine]
methotrimeprazine maleate *CNS depressant; neuroleptic*
methoxamine INN *adrenergic; vasoconstrictor; vasopressor for hypotensive shock during surgery* [also: methoxamine HCl]
methoxamine HCl USP *adrenergic; vasoconstrictor; vasopressor for hypo-*

tensive shock during surgery [also: methoxamine]
methoxiflurane [see: methoxyflurane]
methoxsalen (8-methoxsalen) USP *repigmentation agent for vitiligo; antipsoriatic; palliative treatment for cutaneous T-cell lymphoma (CTCL); investigational (orphan) for diffuse systemic sclerosis and cardiac allografts* ② **methixene**
methoxy polyethylene glycol [see: polyethylene glycol monomethyl ether]
2-methoxyestradiol *investigational (orphan) for multiple myeloma*
methoxyfenoserpin [see: mefeserpine]
methoxyflurane USAN, USP, INN, BAN *inhalation general anesthetic*
methoxyphedrine INN
p-**methoxyphenacyl** [see: anisatil]
methoxyphenamine INN [also: methoxyphenamine HCl]
methoxyphenamine HCl USP [also: methoxyphenamine]
4-methoxyphenol [see: mequinol]
o-**methoxyphenyl salicylate acetate** [see: guacetisal]
methoxypromazine maleate [see: methopromazine]
8-methoxypsoralen (8-MOP) [see: methoxsalen]
5-methoxyresorcinol [see: flamenol]
methphenoxydiol [see: guaifenesin]
methscopolamine bromide USP *GI antispasmodic; peptic ulcer adjunct* [also: hyoscine methobromide]
methscopolamine nitrate *anticholinergic*
methsuximide USP, BAN *succinimide anticonvulsant for absence (petit mal) seizures* [also: mesuximide]
methyclothiazide USAN, USP, INN *diuretic; antihypertensive 2.5, 5 mg oral*
methydromorphine [see: methyldihydromorphine]
methyl alcohol NF *solvent*
methyl benzoquate BAN *coccidiostat for poultry* [also: nequinate]
methyl cresol [see: cresol]
methyl cysteine [see: mecysteine]

methyl p-hydroxybenzoate [see: methylparaben]

methyl isobutyl ketone NF *alcohol denaturant*

methyl nicotinate USAN

methyl palmoxirate USAN *antidiabetic*

methyl phthalate [see: dimethyl phthalate]

methyl salicylate NF *flavoring agent; counterirritant; topical anesthetic*

methyl sulfoxide [see: dimethyl sulfoxide]

methyl violet [see: gentian violet]

l-methylaminoethanolcatechol [see: epinephrine]

methylaminopterin [see: methotrexate]

methylandrostenediol [see: methandriol]

methylatropine nitrate USAN *anticholinergic* [also: atropine methonitrate]

methylbenactyzium bromide INN

methylbenzethonium chloride USP, INN *topical anti-infective/antiseptic*

α-methylbenzylhydrazine [see: mebanazine]

methylcarbamate of salicylanilide [see: anilamate]

methyl-CCNU (chloroethyl-cyclohexyl-nitrosourea) [see: semustine]

methylcellulose USP, INN *ophthalmic moisturizer; suspending and viscosity-increasing agent; bulk laxative*

methylcellulose, propylene glycol ether of [see: hydroxypropyl methylcellulose]

methylchromone INN, BAN

N-methyl-D-aspartate (NMDA) *an endogenous neurotransmitter similar to glutamate; an NMDA inhibitor blocks the action of glutamate, which can overstimulate the receptors and become neurotoxic in excessive amounts, causing various dementias and CNS disorders*

methyldesorphine INN, BAN

methyldigoxin [see: metildigoxin]

methyldihydromorphine INN

methyldihydromorphinone HCl [see: metopon]

methyldinitrobenzamide [see: dinitolmide]

methyldioxatrine [see: meletimide]

N-methyldiphenethylamine [see: demelverine]

α-methyl-DL-thyroxine ethyl ester [see: etiroxate]

methyldopa USAN, USP, INN, BAN, JAN *centrally acting antiadrenergic antihypertensive* 250, 500 mg oral Ⓓ levodopa

α-methyldopa [now: methyldopa]

methyldopate BAN *centrally acting antiadrenergic antihypertensive* [also: methyldopate HCl]

methyldopate HCl USAN, USP *centrally acting antiadrenergic antihypertensive* [also: methyldopate] 50 mg/mL injection

methylene blue (MB) USP *antimethemoglobinemic; GU antiseptic; antidote to cyanide poisoning; diagnostic aid for gastric secretions* [also: methylthioninium chloride] 65 mg oral; 10 mg/mL injection

methylene chloride NF *solvent*

methylene diphosphonate (MDP) [now: medronate disodium]

methylenedioxyamphetamine (MDA) [see: MDMA, MDEA]

3,4-methylenedioxyethamphetamine (MDEA) [q.v.]

3,4-methylenedioxymethamphetamine (MDMA) [q.v.]

6-methyleneoxytetracycline (MOTC) [see: methacycline]

methylenprednisolone [see: prednylidene]

methylergometrine INN *oxytocic* [also: methylergonovine maleate]

methylergometrine maleate [see: methylergonovine maleate]

methylergonovine maleate USP *oxytocic for induction of labor, control of postpartum uterine atony, and postpartum hemorrhage* [also: methylergometrine]

methylergonovinium bimaleate [see: methylergonovine maleate]

methylergotamine [see: metergotamine]

methylestrenolone [see: normethandrone]

methyl-GAG (methylglyoxal-*bis*-guanylhydrazone) [see: mitoguazone]

methylglyoxal-*bis*-guanylhydrazone (methyl-GAG; MGBG) [see: mitoguazone]

1-methylhexylamine [see: tuaminoheptane]

1-methylhexylamine sulfate [see: tuaminoheptane sulfate]

N-methylhydrazine [see: procarbazine]

Methylin tablets, chewable tablets, oral liquid ℞ *CNS stimulant for attention-deficit hyperactivity disorder (ADHD) and narcolepsy* [methylphenidate HCl] 5, 10, 20 mg; 2.5, 5, 10 mg; 5, 10 mg/5 mL

Methylin ER extended-release tablets ℞ *CNS stimulant for attention-deficit hyperactivity disorder (ADHD) and narcolepsy* [methylphenidate HCl] 10, 20 mg

methylmorphine [see: codeine]

methyl-nitro-imidazole [see: carnidazole]

methylnortestosterone [see: normethandrone]

methylparaben USAN, NF *antifungal agent; preservative*

methylparaben sodium USAN, NF *antimicrobial preservative*

methylparafynol [see: meparfynol]

methylpentynol INN, BAN

methylperidol [see: moperone]

(+)-methylphenethylamine [see: dextroamphetamine]

(−)-methylphenethylamine [see: levamphetamine]

methylphenethylamine HCl [see: amphetamine HCl]

methylphenethylamine phosphate [see: amphetamine phosphate]

(−)-methylphenethylamine succinate [see: levamfetamine succinate]

methylphenethylamine sulfate [see: amphetamine sulfate]

(+)-methylphenethylamine sulfate [see: dextroamphetamine sulfate]

methylphenidate INN, BAN *CNS stimulant for attention-deficit hyperac-tivity disorder (ADHD) and narcolepsy; also abused as a street drug* [also: methylphenidate HCl]

methylphenidate HCl (MPH) USP, JAN *CNS stimulant for attention-deficit hyperactivity disorder (ADHD) and narcolepsy; also abused as a street drug* [also: methylphenidate] 5, 10, 20 mg oral

methylphenobarbital INN *anticonvulsant; sedative* [also: mephobarbital; methylphenobarbitone]

methylphenobarbitone BAN *anticonvulsant; sedative* [also: mephobarbital; methylphenobarbital]

d-methylphenylamine sulfate [see: dextroamphetamine sulfate]

methylphytyl napthoquinone [see: phytonadione]

methylprednisolone USP, INN, BAN, JAN *corticosteroid; anti-inflammatory; immunosuppressant* 4, 8, 16 mg oral

methylprednisolone aceponate INN

methylprednisolone acetate USP, JAN *corticosteroid; anti-inflammatory; immunosuppressant* 20, 40, 80 mg/mL injection

methylprednisolone hemisuccinate USP *corticosteroid; anti-inflammatory*

methylprednisolone sodium phosphate USAN *corticosteroid; anti-inflammatory* 40, 125, 500, 1000 mg/vial injection

methylprednisolone sodium succinate USP, JAN *corticosteroid; anti-inflammatory; immunosuppressant*

methylprednisolone suleptanate USAN, INN *corticosteroid; anti-inflammatory*

methylpromazine

4-methylpyrazole (4-MP) [see: fomepizole]

methylrosaniline chloride [now: gentian violet]

methylrosanilinium chloride INN *topical anti-infective* [also: gentian violet]

methylscopolamine bromide [see: methscopolamine bromide]

methylsulfate USP *combining name for radicals or groups* [also: metilsulfate]

methylsulfonylmethane (MSM)
*natural source of sulfur; promotes an
increase in collagen and the endogenous
antioxidant glutathione*

methyltestosterone USP, INN, BAN
*oral/parenteral androgen for hypogo-
nadism or testosterone deficiency in
men, delayed puberty in boys, and
metastatic breast cancer in women; also
abused as a street drug* 10, 25 mg oral

methyltheobromine [see: caffeine]

methylthionine chloride [see: methylene blue]

methylthionine HCl [see: methylene
blue]

methylthioninium chloride INN *antimethemoglobinemic; antidote to cyanide poisoning* [also: methylene blue]

methylthiouracil USP, INN

methyltrienolone [see: metribolone]

methynodiol diacetate USAN *progestin* [also: metynodiol]

methyprylon USP, INN *sedative; hypnotic* [also: methyprylone]

methyprylone BAN *sedative* [also:
methyprylon]

methyridene BAN [also: metyridine]

methysergide USAN, INN, BAN
*migraine-specific vasoconstrictor and
peripheral serotonin antagonist for the
prophylaxis of vascular headaches*

methysergide maleate USP *migraine-
specific vasoconstrictor and peripheral
serotonin antagonist for the prophylaxis
of vascular headaches*

metiamide USAN, INN *antagonist to histamine H_2 receptors*

metiapine USAN, INN *antipsychotic*

metiazinic acid INN

metibride INN

meticillin INN *penicillinase-resistant
penicillin antibiotic* [also: methicillin
sodium]

meticillin sodium *penicillinase-resistant penicillin antibiotic* [see: methicillin sodium]

Meticorten tablets ℞ *corticosteroid;
anti-inflammatory; immunosuppressant*
[prednisone] 1 mg

meticrane INN

metildigoxin INN

metilsulfate INN *combining name for
radicals or groups* [also: methylsulfate]

Metimyd eye drop suspension, ophthalmic ointment ℞ *corticosteroidal
anti-inflammatory; antibiotic* [prednis-
olone acetate; sulfacetamide sodium]
0.5%•10%

metindizate INN [also: methindizate]

metioprim USAN, INN, BAN *antibacterial*

metioxate INN

metipirox INN

metipranolol USAN, INN, BAN *topical
antiglaucoma agent (β-blocker)*

metipranolol HCl *topical antiglaucoma
agent (β-blocker)* 0.3% eye drops

metiprenaline INN

metirosine INN *antihypertensive* [also:
metyrosine]

metisazone INN *antiviral* [also: methis-
azone]

metitepine INN

metixene INN *smooth muscle relaxant*
[also: methixene HCl]

metixene HCl [see: methixene HCl]

metizoline INN *adrenergic; vasoconstrictor* [also: metizoline HCl]

metizoline HCl USAN *adrenergic; vasoconstrictor* [also: metizoline]

metkefamide INN *analgesic* [also: metkephamid acetate]

metkefamide acetate [see: metkephamid acetate]

metkephamid acetate USAN *analgesic*
[also: metkefamide]

metochalcone INN

metocinium iodide INN

metoclopramide INN, BAN, JAN *antiemetic for chemotherapy; GI stimulant;
antidopaminergic; radiosensitizer* [also:
metoclopramide HCl]

metoclopramide HCl USAN, USP, JAN
*antiemetic for chemotherapy; GI stimu-
lant; antidopaminergic; radiosensitizer*
[also: metoclopramide] 5, 10 mg
oral; 5, 10 mg/5 mL oral; 5 mg/mL
injection

**metoclopramide monohydrochlo-
ride monohydrate** [see: metoclopramide HCl]

metocurine iodide USAN, USP *neuromuscular blocker; muscle relaxant* 2 mg/mL injection

metofenazate INN

metofoline INN *analgesic* [also: metopholine]

metogest USAN, INN *hormone*

metolazone USAN, INN *antihypertensive; diuretic* 2.5, 5, 10 mg oral ⧉ metaxalone

metomidate INN, BAN

metopimazine USAN, INN *antiemetic*

Metopirone softgels ℞ *diagnostic aid for pituitary function* [metyrapone] 250 mg ⧉ metyrapone

metopon INN

metopon HCl [see: metopon]

metoprine USAN *antineoplastic*

metoprolol USAN, INN, BAN *antihypertensive; antiadrenergic (β-receptor)* ⧉ metaproterenol

metoprolol fumarate USAN *antihypertensive; antiadrenergic (β-receptor)*

metoprolol succinate USAN *antianginal; antihypertensive; antiadrenergic (β-receptor)*

metoprolol tartrate USAN, USP *antihypertensive; antiadrenergic (β-receptor)* 25, 50, 100 mg oral; 1 mg/mL injection

metoprolol tartrate & hydrochlorothiazide *antihypertensive; β-blocker; diuretic* 50•25, 100•25, 100•50 mg oral

metoquizine USAN, INN *anticholinergic*

metoserpate INN *veterinary sedative* [also: metoserpate HCl]

metoserpate HCl USAN *veterinary sedative* [also: metoserpate]

metostilenol INN

metoxepin INN

metoxiestrol [see: moxestrol]

metrafazoline INN

metralindole INN

metrazifone INN

metreleptin USAN, INN *metabolic regulator for obesity*

metrenperone USAN, INN, BAN *veterinary myopathic*

metribolone INN

metrifonate USAN, INN *veterinary anthelmintic; investigational (NDA filed) acetylcholinesterase inhibitor for Alzheimer dementia* [also: trichlorfon; metriphonate]

metrifudil INN

metriphonate BAN *veterinary anthelmintic* [also: trichlorfon; metrifonate]

metrizamide USAN, INN *parenteral radiopaque contrast medium (48.25% iodine)*

metrizoate sodium USAN *radiopaque contrast medium* [also: sodium metrizoate]

Metro I.V. ready-to-use injection ℞ *antibiotic; antiprotozoal; amebicide* [metronidazole] 500 mg/100 mL

MetroCream; MetroGel; MetroLotion ℞ *antibiotic for rosacea (orphan); investigational (orphan) for decubitus ulcers and perioral dermatitis* [metronidazole] 0.75%

MetroGel gel ℞ *antibacterial for rosacea* [metronidazole] 1%

MetroGel Vaginal gel ℞ *antibacterial for bacterial vaginosis* [metronidazole] 0.75%

metronidazole USAN, USP, INN, BAN *antibiotic; antiprotozoal/amebicide; acne rosacea treatment (orphan); investigational (orphan) for decubitus ulcers and perioral dermatitis* 250, 375, 500, 750 mg oral; 500 mg/100 mL injection; 0.75% topical

metronidazole benzoate *antiprotozoal (Trichomonas)*

metronidazole HCl USAN *antibiotic; antiprotozoal; amebicide*

metronidazole phosphate USAN *antibacterial; antiprotozoal*

MET-Rx food bar, powder for drink OTC *enteral nutritional therapy* 100 g; 72 g

Metubine Iodide IV injection (discontinued 2004) ℞ *neuromuscular blocker; anesthesia adjunct* [metocurine iodide] 2 mg/mL

metuclazepam [see: metaclazepam]

meturedepa USAN, INN *antineoplastic*

metynodiol INN *progestin* [also: methynodiol diacetate]

metynodiol diacetate [see: methyno-diol diacetate]

metyrapone USAN, USP, INN *diagnostic aid for pituitary function* 🔄 Metopirone; metyrosine

metyrapone tartrate USAN *pituitary function test*

metyridine INN [also: methyridene]

metyrosine USAN, USP *antihypertensive; pheochromocytomic agent* 🔄 metyrapone

Mevacor tablets ℞ *HMG-CoA reductase inhibitor for hypercholesterolemia and atherosclerosis; also for primary prevention of coronary heart disease* [lovastatin] 10, 20, 40 mg

mevastatin INN

mevinolin [now: lovastatin]

mexafylline INN

mexazolam INN

mexenone INN, BAN

mexiletine INN, BAN *antiarrhythmic* [also: mexiletine HCl]

mexiletine HCl USAN, USP *antiarrhythmic* [also: mexiletine]

mexiprostil INN

Mexitil capsules ℞ *antiarrhythmic* [mexiletine HCl] 150, 200, 250 mg

mexoprofen INN

mexrenoate potassium USAN, INN *aldosterone antagonist*

Mexsana Medicated powder OTC *topical diaper rash treatment* [kaolin; zinc oxide; eucalyptus oil; camphor; corn starch]

mezacopride INN

mezepine INN

mezereon (*Daphne mezereum*) bark *medicinal herb used as a cathartic, diuretic, emetic, and rubefacient; eating the berries can be fatal, and people have been poisoned by eating birds that ate the berries*

mezilamine INN

Mezlin powder for IV or IM injection (discontinued 2004) ℞ *extended-spectrum penicillin antibiotic* [mezlocillin sodium] 1, 2, 3, 4, 20 g/vial 🔄 Meclan

mezlocillin USAN, INN *extended-spectrum penicillin antibiotic*

mezlocillin sodium USP *extended-spectrum penicillin antibiotic*

MF (methotrexate [with leucovorin rescue], fluorouracil) *chemotherapy protocol for breast cancer*

MF (mitomycin, fluorouracil) *chemotherapy protocol*

MFP (melphalan, fluorouracil, medroxyprogesterone acetate) *chemotherapy protocol*

MG Cold Sore Formula solution OTC *topical oral anesthetic; antipruritic/counterirritant* [lidocaine; menthol] 2•1%

MG217 Medicated conditioner (discontinued 2003) OTC *antipsoriatic; antiseborrheic* [coal tar solution] 2%

MG217 Medicated ointment OTC *antipsoriatic; antiseborrheic; antifungal; keratolytic* [coal tar solution; colloidal sulfur; salicylic acid] 2%• 1.1%•1.5%

MG217 Medicated shampoo (discontinued 2003) OTC *antipsoriatic; antiseborrheic; antifungal; keratolytic* [coal tar solution; salicylic acid] 5%•2%

MG217 Medicated Tar lotion, ointment OTC *antipsoriatic; antiseborrheic* [coal tar solution] 1%; 2%

MG217 Medicated Tar shampoo OTC *antiseborrheic; antipsoriatic; antipruritic; antibacterial* [coal tar] 3%

MG217 Medicated Tar-Free shampoo OTC *antiseborrheic; keratolytic* [sulfur; salicylic acid] 5%•3%

MG217 Sal-Acid ointment OTC *antipsoriatic; keratolytic* [salicylic acid] 3%

MG400 shampoo OTC *antiseborrheic; keratolytic* [salicylic acid; sulfur] 3%•5%

MGA (melengestrol acetate) [q.v.]

MGBG (methylglyoxal-*bis*-guanyl-hydrazone) [see: mitoguazone]

MGW (magnesium sulfate + glycerin + water) enema [q.v.]

MHP-A tablets ℞ *urinary antibiotic; antiseptic; analgesic; antispasmodic* [methenamine; phenyl salicylate; methylene blue; benzoic acid; atropine sulfate; hyoscyamine sulfate] 40.8•18.1•5.4•4.5•0.03•0.03 mg

Miacalcin nasal spray ℞ *calcium regulator for postmenopausal osteoporosis (only)* [calcitonin (salmon)] 200 IU/0.09 mL dose

Miacalcin subcu or IM injection ℞ *calcium regulator for Paget disease (orphan), hypercalcemia, and postmenopausal osteoporosis* [calcitonin (salmon)] 200 IU/mL

Mi-Acid gelcaps OTC *antacid* [calcium carbonate; magnesium carbonate] 311•232 mg

Mi-Acid; Mi-Acid II oral liquid OTC *antacid; antiflatulent* [aluminum hydroxide; magnesium hydroxide; simethicone] 200•200•20 mg/5 mL; 400•400•40 mg/5 mL

mianserin INN, BAN *serotonin inhibitor; antihistamine* [also: mianserin HCl]

mianserin HCl USAN, JAN *serotonin inhibitor; antihistamine* [also: mianserin]

mibefradil INN *vasodilator and calcium channel blocker for hypertension and chronic stable angina* [also: mibefradil dihydrochloride]

mibefradil dihydrochloride USAN *vasodilator and calcium channel blocker for hypertension and chronic stable angina* [also: mibefradil]

M¹³¹IBG [now: iobenguane sulfate I 131]

MIBG-I-123 [see: iobenguane sulfate I 123]

mibolerone USAN, INN *anabolic; androgen*

micafungin sodium *systemic echinocandin antifungal for esophageal candidiasis and Candida prophylaxis*

Micanol ⓒ cream OTC *antipsoriatic* [anthralin] 1%, 3%

Micardis tablets ℞ *long-acting antihypertensive; angiotensin II receptor antagonist* [telmisartan] 20, 40, 80 mg

Micardis HCT tablets ℞ *long-acting antihypertensive; angiotensin II receptor antagonist; diuretic* [telmisartan; hydrochlorothiazide] 40•12.5, 80•12.5, 80•25 mg

Micardis Plus ⓒ tablets ℞ *long-acting antihypertensive; angiotensin II recep-*

tor antagonist; diuretic [telmisartan; hydrochlorothiazide] 80•12.5 mg

Micatin cream, powder, spray powder, spray liquid OTC *antifungal* [miconazole nitrate] 2%

MICE (mesna [rescue], ifosfamide, carboplatin, etoposide) *chemotherapy protocol for osteosarcoma and lung cancer* [also: ICE]

micinicate INN

Miconal cream ℞ *topical antipsoriatic* [anthralin] 1%

miconazole USP, INN, BAN, JAN *fungicidal*

Miconazole 7 vaginal suppositories OTC *antifungal* [miconazole nitrate] 100 mg

miconazole nitrate USAN, USP, JAN *antifungal* 2% topical

Micrainin tablets ℞ *analgesic; antipyretic; anti-inflammatory; anxiolytic; sedative* [aspirin; meprobamate] 325•200 mg

MICRhoGAM IM injection, prefilled syringes ℞ *obstetric Rh factor immunity suppressant* [Rh₀(D) immune globulin (gamma globulin)] 50 μg (5%) ⑫ microgram

microbubble contrast agent *investigational (orphan) neurosonographic diagnostic aid for intracranial tumors*

Microcaps (trademarked dosage form) *fast-melting tablets*

microcrystalline cellulose [see: cellulose, microcrystalline]

microcrystalline wax [see: wax, microcrystalline]

microfibrillar collagen hemostat (MCH) *topical local hemostatic*

Microgestin Fe 1/20; Microgestin Fe 1.5/30 tablets (in packs of 28) ℞ *monophasic oral contraceptive; iron supplement* [norethindrone acetate; ethinyl estradiol; ferrous fumarate] 1 mg•20 μg•75 mg; 1.5 mg•30 μg•75 mg

Micro-K; Micro-K 10 Extencaps (controlled-release capsules) ℞ *potassium supplement* [potassium chloride] 600 mg (8 mEq K); 750 mg (10 mEq K)

Micro-K LS extended-release powder for oral solution ℞ *potassium supplement* [potassium chloride] 20 mEq K/pkt.

MicroKlenz topical liqid OTC *antiseptic wound cleanser* [acemannan]

Microlipid emulsion OTC *dietary fat supplement* [safflower oil] 50%

Micronase tablets ℞ *sulfonylurea antidiabetic* [glyburide] 1.25, 2.5, 5 mg

microNefrin solution for inhalation OTC *sympathomimetic bronchodilator for bronchial asthma and COPD* [racepinephrine HCl] 2.25%

micronized aluminum *astringent*

Micronized Glyburide tablets ℞ *sulfonylurea antidiabetic* [glyburide] 1.5, 3 mg

micronomicin INN

Micronor [see: Ortho Micronor]

Microstix-3 reagent strips for professional use *in vitro diagnostic aid for nitrate, uropathogens, or bacteria in the urine*

MicroTrak Chlamydia trachomatis slide test for professional use *in vitro diagnostic aid for* Chlamydia trachomatis

MicroTrak HSV 1/HSV 2 Culture Identification/Typing Test culture test for professional use *in vitro diagnostic aid for herpes simplex virus in tissue cultures*

MicroTrak HSV 1/HSV 2 Direct Specimen Identification/Typing Test slide test for professional use *in vitro diagnostic aid for herpes simplex virus in external lesions*

MicroTrak Neisseria gonorrhoeae Culture Confirmation Test reagent kit for professional use *in vitro diagnostic aid for* Neisseria gonorrhoeae

Microzide capsules ℞ *once-daily antihypertensive; thiazide diuretic* [hydrochlorothiazide] 12.5 mg ⊉ Maxzide

mictine [see: aminometradine]

midaflur USAN, INN *sedative*

midaglizole INN

midalcipran [see: milnacipran]

midamaline INN

Midamor tablets ℞ *antihypertensive; potassium-sparing diuretic* [amiloride HCl] 5 mg

midazogrel INN

midazolam INN, BAN, JAN *short-acting benzodiazepine general anesthetic* [also: midazolam HCl]

midazolam HCl USAN *short-acting benzodiazepine general anesthetic* [also: midazolam] 1, 5 mg/mL injection

midazolam maleate USAN *intravenous anesthetic*

Midchlor capsules (discontinued 2000) ℞ *cerebral vasoconstrictor and analgesic for vascular and tension headaches; "possibly effective" for migraine headaches* [isometheptene mucate; dichloralphenazone; acetaminophen] 65•100•325 mg

midecamycin INN

midodrine INN, BAN *antihypotensive; vasoconstrictor; vasopressor for orthostatic hypotension (OH)* [also: midodrine HCl]

midodrine HCl USAN, JAN *antihypotensive; vasoconstrictor; vasopressor for orthostatic hypotension (orphan)* [also: midodrine] 2.5, 5, 10 mg oral

Midol, Maximum Strength Cramp Formula tablets OTC *analgesic; antiarthritic; antipyretic; nonsteroidal anti-inflammatory drug (NSAID)* [ibuprofen] 200 mg

Midol Extended Relief caplets OTC *analgesic; antiarthritic; antipyretic; nonsteroidal anti-inflammatory drug (NSAID)* [naproxen sodium] 220 mg (=200 mg base)

Midol Maximum Strength Menstrual caplets, gelcaps OTC *analgesic; anti-inflammatory; antihistaminic sleep aid* [acetaminophen; caffeine; pyrilamine maleate] 500•60•15 mg

Midol PM caplets OTC *analgesic; antipyretic; antihistaminic sleep aid* [acetaminophen; diphenhydramine] 500•25 mg

Midol PMS caplets, gelcaps OTC *analgesic; anti-inflammatory; diuretic; antihistaminic sleep aid* [acetaminophen;

pamabrom; pyrilamine maleate] 500•25•15 mg

Midol Teen caplets OTC *analgesic; anti-inflammatory; diuretic* [acetaminophen; pamabrom] 500•25 mg

Midrin capsules ℞ *cerebral vasoconstrictor and analgesic for vascular and tension headaches; "possibly effective" for migraine headaches* [isomeptene mucate; dichloralphenazone; acetaminophen] 65•100•325 mg ⑨ Mydfrin

Midstream Pregnancy Test kit for home use *in vitro diagnostic aid; urine pregnancy test*

MIFA (mitomycin, fluorouracil, Adriamycin) *chemotherapy protocol*

mifarmonab [see: imciromab pentetate]

Mifegyne (European name for U.S. product Mifeprex)

mifentidine INN

Mifeprex tablets ℞ *abortifacient; postcoital contraceptive; progesterone antagonist; also used for uterine leiomyomata* [mifepristone] 200 mg (note: not available to pharmacies; must be obtained from a physician in an office, clinic, or hospital setting)

mifepristone USAN, INN, BAN *progesterone antagonist; abortifacient; postcoital contraceptive; investigational (Phase III) GR-II antagonist to reduce abnormal cortisol release in psychotic major depression*

mifobate USAN, INN *antiatherosclerotic*

miglitol USAN, INN, BAN *antidiabetic agent for type 2 diabetes; alpha-glucosidase inhibitor that delays the digestion of dietary carbohydrates*

miglustat *glucosylceramide synthase inhibitor; substrate reduction therapy (SRT) to reduce the glycosphingolipid (GSL) production in type I Gaucher disease*

mignonette, Jamaica *medicinal herb* [see: henna (Lawsonia)]

Migranal nasal spray ℞ *rapid-acting antimigraine agent* [dihydroergotamine mesylate] 0.05 mg/spray

Migratine capsules ℞ *cerebral vasoconstrictor and analgesic for vascular and tension headaches; "possibly effective" for migraine headaches* [isomeptene mucate; dichloralphenazone; acetaminophen] 65•100•325 mg

mikamycin INN, BAN

MiKasome ℞ *investigational (Phase II) antibiotic liposomal formulation for complicated urinary tract infections and AIDS-related mycobacterial infections* [amikacin]

milacemide INN *anticonvulsant; antidepressant* [also: milacemide HCl]

milacemide HCl USAN *anticonvulsant; antidepressant* [also: milacemide]

milameline HCl USAN *partial muscarinic agonist for Alzheimer disease*

mild silver protein [see: silver protein, mild]

milenperone USAN, INN, BAN *antipsychotic*

Miles Nervine caplets OTC *antihistaminic sleep aid* [diphenhydramine HCl] 25 mg

milfoil *medicinal herb* [see: yarrow]

milipertine USAN, INN *antipsychotic*

milk ipecac *medicinal herb* [see: birthroot; dogbane]

milk of bismuth [see: bismuth, milk of]

milk of magnesia [see: magnesia, milk of]

Milk of Magnesia-Cascara, Concentrated oral suspension OTC *antacid; saline/stimulant laxative* [milk of magnesia; aromatic cascara fluidextract; alcohol 7%] 30•5 mL/15 mL

milk thistle (Silybum marianum) seeds *medicinal herb for Amanita mushroom poisoning, bronchitis, gallbladder disorders, hemorrhage, liver damage, peritonitis, spleen disorders, stomach disorders, and varicose veins*

milkweed (Asclepias syriaca) roots *medicinal herb used as a diuretic, emetic, purgative, and tonic*

milnacipran INN *investigational (Phase III) serotonin and norepinephrine reuptake inhibitor for depression and fibromyalgia syndrome*

milodistim USAN *antineutropenic; hematopoietic stimulant; granulocyte mac-*

rophage colony-stimulating factor (GM-CSF) + interleukin 3

Milontin Kapseals (capsules) (discontinued 2002) ℞ succinimide anticonvulsant [phensuximide] 500 mg ▣ Dilantin; Miltown; Mylanta

miloxacin INN

milrinone USAN, INN, BAN cardiotonic

milrinone lactate vasodilator for congestive heart failure 1 mg/mL injection

miltefosine INN

Miltown tablets ℞ anxiolytic; also abused as a street drug [meprobamate] 200, 400 mg ▣ Milontin

Miltown-600 tablets (discontinued 2001) ℞ anxiolytic; also abused as a street drug [meprobamate] 600 mg ▣ Milontin

milverine INN

mimbane INN analgesic [also: mimbane HCl]

mimbane HCl USAN analgesic [also: mimbane]

minalrestat USAN aldose reductase inhibitor for diabetic neuropathy and other long-term diabetic complications

minaprine USAN, INN, BAN psychotropic

minaprine HCl USAN antidepressant

minaxolone USAN, INN anesthetic

mindodilol INN

mindolic acid [see: clometacin]

mindoperone INN

MINE (mesna [rescue], ifosfamide, Novantrone, etoposide) chemotherapy protocol for non-Hodgkin lymphoma

MINE-ESHAP (alternating cycles of MINE and ESHAP) chemotherapy protocol for non-Hodgkin lymphoma

minepentate INN, BAN

Mineral Ice [see: Therapeutic Mineral Ice]

mineral oil USP emollient/protectant; laxative; solvent

mineral oil, light NF tablet and capsule lubricant; vehicle

mineralocorticoids a class of adrenal cortical steroids that are used for partial replacement therapy in adrenocortical insufficiency

Mini Two-Way Action tablets OTC bronchodilator; decongestant; expectorant [ephedrine HCl; guaifenesin] 12.5•200, 25•200 mg

MiniAdFVIII ℞ investigational (orphan) agent for hemophilia A [adenovirus-based vector Factor VIII complementary DNA to somatic cells]

mini-BEAM (BCNU, etoposide, ara-C, melphalan) chemotherapy protocol for Hodgkin lymphoma

mini-COAP (cyclophosphamide, Oncovin, ara-C, prednisone) chemotherapy protocol

Minidyne solution OTC broad-spectrum antimicrobial [povidone-iodine] 10%

Min-I-Mix (delivery system) dual-chambered prefilled syringe

Minipress capsules ℞ antihypertensive; α_1-adrenergic blocker [prazosin HCl] 1, 2, 5 mg

Minirin nasal spray ℞ posterior pituitary hormone for hemophilia A (orphan), von Willebrand disease (orphan), central diabetes insipidus, and nocturnal enuresis [desmopressin acetate; chlorobutanol] 10•500 µg/dose

Minitran transdermal patch ℞ antianginal; vasodilator [nitroglycerin] 9, 18, 36, 54 mg (0.1, 0.2, 0.4, 0.6 mg/hr.)

Minit-Rub OTC analgesic; counterirritant [methyl salicylate; menthol; camphor] 15%•3.5%•2.3%

Minizide 1; Minizide 2; Minizide 5 capsules ℞ antihypertensive; α-blocker; diuretic [prazosin HCl; polythiazide] 1•0.5 mg; 2•0.5 mg; 5•0.5 mg

Minocin pellet-filled capsules, oral suspension ℞ tetracycline antibiotic [minocycline HCl] 50, 100 mg; 50 mg/5 mL ▣ Indocin; Mithracin; niacin

Minocin powder for IV injection ℞ tetracycline antibiotic [minocycline] 100 mg/vial ▣ Indocin; Mithracin; niacin

minocromil USAN, INN, BAN prophylactic antiallergic

minocycline USAN, INN, BAN gram-negative and gram-positive bacteriostatic; antirickettsial

minocycline HCl USP *gram-negative and gram-positive bacteriostatic; antirickettsial; adjunct to scaling and root planing for periodontitis* 50, 75, 100 mg oral

Minox ⒸⒶⓃ *topical solution* OTC *hair growth stimulant* [minoxidil] 2%

minoxidil USAN, USP, INN, BAN *antihypertensive; peripheral vasodilator; hair growth stimulant* 2.5, 10 mg oral

Minoxidil for Men *topical solution* OTC *hair growth stimulant* [minoxidil; alcohol 60%] 2%, 5%

mint; lamb mint; mackerel mint; Our Lady's mint *medicinal herb* [see: spearmint]

mint, brandy; lamb mint *medicinal herb* [see: peppermint]

mint, mountain *medicinal herb* [see: marjoram; Oswego tea]

mint, squaw *medicinal herb* [see: pennyroyal]

Mintezol *chewable tablets, oral suspension* R *anthelmintic for strongyloidiasis (threadworm), larva migrans, and trichinosis* [thiabendazole] 500 mg; 500 mg/5 mL

Mintox *chewable tablets, oral suspension* OTC *antacid* [aluminum hydroxide; magnesium hydroxide] 200•200 mg; 225•200 mg/5 mL

Mintox Plus *oral liquid* OTC *antacid; antiflatulent* [aluminum hydroxide; magnesium hydroxide; simethicone] 500•450•40 mg/5 mL

Minute-Gel R *topical dental caries preventative* [acidulated phosphate fluoride] 1.23%

✳ **Miochol-E** *solution* R *direct-acting miotic for ophthalmic surgery* [acetylcholine chloride] 1:100

mioflazine INN, BAN *coronary vasodilator* [also: mioflazine HCl]

mioflazine HCl USAN *coronary vasodilator* [also: mioflazine]

Miostat *solution* R *direct-acting miotic for ophthalmic surgery* [carbachol] 0.01%

miotics *a class of drugs that cause the pupil of the eye to contract*

mipafilcon A USAN *hydrophilic contact lens material*

mipimazole INN

Miradon *tablets* (discontinued 2003) R *indanedione-derivative anticoagulant* [anisindione] 50 mg

MiraFlow *solution* OTC *cleaning solution for hard or soft contact lenses*

MiraForte [see: Super MiraForte with Chrysin]

MiraLax *powder for oral solution* R *hyperosmotic laxative; pre-procedure bowel evacuant* [polyethylene glycol 3350] 17 g/dose

Mirapex *tablets* R *dopamine agonist; antiparkinsonian* [pramipexole dihydrochloride] 0.125, 0.25, 0.5, 1, 1.5 mg

Miraphen PSE *extended-release tablets* R *decongestant; expectorant* [pseudoephedrine HCl; guaifenesin] 120•600 mg

MiraSept Step 2 *solution* OTC *rinsing/storage solution for soft contact lenses* [sodium chloride (preserved saline solution)]

MiraSept System *solutions* OTC *two-step chemical disinfecting system for soft contact lenses* [hydrogen peroxide based] 3%

Mircette *tablets* (in packs of 28) R *biphasic oral contraceptive* [desogestrel; ethinyl estradiol]
Phase 1 (21 days): 150•20 μg;
Phase 2 (5 days): 0•10 μg

Mirena *intrauterine device* (IUD) R *long-term (5 year) contraceptive insert* [levonorgestrel] 20 μg/day

Mireze ⒸⒶⓃ *eye drops* (name changed to Alocril in 2001)

mirfentanil INN *analgesic* [also: mirfentanil HCl]

mirfentanil HCl USAN *analgesic* [also: mirfentanil]

mirincamycin INN *antibacterial; antimalarial* [also: mirincamycin HCl]

mirincamycin HCl USAN *antibacterial; antimalarial* [also: mirincamycin]

mirisetron maleate USAN *anxiolytic*

miristalkonium chloride INN

miroprofen INN

mirosamicin INN

mirostipen USAN *myeloprotectant*

mirtazapine USAN, INN *tetracyclic antidepressant; serotonin 5-HT$_{1A}$ agonist* 7.5, 15, 30, 45 mg oral

misonidazole USAN, INN *antiprotozoal* (*Trichomonas*)

misoprostol USAN, INN, BAN *prevents NSAID-induced gastric ulcers; has been used for cervical ripening and induction of labor; use by pregnant women can cause abortion, premature birth, or birth defects* 100, 200 μg oral

Mission Prenatal; Mission Prenatal F.A.; Mission Prenatal H.P. tablets OTC *vitamin/iron supplement* [multiple vitamins; ferrous gluconate; folic acid] ±•30•0.4 mg; ±•30•0.8 mg; ±•30•0.8 mg

Mission Prenatal Rx tablets ℞ *vitamin/calcium/iron supplement* [multiple vitamins; calcium; iron; folic acid] ±•175•29.5•1 mg

Mission Surgical Supplement tablets OTC *vitamin/iron supplement* [multiple vitamins; ferrous gluconate] ±•27 mg

mistletoe (*Phoradendron flavescens; P. serotinum; P. tomentosum; Viscum album*) plant *medicinal herb for cancer, chorea, epilepsy, hypertension, internal hemorrhages, menstrual disorders, nervousness, poor circulation, and spleen disorders; not generally regarded as safe and effective for ingestion as it is highly toxic*

Mistometer (trademarked form) *metered-dose inhalation aerosol*

Mitchella repens *medicinal herb* [see: squaw vine]

Mithracin powder for IV infusion (discontinued 2002) ℞ *antibiotic antineoplastic for malignant testicular tumors* [plicamycin] 2.5 mg ⊡ Minocin

mithramycin [now: plicamycin] ⊡ mitomycin

mitindomide USAN, INN *antineoplastic*

mitobronitol INN, BAN

mitocarcin USAN, INN *antineoplastic*

mitoclomine INN, BAN

mitocromin USAN *antineoplastic*

mitoflaxone INN

mitogillin USAN, INN *antineoplastic*

mitoguazone INN *investigational antineoplastic for multiple myeloma and head, esophagus, and prostate cancer; investigational (orphan) for non-Hodgkin lymphoma*

mitolactol INN *investigational (orphan) antineoplastic for brain tumors and recurrent or metastatic cervical squamous cell carcinoma*

mitomalcin USAN, INN *antineoplastic*

mitomycin USAN, USP, INN, BAN *antibiotic antineoplastic for disseminated adenocarcinoma of the stomach or pancreas; investigational (orphan) for refractory glaucoma and glaucoma surgery* 5, 20, 40 mg injection ⊡ mithramycin; Mutamycin

mitomycin C (MTC) [see: mitomycin]

mitonafide INN

mitopodozide INN, BAN

mitoquidone INN, BAN

mitosper USAN, INN *antineoplastic*

mitotane USAN, USP, INN *antibiotic antineoplastic for inoperable adrenal cortical carcinoma and Cushing syndrome*

mitotenamine INN, BAN

mitotic inhibitors *a class of antineoplastics that inhibit cell division (mitosis)*

mitoxantrone INN *antibiotic antineoplastic* [also: mitoxantrone HCl; mitozantrone]

mitoxantrone HCl USAN *antibiotic antineoplastic for prostate cancer and acute nonlymphocytic leukemia (ANLL) (orphan); immunomodulator for progressive and relapsing-remitting multiple sclerosis* [also: mitoxantrone; mitozantrone]

mitozantrone BAN *antineoplastic* [also: mitoxantrone HCl; mitoxantrone]

mitozolomide INN, BAN

Mitran capsules (discontinued 2003) ℞ *benzodiazepine anxiolytic; sedative* [chlordiazepoxide HCl] 10 mg

Mitrolan chewable tablets (discontinued 2004) OTC *bulk laxative; antidiarrheal* [calcium polycarbophil] 625 mg

mitronal [see: cinnarizine]

mitumomab USAN *antineoplastic monoclonal antibody for* G_{D3} *ganglioside–expressing tumors; investigational (Phase III) for small cell lung cancer*

Mivacron IV infusion ℞ *muscle relaxant; adjunct to anesthesia* [mivacurium chloride] 0.5, 2 mg/mL

mivacurium chloride USAN, INN, BAN *neuromuscular blocking agent*

mivobulin isethionate USAN *antineoplastic; mitotic inhibitor; tubulin binder*

Mixed E 400; Mixed E 1000 softgels OTC *vitamin supplement* [vitamin E] 400 IU; 1000 IU

mixed respiratory vaccine (MRV) *active bacterin for respiratory tract infections*

mixed tocopherols [see: vitamin E]

mixidine USAN, INN *coronary vasodilator*

Mix-O-Vial (trademarked packaging form) *two-compartment vial*

mizoribine INN

MK-826 *investigational (NDA filed) broad-spectrum carbapenem antibiotic*

MKC-442 *investigational (Phase III) non-nucleoside reverse transcriptase inhibitor (NNRTI) for HIV and AIDS*

MM (mercaptopurine, methotrexate) *chemotherapy protocol*

MMOPP (methotrexate, mechlorethamine, Oncovin, procarbazine, prednisone) *chemotherapy protocol*

MMP (matrix metalloproteinase) inhibitors [q.v.]

MMR (measles, mumps & rubella vaccines) [q.v.]

M-M-R II powder for subcu injection ℞ *measles, mumps, and rubella vaccine* [measles, mumps, and rubella virus vaccine, live] 0.5 mL

MOB (mechlorethamine, Oncovin, bleomycin) *chemotherapy protocol*

MOB-III (mitomycin, Oncovin, bleomycin, cisplatin) *chemotherapy protocol*

Moban oral concentrate (discontinued 2003) ℞ *conventional (typical) dihydroindolone antipsychotic for schizophrenia* [molindone HCl] 20 mg/mL ⊡ Mobidin; Modane

Moban tablets ℞ *conventional (typical) dihydroindolone antipsychotic for schizophrenia* [molindone HCl] 5, 10, 25, 50 mg ⊡ Mobidin; Modane

mobecarb INN

mobenzoxamine INN

Mobic tablets, oral suspension ℞ *once-daily analgesic, antipyretic, and antiarthritic for osteoarthritis and rheumatoid arthritis; COX-2 inhibitor; nonsteroidal anti-inflammatory drug (NSAID)* [meloxicam] 7.5, 15 mg; 7.5 mg/5 mL

Mobicox ⒸⒶ⒩ tablets ℞ *once-daily analgesic, antiarthritic, and antipyretic; COX-2 inhibitor; nonsteroidal anti-inflammatory drug (NSAID)* [meloxicam] 7.5, 15 mg

Mobidin tablets ℞ *analgesic; antipyretic; anti-inflammatory; antirheumatic* [magnesium salicylate] 600 mg ⊡ Moban

Mobigesic tablets OTC *analgesic; antipyretic; anti-inflammatory; antihistaminic sleep aid* [magnesium salicylate; phenyltoloxamine citrate] 325•30 mg

Mobist ℞ *investigational neuroprotectant*

Mobisyl Creme OTC *topical analgesic* [trolamine salicylate] 10%

MOBP (mitomycin, Oncovin, bleomycin, Platinol) *chemotherapy protocol for cervical cancer*

moccasin snake antivenin [see: antivenin (Crotalidae) polyvalent]

mocimycin INN

mociprazine INN

mock pennyroyal *medicinal herb* [see: pennyroyal]

moclobemide USAN, INN, BAN *antidepressant; MAO inhibitor*

moctamide INN

Moctanin biliary infusion (discontinued 2005) ℞ *anticholelithogenic for dissolution of cholesterol gallstones (orphan)* [monoctanoin]

modafinil USAN, INN *analeptic for excessive daytime sleepiness due to narcolepsy (orphan), obstructive sleep apnea, or shift work sleep disorder (SWSD); also used for fatigue associated with multiple sclerosis*

modaline INN *antidepressant* [also: modaline sulfate]

modaline sulfate USAN *antidepressant* [also: modaline]

Modane enteric-coated tablets OTC *stimulant laxative* [bisacodyl] 5 mg ℞ Moban; Mudrane

Modane Bulk powder (discontinued 2003) OTC *bulk laxative* [psyllium husk] 3.4 g/tsp.

Modane Soft capsules (discontinued 2003) OTC *laxative; stool softener* [docusate sodium] 100 mg

modecainide USAN, INN *antiarrhythmic*

Modecate Ⓒ subcu or IM injection ℞ *conventional (typical) phenothiazine antipsychotic for schizophrenia and psychotic disorders; used for prolonged parenteral neuroleptic therapy* [fluphenazine decanoate] 25, 100 mg/mL

Modicon tablets (in Dialpaks and Veridates of 28) ℞ *monophasic oral contraceptive* [norethindrone; ethinyl estradiol] 0.5 mg•35 μg ℞ Mylicon

modified Bagshawe protocol *chemotherapy protocol* [see: CHAMOCA]

modified bovine lung surfactant extract [see: beractant]

modified Burow solution [see: aluminum acetate solution]

modified cellulose gum [now: croscarmellose sodium]

modified Shohl solution (sodium citrate & citric acid) *urinary alkalinizer; compounding agent*

Modiodal (foreign name for U.S. product Provigil)

Moditen Enanthate Ⓒ subcu or IM injection ℞ *conventional (typical) phenothiazine antipsychotic for schizophrenia and psychotic disorders* [fluphenazine enanthate] 25 mg/mL

Moditen HCl Ⓒ tablets ℞ *conventional (typical) phenothiazine antipsychotic for schizophrenia and psychotic disorders* [fluphenazine HCl] 10 mg

Modural powder OTC *carbohydrate caloric supplement* [glucose polymers]

Moduretic tablets ℞ *antihypertensive; diuretic* [amiloride HCl; hydrochlorothiazide] 5•50 mg

moexipril INN, BAN *antihypertensive; angiotensin-converting enzyme (ACE) inhibitor*

moexipril HCl USAN *antihypertensive; angiotensin-converting enzyme (ACE) inhibitor* 7.5, 15 mg oral

moexiprilat INN

MOF (MeCCNU, Oncovin, fluorouracil) *chemotherapy protocol*

mofebutazone INN

mofedione [see: oxazidione]

mofegiline INN *antiparkinsonian* [also: mofegiline HCl]

mofegiline HCl USAN *antiparkinsonian* [also: mofegiline]

mofetil USAN, INN *combining name for radicals or groups*

mofloverine INN

mofoxime INN

MOF-STREP; MOF-Strep (MeCCNU, Oncovin, fluorouracil, streptozocin) *chemotherapy protocol*

Mogadon (approved in Canada and Europe) ℞ *investigational benzodiazepine tranquilizer; anxiolytic; anticonvulsant; hypnotic* [nitrazepam]

moguisteine INN

Moist Again vaginal gel OTC *lubricant* [glycerin; aloe vera]

Moi-Stir oral spray, Swabsticks OTC *saliva substitute* ℞ moisture

Moisture Drops eye drops OTC *ophthalmic moisturizer/lubricant* [hydroxypropyl methylcellulose] 0.5%

Moisture Eyes eye drops OTC *ocular moisturizer/lubricant* [propylene glycol] 0.95%

molfarnate INN

molgramostim USAN, INN, BAN *antineutropenic; hematopoietic stimulant; investigational (Phase II/III) cytokine to AIDS*

molinazone USAN, INN *analgesic*

molindone INN *conventional (typical) dihydroindolone antipsychotic for schizophrenia* [also: molindone HCl]

molindone HCl USAN *conventional (typical) dihydroindolone antipsychotic for schizophrenia* [also: molindone]

Mollifene Ear Wax Removing Formula drops OTC *agent to emulsify and disperse ear wax* [carbamide peroxide] 6.5%

molracetam INN

molsidomine USAN, INN *antianginal; coronary vasodilator*

molybdenum *element* (Mo)

Molypen IV injection ℞ *intravenous nutritional therapy* [ammonium molybdate tetrahydrate] 25 μg/mL

Momentum caplets OTC *analgesic; antipyretic; anti-inflammatory; antihistamine* [aspirin; phenyltoloxamine citrate] 500•15 mg

Momentum Muscular Backache Formula caplets OTC *analgesic; antipyretic; anti-inflammatory* [magnesium salicylate] 580 mg

mometasone INN, BAN *topical corticosteroidal anti-inflammatory* [also: mometasone furoate]

mometasone furoate USAN *topical corticosteroidal anti-inflammatory; oral inhalation aerosol for chronic asthma; nasal aerosol for allergic rhinitis and nasal polyps* [also: mometasone] 0.1% topical

Momordica charantia medicinal herb [see: bitter melon]

MOMP (mechlorethamine, Oncovin, methotrexate, prednisone) *chemotherapy protocol*

Monafed sustained-release tablets (discontinued 2002) ℞ *expectorant* [guaifenesin] 600 mg

Monafed DM tablets (discontinued 2002) ℞ *antitussive; expectorant* [dextromethorphan hydrobromide; guaifenesin] 30•600 mg

monalazone disodium INN

monalium hydrate [see: magaldrate]

Monarc-M powder for IV injection ℞ *antihemophilic* [antihemophilic factor VIII, solvent/detergent-treated and monoclonal purified] 10–15 IU

Monarda didyma medicinal herb [see: Oswego tea]

Monarda fistulosa medicinal herb [see: wild bergamot]

Monarda punctata medicinal herb [see: horsemint]

monascus yeast (*Monascus purpureus*) *natural remedy for gastric disorders, indigestion, lowering cholesterol, and poor circulation*

monatepil INN *antianginal; antihypertensive* [also: monatepil maleate]

monatepil maleate USAN *antianginal; antihypertensive* [also: monatepil]

monensin USAN, INN *antiprotozoal; antibacterial; antifungal*

Monistat cream OTC *antifungal* [miconazole nitrate] 2%

Monistat 1 vaginal ointment in prefilled applicator OTC *antifungal* [tioconazole] 6.5%

Monistat 1 Combination Pack vaginal inserts + cream OTC *antifungal* [miconazole nitrate] 200 mg + 2%

Monistat 1-Day vaginal ointment in prefilled applicator OTC *antifungal* [tioconazole] 6.5%

Monistat 3 vaginal cream, combination pack (vaginal inserts + cream), cream combination pak (vaginal cream in prefilled applicators + external cream) OTC *antifungal* [miconazole nitrate] 2%; 200 mg + 2%; 4% + 2%

Monistat 3 vaginal inserts (discontinued 2001) OTC *antifungal* [miconazole nitrate] 200 mg

Monistat 7 vaginal inserts, vaginal cream, combination pack (inserts + cream) OTC *antifungal* [miconazole nitrate] 100 mg; 2%; 100 mg + 2%

Monistat Dual-Pak vaginal inserts + cream (name changed to Monistat 1 Combination Pack in 2001)

Monistat-Derm cream ℞ *antifungal* [miconazole nitrate] 2%

mono- & di-acetylated monoglycerides NF *plasticizer*

mono- & di-glycerides NF *emulsifying agent*

monoamine oxidase inhibitors (MAOIs) *a class of antidepressants that increase CNS monoamine neurotransmitters (epinephrine, norepinephrine, and serotonin)*

monobactams *a class of bactericidal antibiotics effective against gram-negative aerobic pathogens*

monobasic potassium phosphate [see: potassium phosphate, monobasic]

monobasic sodium phosphate [see: sodium phosphate, monobasic]

monobenzone USP, INN *depigmenting agent for vitiligo*

monobenzyl ether of hydroquinone [see: monobenzone]

monobromated camphor [see: camphor, monobromated]

Monocal tablets OTC *calcium/fluoride supplement* [calcium; fluoride] 250•3 mg

monocalcium phosphate [see: calcium phosphate, dibasic]

Monocaps tablets OTC *vitamin/mineral/iron supplement* [multiple vitamins & minerals; ferrous fumarate; folic acid; biotin] ±•14 mg•0.1 mg•15 μg ② Monoclate; Monoket

Mono-Chlor topical liquid ℞ *cauterant; keratolytic* [monochloroacetic acid] 80%

monochloroacetic acid *strong keratolytic/cauterant*

monochlorothymol [see: chlorothymol]

monochlorphenamide [see: clofenamide]

Monocid powder for IV or IM injection (discontinued 2004) ℞ *cephalosporin antibiotic* [cefonicid sodium] 1, 10 g ② Monocete

Monoclate P powder for IV injection ℞ *antihemophilic to correct coagulation deficiency* [antihemophilic factor concentrate, recombinant] ② Monocaps; Monoket

monoclonal antibody 5A8 to CD4 *investigational (orphan) for post-exposure prophylaxis to occupational HIV exposure*

monoclonal antibody 7E3 [see: abciximab]

monoclonal antibody B43.13 *investigational (orphan) for epithelial ovarian cancer*

monoclonal antibody to CD22 antigen on B-cells, radiolabeled [now: epratuzumab]

monoclonal antibody to CEA, humanized [now: labetuzumab]

monoclonal antibody to cytomegalovirus, human *investigational (orphan) prophylaxis for CMV retinitis and CMV disease in solid organ transplants*

monoclonal antibody E5 [now: edobacomab]

monoclonal antibody to hepatitis B virus, human *investigational (orphan) hepatitis B prophylaxis for liver transplant*

monoclonal antibody LL2, humanized [now: epratuzumab]

monoclonal antibody to lupus nephritis *investigational (orphan) for immunization against lupus nephritis*

monoclonal antibody PM-81 *investigational (orphan) for acute myelogenous leukemia*

monoclonal antibody PM-81 & AML-2-23 *investigational (orphan) for bone marrow transplant for acute myelogenous leukemia*

monoclonal factor IX [see: factor IX complex]

Monocor ⒸⒶⓃ film-coated tablets ℞ *antihypertensive; antiadrenergic (β-blocker)* [bisoprolol fumarate] 5, 10 mg

monoctanoin USAN, BAN *anticholelithogenic for dissolution of cholesterol gallstones* (orphan)

monoctanoin component A
monoctanoin component B
monoctanoin component C
monoctanoin component D

Mono-Diff reagent kit for professional use *in vitro diagnostic aid for mononucleosis*

Monodox capsules ℞ *tetracycline antibiotic* [doxycycline monohydrate] 50, 100 mg

Mono-Drop (trademarked delivery system) *prefilled eye drop dispenser*

monoethanolamine NF *surfactant*

monoethanolamine oleate INN *sclerosing agent* [also: ethanolamine oleate]

Mono-Gesic film-coated tablets (discontinued 2004) ℞ *analgesic; antipyretic; anti-inflammatory; antirheumatic* [salsalate] 750 mg

Monoket tablets ℞ *antianginal; vasodilator* [isosorbide mononitrate] 10, 20 mg ② Monocete

Mono-Latex reagent kit for professional use *in vitro diagnostic aid for mononucleosis*

monolaurin *investigational (Phase III, orphan) for nonbullous congenital ichthyosiform erythroderma*

monometacrine INN

Mononessa tablets (in packs of 28) ℞ *monophasic oral contraceptive* [norgestimate; ethinyl estradiol] 0.25 mg• 35 μg

Mononine powder for IV infusion ℞ *antihemophilic for factor IX deficiency (hemophilia B; Christmas disease) (orphan)* [factor IX concentrate] 100 IU/mL

monooctanoin [see: monoctanoin]

monophenylbutazone [see: mofebutazone]

monophosphothiamine INN

Mono-Plus reagent kit for professional use *in vitro diagnostic aid for mononucleosis*

monopotassium 4-aminosalicylate [see: aminosalicylate potassium]

monopotassium carbonate [see: potassium bicarbonate]

monopotassium D-gluconate [see: potassium gluconate]

monopotassium monosodium tartrate tetrahydrate [see: potassium sodium tartrate]

monopotassium phosphate [see: potassium phosphate, monobasic]

Monopril tablets ℞ *antihypertensive; angiotensin-converting enzyme (ACE) inhibitor; adjunctive treatment for CHF* [fosinopril sodium] 10, 20, 40 mg

Monopril-HCT tablets ℞ *antihypertensive; angiotensin-converting enzyme (ACE) inhibitor; diuretic* [fosinopril sodium; hydrochlorothiazide] 10• 12.5, 20•12.5 mg

monosodium *p*-aminohippurate [see: aminohippurate sodium]

monosodium 4-aminosalicylate dihydrate [see: aminosalicylate sodium]

monosodium carbonate [see: sodium bicarbonate]

monosodium D-gluconate [see: sodium gluconate]

monosodium D-thyroxine hydrate [see: dextrothyroxine sodium]

monosodium glutamate NF *flavoring agent; perfume*

monosodium L-ascorbate [see: sodium ascorbate]

monosodium L-thyroxine hydrate [see: levothyroxine sodium]

monosodium phosphate dihydrate [see: sodium phosphate, monobasic]

monosodium phosphate monohydrate [see: sodium phosphate, monobasic]

monosodium salicylate [see: sodium salicylate]

monosodium sulfite [see: sodium bisulfite]

Monospot slide test for professional use *in vitro diagnostic aid for mononucleosis*

monostearin [see: glyceryl monostearate]

Monosticon Dri-Dot slide test for professional use *in vitro diagnostic aid for mononucleosis*

monosulfiram BAN [also: sulfiram]

Mono-Sure slide test for professional use *in vitro diagnostic aid for mononucleosis*

Mono-Test slide test for professional use *in vitro diagnostic aid for mononucleosis*

monothioglycerol NF *preservative*

Monotropa uniflora *medicinal herb* [see: fit root]

Mono-Vacc Test (O.T.) single-use intradermal puncture test device (discontinued 2002) *tuberculosis skin test* [old tuberculin] 5 U

Monovial (trademarked delivery system) *single-use vial with transfer needle set*

monoxerutin INN

Monsel solution [see: ferric subsulfate]

montelukast sodium USAN *leukotriene receptor inhibitor for allergic rhinitis and the prophylaxis and chronic treatment of asthma*

monteplase INN

montirelin INN

montmorillonite (redmond clay) *natural remedy for bug bites and stings and other skin problems*

Monuril (foreign name for U.S. product Monurol)

Monurol granules for oral solution ℞ *broad-spectrum bactericidal antibiotic for urinary tract infections* [fosfomycin tromethamine] 3 g/pkt.

moose elm *medicinal herb* [see: slippery elm]

8-MOP capsules ℞ *systemic psoralens for psoriasis, repigmentation of idiopathic vitiligo, and cutaneous T-cell lymphoma (CTCL); used to increase tolerance to sunlight and enhance pigmentation* [methoxsalen] 10 mg

MOP (mechlorethamine, Oncovin, prednisone) *chemotherapy protocol*

MOP (mechlorethamine, Oncovin, procarbazine) *chemotherapy protocol for pediatric brain tumors*

8-MOP (8-methoxypsoralen) [see: methoxsalen]

MOP-BAP (mechlorethamine, Oncovin, procarbazine, bleomycin, Adriamycin, prednisone) *chemotherapy protocol*

moperone INN

mopidamol INN

mopidralazine INN

MOPP (mechlorethamine, Oncovin, procarbazine, prednisone) *chemotherapy protocol for Hodgkin lymphoma and brain cancer (medulloblastoma)*

MOPP (mustine HCl, Oncovin, procarbazine, prednisone) *chemotherapy protocol*

MOPP/ABV (mechlorethamine, Oncovin, procarbazine, prednisone, Adriamycin, bleomycin, vinblastine) *chemotherapy protocol for Hodgkin lymphoma*

MOPP/ABVD (alternating cycles of MOPP and ABVD) *chemotherapy protocol for Hodgkin lymphoma*

MOPP-BLEO; MOPP-Bleo (mechlorethamine, Oncovin, procarbazine, prednisone, bleomycin) *chemotherapy protocol*

MOPPHDB (mechlorethamine, Oncovin, procarbazine, prednisone, high-dose bleomycin) *chemotherapy protocol*

MOPPLDB (mechlorethamine, Oncovin, procarbazine, prednisone, low-dose bleomycin) *chemotherapy protocol*

MOPr (mechlorethamine, Oncovin, procarbazine) *chemotherapy protocol*

moprolol INN

moquizone INN

moracizine INN, BAN *antiarrhythmic* [also: moricizine]

morantel INN *anthelmintic* [also: morantel tartrate]

morantel tartrate USAN *anthelmintic* [also: morantel]

Moranyl (available only from the Centers for Disease Control) ℞ *antiparasitic for African trypanosomiasis and onchocerciasis* [suramin sodium]

morazone INN, BAN

morclofone INN

More-Dophilus powder OTC *probiotic; dietary supplement; fever blister treatment; not generally regarded as safe and effective as an antidiarrheal* [Lactobacillus acidophilus] 4 billion CFU/g

morforex INN

moricizine USAN *antiarrhythmic* [also: moracizine]

moricizine HCl *antiarrhythmic for severe ventricular arrhythmias*

morinamide INN

Morinda citrifolia medicinal herb [see: noni]

Mormon tea medicinal herb [see: ephedra]

morniflumate USAN, INN anti-inflammatory

morning glory (Ipomoea violacea) seeds contain lysergic acid amide, chemically similar to LSD, which produce hallucinations when ingested as a street drug [see also: LSD]

morocromen INN

moroxydine INN, BAN

morphazinamide [see: morinamide]

Morphelan (name changed to Avinza upon marketing release in 2002)

morpheridine INN, BAN

morphine BAN narcotic analgesic; widely abused as a street drug, which leads to dependence [also: morphine sulfate]

morphine dinicotinate ester [see: nicomorphine]

morphine HCl USP narcotic analgesic preferred in Germany and England; widely abused as a street drug, which leads to dependence

Morphine LP ⓒ epidural injection ℞ narcotic analgesic [morphine sulfate] 0.5, 1 mg/mL

morphine sulfate (MS) USP narcotic analgesic preferred in the U.S.; intraspinal microinfusion for intractable chronic pain (orphan); widely abused as a street drug, which leads to dependence [also: morphine] 15, 30, 60 mg oral; 10, 20 mg/5 mL oral; 0.5, 1, 2, 4, 5, 8, 10, 15, 25, 30, 50 mg/mL injection; 5, 10, 20, 30 mg rectal

4-morpholinecarboximidoylguanidine [see: moroxydine]

2-morpholinoethylrutin [see: ethoxazorutoside]

3-morpholinosydnoneimine [see: linsidomine]

morpholinyl succinimide [see: morsuximide]

morpholinylethyl morphine [see: pholcodine]

morrhuate sodium USP sclerosing agent for varicose veins [also: sodium morrhuate] 50 mg/mL injection

morsuximide INN

morsydomine [see: molsidomine]

mortification root medicinal herb [see: marsh mallow]

Morton Salt Substitute; Morton Seasoned Salt Substitute OTC salt substitute [potassium chloride] 64 mEq K/5 g; 56 mEq K/5 g

Morus nigra; M. rubra medicinal herb [see: mulberry]

Moschus moschiferus natural remedy [see: deer musk]

Mosco topical liquid OTC keratolytic [salicylic acid in flexible collodion] 17.6%

mosquito plant medicinal herb [see: pennyroyal]

motapizone INN

MOTC (methyleneoxytetracycline) [see: methacycline]

motexafin gadolinium USAN investigational (Phase III) radiosensitizer for brain metastases

motexafin lutetium USAN investigational photo-antineoplastic for recurrent breast cancer; investigational photoangioplastic for atherosclerosis; investigational (Phase I/II) photosensitizer for ophthalmic therapy and imaging

mother of thyme medicinal herb [see: thyme]

motherwort (Leonurus cardiaca) flowering tops and leaves medicinal herb used as an antispasmodic, astringent, calmative, cardiac, emmenagogue, hepatic, laxative, nervine, and stomachic

Motilium ⓒ film-coated tablets ℞ antiemetic for diabetic gastroparesis and chronic gastritis (investigational (NDA filed) in the U.S.) [domperidone maleate] 10 mg

Motofen tablets ℞ antidiarrheal [difenoxin HCl; atropine sulfate] 1•0.025 mg

motrazepam INN

motretinide USAN, INN keratolytic

Motrin tablets ℞ *analgesic; antiarthritic; antipyretic; nonsteroidal anti-inflammatory drug (NSAID)* [ibuprofen] 400, 600, 800 mg

Motrin, Children's chewable tablets, oral suspension OTC *analgesic; antiarthritic; antipyretic; nonsteroidal anti-inflammatory drug (NSAID)* [ibuprofen] 50 mg; 100 mg/5 mL

Motrin, Infants' oral drops OTC *analgesic; antipyretic; nonsteroidal anti-inflammatory drug (NSAID)* [ibuprofen] 40 mg/mL

Motrin, Junior Strength tablets, chewable tablets OTC *analgesic; antiarthritic; antipyretic; nonsteroidal anti-inflammatory drug (NSAID)* [ibuprofen] 100 mg

Motrin Children's Cold oral suspension OTC *decongestant; analgesic; antipyretic* [pseudoephedrine HCl; ibuprofen] 15•100 mg/5 mL

Motrin IB tablets, gelcaps OTC *analgesic, antiarthritic; antipyretic; nonsteroidal anti-inflammatory drug (NSAID)* [ibuprofen] 200 mg

Motrin IB Sinus caplets (name changed to Motrin Sinus Headache in 2002)

Motrin Migraine Pain caplets OTC *analgesic; nonsteroidal anti-inflammatory drug (NSAID)* [ibuprofen] 200 mg

Motrin Sinus Headache caplets OTC *decongestant; analgesic* [pseudoephedrine HCl; ibuprofen] 30•200 mg

mountain ash *(Sorbus americana; S. aucuparia)* fruit *medicinal herb used as an aperient, astringent, and diuretic*

mountain balm *medicinal herb* [see: yerba santa]

mountain box; mountain cranberry *medicinal herb* [see: uva ursi]

mountain laurel *(Kalmia latifolia)* leaves *medicinal herb used as an astringent and sedative*

mountain mahogany *medicinal herb* [see: birch]

mountain mint *medicinal herb* [see: marjoram; Oswego tea]

mountain snuff; mountain tobacco *medicinal herb* [see: arnica]

mountain sorrel *medicinal herb* [see: wood sorrel]

mountain strawberry *medicinal herb* [see: strawberry]

mountain sumach *medicinal herb* [see: sumach]

mountain sweet *medicinal herb* [see: New Jersey tea]

mountain tea *medicinal herb* [see: wintergreen]

mouse ear *(Hieracium pilosella)* plant *medicinal herb used as an astringent, cholagogue, and diuretic*

MouthKote oral spray OTC *saliva substitute*

MouthKote O/R mouthwash OTC *anesthetic and antimicrobial throat irrigation* [benzyl alcohol; menthol]

MouthKote O/R oral solution OTC *topical antihistamine* [diphenhydramine] 1.25%

MouthKote P/R oral solution, ointment (discontinued 2004) OTC *topical antihistamine* [diphenhydramine HCl] 1.25%; 25%

mouthroot *medicinal herb* [see: gold thread]

moveltipril INN

moxadolen INN

moxalactam disodium USAN, USP *bactericidal antibiotic* [also: latamoxef]

moxantrazole [now: teloxantrone HCl]

moxaprindine INN

moxastine INN

moxaverine INN, BAN

moxazocine USAN, INN *analgesic; antitussive*

moxestrol INN

moxicoumone INN

moxidectin USAN, INN *veterinary antiparasitic*

moxifloxacin HCl USAN *broad-spectrum fluoroquinolone antibiotic*

moxilubant maleate USAN *leukotriene B$_4$ receptor antagonist for rheumatoid arthritis and psoriasis*

moxipraquine INN, BAN

moxiraprine INN

moxisylyte INN [also: thymoxamine]

moxnidazole USAN, INN *antiprotozoal (Trichomonas)*

moxonidine USAN, INN *centrally acting sympatholytic for hypertension, congestive heart failure, and type 2 diabetes*

M-oxy tablets ℞ *narcotic analgesic* [oxycodone HCl] 5 mg

MP (melphalan, prednisone) *chemotherapy protocol for multiple myeloma*

MP (mitoxantrone, prednisone) *chemotherapy protocol for prostate cancer*

4-MP (4-methylpyrazole) [see: fomepizole]

6-MP (6-mercaptopurine) [see: mercaptopurine]

MPA (medroxyprogesterone acetate) [q.v.]

MPA (mycophenolic acid) [q.v.]

MPF [see: Mucoprotective Factor]

m-PFL (methotrexate, Platinol, fluorouracil, leucovorin [rescue]) *chemotherapy protocol*

MPH (methylphenidate HCl) [q.v.]

MPL (melphalan) [q.v.]

MPL + PRED (melphalan, prednisone) *chemotherapy protocol*

M-Prednisol-40; M-Prednisol-80 intralesional, soft tissue, and IM injection (discontinued 2004) ℞ *corticosteroid; anti-inflammatory; immunosuppressant* [methylprednisolone acetate] 40 mg/mL; 80 mg/mL

MRV (mixed respiratory vaccine) [q.v.]

M-R-Vax II powder for subcu injection (discontinued 2004) ℞ *measles and rubella vaccine* [measles and rubella virus vaccine, live] 0.5 mL

MS (magnesium salicylate) [q.v.]

MS (morphine sulfate) [q.v.]

MS Contin controlled-release tablets ℞ *narcotic analgesic; preoperative sedative and anxiolytic* [morphine sulfate] 15, 30, 60, 100, 200 mg

MSD Enteric-Coated ASA ⓒᴬᴺ tablets OTC *analgesic; antipyretic; anti-inflammatory; antirheumatic* [aspirin] 325, 650 mg

MSIR capsules (discontinued 2003) ℞ *narcotic analgesic; preoperative sedative and anxiolytic* [morphine sulfate] 15, 30 mg

MSIR tablets (discontinued 2005) ℞ *narcotic analgesic; preoperative sedative and anxiolytic* [morphine sulfate] 15, 30 mg

MSIR oral solution, oral concentrate ℞ *narcotic analgesic; preoperative sedative and anxiolytic* [morphine sulfate] 10, 20 mg/5 mL; 20 mg/mL

MSM (methylsulfonylmethane) *natural source of sulfur; promotes an increase in collagen and the endogenous antioxidant glutathione*

MSTA (Mumps Skin Test Antigen) intradermal injection ℞ *diagnostic aid to assess immune system competency (not effective in testing immunity to mumps virus)* [mumps skin test antigen] 0.1 mL (4 U/0.1 mL)

MT6 (mercaptomerin) [q.v.]

M-Tabs (trademarked form) *orally disintegrating tablets*

MTC (mitomycin C) [see: mitomycin]

M.T.E.-4; M.T.E.-5; M.T.E.-6; M.T.E.-7; M.T.E.-4 Concentrated; M.T.E.-5 Concentrated; M.T.E.-6 Concentrated IV injection ℞ *intravenous nutritional therapy* [multiple trace elements (metals)]

mTHPC [see: temoporfin]

MTX (methotrexate) [q.v.]

MTX + MP + CTX (methotrexate, mercaptopurine, cyclophosphamide) *chemotherapy protocol*

MTX/6-MP (methotrexate, mercaptopurine) *chemotherapy protocol for acute lymphocytic leukemia (ALL); the ongoing continuation protocol* [also: 1DMTX/6-MP (the first-day initiation protocol)]

MTX/6-MP/VP (methotrexate, mercaptopurine, vincristine, prednisone) *chemotherapy protocol for acute lymphocytic leukemia (ALL)*

MTX-CDDPAdr (methotrexate [with leucovorin rescue], CDDP,

Adriamycin) *chemotherapy protocol for pediatric osteosarcoma*

Mucinex dual-release tablets OTC *expectorant* [guaifenesin] 600 (100 mg immediate release, 500 mg extended release)

Mucinex DM extended-release tablets OTC *antitussive; expectorant* [dextromethorphan hydrobromide; guaifenesin] 30•600, 60•1200 mg

Muco-Fen; Muco-Fen 800; Muco-Fen 1200 timed-release tablets (discontinued 2004) ℞ *expectorant* [guaifenesin] 1000 mg; 800 mg; 1200 mg

Muco-Fen DM sustained-release tablets ℞ *antitussive; expectorant* [dextromethorphan hydrobromide; guaifenesin] 60•1000 mg

Muco-Fen LA timed-release tablets (discontinued 2002) ℞ *expectorant* [guaifenesin] 600 mg

mucoid exopolysaccharide *Pseudomonas* **hyperimmune globulin (MEPIG)** *investigational (orphan) for pulmonary infections of cystic fibrosis*

mucolytics *a class of respiratory inhalant drugs that destroy or inhibit mucin*

Mucomyst solution for nebulization or intratracheal instillation ℞ *mucolytic* [acetylcysteine sodium] 10%, 20%

Mucomyst 10 IV ℞ *investigational (orphan) for severe acetaminophen overdose* [acetylcysteine]

Mucoprotective Factor (MPF) (trademarked ingredient) *aromatic flavored syrup* [eriodictyon]

Mucosil-10; Mucosil-20 solution for nebulization or intratracheal instillation (discontinued 2004) ℞ *mucolytic* [acetylcysteine sodium] 10%; 20%

Mudrane tablets ℞ *antiasthmatic; bronchodilator; decongestant; expectorant; sedative* [aminophylline; ephedrine HCl; potassium iodide; phenobarbital] 111•16•195•8 mg ⓑ Modane

Mudrane GG tablets ℞ *antiasthmatic; decongestant; expectorant; sedative* [theophylline; ephedrine HCl; guaifenesin; phenobarbital] 111•16•100•8 mg

Mudrane GG-2 tablets ℞ *antiasthmatic; bronchodilator; expectorant* [theophylline; guaifenesin] 111•100 mg

mugwort (Artemisia vulgaris) root and plant *medicinal herb used as a diaphoretic, emmenagogue, and laxative*

muira puama (Ptychopetalum olacoides) stem *medicinal herb used as an aphrodisiac and treatment for impotence in South America; clinical trials in France confirm these effects*

mulberry (Morus nigra; M. rubra) bark *medicinal herb used as an anthelmintic and cathartic*

mullein (Verbascum nigrum; V. phlomoides; V. thapsiforme; V. thapsus) plant *medicinal herb for asthma, bleeding in bowel and lungs, bronchitis, bruises, cough, croup, diarrhea, earache, gout, hemorrhoids, insomnia, lymphatic system, nervousness, pain, pleurisy, sinus congestion, and tuberculosis*

MulTE-Pak-4; MulTE-Pak-5 IV injection ℞ *intravenous nutritional therapy* [multiple trace elements (metals)]

Multi 75 timed-release tablets OTC *vitamin/mineral supplement* [multiple vitamins & minerals; folic acid; biotin] ±•0.4•± mg

Multi Vit with Iron drops OTC *vitamin/iron supplement* [multiple vitamins; iron] ±•10 mg/mL

Multi Vitamin Concentrate injection ℞ *parenteral vitamin supplement* [multiple vitamins]

Multi-12; Multi-12 Pediatric ⓒᴬᴺ IV infusion ℞ *vitamin supplement* [multiple vitamins]

Multi-Day tablets OTC *vitamin supplement* [multiple vitamins; folic acid] ±•0.4 mg

Multi-Day Plus Iron tablets OTC *vitamin/iron supplement* [multiple vitamins; iron; folic acid] ±•18•0.4 mg

Multi-Day Plus Minerals tablets OTC *vitamin/mineral/iron supplement* [multiple vitamins & minerals; iron; folic acid; biotin] ±•18 mg•0.4 mg•30 µg

Multi-Day with Calcium and Extra Iron tablets OTC *vitamin/calcium/iron supplement* [multiple vitamins; calcium; iron; folic acid] ≟•≟•27•0.4 mg

Multifol caplets ℞ *vitamin/calcium/iron supplement* [multiple vitamins; calcium; iron (as ferrous fumarate); folic acid] ≟•125•65•1 mg

MultiKine injection ℞ *investigational (Phase III) antineoplastic for prostate cancer; investigational (Phase I) immunotherapeutic agent for HIV and HPV infections* [multiple leukocytes and interleukins]

Multilex; Multilex-T & M tablets OTC *vitamin/mineral/iron supplement* [multiple vitamins & minerals; iron] ≟•15 mg

Multilyte-20; Multilyte-40 IV admixture ℞ *intravenous electrolyte therapy* [combined electrolyte solution]

Multi-Mineral tablets OTC *mineral supplement* [multiple minerals]

Multiple Trace Element; Multiple Trace Element Concentrated; Multiple Trace Element Pediatric IV injection (discontinued 2003) ℞ *intravenous nutritional therapy* [multiple trace elements (metals)]

Multiple Trace Element Neonatal; Multiple Trace Element with Selenium; Multiple Trace Element with Selenium Concentrated IV injection ℞ *intravenous nutritional therapy* [multiple trace elements (metals)]

Multistix; Multistix 2; Multistix 7; Multistix 8 SG; Multistix 9; Multistix 9 SG; Multistix 10 SG; Multistix SG reagent strips OTC *in vitro diagnostic aid for multiple urine products*

Multistix PRO reagent strips for professional use ℞ *in vitro diagnostic aid for urine protein/creatinine ratio*

Multitest CMI single-use intradermal skin test device (discontinued 2004) ℞ *skin test for multiple allergen sensitivity* [skin test antigens (seven different); glycerin (one for test control)]

Multitrace-5 Concentrate IV injection ℞ *intravenous nutritional therapy* [multiple trace elements (metals)]

multivitamin infusion, neonatal formula *investigational (orphan) total parenteral nutrition for very low birth-weight infants*

Multi-Vitamin Mineral with Beta-Carotene tablets OTC *vitamin/mineral/iron supplement* [multiple vitamins & minerals; ferrous fumarate; folic acid; biotin] ≟•27•0.4•0.45 mg

Multivitamin with Fluoride drops ℞ *pediatric vitamin supplement and dental caries preventative* [multiple vitamins; fluoride] ≟•0.25, ≟•0.5 mg/mL

Multivitamins capsules OTC *vitamin supplement* [multiple vitamins]

Mulvidren-F Softabs (chewable tablets) ℞ *pediatric vitamin supplement and dental caries preventative* [multiple vitamins; fluoride] ≟•1 mg

mumps skin test antigen (MSTA) USP *diagnostic aid to assess immune system competency*

mumps vaccine [see: mumps virus vaccine, inactivated]

mumps virus vaccine, inactivated NF

mumps virus vaccine, live USP *active immunizing agent for mumps*

Mumpsvax powder for subcu injection ℞ *mumps vaccine* [mumps virus vaccine, live] 0.5 mL

mupirocin USAN, INN, BAN *topical antibiotic* 2% topical

mupirocin calcium USAN *topical antibiotic* (base=93%)

muplestim USAN *progenitor cell stimulator for neutropenia and thrombocytopenia*

murabutide INN

muraglitazar *peroxisome proliferator–activated receptor (PPAR) alpha/gamma agonist; antidiabetic to control blood glucose levels, lower triglycerides, and raise HDL*

Murine eye drops OTC *ophthalmic moisturizer/lubricant* [polyvinyl alcohol] 0.5%

Murine Ear Drops OTC *agent to emulsify and disperse ear wax* [carbamide peroxide; alcohol] 6.5%•6.3%

Murine Plus eye drops OTC *topical ophthalmic decongestant and vasoconstrictor* [tetrahydrozoline HCl] 0.05%

Muro 128 eye drops, ophthalmic ointment OTC *corneal edema-reducing agent* [sodium chloride (hypertonic saline solution)] 2%, 5%; 5%

murocainide INN

Murocel eye drops OTC *ophthalmic moisturizer/lubricant* [methylcellulose] 1%

Murocoll-2 eye drops ℞ *cycloplegic; mydriatic* [scopolamine hydrobromide; phenylephrine HCl] 0.3%•10%

murodermin INN

muromonab-CD3 USAN, INN *immunosuppressive monoclonal antibody (MAb) for renal, hepatic, and cardiac transplants*

Muroptic-5 eye drops OTC *corneal edema-reducing agent* [sodium chloride (hypertonic saline solution)] 5%

muscarinic agonists *a class of investigational analgesics*

Muse single-use intraurethral suppository ℞ *vasodilator for erectile dysfunction* [alprostadil] 125, 150, 500, 1000 μg

musk *natural remedy* [see: deer musk]

mustaral oil [see: allyl isothiocyanate]

mustard (Brassica alba; Sinapis alba) seeds and oil *medicinal herb for indigestion and liver and lung disorders; also used as an appetizer, diuretic, emetic, and soak for aching feet, arthritis, and rheumatism*

mustard oil [see: allyl isothiocyanate]

Mustargen powder for IV or intracavitary injection ℞ *nitrogen mustard-type alkylating antineoplastic for multiple carcinomas, lymphomas and leukemias, mycosis fungoides, and polycythemia vera* [mechlorethamine HCl] 10 mg

Musterole Deep Strength Rub OTC *analgesic; counterirritant* [methyl salicylate; methyl nicotinate; menthol] 30%•0.5%•3%

Musterole Extra Strength OTC *topical analgesic; counterirritant* [camphor; menthol] 5%•3%

mustine BAN *nitrogen mustard-type alkylating antineoplastic* [also: mechlorethamine HCl; chlormethine; nitrogen mustard N-oxide HCl]

mustine HCl [see: mechlorethamine HCl]

Mutamycin powder for IV injection ℞ *antibiotic antineoplastic for disseminated adenocarcinoma of the stomach or pancreas* [mitomycin] 5, 20, 40 mg
🔊 mitomycin

muzolimine USAN, INN *diuretic; antihypertensive*

MV (mitomycin, vinblastine) *chemotherapy protocol for breast cancer*

MV (mitoxantrone, VePesid) *chemotherapy protocol for acute myelocytic leukemia (ALL)*

MVAC; M-VAC (methotrexate, vinblastine, Adriamycin, cisplatin) *chemotherapy protocol for bladder cancer*

M-Vax ℞ *investigational (Phase III, orphan) theraccine for postsurgical stage III malignant melanoma* [DNP-conjugated tumor vaccine]

MVF (mitoxantrone, vincristine, fluorouracil) *chemotherapy protocol*

M.V.I. Neonatal IV infusion ℞ *investigational (orphan) total parenteral nutrition for very low birthweight infants* [multiple vitamins]

M.V.I. Pediatric injection ℞ *parenteral vitamin supplement* [multiple vitamins; folic acid; biotin] ≛•140•20 μg/5 mL

M.V.I.-12 injection ℞ *parenteral vitamin supplement* [multiple vitamins; folic acid; biotin] ≛•400•60 μg/5 mL

M.V.M. capsules OTC *vitamin/mineral/iron supplement* [multiple vitamins & minerals; iron; folic acid; biotin] ≛•3.6 mg•0.08 mg•160 μg

MVP (mitomycin, vinblastine, Platinol) *chemotherapy protocol for non–small cell lung cancer (NSCLC)*

MVPP (mechlorethamine, vinblastine, procarbazine, prednisone) *chemotherapy protocol for Hodgkin lymphoma*

MVT (mitoxantrone, VePesid, thiotepa) *chemotherapy protocol*

MVVPP (mechlorethamine, vincristine, vinblastine, procarbazine, prednisone) *chemotherapy protocol*

Myadec tablets OTC *vitamin/mineral/iron supplement* [multiple vitamins & minerals; iron; folic acid; biotin] ± • 18 mg•0.4 mg•30 μg

Myambutol film-coated tablets ℞ *tuberculostatic* [ethambutol HCl] 100, 400 mg ⊡ Nembutal

Mycamine powder for IV infusion ℞ *antifungal for esophageal candidiasis and* Candida *prophylaxis* [micafungin sodium] 50 mg/dose

Mycelex cream, solution (discontinued 2000) ℞ *topical antifungal* [clotrimazole] 1%

Mycelex troches ℞ *antifungal; oral candidiasis prophylaxis or treatment* [clotrimazole] 10 mg

Mycelex OTC cream, solution (discontinued 2000) OTC *topical antifungal* [clotrimazole] 1%

Mycelex Twin Pack vaginal inserts + cream (discontinued 2001) ℞ *antifungal* [clotrimazole] 500 mg; 1%

Mycelex-3 vaginal cream in prefilled applicator OTC *antifungal* [butoconazole nitrate] 2%

Mycelex-7 vaginal cream, combination pack (vaginal inserts + cream) OTC *antifungal* [clotrimazole] 1%; 100 mg + 1%

Mycelex-7 vaginal inserts (discontinued 2001) OTC *antifungal* [clotrimazole] 100 mg

Mycelex-G vaginal inserts (discontinued 2001) ℞ *antifungal* [clotrimazole] 500 mg

Mycifradin Sulfate oral solution ℞ *aminoglycoside antibiotic* [neomycin sulfate] 125 mg/5 mL

Myciguent ointment, cream (discontinued 2003) OTC *antibiotic* [neomycin sulfate] 3.5 mg/g

Mycinaire Saline Mist nasal spray OTC *nasal moisturizer* [sodium chloride (saline solution)] 0.65%

Mycinette throat spray OTC *topical anesthetic; oral antiseptic; astringent* [phenol; alum] 1.4%•0.3%

Mycinettes lozenges OTC *topical oral anesthetic* [benzocaine] 15 mg

"mycins" *brief term for a class of antibiotics derived from various strains of the fungus-like bacteria* Streptomyces, *or their synthetic analogues, whose generic names end in "mycin," such as lincomycin* [properly called: aminoglycosides]

Myci-Spray nasal spray OTC *nasal decongestant; antihistamine* [phenylephrine HCl; pyrilamine maleate] 0.25%•0.15%

Mycitracin Plus ointment (discontinued 2001) OTC *topical antibiotic; local anesthetic* [polymyxin B sulfate; neomycin sulfate; bacitracin; lidocaine] 5000 U•3.5 mg•500 U•40 mg per g

Mycitracin Triple Antibiotic ointment (discontinued 2001) OTC *topical antibiotic* [polymyxin B sulfate; neomycin sulfate; bacitracin] 5000 U•3.5 mg•500 U per g

mycobacterial cell wall complex (MCC) [see: urocidin]

Mycobacterium avium sensitin RS-10 *investigational (orphan) diagnostic aid for* Mycobacterium avium *infection in immunocompromised patients*

Myco-Biotic II cream ℞ *topical corticosteroidal anti-inflammatory; antifungal* [triamcinolone acetonide; neomycin sulfate; nystatin] 0.1%• 0.5%•100 000 U per g

Mycobutin capsules ℞ *antiviral/antibacterial for prevention of* Mycobacterium avium *complex (MAC) in advanced HIV patients (orphan)* [rifabutin] 150 mg

Mycocide NS solution OTC *topical antiseptic* [benzalkonium chloride]

Mycogen II cream, ointment ℞ *topical corticosteroidal anti-inflammatory; antifungal* [triamcinolone acetonide; nystatin] 0.1%•100 000 U per g

Mycolog-II cream, ointment ℞ *topical corticosteroidal anti-inflammatory; antifungal* [triamcinolone acetonide; nystatin] 0.1%•100 000 U per g

Myconel cream ℞ *topical corticosteroidal anti-inflammatory; antifungal* [triamcinolone acetonide; nystatin] 0.1%•100 000 U per g

mycophenolate mofetil USAN *purine biosynthesis inhibitor; immunosuppressant for allogenic renal, hepatic, or cardiac transplants*

mycophenolate mofetil HCl USAN *immunosuppressant for allogenic renal, hepatic, or cardiac transplants; purine biosynthesis inhibitor*

mycophenolic acid (MPA) USAN, INN *antineoplastic; immunosuppressant for allogenic renal, hepatic, or cardiac transplants*

Mycostatin cream, ointment, powder ℞ *antifungal* [nystatin] 100 000 U/g; 100 000 U/g; 100 000 U/g

Mycostatin film-coated tablets ℞ *systemic antifungal* [nystatin] 500 000 U

Mycostatin oral suspension (discontinued 2004) ℞ *antifungal; oral candidiasis treatment* [nystatin] 100 000 U/mL

Mycostatin Pastilles (troches) ℞ *antifungal; oral candidiasis treatment* [nystatin] 200 000 U

Mycostatin vaginal inserts (discontinued 2001) ℞ *topical antifungal* [nystatin] 100 000 U

Myco-Triacet II cream, ointment ℞ *topical corticosteroidal anti-inflammatory; antifungal* [triamcinolone acetonide; nystatin] 0.1%•100 000 U per g

mydeton [see: tolperisone]

Mydfrin 2.5% eye drops ℞ *topical ophthalmic decongestant and vasoconstrictor; mydriatic* [phenylephrine HCl] 2.5% ② Midrin; Myfedrine

Mydriacyl Drop-Tainers (eye drops) ℞ *cycloplegic; mydriatic* [tropicamide] 0.5%, 1%

mydriatics *a class of drugs that cause the pupil of the eye to dilate*

myelin *investigational (orphan) for multiple sclerosis*

myeloid progenitor inhibitory factor 1 (MPIF-1) [see: mirostipen]

myelosan [see: busulfan]

myfadol INN

Myfortic film-coated delayed-release tablets ℞ *immunosuppressant for allogenic renal, hepatic, or cardiac transplants* [mycophenolic acid] 180, 360 mg

Mygel; Mygel II oral suspension OTC *antacid; antiflatulent* [aluminum hydroxide; magnesium hydroxide; simethicone] 200•200•20 mg/5 mL; 400•400•40 mg/5 mL

Mykrox tablets ℞ *antihypertensive; diuretic* [metolazone] 0.5 mg

Mylagen gelcaps OTC *antacid* [calcium carbonate; magnesium carbonate] 311•232 mg

Mylagen; Mylagen II oral liquid OTC *antacid; antiflatulent* [aluminum hydroxide; magnesium hydroxide; simethicone] 200•200•20 mg/5 mL; 400•400•40 mg/5 mL

Mylanta chewable tablets, oral liquid OTC *antacid; antiflatulent* [aluminum hydroxide; magnesium hydroxide; simethicone] 200•200•20, 400•400•40 mg; 200•200•20, 400•400•40 mg/5 mL ② Dilantin; Milontin

Mylanta gelcaps OTC *antacid* [calcium carbonate; magnesium carbonate] 311•232 mg

Mylanta lozenges OTC *antacid* [calcium carbonate] 600 mg

Mylanta, Children's oral liquid, chewable tablets OTC *antacid* [calcium carbonate] 400 mg/5 mL; 400 mg

Mylanta AR ("acid reducer") tablets OTC *histamine H_2 antagonist for heartburn and acid indigestion* [famotidine] 10 mg

Mylanta Gas chewable tablets OTC *antiflatulent* [simethicone] 40, 80, 125 mg

Mylanta Supreme oral liquid OTC *antacid* [calcium carbonate; magnesium hydroxide] 400•135 mg/5 mL

Myleran tablets ℞ *alkylating antineoplastic for chronic myelogenous leukemia (CML)* [busulfan] 2 mg ② Mylicon

Mylicon drops OTC *antiflatulent* [simethicone] 40 mg/0.6 mL ② Modicon; Myleran

Mylinax ℞ *investigational (orphan) agent for chronic progressive multiple sclerosis* [cladribine]

Mylocel film-coated caplets ℞ *antineoplastic for melanoma, squamous cell carcinoma, myelocytic leukemia, and ovarian cancer* [hydroxyurea] 1000 mg

Myloral ℞ *investigational (Phase III) oral treatment for multiple sclerosis* [bovine myelin]

Mylotarg powder for IV injection ℞ *antibody-targeted chemotherapy agent for acute myeloid leukemia (orphan)* [gemtuzumab ozogamicin] 5 mg/vial

Mylovenge ℞ *investigational (orphan) agent for multiple myeloma* [antigen-presenting cells pulsed with tumor immunoglobulin idiotype]

Myminic Expectorant oral liquid (discontinued 2002) OTC *decongestant; expectorant* [phenylpropanolamine HCl; guaifenesin; alcohol 5%] 12.5•100 mg/5 mL

Myminicol oral liquid (discontinued 2002) OTC *antitussive; decongestant; antihistamine* [dextromethorphan hydrobromide; phenylpropanolamine HCl; chlorpheniramine maleate] 10•12.5•2 mg/5 mL

Mynatal capsules ℞ *vitamin/mineral/calcium/iron supplement* [multiple vitamins & minerals; calcium; iron; folic acid; biotin] ±•300•65•1•0.03 mg

Mynatal FC caplets ℞ *vitamin/mineral/calcium/iron supplement* [multiple vitamins & minerals; calcium; iron; folic acid; biotin] ±•250•60•1•0.03 mg

Mynatal P.N. captabs ℞ *vitamin/calcium/iron supplement* [multiple vitamins; calcium; iron; folic acid] ±• 125•60•1 mg

Mynatal P.N. Forte caplets ℞ *vitamin/mineral/calcium/iron supplement* [multiple vitamins & minerals; calcium; iron; folic acid] ±•250•60•1 mg

Mynatal Rx caplets ℞ *vitamin/mineral/calcium/iron supplement* [multiple vitamins & minerals; calcium; iron; folic acid; biotin] ±•200•60•1•0.03 mg

Mynate 90 Plus delayed-release caplets ℞ *vitamin/calcium/iron supplement* [multiple vitamins; calcium; iron; folic acid] ±•250•90•1 mg

Myobloc injection ℞ *neurotoxin complex for symptomatic treatment of cervical dystonia (orphan)* [botulinum toxin, type B] 5000 U/mL

Myochrysine IM injection ℞ *antirheumatic* [gold sodium thiomalate] 50 mg/mL

Myocide NS solution OTC *topical antiseptic* [benzalkonium chloride]

Myoflex Creme OTC *topical analgesic* [trolamine salicylate] 10%

Myolin IV or IM injection ℞ *skeletal muscle relaxant* [orphenadrine citrate] 30 mg/mL

Myotonachol tablets (discontinued 2001) ℞ *cholinergic urinary stimulant for postsurgical and postpartum urinary retention* [bethanechol chloride] 10, 25 mg

Myoview ℞ *cardiovascular imaging aid* [technetium Tc 99m tetrofosmin]

Myphetane DC Cough syrup (discontinued 2002) ℞ *narcotic antitussive; decongestant; antihistamine* [codeine phosphate; phenylpropanolamine HCl; brompheniramine maleate; alcohol 1.2%] 10•12.5•2 mg/5 mL

Myphetane DX Cough syrup (discontinued 2002) ℞ *antitussive; decongestant; antihistamine* [dextromethorphan hydrobromide; pseudoephedrine HCl; brompheniramine maleate; alcohol 1%] 10•30• 2 mg/ 5 mL

Myrac film-coated tablets ℞ *tetracycline antibiotic* [minocycline HCl] 50, 75, 100 mg

myralact INN, BAN

Myrica cerifera medicinal herb [see: bayberry]

myricodine [see: myrophine]

Myristica fragrans medicinal herb [see: nutmeg; mace]

myristica oil [see: nutmeg oil]

myristyl alcohol NF *stiffening agent*

myristyltrimethylammonium bromide *antiseborrheic*

myrophine INN, BAN

Myroxylon balsamum; M. pereirae medicinal herb [see: Peruvian balsam]

myrrh *(Commiphora abssynica; C. molmol; C. myrrha)* seeds *medicinal herb for bad breath, bronchitis, cancer, constipation, hay fever, hemorrhoids, leprosy, lung diseases, mouth and skin sores, sore throat, syphilis, and stimulating menses; also used as an antiseptic and astringent*

myrtecaine INN

Myrtilli fructus medicinal herb [see: bilberry]

myrtle medicinal herb [see: periwinkle]

myrtle, bog medicinal herb [see: buckbean]

myrtle, wax medicinal herb [see: bayberry]

myrtle flag; grass myrtle; sweet myrtle medicinal herb [see: calamus]

Mysoline oral suspension (discontinued 2004) ℞ *anticonvulsant for grand mal, psychomotor, or focal epileptic seizures* [primidone] 250 mg/5 mL

Mysoline tablets ℞ *anticonvulsant for grand mal, psychomotor, or focal epileptic seizures* [primidone] 50, 250 mg

myspamol [see: proquamezine]

Mytelase caplets ℞ *anticholinesterase muscle stimulant; myasthenia gravis* treatment [ambenonium chloride] 10 mg

Mytrex cream, ointment (discontinued 2004) ℞ *corticosteroidal anti-inflammatory; antifungal* [triamcinolone acetonide; nystatin] 0.1% • 100 000 U/g

Mytussin syrup (discontinued 2002) OTC *expectorant* [guaifenesin; alcohol 3.5%] 100 mg/5 mL

Mytussin AC Cough syrup ℞ *narcotic antitussive; expectorant* [codeine phosphate; guaifenesin; alcohol 3.5%] 10 • 100 mg/5 mL

Mytussin DAC syrup (discontinued 2002) ℞ *narcotic antitussive; decongestant; expectorant* [codeine phosphate; pseudoephedrine HCl; guaifenesin; alcohol 1.7%] 10 • 30 • 100 mg/5 mL

Mytussin DM syrup OTC *antitussive; expectorant* [dextromethorphan hydrobromide; guaifenesin] 10 • 100 mg/5 mL

myuizone [see: thioacetazone; thiacetazone]

My-Vitalife capsules OTC *vitamin/mineral/calcium/iron supplement* [multiple vitamins & minerals; calcium; iron; folic acid; biotin] $\triangleq$ • 130 • 27 • 0.4 • 0.03 mg

MZM tablets ℞ *carbonic anhydrase inhibitor for glaucoma* [methazolamide] 25, 50 mg

MZM (methazolamide) [q.v.]

M-Zole 3 Combination Pack vaginal suppositories + cream OTC *antifungal* [miconazole nitrate] 200 mg; 2%

M-Zole 7 Dual Pack vaginal suppositories + cream OTC *antifungal* [miconazole nitrate] 100 mg; 2%

N₂ (nitrogen) [q.v.]

N-3 polyunsaturated fatty acids [see: doconexent; icosapent; omega-3 marine triglycerides]

Na PCA; sodium PCA (sodium pyrrolidone carboxylic acid) [q.v.]

²²Na [see: sodium chloride Na 22]

nabazenil USAN, INN *anticonvulsant*

Nabi-HB IM injection ℞ *immunizing agent following exposure to hepatitis B surface antigen* [hepatitis B immune globulin] 1, 5 mL

nabilone USAN, INN, BAN *minor tranquilizer*

nabitan INN *analgesic* [also: nabitan HCl]

nabitan HCl USAN *analgesic* [also: nabitan]

nabotate INN *antiglaucoma agent; antinauseant* [also: nabotate HCl]

nabotate HCl USAN *antiglaucoma agent; antinauseant* [also: nabotate]

nabumetone USAN, INN, BAN *antiarthritic; nonsteroidal anti-inflammatory drug (NSAID)* 500, 750 mg oral

nabutan HCl [now: nabitan HCl]

NAC (N-acetyl cysteine) *natural source of cysteine; promotes an increase in the endogenous antioxidant glutathione* [also see: acetylcysteine]

NAC (nitrogen mustard, Adriamycin, CCNU) *chemotherapy protocol*

nacartocin INN

NaCl (sodium chloride) [q.v.]

NAD (nicotinamide-adenine dinucleotide) [see: nadide]

nadide USAN, INN *antagonist to alcohol and narcotics*

nadisan [see: carbutamide]

nadolol USAN, USP, INN, BAN *antianginal; antihypertensive; antiadrenergic (β-blocker)* 20, 40, 80, 120, 160 mg oral ② Nandol

nadoxolol INN

nadroparin calcium INN, BAN *anticoagulant; low molecular weight heparin*

naepaine HCl NF

nafamostat INN *anticoagulant; antifibrinolytic* [also: nafamostat mesylate; nafamostat mesilate]

nafamostat mesilate JAN *anticoagulant; antifibrinolytic* [also: nafamostat mesylate; nafamostat]

nafamostat mesylate USAN *anticoagulant; antifibrinolytic* [also: nafamostat; nafamostat mesilate]

nafarelin INN, BAN *luteinizing hormone-releasing hormone (LHRH) agonist* [also: nafarelin acetate]

nafarelin acetate USAN *luteinizing hormone-releasing hormone (LHRH) agonist for central precocious puberty (orphan) and endometriosis* [also: nafarelin]

Nafazair eye drops ℞ *topical ophthalmic decongestant and vasoconstrictor* [naphazoline HCl] 0.1%

nafazatrom INN, BAN

nafcaproic acid INN

nafcillin INN *penicillinase-resistant penicillin antibiotic* [also: nafcillin sodium]

nafcillin sodium USP *penicillinase-resistant penicillin antibiotic* [also: nafcillin] 1, 2 g IV infusion

nafenodone INN

nafenopin USAN, INN *antihyperlipoproteinemic*

nafetolol INN

nafimidone INN *anticonvulsant* [also: nafimidone HCl]

nafimidone HCl USAN *anticonvulsant* [also: nafimidone]

nafiverine INN

naflocort USAN, INN *topical adrenocortical steroid*

nafomine INN *muscle relaxant* [also: nafomine malate]

nafomine malate USAN *muscle relaxant* [also: nafomine]

nafoxadol INN

nafoxidine HCl USAN, INN *antiestrogen*

nafronyl oxalate USAN *vasodilator* [also: naftidrofuryl]

naftalofos USAN, INN *veterinary anthelmintic*

naftazone INN, BAN

naftidrofuryl INN *vasodilator* [also: nafronyl oxalate]

naftifine INN, BAN *broad-spectrum antifungal* [also: naftifine HCl]

naftifine HCl USAN *broad-spectrum antifungal* [also: naftifine]

Naftin cream, gel ℞ *topical antifungal* [naftifine HCl] 1%

naftopidil INN

naftoxate INN

naftypramide INN *antibacterial*

Naganol (available only from the Centers for Disease Control) ℞ *antiparasitic for African trypanosomiasis and onchocerciasis* [suramin sodium]

naganol [see: suramin sodium]

NaGHB (sodium gamma hydroxybutyrate) [see: gamma hydroxybutyrate (GHB); sodium oxybate]

Naglazyme IV infusion ℞ *recombinant human enzyme for the treatment of mucopolysaccharidosis VI (MPS VI; Maroteaux-Lamy syndrome)* [galsulfase] 1 mg/mL

nagrestipen USAN *stem cell inhibitory protein*

nalazosulfamide [see: salazosulfamide]

nalbuphine INN, BAN *narcotic agonist-antagonist analgesic for moderate to severe pain; adjunct to obstetric and surgical analgesia* [also: nalbuphine HCl]

nalbuphine HCl USAN *narcotic agonist-antagonist analgesic for moderate to severe pain; adjunct to obstetric and surgical analgesia* [also: nalbuphine] 10, 20 mg/mL injection

Naldecon sustained-release tablets, syrup, pediatric syrup, pediatric drops (discontinued 2001) ℞ *decongestant; antihistamine* [phenylpropanolamine HCl; phenylephrine HCl; chlorpheniramine maleate; phenyltoloxamine citrate] 40•10•5•15 mg; 20•5•2.5•7.5 mg/5 mL; 5•1.25•0.5•2 mg/5 mL; 5•1.25•0.5•2 mg/mL 🔊 Nalfon

Naldecon CX Adult oral liquid (discontinued 2002) ℞ *narcotic antitussive; decongestant; expectorant* [codeine phosphate; phenylpropanolamine HCl; guaifenesin] 10•12.5•200 mg/5 mL

Naldecon DX children's syrup, pediatric drops (discontinued 2002) OTC *pediatric antitussive, decongestant, and expectorant* [dextromethorphan hydrobromide; phenylpropanolamine HCl; guaifenesin] 5•6.25•100 mg/5 mL; 5•6.25•50 mg/mL

Naldecon DX Adult oral liquid (discontinued 2002) OTC *antitussive; decongestant; expectorant* [dextromethorphan hydrobromide; phenylpropanolamine HCl; guaifenesin] 10•12.5•200 mg/5 mL

Naldecon EX children's syrup, pediatric drops (discontinued 2002) OTC *decongestant; expectorant* [phenylpropanolamine HCl; guaifenesin] 6.25•100 mg/5 mL; 6.25•50 mg/mL

Naldecon Senior DX oral liquid (discontinued 2003) OTC *antitussive; expectorant* [dextromethorphan hydrobromide; guaifenesin] 20•400 mg/10 mL

Naldecon Senior EX oral liquid OTC *expectorant* [guaifenesin] 200 mg/5 mL

Naldelate syrup, pediatric syrup (discontinued 2001) ℞ *decongestant; antihistamine; sleep aid* [phenylpropanolamine HCl; phenylephrine HCl; chlorpheniramine maleate; phenyltoloxamine citrate] 20•5•2.5•7.5 mg/5 mL; 5•1.25•0.5•2 mg/5 mL

Naldelate DX Adult oral liquid (discontinued 2002) OTC *antitussive; decongestant; expectorant* [dextromethorphan hydrobromide; phenylpropanolamine HCl; guaifenesin] 10•12.5•200 mg/5 mL

Nalex Expectorant oral liquid ℞ *narcotic antitussive; decongestant; expectorant* [hydrocodone bitartrate; pseudoephedrine HCl; guaifenesin; alcohol 12.5%] 5•60•200 mg/5 mL

Nalex-A caplets, oral liquid ℞ *decongestant; antihistamine; sleep aid* [phenylephrine HCl; chlorpheniramine maleate; phenyltoloxamine citrate] 20•4•40 mg; 5•2.5•7.5 mg/5 mL

Nalex-A 12 oral suspension ℞ *decongestant; antihistamine; sleep aid* [phenylephrine HCl; chlorpheniramine maleate; phenyltoloxamine citrate] 5•2•12.5 mg/5 mL

Nalex-DH oral liquid ℞ *narcotic antitussive; decongestant* [hydrocodone bitartrate; phenylephrine HCl] 2.5•5 mg/5 mL

Nalfon Pulvules (capsules) ℞ *analgesic; antiarthritic; nonsteroidal anti-inflam-*

matory drug (NSAID) [fenoprofen calcium] 200, 300 mg ☑ Naldecon

Nalgest sustained-release tablets, syrup, pediatric syrup, pediatric drops (discontinued 2001) ℞ *decongestant; antihistamine* [phenylpropanolamine HCl; phenylephrine HCl; chlorpheniramine maleate; phenyltoloxamine citrate] 40•10•5•15 mg; 20•5•2.5•7.5 mg/5 mL; 5•1.25•0.5•2 mg/5 mL; 5•1.25•0.5•2 mg/mL

nalidixane [see: nalidixic acid]

nalidixate sodium USAN *antibacterial*

nalidixic acid USAN, USP, INN *urinary antibiotic*

Nallpen powder for IV or IM injection (discontinued 2002) ℞ *penicillinase-resistant penicillin antibiotic* [nafcillin sodium] 0.5, 1, 2, 10 g

nalmefene USAN, INN, BAN *narcotic antagonist; antidote to opioid overdose*

nalmefene HCl *narcotic antagonist; antidote to opioid overdose; postanesthesia "stir-up"*

nalmetrene [now: nalmefene]

nalmexone INN *analgesic; narcotic antagonist* [also: nalmexone HCl]

nalmexone HCl USAN *analgesic; narcotic antagonist* [also: nalmexone]

nalorphine INN [also: nalorphine HCl]

nalorphine HCl USP [also: nalorphine]

naloxiphane tartrate [see: levallorphan tartrate]

naloxone INN, BAN *narcotic antagonist* [also: naloxone HCl]

naloxone HCl USAN, USP, JAN *narcotic antagonist* [also: naloxone] 0.02, 0.4 mg/mL injection

naloxone HCl & buprenorphine HCl *investigational (orphan) for opiate addictions*

naloxone HCl & pentazocine *narcotic agonist-antagonist analgesic* 0.5•50 mg oral

naltrexone USAN, INN, BAN *narcotic antagonist*

naltrexone HCl *narcotic antagonist for opiate blockage and maintenance in formerly opiate-dependent individuals (orphan); treatment for alcoholism;*

investigational (Phase III) for irritable bowel syndrome (IBS) 50 mg oral

Namenda film-coated caplets, oral solution *NMDA (N-methyl-D-aspartate) antagonist for Alzheimer disease; investigational (Phase III) neuroprotective agent for diabetic neuropathy, vascular dementia, Parkinson disease, and AIDS dementia* [memantine HCl] 5, 10 mg; 2 mg/mL

naminterol INN

[¹³N]ammonia [see: ammonia N 13]

namoxyrate USAN, INN *analgesic*

namuron [see: cyclobarbitone]

nanafrocin INN

nandrolone BAN *anabolic* [also: nandrolone cyclotate]

nandrolone cyclotate USAN *anabolic* [also: nandrolone]

nandrolone decanoate USAN, USP *androgen/anabolic steroid for anemia of renal insufficiency; also used for AIDS-wasting syndrome; sometimes abused as a street drug* 100, 200 mg/mL injection (in oil)

nandrolone phenpropionate USP *androgen/anabolic steroid for metastatic breast cancer in women; sometimes abused as a street drug*

naniopine [see: nanofin]

NanobacTEST-S for professional use *blood serum test for the presence of nanobacterial antigens and antibodies*

NanobacTEST-U/A for professional use *rapid screening urine test for the presence of live, uncalcified nanobacteria by visual color comparison* [ELISA test]

nanofin INN

nanterinone INN, BAN

nantradol INN *analgesic* [also: nantradol HCl]

nantradol HCl USAN *analgesic* [also: nantradol]

NAPA (N-acetyl-*p*-aminophenol) [see: acetaminophen]

NAPA (N-acetyl-procainamide) [q.v.]

napactadine INN *antidepressant* [also: napactadine HCl]

napactadine HCl USAN *antidepressant* [also: napactadine]

napadisilate INN *combining name for radicals or groups* [also: napadisylate]

napadisylate BAN *combining name for radicals or groups* [also: napadisilate]

napamezole INN *antidepressant* [also: napamezole HCl]

napamezole HCl USAN *antidepressant* [also: napamezole]

Na-PCA topical spray OTC *natural skin moisturizing factor; humectant* [sodium pyrrolidone carboxylic acid; aloe vera]

naphazoline INN, BAN *topical ophthalmic decongestant and vasoconstrictor; nasal decongestant* [also: naphazoline HCl; naphazoline nitrate]

naphazoline HCl USP *topical ophthalmic decongestant and vasoconstrictor; nasal decongestant* [also: naphazoline; naphazoline nitrate] 0.1% eye drops

naphazoline HCl & antazoline phosphate *topical ocular decongestant and antihistamine* 0.05%•0.5%

naphazoline HCl & pheniramine maleate *topical ocular decongestant and antihistamine* 0.025%•0.3% eye drops

naphazoline nitrate JAN *topical ocular vasoconstrictor; nasal decongestant* [also: naphazoline HCl; naphazoline]

Naphazoline Plus eye drops OTC *topical ophthalmic decongestant and antihistamine* [naphazoline HCl; pheniramine maleate] 0.025%•0.3%

Naphcon eye drops OTC *topical ophthalmic decongestant and vasoconstrictor* [naphazoline HCl] 0.012%

Naphcon Forte Drop-Tainers (eye drops) ℞ *topical ophthalmic decongestant and vasoconstrictor* [naphazoline HCl] 0.1%

Naphcon-A Drop-Tainers (eye drops) OTC *topical ophthalmic decongestant and antihistamine* [naphazoline HCl; pheniramine maleate] 0.025%•0.3%

Naphoptic-A eye drops ℞ *topical ophthalmic decongestant and antihistamine* [naphazoline HCl; pheniramine maleate] 0.025%•0.3%

2-naphthol [see: betanaphthol]

naphthonone INN

naphthypramide [see: naftypramide]

Naphuride (available only from the Centers for Disease Control) ℞ *antiparasitic for African trypanosomiasis and onchocerciasis* [suramin sodium]

napirimus INN

napitane mesylate USAN *antidepressant; α-adrenergic blocker; norepinephrine uptake antagonist*

Naprelan controlled-release tablets ℞ *once-daily analgesic and antiarthritic; nonsteroidal anti-inflammatory drug (NSAID)* [naproxen sodium] 412.5, 550 mg (=375, 500 mg base)

naprodoxime INN

Naprosyn tablets, oral suspension ℞ *analgesic; antiarthritic; nonsteroidal anti-inflammatory drug (NSAID)* [naproxen] 250, 375, 500 mg; 125 mg/5 mL ⊘ Meprospan; Natacyn

Naprosyn EC [see: EC-Naprosyn]

naproxen USAN, USP, INN, BAN, JAN *analgesic; antiarthritic; nonsteroidal anti-inflammatory drug (NSAID)* 250, 375, 500 mg oral; 125 mg/5 mL oral

naproxen sodium USAN, USP *analgesic; antiarthritic; antipyretic; nonsteroidal anti-inflammatory drug (NSAID)* (base=91%) 220, 275, 550 mg oral

naproxol USAN, INN *anti-inflammatory; analgesic; antipyretic*

napsagatran USAN, INN *antithrombotic*

napsilate INN *combining name for radicals or groups* [also: napsylate]

napsylate USAN, BAN *combining name for radicals or groups* [also: napsilate]

Naqua tablets ℞ *diuretic; antihypertensive* [trichlormethiazide] 2, 4 mg

naranol INN *antipsychotic* [also: naranol HCl]

naranol HCl USAN *antipsychotic* [also: naranol]

narasin USAN, INN, BAN *coccidiostat; veterinary growth stimulant*

naratriptan INN, BAN *vascular serotonin 5-HT$_{1D}$ receptor agonist for the acute treatment of migraine* [also: naratriptan HCl]

naratriptan HCl USAN *vascular serotonin 5-HT$_{1D}$ receptor agonist for the* *acute treatment of migraine* [also: naratriptan]

Narcan IV, IM, or subcu injection ℞ *narcotic antagonist for opiate dependence or overdose; hypotension treatment* [naloxone HCl] 0.4 mg/mL ☒ Marcaine

Narcan neonatal injection (discontinued 2003) ℞ *narcotic antagonist for opiate dependence* [naloxone HCl] 0.02 mg/mL ☒ Marcaine

narcotic agonist-antagonists *a class of opioid or morphine-like analgesics with lower abuse potential than pure narcotic agonist analgesics*

narcotic agonists; narcotics *a class of opioid or morphine-like analgesics that relieve pain and induce sleep*

narcotine [see: noscapine]

narcotine HCl [see: noscapine HCl]

nard *medicinal herb* [see: spikenard]

Nardil sugar-coated tablets ℞ *antipsychotic; monoamine oxidase inhibitor (MAOI) for treatment-resistant atypical depression* [phenelzine sulfate] 15 mg ☒ Norinyl

Naropin injection ℞ *long-acting local or regional anesthetic for surgery; epidural block for cesarean section* [ropivacaine HCl] 0.2%, 0.5%, 0.75%, 1%

narrow dock *medicinal herb* [see: yellow dock]

Nasabid prolonged-action capsules (discontinued 2002) ℞ *decongestant; expectorant* [pseudoephedrine HCl; guaifenesin] 90•250 mg

Nasabid SR long-acting tablets ℞ *decongestant; expectorant* [pseudoephedrine HCl; guaifenesin] 90•600 mg

Nasacort nasal spray (discontinued 2003) ℞ *corticosteroidal anti-inflammatory for seasonal or perennial rhinitis* [triamcinolone acetonide] 55 μg/dose

Nasacort AQ metered-dose aerosol ℞ *corticosteroidal anti-inflammatory for seasonal or perennial rhinitis* [triamcinolone acetonide] 55 μg/dose

Nasacort HFA pressurized metered-dose inhaler (pMDI) with a CFC-free propellant ℞ *corticosteroidal anti-inflammatory for seasonal or perennial rhinitis* [triamcinolone acetonide] 55 μg/dose

NāSal nasal spray, nose drops OTC *nasal moisturizer* [sodium chloride (saline solution)] 0.65%

Nasal Decongestant pediatric oral drops OTC *nasal decongestant* [pseudoephedrine HCl] 7.5 mg/0.8 mL

Nasal Decongestant spray OTC *nasal decongestant* [oxymetazoline HCl] 0.05%

Nasal Decongestant, Children's Non-Drowsy oral liquid OTC *nasal decongestant* [pseudoephedrine HCl] 15 mg/5 mL

Nasal Decongestant Sinus Non-Drowsy tablets OTC *decongestant; analgesic; antipyretic* [pseudoephedrine HCl; acetaminophen] 30•500 mg

Nasal Jelly ointment (discontinued 2002) OTC *nasal moisturizer* [phenol; camphor; menthol; eucalyptus oil; oil of lavender]

Nasal Moist nasal spray OTC *nasal moisturizer* [sodium chloride (saline solution)] 0.65%

Nasal Relief nasal spray OTC *nasal decongestant* [oxymetazoline HCl] 0.05%

Nasal Spray OTC *nasal moisturizer* [sodium chloride (saline solution)]

NasalCrom nasal spray OTC *anti-inflammatory/mast cell stabilizer for the prophylaxis of allergic rhinitis; treatment for mastocytosis (orphan)* [cromolyn sodium] 4% (5.2 mg/dose)

NasalCrom, Children's nasal spray (discontinued 2003) OTC *anti-inflammatory/mast cell stabilizer for the prophylaxis of allergic rhinitis* [cromolyn sodium] 4% (5.2 mg/dose)

NasalCrom A nasal spray + tablets OTC *anti-inflammatory/mast cell stabilizer for the prophylaxis of allergic rhinitis; antihistamine* [cromolyn sodium;

chlorpheniramine maleate] 4% (5.2 mg/dose); 4 mg

NasalCrom CA nasal spray + tablets OTC *anti-inflammatory/mast cell stabilizer for the prophylaxis of allergic rhinitis; decongestant; analgesic* [cromolyn sodium; pseudoephedrine HCl; acetaminophen] 4% (5.2 mg/dose); 30 mg•500 mg

Nasal-Ease with Zinc nasal gel OTC *nasal moisturizer and anti-infective* [zinc acetate]

Nasal-Ease with Zinc Gluconate nasal spray OTC *nasal moisturizer and anti-infective* [zinc gluconate]

Nasalide nasal spray (discontinued 2004) ℞ *corticosteroidal anti-inflammatory for seasonal or perennial rhinitis* [flunisolide] 0.025% (25 μg/dose)

Nasarel metered dose nasal spray ℞ *corticosteroidal anti-inflammatory for seasonal or perennial rhinitis* [flunisolide] 0.025% (29 μg/dose) ☒ Nizoral

Nasatab LA long-acting film-coated caplets ℞ *decongestant; expectorant* [pseudoephedrine HCl; guaifenesin] 120•500 mg

Nascobal nasal gel in metered-dose applicator, nasal spray ℞ *maintenance administration following intramuscular vitamin B₁₂ therapy* [cyanocobalamin] 500 μg/0.1 mL dose

NASHA (non-animal stabilized hyaluronic acid) [see: hyaluronic acid]

Nashville rabbit antithymocyte serum [see: lymphocyte immune globulin, antithymocyte]

Nashville Rabbit Antithymocyte Serum ℞ *investigational (orphan) passive immunizing agent to prevent allograft rejection of solid organ and bone marrow transplants* [antithymocyte globulin, rabbit]

Nasonex nasal spray ℞ *corticosteroid for the prophylaxis and treatment of seasonal and perennial allergic rhinitis; treatment for nasal polyps* [mometasone furoate] 0.05% (50 μg/dose)

Nasop orally disintegrating tablets ℞ *nasal decongestant* [phenylephrine HCl] 10 mg

Nasturtium officinale *medicinal herb* [see: watercress]

NataChew chewable tablets ℞ *prenatal vitamin/mineral supplement* [multiple vitamins & minerals; ferrous fumarate; folic acid] ±•29•1 mg

Natacyn eye drop suspension ℞ *ophthalmic antifungal agent* [natamycin] 5% ☒ Naprosyn

NataFort film-coated tablets ℞ *prenatal vitamin/iron supplement* [multiple vitamins; ferrous sulfate; folic acid] ±•60•1 mg

NatalCare Plus; NatalCare Three film-coated tablets ℞ *vitamin/mineral/calcium/iron supplement* [multiple vitamins & minerals; calcium; iron; folic acid] ±•200•27•1 mg

Natalins tablets (discontinued 2001) OTC *vitamin/calcium/iron supplement* [multiple vitamins; calcium; iron; folic acid] ±•200•30•0.5 mg

Natalins Rx tablets (name changed to Enfamil Natalins Rx in 2001)

natalizumab *humanized monoclonal antibody (huMAb) anti-inflammatory for treatment of multiple sclerosis; investigational (Phase III) for Crohn disease and rheumatoid arthritis; withdrawn from the market in 2005 due to safety concerns*

natamycin USAN, USP, INN, BAN *ophthalmic fungicidal antibiotic* [also: pimaricin]

Natarex Prenatal tablets ℞ *vitamin/calcium/iron supplement* [multiple vitamins; calcium; iron; folic acid; biotin] ±•200•60•1•0.03 mg

NataTab CFe; NataTab FA; NataTab Rx film-coated tablets ℞ *prenatal vitamin/mineral supplement* [multiple vitamins & minerals]

nateglinide USAN *amino acid–derivative; oral antidiabetic agent that stimulates the release of insulin from the pancreas for type 2 diabetes*

Natelle-EZ caplets ℞ *vitamin/mineral/ calcium/iron supplement* [multiple vitamins & minerals; calcium; iron; folic acid biotin] ± • 100 • 25 • 1 • 0.3 mg

Natrecor powder for IV injection ℞ *human B-type natriuretic peptide (hBNP); vasodilator for acute congestive heart failure* [nesiritide citrate] 1.58 mg/vial

Natru-Vent nasal spray OTC *nasal decongestant* [xylometazoline HCl] 0.05%, 0.1%

Natural Fiber Laxative powder OTC *bulk laxative* [psyllium hydrophilic mucilloid] 3.4 g/dose

natural killer cell stimulatory factor [see: edodekin alfa]

Naturalyte oral solution OTC *electrolyte replacement* [sodium, potassium, and chloride electrolytes] 240 mL, 1 L

Nature Throid tablets ℞ *thyroid replacement therapy for hypothyroidism or thyroid cancer* [thyroid, desiccated (porcine)] 32.4, 64.8, 129.6, 194.4 mg

Nature's Choice ⒸⒶⓃ powder for oral solution OTC *vitamin/mineral/calcium/ iron supplement* [multiple vitamins & minerals; calcium; iron; folic acid; biotin] ± • 500 • 4 • 0.08 • 0.06 mg

Nature's Remedy tablets OTC *stimulant laxative* [cascara sagrada; aloe] 150 • 100 mg

Nature's Tears eye drops OTC *ophthalmic moisturizer/lubricant* [hydroxypropyl methylcellulose] 0.4%

Naturetin tablets ℞ *antihypertensive; diuretic* [bendroflumethiazide] 5 mg

Naturvus hydrophilic contact lens material [hefilcon B]

Nausea Relief oral solution OTC *antiemetic for nausea associated with influenza, morning sickness, motion sickness, inhalation anesthesia, or food and drink indiscretions* [phosphorated carbohydrate solution (dextrose, fructose, and phosphoric acid)] 1.87 g• 1.87 g•21.5 mg per dose

Nausetrol oral solution OTC *antiemetic for nausea associated with influenza, morning sickness, motion sickness,* *inhalation anesthesia, or food and drink indiscretions* [phosphorated carbohydrate solution (fructose, dextrose, and orthophosphoric acid)] 118 mL (1870•1870•21.5 mg)

Navane capsules ℞ *conventional (typical) thioxanthene antipsychotic for schizophrenia* [thiothixene] 1, 2, 5, 10, 20 mg

Navane oral concentrate ℞ *conventional (typical) thioxanthene antipsychotic for schizophrenia* [thiothixene HCl] 5 mg/mL

Navelbine IV injection ℞ *antineoplastic for Hodgkin disease and lung, breast and ovarian cancer* [vinorelbine tartrate] 10 mg/mL

naxagolide INN *antiparkinsonian; dopamine agonist* [also: naxagolide HCl]

naxagolide HCl USAN *antiparkinsonian; dopamine agonist* [also: naxagolide]

naxaprostene INN

naxifylline USAN *treatment of edema due to congestive heart failure*

9-NC (9-nitrocamptothecin) [see: rubitecan]

ND Clear sustained-release capsules ℞ *decongestant; antihistamine* [pseudoephedrine HCl; chlorpheniramine maleate] 120•8 mg

ND-Gesic tablets (discontinued 2002) OTC *decongestant; antihistamine; analgesic* [phenylephrine HCl; chlorpheniramine maleate; pyrilamine maleate; acetaminophen] 5•2•12.5•300 mg

NE-1530 *investigational (Phase II) agent for the prevention of otitis media (clinical trials discontinued 1999)*

nealbarbital INN [also: nealbarbitone]

nealbarbitone BAN [also: nealbarbital]

nebacumab USAN, INN, BAN *antiendotoxin monoclonal antibody; investigational (orphan) for gram-negative bacteremia in endotoxin shock*

Nebcin IV or IM injection, pediatric injection, powder for injection ℞ *aminoglycoside antibiotic* [tobramycin sulfate] 10, 40 mg/mL; 10 mg/mL; 1.2 g

nebidrazine INN

nebivolol USAN, INN *investigational (NDA filed) antihypertensive (selective β₁-blocker)*

nebracetam INN

nebramycin USAN, INN *antibacterial*

nebramycin factor 6 [see: tobramycin]

NebuPent inhalation aerosol ℞ *antiprotozoal; treatment and prophylaxis of* Pneumocystis carinii *pneumonia (orphan)* [pentamidine isethionate] 300 mg

Necon 0.5/35; Necon 1/35 tablets (in packs of 21 or 28) ℞ *monophasic oral contraceptive* [norethindrone; ethinyl estradiol] 0.5 mg•35 μg; 1 mg•35 μg

Necon 1/50 tablets (in packs of 21 or 28) ℞ *monophasic oral contraceptive* [norethindrone; mestranol] 1 mg• 50 μg

Necon 10/11 tablets (in packs of 21 or 28) ℞ *biphasic oral contraceptive* [norethindrone; ethinyl estradiol] Phase 1 (10 days): 500•35 μg; Phase 2 (11 days): 1000•35 μg

Necon 7/7/7 tablets (in packs of 28) ℞ *triphasic oral contraceptive* [norethindrone; ethinyl estradiol] Phase 1 (7 days): 500•35 μg; Phase 2 (7 days): 750•35 μg; Phase 3 (7 days): 1000•35 μg

nedocromil USAN, INN, BAN *antiinflammatory; prophylactic antiallergic; mast cell stabilizer*

nedocromil calcium USAN *antiinflammatory; prophylactic antiallergic; mast cell stabilizer*

nedocromil sodium USAN *anti-inflammatory; mast cell stabilizer; antiasthmatic; prophylactic antiallergic*

neem tree (*Azadirachta indica*) fruit, leaves, root, and oil *medicinal herb for contraception, diabetes, heart disease, malaria, skin diseases, ulcers, and worms; also used as a pesticide and insect repellent; not generally regarded as safe and effective for infants as it may cause death*

nefazodone INN *antidepressant; selective serotonin and norepinephrine reup-* *take inhibitor (SSNRI)* [also: nefazodone HCl]

nefazodone HCl USAN *antidepressant; selective serotonin and norepinephrine reuptake inhibitor (SSNRI)*; discontinued 2004 due to safety concerns [also: nefazodone] 50, 100, 150, 200, 250 mg oral

neflumozide INN *antipsychotic* [also: neflumozide HCl]

neflumozide HCl USAN *antipsychotic* [also: neflumozide]

nefocon A USAN *hydrophobic contact lens material*

nefopam INN *analgesic* [also: nefopam HCl]

nefopam HCl USAN *analgesic* [also: nefopam]

nefrolan [see: clorexolone]

NegGram caplets, oral suspension ℞ *urinary antibiotic* [nalidixic acid] 500 mg; 250 mg/5 mL

nelarabine USAN *antineoplastic for T-cell and B-cell lymphomas*

neldazosin INN

nelezaprine INN *muscle relaxant* [also: nelezaprine maleate]

nelezaprine maleate USAN *muscle relaxant* [also: nelezaprine]

nelfilcon A USAN *hydrophilic contact lens material*

nelfinavir mesylate USAN *antiretroviral; protease inhibitor for HIV-1 infection*

Nelova 0.5/35E; Nelova 1/35E tablets (in packs of 21 or 28) (discontinued 2001) ℞ *monophasic oral contraceptive* [norethindrone; ethinyl estradiol] 0.5 mg•35 μg; 1 mg•35 μg

Nelova 1/50M tablets (in packs of 21 or 28) (discontinued 2001) ℞ *monophasic oral contraceptive* [norethindrone; mestranol] 1 mg•50 μg

Nelova 10/11 tablets (in packs of 21 and 28) (discontinued 2001) ℞ *biphasic oral contraceptive* [norethindrone; ethinyl estradiol] Phase 1 (10 days): 0.5 mg•35 μg; Phase 2 (11 days): 1 mg•35 μg

nemadectin USAN, INN *veterinary antiparasitic*

nemazoline INN *nasal decongestant* [also: nemazoline HCl]

nemazoline HCl USAN *nasal decongestant* [also: nemazoline]

Nembutal elixir ℞ *sedative; hypnotic; also abused as a street drug* [pentobarbital] 20 mg/5 mL ⊡ Myambutal

Nembutal Sodium capsules, IV or IM injection, suppositories ℞ *sedative; hypnotic; also abused as a street drug* [pentobarbital sodium] 50, 100 mg; 50 mg/mL; 30, 60, 120, 200 mg

neoarsphenamine NF, INN

Neo-Calglucon syrup (discontinued 2002) OTC *calcium supplement* [calcium glubionate] 1.8 g/5 mL

neocarzinostatin [now: zinostatin]

Neocate One + ready-to-use oral liquid OTC *pediatric enteral nutritional therapy* [lactose-free formula] 237 mL

Neocera (trademarked ingredient) *suppository base* [polyethylent glycol 400, 1450, and 8000; polysorbate 60]

neocid [see: chlorophenothane]

neocinchophen NF, INN

NeoDecadron Ocumeter (eye drops), ophthalmic ointment ℞ *topical ophthalmic corticosteroidal anti-inflammatory; antibiotic* [dexamethasone sodium phosphate; neomycin sulfate] 0.1%•0.35%; 0.05%•0.35%

Neo-Dexair eye drops ℞ *topical ophthalmic corticosteroidal anti-inflammatory; antibiotic* [dexamethasone sodium phosphate; neomycin sulfate] 0.1%•0.35%

Neo-Dexameth eye drops ℞ *topical ophthalmic corticosteroidal anti-inflammatory; antibiotic* [dexamethasone sodium phosphate; neomycin sulfate] 0.1%•0.35%

Neo-Diaral capsules OTC *antidiarrheal* [loperamide] 2 mg

neodymium *element (Nd)*

Neo-fradin oral solution ℞ *aminoglycoside antibiotic* [neomycin sulfate] 125 mg/5 mL

Neoloid oral emulsion OTC *stimulant laxative* [castor oil] 36.4%

Neomark ℞ *investigational (NDA filed, orphan) radiosensitizer for primary brain tumors* [broxuridine]

neo-mercazole [see: carbimazole]

Neomixin ointment (discontinued 2001) OTC *topical antibiotic* [polymyxin B sulfate; neomycin sulfate; bacitracin zinc] 5000 U•3.5 mg•400 U per g ⊡ neomycin

neomycin INN, BAN *antibacterial* [also: neomycin palmitate] ⊡ Neomixin

neomycin B [see: framycetin]

neomycin palmitate USAN *antibacterial* [also: neomycin]

neomycin sulfate USP *aminoglycoside antibiotic* 500 mg oral

neomycin sulfate & polymyxin B sulfate & bacitracin zinc *topical antibiotic* 5 mg•10 000 U•400 U per g ophthalmic

neomycin sulfate & polymyxin B sulfate & dexamethasone *topical ophthalmic antibiotic and corticosteroidal anti-inflammatory* 0.35%•10 000 U/mL•0.1% eye drops

neomycin sulfate & polymyxin B sulfate & gramicidin *topical antibiotic* 1.75 mg•10 000 U•0.025 mg per mL eye drops

neomycin sulfate & polymyxin B sulfate & hydrocortisone *topical ophthalmic antibiotic and corticosteroidal anti-inflammatory* 0.35%•10 000 U/mL•1% eye drops

neomycin undecenoate [see: neomycin undecylenate]

neomycin undecylenate USAN *antibacterial; antifungal*

neon *element (Ne)*

Neopap suppositories OTC *analgesic; antipyretic* [acetaminophen] 125 mg

neopenyl [see: clemizole penicillin]

neoquate [see: nequinate]

Neoral gelcaps, oral solution ℞ *immunosuppressant for allogenic kidney, liver, and heart transplants (orphan), rheumatoid arthritis, and psoriasis* [cyclosporine; alcohol 11.9%] 25, 100 mg; 100 mg/mL

Neosar powder for IV injection ℞ *nitrogen mustard-type alkylating antineoplastic for multiple leukemias, lymphomas, blastomas, sarcomas, and organ cancers* [cyclophosphamide] 100 mg

Neosol orally disintegrating tablets ℞ *GI/GU antispasmodic; antiparkinsonian; anticholinergic "drying agent" for allergic rhinitis and hyperhidrosis* [hyoscyamine sulfate] 0.125 mg

Neosporin cream (discontinued 2001) OTC *antibiotic* [polymyxin B sulfate; neomycin sulfate] 10 000 U•3.5 mg per g

Neosporin Drop Dose (eye drops) ℞ *antibiotic* [polymyxin B sulfate; neomycin sulfate; gramicidin] 10 000 U•1.75 mg•0.025 mg per mL

Neosporin ointment (discontinued 2001) OTC *antibiotic* [polymyxin B sulfate; neomycin sulfate; bacitracin] 10 000 U•3.5 mg•500 U per g

Neosporin ophthalmic ointment ℞ *antibiotic* [polymyxin B sulfate; neomycin sulfate; bacitracin zinc] 10 000 U•5 mg•400 U per g

Neosporin AF cream, spray liquid OTC *antifungal* [miconazole nitrate] 2%

Neosporin G.U. Irrigant solution ℞ *antibiotic* [neomycin sulfate; polymyxin B sulfate] 40 mg•200 000 U per mL

Neosporin Original ointment OTC *antibiotic* [polymyxin B sulfate; neomycin sulfate; bacitracin zinc] 5000 U•3.5 mg•400 U per g

Neosporin Plus cream (discontinued 2001) OTC *antibiotic; local anesthetic* [polymyxin B sulfate; neomycin; lidocaine] 10 000 U•3.5 mg•40 mg per g

Neosporin Plus ointment (discontinued 2001) OTC *antibiotic; local anesthetic* [polymyxin B sulfate; bacitracin zinc; neomycin; lidocaine] 10 000 U•500 U•3.5 mg•40 mg per g

Neosporin Plus Pain Relief cream OTC *antibiotic; local anesthetic* [polymyxin B sulfate; neomycin sulfate; pramoxine HCl] 10 000 U•3.5 mg•10 mg per g

Neosporin Plus Pain Relief ointment OTC *antibiotic; local anesthetic* [polymyxin B sulfate; neomycon sulfate; bacitracin zinc; pramoxine HCl] 10 000 U•3.5 mg•500 U•10 mg per g

neostigmine BAN *cholinergic/anticholinesterase muscle stimulant* [also: neostigmine bromide]

neostigmine bromide USP, INN, BAN *cholinergic/anticholinesterase muscle stimulant* [also: neostigmine] 15 mg oral

neostigmine methylsulfate USP *cholinergic/anticholinesterase muscle stimulant; urinary stimulant for postsurgical urinary retention; treatment for myasthenia gravis; antidote to neuromuscular blockers* 1:1000 (1 mg/mL), 1:2000 (0.5 mg/mL) injection

Neostrata Skin Lightening gel OTC *hyperpigmentation bleaching agent* [hydroquinone] 2%

Neo-Synephrine eye drops, viscous solution ℞ *topical ophthalmic decongestant and vasoconstrictor; mydriatic* [phenylephrine HCl] 2.5%, 10%; 10%

Neo-Synephrine IV, IM, or subcu injection ℞ *vasopressor for hypotensive or cardiac shock* [phenylephrine HCl] 1% (10 mg/mL)

Neo-Synephrine nasal spray, nose drops (multiple name changes in 2002) OTC *nasal decongestant* [phenylephrine HCl] 0.25%, 0.5%, 1%; 0.125%, 0.25%, 0.5%, 1%

Neo-Synephrine 4-Hour Mild Formula nasal spray OTC *nasal decongestant* [phenylephrine HCl] 0.25%

Neo-Synephrine 4-Hour Regular Strength; Neo-Synephrine 4-Hour Extra Strength nasal spray, nose drops OTC *nasal decongestant* [phenylephrine HCl] 0.5%; 1%

Neo-Synephrine 12-Hour; Neo-Synephrine 12-Hour Extra Moisturizing nasal spray OTC *nasal decongestant* [oxymetazoline HCl] 0.05%

Neo-Tabs tablets ℞ *aminoglycoside antibiotic* [neomycin sulfate] 500 mg

NeoTect kit for injection preparation ℞ *radiopharmaceutical imaging agent for lung cancer; investigational (NDA filed) for malignant melanoma and neuroendocrine disorders* [depreotide]

Neotrace-4 IV injection ℞ *intravenous nutritional therapy* [multiple trace elements (metals)]

Neotricin HC ophthalmic ointment ℞ *topical ophthalmic corticosteroidal anti-inflammatory; antibiotic* [hydrocortisone acetate; neomycin sulfate; bacitracin zinc; polymyxin B sulfate] 1%•3.5%•400 U/g•10 000 U/g

Neovastat ℞ *investigational (Phase III) shark cartilage–based angiogenesis inhibitor for osteoarthritis, rheumatoid arthritis, and various cancers; investigational (orphan) for renal cell carcinoma* [AE-941 (code name—generic name not yet assigned)] ⊡ Novastan

nepafenac USAN *topical ophthalmic anti-inflammatory and analgesic*

Nepeta cataria *medicinal herb* [see: catnip]

Nephplex Rx tablets ℞ *vitamin/zinc supplement* [multiple B vitamins; ascorbic acid; folic acid; biotin; zinc] ±•60•1•0.3•12.5 mg

NephrAmine 5.4% IV infusion ℞ *nutritional therapy for renal failure* [multiple essential amino acids; electrolytes]

nephritics *a class of agents that affect the kidney (a term used in folk medicine)*

Nephro-Calci tablets OTC *calcium supplement* [calcium carbonate] 1500 mg (600 mg Ca)

Nephrocaps capsules ℞ *vitamin supplement* [multiple B vitamins; vitamin C; folic acid; biotin] ±•100 mg•1 mg•150 µg

Nephro-Fer tablets OTC *hematinic; iron supplement* [ferrous fumarate (source of iron)] 350 mg (115 mg)

Nephro-Fer Rx film-coated tablets (discontinued 2004) ℞ *hematinic* [ferrous fumarate; folic acid] 106.9•1 mg

Nephron solution for inhalation OTC *sympathomimetic bronchodilator* [racepinephrine HCl] 2.25%

Nephron FA tablets ℞ *hematinic* [ferrous fumarate; multiple B vitamins; ascorbic acid; folic acid; biotin; docusate sodium] 66.6•±•40•1•0.3• 75 mg

Nephro-Vite Rx film-coated tablets ℞ *vitamin supplement* [multiple B vitamins; vitamin C; folic acid; biotin] ±•60 mg•1 mg•300 µg

Nephro-Vite Rx + Fe film-coated tablets (discontinued 2004) ℞ *hematinic* [ferrous fumarate; multiple B vitamins; ascorbic acid; folic acid; biotin] 100•±•60•1•0.3 mg

Nephro-Vite Vitamin B Complex and C Supplement tablets OTC *vitamin supplement* [multiple B vitamins; vitamin C; folic acid; biotin] ±•60•0.8•0.3 mg

Nephrox oral suspension OTC *antacid; laxative* [aluminum hydroxide; mineral oil 10%] 320 mg/5 mL

nepicastat HCl USAN *dopamine β-hydroxylase inhibitor for congestive heart failure*

Nepro oral liquid OTC *enteral nutritional therapy for acute or chronic renal failure* [lactose-free formula] 240 mL

neptamustine INN *antineoplastic* [also: pentamustine]

Neptazane tablets (discontinued 2004) ℞ *carbonic anhydrase inhibitor for glaucoma* [methazolamide] 25, 50 mg

neptunium *element (Np)*

nequinate USAN, INN *coccidiostat for poultry* [also: methyl benzoquate]

neramexane *investigational (Phase III) NMDA (N-methyl-D-aspartate)-receptor antagonist for Alzheimer disease*

neraminol INN

nerbacadol INN

nerelimomab USAN *monoclonal antibody; investigational (Phase III) cytokine modulator for septic shock*

neridronic acid INN

Nerium indicum; N. oleander *medicinal herb* [see: oleander]

nervines *a class of agents that have a calming or soothing effect on the nerves (a term used in folk medicine)*

Nervocaine 1% injection (discontinued 2002) ℞ *injectable local anesthetic* [lidocaine HCl] 1%

Nesacaine; Nesacaine MPF injection ℞ *local anesthetic; central or peripheral nerve block, including lumbar and epidural block* [chloroprocaine HCl] 1%, 2%; 2%, 3%

nesapidil INN

nesiritide USAN *human B-type natriuretic peptide (hBNP); vasodilator for acute congestive heart failure*

nesiritide citrate *human B-type natriuretic peptide (hBNP); vasodilator for acute congestive heart failure*

nesosteine INN

Nestabs tablets (name changed to Vitelle Nestabs OTC in 2000)

Nestabs CBF; Nestabs FA tablets ℞ *vitamin/calcium/iron supplement for pregnancy and lactation* [multiple vitamins; calcium; iron; folic acid] ≛•200•50•1 mg; ≛•200•29•1 mg

Nestlé Good Start [see: Good Start]

Nestle VHC 2.25 oral liquid OTC *enteral nutritional therapy* [lactose-free formula]

Nestrex tablets (name changed to Vitelle Nestrex in 2001)

nethalide [see: pronetalol]

netilmicin INN, BAN *aminoglycoside antibiotic* [also: netilmicin sulfate]

netilmicin sulfate USAN, USP *aminoglycoside antibiotic* [also: netilmicin]

netobimin USAN, INN, BAN *veterinary anthelmintic*

netrafilcon A USAN *hydrophilic contact lens material*

Netromicina (Mexican name for U.S. product Netromycin)

Netromycin IV or IM injection (discontinued 2003) ℞ *aminoglycoside antibiotic* [netilmicin sulfate] 100 mg/mL

nettle *(Urtica dioica; U. urens)* leaves and root *medicinal herb for blood cleansing, bronchitis, diarrhea,* edema, hypertension, bleeding, and rheumatism; competitively binds to sex hormone–binding globulin (SHBG) to increase the level of free testosterone

nettle, hemp; bee nettle; dog nettle; hemp dead nettle *medicinal herb* [see: hemp nettle]

nettle flowers; dead nettle; stingless nettle; white nettle *medicinal herb* [see: blind nettle]

Neulasta subcu injection in prefilled syringe ℞ *hematopoietic stimulant for severe chronic neutropenia following cancer chemotherapy* [pegfilgrastim] 6 mg/0.6 mL

Neumega subcu injection ℞ *platelet growth factor for prevention of thrombocytopenia following chemotherapy or radiation* (orphan) [oprelvekin] 5 mg

Neupogen IV or subcu injection, prefilled syringes ℞ *hematopoietic stimulant for severe chronic neutropenia* (orphan); *investigational (Phase III, orphan) cytokine for AIDS-related cytomegalovirus retinitis; investigational (orphan) for myelodysplastic syndrome* [filgrastim] 300 μg/mL; 300, 480 μg

Neupro transdermal patch ℞ *investigational (NDA filed) transdermal dopamine D₂ agonist for Parkinson disease and restless leg syndrome* [rotigotine]

neural dopaminergic cells (or precursors), porcine fetal *investigational (orphan) intracerebral implant for stage 4 and 5 Parkinson disease*

neural gabaergic cells (or precursors), porcine fetal *investigational (orphan) intracerebral implant for Huntington disease*

Neuramate tablets (discontinued 2001) ℞ *anxiolytic* [meprobamate] 400 mg

NeuRecover-DA; NeuRecover-SA capsules OTC *dietary supplement* [multiple vitamins & minerals; multiple amino acids; folic acid] ≛•0.067 mg; ≛•0.067 mg

NeuRecover-LT capsules (discontinued 2001) OTC *dietary supplement* [multiple vitamins & minerals; multiple amino acids; folic acid] ≛•0.03 mg

Neurelan *investigational (orphan) agent for multiple sclerosis and spinal cord injury* [fampridine]

Neurobloc (name changed to Myobloc upon marketing release in 2001)

Neurodep injection ℞ *parenteral vitamin therapy* [multiple B vitamins; vitamin C] ≛•50 mg/mL

Neurodep-Caps capsules OTC *vitamin supplement* [vitamins B$_1$, B$_6$, and B$_{12}$] 125•125•1 mg

Neurolite injection ℞ *imaging aid for SPECT brain scans* [technetium Tc 99m bicisate]

Neurontin capsules, film-coated caplets, oral solution ℞ *anticonvulsant for partial-onset seizures; treatment for postherpetic neuralgia; investigational (orphan) for amyotrophic lateral sclerosis* [gabapentin] 100, 300, 400 mg; 600, 800 mg; 250 mg/5 mL

neurosin [see: calcium glycerophosphate]

NeuroSlim capsules OTC *dietary supplement* [multiple vitamins & minerals; multiple amino acids; folic acid; biotin] ≛•0.066•0.05 mg

neurotrophic growth factor [see: methionyl neurotrophic factor]

neurotrophin-1 *investigational (orphan) for motor neuron disease and amyotrophic lateral sclerosis*

neustab [see: thioacetazone; thiacetazone]

Neut IV or subcu injection ℞ *pH buffer for metabolic acidosis; urinary alkalinizer* [sodium bicarbonate] 4% (0.48 mEq Na/mL)

Neutra-Caine liquid ℞ *mixed with injectable local anesthetics to reduce stinging pain at the injection site* [sodium bicarbonate] 7.5%

NeutraGard Advanced dental gel ℞ *topical caries preventative* [sodium fluoride] 1.1%

neutral acriflavine [see: acriflavine]

Neutral C ⓒᴬᴺ capsules OTC *vitamin C supplement* [calcium polyascorbate; lemon bioflavonoids; echinacea] 600•≛•≛ mg

Neutral C + CoEnzyme Q10 ⓒᴬᴺ capsules OTC *vitamin/mineral supplement* [multiple vitamins; multiple minerals; calcium ascorbate; coenzyme Q10; folic acid] ≛•≛•320•10•0.5 mg

neutral insulin INN, BAN, JAN *antidiabetic* [also: insulin, neutral]

Neutralca-S ⓒᴬᴺ oral suspension OTC *antacid* [aluminum hydroxide; magnesium hydroxide] 200•200 mg/5 mL

neutramycin USAN, INN *antibacterial*

Neutra-Phos powder for oral solution OTC *phosphorus supplement* [monobasic sodium phosphate; monobasic potassium phosphate; dibasic sodium phosphate; dibasic potassium phosphate] 250 mg P/pkt.

Neutra-Phos-K powder for oral solution OTC *phosphorus supplement* [monobasic potassium phosphate; dibasic potassium phosphate] 250 mg P/pkt.

NeuTrexin powder for IV injection ℞ *antiprotozoal for AIDS-related* Pneumocystis carinii *pneumonia (orphan); investigational (orphan) antineoplastic for multiple cancers* [trimetrexate glucuronate] 25 mg

neutroflavine [see: acriflavine]

Neutrogena Acne Mask (discontinued 2003) OTC *keratolytic cleansing mask for acne* [benzoyl peroxide] 5%

Neutrogena Antiseptic Cleanser for Acne-Prone Skin topical liquid OTC *cleanser for acne* [benzethonium chloride]

Neutrogena Body lotion, oil OTC *moisturizer; emollient*

Neutrogena Clear Pore topical liquid OTC *keratolytic cleansing mask for acne* [benzoyl peroxide] 3.5%

Neutrogena Drying gel OTC *topical astringent and antiseptic for acne* [hamamelis water; isopropyl alcohol]

Neutrogena Moisture lotion OTC *moisturizer; emollient*

Neutrogena Non-Drying Cleansing lotion OTC *soap-free therapeutic skin cleanser*

Nevanac

Neutrogena Norwegian Formula Hand cream OTC *moisturizer; emollient*

Neutrogena Oil-Free Acne Wash topical liquid OTC *keratolytic cleanser for acne* [salicylic acid] 2%

Neutrogena Soap; Neutrogena Cleansing for Acne-Prone Skin; Neutrogena Baby Cleansing Formula Soap; Neutrogena Dry Skin Soap; Neutrogena Oily Skin Soap bar OTC *therapeutic skin cleanser*

Neutrogena T/Derm topical oil (discontinued 2003) OTC *antipsoriatic; antiseborrheic* [coal tar] 5%

Neutrogena T/Gel shampoo, conditioner (discontinued 2003) OTC *antiseborrheic; antipsoriatic; antipruritic; antibacterial* [coal tar] 2%; 1.5%

Neutrogena T/Gel Original shampoo OTC *antiseborrheic; antipsoriatic; antipruritic; antibacterial* [coal tar extract] 2%

Neutrogena T/Sal shampoo OTC *antiseborrheic; antipsoriatic; antipruritic; antibacterial* [salicylic acid; coal tar] 2%•2%

nevirapine USAN, INN *antiviral nonnucleoside reverse transcriptase inhibitor (NNRTI) for HIV-1*

Nevis tablets ℞ *investigational (NDA filed) synthetic progestin/estrogen; hormone replacement therapy for postmenopausal symptoms* [norethindrone acetate; ethinyl estradiol] 1 mg•5 μg

New Jersey tea (*Ceanothus americanus*) root bark *medicinal herb used as an astringent, expectorant, and sedative*

New Zealand green-lipped mussel (*Perna canaliculus*) freeze-dried body or gonads *natural treatment for osteoarthritis and rheumatoid arthritis*

new-estranol 1 [see: diethylstilbestrol]

new-oestranol 1 [see: diethylstilbestrol]

new-oestranol 11 [see: diethylstilbestrol dipropionate]

NewPaks (trademarked delivery form) *ready-to-use closed system containers*

New-Skin topical liquid, spray OTC *skin protectant; antiseptic* [hydroxyquinoline]

nexeridine INN *analgesic* [also: nexeridine HCl]

nexeridine HCl USAN *analgesic* [also: nexeridine]

Nexium delayed-release enteric-coated pellets in capsules ℞ *proton pump inhibitor for gastric and duodenal ulcers, erosive esophagitis, GERD, and other gastroesophageal disorders* [esomeprazole magnesium] 20, 40 mg

Nexium I.V. powder for infusion ℞ *proton pump inhibitor for short-term treatment in patients who cannot take the drug orally* [esomeprazole magnesium] 20, 40 mg/dose

Nexrutine capsules OTC *dietary supplement; selective COX-2 inhibitor; anti-inflammatory; antipyretic* [Phellodendron amurense extract] 250 mg

NFL (Novantrone, fluorouracil, leucovorin [rescue]) *chemotherapy protocol for breast cancer*

NG-29 *investigational (orphan) diagnostic aid for pituitary release of growth hormone*

N.G.T. cream ℞ *topical corticosteroidal anti-inflammatory; antifungal* [triamcinolone acetonide; nystatin] 0.1%•100 000 U per g

niacin (vitamin B₃) USP *water-soluble vitamin; peripheral vasodilator; antihyperlipidemic* [also: nicotinic acid] 50, 100, 125, 250, 400, 500 mg oral ⑤ Minocin

niacinamide (vitamin B₃) USP *water-soluble vitamin; enzyme cofactor* [also: nicotinamide] 100, 500 mg oral

niacinamide hydroiodide *expectorant*

Niacor immediate-release tablets (discontinued 2005) ℞ *vitamin B₃ therapy; peripheral vasodilator; antihyperlipidemic for hypertriglyceridemia (types IV and V hyperlipidemia)* [niacin] 500 mg

nialamide NF, INN

niaprazine INN

Niaspan extended-release caplets ℞ *peripheral vasodilator; antihyperlipidemic; vitamin B$_3$* [niacin] 500, 750, 1000 mg

NiaStase ⒸⒶⓃ powder for IV injection ℞ *recombinant coagulation Factor VII for hemophilia A and B* [eptacog alfa (activated)] 1.2, 2.4, 4.8 mg/vial

nibroxane USAN, INN *topical antimicrobial*

Nicabate (European name for U.S. product Nicoderm)

nicafenine INN

nicainoprol INN

nicametate INN, BAN

nicaraven INN

nicarbazin BAN

nicardipine INN, BAN *vasodilator; calcium channel blocker* [also: nicardipine HCl]

nicardipine HCl USAN *antianginal; antihypertensive; vasodilator; calcium channel blocker* [also: nicardipine] 20, 30 mg oral

NicCheck I reagent strips *in vitro diagnostic aid for urine nicotine, used to determine the smoking status of the subject*

NicCheck II reagent strips *investigational in vitro diagnostic aid for urine nicotine, used to determine exposure to passive cigarette smoke*

N'Ice throat spray OTC *topical analgesic; counterirritant; mild local anesthetic* [menthol] 0.12%

N'Ice; N'Ice 'n Clear lozenges OTC *topical oral analgesic; counterirritant; mild local anesthetic* [menthol] 5 mg

N'Ice Vitamin C Drops (lozenges) OTC *vitamin C supplement* [ascorbic acid; menthol] 60• ? mg

nicergoline USAN, INN *vasodilator*

niceritrol INN, BAN

nicethamide BAN [also: nikethamide]

niceverine INN

nickel *element (Ni)*

niclofolan INN, BAN

niclosamide USAN, INN *anthelmintic for cestodiasis (tapeworm)*

nicoboxil INN

nicoclonate INN

nicocodine INN, BAN

nicocortonide INN

Nicoderm CQ Step 1; Nicoderm CQ Step 2; Nicoderm CQ Step 3 transdermal patch OTC *smoking deterrent; nicotine withdrawal aid* [nicotine] 21 mg/day; 14 mg/day; 7 mg/day

nicodicodine INN, BAN

nicoduozide (isoniazid + nicothiazone)

nicofibrate INN

nicofuranose INN

nicofurate INN

nicogrelate INN

Nicomide tablets ℞ *vitamin/mineral supplement* [nicotinamide; zinc oxide; cupric oxide; folic acid] 750• 25•1.5•0.5 mg

nicomol INN

nicomorphine INN, BAN

nicopholine INN

nicorandil USAN, INN *coronary vasodilator*

Nicorette chewing gum OTC *smoking deterrent; nicotine withdrawal aid* [nicotine polacrilex] 2, 4 mg

Nicorette Plus ⒸⒶⓃ chewing pieces OTC *smoking deterrent; nicotine withdrawal aid* [nicotine polacrilex] 4 mg

Nicosyn lotion ℞ *antibiotic for acne* [sulfacetamide sodium; sulfur] 10%•5%

nicothiazone INN

nicotinaldehyde thiosemicarbazone [see: nicothiazone]

nicotinamide (vitamin B$_3$) INN, BAN, JAN *water-soluble vitamin; enzyme cofactor* [also: niacinamide]

nicotinamide-adenine dinucleotide (NAD) [now: nadide]

nicotine *a very poisonous alkaloid used as an insecticide and external parasiticide; the active principle in tobacco; smoking cessation aid* [also see: tobacco] 7, 14, 21 mg/day transdermal

nicotine bitartrate USAN *smoking cessation aid*

nicotine & mecamylamine HCl *investigational (Phase III) transdermal patch for smoking cessation*

nicotine polacrilex USAN *smoking deterrent; nicotine withdrawal aid* 2, 4 mg oral

nicotine resin complex [see: nicotine polacrilex]

Nicotinex elixir (discontinued 2004) OTC *vitamin B₃ supplement; antihyperlipidemic* [niacin] 50 mg/5 mL

nicotinic acid (vitamin B₃) INN, BAN, JAN *water-soluble vitamin; peripheral vasodilator; antihyperlipidemic* [also: niacin] 50, 100, 125, 250, 400, 500 mg oral

nicotinic acid amide [see: niacinamide]

nicotinic acid 1-oxide [see: oxiniacic acid]

nicotinohydroxamic acid [see: nicoxamat]

6-nicotinoyl dihydrocodeine [see: nicodicodine]

6-nicotinoylcodeine [see: nicocodine]

4-nicotinoylmorpholine [see: nicopholine]

nicotinyl alcohol USAN, BAN *peripheral vasodilator*

nicotinyl tartrate

Nicotrol oral inhaler ℞ *smoking deterrent; nicotine withdrawal aid* [nicotine] 10 mg (4 mg delivered) per cartridge

Nicotrol NS nasal spray ℞ *smoking deterrent; nicotine withdrawal aid* [nicotine] 0.5 mg/spray

Nicotrol Step 1; Nicotrol Step 2; Nicotrol Step 3 transdermal patch OTC *smoking deterrent; nicotine withdrawal aid* [nicotine] 15 mg/day; 10 mg/day; 5 mg/day

nicotylamide [see: niacinamide]

nicoumalone BAN [also: acenocoumarol]

nicoxamat INN

nictiazem INN

nictindole INN

Nidagel ⒸⒶⓃ vaginal gel ℞ *antibacterial for bacterial vaginosis* [metronidazole] 0.75%

Nidran ℞ *alkylating antineoplastic* [nimustin HCl]

nidroxyzone INN

Nifediac CC film-coated extended-release tablets ℞ *antianginal; antihypertensive; calcium channel blocker* [nifedipine] 30, 60, 90 mg

Nifedical XL film-coated sustained-release tablets ℞ *antianginal; antihypertensive; calcium channel blocker* [nifedipine] 30, 60 mg

nifedipine USAN, USP, INN, BAN *antianginal; antihypertensive; coronary vasodilator; calcium channel blocker; investigational (orphan) for interstitial cystitis* 10, 20, 30, 60, 90 mg oral

nifenalol INN

nifenazone INN, BAN

Niferex tablets, elixir OTC *hematinic; iron supplement* [polysaccharide-iron complex] 50 mg Fe; 100 mg Fe/5 mL

Niferex-150 capsules OTC *hematinic; vitamin/iron supplement* [polysaccharide-iron complex; vitamin C] 150 mg Fe•50 mg

Niferex-150 Forte capsules ℞ *hematinic* [polysaccharide-iron complex; cyanocobalamin; folic acid] 150 mg Fe•25 μg•1 mg

Niferex-PN film-coated tablets ℞ *prenatal vitamin/iron supplement* [polysaccharide-iron complex; multiple vitamins & minerals; folic acid] 60• ≛•1 mg

Niferex-PN Forte film-coated tablets ℞ *prenatal vitamin/mineral/calcium/iron supplement* [multiple vitamins & minerals; calcium; polysaccharide-iron complex; folic acid] ≛•250• 60•1 mg

niflumic acid INN

nifluridide USAN *ectoparasiticide*

nifungin USAN, INN

nifuradene USAN, INN *antibacterial*

nifuralazine [see: furalazine]

nifuraldezone USAN, INN *antibacterial*

nifuralide INN

nifuramizone [see: nifurethazone]

nifuratel USAN, INN *antibacterial; antifungal; antiprotozoal (Trichomonas)*

nifuratrone USAN, INN *antibacterial*

nifurazolidone [see: furazolidone]

nifurdazil USAN, INN *antibacterial*

nifurethazone INN

nifurfoline INN

nifurhydrazone [see: nihydrazone]

nifurimide USAN, INN *antibacterial*

nifurizone INN

nifurmazole INN

nifurmerone USAN, INN *antifungal*

nifuroquine INN

nifuroxazide INN

nifuroxime NF, INN

nifurpipone (NP) INN

nifurpirinol USAN, INN *antibacterial*

nifurprazine INN

nifurquinazol USAN, INN *antibacterial*

nifursemizone USAN, INN *antiprotozoal for poultry (Histomonas)*

nifursol USAN, INN *antiprotozoal for poultry (Histomonas)*

nifurthiazole USAN, INN *antibacterial*

nifurthiline [see: thiofuradene]

nifurtimox INN, BAN (available only from Centers for Disease Control and Prevention) *investigational anti-infective for Chagas disease*

nifurtoinol INN

nifurvidine INN

nifurzide INN

Night Time Cold/Flu Relief oral liquid (discontinued 2002) OTC *antitussive; decongestant; antihistamine; analgesic* [dextromethorphan hydrobromide; pseudoephedrine HCl; doxylamine succinate; acetaminophen; alcohol 10%] 30•60•12.5•1000 mg/30 mL

nightshade; nightshade vine *medicinal herb* [see: bittersweet nightshade]

nightshade, American *medicinal herb* [see: pokeweed]

nightshade, deadly *medicinal herb* [see: belladonna]

nightshade, fetid; stinking nightshade *medicinal herb* [see: henbane]

nightshade, three-leaved *medicinal herb* [see: birthroot]

Night-Time Effervescent Cold tablets for oral solution (discontinued 2002) OTC *decongestant; antihistamine; analgesic; antipyretic* [phenylpropanol-

amine HCl; diphenhydramine citrate; aspirin] 15•38.33•325 mg

Nighttime Sleep Aid tablets (discontinued 2002) OTC *antihistaminic sleep aid* [diphenhydramine HCl] 50 mg

NightTime TheraFlu powder for oral solution (discontinued 2002) OTC *antitussive; decongestant; antihistamine; analgesic* [dextromethorphan hydrobromide; pseudoephedrine HCl; chlorpheniramine maleate; acetaminophen] 30•60•4•1000 mg/pkt. ⊡ Thera-Flur

niguldipine INN

nihydrazone INN

nikethamide NF, INN [also: nicethamide]

Nilandron tablets ℞ *antiandrogen antineoplastic for metastatic prostate cancer* [nilutamide] 50, 150 mg

nileprost INN

nilestriol INN *estrogen* [also: nylestriol]

nilprazole INN

Nilstat cream, ointment ℞ *antifungal* [nystatin] 100 000 U/g ⊡ Nitrostat; nystatin

Nilstat oral suspension, powder for oral suspension ℞ *antifungal; oral candidiasis treatment* [nystatin] 100 000 U/mL; 150 million, 500 million, 1 billion, 2 billion U

niludipine INN

nilutamide USAN, INN, BAN *antiandrogen antineoplastic adjunct to surgical or chemical castration for metastatic prostate cancer*

nilvadipine USAN, INN, JAN *calcium channel antagonist*

nimazone USAN, INN *anti-inflammatory*

Nimbex IV infusion ℞ *nondepolarizing neuromuscular blocking agent for anesthesia* [cisatracurium besylate] 2, 10 mg/mL

Nimbus; Nimbus Quick Strip test kit for home use *in vitro diagnostic aid; urine pregnancy test* [monoclonal antibody-based enzyme immunoassay]

Nimbus Plus test kit for professional use *in vitro diagnostic aid; urine pregnancy test*

nimesulide INN, BAN

nimetazepam INN

nimidane USAN, INN *veterinary acaricide*

nimodipine USAN, INN, BAN *vasodilator; calcium channel blocker for subarachnoid hemorrhage (SAH)*

nimorazole INN, BAN

Nimotop soft liquid-filled capsules R *calcium channel blocker for subarachnoid hemorrhage (SAH)* [nimodipine] 30 mg

nimustine INN *alkylating neoplastic*

nimustine HCl *alkylating neoplastic*

niobium *element (Nb)*

niometacin INN

Nion B Plus C caplets OTC *vitamin supplement* [multiple B vitamins; vitamin C] ± •300 mg

Nipent powder for IV injection R *antibiotic antineoplastic for hairy cell leukemia (orphan); investigational (orphan) for chronic lymphocytic leukemia and cutaneous T-cell lymphoma; investigational (Phase III) for AIDS-related non-Hodgkin lymphoma* [pentostatin] 10 mg

niperotidine INN

nipradilol INN

Nipride *brand discontinued 1992* [see: sodium nitroprusside]

niprofazone INN

Niravam orally disintegrating tablets R *benzodiazepine anxiolytic; sedative; treatment for panic disorders and agoraphobia* [alprazolam] 0.25, 0.5, 1, 2 mg

niridazole USAN, INN *antischistosomal*

nisbuterol INN *bronchodilator* [also: nisbuterol mesylate]

nisbuterol mesylate USAN *bronchodilator* [also: nisbuterol]

nisin *investigational agent for severe colonic bacterial infections*

nisobamate USAN, INN *minor tranquilizer*

nisoldipine USAN, INN, BAN, JAN *coronary vasodilator; calcium channel blocker for hypertension*

nisoxetine USAN, INN *antidepressant*

nisterime INN *androgen* [also: nisterime acetate]

nisterime acetate USAN *androgen* [also: nisterime]

nitarsone USAN, INN *antiprotozoal (Histomonas)*

nitazoxanide (NTZ) INN *antiprotozoal for pediatric diarrhea due to* Cryptosporidium parvum *and* Giardia lamblia *infections; investigational (orphan) for AIDS-related diarrhea*

Nite Time Children's Liquid OTC *antitussive; decongestant; antihistamine* [dextromethorphan hydrobromide; pseudoephedrine HCl; chlorpheniramine maleate] 15•30•2 mg/15 mL

Nite Time Cold Formula for Adults oral liquid OTC *antitussive; decongestant; antihistamine; analgesic* [dextromethorphan hydrobromide; pseudoephedrine HCl; doxylamine succinate; acetaminophen; alcohol 10%] 30•60•12.5•1000 mg/30 mL

nithiamide USAN *veterinary antibacterial* [also: aminitrozole; acinitrazole]

nitisinone *adjunctive treatment for hereditary tyrosinemia type 1 (HT-1), a pediatric liver disease (orphan)*

nitracrine INN

nitrafudam INN *antidepressant* [also: nitrafudam HCl]

nitrafudam HCl USAN *antidepressant* [also: nitrafudam]

nitralamine HCl USAN *antifungal*

nitramisole INN *anthelmintic* [also: nitramisole HCl]

nitramisole HCl USAN *anthelmintic* [also: nitramisole]

nitraquazone INN

nitrates *a class of antianginal agents that cause the relaxation of vascular smooth muscles*

nitratophenylmercury [see: phenylmercuric nitrate]

nitrazepam USAN, INN, BAN, JAN *investigational benzodiazepine sedative; anxiolytic; anticonvulsant; hypnotic*

Nitrazine paper for professional use (discontinued 2002) *in vitro diagnostic aid for urine pH determination*

nitre, sweet spirit of [see: ethyl nitrite]

nitrefazole INN, BAN

Nitrek transdermal patch ℞ *antianginal; vasodilator* [nitroglycerin] 22.4, 44.8, 67.2 mg (0.2, 0.4, 0.6 mg/hr.)

nitrendipine USAN, INN, BAN, JAN *investigational (NDA filed) antihypertensive; calcium channel blocker*

nitric acid NF *acidifying agent*

nitric oxide *inhalation gas for neonatal hypoxic respiratory failure due to persistent pulmonary hypertension (orphan); investigational (orphan) for acute adult respiratory distress syndrome; investigational to prevent reperfusion injury following lung transplants*

nitricholine perchlorate INN

p-nitrobenzenearsonic acid [see: nitarsone]

Nitro-Bid ointment ℞ *antianginal; vasodilator* [nitroglycerin] 2% (15 mg/inch) ⧫ Nicobid

Nitro-Bid IV infusion ℞ *antianginal; vasodilator; perioperative antihypertensive; for congestive heart failure with myocardial infarction* [nitroglycerin] 5 mg/mL

9-nitrocamptothecin (9-NC) [now: rubitecan]

nitroclofene INN

nitrocycline USAN, INN *antibacterial*

nitrodan USAN, INN *anthelmintic*

Nitrodisc transdermal patch ℞ *antianginal; vasodilator* [nitroglycerin] 16, 24, 32 mg (0.2, 0.3, 0.4 mg/hr.)

Nitro-Dur transdermal patch ℞ *antianginal; vasodilator* [nitroglycerin] 20, 40, 60, 80, 120, 160 mg (0.1, 0.2, 0.3, 0.4, 0.6, 0.8 mg/hr.)

nitroethanolamine [see: aminoethyl nitrate]

nitrofuradoxadone [see: furmethoxadone]

nitrofural INN *broad-spectrum bactericidal; adjunct to burn treatment* [also: nitrofurazone]

nitrofurantoin USP, INN *urinary antibiotic* 50, 100 mg oral

nitrofurantoin sodium *urinary antibiotic*

nitrofurazone USP, BAN *broad-spectrum bactericidal; adjunct to burn treatment*

and skin grafting [also: nitrofural] 0.2% topical

nitrofurmethone [see: furaltadone]

nitrofuroxizone [see: nidroxyzone]

Nitrogard transmucosal extended-release tablets ℞ *antianginal; vasodilator* [nitroglycerin] 2, 3 mg

nitrogen (N_2) NF *air displacement agent; element (N)*

nitrogen monoxide [see: nitrous oxide]

nitrogen mustard N-oxide HCl JAN *alkylating antineoplastic* [also: mechlorethamine HCl; chlormethine; mustine]

nitrogen mustards *a class of alkylating antineoplastics*

nitrogen oxide (N_2O) [see: nitrous oxide]

nitroglycerin USP *coronary vasodilator; antianginal; antihypertensive* [also: glyceryl trinitrate] 0.3, 0.4, 0.6 mg sublingual; 2.5, 6.5, 9 mg oral; 5 mg/mL injection; 0.1, 0.2, 0.4, 0.6 mg/hr. transdermal; 2% topical ⧫ Nitroglyn

Nitroglyn extended-release capsules (discontinued 2004) ℞ *antianginal; vasodilator* [nitroglycerin] 2.5, 6.5, 9, 13 mg ⧫ nitroglycerin

nitrohydroxyquinoline [see: nitroxoline]

Nitrol ointment, Appli-Kit (ointment & adhesive dosage covers) (discontinued 2003) ℞ *antianginal; vasodilator* [nitroglycerin] 2% (15 mg/inch)

Nitrolan oral liquid OTC *enteral nutritional therapy* [lactose-free formula]

Nitrolingual Pumpspray CFC-free translingual aerosol ℞ *antianginal; vasodilator* [nitroglycerin] 0.4 mg/spray

nitromannitol [see: mannitol hexanitrate]

nitromersol USP *topical anti-infective*

nitromide USAN *coccidiostat for poultry; antibacterial*

nitromifene INN

nitromifene citrate USAN *antiestrogen*

NitroMist translingual aerosol ℞ *investigational (NDA filed) antianginal; vasodilator* [nitroglycerin]

Nitrong sustained-release tablets (discontinued 2004) ℞ *antianginal; vasodilator* [nitroglycerin] 2.6, 6.5, 9 mg

Nitropress powder for IV injection, flip-top vials ℞ *vasodilator for hypertensive emergency* [sodium nitroprusside] 50 mg/dose

nitroprusside sodium [see: sodium nitroprusside]

NitroQuick sublingual tablets ℞ *antianginal; vasodilator* [nitroglycerin] 0.3, 0.4, 0.6 mg (1/200, 1/150, 1/100 gr.)

nitroscanate USAN, INN *veterinary anthelmintic*

nitrosoureas *a class of alkylating antineoplastics*

Nitrostat sublingual tablets ℞ *antianginal; vasodilator* [nitroglycerin] 0.3, 0.4, 0.6 mg (1/200, 1/150, 1/100 gr.)

nitrosulfathiazole INN [also: paranitrosulfathiazole]

NitroTab sublingual tablets ℞ *antianginal; vasodilator* [nitroglycerin] 0.3, 0.4, 0.6 mg (1/200, 1/150, 1/100 gr.)

Nitro-Time extended-release capsules ℞ *antianginal; vasodilator* [nitroglycerin] 2.5, 6.5, 9 mg

nitrous acid, sodium salt [see: sodium nitrite]

nitrous oxide (N₂O) USP *a weak inhalation general anesthetic; sometimes abused as a street drug to create a dreamy or floating sensation*

nitroxinil INN

nitroxoline INN, BAN

nivacortol INN *corticosteroid; antiinflammatory* [also: nivazol]

nivadipine [see: nilvadipine]

nivaquine [see: chloroquine phosphate]

nivazol USAN *corticosteroid; anti-inflammatory* [also: nivacortol]

Nivea After Tan; Nivea Moisturizing; Nivea Moisturizing Extra Enriched lotion OTC *moisturizer; emollient*

Nivea Moisturizing; Nivea Skin oil OTC *moisturizer; emollient*

Nivea Moisturizing Creme Soap bar OTC *therapeutic skin cleanser*

Nivea Ultra Moisturizing Creme OTC *moisturizer; emollient*

nivimedone sodium USAN *antiallergic*

Nix creme rinse OTC *pediculicide for lice; scabicide* [permethrin; alcohol 20%] 1%

nixylic acid INN

nizatidine USAN, USP, INN, BAN, JAN *histamine H₂ antagonist for gastric and duodenal ulcers* 150, 300 mg oral

nizofenone INN

Nizoral cream (discontinued 2003) ℞ *antifungal* [ketoconazole] 2%

Nizoral shampoo ℞ *antifungal* [ketoconazole] 2% ☑ Nasarel

Nizoral tablets ℞ *systemic imidazole antifungal* [ketoconazole] 200 mg ☑ Nasarel

Nizoral A-D shampoo OTC *antifungal for dandruff* [ketoconazole] 1% ☑ Nasarel

NMDA (N-methyl-D-aspartate) [q.v.]

N-Multistix; N-Multistix SG reagent strips *in vitro diagnostic aid for multiple urine products*

NN-622 *investigational (Phase III) dual-acting insulin sensitizer for type 2 diabetes*

NNRTIs (non-nucleoside reverse transcriptase inhibitors) [see: reverse transcriptase inhibitors]

No Pain-HP roll-on OTC *topical analgesic* [capsaicin] 0.075%

nobelium *element (No)*

noberastine USAN, INN, BAN *antihistamine*

noble yarrow *medicinal herb* [see: yarrow]

nocebo effect [L. I will harm] *a perceived adverse effect from an inert substance* [compare to: placebo effect]

nocloprost INN

nocodazole USAN, INN *antineoplastic*

nodding wakerobin *medicinal herb* [see: birthroot]

NōDōz chewable tablets (discontinued 2001) OTC *CNS stimulant; analeptic* [caffeine] 100 mg

NōDōz coated caplets OTC *CNS stimulant; analeptic* [caffeine] 200 mg

nofecainide INN

nofetumomab merpentan *monoclonal antibody imaging agent for small cell lung cancer*

nogalamycin USAN, INN *antineoplastic*

No-Hist capsules (discontinued 2002) ℞ *nasal decongestant* [phenylephrine HCl; phenylpropanolamine HCl; pseudoephedrine HCl] 5•40•40 mg

Nolahist tablets OTC *nonselective piperidine antihistamine for allergic rhinitis* [phenindamine tartrate] 25 mg

Nolamine timed-release tablets (discontinued 2001) ℞ *decongestant; antihistamine* [phenylpropanolamine HCl; chlorpheniramine maleate; phenindamine tartrate] 50•4•24 mg

nolatrexed dihydrochloride *thymidylate synthase inhibitor that disrupts DNA replication; investigational (Phase III) for inoperable primary liver cancer*

nolinium bromide USAN, INN *antisecretory; antiulcerative*

Nolvadex tablets ℞ *antiestrogen antineoplastic for advanced postmenopausal breast cancer; also for breast cancer prevention in high-risk patients* [tamoxifen citrate] 10, 20 mg

nomegestrol INN

nomelidine INN

nomifensine INN *antidepressant* [also: nomifensine maleate]

nomifensine maleate USAN *antidepressant* [also: nomifensine]

nonabine INN, BAN

nonabsorbable surgical suture [see: suture, nonabsorbable surgical]

nonachlazine [now: azaclorzine HCl]

nonacog alfa USAN, INN *synthetic human blood coagulation factor IX; antihemophilic for hemophilia B and Christmas disease (orphan)* [also: factor IX complex]

nonanedioic acid [see: azelaic acid]

nonaperone INN

nonapyrimine INN

nonathymulin INN

nondestearinated cod liver oil [see: cod liver oil, nondestearinated]

Non-Drowsy Allergy Relief for Kids syrup OTC *nonsedating antihistamine for allergic rhinitis* [loratadine] 5 mg/5 mL

Non-Habit Forming Stool Softener capsules OTC *laxative; stool softener* [docusate sodium] 100 mg

noni (Morinda citrifolia) berries *medicinal herb for arthritis, bacterial infections, diabetes, drug addiction, headache, hypertension, liver and skin disorders, pain, and slowing aging; also used as an antioxidant*

nonionic contrast media *a class of newer radiopaque agents that, in general, have a low osmolar concentration of iodine (the contrast agent), which corresponds to a lower incidence of adverse reactions* [also called: low osmolar contrast media (LOCM)]

nonivamide INN

non-nucleoside reverse transcriptase inhibitors (NNRTIs) [see: reverse transcriptase inhibitors]

nonoxinol 4 INN *surfactant* [also: nonoxynol 4]

nonoxinol 9 INN *wetting and solubilizing agent; spermaticide* [also: nonoxynol 9]

nonoxinol 15 INN *surfactant* [also: nonoxynol 15]

nonoxinol 30 INN *surfactant* [also: nonoxynol 30]

nonoxynol 4 USAN *surfactant* [also: nonoxinol 4]

nonoxynol 9 USAN, USP *wetting and solubilizing agent; spermicide* [also: nonoxinol 9]

nonoxynol 10 NF *surfactant*

nonoxynol 15 USAN *surfactant* [also: nonoxinol 15]

nonoxynol 30 USAN *surfactant* [also: nonoxinol 30]

nonsteroidal anti-inflammatory drugs (NSAIDs) *a class of anti-inflammatory drugs that have analgesic and antipyretic effects*

nonylphenoxypolyethoxyethanol [see: nonoxynol 4, 9, 15, & 30]

Nootropil ℞ *cognition adjuvant; investigational (orphan) for myoclonus* [piracetam]

nopal plant *medicinal herb for cleansing the lymphatic system, diabetes, digestion, obesity, neutralizing toxins, and preventing arteriosclerosis*

Nora-BE tablets (in packs of 28) ℞ *oral contraceptive (progestin only)* [norethindrone] 0.35 mg

noracymethadol INN *analgesic* [also: noracymethadol HCl]

noracymethadol HCl USAN *analgesic* [also: noracymethadol]

noradrenaline bitartrate [see: norepinephrine bitartrate]

noramidopyrine methanesulfonate sodium [see: dipyrone]

norandrostenolone phenylpropionate [see: nandrolone phenpropionate]

norbolethone USAN *anabolic* [also: norboletone]

norboletone INN *anabolic* [also: norbolethone]

norbudrine INN [also: norbutrine]

norbutrine BAN [also: norbudrine]

norclostebol INN

Norco tablets ℞ *narcotic analgesic and antitussive* [hydrocodone bitartrate; acetaminophen] 5•325, 7.5•325, 10•325 mg

norcodeine INN, BAN

Norcuron powder for IV injection ℞ *nondepolarizing neuromuscular blocker; adjunct to anesthesia* [vecuronium bromide] 10, 20 mg/vial

norcycline [see: sancycline]

nordazepam INN

nordefrin HCl NF

Nordette tablets (in Pilpaks of 21 or 28) ℞ *monophasic oral contraceptive; emergency postcoital contraceptive* [levonorgestrel; ethinyl estradiol] 0.15 mg•30 µg

nordinone INN

NordiPen (trademarked device) *subcu self-injector for Norditropin*

Norditropin powder for subcu injection, prefilled cartridges for NordiPen (self-injection device) ℞ *growth hormone for adults or children with congenital or endogenous growth hor-*

mone deficiency, children with Turner syndrome or renal-induced growth failure [somatropin] 4, 8 mg (12, 24 IU) per vial; 5, 10, 15 mg (15, 30, 45 IU) per 1.5 mL cartridge

Norditropin NordiFlex self-injector ℞ *growth hormone for adults or children with congenital or endogenous growth hormone deficiency, children with Turner syndrome or renal-induced growth failure* [somatropin] 5, 15 mg

Norel capsules (discontinued 2001) ℞ *decongestant; expectorant* [phenylephrine HCl; phenylpropanolamine HCl; guaifenesin] 5•45•200 mg

Norel DM oral liquid ℞ *pediatric decongestant, antihistamine, and expectorant* [phenylephrine HCl; chlorpheniramine maleate; dextromethorphan hydrobromide] 10•4•15 mg/5 mL

Norel LA extended-release tablets ℞ *decongestant; antihistamine* [phenylephrine HCl; carbinoxamine maleate] 40•8 mg

Norel Plus capsules (discontinued 2002) ℞ *decongestant; antihistamine; analgesic* [phenylpropanolamine HCl; chlorpheniramine maleate; phenyltoloxamine dihydrogen citrate; acetaminophen] 25•4•25•325 mg

norelgestromin USAN *investigational progestin-type contraceptive*

norephedrine HCl [see: phenylpropanolamine HCl]

norepinephrine INN *adrenergic; vasoconstrictor; vasopressor for shock* [also: norepinephrine bitartrate]

norepinephrine bitartrate USAN, USP *adrenergic; vasoconstrictor; vasopressor for acute hypotensive shock* [also: norepinephrine] 1 mg/mL injection

norethandrolone NF, INN

norethindrone USP *progestin for amenorrhea, abnormal uterine bleeding, and endometriosis* [also: norethisterone]

norethindrone acetate USP *progestin for amenorrhea, abnormal uterine bleeding, and endometriosis* 5 mg oral

norethisterone INN, BAN, JAN *progestin* [also: norethindrone]

norethynodrel USAN, USP *progestin* [also: noretynodrel]

noretynodrel INN *progestin* [also: norethynodrel]

noreximide INN

norfenefrine INN

Norflex sustained-release tablets, IV or IM injection ℞ *skeletal muscle relaxant* [orphenadrine citrate] 100 mg; 30 mg/mL

norfloxacin USAN, USP, INN, BAN, JAN *broad-spectrum fluoroquinolone antibiotic*

norfloxacin succinil INN

norflurane USAN, INN *inhalation anesthetic*

Norforms vaginal suppositories OTC *feminine deodorant* [polyethylene glycol]

Norgesic; Norgesic Forte tablets ℞ *skeletal muscle relaxant; analgesic* [orphenadrine citrate; aspirin; caffeine] 25•385•30 mg; 50•770•60 mg

norgesterone INN

norgestimate USAN, INN, BAN *progestin*

norgestomet USAN, INN *progestin*

norgestrel USAN, USP, INN *progestin*

d-norgestrel *(incorrect enantiomer designation)* [now: levonorgestrel]

D-norgestrel [see: levonorgestrel]

norgestrienone INN

Norinyl 1 + 35 tablets (in Wallettes of 28) ℞ *monophasic oral contraceptive* [norethindrone; ethinyl estradiol] 1 mg•35 μg 🖉 Nardil

Norinyl 1 + 50 tablets (in Wallettes of 28) ℞ *monophasic oral contraceptive* [norethindrone; mestranol] 1 mg•50 μg

Norisodrine with Calcium Iodide syrup (discontinued 2002) ℞ *bronchodilator; expectorant* [isoproterenol sulfate; calcium iodide; alcohol 6%] 3•150 mg

Noritate cream ℞ *antibiotic for rosacea* [metronidazole] 1%

norletimol INN

norleusactide INN [also: pentacosactride]

norlevorphanol INN, BAN

norlupinanes *a class of antibiotics* [also called: quinolizidines]

½ normal saline (½ NS; 0.45% sodium chloride) *electrolyte replacement*

normal saline (NS; 0.9% sodium chloride) *electrolyte replacement* [also: saline solution]

normal serum albumin [see: albumin, human]

Normaline tablets OTC *sodium chloride replacement; dehydration preventative* [sodium chloride] 250 mg

normethadone INN, BAN

normethandrolone [see: normethandrone]

normethandrone INN

normethisterone [see: normethandrone]

Normodyne film-coated tablets (discontinued 2004) ℞ *antihypertensive; antiadrenergic (α- and β-blocker)* [labetalol HCl] 100, 200, 300 mg

Normodyne IV infusion ℞ *antihypertensive; antiadrenergic (α- and β-blocker)* [labetalol HCl] 5 mg/mL

normorphine INN, BAN

Normosol-M IV infusion ℞ *intravenous electrolyte therapy* [combined electrolyte solution] 1000 mL

Normosol-M and 5% Dextrose; Normosol-R and 5% Dextrose IV infusion ℞ *intravenous nutritional/ electrolyte therapy* [combined electrolyte solution; dextrose]

Normosol-R; Normosol-R pH 7.4 IV infusion ℞ *intravenous electrolyte therapy* [combined electrolyte solution]

Noroxin film-coated tablets ℞ *broad-spectrum fluoroquinolone antibiotic* [norfloxacin] 400 mg

Norpace capsules ℞ *antiarrhythmic* [disopyramide phosphate] 100, 150 mg

Norpace CR controlled-release capsules ℞ *antiarrhythmic* [disopyramide phosphate] 100, 150 mg

norpipanone INN, BAN

Norplant implantable Silastic capsules (discontinued 2003) ℞ *long-term (5-*

year) contraceptive system [levonorgestrel] 216 mg (6 capsules × 36 mg)

Norpramin film-coated tablets ℞ *tricyclic antidepressant* [desipramine HCl] 10, 25, 50, 75, 100, 150 mg ② imipramine

norpseudoephedrine [see: cathine]

Nor-QD tablets (in packs of 28) ℞ *oral contraceptive (progestin only)* [norethindrone] 0.35 mg

nortestosterone phenylpropionate [see: nandrolone phenpropionate]

Nor-Tet capsules ℞ *broad-spectrum antibiotic* [tetracycline HCl] 250, 500 mg

nortetrazepam INN

Nortrel 0.5/35; Nortrel 1/35 tablets (in packs of 21 or 28) ℞ *monophasic oral contraceptive* [norethindrone; ethinyl estradiol] 0.5 mg•35 μg; 1 mg•35 μg

nortriptyline HCl USAN, USP, INN *tricyclic antidepressant* [10, 25, 50, 75 mg oral; 10 mg/5 mL oral] ② amitriptyline

Norvasc tablets ℞ *antianginal; antihypertensive; calcium channel blocker* [amlodipine] 2.5, 5, 10 mg

norvinisterone INN

norvinodrel [see: norgesterone]

Norvir soft capsules, oral solution ℞ *antiviral protease inhibitor for HIV infection* [ritonavir] 100 mg; 80 mg/mL

Norway pine; Norway spruce *medicinal herb* [see: spruce]

Norwich tablets OTC *analgesic; antipyretic; anti-inflammatory; antirheumatic* [aspirin] 325, 500 mg

Norzine IM injection, suppositories, tablets ℞ *antiemetic* [thiethylperazine maleate] 5 mg/mL; 10 mg; 10 mg

nosantine INN, BAN

noscapine USP, INN *antitussive*

noscapine HCl NF

Nose Better gel OTC *emollient; moisturizer; protectant; counterirritant* [allantoin; camphor; menthol] 0.5%•0.75%•0.5%

nosebleed *medicinal herb* [see: yarrow]

nosiheptide USAN, INN *veterinary growth stimulant*

Nōstril; Children's Nōstril nasal spray (discontinued 2002) OTC *nasal decongestant* [phenylephrine HCl] 0.5%; 0.25%

Nōstrilla 12-Hour nasal spray OTC *nasal decongestant* [oxymetazoline HCl] 0.05%

notensil maleate [see: acepromazine]

Notuss PD oral liquid ℞ *narcotic antitussive; decongestant; antihistamine* [hydrocodone bitartrate; phenylephrine HCl; dexchlorpheniramine maleate] 4•5•2 mg/5 mL

Nouriva Repair cream OTC *emollient/protectant* [petrolatum; paraffin; mineral oil]

NovaCare film-coated tablets ℞ *prenatal vitamin/mineral/calcium/iron supplement* [multiple vitamins & minerals; calcium; iron; folic acid] ≛•250•40•1 mg

Novacet lotion ℞ *acne treatment* [sulfacetamide sodium; sulfur] 10%•5%

Novacort gel ℞ *corticosteroidal anti-inflammatory; local anesthetic* [hydrocortisone acetate; pramoxine] 2%•1%

Nova-Dec tablets OTC *vitamin/mineral/iron supplement* [multiple vitamins & minerals; iron; folic acid; biotin] ≛•30 mg•0.4 mg•30 μg

Novafed A sustained-release capsules (discontinued 2002) ℞ *decongestant; antihistamine* [pseudoephedrine HCl; chlorpheniramine maleate] 120•8 mg

Novagest Expectorant with Codeine oral liquid (discontinued 2002) ℞ *narcotic antitussive; decongestant; expectorant* [codeine phosphate; pseudoephedrine HCl; guaifenesin; alcohol 1.4%] 10•30•100 mg/5 mL

Novahistine DH syrup ℞ *narcotic antitussive; decongestant; antihistamine* [codeine phosphate; pseudoephedrine HCl; chlorpheniramine maleate; alcohol 5%] 10•30•2 mg/5 mL

Novahistine DMX oral liquid OTC *antitussive; decongestant; expectorant* [dextromethorphan hydrobromide; pseudoephedrine HCl; guaifenesin; alcohol 5%] 10•30•100 mg/5 mL

novamidon [see: aminopyrine]

Novamine; Novamine 15% IV infusion ℞ *total parenteral nutrition; peripheral parenteral nutrition* [multiple essential and nonessential amino acids]

Novamoxin ⓒ capsules, chewable tablets, oral suspension ℞ *aminopenicillin antibiotic* [amoxicillin trihydrate] 250, 500 mg; 125, 250 mg; 125, 250 mg/5 mL

Novantrone IV infusion ℞ *antibiotic antineoplastic for prostate cancer and acute nonlymphocytic leukemia (ANLL) (orphan); immunomodulator for progressive and relapsing-remitting multiple sclerosis* [mitoxantrone HCl] 2 mg/mL

Novarel powder for IM injection ℞ *gonad-stimulating hormone for prepubertal cryptorchidism and hypogonadism; ovulation stimulant; testosterone stimulant* [chorionic gonadotropin] 1000 U/mL

Novasal film-coated tablets ℞ *analgesic; antipyretic; anti-inflammatory* [magnesium salicylate tetrahydrate] 600 mg

Novasen ⓒ enteric-coated tablets OTC *analgesic; antipyretic; anti-inflammatory; antirheumatic* [aspirin] 325, 650 mg

NovaSource Renal oral liquid OTC *nutritional therapy for renal failure* [multiple vitamins & minerals] 237 mL/pkt.

novel (atypical) antipsychotics *a class of agents with a high affinity to the serotonin receptors and varying degrees of affinity to other neurotransmitter receptors; "atypical" due to the low incidence of extrapyramidal side effects (EPS)* [compare to: conventional (typical) antipsychotics]

Novo-Amiodarone ⓒ tablets ℞ *antiarrhythmic* [amiodarone HCl] 200 mg

novobiocin INN, BAN *bacteriostatic antibiotic* [also: novobiocin calcium]

novobiocin calcium USP *bacteriostatic antibiotic* [also: novobiocin]

novobiocin sodium USP *bacteriostatic antibiotic*

Novocain injection ℞ *injectable local anesthetic for central or peripheral nerve block* [procaine HCl] 1%, 10%

Novo-Cefaclor ⓒ capsules ℞ *cephalosporin antibiotic* [cefaclor] 250, 500 mg

Novo-Cefadroxil ⓒ capsules ℞ *cephalosporin antibiotic* [cefadroxil] 500 mg

Novo-Clonazepam ⓒ tablets ℞ *anticonvulsant* [clonazepam] 0.5, 2 mg

Novo-Cyproterone ⓒ tablets ℞ *antiandrogen antineoplastic for advanced prostatic carcinoma* [cyproterone acetate] 50 mg

Novo-Difenac-K ⓒ tablets ℞ *analgesic; antiarthritic; nonsteroidal anti-inflammatory drug (NSAID)* [diclofenac potassium] 50 mg

Novo-Diltiazem CD ⓒ (once daily) controlled-delivery capsules ℞ *antihypertensive; antianginal; antiarrhythmic; calcium channel blocker* [diltiazem HCl] 120, 180, 240, 300 mg

Novo-Divalproex ⓒ enteric-coated tablets ℞ *anticonvulsant* [divalproex sodium] 125, 250, 500 mg

Novo-Domperidone ⓒ film-coated tablets ℞ *antiemetic for diabetic gastroparesis and chronic gastritis* [domperidone maleate] 10 mg

Novo-Fluvoxamine ⓒ tablets ℞ *selective serotonin reuptake inhibitor (SSRI) for depression and obsessive-compulsive disorder (OCD)* [fluvoxamine maleate] 50, 100 mg

Novo-Gemfibrozil ⓒ capsules, tablets ℞ *antihyperlipidemic for hypertriglyceridemia and coronary heart disease* [gemfibrozil] 300 mg; 600 mg

Novo-Glyburide ⓒ tablets ℞ *sulfonylurea antidiabetic* [glyburide] 2.5, 5 mg

Novo-Hydrazide ⓒ tablets ℞ *antihypertensive; diuretic* [hydrochlorothiazide] 25, 50 mg

Novo-Ketoconazole ⓒ tablets ℞ *broad-spectrum antifungal* [ketoconazole] 200 mg

Novolin 70/30 vials for subcu injection OTC *antidiabetic* [isophane human insulin (rDNA); human insulin (rDNA)] 100 U/mL

Novolin 70/30 PenFill NovoPen cartridge OTC *antidiabetic* [isophane human insulin (rDNA); human insulin (rDNA)] 150 U/1.5 mL, 300 U/3 mL

Novolin 70/30 Prefilled syringes OTC *antidiabetic* [isophane human insulin (rDNA); human insulin (rDNA)] 150 U/1.5 mL

Novolin ge 10/90 PenFill ⓒⒶⓃ NovoPen cartridges OTC *antidiabetic* [human insulin (rDNA); isophane human insulin (rDNA)] 3 mL

Novolin ge 20/80 PenFill ⓒⒶⓃ NovoPen cartridges OTC *antidiabetic* [human insulin (rDNA); isophane human insulin (rDNA)] 3 mL

Novolin ge 30/70 ⓒⒶⓃ vials for subcu injection OTC *antidiabetic* [human insulin (rDNA); isophane human insulin (rDNA)] 100 U/mL; 1.5, 3 mL

Novolin ge 30/70 PenFill ⓒⒶⓃ NovoPen cartridges OTC *antidiabetic* [human insulin (rDNA); isophane human insulin (rDNA)] 100 U/mL; 1.5, 3 mL

Novolin ge 40/60 PenFill ⓒⒶⓃ NovoPen cartridges OTC *antidiabetic* [human insulin (rDNA); isophane human insulin (rDNA)] 3 mL

Novolin ge 50/50 PenFill ⓒⒶⓃ NovoPen cartridges OTC *antidiabetic* [human insulin (rDNA); isophane human insulin (rDNA)] 3 mL

Novolin ge Lente ⓒⒶⓃ vials for subcu injection OTC *antidiabetic* [human insulin zinc (rDNA)] 100 U/mL

Novolin ge NPH ⓒⒶⓃ vials for subcu injection OTC *antidiabetic* [isophane human insulin (rDNA)] 100 U/mL; 1.5, 3 mL

Novolin ge NPH PenFill ⓒⒶⓃ NovoPen cartridges OTC *antidiabetic* [isophane human insulin (rDNA)] 100 U/mL; 1.5, 3 mL

Novolin ge Toronto ⓒⒶⓃ vials for subcu injection OTC *antidiabetic* [human insulin (rDNA)] 100 U/mL; 1.5, 3 mL

Novolin ge Toronto PenFill ⓒⒶⓃ NovoPen cartridges OTC *antidiabetic* [human insulin (rDNA)] 100 U/mL; 1.5, 3 mL

Novolin ge Ultralente ⓒⒶⓃ vials for subcu injection OTC *antidiabetic* [human insulin zinc (rDNA)] 100 U/mL

Novolin L vials for subcu injection (discontinued 2003) OTC *antidiabetic* [insulin zinc, human (rDNA)] 100 U/mL

Novolin N vials for subcu injection OTC *antidiabetic* [isophane human insulin (rDNA)] 100 U/mL

Novolin N PenFill NovoPen cartridge OTC *antidiabetic* [isophane human insulin (rDNA)] 150 U/1.5 mL, 300 U/3 mL

Novolin N Prefilled syringes OTC *antidiabetic* [isophane human insulin (rDNA)] 150 U/1.5 mL

Novolin R vials for subcu injection OTC *antidiabetic* [human insulin (rDNA)] 100 U/mL

Novolin R PenFill NovoPen cartridges OTC *antidiabetic* [human insulin (rDNA)] 150 U/1.5 mL, 300 U/3 mL

Novolin R Prefilled syringes OTC *antidiabetic* [human insulin (rDNA)] 150 U/1.5 mL

NovoLog vials for subcu injection ℞ *rapid-acting insulin analogue for diabetes* [human insulin aspart (rDNA)] 100 U/mL

NovoLog FlexPen self-injector ℞ *rapid-acting insulin analogue for diabetes* [human insulin aspart (rDNA)] 300 U/3 mL

NovoLog Mix 70/30 FlexPen self-injector ℞ *rapid-acting insulin analogue for diabetes* [insulin aspart protamine; insulin aspart] 70%•30%

NovoLog Mix 70/30 PenFill NovoPen cartridges ℞ *rapid-acting insulin analogue for diabetes* [insulin aspart protamine; insulin aspart] 70%•30%

NovoLog PenFill NovoPen cartridges ℞ *rapid-acting insulin analogue for dia-*

betes [human insulin aspart (rDNA)] 300 U/3 mL

Novo-Lorazem Ⓒ tablets ℞ *benzodiazepine anxiolytic* [lorazepam] 0.5, 1, 2 mg

Novo-Medrone Ⓒ tablets ℞ *progestin for secondary amenorrhea, abnormal uterine bleeding, and endometrial hyperplasia* [medroxyprogesterone acetate] 2.5, 5, 10 mg

Novo-Metformin Ⓒ film-coated tablets ℞ *biguanide antidiabetic* [metformin HCl] 500, 850 mg

Novo-Metoprol Ⓒ tablets, film-coated caplets ℞ *antihypertensive; antianginal; antiadrenergic (β-blocker)* [metoprolol tartrate] 50, 100 mg

Novo-Moclobemide Ⓒ tablets ℞ *antidepressant* [moclobemide] 100, 150, 300 mg

Novo-Naprox Ⓒ tablets ℞ *analgesic; antiarthritic; nonsteroidal anti-inflammatory drug (NSAID)* [naproxen] 125, 250, 375, 500 mg

Novo-Naprox SR Ⓒ sustained-release tablets ℞ *analgesic; antiarthritic; nonsteroidal anti-inflammatory drug (NSAID)* [naproxen] 750 mg

Novo-Naprox-EC Ⓒ enteric-coated tablets ℞ *analgesic; antiarthritic; nonsteroidal anti-inflammatory drug (NSAID)* [naproxen] 250, 375, 500 mg

Novo-Nizatidine Ⓒ capsules ℞ *histamine H₂ antagonist for treatment of gastric and duodenal ulcers* [nizatidine] 150, 300 mg

Novo-Norfloxacin Ⓒ tablets ℞ *broad-spectrum fluoroquinolone antibiotic* [norfloxacin] 400 mg

NovoNorm (European name for U.S. product **Prandin**)

Novopaque oral/rectal suspension (discontinued 2001) ℞ *radiopaque contrast medium for gastrointestinal imaging* [barium sulfate] 60%

NovoPen 1.5; NovoPen Junior pre-filled reusable syringe *uses Novolin PenFill cartridges and NovoFine 30-gauge disposable needles* [insulin (several types available)] 1–40 U/injection

Novo-Ranidine Ⓒ film-coated tablets ℞ *histamine H₂ antagonist for gastric and duodenal ulcers* [ranitidine HCl] 150, 300 mg

NovoRapid Ⓒ vials for subcu injection ℞ *rapid-acting insulin analogue for diabetes* [insulin aspart, human (rDNA)] 100 U/mL

Novo-Salmol Ⓒ tablets ℞ *sympathomimetic bronchodilator* [salbutamol sulfate] 2, 4 mg

Novo-Semide Ⓒ tablets ℞ *antihypertensive; loop diuretic* [furosemide] 20, 40, 80 mg

Novo-Sertraline Ⓒ capsules ℞ *selective serotonin reuptake inhibitor (SSRI) for depression* [sertraline HCl] 25, 50, 100 mg

NovoSeven powder for IV injection ℞ *coagulant for hemophilia A and B (orphan)* [factor VIIa, recombinant] 1.2, 2.4, 4.8 mg/vial

Novo-Terazosin Ⓒ tablets ℞ *antihypertensive (α-blocker); treatment for benign prostatic hyperplasia (BPH)* [terazosin HCl] 1, 2, 5, 10 mg

Novo-Timol Ⓒ eye drops (discontinued 2001) ℞ *topical antiglaucoma agent (β-blocker)* [timolol maleate] 0.25%, 0.5%

Novo-Triptyn Ⓒ tablets ℞ *tricyclic antidepressant* [amitriptyline HCl] 10, 25, 50 mg

Novoxapam Ⓒ tablets ℞ *benzodiazepine anxiolytic* [oxazepam] 10, 15, 30 mg

NOVP (Novantrone, Oncovin, vinblastine, prednisone) *chemotherapy protocol for Hodgkin lymphoma*

noxiptiline INN [also: noxiptyline]

noxiptyline BAN [also: noxiptiline]

noxythiolin BAN [also: noxytiolin]

noxytiolin INN [also: noxythiolin]

NP (nifurpipone) [q.v.]

NPH (neutral protamine Hagedorn) insulin [see: insulin, isophane]

NPH Iletin II vials for subcu injection (discontinued 2005) OTC *antidiabetic* [isophane insulin (pork)] 100 U/mL

NRTIs (nucleoside reverse transcriptase inhibitors) [see: reverse transcriptase inhibitors]

NS (normal saline) [q.v.]

NSAIDs (nonsteroidal anti-inflammatory drugs) [q.v.] Ⓡ InFeD

NTBC *investigational (orphan) for tyrosinemia type I*

NTZ (nitazoxanide) [q.v.]

NTZ Long Acting nasal spray, nose drops (discontinued 2002) OTC *nasal decongestant* [oxymetazoline HCl] 0.05%

Nubain IV, IM, or subcu injection ℞ *narcotic agonist-antagonist analgesic for moderate to severe pain; adjunct to obstetric and surgical analgesia* [nalbuphine HCl] 10, 20 mg/mL

Nu-Beclomethasone Ⓒᴬᴺ nasal spray ℞ *corticosteroidal anti-inflammatory for chronic asthma and rhinitis* [beclomethasone dipropionate] 50 μg/ metered dose

nucleoside reverse transcriptase inhibitors (NRTI) *a class of antiretroviral drugs that inhibits the activity of reverse transcriptase (polymerase) in viral cells, causing a termination of DNA chain elongation, which prevents replication of the cells* [see: reverse transcriptase inhibitors]

nuclomedone INN

nuclotixene INN

Nucofed capsules, syrup ℞ *narcotic antitussive; decongestant* [codeine phosphate; pseudoephedrine HCl] 20•60 mg; 20•60 mg/5 mL

Nucofed Expectorant syrup (discontinued 2002) ℞ *narcotic antitussive; decongestant; expectorant* [codeine phosphate; pseudoephedrine HCl; guaifenesin; alcohol 12.5%] 20•60• 200 mg/5 mL

Nucofed Pediatric Expectorant syrup ℞ *narcotic antitussive; decongestant; expectorant* [codeine phosphate; pseudoephedrine HCl; guaifenesin; alcohol 6%] 10•30•100 mg/5 mL

Nucotuss Expectorant oral liquid (discontinued 2002) ℞ *narcotic anti-*

tussive; decongestant; expectorant [codeine phosphate; pseudoephedrine HCl; guaifenesin; alcohol 12.5%] 20•60•200 mg/5 mL

Nucotuss Pediatric Expectorant oral liquid ℞ *narcotic antitussive; decongestant; expectorant* [codeine phosphate; pseudoephedrine HCl; guaifenesin; alcohol 6%] 10•30•100 mg/5 mL

Nu-Diltiaz-CD Ⓒᴬᴺ capsules ℞ *antihypertensive; antianginal* [diltiazem HCl] 120, 180, 240 mg

Nu-Divalproex Ⓒᴬᴺ tablets ℞ *anticonvulsant* [divalproex sodium] 125, 250, 500 mg

Nu-Enalapril Ⓒᴬᴺ tablets ℞ *antihypertensive; angiotensin-converting enzyme (ACE) inhibitor* [enalapril maleate]

nufenoxole USAN, INN *antiperistaltic*

Nu-Fluvoxamine Ⓒᴬᴺ tablets ℞ *selective serotonin reuptake inhibitor (SSRI) for depression and obsessive-compulsive disorder (OCD)* [fluvoxamine maleate]

Nuhist pediatric oral suspension ℞ *decongestant; antihistamine* [phenylephrine tannate; chlorpheniramine tannate] 5•4.5 mg/5 mL

Nu-Iron elixir (discontinued 2005) OTC *hematinic; iron supplement* [polysaccharide-iron complex] 100 mg Fe/5 mL

Nu-Iron 150 capsules OTC *hematinic; iron supplement* [polysaccharide-iron complex] 150 mg Fe

Nu-Iron Plus elixir ℞ *hematinic* [polysaccharide-iron complex; cyanocobalamin; folic acid] 300 mg•75 μg• 3 mg per 15 mL

Nu-Iron V film-coated tablets ℞ *vitamin/iron supplement* [polysaccharide-iron complex; multiple vitamins; folic acid] 60•±•1 mg

Nu-knit (trademarked form) *oxidized cellulose hemostatic pad*

NuLev orally disintegrating tablets ℞ *GI/GU antispasmodic; antiparkinsonian; anticholinergic "drying agent" for allergic rhinitis* [hyoscyamine sulfate] 0.125 mg

NuLytely powder for oral solution ℞ *pre-procedure bowel evacuant* [polyethylene glycol–electrolyte solution (PEG 3350)] 60, 105 g/L

Nu-Moclobemide ⊛ tablets ℞ *antidepressant* [moclobemide] 100, 150 mg

Numorphan IV, IM, or subcu injection, suppositories ℞ *narcotic analgesic; preoperative support of anesthesia; investigational (orphan) for intractable pain in narcotic-tolerant patients* [oxymorphone HCl] 1, 1.5 mg/mL; 5 mg

Numzident gel OTC *topical oral anesthetic* [benzocaine] 10%

Numzit Teething gel OTC *topical oral anesthetic* [benzocaine] 7.5%

Numzit Teething lotion OTC *topical oral anesthetic* [benzocaine; alcohol 12.1%] 0.2%

Nu-Natal Advanced film-coated tablets ℞ *vitamin/mineral/calcium/iron supplement; stool softener* [multiple vitamins & minerals; calcium; iron; folic acid; docusate sodium] ≟ • 200•90•1•50 mg

Nupercainal cream (discontinued 2005) OTC *topical local anesthetic* [dibucaine] 0.5%

Nupercainal ointment OTC *topical local anesthetic* [dibucaine] 1%

Nupercainal rectal suppositories OTC *emollient; astringent* [cocoa butter; zinc oxide] 2.1•0.25 g

Nuprin tablets, caplets OTC *analgesic; antiarthritic; antipyretic; nonsteroidal anti-inflammatory drug (NSAID)* [ibuprofen] 200 mg

Nuprin Backache caplets OTC *analgesic; antipyretic; anti-inflammatory* [magnesium salicylate] 580 mg

Nu-Prochlor ⊛ film-coated tablets ℞ *conventional (typical) phenothiazine antipsychotic for schizophrenia; anxiolytic; antiemetic for nausea and vomiting; also used for acute treatment of migraine headaches* [prochlorperazine bimaleate] 5, 10 mg

Nuquin HP cream ℞ *hyperpigmentation bleaching agent* [hydroquinone (in a sunscreen base)] 4%

Nuquin HP gel (discontinued 2003) ℞ *hyperpigmentation bleaching agent* [hydroquinone (in a sunscreen base)] 4%

Nuromax IV injection (discontinued 2004) ℞ *nondepolarizing neuromuscular blocker; adjunct to anesthesia* [doxacurium chloride] 1 mg/mL

Nursette (trademarked form) *prefilled disposable bottle*

Nu-Salt OTC *salt substitute* [potassium chloride] 68 mEq K/5 g

nut, oil *medicinal herb* [see: butternut]

Nu-Tears eye drops OTC *ophthalmic moisturizer/lubricant* [polyvinyl alcohol] 1.4%

Nu-Tears II eye drops OTC *ophthalmic moisturizer/lubricant* [polyvinyl alcohol; polyethylene glycol 400] 1%•1%

Nu-Timolol ⊛ tablets ℞ *antihypertensive; antiadrenergic (β-blocker); migraine prophylaxis* [timolol maleate] 5, 10, 20 mg

nutmeg (Myristica fragrans) seed and aril *medicinal herb for diarrhea, flatulence, inducing expectoration, insomnia, mouth sores, rheumatism, salivary stimulation, and stimulating menstruation*

nutmeg oil NF

Nutracort cream ℞ *topical corticosteroidal anti-inflammatory* [hydrocortisone] 1%

Nutraderm cream, lotion OTC *moisturizer; emollient*

Nutraderm OTC *lotion base*

Nutraderm Bath Oil OTC *bath emollient*

Nutraloric powder OTC *enteral nutritional therapy* [milk-based formula]

Nutrament oral liquid OTC *enteral nutritional therapy* 12 oz. cans

Nutramigen oral liquid, powder for oral liquid OTC *hypoallergenic infant food* [enzymatically hydrolyzed protein formula]

Nutraplus cream, lotion OTC *moisturizer; emollient; keratolytic* [urea] 10%

Nutra-Soothe bath oil OTC *bath emollient* [colloidal oatmeal; light mineral oil]

Nutren 1.0 oral liquid OTC *enteral nutritional therapy* [lactose-free formula]

Nutren 1.5 oral liquid OTC *enteral nutritional therapy* [lactose-free formula]

Nutren 2.0 ready-to-use oral liquid OTC *enteral nutritional therapy* [lactose-free formula]

Nutr-E-Sol oral liquid OTC *vitamin supplement* [vitamin E] 133 IU/5 mL

Nutricon tablets OTC *vitamin/mineral/calcium/iron supplement* [multiple vitamins & minerals; calcium; iron; folic acid; biotin] ± • 200 • 20 • 0.4 • 0.15 mg

Nutrifac ZX caplets ℞ *vitamin/mineral supplement* [multiple vitamins & minerals; folic acid; biotin] ± • 1 • 0.2 mg

NutriFocus ready-to-use oral liquid OTC *enteral nutritional therapy* [milk-based formula] 237 mL cans

NutriHeal ready-to-use oral liquid OTC *enteral nutritional therapy* [milk-based formula] 250 mL cans

Nutrilan ready-to-use oral liquid OTC *enteral nutritional therapy* [lactose-free formula]

Nutrilyte; Nutrilyte II IV admixture ℞ *intravenous electrolyte therapy* [combined electrolyte solution]

Nutrineal Peritoneal Dialysis Solution with 1.1% Amino Acid ℞ *investigational (orphan) nutritional supplement for continuous ambulatory peritoneal dialysis patients*

Nutropin powder for subcu injection ℞ *growth hormone for adults or children with congenital or endogenous growth hormone deficiency, children with Turner syndrome or renal-induced growth failure, or AIDS-wasting syndrome (orphan)* [somatropin] 5, 10 mg (13, 26 IU)/vial

Nutropin AQ subcu injection, Pen (prefilled syringe) ℞ *growth hormone for congenital or renal-induced growth failure and Turner syndrome (orphan); investigational (orphan) for severe burns* [somatropin] 10 mg (30 IU)/vial, 10 mg (30 IU)/2 mL cartridge

Nutropin Depot sustained-release injection (discontinued 2004) ℞

once- or twice-monthly doseform [somatropin] 13.5, 18, 22.5 mg

Nutrox capsules OTC *dietary supplement* [multiple vitamins & minerals; multiple amino acids]

Nu-Valproic ⒸⒶⓃ capsules ℞ *anticonvulsant* [valproic acid] 250 mg

NuvaRing vaginal ring ℞ *self-administered one-month contraceptive insert* [ethinyl estradiol; etonogestrel] 15 • 120 μg/day

nuvenzepine INN

Nuvion ℞ *investigational monoclonal antibody for organ transplants, autoimmune diseases, and other T lymphocyte disorders* [visilizumab]

nyctal [see: carbromal]

nydrane [see: benzchlorpropamid]

Nydrazid IM injection ℞ *tuberculostatic* [isoniazid] 100 mg/mL

nylestriol USAN *estrogen* [also: nilestriol]

nylidrin HCl USP *peripheral vasodilator* [also: buphenine]

Nymphaea odorata medicinal herb [see: white pond lilly]

NyQuil Cold/Cough Relief, Children's oral liquid OTC *antitussive; decongestant; antihistamine* [dextromethorphan hydrobromide; pseudoephedrine HCl; chlorpheniramine maleate] 15 • 30 • 2 mg/15 mL

NyQuil Cough syrup OTC *antitussive; antihistamine* [dextromethorphan hydrobromide; doxylamine succinate] 30 • 12.5 mg/30 mL

NyQuil Hot Therapy powder for oral solution (discontinued 2002) OTC *antitussive; decongestant; antihistamine; analgesic* [dextromethorphan hydrobromide; pseudoephedrine HCl; doxylamine succinate; acetaminophen] 30 • 60 • 12.5 • 1000 mg/pkt.

NyQuil LiquiCaps (name changed to NyQuil Multi-Symptom Cold & Flu Relief in 2002)

NyQuil Multi-Symptom Cold & Flu Relief LiquiCaps (liquid-filled capsules) OTC *antitussive; decongestant; antihistamine; analgesic* [dextromethorphan hydrobromide; pseudoephedrine

HCl; doxylamine succinate; aceta-
minophen] 10•30•6.25•250 mg

**NyQuil Multisymptom Cold/Flu
Relief** oral liquid OTC *antitussive;
decongestant; antihistamine; analgesic*
[dextromethorphan hydrobromide;
pseudoephedrine HCl; doxylamine
succinate; acetaminophen; alcohol
10%] 30•60•12.5•1000 mg/30 mL

**NyQuil Nighttime Cold/Flu Medi-
cine** oral liquid (discontinued 2002)
OTC *antitussive; decongestant; antihistamine; analgesic* [dextromethorphan
hydrobromide; pseudoephedrine
HCl; doxylamine succinate; acetaminophen; alcohol 25%] 5•10•
1.25•167 mg/5 mL

nystatin USAN, INN, BAN, JAN *polyene
antifungal* 500 000 U/mL oral;
100 000 mg vaginal; 100 000 U/g
topical ⚗ Nilstat; Nitrostat

Nystex cream, ointment (discontinued 2003) ℞ *antifungal* [nystatin]
100 000 U/g

Nystex oral suspension (discontinued
2003) ℞ *antifungal; oral candidiasis
treatment* [nystatin] 100 000 U/mL

Nystop powder ℞ *topical antifungal*
[nystatin] 100 000 U/g

Nytcold Medicine oral liquid (discontinued 2002) OTC *antitussive;
decongestant; antihistamine; analgesic*
[dextromethorphan hydrobromide;
pseudoephedrine HCl; doxylamine
succinate; acetaminophen; alcohol
25%] 5•10•1.25•167 mg/5 mL

Nytol tablets OTC *antihistaminic sleep aid*
[diphenhydramine HCl] 25, 50 mg

**NZGLM (New Zealand green-
lipped mussel)** [q.v.]

O₂ (oxygen) [q.v.]

oak *medicinal herb* [see: white oak]

OAP (Oncovin, ara-C, prednisone)
chemotherapy protocol

oatmeal, colloidal *demulcent*

oats (Avena sativa) grain and straw
*medicinal herb for dry itchy skin, hyper-
lipidemia, indigestion, insomnia, nervousness, opium addiction, reducing
the desire to smoke, and strengthening
the heart*

obecalp *placebo (spelled backward)* [q.v.]

Obenix capsules (discontinued 2001)
℞ *anorexiant; CNS stimulant* [phen-
termine HCl] 37.5 mg

obidoxime chloride USAN, INN *cholinesterase reactivator*

oblimersen sodium *investigational
(NDA filed) antisense therapy for lung
cancer and chronic lymphocytic leukemia*

Obstetrix-100 tablets ℞ *prenatal vita-
min/mineral/calcium/iron supplement;
stool softener* [multiple vitamins; cal-

cium; iron; folic acid; zinc; docusate
sodium] ±•250•100•1•25•50 mg

Obtrex tablets ℞ *prenatal vitamin/min-
eral supplement; stool softener* [multi-
ple vitamins and minerals; docusate
sodium] ±•50 mg

O-Cal f.a. tablets ℞ *vitamin/mineral/cal-
cium/iron supplement and dental caries
preventative* [multiple vitamins & minerals; calcium; iron; folic acid; sodium
fluoride] ±•200•66•1•1.1 mg

O-Cal Prenatal tablets ℞ *vitamin/min-
eral/calcium/iron supplement* [multiple
vitamins & minerals; calcium; iron;
folic acid] ±•200•15•1 mg

ocaperidone USAN, INN, BAN *antipsychotic*

Occlusal-HP topical liquid OTC *keratolytic* [salicylic acid in polyacrylic
vehicle] 17%

Occucoat ophthalmic solution ℞ *ophthalmic surgical aid* [hydroxypropyl
methylcellulose] 2%

Ocean; Ocean for Kids nasal spray OTC *nasal moisturizer* [sodium chloride (saline solution)] 0.65%

ocfentanil INN *narcotic analgesic* [also: ocfentanil HCl]

ocfentanil HCl USAN *narcotic analgesic* [also: ocfentanil]

ociltide INN

Ocimum basilicum medicinal herb [see: basil]

ocinaplon USAN *anxiolytic*

OCL oral solution Rx *pre-procedure bowel evacuant* [polyethylene glycol–electrolyte solution (PEG 3350)] 60 g/L

ocrase INN

ocrilate INN *tissue adhesive* [also: ocrylate]

ocrylate USAN *tissue adhesive* [also: ocrilate]

OCT (22-oxacalcitriol) [see: maxacalcitol]

octabenzone USAN, INN *ultraviolet screen*

octacaine INN

octacosactrin BAN [also: tosactide]

octacosanol *natural extract of wheat germ used to treat hypercholesterolemia; effective for lowering LDL-cholesterol, raising HDL-cholesterol, stopping the formation of arterial lesions and plaque deposits, and inhibiting clot formation*

octadecafluorodecehydronaphthalene [see: perflunafene]

octadecanoic acid, calcium salt [see: calcium stearate]

octadecanoic acid, sodium salt [see: sodium stearate]

octadecanoic acid, zinc salt [see: zinc stearate]

1-octadecanol [see: stearyl alcohol]

9-octadecenylamine hydrofluoride [see: dectaflur]

octafonium chloride INN

Octagam IV infusion Rx *passive immunizing agent for primary immune deficient diseases and severe combined immunodeficiencies* [immune globulin] 5% in 1, 2.5, 5, 10 g bottles

Octamide PFS IV or IM injection Rx *antiemetic for chemotherapy; GI stimulant; peristaltic* [metoclopramide HCl] 5 mg/mL

octamoxin INN

octamylamine INN

octanoic acid USAN, INN *antifungal*

octapinol INN

octastine INN

octatropine methylbromide INN, BAN *anticholinergic; peptic ulcer adjunct* [also: anisotropine methylbromide]

octatropone bromide [see: anisotropine methylbromide]

octaverine INN, BAN

octazamide USAN, INN *analgesic*

octenidine INN, BAN *topical anti-infective* [also: octenidine HCl]

octenidine HCl USAN *topical anti-infective* [also: octenidine]

octenidine saccharin USAN *dental plaque inhibitor*

Octicare ear drops, ear drop suspension Rx *topical corticosteroidal anti-inflammatory; antibiotic* [hydrocortisone; neomycin sulfate; polymyxin B sulfate] 1%•5 mg•10 000 U per mL

octicizer USAN *plasticizer*

octil INN *combining name for radicals or groups*

octimibate INN

octinoxate USAN *ultraviolet B sunscreen*

octisalate USAN *ultraviolet sunscreen*

octisamyl [see: octamylamine]

Octocaine HCl injection Rx *injectable local anesthetic* [lidocaine HCl; epinephrine] 2%•1:50 000, 2%•1:100 000

octoclothepine [see: clorotepine]

octocrilene INN *ultraviolet screen* [also: octocrylene]

octocrylene USAN *ultraviolet screen* [also: octocrilene]

octodecactide [see: codactide]

octodrine USAN, INN *adrenergic; vasoconstrictor; local anesthetic*

octopamine INN

octotiamine INN

octoxinol INN *surfactant/wetting agent* [also: octoxynol 9]

octoxynol 9 USAN, NF *surfactant/wetting agent; spermicide* [also: octoxinol]

OctreoScan powder for injection ℞ *radiopaque contrast medium* [oxidron-ate sodium] 2 mg

OctreoScan 111 injection ℞ *radioactive imaging agent for SPECT scans of neuroendocrine tumors* [indium In 111 pentetreotide] 10 μg/vial

octreotide USAN, INN, BAN *gastric antisecretory*

octreotide acetate USAN *gastric antisecretory for acromegaly and severe diarrhea due to VIPomas and other tumors (orphan)*

octreotide pamoate USAN *antineoplastic*

octriptyline INN *antidepressant* [also: octriptyline phosphate]

octriptyline phosphate USAN *antidepressant* [also: octriptyline]

octrizole USAN, INN *ultraviolet screen*

octyl methoxycinnamate [see: octinoxate]

octyl salicylate [see: octisalate]

S-octyl thiobenzoate [see: tioctilate]

octyl-2-cyanoacrylate [see: ocrylate]

octyldodecanol NF *oleaginous vehicle*

OcuCaps caplets OTC *vitamin/mineral supplement* [vitamins A, C, and E; multiple minerals] 5000 IU•400 mg•182 mg• ±

OcuClear eye drops OTC *topical ophthalmic decongestant and vasoconstrictor* [oxymetazoline HCl] 0.025%

OcuCoat prefilled syringe OTC *ophthalmic surgical aid* [hydroxypropyl methylcellulose] 2%

OcuCoat; OcuCoat PF eye drops OTC *ophthalmic moisturizer/lubricant* [hydroxypropyl methylcellulose] 0.8%

Ocudose (trademarked delivery device) *single-use eye drop dispenser*

Ocufen eye drops ℞ *topical ophthalmic nonsteroidal anti-inflammatory drug (NSAID); intraoperative miosis inhibitor* [flurbiprofen sodium] 0.03%

ocufilcon A USAN *hydrophilic contact lens material*

ocufilcon B USAN *hydrophilic contact lens material*

ocufilcon C USAN *hydrophilic contact lens material*

ocufilcon D USAN *hydrophilic contact lens material*

ocufilcon F USAN *hydrophilic contact lens material*

Ocuflox eye drops ℞ *topical fluoroquinolone antibiotic for bacterial conjunctivitis and corneal ulcers (orphan)* [ofloxacin] 0.3%

Ocumeter (trademarked delivery device) *prefilled eye drop dispenser*

Ocupress eye drops ℞ *antiglaucoma agent (β-blocker)* [carteolol HCl] 1%

Ocusert Pilo-20; Ocusert Pilo-40 continuous-release ocular wafer ℞ *topical antiglaucoma agent; direct-acting miotic* [pilocarpine] 20 μg/hr.; 40 μg/hr.

OCuSOFT solution, pads OTC *eyelid cleanser for blepharitis or contact lenses*

OCuSoft VMS film-coated tablets OTC *vitamin/mineral supplement* [vitamins A, C, and E; multiple minerals] 5000 IU•60 mg•30 mg• ±

Ocusulf-10 eye drops ℞ *antibiotic* [sulfacetamide sodium] 10%

Ocutricin ophthalmic ointment ℞ *topical ophthalmic antibiotic* [polymyxin B sulfate; neomycin sulfate; bacitracin zinc] 10 000 U•3.5 mg•400 U per g

Ocuvite; Ocuvite PreserVision film-coated tablets OTC *vitamin/mineral supplement* [vitamins A, C, and E; multiple minerals] 5000 IU•60 mg•30 IU• ±; 7160 IU•113 mg•100 IU• ±

Ocuvite Extra tablets OTC *vitamin/mineral supplement* [vitamins A, C, and E; multiple B vitamins; multiple minerals; lutein] 1000 IU•300 mg•100 IU• ± • ± •2 mg

Ocuvite Lutein capsules OTC *vitamin/mineral supplement* [vitamins C and E; multiple minerals; lutein] 60 mg•30 IU• ± •6 mg

Odor Free ArthriCare [see: ArthriCare, Odor Free]

Oenothera biennis *medicinal herb* [see: evening primrose]

OEP (oil of evening primrose) [see: evening primrose]

Oesclim ⓒ transdermal patch ℞ *estrogen replacement therapy for post-menopausal symptoms* [estradiol-17β hemihydrate] 25, 50 μg/day

Oesto-Mins powder OTC *vitamin/mineral supplement* [vitamins C and D; calcium; magnesium; potassium] 500 mg•100 IU•250 mg•250 mg•45 mg per 4.5 g

oestradiol BAN *estrogen replacement therapy for the treatment of postmeno-pausal disorders and prevention of post-menopausal osteoporosis; palliative therapy for prostatic and breast cancers* [also: estradiol]

oestradiol benzoate BAN [also: estradiol benzoate]

oestradiol valerate BAN *estrogen* [also: estradiol valerate]

oestriol succinate BAN *estrogen* [also: estriol; estriol succinate]

oestrogenine [see: diethylstilbestrol]

oestromenin [see: diethylstilbestrol]

oestrone BAN *estrogen replacement therapy for postmenopausal disorders; palliative therapy for prostatic and breast cancers* [also: estrone]

Off-Ezy Corn & Callus Remover kit (topical liquid + cushion pads) OTC *keratolytic* [salicylic acid in a collodion-like vehicle] 17%

Off-Ezy Wart Remover topical liquid OTC *keratolytic* [salicylic acid in a collodion-like vehicle] 17%

ofloxacin USAN, INN, BAN, JAN *broad-spectrum fluoroquinolone antibiotic; topical corneal ulcer treatment* (orphan) 200, 300, 400 mg oral; 0.3% eye drops

ofornine USAN, INN *antihypertensive*

oftasceine INN

Ogen tablets ℞ *bioidentical human estrogen replacement therapy for the treatment of postmenopausal symptoms and prevention of postmenopausal osteoporosis* [estrone (from estropipate)] 0.625 (0.75), 1.25 (1.5), 2.5 (3) mg

Ogen Vaginal cream ℞ *natural estrogen replacement for postmenopausal atrophic vaginitis* [estropipate] 1.5 mg/g

Ogestrel 0.5/50 tablets (in packs of 28) ℞ *monophasic oral contraceptive; emergency postcoital contraceptive* [norgestrel; ethinyl estradiol] 0.5 mg•50 μg

oglufanide disodium USAN *immuno-modulator; investigational (Phase III) angiogenesis inhibitor antineoplastic for Kaposi sarcoma and solid tumor cancers*

oidiomycin *diagnostic aid for cell-mediated immunity; extract of the Oidio-mycetes fungus family*

oil nut *medicinal herb* [see: butternut]

oil of evening primrose (OEP) [see: evening primrose]

oil of mustard [see: allyl isothiocyanate]

Oil of Olay Foaming Face Wash topical liquid OTC *cleanser for acne*

oil ricini [see: castor oil]

Oilatum Soap bar OTC *therapeutic skin cleanser*

ointment, hydrophilic USP *ointment base; oil-in-water emulsion*

ointment, white USP *oleaginous ointment base*

ointment, yellow USP *ointment base*

olaflur USAN, INN, BAN *dental caries prophylactic*

olamine USAN, INN *combining name for radicals or groups*

olanexidine HCl USAN *topical antibiotic for nosocomial or wound infections*

olanzapine USAN, INN *novel (atypical) thienobenzodiazepine antipsychotic for schizophrenia and manic episodes of a bipolar disorder; also used for obsessive-compulsive disorder (OCD) and agitation or psychosis due to Alzheimer or other dementias*

olaquindox INN, BAN

old man's beard *medicinal herb* [see: fringe tree; woodbine]

old tuberculin (OT) [see: tuberculin]

Olea europaea medicinal herb [see: olive]

oleander (Nerium indicum; N. oleander) plant *medicinal herb for asthma, cancer, corns, epilepsy, and heart disease; not generally regarded as safe and effective in any form as it is very toxic*

oleandomycin INN [also: oleandomycin phosphate]

oleandomycin, triacetate ester [see: troleandomycin]

oleandomycin phosphate NF [also: oleandomycin]

oleic acid NF emulsion adjunct

oleic acid I 125 USAN radioactive agent

oleic acid I 131 USAN radioactive agent

oleovitamin A [now: vitamin A]

oleovitamin A & D USP source of vitamins A and D

oleovitamin D, synthetic [now: ergocalciferol]

olethytan 20 [see: polysorbate 80]

oletimol INN

oleum caryophylii [see: clove oil]

oleum gossypii seminis [see: cottonseed oil]

oleum maydis [see: corn oil]

oleum ricini [see: castor oil]

oleyl alcohol NF emulsifying agent; emollient

oligomycin D [see: rutamycin]

olive (Olea europaea) leaves, bark, and fruit medicinal herb used as an antiseptic, astringent, cholagogue, demulcent, emollient, febrifuge, hypoglycemic, laxative, and tranquilizer

olive, spurge; spurge laurel medicinal herb [see: mezereon]

olive oil NF pharmaceutic aid

olivomycin INN

olmesartan USAN antihypertensive; angiotensin II receptor antagonist

olmesartan medoxomil USAN, INN antihypertensive; angiotensin II receptor antagonist

olmidine INN

olopatadine INN antiallergic; antiasthmatic

olopatadine HCl USAN antiallergic; antiasthmatic; ophthalmic antihistamine and mast cell stabilizer

olpimedone INN

olsalazine INN, BAN GI anti-inflammatory [also: olsalazine sodium]

olsalazine sodium USAN GI anti-inflammatory; treatment of ulcerative colitis [also: olsalazine]

oltipraz INN

Olux topical foam ℞ corticosteroidal anti-inflammatory for scalp dermatoses and plaque psoriasis [clobetasol propionate; alcohol 60%] 0.05%

olvanil USAN, INN analgesic

OM 401 investigational (orphan) for sickle cell disease

omaciclovir USAN antiviral DNA polymerase inhibitor for herpes zoster

Omacor ℞ adjunct to diet restriction for hypertriglyceridemia [omega-3 acid ethyl esters]

OMAD (Oncovin, methotrexate/citrovorum factor, Adriamycin, dactinomycin) chemotherapy protocol

omalizumab recombinant humanized monoclonal antibody (rhuMAb) to immunoglobulin E (anti-IgE) for treatment of moderate to severe asthma

omapatrilat vasopeptidase inhibitor (VPI); investigational (NDA filed) endopeptidase and angiotensin-converting enzyme (ACE) inhibitor for hypertension and congestive heart failure

omega-3 acid ethyl esters ethyl esters of docosahexaenoic acid (q.v.) and eicosapentaenoic acid (q.v.); adjunct to diet restriction for hypertriglyceridemia

omega-3 fatty acids [see: docosahexaenoic acid; doconexent; eicosapentaenoic acid; icosapent]

omega-3 fatty acids with all double bonds in the cis configuration investigational (orphan) preventative for organ graft rejection

omega-3 marine triglycerides BAN [12% docosahexaenoic acid (q.v.) + 18% eicosapentaenoic acid (q.v.)]

omeprazole USAN, INN, BAN, JAN proton pump inhibitor for gastric and duodenal ulcers, erosive esophagitis, GERD, upper GI bleeding, and other gastroesophageal disorders 10, 20 mg oral

omeprazole magnesium USAN proton pump inhibitor for gastric and duodenal ulcers, erosive esophagitis, GERD, and other gastroesophageal disorders (base= 97%)

omeprazole sodium USAN *gastric anti-secretory*

omidoline INN

Omnicef capsules, oral suspension ℞ *cephalosporin antibiotic* [cefdinir] 300 mg; 125, 250 mg/5 mL

OmniHIB powder for IM injection, prefilled syringes ℞ *Haemophilus influenzae type b (HIB) vaccine* [Hemophilus b conjugate vaccine; tetanus toxoid] 10•24 μg/0.5 mL

OMNIhist L.A. long-acting tablets ℞ *decongestant; antihistamine; anticholinergic to dry mucosal secretions* [phenylephrine HCl; chlorpheniramine maleate; methscopolamine nitrate] 20•8•2.5 mg

Omnipaque injection ℞ *radiopaque contrast medium* [iohexol (46.36% iodine)] 302, 388, 518, 647, 755 mg/mL (140, 180, 240, 300, 350 mg/mL)

Omnipaque injection (discontinued 2001) ℞ *radiopaque contrast medium* [iohexol (46.36% iodine)] 453 mg/mL (210 mg/mL)

Omnipen capsules, powder for oral suspension (discontinued 2002) ℞ *aminopenicillin antibiotic* [ampicillin] 250, 500 mg; 125, 250 mg/5 mL ② Unipen

Omnipen-N powder for IV or IM injection (discontinued 2002) ℞ *aminopenicillin antibiotic* [ampicillin sodium] 125, 250, 500 mg, 1, 2, 10 g

Omniscan IV injection ℞ *MRI contrast medium* [gadodiamide] 287 mg/mL

omoconazole INN *antifungal*

omoconazole nitrate USAN *antifungal*

omonasteine INN

OMS Concentrate drops (discontinued 2001) ℞ *narcotic analgesic* [morphine sulfate] 20 mg/mL

onapristone INN *investigational antineoplastic for hormone-dependent cancers*

Oncaspar IV or IM injection ℞ *antineoplastic for acute lymphocytic leukemia (orphan) and acute lymphoblastic leukemia* [pegaspargase] 750 IU/mL

Oncet capsules (discontinued 2002) ℞ *narcotic antitussive; analgesic* [hydrocodone bitartrate; acetaminophen] 5•500 mg

Oncocine-HspE7 ℞ *investigational (Phase I) agent for cervical cancer*

Onconase ℞ *investigational (Phase III) treatment for pancreatic, breast, colorectal, prostate, and small cell lung cancers* [ranpirnase]

Oncophage ℞ *investigational (Phase III, orphan) antineoplastic for renal cell carcinoma and metastatic melanoma* [gp96 heat shock protein-peptide complex]

OncoScint CR/OV ℞ *radiodiagnostic imaging aid for ovarian (orphan) and colorectal cancer* [indium In 111 satumomab pendetide]

Onco-TCS *investigational (Phase III) antineoplastic for advanced non-Hodgkin lymphoma* [vincristine liposomal]

OncoTICE ⓒⒶⓃ powder for intravesical instillation ℞ *antineoplastic for urinary bladder cancer* [BCG vaccine, Tice strain] 50 mg

Oncovin IV injection, Hyporets (prefilled syringes) ℞ *antineoplastic for lung and breast cancers, various leukemias, lymphomas, and sarcomas* [vincristine sulfate] 1 mg/mL ② Ancobon

Oncovite tablets OTC *vitamin supplement* [multiple vitamins]

ondansetron INN, BAN *serotonin 5-HT₃ receptor antagonist; antiemetic for nausea following chemotherapy, radiation, or surgery* [also: ondansetron HCl]

ondansetron HCl USAN *serotonin 5-HT₃ receptor antagonist; antiemetic for nausea following chemotherapy, radiation, or surgery* [also: ondansetron] 4, 8 mg oral

Ondrox sustained-release tablets OTC *vitamin/mineral/calcium supplement* [multiple vitamins & minerals; multiple amino acids; calcium; folic acid; biotin] ±•±•50•0.2•0.015 mg

1+1-F Creme ℞ *topical corticosteroidal anti-inflammatory; antifungal; antibacterial; local anesthetic* [hydrocortisone; clioquinol; pramoxine] 1%•3%•1%

1% HC ointment ℞ *topical corticosteroidal anti-inflammatory* [hydrocortisone] 1%

One Touch reagent strips for home use *in vitro diagnostic aid for blood glucose*

109.881 *investigational (Phase III) taxoid for breast cancer*

166Ho-DOTMP *investigational (orphan) for multiple myeloma*

One-A-Day 55 Plus tablets OTC *geriatric vitamin/mineral supplement* [multiple vitamins & minerals; folic acid; biotin] ≐•400•30 μg

One-A-Day Essential tablets OTC *vitamin supplement* [multiple vitamins; folic acid] ≐•400 μg

One-A-Day Extras Antioxidant softgel capsules OTC *vitamin/mineral supplement* [vitamins A, C, and E; multiple minerals] 5000 IU•250 mg•200 IU•≐

One-A-Day Kids chewable tablets OTC *vitamin/mineral/iron supplement* [multiple vitamins & minerals; iron; folic acid; biotin] ≐•18•0.4•0.03 mg

One-A-Day Kids Scooby-Doo! Fizzy Vites chewable tablets OTC *vitamin/mineral/calcium/iron supplement* [multiple vitamins & minerals; calcium; iron (as ferrous fumarate); folic acid; biotin] ≐•50•9•0.2•0.02 mg

One-A-Day Maximum Formula tablets OTC *vitamin/mineral/iron supplement* [multiple vitamins & minerals; iron; folic acid; biotin] ≐•18•0.4•0.03 mg

One-A-Day Men's Vitamins tablets OTC *vitamin supplement* [multiple vitamins; folic acid] ≐•400 μg

One-A-Day WeightSmart tablets OTC *vitamin/mineral/calcium/iron supplement* [multiple vitamins & minerals; calcium; iron (as ferrous fumarate); folic acid] ≐•300•18•0.4 mg

One-A-Day Women's Formula tablets OTC *vitamin/calcium/iron supplement* [multiple vitamins; calcium; iron; folic acid] ≐•450•27•0.4 mg

One-Alpha Ⓒᴬᴺ capsules, oral solution, IV injection ℞ *vitamin D therapy;* *calcium regulator for hypocalcemia and osteodystrophy of chronic renal dialysis and hyperparathyroidism of chronic renal failure* [alfacalcidol] 0.25, 0.5, 1 μg; 0.2 μg/mL; 2 μg/mL

1-alpha-D2 *investigational (Phase III) for secondary hyperparathyroidism in hemodialysis patients*

one.click (trademarked device) *subcutaneous auto-injector*

1DMTX/6-MP (methotrexate [with leucovorin rescue], mercaptopurine) *chemotherapy protocol for acute lymphocytic leukemia (ALL); the first-day initiation protocol* [also: MTX/6-MP (the ongoing continuation protocol)]

One-Tablet-Daily OTC *vitamin supplement* [multiple vitamins; folic acid] ≐•400 μg

One-Tablet-Daily with Iron OTC *vitamin/iron supplement* [multiple vitamins; iron; folic acid] ≐•18•0.4 mg

One-Tablet-Daily with Minerals OTC *vitamin/mineral/iron supplement* [multiple vitamins & minerals; iron; folic acid; biotin] ≐•18•0.4•0.03 mg

onion (Allium cepa) bulb *medicinal herb used as an anthelmintic, antiseptic, antispasmodic, carminative, diuretic, expectorant, and stomachic*

Onkolox ℞ *investigational (orphan) agent for renal cell carcinoma* [coumarin]

Ontak frozen solution for IV injection ℞ *antineoplastic for recurrent or persistent cutaneous T-cell lymphoma (orphan)* [denileukin diftitox] 150 μg/mL

ontazolast USAN *antiasthmatic; leukotriene biosynthesis inhibitor*

ontianil INN

Onxol IV infusion ℞ *antineoplastic for AIDS-related Kaposi sarcoma (orphan), breast and ovarian cancers, and non–small cell lung cancer (NSCLC)* [paclitaxel] 6 mg/mL

Ony-Clear topical solution OTC *antifungal* [benzalkonium chloride] 1%

OP-1 (osteogenic protein-1) [q.v.]

OPA (Oncovin, prednisone, Adriamycin) *chemotherapy protocol for pediatric Hodgkin lymphoma*

OPAL (Oncovin, prednisone, L-asparaginase) *chemotherapy protocol*

Opcon-A eye drops OTC *topical ophthalmic decongestant, antihistamine, and lubricant* [naphazoline HCl; pheniramine maleate; hydroxypropyl methylcellulose] 0.027%•0.315%•0.5%

OPEN (Oncovin, prednisone, etoposide, Novantrone) *chemotherapy protocol*

Operand solution, prep pads, swab sticks, surgical scrub, perineal wash concentrate, aerosol, Iofoam skin cleanser, ointment OTC *broad-spectrum antimicrobial* [povidone-iodine] 1%; 1%; 1%; 7.5%; 1%; 0.5%; 1%; 1%

Operand Douche concentrate OTC *antiseptic/germicidal; vaginal cleanser and deodorizer* [povidone-iodine]

Ophthalgan eye drops (discontinued 2003) ℞ *corneal edema-reducing and clearing agent* [glycerin]

Ophthetic eye drops ℞ *topical ophthalmic anesthetic* [proparacaine HCl] 0.5%

Ophthifluor antecubital venous injection ℞ *ophthalmic diagnostic agent* [fluorescein sodium] 10%

opiniazide INN

opipramol INN *antidepressant; antipsychotic* [also: opipramol HCl]

opipramol HCl USAN *antidepressant; antipsychotic* [also: opipramol]

opium USP *narcotic analgesic; antiperistaltic; used in neonatal opioid withdrawal programs; widely abused as a street drug, which is highly addictive* 10 mg/mL oral

opium, powdered USP *narcotic analgesic*

Oplopanax horridus *medicinal herb* [see: devil's club]

Oporia ℞ *second-generation selective estrogen receptor modulator (SERM); investigational (NDA filed) for osteoporosis and the reduction of LDL cholesterol; investigational (Phase III) for breast cancer* [lasofoxifene tartrate]

OPP (Oncovin, procarbazine, prednisone) *chemotherapy protocol*

OPPA (Oncovin, prednisone, procarbazine, Adriamycin) *chemotherapy protocol for pediatric Hodgkin lymphoma*

oprelvekin USAN *platelet growth factor for prevention of thrombocytopenia following chemotherapy or radiation (orphan)* [also: interleukin 11, recombinant human]

Opteform moldable bone paste ℞ *human allograft material for orthopedic surgery* [demineralized bone powder; cortical bone chips]

Opticare PMS tablets OTC *vitamin/mineral supplement; digestive enzymes* [multiple vitamins & minerals; iron; folic acid; biotin; amylase; protease; lipase] ±•2.5 mg•0.033 mg•10.4 μg•2500 U•2500 U•200 U

Opti-Clean solution OTC *cleaning solution for hard, soft, or rigid gas permeable contact lenses*

Opti-Clean II solution OTC *cleaning solution for hard or soft contact lenses*

Opti-Clean II Especially for Sensitive Eyes solution OTC *cleaning solution for rigid gas permeable contact lenses*

OptiClik (trademarked insulin delivery device) *refillable subcu injector*

Opticrom 4% eye drops ℞ *ophthalmic mast cell stabilizer for vernal keratoconjunctivitis (orphan)* [cromolyn sodium]

Opticyl eye drops ℞ *cycloplegic; mydriatic* [tropicamide] 0.5%, 1%

Opti-Free solution OTC *chemical disinfecting solution for soft contact lenses* [note: one of four different products with the same name]

Opti-Free solution OTC *rewetting solution for soft contact lenses* [note: one of four different products with the same name]

Opti-Free solution OTC *surfactant cleaning solution for soft contact lenses* [note: one of four different products with the same name]

Opti-Free tablets OTC *enzymatic cleaner for soft contact lenses* [pork pancreatin] [note: one of four different products with the same name]

Opti-Free Express Multi-Purpose solution OTC *for soft contact lenses*

Optigene ophthalmic solution OTC *extraocular irrigating solution* [sterile isotonic solution]

Optigene 3 eye drops OTC *topical ophthalmic decongestant and vasoconstrictor* [tetrahydrozoline HCl] 0.05%

Optilets-500 Filmtabs (film-coated tablets) OTC *vitamin supplement* [multiple vitamins]

Optilets-M-500 Filmtabs (film-coated tablets) OTC *vitamin/mineral/iron supplement* [multiple vitamins & minerals; iron] ± • 20 mg

OptiMARK IV injection ℞ *MRI contrast medium for imaging of the brain, head, and spine and liver structure and vascularity* [gadoversetamide] 330.9 mg

Optimental oral liquid OTC *enteral nutritional therapy* 237 mL

Optimine tablets (discontinued 2002) ℞ *piperidine antihistamine for allergic rhinitis and chronic urticaria* [azatadine maleate] 1 mg

Optimmune ℞ *investigational (orphan) tear stimulant for severe keratoconjunctivitis sicca in Sjögren syndrome* [cyclosporine]

Optimoist oral spray (discontinued 2003) OTC *saliva substitute*

Optimox Prenatal tablets OTC *vitamin/mineral/calcium/iron supplement* [multiple vitamins & minerals; calcium; iron; folic acid] ± • 100 • 5 • 0.133 mg

Opti-One solution OTC *rewetting solution for soft contact lenses*

Opti-One Multi-Purpose solution OTC *chemical disinfecting solution for soft contact lenses*

OptiPen One (trademarked insulin delivery device) *cartridge-type subcu injector*

OptiPranolol eye drops ℞ *topical antiglaucoma agent (β-blocker)* [metipranolol HCl] 0.3%

Optiray 160; Optiray 240; Optiray 300; Optiray 320; Optiray 350 injection ℞ *radiopaque contrast medium* [ioversol (47.3% iodine)] 339 mg/mL (160 mg/mL); 509 mg/mL (240 mg/mL); 636 mg/mL (300 mg/mL); 678 mg/mL (320 mg/mL); 741 mg/mL (350 mg/mL)

Opti-Soft Especially for Sensitive Eyes solution OTC *rinsing/storage solution for soft contact lenses* [sodium chloride (preserved saline solution)]

Optison injectable suspension (discontinued 2005) *ultrasound contrast medium for cardiac imaging; investigational (Phase III) diagnostic aid for infertility due to obstructed fallopian tubes* [perflutren] 3 mL

Opti-Tears solution OTC *rewetting solution for hard or soft contact lenses*

Optivar eye drops ℞ *selective H_1 antagonist; antihistamine; mast cell stabilizer* [azelastine HCl] 0.05%

Optivite P.M.T. tablets OTC *geriatric vitamin/mineral supplement* [multiple vitamins & minerals; folic acid; biotin] ± • 30 • ≗ μg

OptiZen eye drops OTC *ophthalmic moisturizer/lubricant* [polysorbate 80] 0.5%

Opti-Zyme Enzymatic Cleaner Especially for Sensitive Eyes tablets OTC *enzymatic cleaner for soft or rigid gas permeable contact lenses* [pork pancreatin]

Optrin ℞ *investigational (Phase I/II) photodynamic therapy for age-related macular degeneration* [motexafin lutetium]

Optro ℞ *investigational agent for chronic anemia* [human hemoglobin, recombinant]

OPV (oral poliovirus vaccine) [see: poliovirus vaccine, live oral]

ORA5 topical liquid OTC *oral anti-infective* [copper sulfate; iodine; potassium iodide]

Orabase gel OTC *mucous membrane anesthetic* [benzocaine] 15%

Orabase Baby gel OTC *topical oral anesthetic* [benzocaine] 7.5%

Orabase HCA oral paste ℞ *topical corticosteroidal anti-inflammatory* [hydrocortisone acetate] 0.5%

Orabase Lip Healer cream OTC *topical oral anesthetic; antipruritic/counterirritant; vulnerary* [benzocaine; menthol; allantoin] 5%•0.5%•1.5%

Orabase Soothe-N-Seal topical liquid OTC *mucous membrane sealant and protectant for canker and mouth sores* [cyanoacrylate]

Orabase-B oral paste OTC *topical oral anesthetic* [benzocaine] 20% ☑ Orinase

Orabase-Plain oral paste OTC *relief from minor oral irritations* [plasticized hydrocarbon gel]

Oracea ℞ *tetracycline antibiotic; investigational (Phase III) once-daily treatment for rosacea* [doxycycline]

Oracit solution ℞ *urinary alkalinizing agent* [sodium citrate; citric acid] 490•640 mg/5 mL

Oragrafin Sodium capsules (discontinued 2001) ℞ *radiopaque contrast medium for cholecystography* [ipodate sodium (61.4% iodine)] 500 mg (307 mg)

Orajel topical liquid OTC *mucous membrane anesthetic* [benzocaine; alcohol 44.2%] 20%

Orajel; Orajel Brace-aid; Orajel/d; Denture Orajel; Baby Orajel; Baby Orajel Nighttime Formula gel OTC *mucous membrane anesthetic* [benzocaine] 20%; 20%; 10%; 10%; 7.5%; 10%

Orajel Mouth-Aid topical liquid, gel OTC *mucous membrane anesthetic* [benzocaine] 20%

Orajel Perioseptic oral liquid OTC *topical anti-inflammatory and anti-infective for braces* [carbamide peroxide] 15%

Orajel P.M. Nighttime Formula Toothache Pain Relief cream OTC *mucous membrane anesthetic* [benzocaine] 20%

Orajel Tooth & Gum Cleanser, Baby gel OTC *removes plaque-like film* [poloxamer 407; simethicone] 2%•0.12%

Oral Wound Rinse mouthwash OTC *hydrogel wound treatment* [acemannan]

Oralease ℞ *investigational (Phase III) analgesic for pain due to oral ulcers*

Oralet (trademarked dosage form) *oral lozenge/lollipop*

Oralgen; Oralin ⓒ ℞ *investigational (Phase II/III) oral insulin formulation*

Oralone Dental paste ℞ *topical corticosteroidal anti-inflammatory* [triamcinolone acetonide] 0.1%

Oramorph SR sustained-release tablets ℞ *narcotic analgesic* [morphine sulfate] 15, 30, 60, 100 mg

orange flower oil NF *flavoring agent; perfume*

orange flower water NF

orange oil NF

orange peel tincture, sweet NF

orange root *medicinal herb* [see: goldenseal]

orange spirit, compound NF

orange swallow wort *medicinal herb* [see: pleurisy root]

orange syrup NF

Orap tablets ℞ *antispasmodic/antidyskinetic for Tourette syndrome* [pimozide] 1, 2 mg (4 mg available in Canada)

Oraphen-PD elixir OTC *analgesic; antipyretic* [acetaminophen] 120 mg/5 mL

Orapred oral solution ℞ *corticosteroid; anti-inflammatory* [prednisolone sodium phosphate; alcohol 2%] 20.2 mg/5 mL (15 mg prednisolone/5 mL)

OraQuick Advance HIV-1/2 Antibody Test reagent kit for professional use ℞ *in vitro diagnostic aid for HIV-1 and HIV-2 antibodies in oral fluid, whole blood, or plasma*

OraQuick Rapid HIV-1 Antibody Test reagent kit for home use *in vitro diagnostic aid for HIV-1 and HIV-2 antibodies in a fingerstick blood sample and HIV-1 antibodies in oral fluid*

Orarinse ℞ *investigational (Phase II) mucositis treatment*

orarsan [see: acetarsone] ☑ Oracin; Orasone

Orasept throat spray OTC *topical oral anesthetic; antiseptic* [benzocaine;

methylbenzethonium chloride] 0.996%•1.037%

Orasept topical liquid OTC *oral astringent; antiseptic* [tannic acid; methylbenzethonium chloride; alcohol 53.31%] 12.16%•1.53%

Orasol topical liquid OTC *oral anesthetic; antipruritic/counterirritant; antiseptic* [benzocaine; phenol; alcohol 70%] 6.3%•0.5%

Orasone tablets ℞ *corticosteroid; antiinflammatory; immunosuppressant* [prednisone] 1, 5, 10, 20, 50 mg ☒ Oracin; orarsan

OraSure reagent kit for home use *in vitro diagnostic aid for HIV antibodies*

OraSure HIV-1 reagent kit for professional use *in vitro diagnostic aid for HIV antibodies using oral mucosal transudate* [single-sample, three-test kit: two ELISA assays + Western Blot assay]

Orathecin capsules ℞ *investigational (Phase III) antineoplastic for pancreatic cancer* [rubitecan]

orazamide INN

Orazinc capsules, tablets OTC *zinc supplement* [zinc sulfate] 220 mg; 110 mg

orbofiban acetate USAN *platelet aggregation inhibitor; fibrinogen receptor antagonist*

orbutopril INN

OrCel ℞ *investigational bilayered cellular matrix for acute and chronic diabetic foot ulcers* [collagen sponge seeded with allogenic dermal and epidermal cells]

orchanet *medicinal herb* [see: henna (Alkanna)]

orciprenaline INN, BAN *bronchodilator* [also: metaproterenol polistirex]

orciprenaline polistirex [see: metaproterenol polistirex]

orciprenaline sulfate [see: metaproterenol sulfate]

orconazole INN *antifungal* [also: orconazole nitrate]

orconazole nitrate USAN *antifungal* [also: orconazole]

Ordrine AT extended-release capsules (discontinued 2002) ℞ *antitussive; decongestant* [caramiphen edisylate; phenylpropanolamine HCl] 40•75 mg

oregano *medicinal herb* [see: marjoram]

Oregon grape *(Mahonia aquifolium)* rhizome and root *medicinal herb for acne, blood disorders, eczema, jaundice, liver disorders, promoting digestion, psoriasis, and staphylococcal infections*

orestrate INN

orestrol [see: diethylstilbestrol dipropionate]

Oretic tablets ℞ *antihypertensive; diuretic* [hydrochlorothiazide] 25, 50 mg ☒ Oreton

Oreton Methyl tablets, buccal tablets (discontinued 2001) ℞ *androgen for hypogonadism or testosterone deficiency in men, delayed puberty in boys, and metastatic breast cancer in women; also abused as a street drug* [methyltestosterone] 10 mg ☒ Oretic

Orexin chewable tablets OTC *vitamin supplement* [vitamins B_1, B_6, and B_{12}] 8.1 mg•4.1 mg•25 µg

Orfadin capsules ℞ *adjunctive treatment for hereditary tyrosinemia type 1 (HT-1), a pediatric liver disease* (orphan) [nitisinone] 2, 5, 10 mg

Organidin NR tablets, oral liquid ℞ *expectorant* [guaifenesin] 200 mg; 100 mg/5 mL

organoclay [see: bentoquatam]

Organan deep subcu injection (discontinued 2004) ℞ *anticoagulant/antithrombotic for prevention of deep vein thrombosis (DVT) following hip replacement surgery* [danaparoid sodium] 750 anti-Xa U/0.6 mL

orgotein USAN, INN, BAN *anti-inflammatory; antirheumatic; investigational (orphan) for amyotrophic lateral sclerosis and to prevent donor organ reperfusion injury* [previously known as superoxide dismutase (SOD)]

orgotein, recombinant human *investigational (orphan) for bronchopulmonary dysplasia of premature neonates*

orienticine A; orienticine D [see: orientiparcin]

orientiparcin INN [a mixture of orienticine A and orienticine D]

Origanum vulgare medicinal herb [see: marjoram]

Orimune oral suspension (discontinued 2004) ℞ *poliomyelitis vaccine* [poliovirus vaccine, live oral trivalent] 0.5 mL

Orinase tablets ℞ *sulfonylurea antidiabetic* [tolbutamide] 500 mg ⑤ Orabase; Ornade; Ornex; Tolinase

Orinase Diagnostic powder for IV injection ℞ *in vivo diagnostic aid for pancreas function and diabetes* [tolbutamide sodium] 1 g

oritavancin diphosphate USAN *antibiotic; peptidoglycan synthesis inhibitor*

Orlaam IV injection (discontinued 2004) ℞ *narcotic analgesic for management of opiate addiction* (orphan) [levomethadyl acetate HCl] 10 mg/mL

orlipastat [see: orlistat]

orlistat USAN, INN *lipase inhibitor to suppress the absorption of dietary fats, leading to weight loss; preventative for type 2 diabetes*

ormaplatin USAN *antineoplastic*

ormetoprim USAN, INN *antibacterial*

Ornade Spansules (sustained-release capsules) (discontinued 2001) ℞ *decongestant; antihistamine* [phenylpropanolamine HCl; chlorpheniramine maleate] 75•12 mg ⑤ Orinase; Ornex

Ornex No Drowsiness caplets OTC *decongestant; analgesic; antipyretic* [pseudoephedrine HCl; acetaminophen] 30•325, 30•500 mg ⑤ Orex; Orinase; Ornade

ornidazole USAN, INN *anti-infective*

Ornidyl IV injection concentrate ℞ *antiprotozoal for* Trypanosoma brucei gambiense *(sleeping sickness) infection* (orphan); *investigational* (orphan) *for AIDS-related* Pneumocystis carinii *pneumonia* [eflornithine HCl] 200 mg/mL

ornipressin INN

ornithine (L-ornithine) INN

ornithine vasopressin [see: ornipressin]

ornoprostil INN

Oros (trademarked delivery system) *patterned-release tablets*

orotic acid INN

orotirelin INN

orpanoxin USAN, INN *anti-inflammatory*

orphenadrine citrate [see: orphenadrine citrate]

orphenadrine INN, BAN *skeletal muscle relaxant; antihistamine* [also: orphenadrine citrate]

orphenadrine citrate USP *skeletal muscle relaxant; antihistamine* [also: orphenadrine] 100 mg oral; 30 mg/mL injection

orphenadrine HCl *anticholinergic; antiparkinsonian*

Orphengesic; Orphengesic Forte tablets ℞ *skeletal muscle relaxant; analgesic* [orphenadrine citrate; aspirin; caffeine] 25•385•30 mg; 50•770•60 mg

orpressin [see: ornipressin]

orris root (Iris florentina) medicinal herb used as a diuretic and stomachic

ortetamine INN

orthesin [see: benzocaine]

Ortho 0.5/35; Ortho 1/35 Ⓐ tablets (in 21 or 28 packs) ℞ *monophasic oral contraceptive* [norethindrone; ethinyl estradiol] 0.5 mg•35 μg; 1 mg•35 μg

Ortho 7/7/7 Ⓐ tablets (in 21 or 28 packs) ℞ *triphasic oral contraceptive* [norethindrone; ethinyl estradiol] Phase 1 (7 days): 0.5 mg•35 μg; Phase 2 (7 days): 0.75 mg•35 μg; Phase 3 (7 days): 1 mg•35 μg

Ortho Dienestrol vaginal cream (discontinued 2003) ℞ *estrogen replacement for postmenopausal atrophic vaginitis* [dienestrol] 0.01%

Ortho Evra transdermal patch ℞ *once-weekly contraceptive* [norelgestromin; ethinyl estradiol] 150•20 μg/day

Ortho Micronor tablets (in Dialpaks of 28) ℞ *oral contraceptive (progestin only)* [norethindrone] 0.35 mg

Ortho Tri-Cyclen tablets (in Dial-paks and Veridates of 28) ℞ *triphasic oral contraceptive; treatment for acne vulgaris in females* [norgestimate; ethinyl estradiol]
Phase 1 (7 days): 180•35 μg;
Phase 2 (7 days): 215•35 μg;
Phase 3 (7 days): 250•35 μg

Ortho Tri-Cyclen Lo tablets (in Dialpaks and Veridates of 28) ℞ *triphasic oral contraceptive* [norgestimate; ethinyl estradiol]
Phase 1 (7 days): 180•25 μg;
Phase 2 (7 days): 215•25 μg;
Phase 3 (7 days): 250•25 μg

Ortho-Cept tablets (in Dialpaks and Veridates of 28) ℞ *monophasic oral contraceptive* [desogestrel; ethinyl estradiol] 0.15 mg•30 μg

Orthoclone OKT3 IV injection ℞ *immunosuppressant for renal, cardiac, and hepatic transplants* [muromonab-CD3] 5 mg/5 mL ☒ Ortho-Creme

orthocresol NF

Ortho-Cyclen tablets (in Dialpaks and Veridates of 28) ℞ *monophasic oral contraceptive* [norgestimate; ethinyl estradiol] 0.25 mg•35 μg

Ortho-Est tablets ℞ *bioidentical human estrogen replacement therapy for the treatment of postmenopausal symptoms and prevention of postmenopausal osteoporosis* [estrone (from estropipate)] 0.625 (0.75), 1.25 (1.5) mg

Ortho-Gynol vaginal gel OTC *spermicidal contraceptive (for use with a diaphragm)* [octoxynol 9] 1%

Ortho-Novum 1/35 tablets (in Dialpaks and Veridates of 28) ℞ *monophasic oral contraceptive* [norethindrone; ethinyl estradiol] 1 mg•35 μg

Ortho-Novum 1/50 tablets (in Dialpaks of 28) ℞ *monophasic oral contraceptive* [norethindrone; mestranol] 1 mg•50 μg

Ortho-Novum 7/7/7 tablets (in Dialpaks and Veridates of 28) ℞ *triphasic oral contraceptive* [norethindrone; ethinyl estradiol]
Phase 1 (7 days): 500•35 μg;
Phase 2 (7 days): 750•35 μg;
Phase 3 (7 days): 1000•35 μg

Ortho-Novum 10/11 tablets (in Dialpaks of 28) ℞ *biphasic oral contraceptive* [norethindrone; ethinyl estradiol]
Phase 1 (10 days): 500•35 μg;
Phase 2 (11 days): 1000•35 μg

Ortho-Prefest [see: Prefest]

orthotolidine

Orthovisc intra-articular injection in single-use vials ℞ *viscoelastic lubricant and "shock absorber" for osteoarthritis of the knee* [hyaluronan] 30 mg

OrthoWash oral rinse ℞ *dental caries preventative* [sodium fluoride (as acidulated phosphate solution)] 0.044%

Orthoxicol Cough syrup (discontinued 2002) OTC *antitussive; decongestant; antihistamine* [dextromethorphan hydrobromide; phenylpropanolamine HCl; chlorpheniramine maleate; alcohol 8%] 6.7•8.3•1.3 mg/5 mL

Orudis capsules (discontinued 2004) ℞ *analgesic; antiarthritic; nonsteroidal anti-inflammatory drug (NSAID)* [ketoprofen] 25, 50, 75 mg

Orudis KT tablets OTC *analgesic; antiarthritic; antipyretic; nonsteroidal anti-inflammatory drug (NSAID)* [ketoprofen] 12.5 mg

Oruvail sustained-release pellets in capsules ℞ *once-daily antiarthritic; nonsteroidal anti-inflammatory drug (NSAID)* [ketoprofen] 100, 150, 200 mg

oryzanol A, B, and C *medicinal herb* [see: rice bran oil]

osalmid INN

osarsal [see: acetarsone]

Os-Cal 250+D; Os-Cal 500+D film-coated tablets OTC *dietary supplement* [calcium (as carbonate); vitamin D] 250 mg•125 IU; 500 mg•200 IU

Os-Cal 500 tablets, chewable tablets OTC *calcium supplement* [calcium carbonate] 1250 mg (500 mg Ca)

Os-Cal Fortified tablets OTC *vitamin/mineral/calcium/iron supplement* [multiple vitamins & minerals; calcium (as carbonate); iron (as ferrous fumarate)] ≙•250•5 mg

Os-Cal Ultra tablets OTC *vitamin/mineral/calcium supplement* [multiple vitamins & minerals; calcium (as carbonate)] ±•600 mg

oseltamivir phosphate USAN *antiviral neuraminidase inhibitor for influenza A and B*

osmadizone INN

Osmitrol IV infusion ℞ *antihypertensive; osmotic diuretic* [mannitol] 5%, 10%, 15%, 20%

osmium *element (Os)*

Osmoglyn solution ℞ *osmotic diuretic* [glycerin] 50%

Osmolite; Osmolite HN oral liquid OTC *enteral nutritional therapy* [lactose-free formula]

Osmorhiza longistylis medicinal herb [see: sweet cicely]

osmotic diuretics *a class of diuretics that increase excretion of sodium and chloride and decrease tubular absorption of water*

Osmunda cinnamomea; O. regalis medicinal herb [see: buckhorn brake]

OspA [see: lipoprotein OspA, recombinant]

Ostac ⒸⒶⓃ capsules, IV infusion ℞ *bisphosphonate bone resorption inhibitor for hypercalcemia of malignancy and osteolysis due to bone metastasis of malignant tumors* [clodronate disodium] 400 mg; 30 mg/mL

Osteocalcin subcu or IM injection ℞ *calcium regulator for hypercalcemia, Paget disease, and postmenopausal osteoporosis* [calcitonin (salmon)] 200 IU/mL

Osteo-D ℞ *calcium regulator; investigational (orphan) for familial hypophosphatemic rickets* [secalciferol]

Osteofil injectable bone paste ℞ *human allograft material for orthopedic surgery* [demineralized bone powder]

OsteoMax effervescent powder for oral solution OTC *dietary supplement* [calcium citrate; vitamin D; magnesium] 500 mg•200 IU•200 mg

Osteo-Mins powder OTC *dietary supplement* [multiple minerals; vitamins C and D] ±•500 mg•100 IU

Ostiderm lotion OTC *for hyperhidrosis and bromhidrosis* [aluminum sulfate; zinc oxide] 14.5•? mg/g

Ostiderm roll-on OTC *for hyperhidrosis and bromhidrosis* [aluminum chlorohydrate; camphor; alcohol] ?•?•?

ostreogrycin INN, BAN

osvarsan [see: acetarsone]

Oswego tea *(Monarda didyma)* leaves and flowers *medicinal herb used as a calmative, rubefacient, and stimulant*

OT (old tuberculin) [see: tuberculin]

Otic Domeboro ear drops ℞ *antibacterial; antifungal* [acetic acid; aluminum acetate] 2%•?

Otic-Care ear drops, otic suspension ℞ *topical corticosteroidal anti-inflammatory; antibiotic* [hydrocortisone; neomycin sulfate; polymyxin B sulfate] 1%•5 mg•10 000 U per mL

otilonium bromide INN, BAN

Oti-Med ear drops ℞ *topical corticosteroidal anti-inflammatory; antibacterial; topical local anesthetic* [hydrocortisone; chloroxylenol; pramoxine HCl] 10•1•10 mg/mL

otimerate sodium INN

OtiTricin otic suspension ℞ *topical corticosteroidal anti-inflammatory; antibiotic* [hydrocortisone; neomycin sulfate; polymyxin B sulfate] 1%•5 mg•10 000 U per mL

Otobiotic Otic ear drops ℞ *topical corticosteroidal anti-inflammatory; antibiotic* [hydrocortisone; polymyxin B sulfate] 0.5%•10 000 U per mL ⓠ Urobiotic

Otocain ear drops ℞ *topical local anesthetic* [benzocaine] 20%

Otocalm ear drops ℞ *topical local anesthetic; analgesic* [benzocaine; antipyrine] 1.4%•5.4%

Otocort ear drops, otic suspension ℞ *topical corticosteroidal anti-inflammatory; antibiotic* [hydrocortisone; neomycin sulfate; polymyxin B sulfate] 1%•5 mg•10 000 U per mL

Otomar-HC ear drops ℞ *topical corti-costeroidal anti-inflammatory; local anesthetic; antibacterial* [hydrocorti-sone; pramoxine HCl; chloroxyle-nol] 10•10•1 mg/mL

Otomycet-HC ear drops ℞ *topical cor-ticosteroidal anti-inflammatory; anti-bacterial; antifungal* [hydrocortisone; acetic acid] 1%•2%

Otomycin-HPN Otic ear drops ℞ *topical corticosteroidal anti-inflamma-tory; antibiotic* [hydrocortisone; neo-mycin sulfate; polymyxin B sulfate] 1%•5 mg•10 000 U per mL

Otosporin ear drops ℞ *topical cortico-steroidal anti-inflammatory; antibiotic* [hydrocortisone; neomycin sulfate; polymyxin B sulfate] 1%•5 mg•10 000 U per mL

Otrivin nasal spray, nose drops, pedi-atric nose drops OTC *nasal deconges-tant* [xylometazoline HCl] 0.1%; 0.1%; 0.05% ℞ Lotrimin

ouabain USP

Our Lady's mint *medicinal herb* [see: spearmint]

Outgro solution OTC *pain relief for ingrown toenails* [tannic acid; chloro-butanol; isopropyl alcohol 83%] 25%•5%

Ovace foam ℞ *antibiotic for acute and chronic seborrheic dermatitis and secon-dary bacterial infections of the scalp and skin* [sulfacetamide sodium] 10%

ovandrotone albumin INN, BAN

O-Vax ℞ *investigational (Phase III, orphan) therapeutic vaccine for adjuvant treatment of ovarian cancer* [autolo-gous cell (AC) vaccine] ℞ Ovarex

Ovcon-35 caplets, chewable tablets (in packs of 21 or 28) ℞ *monophasic oral contraceptive* [norethindrone; ethinyl estradiol] 0.4 mg•35 μg

Ovcon-50 caplets (in packs of 28) ℞ *monophasic oral contraceptive* [norethin-drone; ethinyl estradiol] 1 mg•50 μg

Ovide lotion ℞ *pediculicide for lice* [malathion; isopropyl alcohol 78%] 0.5%

Ovidrel prefilled syringes for subcu injection ℞ *fertility stimulant for anovulatory women; adjuvant therapy for cryptorchidism* [choriogonadotro-pin alfa] 250 μg/0.5 mL

ovine corticotropin-releasing hor-mone [see: corticorelin ovine triflu-tate]

Ovitrelle (European name for U.S. product **Ovidrel**)

Ovoid (trademarked dosage form) *sugar-coated tablet*

Ovral tablets (in Pilpaks of 21 and 28) ℞ *monophasic oral contraceptive; emer-gency postcoital contraceptive* [norges-trel; ethinyl estradiol] 0.5 mg•50 μg

Ovrette tablets (in Pilpaks of 28) ℞ *oral contraceptive (progestin only)* [norgestrel] 0.075 mg

OvuGen test kit (discontinued 2004) *in vitro diagnostic aid to predict ovula-tion time*

OvuKIT Self-Test kit for home use (discontinued 2004) *in vitro diagnos-tic aid to predict ovulation time*

Ovulation Scope kit for home use *in vitro diagnostic aid to predict ovulation time from a saliva sample*

OvuLite kit for home use *in vitro diag-nostic aid to predict ovulation time from a saliva sample*

OvuQuick Self-Test kit for home use (discontinued 2004) *in vitro diagnos-tic aid to predict ovulation time*

[¹⁵O]water [see: water O 15]

ox bile extract [see: bile salts]

oxabolone cipionate INN

oxabrexine INN

22-oxacalcitriol (OCT) [see: maxa-calcitol]

oxaceprol INN

oxacillin INN *penicillinase-resistant peni-cillin antibiotic* [also: oxacillin sodium]

oxacillin sodium USAN, USP *penicilli-nase-resistant penicillin antibiotic* [also: oxacillin] 250 mg/5 mL oral; 0.5, 1, 2, 10 g IV injection

oxadimedine INN

oxadimedine HCl [see: oxadimedine]

oxadoddy *medicinal herb* [see: Culver root]

oxaflozane INN

oxaflumazine INN

oxafuradene [see: nifuradene]

oxagrelate USAN, INN *platelet antiaggregatory agent*

oxalinast INN

oxaliplatin USAN, INN *alkylating antineoplastic for metastatic ovarian and colorectal cancers (orphan); investigational (Phase III) for pancreatic cancer*

Oxalis acetosella *medicinal herb* [see: wood sorrel]

oxamarin INN *hemostatic* [also: oxamarin HCl]

oxamarin HCl USAN *hemostatic* [also: oxamarin]

oxametacin INN

oxamisole INN *immunoregulator* [also: oxamisole HCl]

oxamisole HCl USAN *immunoregulator* [also: oxamisole]

oxamniquine USAN, USP, INN *antischistosomal; anthelmintic for schistosomiasis (flukes)*

oxamphetamine hydrobromide [see: hydroxyamphetamine hydrobromide]

oxamycin [see: cycloserine]

oxanamide INN

Oxandrin caplets ℞ *anabolic steroid for bone pain due to osteoporosis; investigational (Phase III, orphan) for AIDS-wasting syndrome; investigational (orphan) for muscular dystrophy and alcoholic hepatitis; also abused as a street drug to increase muscle mass* [oxandrolone] 2.5, 10 mg

Oxandrin gel ℞ *investigational (Phase II) steroid for AIDS-wasting syndrome* [oxandrolone]

oxandrolone USAN, USP, INN, BAN, JAN *anabolic steroid for bone pain due to osteoporosis; investigational (Phase III, orphan) for AIDS-wasting syndrome; investigational (orphan) for muscular dystrophy and alcoholic hepatitis; also abused as a street drug to increase muscle mass*

oxantel INN *anthelmintic* [also: oxantel pamoate]

oxantel pamoate USAN *anthelmintic* [also: oxantel]

oxantrazole HCl [see: piroxantrone HCl]

oxapadol INN

oxapium iodide INN

oxaprazine

oxapropanium iodide INN

oxaprotiline INN *antidepressant* [also: oxaprotiline HCl]

oxaprotiline HCl USAN *antidepressant* [also: oxaprotiline]

oxaprozin USAN, INN, BAN *antiarthritic; nonsteroidal anti-inflammatory drug (NSAID)* 600 mg oral

oxaprozin potassium *antiarthritic; nonsteroidal anti-inflammatory drug (NSAID) (base=88.5%)*

oxarbazole USAN, INN *antiasthmatic*

oxarutine [see: ethoxazorutoside]

oxatomide USAN, INN *antiallergic; antiasthmatic*

oxazafone INN

oxazepam USAN, USP, INN *benzodiazepine anxiolytic; sedative; alcohol withdrawal aid* 10, 15, 30 mg oral

oxazidione INN

oxazolam INN

oxazolidin [see: oxyphenbutazone]

oxazolidinediones *a class of anticonvulsants (no longer used)*

oxazorone INN

oxcarbazepine INN *anticonvulsant for partial seizures in adults or children*

oxdralazine INN

oxeladin INN, BAN

oxendolone USAN, INN *antiandrogen for benign prostatic hypertrophy*

oxepinac INN

oxerutins BAN

oxetacaine INN *topical anesthetic* [also: oxethazaine]

oxetacillin INN

2-oxetanone [see: propiolactone]

oxethazaine USAN, BAN *topical anesthetic* [also: oxetacaine]

oxetorone INN *migraine-specific analgesic* [also: oxetorone fumarate]

oxetorone fumarate USAN *migraine-specific analgesic* [also: oxetorone]

Oxeze Ⓒⓐⓝ Turbuhaler (dry powder in a metered-dose inhaler) ℞ *twice-daily bronchodilator for asthma* [formoterol fumarate] 6, 12 μg/dose

oxfenamide [see: oxiramide]

oxfendazole USAN, INN *anthelmintic*

oxfenicine USAN, INN, BAN *vasodilator*

oxibendazole USAN, INN *anthelmintic*

oxibetaine INN

oxibuprocaine chloride [see: benoxinate HCl]

oxichlorochine sulfate [see: hydroxychloroquine sulfate]

oxicinchophen [see: oxycinchophen]

oxiconazole INN, BAN *broad-spectrum topical antifungal* [also: oxiconazole nitrate]

oxiconazole nitrate USAN *broad-spectrum topical antifungal* [also: oxiconazole]

oxicone [see: oxycodone]

oxidized cellulose [see: cellulose, oxidized]

oxidized cholic acid [see: dehydrocholic acid]

oxidized regenerated cellulose [see: cellulose, oxidized regenerated]

oxidopamine USAN, INN *ophthalmic adrenergic*

oxidronate sodium *parenteral radiopaque contrast medium*

oxidronic acid USAN, INN, BAN *calcium regulator*

oxifenamate [see: hydroxyphenamate]

oxifentorex INN

Oxi-Freeda tablets OTC *dietary supplement* [multiple vitamins & minerals; multiple amino acids]

oxifungin INN *antifungal* [also: oxifungin HCl]

oxifungin HCl USAN *antifungal* [also: oxifungin]

oxilorphan USAN, INN *narcotic antagonist*

oximetazoline HCl [see: oxymetazoline HCl]

oximetholone [see: oxymetholone]

oximonam USAN, INN *antibacterial*

oximonam sodium USAN *antibacterial*

oxindanac INN

oxiniacic acid INN

oxiperomide USAN, INN *antipsychotic*

oxipertine [see: oxypertine]

oxipethidine [see: hydroxypethidine]

oxiphenbutazone [see: oxyphenbutazone]

oxiphencyclimine chloride [see: oxyphencyclimine HCl]

Oxipor VHC lotion OTC *antipsoriatic; antiseborrheic; keratolytic* [coal tar; alcohol 79%] 5%

Oxiprim ℞ *investigational (NDA filed) xanthine oxidase inhibitor for hyperuricemia* [oxypurinol sodium]

oxiprocaine [see: hydroxyprocaine]

oxiprogesterone caproate [see: hydroxyprogesterone caproate]

oxipurinol INN *xanthine oxidase inhibitor* [also: oxypurinol]

oxiracetam INN, BAN *investigational treatment for Alzheimer disease*

oxiramide USAN, INN *antiarrhythmic*

oxisopred INN

Oxistat cream, lotion ℞ *broad-spectrum topical antifungal* [oxiconazole nitrate] 1%

oxistilbamidine isethionate [see: hydroxystilbamidine isethionate]

oxisuran USAN, INN *antineoplastic*

oxitefonium bromide INN

oxitetracaine [see: hydroxytetracaine]

oxitetracycline [see: oxytetracycline]

oxitriptan INN

oxitriptyline INN

oxitropium bromide INN, BAN

Oxizole Ⓒⓐⓝ cream, lotion ℞ *broad-spectrum topical antifungal* [oxiconazole nitrate] 1%

oxmetidine INN, BAN *antagonist to histamine H_2 receptors* [also: oxmetidine HCl]

oxmetidine HCl USAN *antagonist to histamine H_2 receptors* [also: oxmetidine]

oxmetidine mesylate USAN *antagonist to histamine H_2 receptors*

oxodipine INN

oxogestone INN *progestin* [also: oxogestone phenpropionate] oxogestone phenpropionate USAN *progestin* [also: oxogestone]

oxoglurate INN *combining name for radicals or groups*

oxolamine INN

oxolinic acid USAN, INN *antibacterial*

oxomemazine INN

oxonazine INN

4-oxopentanoic acid, calcium salt [see: calcium levulinate]

oxophenarsine INN [also: oxophenarsine HCl]

oxophenarsine HCl USP [also: oxophenarsine]

5-oxoproline [see: pidolic acid]

oxoprostol INN, BAN

oxozepam [see: oxazepam]

oxpentifylline BAN *peripheral vasodilator; hemorheologic agent* [also: pentoxifylline]

oxpheneridine INN

oxprenoate potassium INN

oxprenolol INN *coronary vasodilator* [also: oxprenolol HCl]

oxprenolol HCl USAN, USP *coronary vasodilator* [also: oxprenolol]

Oxsoralen lotion R *psoralens for repigmentation of idiopathic vitiligo* [methoxsalen] 1%

Oxsoralen-Ultra gelcaps R *systemic psoralens for the treatment of severe recalcitrant psoriasis* [methoxsalen] 10 mg

oxtriphylline USP *bronchodilator* [also: choline theophyllinate] 100, 200 mg oral; 50, 100 mg/5 mL oral

Oxy 5 for Sensitive Skin, Advanced Formula; Advanced Formula Oxy for Sensitive Skin gel (discontinued 2003) OTC *keratolytic for acne* [benzoyl peroxide] 5%; 2.5%

Oxy 5 Tinted lotion (discontinued 2003) OTC *keratolytic for acne* [benzoyl peroxide] 5%

Oxy 10 Advanced Formula gel (discontinued 2003) OTC *keratolytic for acne* [benzoyl peroxide] 10%

Oxy Medicated Cleanser & Pads OTC *keratolytic cleanser for acne* [salicylic acid; alcohol] 0.5%•22%, 0.5%•40%, 2%•50%

Oxy Medicated Soap bar OTC *medicated cleanser for acne* [triclosan] 1%

Oxy Night Watch; Oxy Night Watch for Sensitive Skin lotion OTC *keratolytic for acne* [salicylic acid] 2%; 1%

Oxy Oil-Free Acne Wash topical liquid OTC *keratolytic for acne* [benzoyl peroxide] 10%

oxybenzone USAN, USP, INN *ultraviolet screen*

oxybuprocaine INN, BAN *topical anesthetic* [also: benoxinate HCl; oxybuprocaine HCl]

oxybuprocaine HCl JAN *topical anesthetic* [also: benoxinate HCl; oxybuprocaine]

oxybutynin USAN, INN, BAN *anticholinergic; smooth muscle relaxant; urinary antispasmodic* [also: oxybutynin chloride]

oxybutynin chloride USAN, USP *anticholinergic; smooth muscle relaxant; urinary antispasmodic for urge urinary incontinence and frequency* [also: oxybutynin] 5 mg oral; 5 mg/5 mL oral

Oxycel pads, pledgets, strips R *local hemostat for surgery* [cellulose, oxidized]

oxychlorosene USAN *topical anti-infective*

oxychlorosene sodium USAN *topical anti-infective*

oxycinchophen INN, BAN

oxyclipine INN *anticholinergic* [also: propenzolate HCl]

oxyclipine HCl [see: propenzolate HCl]

oxyclozanide INN, BAN

Oxycocet ⒸⒶⓃ tablets R *narcotic analgesic* [oxycodone HCl; acetaminophen] 5•325 mg

oxycodone USAN, INN, BAN *narcotic analgesic; also abused as a street drug* ⊡ Roxicodone

oxycodone HCl USAN, USP *narcotic analgesic; also abused as a street drug* 5, 10, 15, 20, 30, 40, 80 mg oral; 5 mg/5 mL oral; 20 mg/mL oral drops ⊡ OxyContin, Roxicodone

oxycodone HCl & acetaminophen *narcotic analgesic* 7.5•325, 7.5•500, 10•325, 10•650 mg oral

oxycodone terephthalate USP *narcotic analgesic; also abused as a street drug* ⊡ Roxicodone

OxyContin controlled-release tablets ℞ *narcotic analgesic* [oxycodone HCl] 10, 20, 40, 80 mg

Oxydess II tablets ℞ *CNS stimulant; amphetamine* [dextroamphetamine sulfate] 10 mg

oxydimethylquinazine [see: antipyrine]

oxydipentonium chloride INN

Oxydose oral drops ℞ *narcotic analgesic* [oxycodone HCl] 20 mg/mL

oxyethyltheophylline [see: etofylline]

OxyFast oral drops ℞ *narcotic analgesic* [oxycodone HCl] 20 mg/mL

oxyfedrine INN, BAN

oxyfenamate INN *minor tranquilizer* [also: hydroxyphenamate]

oxyfilcon A USAN *hydrophilic contact lens material*

oxygen (O₂) USP *medicinal gas; element (O)*

oxygen, polymeric *investigational (orphan) for sickle cell anemia*

oxygen 93 percent USP *medicinal gas*

OxyIR immediate-release capsules ℞ *narcotic analgesic* [oxycodone HCl] 5 mg

oxymesterone INN, BAN

oxymetazoline INN, BAN *topical ocular vasoconstrictor; nasal decongestant* [also: oxymetazoline HCl] ⊡ oxymetholone

oxymetazoline HCl USAN, USP *topical ocular vasoconstrictor; nasal decongestant* [also: oxymetazoline] 0.05% nasal

oxymetholone USAN, USP, INN, BAN *androgen; anabolic steroid for anemia; also abused as a street drug* ⊡ oxymetazoline; oxymorphone

oxymethylene urea [see: polynoxylin]

oxymorphone INN, BAN *narcotic analgesic* [also: oxymorphone HCl] ⊡ oxymetholone

oxymorphone HCl USP *narcotic analgesic; investigational (orphan) for intrac-* table pain in narcotic-tolerant patients [also: oxymorphone]

oxypendyl INN

oxypertine USAN, INN *antidepressant*

oxyphenbutazone USP, INN *antiinflammatory; antirheumatic; antipyretic; analgesic*

oxyphencyclimine INN *anticholinergic* [also: oxyphencyclimine HCl]

oxyphencyclimine HCl USP *peptic ulcer adjunct* [also: oxyphencyclimine]

oxyphenhydrazine [see: carsalam]

oxyphenisatin BAN *laxative* [also: oxyphenisatin acetate; oxyphenisatine]

oxyphenisatin acetate USAN *laxative* [also: oxyphenisatine; oxyphenisatin]

oxyphenisatine INN *laxative* [also: oxyphenisatin acetate; oxyphenisatin]

oxyphenonium bromide

oxyphylline [see: etofylline]

oxypurinol USAN *xanthine oxidase inhibitor for hyperuricemia; metabolite of allopurinol* [also: oxipurinol]

oxypurinol sodium *investigational (NDA filed) xanthine oxidase inhibitor for hyperuricemia; metabolite of allopurinol*

oxypyrronium bromide INN

oxyquinoline USAN *disinfectant/antiseptic*

oxyquinoline benzoate [see: benzoxiquine]

oxyquinoline sulfate USAN, NF *complexing agent*

oxyridazine INN

Oxysept solution + tablets OTC *two-step chemical disinfecting system for soft contact lenses* [hydrogen peroxide-based] 3%

Oxysept 2 solution OTC *rinsing/storage solution for soft contact lenses* [sodium chloride (saline solution)]

oxysonium iodide INN

oxytetracycline USP, INN *broad-spectrum tetracycline antibiotic; antirickettsial*

oxytetracycline calcium USP *tetracycline antibiotic; antirickettsial*

oxytetracycline HCl USP *tetracycline antibiotic; antirickettsial*

oxytocics *a class of posterior pituitary hormones that stimulate contraction of the myometrium (uterine muscle)*

oxytocin USP, INN *posterior pituitary hormone; oxytocic for induction of labor* 10 U/mL injection

Oxytrol transdermal patch ℞ *urinary antispasmodic for urge urinary incontinence and frequency* [oxybutynin chloride] 36 mg (3.9 mg/day)

Oxyzal Wet Dressing topical liquid OTC *antiseptic dressing for minor infections* [oxyquinoline sulfate; benzalkonium chloride]

Oysco 500 chewable tablets OTC *calcium supplement* [calcium carbonate] 1250 mg (500 mg Ca)

Oyst-Cal 500 film-coated tablets OTC *calcium supplement* [calcium carbonate] 1250 mg (500 mg Ca)

Oyst-Cal-D film-coated tablets OTC *dietary supplement* [calcium carbonate; vitamin D] 250 mg•125 IU

Oyster Calcium tablets OTC *dietary supplement* [calcium carbonate; vitamins A and D] 375 mg•800 IU•200 IU

Oyster Calcium 500 + D tablets OTC *dietary supplement* [calcium carbonate; vitamin D] 500 mg•125 IU

Oyster Calcium with Vitamin D tablets OTC *dietary supplement* [calcium carbonate; vitamin D] 250 mg•125 IU

Oyster Shell Calcium tablets OTC *calcium supplement* [calcium carbonate] 1250 mg (500 mg Ca)

Oyster Shell Calcium with Vitamin D tablets OTC *dietary supplement* [calcium carbonate; vitamin D] 250 mg•125 IU

Oystercal 500 tablets (discontinued 2002) OTC *calcium supplement* [calcium carbonate] 1250 mg (500 mg Ca)

Oystercal-D 250 tablets OTC *dietary supplement* [calcium carbonate; vitamin D] 250 mg•125 IU

oz; gamma-oz *medicinal herb* [see: rice bran oil]

ozagrel INN *investigational antiasthmatic* [also: ozagrel sodium]

ozagrel sodium JAN *investigational antiasthmatic* [also: ozagrel]

ozolinone USAN, INN *diuretic*

P

P & S shampoo OTC *antiseborrheic; keratolytic* [salicylic acid] 2%

P & S topical liquid OTC *antimicrobial hair dressing* [phenol]

P & S Plus gel (discontinued 2003) OTC *antipsoriatic; antiseborrheic; keratolytic* [coal tar solution; salicylic acid] 8%•2%

p30 protein [see: ranpirnase]

^{32}P [see: chromic phosphate P 32]

^{32}P [see: polymetaphosphate P 32]

^{32}P [see: sodium phosphate P 32]

p53 adenoviral gene *investigational (Phase III) gene therapy for head and neck cancer* [also: adenoviral p53 gene]

P_1E_1; P_2E_1; P_4E_1; P_6E_1 Drop-Tainers (eye drops) (discontinued 2004) ℞ *antiglaucoma agent* [pilocarpine HCl; epinephrine bitartrate] 1%•1%; 2%•1%; 4%•1%; 6%•1%

PAB (para-aminobenzoate) [see: aminobenzoic acid]

PABA (para-aminobenzoic acid) [now: aminobenzoic acid]

PABA sodium [see: aminobenzoate sodium]

PAB-Esc-C (Platinol, Adriamycin, bleomycin, escalating doses of cyclophosphamide) *chemotherapy protocol*

pabestrol D [see: diethylstilbestrol dipropionate]

PAC; PAC-I (Platinol, Adriamycin, cyclophosphamide) *chemotherapy* *protocol for ovarian and endometrial cancer; "I" stands for "Indiana protocol," used for ovarian cancer only*

P-A-C Analgesic tablets OTC *analgesic; antipyretic; anti-inflammatory* [aspirin; caffeine] 400•32 mg

PACE (Platinol, Adriamycin, cyclophosphamide, etoposide) *chemotherapy protocol*

Pacerone tablets ℞ *antiarrhythmic for acute ventricular tachycardia and fibrillation (orphan)* [amiodarone HCl] 100, 200 mg

PA-CI (Adriamycin, cisplatin) *chemotherapy protocol for pediatric hepatoblastoma*

Pacis powder for intravesical instillation (discontinued 2004) ℞ *antineoplastic for urinary bladder cancer* [BCG vaccine, Montreal strain] 120 mg (2.4–12 × 10^8 CFU)

Packer's Pine Tar shampoo (discontinued 2003) OTC *antiseborrheic; antipsoriatic; antipruritic; antibacterial* [pine tar]

Packer's Pine Tar soap OTC *antiseborrheic; antipsoriatic; antipruritic; antibacterial* [pine tar]

paclitaxel USAN, INN, BAN *antineoplastic for AIDS-related Kaposi sarcoma (orphan), breast and ovarian cancers, and non–small cell lung cancer* 6 mg/mL injection

paclitaxel & carboplatin & etoposide *chemotherapy protocol for primary adenocarcinoma and small cell lung cancer (SCLC)*

paclitaxel & trastuzumab *chemotherapy protocol for breast cancer*

paclitaxel & vinorelbine tartrate *chemotherapy protocol for breast cancer*

pacrinolol INN

pactimibe *acyl-CoA cholesterol acyltransferase (ACAT) inhibitor; investigational (Phase III) antiatherosclerotic; keeps cholesterol from sticking to artery walls*

padimate INN *ultraviolet screen* [also: padimate A]

padimate A USAN *ultraviolet screen* [also: padimate]

padimate O USAN *ultraviolet screen*

Paeonia officinalis medicinal herb [see: peony]

pafenolol INN

paflufocon A USAN *hydrophobic contact lens material*

paflufocon B USAN *hydrophobic contact lens material*

paflufocon C USAN *hydrophobic contact lens material*

paflufocon D USAN *hydrophobic contact lens material*

paflufocon E USAN *hydrophobic contact lens material*

pagoclone USAN *nonsedating anxiolytic; investigational (Phase III) for panic disorder; investigational (Phase II) for generalized anxiety disorder*

PAH (para-aminohippurate) [see: aminohippuric acid]

PAHA (para-aminohippuric acid) [see: aminohippuric acid]

Pain Bust-R II cream OTC *analgesic; counterirritant* [methyl salicylate; menthol] 17%•12%

Pain Doctor cream OTC *analgesic; topical anesthetic; antipruritic* [capsaicin; methyl salicylate; menthol] 0.025%•25%•10%

Pain Gel Plus OTC *topical analgesic; counterirritant* [menthol] 4%

Painaid tablets OTC *analgesic; antipyretic; anti-inflammatory* [acetaminophen; aspirin; salicylamide; caffeine] 110•162•152•32.4 mg

Painaid BRF (Back Relief Formula) tablets OTC *analgesic; antipyretic; anti-inflammatory* [magnesium salicylate tetrahydrate; acetaminophen] 250•250 mg

Painaid ESF (Extra Strength Formula) tablets OTC *analgesic; antipyretic; anti-inflammatory* [aspirin; caffeine] 250•250•65 mg

Painaid PMF (Premenstrual Formula) tablets OTC *analgesic; antipyretic; diuretic* [acetaminophen; pamabrom] 500•25 mg

paint, Indian *medicinal herb* [see: bloodroot]

paint, yellow Indian *medicinal herb* [see: goldenseal]

paint root, red *medicinal herb* [see: bloodroot]

Pain-X gel OTC *topical analgesic; counterirritant* [capsaicin; menthol; camphor] 0.05%•5%•4%

PALA disodium [see: sparfosate sodium]

palatrigine INN, BAN

Palcaps 10; Palcaps 20 delayed-release capsules R *porcine-derived digestive enzymes* [lipase; protease; amylase] 10 000•37 500•33 200 USP units; 20 000•75 000•66 400 USP units

paldimycin USAN, INN *antibacterial*

paldimycin A [see: paldimycin]

paldimycin B [see: paldimycin]

pale gentian *medicinal herb* [see: gentian]

palestrol [see: diethylstilbestrol]

Palgic tablets, oral liquid R *antihistamine* [carbinoxamine maleate] 4 mg; 4 mg/5 mL

Palgic-D extended-release caplets R *decongestant; antihistamine* [pseudoephedrine HCl; carbinoxamine maleate] 80•8 mg

Palgic-DS pediatric syrup R *decongestant; antihistamine* [pseudoephedrine HCl; carbinoxamine maleate] 30•2 mg/5 mL

palifermin *keratinocyte growth factor (KGF) for radiation- and chemotherapy-induced oral mucositis*

palinavir USAN *antiviral; HIV-1 protease inhibitor*

palinum [see: cyclobarbitone]

palivizumab *monoclonal antibody for prophylaxis of respiratory syncytial virus (RSV) in infants*

palladium *element (Pd)*

Palladone extended-release pellets in capsules (withdrawn from the market in 2005 due to safety concerns) R *narcotic analgesic* [hydromorphone HCl] 12, 16, 24, 32 mg

palm, dwarf; dwarf palmetto; pan palm *medicinal herb* [see: saw palmetto]

palmidrol INN

Palmitate-A 5000 tablets OTC *vitamin supplement* [vitamin A palmitate] 5000 IU

palmitic acid USAN *ultrasound contrast medium for echocardiography*

palmoxirate sodium USAN *antidiabetic* [also: palmoxiric acid]

palmoxiric acid INN *antidiabetic* [also: palmoxirate sodium]

palonosetron HCl USAN *selective serotonin 5-HT₃ antagonist; antiemetic for chemotherapy-induced nausea and vomiting (CINV)*

PALS coated tablets OTC *systemic deodorant for ostomy, breath, and body odors* [chlorophyllin copper complex] 100 mg

PAM; L-PAM (phenylalanine mustard) [see: melphalan]

2-PAM (2-pyridine aldoxime methylchloride) [see: pralidoxime chloride]

pamabrom USAN *nonprescription diuretic*

pamaqueside USAN *hypocholesterolemic; cholesterol absorption inhibitor; antiatherosclerotic*

pamaquine naphthoate NF

pamatolol INN *antiadrenergic (β-receptor)* [also: pamatolol sulfate]

pamatolol sulfate USAN *antiadrenergic (β-receptor)* [also: pamatolol]

Pamelor capsules, oral solution R *tricyclic antidepressant* [nortriptyline HCl] 10, 25, 50, 75 mg; 10 mg/5 mL ⑨ Dymelor; Panlor

pamidronate disodium USAN *bisphosphonate bone resorption inhibitor for Paget disease, hypercalcemia of malignancy, and bone metastases of breast cancer and multiple myeloma* 3, 6, 9 mg/mL injection

pamidronic acid INN, BAN

Pamine; Pamine Forte tablets R *GI antispasmodic; anticholinergic; peptic* *ulcer treatment* [methscopolamine bromide] 2.5 mg; 5 mg

Pamisyl ℞ *investigational (orphan) for ulcerative colitis* [aminosalicylic acid]

pamoate USAN, USP *combining name for radicals or groups* [also: embonate]

Pamprin, Nighttime powder OTC *antihistaminic sleep aid; analgesic* [diphenhydramine HCl; acetaminophen] 50•650 mg

Pamprin Maximum Pain Relief caplets OTC *analgesic; antipyretic; diuretic* [acetaminophen; magnesium salicylate; pamabrom] 250•250•25 mg

Pamprin Multi-Symptom caplets, tablets OTC *analgesic; antipyretic; diuretic; antihistaminic sleep aid* [acetaminophen; pamabrom; pyrilamine maleate] 500•25•15 mg

Pan C Ascorbate; Pan C-500 tablets OTC *vitamin C supplement with multiple bioflavonoids* [vitamin C; citrus bioflavonoids; hesperidin] 200•100•100 mg; 500•100•100 mg

PAN-2400 capsules OTC *digestive enzymes* [lipase; protease; amylase] 9816•60 214•75 900 U

Panacet 5/500 tablets ℞ *narcotic analgesic* [hydrocodone bitartrate; acetaminophen] 5•500 mg

panadiplon USAN, INN *anxiolytic*

Panadol tablets, caplets OTC *analgesic; antipyretic* [acetaminophen] 500 mg

Panadol, Children's chewable tablets, oral liquid OTC *analgesic; antipyretic* [acetaminophen] 80 mg; 160 mg/5 mL

Panadol, Infants' drops OTC *analgesic; antipyretic* [acetaminophen] 100 mg/mL

Panadol, Junior caplets OTC *analgesic; antipyretic* [acetaminophen] 160 mg

Panafil ointment, spray ℞ *proteolytic enzyme for debridement of necrotic tissue; vulnerary; wound deodorant* [papain; urea; chlorophyllin copper complex] 521 700 U/g•10%•0.5%

Panafil White ointment ℞ *topical enzyme for wound debridement; vulnerary* [papain; urea] 10%•10%

Panalgesic cream OTC *analgesic; counterirritant* [methyl salicylate; menthol] 35%•4%

Panalgesic Gold liniment OTC *analgesic; counterirritant; antiseptic* [methyl salicylate; camphor; menthol; alcohol 22%] 55%•3.1%•1.25%

Panasal 5/500 tablets ℞ *narcotic analgesic* [hydrocodone bitartrate; aspirin] 5•500 mg

Panasol-S tablets ℞ *corticosteroid; anti-inflammatory; immunosuppressant* [prednisone] 1 mg ② Panscol

Panatuss DX oral liquid ℞ *decongestant; antihistamine; antitussive; expectorant* [phenylephrine HCl; dexchlorpheniramine maleate; dextromethorphan hydrobromide; guaifenesin] 5•1•15•100 mg/5 mL

Panax ginseng; P. shin-seng **(Korean ginseng)** *medicinal herb* [see: ginseng]

Panax horridum *medicinal herb* [see: devil's club]

Panax pseudoginseng **(Chikusetsu ginseng; Himalayan ginseng; Sanchi ginseng; Zhuzishen)** *medicinal herb* [see: ginseng]

Panax quinquefolia **(American ginseng)** *medicinal herb* [see: ginseng]

Panax spp. *medicinal herb* [see: ginseng]

Panax trifolius **(dwarf ginseng)** *medicinal herb* [see: ginseng]

Pancof syrup ℞ *narcotic antitussive; decongestant; antihistamine* [dihydrocodeine bitartrate; pseudoephedrine HCl; chlorpheniramine maleate] 7.5•15•2 mg/5 mL

Pancof-EXP syrup ℞ *narcotic antitussive; decongestant; expectorant* [dihydrocodeine bitartrate; pseudoephedrine HCl; guaifenesin] 7.5•15•100 mg/5 mL

Pancof-HC oral liquid (discontinued 2002) ℞ *narcotic antitussive; decongestant; antihistamine* [hydrocodone bitartrate; pseudoephedrine HCl; chlorpheniramine maleate] 3•15•2 mg/5 mL

Pancof-PD syrup ℞ *narcotic antitussive; decongestant; antihistamine*

[dihydrocodeine bitartrate; phenylephrine HCl; chlorpheniramine maleate] 3•7.5•2 mg/5 mL

Pancof-XP oral liquid ℞ *narcotic antitussive; decongestant; expectorant* [hydrocodone bitartrate; pseudoephedrine HCl; guaifenesin] 2.5•15•100 mg/5 mL

pancopride USAN, INN *antiemetic; anxiolytic; peristaltic stimulant*

Pancrease; Pancrease MT 4; Pancrease MT 10; Pancrease MT 16; Pancrease MT 20 capsules containing enteric-coated microtablets ℞ *porcine-derived digestive enzymes* [lipase; protease; amylase] 4.5•25•25; 4•12•12; 10•30•30; 16•48•48; 20•44•56 thousand USP units

pancreatin USP *porcine-derived digestive enzymes; a combination of lipase, protease, and amylase*

Pancreatin, 4X; Pancreatin, 8X tablets (discontinued 2002) OTC *porcine-derived digestive enzymes* [pancreatin (lipase; protease; amylase)] 2400 mg (12 000•60 000•60 000 USP units); 7200 mg (22 500•180 000•180 000 USP units)

Pancrecarb MS-4; Pancrecarb MS-8; Pancrecarb MS-16 delayed-release capsules containing enteric-coated microspheres ℞ *porcine-derived digestive enzymes* [lipase; protease; amylase] 4000•25 000•25 000 USP units; 8000•45 000•40 000 USP units; 16 000•52 000•52 000 USP units

pancrelipase USAN, USP *porcine-derived digestive enzymes; a combination of lipase, protease, and amylase* 4.5•25•20, 8•30•30, 16•48•48, 16•60•60 thousand USP units

Pancrezyme 4X tablets (discontinued 2002) OTC *porcine-derived digestive enzymes* [pancreatin (lipase; protease; amylase)] 2400 mg (12 000•60 000•60 000 USP units)

pancuronium bromide USAN, INN *nondepolarizing neuromuscular blocking agent; muscle relaxant; adjunct to* *tracheal intubation for general anesthesia or mechanical ventilation* 1, 2 mg/mL injection

Pandel cream ℞ *corticosteroidal anti-inflammatory* [hydrocortisone probutate] 0.1%

Panfil G capsules, syrup ℞ *antiasthmatic; bronchodilator; expectorant* [dyphylline; guaifenesin] 200•100 mg; 100•50 mg/5 mL

Panglobulin NF powder for IV infusion ℞ *passive immunizing agent for HIV and idiopathic thrombocytopenic purpura (ITP)* [immune globulin] 1, 3, 6, 12 g

Panhematin powder for IV injection ℞ *enzyme inhibitor for recurrent attacks of acute intermittent porphyria* [hemin] 301 mg/vial

panidazole INN, BAN

Panitone-500 tablets OTC *analgesic; antipyretic* [acetaminophen] 500 mg

Panixine DisperDose tablets for oral suspension ℞ *cephalosporin antibiotic* [cephalexin] 125, 250 mg

Panlor DC capsules ℞ *narcotic antitussive; analgesic* [dihydrocodeine bitartrate; acetaminophen; caffeine] 16•356.4•30 mg ⓓ Pamelor

Panlor SS tablets ℞ *narcotic analgesic* [dihydrocodeine bitartrate; acetaminophen; caffeine] 32•712.8•60 mg

PanMist-DM extended-release caplets, syrup ℞ *antitussive; decongestant; expectorant* [dextromethorphan hydrobromide; pseudoephedrine HCl; guaifenesin] 32•48•595 mg; 15•40•100 mg/5 mL

PanMist-JR extended-release caplets ℞ *decongestant; expectorant* [pseudoephedrine HCl; guaifenesin] 48•595 mg

PanMist-LA extended-release caplets ℞ *decongestant; expectorant* [pseudoephedrine HCl; guaifenesin] 85•795 mg

PanMist-S syrup ℞ *decongestant; expectorant* [pseudoephedrine HCl; guaifenesin] 40•200 mg/5 mL

Panmycin capsules (discontinued 2003) ℞ *broad-spectrum antibiotic* [tetracycline HCl] 250 mg

Pannaz sustained-release tablets ℞ *decongestant; antihistamine; anticholinergic to dry mucosal secretions* [pseudoephedrine HCl; carbinoxamine maleate; methscopolamine bromide] 90•8•2.5 mg

Pannaz S syrup ℞ *decongestant; antihistamine; anticholinergic to dry mucosal secretions* [pseudoephedrine HCl; carbinoxamine maleate; methscopolamine nitrate] 15•2•1.25 mg/5 mL

Panocaps; Panocaps MT 16; Panocaps MT 20 delayed-release capsules ℞ *porcine-derived digestive enzymes* [lipase; protease; amylase] 4500•25 000•20 000 USP units; 16 000•48 000•48 000 USP units; 20 000•44 000•56 000 USP units

Panokase tablets ℞ *porcine-derived digestive enzymes* [lipase; protease; amylase] 8000•30 000•30 000 USP units

panomifene INN

Panoxyl cleansing bar OTC *keratolytic for acne* [benzoyl peroxide] 5%, 10% ⊡ Benoxyl

Panoxyl 5; Panoxyl 10 gel ℞ *keratolytic and antiseptic for acne* [benzoyl peroxide; alcohol] 5%•12%; 10%•20%

Panoxyl AQ 2½; Panoxyl AQ 5; Panoxyl AQ 10 gel ℞ *keratolytic for acne* [benzoyl peroxide] 2.5%; 5%; 10%

Panretin capsules ℞ *investigational (Phase III, orphan) treatment for Kaposi sarcoma and acute promyelocytic leukemia (APL)* [alitretinoin]

Panretin gel ℞ *treatment for cutaneous lesions of AIDS-related Kaposi sarcoma (orphan)* [alitretinoin] 0.1%

Panscol lotion, ointment OTC *keratolytic* [salicylic acid] 3% ⊡ Panasol

pansy (Viola tricolor) plant *medicinal herb used as an anodyne, demulcent, diaphoretic, diuretic, expectorant, laxative, and vulnerary*

pantenicate INN

panthenol USAN, USP, INN *B complex vitamin*

D-panthenol [see: dexpanthenol]

Panthoderm cream OTC *antipruritic; vulnerary; emollient* [dexpanthenol] 2%

Panto IV ⒸⒶⓃ powder for injection ℞ *proton pump inhibitor for erosive esophagitis associated with gastroesophageal reflux disease (GERD)* [pantoprazole sodium] 40 mg/vial

Panto IV ⒸⒶⓃ powder for IV injection ℞ *proton pump inhibitor for gastroesophageal reflux disease (GERD) and eradication of* H. pylori *infection* [pantoprazole sodium]

Pantoloc ⒸⒶⓃ enteric-coated tablets ℞ *proton pump inhibitor for erosive esophagitis associated with gastroesophageal reflux disease (GERD)* [pantoprazole sodium] 40 mg

pantoprazole USAN, INN, BAN *proton pump inhibitor for erosive esophagitis associated with gastroesophageal reflux disease (GERD)*

pantoprazole sodium USAN *proton pump inhibitor for erosive esophagitis associated with gastroesophageal reflux disease (GERD) and Zollinger-Ellison syndrome*

pantothenic acid (vitamin B$_5$) BAN *water-soluble vitamin; enzyme A precursor* [also: calcium pantothenate] 92, 200, 500 mg oral

DL-pantothenic acid [see: calcium pantothenate, racemic]

pantothenol [see: dexpanthenol]

pantothenyl alcohol [see: panthenol]

D-pantothenyl alcohol [see: dexpanthenol]

panuramine INN, BAN

Panvac-VF ℞ *investigational (Phase III) antineoplastic vaccine for metastatic pancreatic cancer*

Panzem ℞ *investigational (orphan) for multiple myeloma* [2-methoxyestradiol]

papain USP *topical proteolytic enzyme for debridement of necrotic tissue*

papain & urea & chlorophyllin *proteolytic enzyme for debridement of* necrotic tissue; *vulnerary; wound deodorant* 521 700 U/g•10%•0.5% topical

papaverine BAN *peripheral vasodilator; smooth muscle relaxant; orphan status withdrawn 1996* [also: papaverine HCl]

papaverine HCl USP *peripheral vasodilator; smooth muscle relaxant for cerebral, myocardial, and peripheral ischemias* [also: papaverine] 150 mg oral; 30 mg/mL

papaveroline INN, BAN

papaya (Carica papaya) leaves, fruit, juice, and seeds *medicinal herb for aiding digestion, gas, insect bites, and intestinal worms*

Papaya Enzyme chewable tablets (discontinued 2002) OTC *digestive enzymes* [papain; amylase] 60•60 mg

Papirine ℞ *investigational antiviral*

Paplex Ultra topical solution ℞ *keratolytic* [salicylic acid in flexible collodion] 26%

papoose root *medicinal herb* [see: blue cohosh]

Par Glycerol elixir ℞ *expectorant* [iodinated glycerol] 60 mg/5 mL

Para Special Lice and Nits Ⓒᴬᴺ spray, shampoo OTC *pediculicide* [piperonyl butoxide; bioallethrin] 2.64%•0.66%; 4.4%•1.1%

para-aminobenzoate (PAB) [see: aminobenzoic acid]

Para-Aminobenzoic Acid tablets, powder OTC *"possibly effective" for scleroderma and other skin diseases and Peyronie disease* [aminobenzoic acid] 100, 500 mg; 120 g

para-aminobenzoic acid (PABA) [now: aminobenzoic acid]

para-aminohippurate (PAH) [see: aminohippuric acid]

para-aminohippurate sodium [see: aminohippurate sodium]

para-aminohippuric acid (PAHA) [see: aminohippuric acid]

para-aminosalicylate (PAS) [see: aminosalicylic acid]

para-aminosalicylic acid (PASA) [see: aminosalicylic acid]

Parabolan *brand name for trenbolone hexahydrobenzylcarbonate, a European veterinary anabolic steroid abused as a street drug*

parabromdylamine maleate [see: brompheniramine maleate]

paracetaldehyde [see: paraldehyde]

paracetamol INN, BAN *analgesic; antipyretic* [also: acetaminophen]

parachlorometaxylenol (PCMX) *topical antiseptic; broad-spectrum antibacterial*

parachlorophenol (PCP) USP *topical antibacterial*

parachlorophenol, camphorated USP *topical dental anti-infective*

paracodin [see: dihydrocodeine]

paraffin NF *stiffening agent*

paraffin, liquid [see: mineral oil]

paraffin, synthetic NF *stiffening agent*

Paraflex caplets ℞ *skeletal muscle relaxant* [chlorzoxazone] 250 mg

paraflutizide INN

Parafon Forte DSC caplets ℞ *skeletal muscle relaxant* [chlorzoxazone] 500 mg ② Pantopon

paraformaldehyde USP

Paraguay tea *medicinal herb* [see: yerba maté]

Para-Hist HD oral liquid (discontinued 2002) ℞ *narcotic antitussive; decongestant; antihistamine* [hydrocodone bitartrate; phenylephrine HCl; chlorpheniramine maleate] 1.67•5•2 mg/5 mL

parahydrecin [now: isomerol]

Paral oral liquid, rectal liquid ℞ *sedative; hypnotic* [paraldehyde]

paraldehyde USP *hypnotic; sedative; anticonvulsant* 1 g/mL oral or rectal

paramethadione USP, INN, BAN *anticonvulsant* ② paramethasone

paramethasone INN *corticosteroid; anti-inflammatory* [also: paramethasone acetate] ② paramethadione

paramethasone acetate USAN, USP *corticosteroid; anti-inflammatory* [also: paramethasone]

para-nitrosulfathiazole NF [also: nitrosulfathiazole]

paranyline HCl USAN *anti-inflammatory* [also: renytoline]

parapenzolate bromide USAN, INN *anticholinergic*

Paraplatin injection, powder for IV injection R *alkylating antineoplastic for ovarian and other cancers* [carboplatin] 10 mg/mL; 50, 150, 450 mg

parapropamol INN

pararosaniline embonate INN *antischistosomal* [also: pararosaniline pamoate]

pararosaniline pamoate USAN *antischistosomal* [also: pararosaniline embonate]

parasympathomimetics *a class of agents that produce effects similar to those of the parasympathetic nervous system* [also called: cholinergic agonists]

Parathar powder for IV injection (discontinued 2004) R *in vivo diagnostic aid for parathyroid-induced hypocalcemia (orphan)* [teriparatide acetate] 200 U

parathesin [see: benzocaine]

parathiazine INN

parathyroid USP *hormone*

parathyroid hormone (1-34), biosynthetic human [see: teriparatide]

parathyroid hormone (1-84), recombinant human *investigational (Phase III) agent to increase bone mineral content and density in postmenopausal osteoporosis*

paraxazone INN

parbendazole USAN, INN *anthelmintic*

parconazole INN *antifungal* [also: parconazole HCl]

parconazole HCl USAN *antifungal* [also: parconazole]

Parcopa RapiTab (orally disintegrating tablets) R *antiparkinsonian; dopamine precursor; decarboxylase inhibitor* [carbidopa; levodopa] 10•100, 25•100, 25•250 mg

parecoxib USAN, INN *COX-2 inhibitor; anti-inflammatory; analgesic*

parecoxib sodium USAN *COX-2 inhibitor; anti-inflammatory; analgesic*

Paredrine eye drops R *mydriatic* [hydroxyamphetamine hydrobromide] 1%

paregoric (PG) (a preparation of opium, anise oil, benzoic acid, camphor, alcohol, and glycerin) USP *antiperistaltic; narcotic analgesic; used in neonatal opioid withdrawal programs; sometimes abused as a street drug* 2 mg opium/5 mL oral

Paremyd eye drops R *mydriatic; weak cycloplegic* [hydroxyamphetamine hydrobromide; tropicamide] 1%•0.25%

parenabol [see: boldenone undecylenate]

Parepectolin concentrated oral liquid OTC *GI adsorbent; antidiarrheal* [attapulgite] 600 mg/15 mL

pareptide INN *antiparkinsonian* [also: pareptide sulfate]

pareptide sulfate USAN *antiparkinsonian* [also: pareptide]

parethoxycaine INN

parethoxycaine HCl [see: parethoxycaine]

Par-F tablets R *vitamin/mineral/calcium/iron supplement* [multiple vitamins & minerals; calcium; iron; folic acid] ±•250•60•1 mg

pargeverine INN

Pargluva tablets R *peroxisome proliferator–activated receptor (PPAR) alpha/gamma agonist; antidiabetic to lower blood glucose, lower triglyceride, and raise HDL levels* [muraglitazar] 5 mg

pargolol INN

pargyline INN *antihypertensive* [also: pargyline HCl]

pargyline HCl USAN, USP *antihypertensive* [also: pargyline]

paricalcitol USAN *synthetic vitamin D analogue for osteodystrophy and hyperparathyroidism secondary to chronic renal failure*

paridocaine INN

Parlodel SnapTabs (scored tablets), capsules R *dopamine agonist; antiparkinsonian; lactation preventative; treats acro-*

megaly, infertility, and hypogonadism [bromocriptine mesylate] 2.5 mg; 5 mg

Par-Natal Plus 1 Improved tablets ℞ *vitamin/calcium/iron supplement* [multiple vitamins; calcium; iron; folic acid] ± • 200 • 65 • 1 mg

Parnate film-coated tablets ℞ *monoamine oxidase inhibitor (MAOI) for reactive depression (a major depressive episode without melancholia)* [tranylcypromine sulfate] 10 mg

parodilol INN

parodyne [see: antipyrine]

paroleine [see: mineral oil]

paromomycin INN, BAN *aminoglycoside antibiotic; amebicide* [also: paromomycin sulfate]

Paromomycin ℞ *investigational (orphan) agent for visceral leishmaniasis* [aminosidine]

paromomycin sulfate USP *aminoglycoside antibiotic; amebicide for acute and chronic intestinal amebiasis; investigational (Phase III) for visceral leishmaniasis* [also: paromomycin]

paroxetine USAN, INN, BAN *selective serotonin reuptake inhibitor (SSRI) for depression, obsessive-compulsive disorder, and panic disorder*

paroxetine HCl *selective serotonin reuptake inhibitor (SSRI) for depression, obsessive-compulsive disorder, panic disorder, social anxiety disorder, generalized anxiety disorder, post-traumatic stress disorder, and premenstrual dysphoric disorder* 10, 20, 30, 40 mg oral

paroxetine mesylate *selective serotonin reuptake inhibitor (SSRI) for depression, obsessive-compulsive disorder, and panic disorder*

paroxyl [see: acetarsone]

paroxypropione INN

parpanit HCl [see: caramiphen HCl]

parsalmide INN

parsley (*Petroselinum sativum*) leaves and root *medicinal herb for amenorrhea, bladder infections, blood building and cleansing, body lice, colic, dysmenorrhea, flatulence, gallstones, inducing*

abortion, jaundice, nephritis, prostate disorders, and urinary retention

parsley fern *medicinal herb* [see: tansy]

parsnip, cow; wooly parsnip *medicinal herb* [see: masterwort]

Partaject ℞ *investigational (Phase II/III) intravenous delivery device*

Parthenocissus quinquefolia *medicinal herb* [see: American ivy]

partricin USAN, INN *antifungal; antiprotozoal*

partridge berry *medicinal herb* [see: squaw vine; wintergreen]

Partuss LA long-acting tablets (discontinued 2002) ℞ *decongestant; expectorant* [phenylpropanolamine HCl; guaifenesin] 75 • 400 mg

parvaquone INN, BAN

Parvlex tablets OTC *hematinic* [ferrous fumarate; multiple B vitamins & minerals; vitamin C; folic acid] 100 • ± • 50 • 0.1 mg

PAS (para-aminosalicylate) [see: aminosalicylic acid]

PASA (para-aminosalicylic acid) [see: aminosalicylic acid]

Paser delayed-release granules for oral solution ℞ *treatment for multidrug-resistant tuberculosis (MDR-TB) (orphan)* [aminosalicylic acid] 4 g/pkt.

pasiniazid INN

pasque flower (*Anemone patens*) plant *medicinal herb used as a diaphoretic, diuretic, and rubefacient; not generally regarded as safe and effective due to toxicity*

passion flower (*Passiflora incarnata*) plant *medicinal herb for asthma, bronchitis, eye infections, fever, inflamed hemorrhoids, insomnia, menopause, nervousness, pain related to neurasthenia, and attention-deficit disorder, nervousness, and excitability in children*

Pastilles (dosage form) *troches*

Patanol Drop-Tainers (eye drops) ℞ *topical ophthalmic antihistamine and mast cell stabilizer for allergic conjunctivitis* [olopatadine HCl] 0.1%

PATCO (prednisone, ara-C, thio-guanine, cyclophosphamide, Oncovin) *chemotherapy protocol*

Pathilon film-coated tablets (discontinued 2001) ℞ *peptic ulcer treatment adjunct* [tridihexethyl chloride] 25 mg ☑ Pathocil

Pathocil capsules, powder for oral suspension (discontinued 2002) ℞ *penicillinase-resistant penicillin antibiotic* [dicloxacillin sodium] 250, 500 mg; 62.5 mg/5 mL ☑ Bactocill; Pathilon; Placidyl

patience, garden *medicinal herb* [see: yellow dock]

patience dock *medicinal herb* [see: bistort]

pau d'arco (*Lapacho colorado; L. morado*) inner bark *medicinal herb for boils, blood cleansing, cancer, Candida albicans infections, chlorosis, diabetes, leukemia, skin wounds, syphilis, and pain*

Paullinia cupana; P. sorbilis *medicinal herb* [see: guarana]

paulomycin USAN, INN *antibacterial*

Pausinystalia johimbe *medicinal herb* [see: yohimbe]

pauson *medicinal herb* [see: bloodroot]

Pavabid Plateau Caps (controlled-release capsules) ℞ *peripheral vasodilator; smooth muscle relaxant for cerebral, myocardial, and peripheral ischemias* [papaverine HCl] 150 mg ☑ Pavased

Pavagen TD timed-release capsules ℞ *peripheral vasodilator; smooth muscle relaxant for cerebral, myocardial, and peripheral ischemias* [papaverine HCl] 150 mg

PAVe (procarbazine, Alkeran, Velban) *chemotherapy protocol*

Pavulon IM injection (discontinued 2004) ℞ *nondepolarizing neuromuscular blocking agent; muscle relaxant; adjunct to tracheal intubation for general anesthesia or mechanical ventilation* [pancuronium bromide] 1, 2 mg/mL ☑ Paverolan

pawpaw (*Asimina triloba*) fruit *medicinal herb used as an antimicrobial and antineoplastic*

paxamate INN

Paxarel tablets ℞ *anxiolytic; sedative* [acecarbromal] 250 mg

Paxene ℞ *investigational (Phase III) antineoplastic for AIDS-related Kaposi sarcoma* [paclitaxel]

Paxil film-coated tablets, oral suspension ℞ *selective serotonin reuptake inhibitor (SSRI) for depression, obsessive-compulsive disorder, panic disorder, social anxiety disorder, generalized anxiety disorder, and post-traumatic stress disorder* [paroxetine HCl] 10, 20, 30, 40 mg; 10 mg/5 mL

Paxil CR enteric-coated controlled-release tablets ℞ *selective serotonin reuptake inhibitor (SSRI) for depression, panic disorder, premenstrual dysphoric disorder (PMDD), and social anxiety disorder* [paroxetine HCl] 12.5, 25, 37.5 mg

pazelliptine INN

pazinaclone USAN *anxiolytic*

Pazo Hemorrhoid ointment OTC *temporary relief of hemorrhoidal symptoms; topical vasoconstrictor; counterirritant; astringent* [ephedrine sulfate; camphor; zinc oxide] 0.2%•2%•5%

Pazo Hemorrhoid suppositories OTC *temporary relief of hemorrhoidal symptoms; topical vasoconstrictor; astringent* [ephedrine sulfate; zinc oxide] 3.8• 96.5 mg

pazoxide USAN, INN *antihypertensive*

PBV (Platinol, bleomycin, vinblastine) *chemotherapy protocol*

PBZ tablets (discontinued 2002) ℞ *antihistamine* [tripelennamine HCl] 25, 50 mg

PBZ (pyribenzamine) [see: tripelennamine]

PBZ-SR extended-release tablets (discontinued 2002) ℞ *antihistamine* [tripelennamine HCl] 100 mg

PC (paclitaxel, carboplatin) *chemotherapy protocol for bladder cancer and non–small cell lung cancer (NSCLC)*

PC (paclitaxel, cisplatin) *chemotherapy protocol for non–small cell lung cancer (NSCLC)*

PC (phosphatidylcholine) [see: lecithin]

PC Tar shampoo OTC *antiseborrheic; antipsoriatic; antipruritic; antibacterial* [coal tar] 1%

PCE Dispertabs (delayed-release tablets) ℞ *macrolide antibiotic* [erythromycin] 333, 500 mg

PCE (Platinol, cyclophosphamide, etoposide) *chemotherapy protocol*

PCE (polymer-coated erythromycin) [see: erythromycin]

PCMX (parachlorometaxylenol) [q.v.]

PCOs (procyanidolic oligomers) [q.v.]

PCP (parachlorophenol) [q.v.]

PCP (phenylcyclohexyl piperidine) *a powerful veterinary analgesic/anesthetic widely abused as a hallucinogenic street drug* [medically known as phencyclidine HCl]

PCV (pneumococcal vaccine) [q.v.]

PCV (procarbazine, CCNU, vincristine) *chemotherapy protocol for brain tumors*

PDE III (phosphodiesterase III) inhibitors *a class of platelet aggregation inhibitors*

PDGA (pteroyldiglutamic acid)

PDLA (phosphinicodilactic acid) [see: foscolic acid]

PDP Liquid Protein (discontinued 2001) OTC *dietary supplement* [hydrolyzed protein; L-tryptophan] 15•$\underline{2}$ g/30 mL

PE (paclitaxel, estramustine) *chemotherapy protocol for prostate cancer*

PE (phenylephrine) [q.v.]

PE (polyethylene) [q.v.]

pea, ground squirrel *medicinal herb* [see: twin leaf]

pea, turkey; wild turkey pea *medicinal herb* [see: turkey corn]

peach (Prunus persica) bark and leaves *medicinal herb for bladder disorders, chest congestion, chronic bronchitis, nausea, and water retention*

peanut oil NF *solvent*

PEB (Platinol, etoposide, bleomycin) *chemotherapy protocol*

pecazine INN, BAN

pecazine acetate [see: pecazine]

pecilocin INN, BAN

pecocycline INN

pectin USP *suspending agent; protectant; GI adsorbent*

pectorals *a class of agents that relieve disorders of the respiratory tract, such as expectorants*

Pedameth capsules, oral liquid ℞ *urinary acidifier to control ammonia production* [racemethionine] 200 mg; 75 mg/5 mL

Pedia Relief Decongestant Plus Cough infants' oral drops OTC *antitussive; decongestant* [dextromethorphan hydrobromide; pseudoephedrine HCl] 5•15 mg/1.6 mL

PediaCare Allergy Formula oral liquid OTC *antihistamine* [chlorpheniramine maleate] 1 mg/5 mL

PediaCare Children's Cold & Allergy oral liquid OTC *decongestant; antihistamine* [pseudoephedrine HCl; chlorpheniramine maleate] 30•2 mg/10 mL

PediaCare Children's Long-Lasting Cough Plus Cold oral liquid OTC *antitussive; decongestant* [dextromethorphan hydrobromide; pseudoephedrine HCl] 7.5•15 mg/5 mL

PediaCare Children's Multi-Symptom Cold chewable tablets OTC *pediatric antitussive, decongestant, and antihistamine* [dextromethorphan hydrobromide; pseudoephedrine HCl; chlorpheniramine maleate] 5•15•1 mg

PediaCare Cold-Allergy chewable tablets (discontinued 2002) OTC *pediatric decongestant and antihistamine* [pseudoephedrine HCl; chlorpheniramine maleate] 15•1 mg

PediaCare Cough-Cold pediatric chewable tablets (discontinued 2002) OTC *antitussive; decongestant; antihistamine* [dextromethorphan

hydrobromide; pseudoephedrine HCl; chlorpheniramine maleate] 5•15•1 mg

PediaCare Cough-Cold; PediaCare Multi-Symptom Cold pediatric oral liquid OTC *antitussive; decongestant; antihistamine* [dextromethorphan hydrobromide; pseudoephedrine HCl; chlorpheniramine maleate] 10•30•2 mg/10 mL

PediaCare Fever oral suspension, oral drops OTC *analgesic; antiarthritic; antipyretic; nonsteroidal anti-inflammatory drug (NSAID)* [ibuprofen] 100 mg/5 mL; 40 mg/mL

PediaCare Infant's Decongestant oral drops OTC *nasal decongestant* [pseudoephedrine HCl] 7.5 mg/0.8 mL

PediaCare Infant's Decongestant & Cough oral drops OTC *antitussive; decongestant* [dextromethorphan hydrobromide; pseudoephedrine HCl] 5•15 mg/1.6 mL

PediaCare Infants' Long-Acting Cough oral drops OTC *antitussive* [dextromethorphan hydrobromide] 7.5 mg/0.8 mL

PediaCare NightRest Cough & Cold pediatric oral liquid OTC *antitussive; decongestant; antihistamine* [dextromethorphan hydrobromide; pseudoephedrine HCl; chlorpheniramine maleate] 15•30•2 mg/10 mL

Pediacof pediatric syrup (discontinued 2002) ℞ *narcotic antitussive; decongestant; antihistamine; expectorant* [codeine phosphate; phenylephrine HCl; chlorpheniramine maleate; potassium iodide; alcohol 5%] 5•2.5•0.75•75 mg/5 mL

Pediacon DX children's syrup, pediatric drops (discontinued 2002) OTC *pediatric antitussive, decongestant, and expectorant* [dextromethorphan hydrobromide; phenylpropanolamine HCl; guaifenesin] 5•6.25•100 mg/5 mL; 5•6.25•50 mg/mL

Pediacon EX pediatric drops (discontinued 2002) OTC *decongestant;*

expectorant [phenylpropanolamine HCl; guaifenesin] 6.25•50 mg/mL

Pediaflor drops ℞ *dental caries preventative* [sodium fluoride] 1.1 mg/mL

Pediahist DM oral drops ℞ *decongestant; antihistamine; antitussive* [pseudoephedrine HCl; brompheniramine maleate; dextromethorphan hydrobromide] 15•1•4 mg/mL

Pediahist DM syrup ℞ *decongestant; antihistamine; antitussive; expectorant* [pseudoephedrine HCl; brompheniramine maleate; dextromethorphan hydrobromide; guaifenesin] 30•2•5•50/5 mL

Pedialyte oral solution, freezer pops OTC *electrolyte replacement* [sodium, potassium, and chloride electrolytes]

Pediamist low-pressure nasal spray OTC *nasal moisturizer for children* [sodium chloride (saline solution)]

Pediapred oral solution ℞ *corticosteroid; anti-inflammatory* [prednisolone sodium phosphate] 5 mg/5 mL

Pediarix IM injection ℞ *active immunizing agent for diphtheria, tetanus, pertussis, hepatitis B and D, and three types of poliovirus* [diphtheria & tetanus toxoids & acellular pertussis (DTaP) vaccine; hepatitis B virus vaccine; inactivated poliovirus vaccine Types 1, 2, and 3] 25 Lf•10 Lf•25 µg•10 µg•40 DU•8 DU•32 DU per 0.5 mL dose

PediaSure; PediaSure with Fiber ready-to-use oral liquid OTC *total or supplementary infant feeding*

Pediatex oral liquid ℞ *antihistamine* [carbinoxamine maleate] 1.5 mg/5 mL

Pediatex 12 oral suspension ℞ *antihistamine* [carbinoxamine tannate] 3.6 mg/5 mL

Pediatex-D pediatric oral liquid ℞ *decongestant; antihistamine* [pseudoephedrine HCl; carbinoxamine maleate] 20•2 mg/5 mL

Pediatex-DM pediatric oral liquid ℞ *antitussive; decongestant; antihistamine* [dextromethorphan hydrobromide;

pseudoephedrine HCl; carbinox-amine maleate] 15•15•2 mg/5 mL

Pediatric Electrolyte oral solution OTC *electrolyte replacement* [dextrose; multiple electrolytes] 1 L

pediatric VAC *chemotherapy protocol for pediatric sarcomas* [see: VAC pediatric]

Pediazole oral suspension ℞ *antibiotic* [erythromycin ethylsuccinate; sulfisoxazole acetyl] 200•600 mg/5 mL

Pedi-Boro Soak Paks powder packets OTC *astringent wet dressing (modified Burow solution)* [aluminum sulfate; calcium acetate]

pediculicides *a class of agents effective against head and pubic lice*

Pedi-Dri powder ℞ *topical antifungal* [nystatin] 100 000 U/g

Pediotic ear drop suspension ℞ *topical corticosteroidal anti-inflammatory; antibiotic* [hydrocortisone; neomycin sulfate; polymyxin B sulfate] 1%•5 mg•10 000 U per mL

Pediox pediatric chewable tablets ℞ *decongestant; antihistamine* [pseudoephedrine HCl; chlorpheniramine maleate] 15•2 mg

Pedi-Pro foot powder OTC *antifungal; anhidrotic* [benzalkonium chloride] 1%

Pedituss Cough pediatric syrup (discontinued 2002) ℞ *narcotic antitussive; decongestant; antihistamine; expectorant* [codeine phosphate; phenylephrine HCl; chlorpheniramine maleate; potassium iodide] 5•2.5•0.75•75 mg/5 mL

Pedi-Vit-A Creme OTC *moisturizer; emollient* [vitamin A] 100 000 U/30 g

Pedotic otic suspension ℞ *topical corticosteroidal anti-inflammatory; antibiotic* [hydrocortisone; neomycin sulfate; polymyxin B sulfate] 1%•5 mg•10 000 U per mL

PedTE-Pak-4 IV injection ℞ *intravenous nutritional therapy* [multiple trace elements (metals)]

Pedtrace-4 IV injection ℞ *intravenous nutritional therapy* [multiple trace elements (metals)]

PedvaxHIB IM injection ℞ *pediatric (2–71 months) vaccine for* Haemophilus influenzae *type b (HIB)* [Hemophilus b conjugate vaccine; Neisseria meningitidis OMPC] 7.5•125 μg/dose

pefloxacin USAN, INN, BAN *antibacterial*

pefloxacin mesylate USAN *antibacterial*

PEG (polyethylene glycol) [q.v.]

pegacaristim USAN *megakaryocyte stimulating factor for thrombocytopenia*

PEG-ADA (polyethylene glycol-adenosine deaminase) [see: pegademase bovine]

pegademase INN *adenosine deaminase (ADA) replacement* [also: pegademase bovine]

pegademase bovine USAN *adenosine deaminase (ADA) replacement for severe combined immunodeficiency disease (orphan)* [also: pegademase]

PEG-adenosine deaminase (PEG-ADA) [see: pegademase bovine]

Peganone tablets ℞ *hydantoin anticonvulsant* [ethotoin] 250, 500 mg

pegaptanib sodium *pegylated VEGF (vascular endothelial growth factor) antagonist for neovascular (wet) age-related macular degeneration (AMD); investigational (Phase II) for diabetic retinopathy*

PEG-L-asparaginase [see: pegaspargase]

pegaspargase (PEG-L-asparaginase) USAN, INN *antineoplastic for acute lymphocytic leukemia (orphan) and acute lymphoblastic leukemia*

Pegasys subcu injection, prefilled syringes ℞ *immunomodulator for chronic hepatitis B and C; investigational (orphan) for renal cell carcinoma* [peginterferon alfa-2a] 180 μg/mL

PEG-ES (polyethylene glycol–electrolyte solution) [q.v.]

pegfilgrastim *recombinant human granulocyte colony-stimulating factor (G-CSF) in polyethylene glycol (PEG); hematopoietic stimulant for severe chronic neutropenia following cancer chemotherapy*

PEG-glucocerebrosidase *investigational (orphan) chronic enzyme replacement therapy for Gaucher disease*

peginterferon alfa-2a *immunomodulator for chronic hepatitis C; investigational (orphan) for renal cell carcinoma*

peginterferon alfa-2b *immunomodulator for chronic hepatitis C; investigational (Phase III) for malignant melanoma and chronic myelogenous leukemia*

PEG-interleukin-2 *investigational (Phase II) cytokine for AIDS; investigational (orphan) for primary immunodeficiencies associated with T-cell defects*

PEG-Intron *powder for subcu injection antiviral; long-acting formulation of Intron A for chronic hepatitis C; investigational (Phase III) for malignant melanoma and chronic myelogenous leukemia* [peginterferon alfa-2b] 100, 160, 240, 300 μg/mL

peglicol 5 oleate USAN *emulsifying agent*

pegnartograstim USAN *immunostimulant adjunct to cancer chemotherapy*

pegorgotein USAN, INN *free-radical scavenger; investigational to prevent irreversible brain damage after head trauma*

pegoterate USAN, INN *suspending agent*

pegoxol 7 stearate USAN *emulsifying agent*

PEG-SOD (polyethylene glycol-superoxide dismutase) [see: pegorgotein]

pegvisomant USAN *growth hormone receptor antagonist for acromegaly (orphan)*

pegylated megakaryocyte growth factor [see: megakaryocyte growth and development factor, pegylated, recombinant human]

pelanserin INN *antihypertensive; vasodilator; serotonin adrenergic blocker* [also: pelanserin HCl]

pelanserin HCl USAN *antihypertensive; vasodilator; serotonin adrenergic blocker* [also: pelanserin]

peldesine USAN *purine nucleoside phosphorylase inhibitor for psoriasis; investigational (orphan) for cutaneous T-cell lymphoma; investigational (Phase III) for HIV*

peliomycin USAN, INN *antineoplastic*

pellants *a class of agents that purify or cleanse the system, particularly the blood* [also called: depurants; depuratives]

pelretin USAN, INN *antikeratinizing agent*

pelrinone INN *cardiotonic* [also: pelrinone HCl]

pelrinone HCl USAN *cardiotonic* [also: pelrinone]

PemADD tablets (discontinued 2003) ℞ *CNS stimulant for attention-deficit hyperactivity disorder (ADHD)* [pemoline] 18.75, 37.5, 75 mg

PemADD CT chewable tablets ℞ *CNS stimulant for attention-deficit hyperactivity disorder (ADHD)* [pemoline] 37.5 mg

pemedolac USAN, INN *analgesic*

pemerid INN *antitussive* [also: pemerid nitrate]

pemerid nitrate USAN *antitussive* [also: pemerid]

pemetrexed disodium USAN *folic acid antagonist; inhibitor of thymidylate synthase, dihydrofolate reductase, and glycinamide ribonucleotide formyl transferase; antineoplastic for malignant pleural mesothelioma (MPM) and non–small cell lung cancer (NSCLC)*

pemirolast INN *ophthalmic antiallergic; mast cell stabilizer* [also: pemirolast potassium]

pemirolast potassium USAN *ophthalmic antiallergic; mast cell stabilizer* [also: pemirolast]

pemoline USAN, INN, BAN, JAN *CNS stimulant for attention-deficit hyperactivity disorder (ADHD) and narcolepsy* 18.75, 37.5, 75 mg oral

pempidine INN, BAN

penamecillin USAN, INN, BAN *antibacterial*

penbutolol INN, BAN *antiadrenergic (β-receptor)* [also: penbutolol sulfate]

penbutolol sulfate USAN *antiadrenergic (β-receptor)* [also: penbutolol]

penciclovir USAN, INN, BAN *topical antiviral for recurrent herpes labialis*

penciclovir sodium USAN *antiviral for herpes infections*

pendecamaine INN, BAN

pendiomide [see: azamethonium bromide]

Penecare cream, lotion OTC *moisturizer; emollient* [lactic acid]

Penecort cream, solution ℞ *topical corticosteroidal anti-inflammatory* [hydrocortisone] 1%

penems *a class of broad-spectrum antibiotics*

Penetrex film-coated tablets (discontinued 2002) ℞ *broad-spectrum fluoroquinolone antibiotic* [enoxacin] 200, 400 mg

PenFill (trademarked form) *insulin injector refill cartridge*

penfluridol USAN, INN *antipsychotic*

penflutizide INN

pengitoxin INN

penicillamine USAN, USP, INN *metal chelating agent; antirheumatic* ② penicillin

penicillin aluminum

penicillin benzathine phenoxymethyl [now: penicillin V benzathine]

penicillin calcium USP

penicillin G benzathine USP *natural penicillin antibiotic* [also: benzathine benzylpenicillin; benzathine penicillin; benzylpenicillin benzathine]

penicillin G hydrabamine *natural penicillin antibiotic*

penicillin G potassium USP *natural penicillin antibiotic* [also: benzylpenicillin potassium] 1, 2, 3, 5, 10, 20 million U injection

penicillin G procaine USP *natural penicillin antibiotic* [also: procaine penicillin] 600 000, 1 200 000 U injection

penicillin G redox [see: redox-penicillin G]

penicillin G sodium USP *natural penicillin antibiotic* [also: benzylpenicillin sodium] 5 million U injection

penicillin hydrabamine phenoxymethyl [now: penicillin V hydrabamine]

penicillin N [see: adicillin]

penicillin O [see: almecillin]

penicillin O chloroprocaine

penicillin O potassium

penicillin O sodium

penicillin phenoxymethyl [now: penicillin V]

penicillin potassium G [see: penicillin G potassium]

penicillin potassium phenoxymethyl [now: penicillin V potassium]

penicillin V USAN, USP *natural penicillin antibiotic* [also: phenoxymethylpenicillin]

penicillin V benzathine USAN, USP *natural penicillin antibiotic*

penicillin V hydrabamine USAN, USP *natural penicillin antibiotic*

penicillin V potassium USAN, USP *natural penicillin antibiotic*

Penicillin VK tablets, powder for oral solution ℞ *natural penicillin antibiotic* [penicillin V potassium] 250, 500 mg; 125, 250 mg/5 mL

penicillin-152 potassium [see: phenethicillin potassium] ② penicillamine; Polycillin

penicillinase INN, BAN

penicillinase-resistant penicillins *a subclass of penicillins (q.v.)*

penicillinphenyrazine [see: phenyracillin]

penicillins *a class of bactericidal antibiotics, divided into natural, penicillinase-resistant, aminopenicillin, and extended-spectrum penicillins, and effective against both gram-positive and gram-negative bacteria* [also called: "cillins"]

penidural [see: benzathine penicillin]

penimepicycline INN

penimocycline INN

PenInject (trademarked delivery device) *prefilled self-injection syringe*

penirolol INN

Pen-Kera cream OTC *moisturizer; emollient*

Penlac Nail Lacquer topical solution ℞ *antifungal for onychomycosis* [ciclopirox] 8%

penmesterol INN

pennyroyal (*Hedeoma pulegeoides; Mentha pulegium*) plant *medicinal herb for childbirth pain, colds, colic, fever, gas, inducing abortion and menstruation, mouth sores, respiratory illnesses, and venomous bites; also used as an insect repellent; not generally regarded as safe and effective for ingestion due to toxicity*

penoctonium bromide INN

penprostene INN

penta tea *medicinal herb* [see: jiaogulan]

pentabamate USAN, INN *minor tranquilizer*

Pentacarinat IV or IM injection ℞ *antiprotozoal; treatment and prophylaxis of* Pneumocystis carinii *pneumonia (orphan)* [pentamidine isethionate] 300 mg

Pentacel ℞ *investigational (Phase III) vaccine for diphtheria, pertussis, tetanus (DPT), polio, and* Haemophilus influenzae *type b*

pentacosactride BAN [also: norleusactide]

pentacynium chloride INN

pentacyone chloride [see: pentacynium chloride]

pentaerithritol tetranicotinate [see: niceritrol]

pentaerithrityl tetranitrate INN *vasodilator* [also: pentaerythritol tetranitrate]

pentaerythritol tetranitrate (PETN) USP *coronary vasodilator; antianginal* [also: pentaerithrityl tetranitrate]

pentaerythritol trinitrate [see: pentrinitrol]

pentafilcon A USAN *hydrophilic contact lens material*

pentafluranol INN, BAN

pentagastrin USAN, INN, JAN *gastric secretion indicator*

pentagestrone INN

pentalamide INN, BAN

pentalyte USAN, USP, NF *electrolyte combination*

Pentam 300 IV or IM injection ℞ *antiprotozoal; treatment and prophylaxis of* Pneumocystis carinii *pneumonia (orphan)* [pentamidine isethionate] 300 mg

pentamethazene [see: azamethonium bromide]

pentamethonium bromide INN, BAN

pentamethylenetetrazol [see: pentylenetetrazol]

pentamidine INN, BAN

pentamidine isethionate *antiprotozoal; treatment and prophylaxis of* Pneumocystis carinii *pneumonia (orphan)* 300 mg injection

pentamin [see: azamethonium bromide]

pentamorphone USAN, INN *narcotic analgesic*

pentamoxane INN

pentamoxane HCl [see: pentamoxane]

pentamustine USAN *antineoplastic* [also: neptamustine]

pentanedial [see: glutaral]

pentanitrol [see: pentaerythritol tetranitrate]

pentaphonate

pentapiperide INN

pentapiperium methylsulfate USAN *anticholinergic* [also: pentapiperium metilsulfate]

pentapiperium metilsulfate INN *anticholinergic* [also: pentapiperium methylsulfate]

pentaquine INN [also: pentaquine phosphate]

pentaquine phosphate USP [also: pentaquine]

Pentasa controlled-release capsules ℞ *anti-inflammatory for active ulcerative colitis, proctosigmoiditis, and proctitis* [mesalamine (5-aminosalicylic acid)] 250, 500 mg

pentasodium colistinmethanesulfonate [see: colistimethate sodium]

Pentaspan ℞ *leukapheresis adjunct to improve leukocyte yield (orphan)* [pentastarch]

pentastarch USAN, BAN *leukapheresis adjunct; red cell sedimenting agent;*

centrifugal leukocyte harvesting aid (orphan)

pentavalent gas gangrene antitoxin

Pentazine VC with Codeine oral liquid (discontinued 2002) R *narcotic antitussive; antihistamine* [codeine phosphate; promethazine HCl] 10•6.25 mg/5 mL

pentazocine USAN, USP, INN, BAN *narcotic agonist-antagonist analgesic; also abused as a street drug*

pentazocine HCl USAN, USP *narcotic agonist-antagonist analgesic; also abused as a street drug*

pentazocine HCl & acetaminophen *narcotic analgesic* 25•650 mg oral

pentazocine lactate USAN, USP *narcotic agonist-antagonist analgesic for moderate to severe pain; adjunct to surgical anesthesia; also abused as a street drug*

pentazocine & naloxone HCl *narcotic agonist-antagonist analgesic; also abused as a street drug* 50•0.5 mg oral

pentetate calcium trisodium (Ca-DTPA) USAN *chelating agent for plutonium, americium, and curium; approved to treat contamination from radioactive materials (radiation sickness from "dirty bombs")* [also: calcium trisodium pentetate] 200 mg/mL (1000 mg/dose) injection

pentetate calcium trisodium Yb 169 USAN *radioactive agent*

pentetate disodium [see: pentetic acid, sodium salts]

pentetate indium disodium In 111 USAN *diagnostic aid; radioactive agent*

pentetate monosodium [see: pentetic acid, sodium salts]

pentetate pentasodium [see: pentetic acid, sodium salts]

pentetate tetrasodium [see: pentetic acid, sodium salts]

pentetate trisodium [see: pentetic acid, sodium salts]

pentetate trisodium calcium [see: pentetate calcium trisodium]

pentetate zinc trisodium (Zn-DTPA) *chelating agent for plutonium, ameri-*

cium, and curium; approved to treat contamination from radioactive materials (radiation sickness from "dirty bombs") 200 mg/mL (1000 mg/dose) injection

pentethylcyclanone [see: cyclexanone]

pentetic acid USAN, BAN *diagnostic aid*

pentetic acid, sodium salts *diagnostic aid*

pentetrazol INN [also: pentylenetetrazol]

penthanil diethylenetriamine penta-acetic acid (DTPA) [see: pentetic acid]

penthienate bromide NF

Penthrane liquid for vaporization R *inhalation general anesthetic* [methoxyflurane]

penthrichloral INN, BAN

pentiapine INN *antipsychotic* [also: pentiapine maleate]

pentiapine maleate USAN *antipsychotic* [also: pentiapine]

penticide [see: chlorophenothane]

pentifylline INN, BAN

pentigetide USAN, INN *antiallergic*

pentisomicin USAN, INN *anti-infective*

pentisomide INN

pentizidone INN *antibacterial* [also: pentizidone sodium]

pentizidone sodium USAN *antibacterial* [also: pentizidone]

pentobarbital USP, INN *sedative; hypnotic; also abused as a street drug* [also: pentobarbitone; pentobarbital calcium] ② phenobarbital

pentobarbital calcium JAN *sedative; hypnotic; also abused as a street drug* [also: pentobarbital; pentobarbitone]

pentobarbital sodium USP, JAN *sedative; hypnotic; also abused as a street drug* [also: pentobarbitone sodium] 100 mg oral; 50 mg/mL injection

pentobarbitone BAN *sedative; hypnotic; also abused as a street drug* [also: pentobarbital]

pentobarbitone sodium BAN *sedative; hypnotic; also abused as a street drug* [also: pentobarbital sodium]

Pentolair eye drops R *mydriatic; cycloplegic* [cyclopentolate HCl] 1%

pentolinium tartrate NF [also: pentolonium tartrate]

pentolonium tartrate INN [also: pentolinium tartrate]

pentolonum bitartrate [see: pentolinium tartrate]

pentomone USAN, INN *prostate growth inhibitor*

pentopril USAN, INN *angiotensin-converting enzyme (ACE) inhibitor*

pentorex INN

pentosalen BAN

pentosan polysulfate sodium USAN, INN *urinary tract anti-inflammatory and analgesic for interstitial cystitis (orphan)* [also: pentosan polysulphate sodium]

pentosan polysulphate sodium BAN *urinary tract anti-inflammatory and analgesic* [also: pentosan polysulfate sodium]

Pentostam (available only from the Centers for Disease Control) ℞ *investigational anti-infective for leishmaniasis* [sodium stibogluconate]

pentostatin USAN, INN *antibiotic antineoplastic for hairy cell leukemia (orphan); investigational (orphan) for chronic lymphocytic leukemia and cutaneous T-cell lymphoma; investigational (Phase III) for AIDS-related non-Hodgkin lymphoma*

Pentothal powder for IV injection ℞ *barbiturate general anesthetic* [thiopental sodium] 2%, 2.5% (20, 25 mg/mL) ② pentrinitrol

pentoxifylline USAN, INN *peripheral vasodilator; hemorheologic agent* [also: oxpentifylline] 400 mg oral

pentoxiverine citrate [see: carbetapentane citrate]

pentoxyverine INN [also: carbetapentane citrate]

pentoxyverine citrate [see: carbetapentane citrate]

Pentrax shampoo OTC *antiseborrheic; antipsoriatic; antipruritic; antibacterial* [coal tar] 5%

Pentrax Gold shampoo (discontinued 2003) OTC *antiseborrheic; antipsoriatic; antipruritic; antibacterial* [coal tar] 4%

pentrinitrol USAN, INN *coronary vasodilator* ② Pentothal

***tert*-pentyl alcohol** [see: amylene hydrate]

6-pentyl-*m*-cresol [see: amylmetacresol]

pentylenetetrazol NF [also: pentetrazol]

pentymal [see: amobarbital]

Pen-Vee K tablets, powder for oral solution (discontinued 2002) ℞ *natural penicillin antibiotic* [penicillin V potassium] 250, 500 mg; 125, 250 mg/5 mL

peony (*Paeonia officinalis*) root (other parts are poisonous) *medicinal herb used as an antispasmodic, diuretic, and sedative*

Pepcid film-coated tablets, powder for oral suspension, IV injection, preloaded syringes for IV ℞ *histamine H₂ antagonist for gastric and duodenal ulcers* [famotidine] 20, 40 mg; 40 mg/5 mL; 10 mg/mL; 20 mg

Pepcid AC ("acid controller") tablets, chewable tablets, gelcaps OTC *histamine H₂ antagonist for heartburn and acid indigestion* [famotidine] 10, 20 mg; 10 mg; 10 mg

Pepcid Complete chewable tablets OTC *combination antacid and histamine H₂ antagonist for heartburn and acid indigestion* [calcium carbonate; magnesium hydroxide; famotidine] 800•165•10 mg

Pepcid RPD orally disintegrating tablets ℞ *histamine H₂ antagonist for gastric and duodenal ulcers* [famotidine] 20, 40 mg

pepleomycin [see: peplomycin sulfate]

peplomycin INN *antineoplastic* [also: peplomycin sulfate]

peplomycin sulfate USAN *antineoplastic* [also: peplomycin]

pepper, African red; American red pepper; bird pepper; cayenne pepper; chili pepper; cockspur pepper; garden pepper; red pepper; Spanish pepper *medicinal herb* [see: cayenne]

pepper, Jamaica *medicinal herb* [see: allspice]

pepper, java; tailed pepper *medicinal herb* [see: cubeb]

pepper, water *medicinal herb* [see: knotweed]

pepper, wild *medicinal herb* [see: mezereon]

pepperidge bush *medicinal herb* [see: barberry]

peppermint NF *flavoring agent; perfume*

peppermint (Mentha piperita) leaves *medicinal herb for appetite stimulation, colds, colic, indigestion, fever, gas and heartburn, headache, shock, sore throat, and toothache*

peppermint oil NF *flavoring agent*

peppermint spirit USP *flavoring agent; perfume*

peppermint water NF *flavored vehicle*

pepsin *digestive aid*

pepstatin USAN, INN *pepsin enzyme inhibitor*

Peptamen ready-to-use oral liquid OTC *enteral nutritional therapy for GI impairment*

Peptavlon subcu injection (discontinued 2002) R *in vivo diagnostic aid for gastrointestinal function* [pentagastrin] 250 μg/mL

Peptic Relief chewable tablets, oral liquid OTC *antidiarrheal; antinauseant* [bismuth subsalicylate] 262 mg; 262 mg/15 mL

peptide YY (PYY) *endogenous peptides manufactured in the GI tract postprandially in proportion to the caloric content of a meal; subdivided into PYY 1-36 (PYY-I) and PYY 3-36 (PYY-II); exogenous administration of PYY 3-36 is investigational for weight loss*

Peptinex; Peptinex DT oral liquid OTC *enteral nutritional treatment for patients with GI impairment* [whey protein–based] 8 oz./pkt.

Pepto Diarrhea Control oral solution OTC *antidiarrheal* [loperamide HCl] 1 mg/5 mL

Pepto-Bismol chewable tablets, caplets, oral liquid OTC *antidiarrheal; antinauseant* [bismuth subsalicylate] 262 mg; 262 mg; 262, 524 mg/15 mL

peraclopone INN

peradoxime INN

perafensine INN

peralopride INN

peramivir USAN *neuraminidase inhibitor for influenza A and B virus infections*

peraquinsin INN

perastine INN

peratizole INN, BAN

perbufylline INN

Perchloracap capsules (discontinued 2005) R *radioimaging adjunct* [potassium perchlorate] 200 mg

Percocet tablets R *narcotic analgesic* [oxycodone HCl; acetaminophen] 2.5•325, 5•325, 7.5•325, 7.5•500, 10•325, 10•650 mg

Percodan; Percodan-Demi tablets R *narcotic analgesic; also abused as a street drug* [oxycodone HCl; oxycodone terephthalate; aspirin] 4.5•0.38•325 mg; 2.25•0.19•325 mg ⑫ Decadron

Percogesic tablets OTC *antihistamine; analgesic* [phenyltoloxamine citrate; acetaminophen] 30•325 mg

Percogesic Extra Strength caplets OTC *antihistamine; analgesic* [diphenhydramine HCl; acetaminophen] 12.5•500 mg

Percolone tablets (discontinued 2005) R *narcotic analgesic* [oxycodone HCl] 5 mg

Perdiem granules OTC *bulk laxative* [psyllium] 4.03 g/tsp. ⑫ Pyridium

Perdiem Overnight Relief granules OTC *bulk laxative; stimulant laxative* [psyllium; senna] 3.25•0.74 g/tsp.

Perfect Image ⒸⒶⓃ capsules OTC *chromium supplement* [chromium chloride] 200 μg

Perfectoderm gel (discontinued 2003) OTC *keratolytic for acne* [benzoyl peroxide] 5%

perfilcon A USAN *hydrophilic contact lens material*

perflenapent USAN *ultrasound contrast medium*

perflexane USAN *investigational (NDA filed) ultrasound contrast medium for cardiac imaging*

perflisopent USAN *ultrasound contrast medium*

perfluamine INN, BAN

perflubron USAN, INN *blood substitute; oral MRI contrast medium; investigational (Phase III) agent for pediatric acute respiratory distress syndrome (ARDS); investigational (Phase III) intravascular oxygen carrier to reduce need for blood transfusions in surgery patients*

perflunafene INN, BAN

perflutren USAN *ultrasound contrast medium for cardiac imaging; investigational (Phase III) for gynecologic imaging*

perfomedil INN

perfosfamide USAN *antineoplastic*

pergolide INN, BAN *dopamine agonist; antiparkinsonian* [also: pergolide mesylate]

pergolide mesylate USAN *dopamine agonist; antiparkinsonian; investigational (orphan) for Tourette syndrome* [also: pergolide] 0.05, 0.25, 1 mg oral

Pergonal powder for IM injection ℞ *ovulation stimulant for women; spermatogenesis stimulant for men* [menotropins] 75, 150 IU

perhexiline INN *coronary vasodilator* [also: perhexiline maleate]

perhexiline maleate USAN *coronary vasodilator* [also: perhexiline]

Periactin syrup (discontinued 2001) ℞ *piperidine antihistamine* [cyproheptadine HCl] 2 mg/5 mL ⊡ Taractan

Periactin tablets (discontinued 2002) ℞ *piperidine antihistamine* [cyproheptadine HCl] 4 mg ⊡ Taractan

periciazine INN *phenothiazine antipsychotic* [also: pericyazine]

Peri-Colace capsules, syrup (discontinued 2003) OTC *stimulant laxative; stool softener* [casanthranol; docusate sodium] 30•100 mg; 30•60 mg/15 mL

PeriColace tablets OTC *stimulant laxative; stool softener* [sennosides; docusate sodium] 8.6•50 mg

pericyazine BAN *phenothiazine antipsychotic* [also: periciazine]

Peridex mouth rinse ℞ *antimicrobial; gingivitis treatment; investigational (orphan) for oral mucositis in bone marrow transplant patients* [chlorhexidine gluconate; alcohol 11.6%] 0.12%

Peridin-C tablets OTC *vitamin C supplement with bioflavonoids* [ascorbic acid; hesperidin] 200•200 mg

Peri-Dose softgels (discontinued 2003) OTC *stimulant laxative; stool softener* [casanthranol; docusate sodium] 30•100 mg

perilla (Perilla frutescens) plant *medicinal herb for asthma, inducing sweating, nausea, gastrointestinal spasms, and sunstroke*

perimetazine INN

perindopril USAN, INN, BAN *antihypertensive; angiotensin-converting enzyme (ACE) inhibitor*

perindopril erbumine USAN *antihypertensive; angiotensin-converting enzyme (ACE) inhibitor*

perindoprilat INN, BAN

PerioChip biodegradable polymer implant ℞ *antimicrobial adjunct to scaling and root planing procedures in periodontitis* [chlorhexidine gluconate] 2.5 mg

PerioGard mouth rinse ℞ *antimicrobial; gingivitis treatment* [chlorhexidine gluconate; alcohol 11.6%] 0.12%

PerioMed oral rinse ℞ *dental caries preventative* [stannous fluoride] 0.64%

Periostat capsules (discontinued 2001) ℞ *antibiotic for periodontal disease* [doxycycline hyclate] 20 mg

Periostat tablets ℞ *antibiotic for periodontal disease* [doxycycline hyclate] 20 mg

peripheral vasodilators *a class of cardiovascular drugs that cause dilation of the blood vessels*

Periploca sylvestris *medicinal herb* [see: gymnema]

perisoxal INN

periwinkle (Catharanthus roseus) plant *medicinal herb for cancer, dia-*

betes, diarrhea, insect stings, nervousness, ocular inflammation, and ulcers; not generally regarded as safe and effective for ingestion because of toxicity

perlapine USAN, INN *hypnotic*

Perles (dosage form) *soft gelatin capsule*

permanganic acid, potassium salt
[see: potassium permanganate]

Permapen Isoject (unit dose syringe) for deep IM injection ℞ *natural penicillin antibiotic* [penicillin G benzathine] 1 200 000 U

Permax tablets ℞ *dopamine agonist; antiparkinsonian; investigational (orphan) for Tourette syndrome* [pergolide mesylate] 0.05, 0.25, 1 mg

permethrin USAN, INN, BAN *ectoparasiticide for scabies and lice* 1%, 5% *topical*

Permitil tablets, oral concentrate (discontinued 2002) ℞ *conventional (typical) phenothiazine antipsychotic for schizophrenia and psychotic disorders* [fluphenazine HCl] 2.5, 5, 10 mg; 5 mg/mL

Perna canaliculus *natural remedy* [see: New Zealand green-lipped mussel]

Pernox Scrub; Pernox Lathering Lotion OTC *abrasive cleanser for acne* [sulfur; salicylic acid]

peroxide, dibenzoyl [see: benzoyl peroxide]

Peroxin A 5; Peroxin A 10 gel (discontinued 2003) ℞ *keratolytic for acne* [benzoyl peroxide] 5%; 10%

peroxisome proliferator–activated receptor (PPAR) agonists *a class of agents that increase insulin receptor sensitivity in type 2 diabetes; PPAR-alpha is associated with lower triglyceride and higher HDL levels; PPAR-gamma is associated with lower blood glucose levels*

Peroxyl mouth rinse, oral gel OTC *cleansing of oral wounds* [hydrogen peroxide] 1.5%

perphenazine USAN, INN *conventional (typical) phenothiazine antipsychotic for schizophrenia and psychotic disorders; treatment for nausea and vomiting* 2, 4, 8, 16 mg *oral*; 16 mg/5 mL *oral*

Persa-Gel; Persa-Gel W 5%; Persa-Gel W 10% gel (discontinued 2003) ℞ *keratolytic for acne* [benzoyl peroxide] 5%, 10%; 5%; 10%

Persantine sugar-coated tablets ℞ *platelet aggregation inhibitor* [dipyridamole] 25, 50, 75 mg ⑨ Pertofrane

Persantine IV injection ℞ *diagnostic aid for coronary artery function* [dipyridamole] 10 mg

Persea americana; P. gratissima *medicinal herb* [see: avocado]

Persian bark; Persian berries *medicinal herb* [see: buckthorn]

Persian walnut *medicinal herb* [see: English walnut]

persic oil NF *vehicle*

persilic acid INN

Pertropin capsules (discontinued 2003) OTC *dietary lipotropic agent* [linolenic acid; multiple essential fatty acids] 7 mins.

Pertussin CS; Pertussin ES syrup (discontinued 2002) OTC *antitussive* [dextromethorphan hydrobromide] 3.5 mg/5 mL; 15 mg/5 mL

pertussis immune globulin USP *passive immunizing agent*

pertussis immune human globulin [now: pertussis immune globulin]

pertussis vaccine USP *active immunizing agent*

pertussis vaccine, acellular [see: diphtheria & tetanus toxoids & acellular pertussis (DTaP) vaccine, adsorbed]

pertussis vaccine, component (alternate name for acellular pertussis vaccine) [see: diphtheria & tetanus toxoids & acellular pertussis (DTaP) vaccine, adsorbed]

pertussis vaccine, whole-cell [see: diphtheria & tetanus toxoids & whole-cell pertussis (DTwP) vaccine, adsorbed]

pertussis vaccine adsorbed USP *active immunizing agent*

Peruvian balsam NF *topical protectant; rubefacient*

Peruvian balsam (*Myroxylon balsamum; M. pereirae*) oil *medicinal* *herb for edema, expelling worms, hemostasis, topical infections, and wound healing*

Peruvian bark; yellow Peruvian bark *medicinal herb* [see: quinine]

Peruvian ginseng *medicinal herb* [see: maca]

Petasites hybridus medicinal herb [see: butterbur]

pethidine INN, BAN *narcotic analgesic; also abused as a street drug* [also: meperidine HCl]

pethidine HCl [see: meperidine HCl]

PETN (pentaerythritol tetranitrate) [q.v.]

petrichloral INN

petrolatum USP *ointment base; emollient/ protectant* [also: yellow petrolatum]

petrolatum, hydrophilic USP *absorbent ointment base; topical protectant*

petrolatum, liquid [see: mineral oil]

petrolatum, liquid emulsion [see: mineral oil emulsion]

petrolatum, white USP, JAN *oleaginous ointment base; topical protectant*

petrolatum gauze [see: gauze, petrolatum]

petroleum benzin [see: benzin, petroleum]

petroleum distillate inhalants *vapors from butane, toluene, acetone, benzene, gasoline, etc. which produce psychoactive effects, abused as street drugs* [see also: nitrous oxide; volatile nitrites]

petroleum jelly [see: petrolatum]

Petroselinum sativum medicinal herb [see: parsley]

Peumus boldus medicinal herb [see: boldo]

pexantel INN

Pexeva tablets R *selective serotonin reuptake inhibitor (SSRI) for depression, obsessive-compulsive disorder, and panic disorder* [paroxetine mesylate] 10, 20, 30, 40 mg

pexiganan acetate USAN *investigational (NDA filed) broad-spectrum topical antibiotic for impetigo and diabetic foot ulcers*

PFA (phosphonoformic acid) [see: foscarnet sodium]

Pfaffia paniculata medicinal herb [see: suma]

Pfeiffer's Cold Sore lotion OTC *topical oral anesthetic; analgesic; counterirritant* [gum benzoin; camphor; menthol; eucalyptol; alcohol 85%] 7%•$\frac{?}{•}\frac{?}{•}\frac{?}{•}\frac{?}{}$

Pfizerpen powder for injection R *natural penicillin antibiotic* [penicillin G potassium] 1, 5, 20 million U

PFL (Platinol, fluorouracil, leucovorin [rescue]) *chemotherapy protocol for head, neck, and gastric cancer*

PFT (L-phenylalanine mustard, fluorouracil, tamoxifen) *chemotherapy protocol*

PG (paregoric) [q.v.]

PG (prostaglandin) [q.v.]

PGA (pteroylglutamic acid) [see: folic acid]

PGE$_1$ (prostaglandin E$_1$) [now: alprostadil]

PGE$_2$ (prostaglandin E$_2$) [now: dinoprostone]

PGF$_{2\alpha}$ (prostaglandin F$_{2\alpha}$) [see: dinoprost]

PGF$_{2\alpha}$ (prostaglandin F$_{2\alpha}$) THAM [see: dinoprost tromethamine]

PGI$_2$ (prostaglandin I$_2$) [now: epoprostenol]

PGX (prostaglandin X) [now: epoprostenol]

Phaenicia sericata natural treatment [see: maggots]

Phanadex Cough syrup (discontinued 2002) OTC *antitussive; decongestant; antihistamine; expectorant* [dextromethorphan hydrobromide; phenylpropanolamine HCl; pyrilamine maleate; guaifenesin] 15•25• 40•100 mg/5 mL

Phanatuss DM Cough syrup OTC *antitussive; expectorant* [dextromethorphan hydrobromide; guaifenesin] 20•200 mg/10 mL

phanchinone [see: phanquinone; phanquone]

phanquinone INN [also: phanquone]

phanquone BAN [also: phanquinone]

pharmaceutical glaze [see: glaze, pharmaceutical]

Pharmaflur; Pharmaflur df; Pharmaflur 1.1 chewable tablets ℞ *dental caries preventative* [sodium fluoride] 2.2 mg; 2.2 mg; 1.1 mg

Pharmalgen subcu or IM injection ℞ *venom sensitivity testing (subcu); venom desensitization therapy (IM)* [extracts of honeybee, yellow jacket, yellow hornet, white-faced hornet, mixed vespid, and wasp venom]

Pharmia regina natural treatment [see: maggots]

Pharmorubicin PFS; Pharmorubicin RDF ⓒ injection ℞ *antibiotic antineoplastic* [epirubicin HCl] 2 mg/mL; 10, 20, 50, 150 mg

Phazyme tablets, drops OTC *antiflatulent* [simethicone] 60 mg; 40 mg/0.6 mL ⊘ Pherazine

Phazyme ⓒ oral liquid OTC *antiflatulent* [simethicone] 125 mg/5 mL

Phazyme 95 tablets OTC *antiflatulent* [simethicone] 95 mg

Phazyme 125 softgels OTC *antiflatulent* [simethicone] 125 mg

phebutazine [see: febuverine]

phebutyrazine [see: febuverine]

phemfilcon A USAN *hydrophilic contact lens material*

phenacaine INN [also: phenacaine HCl]

phenacaine HCl USP [also: phenacaine]

phenacemide USP, INN, BAN *anticonvulsant*

phenacetin USP, INN (*withdrawn from market*) ⊘ phenazocine

phenacon [see: fenaclon]

phenactropinium chloride INN, BAN

phenacyl 4-morpholineacetate [see: mobecarb]

N-phenacylhomatropinium chloride [see: phenactropinium chloride]

phenacylpivalate [see: pibecarb]

phenadoxone INN, BAN

Phenadoz suppositories ℞ *antihistamine; sedative; antiemetic; motion sickness relief* [promethazine HCl] 12.5, 25 mg

phenaglycodol INN

Phenahist-TR sustained-release tablets (discontinued 2001) ℞ *decongestant; antihistamine; anticholinergic* [phenylpropanolamine HCl; phenylephrine HCl; chlorpheniramine maleate; hyoscyamine sulfate; atropine sulfate; scopolamine hydrobromide] 50•25•8•0.19•0.04•0.01 mg

phenamazoline INN

phenamazoline HCl [see: phenamazoline]

Phenameth DM syrup (discontinued 2002) ℞ *antitussive; antihistamine* [dextromethorphan hydrobromide; promethazine HCl; alcohol] 15•6.25 mg/5 mL

phenampromide INN

Phenapap tablets OTC *decongestant; analgesic* [pseudoephedrine HCl; acetaminophen] 30•325 mg

Phenapap Sinus Headache & Congestion tablets (discontinued 2002) OTC *decongestant; antihistamine; analgesic* [pseudoephedrine HCl; chlorpheniramine maleate; acetaminophen] 30•2•325 mg

Phenaphen with Codeine No. 3 & No. 4 capsules (discontinued 2004) ℞ *narcotic antitussive; analgesic* [codeine phosphate; acetaminophen] 30•325 mg; 60•325 mg

phenaphthazine

phenarbutal [see: phetharbital]

phenarsone sulfoxylate INN

Phenaseptic throat spray OTC *antipruritic/counterirritant; mild local anesthetic* [phenol] 1.4%

Phenate timed-release tablets (discontinued 2001) ℞ *decongestant; antihistamine; analgesic* [phenylpropanolamine HCl; chlorpheniramine maleate; acetaminophen] 40•4•325 mg

PhenaVent D film-coated caplets ℞ *decongestant; expectorant* [phenylephrine HCl; guaifenesin] 40•1200 mg

PhenaVent LA extended-release capsules ℞ *decongestant; expectorant* [phenylephrine HCl; guaifenesin] 30•400 mg

Phenazo ⒸⒶⓃ tablets ℞ *urinary analgesic* [phenazopyridine HCl] 100, 200 mg

phenazocine INN ▣ phenacetin

phenazocine hydrobromide [see: phenazocine]

phenazone INN, BAN *analgesic* [also: antipyrine]

phenazopyridine INN, BAN *urinary tract analgesic* [also: phenazopyridine HCl]

phenazopyridine HCl USAN, USP *urinary tract analgesic* [also: phenazopyridine] 100, 200 mg oral

Phenazopyridine Plus tablets ℞ *urinary analgesic; antispasmodic; sedative* [phenazopyridine HCl; hyoscyamine hydrobromide; butabarbital] 150•0.3•15 mg

phenbenicillin BAN [also: fenbenicillin]

phenbutazone sodium glycerate USAN *anti-inflammatory*

phenbutrazate BAN [also: fenbutrazate]

phencarbamide USAN *anticholinergic* [also: fencarbamide]

Phenchlor S.H.A. sustained-release tablets (discontinued 2001) ℞ *decongestant; antihistamine; anticholinergic* [phenylpropanolamine HCl; phenylephrine HCl; chlorpheniramine maleate; hyoscyamine sulfate; atropine sulfate; scopolamine hydrobromide] 50•25•8•0.19•0.04•0.01 mg

phencyclidine INN *anesthetic* [also: phencyclidine HCl]

phencyclidine HCl USAN *anesthetic* [also: phencyclidine]

phendimetrazine INN *anorexiant* [also: phendimetrazine tartrate]

phendimetrazine tartrate USP *anorexiant; CNS stimulant* [also: phendimetrazine] 35 mg oral

phenelzine INN, BAN *antidepressant; MAO inhibitor* [also: phenelzine sulfate] ▣ Phenazine; Phenylzin

phenelzine sulfate USP *antidepressant; MAO inhibitor* [also: phenelzine]

phenemal [see: phenobarbital]

Phenerbel-S tablets ℞ *GI anticholinergic; sedative; analgesic* [belladonna alkaloids; phenobarbital; ergotamine tartrate] 0.2•40•0.6 mg

Phenergan tablets, suppositories, injection ℞ *antihistamine; sedative; antiemetic; motion sickness relief* [promethazine HCl] 25, 50 mg; 12.5, 25, 50 mg; 25, 50 mg/mL ▣ Phenaphen; Theragran

Phenergan Fortis syrup (discontinued 2002) ℞ *antihistamine; sedative; antiemetic; motion sickness relief* [promethazine HCl; alcohol 1.5%] 25 mg/5 mL

Phenergan Plain syrup (discontinued 2002) ℞ *antihistamine; sedative; antiemetic; motion sickness relief* [promethazine HCl] 6.25 mg/5 mL

Phenergan VC syrup (discontinued 2004) ℞ *decongestant; antihistamine* [phenylephrine HCl; promethazine HCl; alcohol 7%] 5•6.25 mg/5 mL

Phenergan VC with Codeine syrup (discontinued 2002) ℞ *narcotic antitussive; decongestant; antihistamine* [codeine phosphate; phenylephrine HCl; promethazine HCl; alcohol 7%] 10•5•6.25 mg/5 mL

Phenergan with Codeine syrup (discontinued 2002) ℞ *narcotic antitussive; antihistamine* [codeine phosphate; promethazine HCl; alcohol 7%] 10•6.25 mg/5 mL

Phenergan with Dextromethorphan syrup (discontinued 2002) ℞ *antitussive; antihistamine* [dextromethorphan hydrobromide; promethazine HCl; alcohol 7%] 15•6.25 mg/5 mL

pheneridine INN

phenethanol [see: phenylethyl alcohol]

phenethazine [see: fenethazine]

phenethicillin potassium USP [also: pheneticillin]

phenethyl alcohol BAN *antimicrobial agent* [also: phenylethyl alcohol]

N-phenethylanthranilic acid [see: enfenamic acid]

phenethylazocine bromide [see: phenazocine hydrobromide]

phenethylhydrazine sulfate [see: phenelzine sulfate]

pheneticillin INN [also: phenethicillin potassium]

pheneticillin potassium [see: phenethicillin potassium]

phenetsal [see: acetaminosalol]

pheneturide INN, BAN [also: acetylpheneturide]

Phenex-1 powder OTC *formula for infants with phenylketonuria*

Phenex-2 powder OTC *enteral nutritional therapy for phenylketonuria (PKU)*

phenformin INN, BAN *biguanide hypoglycemic agent* [also: phenformin HCl]

phenformin HCl USP *hypoglycemic agent (removed from market by FDA in 1977, now available as an investigational drug)* [also: phenformin]

phenglutarimide INN, BAN

Phenhist DH with Codeine oral liquid (discontinued 2002) ℞ *narcotic antitussive; decongestant; antihistamine* [codeine phosphate; pseudoephedrine HCl; chlorpheniramine maleate; alcohol 5%] 10•30•2 mg/5 mL

Phenhist Expectorant oral liquid (discontinued 2002) ℞ *narcotic antitussive; decongestant; expectorant* [codeine phosphate; pseudoephedrine HCl; guaifenesin; alcohol 7.5%] 10•30•100 mg/5 mL

phenicarbazide INN

phenidiemal [see: phetharbital]

phenindamine INN *nonselective piperidine antihistamine* [also: phenindamine tartrate]

phenindamine tartrate USAN *nonselective piperidine antihistamine for allergic rhinitis* [also: phenindamine]

phenindione USP, INN *anticoagulant*

pheniodol sodium INN [also: iodoalphionic acid]

pheniprazine INN, BAN

pheniprazine HCl [see: pheniprazine]

pheniramine INN [also: pheniramine maleate]

pheniramine maleate USAN *antihistamine* [also: pheniramine]

pheniramine maleate & naphazoline HCl *topical ocular antihistamine and decongestant* 0.3%•0.025% eye drops

phenisonone hydrobromide

phenmetraline HCl [see: phenmetrazine HCl]

phenmetrazine INN, BAN *anorexiant; CNS stimulant; also abused as a street drug* [also: phenmetrazine HCl]

phenmetrazine HCl USP *anorexiant; CNS stimulant; also abused as a street drug* [also: phenmetrazine]

phenobamate [see: febarbamate]

phenobarbital USP, INN, JAN *anticonvulsant; hypnotic; sedative; also abused as a street drug* [also: phenobarbitone] 15, 30, 60, 100 mg oral; 15, 20 mg/5 mL oral ☒ pentobarbital

phenobarbital sodium USP, INN, JAN *anticonvulsant; hypnotic; sedative; also abused as a street drug* 30, 60, 65, 130 mg/mL injection

phenobarbitone BAN *anticonvulsant; hypnotic; sedative; also abused as a street drug* [also: phenobarbital]

phenobutiodil INN

phenododecinium bromide [see: domiphen bromide]

phenol USP *topical antiseptic/antipruritic; local anesthetic; preservative*

phenol, liquefied USP *topical antipruritic*

phenol, sodium salt [see: phenolate sodium]

phenol red [see: phenolsulfonphthalein]

phenolate sodium USAN *disinfectant*

Phenolated Calamine lotion OTC *poison ivy treatment* [calamine; zinc oxide; phenol] 8%•8%•1%

phenolphthalein USP, INN *stimulant laxative* [banned in all OTC laxatives in 1998]

phenolphthalein, white [see: phenolphthalein]

phenolphthalein, yellow USP *stimulant laxative* [banned in all OTC laxatives in 1998]

phenolsulfonphthalein USP

phenolsulphonate sodium USP

phenomorphan INN, BAN

phenomycilline [see: penicillin V]

phenoperidine INN, BAN

phenopryldiasulfone sodium [see: solasulfone]

Phenoptic eye drops ℞ *topical ophthalmic decongestant and vasoconstrictor; mydriatic* [phenylephrine HCl] 2.5%

Phenoptin ℞ *investigational (Phase III) oral treatment for mild to moderate phenylketonuria* [sapropterin HCl]

phenosulfophthalein [see: phenolsulfonphthalein]

phenothiazine NF, INN *antipsychotic*

phenothiazines *a class of dopamine receptor antagonists with antipsychotic, hypotensive, antiemetic, antispasmodic, and antihistaminic activity*

phenothrin INN, BAN

phenoxazoline HCl [see: fenoxazoline HCl]

Phenoxine tablets (discontinued 2001) OTC *diet aid* [phenylpropanolamine HCl] 25 mg ⊉ Phenazine

phenoxybenzamine INN *antihypertensive* [also: phenoxybenzamine HCl]

phenoxybenzamine HCl USP *antihypertensive; pheochromocytomic agent* [also: phenoxybenzamine]

phenoxymethylpenicillin INN *natural penicillin antibiotic* [also: penicillin V]

phenoxypropazine BAN [also: fenoxypropazine]

phenoxypropylpenicillin [see: propicillin]

phenozolone [see: fenozolone]

phenprobamate INN, BAN

phenprocoumon USAN, USP, INN *anticoagulant*

phenprocumone [see: phenprocoumon]

phenpromethadrine [see: phenpromethamine]

phenpromethamine INN

phenpropamine citrate [see: alverine citrate]

Phenserine ℞ *investigational (Phase II) acetylcholinesterase (AChE) inhibitor to suppress the formation of beta-amyloid precursor protein (beta-APP) and beta-amyloid plaque to delay the progression of Alzheimer disease*

phensuximide USP, INN, BAN *succinimide anticonvulsant*

phentermine USAN, INN *anorexiant; CNS stimulant; an adrenergic isomer of amphetamine* ⊉ phentolamine

phentermine HCl USP *anorexiant; CNS stimulant; the water-soluble form of phentermine for oral administration* 8, 15, 18.75, 30, 37.5 mg oral

phenthiazine [see: phenothiazine]

phentolamine INN, BAN *antihypertensive; pheochromocytomic agent* [also: phentolamine HCl] ⊉ phentermine; Ventolin

phentolamine HCl USP *antihypertensive; pheochromocytomic agent* [also: phentolamine]

phentolamine mesilate INN, JAN *antiadrenergic; antihypertensive; pheochromocytomic agent* [also: phentolamine mesylate]

phentolamine mesylate USP *antihypertensive; α-adrenergic blocker; pheochromocytomic agent; investigational (Phase III) oral treatment for erectile dysfunction* [also: phentolamine mesilate] 5 mg injection

phentolamine methanesulfonate [now: phentolamine mesylate]

Phentrol 2; Phentrol 4; Phentrol 5 capsules ℞ *anorexiant; CNS stimulant* [phentermine HCl] 30 mg

phentydrone

phenyl aminosalicylate USAN, BAN *antibacterial; tuberculostatic* [also: fenamisal]

phenyl salicylate NF *analgesic; not generally regarded as safe and effective as an antidiarrheal*

phenylalanine (L-phenylalanine) USAN, USP, INN *essential amino acid; symbols: Phe, F*

phenylalanine ammonia-lyase *investigational (orphan) for hyperphenylalaninemia*

phenylalanine mustard (PAM) [see: melphalan]

L-phenylalanine mustard (L-PAM) [see: melphalan]

phenylazo diamino pyridine HCl [see: phenazopyridine HCl]

phenylbenzyl atropine [see: xenytropium bromide]

phenylbutazone USP, INN *antirheumatic; anti-inflammatory; antipyretic; analgesic*

phenylbutylpiperadines *a class of dopamine receptor antagonists with conventional (typical) antipsychotic activity* [also called: butyrophenones]

phenylbutyrate sodium [see: sodium phenylbutyrate]

2-phenylbutyrylurea [see: pheneturide; acetylpheneturide]

phenylcarbinol [see: benzyl alcohol]

phenylcinchoninic acid [now: cinchophen]

α-phenyl-*p*-cresol carbamate [see: diphenan]

phenylcyclohexyl piperidine (PCP) [see: PCP; phencyclidine HCl]

2-phenylcyclopentylamine HCl [see: cypenamine HCl]

phenyldimazone [see: normethadone]

Phenyldrine timed-release tablets (discontinued 2001) OTC *diet aid* [phenylpropanolamine HCl] 75 mg

phenylephrine (PE) INN, BAN *nasal decongestant; ocular vasoconstrictor; vasopressor for hypotensive or cardiac shock* [also: phenylephrine HCl]

phenylephrine bitartrate *bronchodilator; vasoconstrictor*

phenylephrine HCl USP *nasal decongestant; ocular vasoconstrictor; vasopressor for hypotensive or cardiac shock* [also: phenylephrine] 0.25%, 0.5%, 1% nose drops or spray; 2.5%, 10% eye drops; 1% injection

phenylephrine HCl & phenylpropanolamine HCl & guaifenesin *nasal decongestant; expectorant* PPA banned in all OTC products in 2001

phenylephrine HCl & promethazine HCl *decongestant; antihistamine* 5•6.25 mg/5 mL oral

phenylephrine tannate *nasal decongestant*

phenylephrine tannate & chlorpheniramine tannate & pyril-

amine tannate *decongestant; antihistamine* 5•2•12.5 mg/5 mL oral

phenylethanol [see: phenylethyl alcohol]

phenylethyl alcohol USP *antimicrobial agent; preservative* [also: phenethyl alcohol]

phenylethylmalonylurea [see: phenobarbital]

Phenylfenesin L.A. extended-action tablets (discontinued 2002) ℞ *decongestant; expectorant* [phenylpropanolamine HCl; guaifenesin] 75•400 mg

Phenylfenesin L.A. long-acting tablets (discontinued 2002) ℞ *decongestant; expectorant* [phenylpropanolamine HCl; guaifenesin] 75•400 mg

Phenyl-Free oral liquid, powder for oral solution OTC *special diet for infants with phenylketonuria (PKU)*

Phenylgesic tablets OTC *antihistamine; analgesic* [phenyltoloxamine citrate; acetaminophen] 30•325 mg

phenylindanedione [see: phenindione]

phenylmercuric acetate NF *antimicrobial agent; preservative*

phenylmercuric borate INN

phenylmercuric chloride NF

phenylmercuric nitrate NF *antimicrobial agent; preservative; topical antiseptic*

phenylone [see: antipyrine]

phenylpropanolamine (PPA) INN, BAN *vasoconstrictor; nasal decongestant; nonprescription diet aid* [also: phenylpropanolamine HCl] banned in all OTC products in 2001

phenylpropanolamine HCl USP *vasoconstrictor; nasal decongestant; nonprescription diet aid* [also: phenylpropanolamine] banned in all OTC products in 2001

phenylpropanolamine HCl & chlorpheniramine maleate *decongestant; antihistamine* [PPA banned in all OTC products in 2001]

phenylpropanolamine HCl & phenylephrine HCl & guaifenesin *nasal decongestant; expectorant* [PPA banned in all OTC products in 2001]

phenylpropanolamine polistirex USAN *adrenergic; vasoconstrictor* banned in all OTC products in 2001

1-phenylsemicarbazide [see: phenicarbazide]

phenylthilone [see: phenythilone]

phenyltoloxamine INN *antihistamine; sleep aid*

phenyltoloxamine citrate *antihistamine; sleep aid*

phenyltriazines *a class of anticonvulsants*

phenyracillin INN

phenyramidol HCl USAN *analgesic; skeletal muscle relaxant* [also: fenyramidol]

Phenytek extended-release capsules Ŗ *once-daily hydantoin anticonvulsant* [phenytoin sodium] 200, 300 mg

phenythilone INN

phenytoin USAN, USP, INN, BAN *hydantoin anticonvulsant* 125 mg/5 mL oral

phenytoin redox [see: redox-phenytoin]

phenytoin sodium USP *hydantoin anticonvulsant* 100 mg oral; 50 mg/mL injection

Pherazine DM syrup (discontinued 2002) Ŗ *antitussive; antihistamine* [dextromethorphan hydrobromide; promethazine HCl; alcohol 7%] 15•6.25 mg/5 mL

Pherazine VC with Codeine syrup (discontinued 2002) Ŗ *narcotic antitussive; decongestant; antihistamine* [codeine phosphate; phenylephrine HCl; promethazine HCl; alcohol 7%] 10•5•6.25 mg/5 mL

Pherazine with Codeine syrup (discontinued 2002) Ŗ *narcotic antitussive; antihistamine* [codeine phosphate; promethazine HCl; alcohol 7%] 10•6.25 mg/5 mL

phetharbital INN

phezathion [see: fezatione]

Phicon cream OTC *topical anesthetic; emollient* [pramoxine HCl; vitamins A and E] 0.5%•7500 IU•2000 IU

Phicon F cream OTC *local anesthetic; antifungal* [pramoxine HCl; undecylenic acid] 0.05%•8%

Phillips' Chewable tablets OTC *antacid* [magnesium hydroxide] 311 mg

Phillips' Liqui-Gels OTC *laxative; stool softener* [docusate sodium] 100 mg

Phillips' Milk of Magnesia; Concentrated Phillips' Milk of Magnesia oral liquid OTC *antacid; saline laxative* [magnesium hydroxide] 400 mg/5 mL; 800 mg/5 mL

pHisoDerm; pHisoDerm for Baby topical liquid OTC *soap-free therapeutic skin cleanser*

pHisoDerm Cleansing Bar (discontinued 2004) OTC *therapeutic skin cleanser*

pHisoHex topical liquid Ŗ *bacteriostatic skin cleanser* [hexachlorophene] 3% ② Fostex

phloropropiophenone [see: flopropione]

pholcodine INN

pholedrine INN, BAN

pholescutol [see: folescutol]

Phoradendron flavescens; P. serotinum; P. tomentosum *medicinal herb* [see: mistletoe]

PhosChol softgels, oral liquid concentrate OTC *lipotropic* [phosphatidylcholine] 565, 900 mg; 3 g/5 mL

phoscolic acid [see: foscolic acid]

Phos-Flur oral rinse Ŗ *topical dental caries preventative* [acidulated phosphate fluoride] 0.44 mg/mL

PhosLo tablets, capsules, gelcaps Ŗ *buffering agent for hyperphosphatemia in end-stage renal disease* (orphan) [calcium acetate] 667 mg; 333.3, 667 mg; 667 mg

Phos-NaK powder for oral solution Ŗ *phosphorus/electrolyte supplement* [phosphorus; potassium; sodium] 250•280•160 mg/pkt.

phosphate salt of tricyclic nucleoside [now: triciribine phosphate]

phosphatidylcholine (PC) [see: lecithin]

phosphatidylserine (PS) *natural agent to improve neural function, maintain brain cell membrane integrity, and pro-*

tect the brain against age-related functional deterioration

phosphinic acid [see: hypophosphorous acid]

2,2'-phosphinicodilactic acid (PDLA) [see: foscolic acid]

Phosphocol P 32 suspension for intracavitary instillation, interstitial injection ℞ *radiopharmaceutical antineoplastic* [chromic phosphate P 32] 10, 15 mCi

phosphocysteamine *investigational (orphan) for cystinosis*

phosphodiesterase III (PDE III) inhibitors *a class of platelet aggregation inhibitors*

Phospholine Iodide powder for eye drops ℞ *antiglaucoma agent; irreversible cholinesterase inhibitor miotic* [echothiophate iodide] 0.125%

phosphonoformic acid (PFA) [see: foscarnet sodium]

phosphonomethoxypropyladenine (PMPA) [see: tenofovir]

phosphorated carbohydrate solution (hyperosmolar solution with phosphoric acid) *antiemetic for nausea associated with influenza, morning sickness, motion sickness, inhalation anesthesia, or food and drink indiscretions*

phosphoric acid NF *solvent; acidifying agent*

phosphoric acid, aluminum salt [see: aluminum phosphate gel]

phosphoric acid, calcium salt [see: calcium phosphate, dibasic]

phosphoric acid, chromium salt [see: chromic phosphate Cr 51 & P 32]

phosphoric acid, diammonium salt [see: ammonium phosphate]

phosphoric acid, dipotassium salt [see: potassium phosphate, dibasic]

phosphoric acid, disodium salt heptahydrate [see: sodium phosphate, dibasic]

phosphoric acid, disodium salt hydrate [see: sodium phosphate, dibasic]

phosphoric acid, magnesium salt [see: magnesium phosphate]

phosphoric acid, monopotassium salt [see: potassium phosphate, monobasic]

phosphoric acid, monosodium salt dihydrate [see: sodium phosphate, monobasic]

phosphoric acid, monosodium salt monohydrate [see: sodium phosphate, monobasic]

phosphorofluoridic acid, disodium salt [see: sodium monofluorophosphate]

phosphorothiolate deoxyribose *investigational (orphan) agent for advanced malignant melanoma*

phosphorus *element (P)*

Phospho-Soda [see: Fleet Phospho-Soda]

phosphothiamine [see: monophosphothiamine]

Photofrin PDT powder for IV injection ℞ *laser light–activated antineoplastic for photodynamic therapy (PDT) of esophageal (orphan) and non–small cell lung cancers (NSCLC); used for ablation of high-grade dysplasia in Barrett esophagus patients; investigational (orphan) for bladder cancer* [porfimer sodium] 75 mg

phoxim INN, BAN

Phrenilin tablets ℞ *analgesic; barbiturate sedative* [acetaminophen; butalbital] 325•50 mg

Phrenilin Forte capsules ℞ *analgesic; barbiturate sedative* [acetaminophen; butalbital] 650•50 mg

PHRT (procarbazine, hydroxyurea, radiotherapy) *chemotherapy protocol*

phthalofyne USAN *veterinary anthelmintic* [also: ftalofyne]

phthalylsulfacetamide NF

phthalylsulfamethizole INN

phthalylsulfathiazole USP, INN

phylcardin [see: aminophylline]

phyllindon [see: aminophylline]

Phyllocontin controlled-release tablets (discontinued 2004) ℞ *antiasthmatic; bronchodilator* [aminophylline] 225 mg

phylloquinone [see: phytonadione]

Phylorinol mouthwash/gargle OTC *topical antipruritic/counterirritant; mild local anesthetic* [phenol] 0.6%

Phylorinol topical liquid OTC *antipruritic/counterirritant; mild local anesthetic; antiseptic; astringent; oral deodorant* [phenol; boric acid; strong iodine solution; chlorophyllin copper complex] 0.6% ● ? ● ? ● ?

physic root *medicinal herb* [see: Culver root]

physiological irrigating solution *for general irrigating, washing and rinsing; not for injection*

Physiolyte topical liquid ℞ *sterile irrigant* [physiological irrigating solution]

PhysioSol topical liquid ℞ *sterile irrigant* [physiological irrigating solution]

physostigmine USP, BAN *reversible cholinesterase inhibitor miotic for glaucoma* ② pyridostigmine; Prostigmin

physostigmine salicylate USP *cholinergic to reverse anticholinergic overdose; investigational (orphan) for Friedreich and other inherited ataxias* 1 mg/mL injection

physostigmine sulfate USP *ophthalmic cholinergic for glaucoma; miotic*

phytate persodium USAN *pharmaceutic aid*

phytate sodium USAN *calcium-chelating agent*

phytic acid [see: fytic acid]

Phytolacca americana; P. decandra; P. rigida *medicinal herb* [see: pokeweed]

phytomenadione (vitamin K₁) INN, BAN *fat-soluble vitamin; prothrombogenic* [also: phytonadione]

phytonadiol sodium diphosphate INN

phytonadione (vitamin K₁) USP, JAN *fat-soluble vitamin; prothrombogenic* [also: phytomenadione] 2 mg/mL injection

PIA (Platinol, ifosfamide, Adriamycin) *chemotherapy protocol*

pibecarb INN

piberaline INN

piboserod HCl USAN, BAN *selective serotonin 5-HT₄ receptor antagonist for irritable bowel syndrome*

pibrozelesin hydrobromide USAN *antineoplastic*

picafibrate INN

picartamide INN

Picea excelsa; P. mariana *medicinal herb* [see: spruce tree]

picenadol INN *analgesic* [also: picenadol HCl]

picenadol HCl USAN *analgesic* [also: picenadol]

picilorex INN

pick purse; pickpocket *medicinal herb* [see: shepherd's purse]

piclamilast USAN *phosphodiesterase type IV inhibitor for asthma*

piclonidine INN

piclopastine INN

picloxydine INN, BAN

picobenzide INN

picodralazine INN

picolamine INN

piconol INN

picoperine INN

picoprazole INN

picotrin INN *keratolytic* [also: picotrin diolamine]

picotrin diolamine USAN *keratolytic* [also: picotrin]

Picovir ℞ *investigational (NDA filed) viral replication inhibitor for viral respiratory infections, including the common cold* [pleconaril]

Picrasma excelsa *medicinal herb* [see: quassia]

picric acid [see: trinitrophenol]

picrotoxin NF

picumast INN, BAN

picumeterol INN, BAN *bronchodilator* [also: picumeterol fumarate]

picumeterol fumarate USAN *bronchodilator* [also: picumeterol]

pidolacetamol INN

pidolic acid INN

pifarnine USAN, INN *gastric antiulcerative*

pifenate INN, BAN

pifexole INN

piflutixol INN

pifoxime INN

pigeonberry *medicinal herb* [see: pokeweed]

piketoprofen INN

Pilagan eye drops (discontinued 2004) ℞ *antiglaucoma agent; direct-acting miotic* [pilocarpine nitrate] 1%, 2%, 4%

pildralazine INN

pilewort *(Erechtites hieracifolia)* plant *medicinal herb used as an astringent and emetic*

Pilocar eye drops ℞ *antiglaucoma agent; direct-acting miotic* [pilocarpine HCl] 0.5%, 1%, 2%, 3%, 4%, 6%

pilocarpine USP, BAN *antiglaucoma agent; ophthalmic cholinergic*

pilocarpine HCl USP *ophthalmic cholinergic; antiglaucoma; miotic; treatment of xerostomia and keratoconjunctivitis sicca due to radiotherapy or Sjögren syndrome (orphan); also for dry mouth* 0.5%, 1%, 2%, 4%, 6%, 8% eye drops; 5 mg oral

pilocarpine nitrate USP *ophthalmic cholinergic; antiglaucoma; miotic*

Pilopine HS ophthalmic gel ℞ *topical antiglaucoma agent; direct-acting miotic* [pilocarpine HCl] 4%

Piloptic-½; Piloptic-1; Piloptic-2; Piloptic-3; Piloptic-4; Piloptic-6 eye drops ℞ *topical antiglaucoma agent; direct-acting miotic* [pilocarpine HCl] 0.5%; 1%; 2%; 3%; 4%; 6%

Pilopto-Carpine eye drops ℞ *topical antiglaucoma agent; direct-acting miotic* [pilocarpine HCl] 4%

Pilostat eye drops ℞ *topical antiglaucoma agent; direct-acting miotic* [pilocarpine HCl] 0.5%, 1%, 2%, 3%, 4%, 6%

Pilpak (trademarked packaging form) *patient compliance package*

Pima syrup ℞ *expectorant* [potassium iodide] 325 mg/5 mL

pimagedine HCl USAN *advanced glycosylation inhibitor for type 1 diabetes; investigational (Phase III) for diabetics in end-stage renal disease*

pimaricin JAN *ophthalmic antibacterial/antifungal antibiotic* [also: natamycin]

pimeclone INN

pimecrolimus USAN, INN *immunosuppressant for atopic dermatitis*

pimefylline INN

pimelautide INN

Pimenta dioica; P. officinalis *medicinal herb* [see: allspice]

pimetacin INN

pimethixene INN

pimetine INN *antihyperlipoproteinemic* [also: pimetine HCl]

pimetine HCl USAN *antihyperlipoproteinemic* [also: pimetine]

pimetixene [see: pimethixene]

pimetremide INN

pimeverine [see: pimetremide]

piminodine INN [also: piminodine esylate]

piminodine esylate NF [also: piminodine]

piminodine ethanesulfonate [see: piminodine esylate]

pimobendan USAN, INN *cardiotonic*

pimonidazole INN, BAN

pimozide USAN, USP, INN, BAN, JAN *antispasmodic/antidyskinetic for Tourette syndrome; diphenylbutylpiperidine antipsychotic; neuroleptic*

pimpernel; small pimpernel *medicinal herb* [see: burnet]

pimpernel, blue *medicinal herb* [see: skullcap]

pimpernel, water *medicinal herb* [see: brooklime]

Pimpinella anisum *medicinal herb* [see: anise]

Pimpinella magna; P. saxifrage *medicinal herb* [see: burnet]

pinacidil USAN, INN *antihypertensive (approved in 1989, but not marketed by the manufacturer)*

pinadoline USAN, INN *analgesic*

pinafide INN

pinaverium bromide INN *GI antispasmodic*

pinazepam INN

pincainide INN

pindolol USAN, USP, INN, BAN *antianginal; antihypertensive; vasodilator; antiadrenergic (β-receptor)* 5, 10 mg oral

pine, Norway *medicinal herb* [see: spruce]

pine, prince's *medicinal herb* [see: pipsissewa]

pine bark extract *natural free radical scavenger for inflammatory collagen disease and peripheral vascular disease; contains 80%–85% procyanidolic oligomers (PCOs)*

pine needle oil NF

pine tar USP

pineapple (Ananas comosus) *fruit medicinal herb for constipation, jaundice, soft tissue inflammation, and topical wound debridement*

Pink Bismuth *oral liquid* OTC *antidiarrheal; antinauseant* [bismuth subsalicylate] 130, 262 mg/15 mL

pinolcaine INN

pinoxepin INN *antipsychotic* [also: pinoxepin HCl]

pinoxepin HCl USAN *antipsychotic* [also: pinoxepin]

Pin-Rid *soft gel capsules, oral liquid* OTC *anthelmintic for ascariasis (roundworm) and enterobiasis (pinworm)* [pyrantel pamoate] 180 mg; 50 mg/mL

Pinus palustris *natural remedy* [see: turpentine]

Pinus strobus *medicinal herb* [see: white pine]

Pin-X *oral liquid* OTC *anthelmintic for ascariasis (roundworm) and enterobiasis (pinworm)* [pyrantel pamoate] 50 mg/mL

pioglitazone INN *thiazolidinedione antidiabetic; increases cellular response to insulin without increasing insulin secretion* [also: pioglitazone HCl]

pioglitazone HCl USAN *thiazolidinedione antidiabetic; increases cellular response to insulin without increasing insulin secretion* [also: pioglitazone]

pipacycline INN

pipamazine INN

pipamperone USAN, INN *antipsychotic*

pipaneperone [see: pipamperone]

pipazetate INN *antitussive* [also: pipazethate]

pipazethate USAN *antitussive* [also: pipazetate]

pipe plant; Dutchman's pipe; Indian pipe *medicinal herb* [see: fit root]

pipebuzone INN

pipecuronium bromide USAN, INN, BAN *nondepolarizing neuromuscular blocking agent; muscle relaxant; adjunct to general anesthesia*

pipemidic acid INN

pipenzolate bromide INN

pipenzolate methylbromide [see: pipenzolate bromide]

pipenzolone bromide [see: pipenzolate bromide]

pipequaline INN

Piper cubeba *medicinal herb* [see: cubeb]

Piper methysticum *medicinal herb* [see: kava kava]

piperacetazine USAN, USP, INN *antipsychotic* ⊉ piperazine

piperacillin INN, BAN *extended-spectrum penicillin antibiotic* [also: piperacillin sodium]

piperacillin sodium USAN, USP, JAN *extended-spectrum penicillin antibiotic* [also: piperacillin] 2, 3, 4 g injection

piperamide INN *anthelmintic* [also: piperamide maleate]

piperamide maleate USAN *anthelmintic* [also: piperamide]

piperamine [see: bamipine]

piperazine USP *anthelmintic for enterobiasis (pinworm) and ascariasis (roundworm)* ⊉ piperacetazine

piperazine calcium edetate INN *anthelmintic* [also: piperazine edetate calcium]

piperazine citrate USP *anthelmintic* 250 mg oral; 500 mg/mL oral

piperazine citrate hydrate [see: piperazine citrate]

piperazine edetate calcium USAN *anthelmintic* [also: piperazine calcium edetate]

piperazine estrone sulfate [now: estropipate]

piperazine hexahydrate [see: piperazine citrate]

piperazine phosphate

piperazine phosphate monohydrate [see: piperazine phosphate]

piperazine theophylline ethanoate [see: acefylline piperazine]

piperidine phosphate

piperidines *a class of antihistamines*

piperidolate INN [also: piperidolate HCl]

piperidolate HCl USP [also: piperidolate]

piperilate [see: pipethanate]

piperine USP *natural pepper extract that increases the absorption of chrysin*

piperocaine INN [also: piperocaine HCl]

piperocaine HCl USP [also: piperocaine]

piperonyl butoxide *pediculicide for lice*

piperoxan INN

piperphenidol HCl

piperylone INN

pipethanate INN

pipobroman USAN, USP, INN *alkylating antineoplastic*

pipoctanone INN

pipofezine INN

piposulfan USAN, INN *antineoplastic*

pipotiazine INN *phenothiazine antipsychotic* [also: pipotiazine palmitate]

pipotiazine palmitate USAN *phenothiazine antipsychotic* [also: pipotiazine]

pipoxizine INN

pipoxolan INN *muscle relaxant* [also: pipoxolan HCl]

pipoxolan HCl USAN *muscle relaxant* [also: pipoxolan]

Pipracil *powder for IV or IM injection (discontinued 2004)* ℞ *extended-spectrum penicillin antibiotic* [piperacillin sodium] 2, 3, 4, 40 g/vial

pipradimadol INN

pipradrol INN [also: pipradrol HCl]

pipradrol HCl NF [also: pipradrol]

pipramadol INN

pipratecol INN

piprinhydrinate INN, BAN

piprocurarium iodide INN

piprofurol INN

piprozolin USAN, INN *choleretic*

pipsissewa (*Chimaphila umbellata*) *plant medicinal herb used as an astringent, diaphoretic, and diuretic*

piquindone INN *antipsychotic* [also: piquindone HCl]

piquindone HCl USAN *antipsychotic* [also: piquindone]

piquizil INN *bronchodilator* [also: piquizil HCl]

piquizil HCl USAN *bronchodilator* [also: piquizil]

piracetam USAN, INN, BAN *cognition adjuvant; investigational (orphan) for myoclonus* ⸬ piroxicam

pirandamine INN *antidepressant* [also: pirandamine HCl]

pirandamine HCl USAN *antidepressant* [also: pirandamine]

pirarubicin INN

piraxelate INN

pirazmonam INN *antimicrobial* [also: pirazmonam sodium]

pirazmonam sodium USAN *antimicrobial* [also: pirazmonam]

pirazofurin INN *antineoplastic* [also: pyrazofurin]

pirazolac USAN, INN, BAN *antirheumatic*

pirbenicillin INN *antibacterial* [also: pirbenicillin sodium]

pirbenicillin sodium USAN *antibacterial* [also: pirbenicillin]

pirbuterol INN *sympathomimetic bronchodilator* [also: pirbuterol acetate]

pirbuterol acetate USAN *sympathomimetic bronchodilator* [also: pirbuterol]

pirbuterol HCl USAN *bronchodilator*

pirdonium bromide INN

pirenoxine INN

pirenperone USAN, INN, BAN *tranquilizer*

pirenzepine INN, BAN *tricyclic benzodiazepine for peptic ulcers* [also: pirenzepine HCl]

pirenzepine HCl USAN, JAN *investigational (NDA filed) tricyclic benzodiazepine for peptic ulcers* [also: pirenzepine]

pirepolol INN

piretanide USAN, INN *diuretic*

pirfenidone USAN, INN *analgesic; anti-inflammatory; antipyretic*

piribedil INN

piribenzyl methylsulfate [see: bevonium metilsulfate]

piridicillin INN *antibacterial* [also: piridicillin sodium]

piridicillin sodium USAN *antibacterial* [also: piridicillin]

piridocaine INN

piridocaine HCl [see: piridocaine]

piridoxilate INN, BAN

piridronate sodium USAN *calcium regulator*

piridronic acid INN

pirifibrate INN

pirinidazole INN

pirinitramide [see: piritramide]

pirinixic acid INN

pirinixil INN

piriprost USAN *antiasthmatic*

piriprost potassium USAN *antiasthmatic*

piriqualone INN

pirisudanol INN

piritramide INN, BAN

piritrexim INN *antiproliferative agent* [also: piritrexim isethionate]

piritrexim isethionate USAN *antiproliferative; orphan status withdrawn 1996* [also: piritrexim]

pirlimycin HCl USAN *antibacterial*

pirlindole INN

pirmagrel USAN, INN *thromboxane synthetase inhibitor*

pirmenol INN *antiarrhythmic* [also: pirmenol HCl]

pirmenol HCl USAN *antiarrhythmic* [also: pirmenol]

pirnabin INN *antiglaucoma agent* [also: pirnabine]

pirnabine USAN *antiglaucoma agent* [also: pirnabin]

piroctone USAN, INN *antiseborrheic*

piroctone olamine USAN *antiseborrheic*

pirodavir USAN, INN, BAN *antiviral*

pirogliride INN *antidiabetic* [also: pirogliride tartrate]

pirogliride tartrate USAN *antidiabetic* [also: pirogliride]

piroheptine INN

pirolate USAN, INN *antiasthmatic*

pirolazamide USAN, INN *antiarrhythmic*

piromidic acid INN

piroxantrone INN *antineoplastic* [also: piroxantrone HCl]

piroxantrone HCl USAN *antineoplastic* [also: piroxantrone]

piroxicam USAN, USP, INN, BAN, JAN *antiarthritic; nonsteroidal anti-inflammatory drug (NSAID)* 10, 20 mg oral ⧄ piracetam

piroxicam β-cyclodextrin [see: piroxicam betadex]

piroxicam betadex USAN *analgesic; antirheumatic; nonsteroidal anti-inflammatory drug (NSAID)*

piroxicam cinnamate USAN *anti-inflammatory*

piroxicam olamine USAN *analgesic; anti-inflammatory*

piroxicillin INN

piroximone USAN, INN, BAN *cardiotonic*

pirozadil INN

pirprofen USAN, INN, BAN *anti-inflammatory*

pirquinozol USAN, INN *antiallergic*

pirralkonium bromide INN

pirroksan [now: proroxan HCl]

pirsidomine USAN, INN *vasodilator*

pirtenidine INN *treatment for gingivitis* [also: pirtenidine HCl]

pirtenidine HCl USAN *treatment for gingivitis* [also: pirtenidine]

pistachio *medicinal herb* [see: witch hazel]

pitch tree, Canada; hemlock pitch tree *medicinal herb* [see: hemlock]

pitcher plant (Sarracenia purpurea) root *medicinal herb used as an astringent, diuretic, and stimulant*

pitenodil INN

Pitocin IV, IM injection ℞ *oxytocic for induction of labor, postpartum bleeding, and incomplete abortion* [oxytocin] 10 U/mL ⧄ Pitressin

pitofenone INN

Pitressin Synthetic IM or subcu injection ℞ *pituitary antidiuretic hormone for diabetes insipidus or prevention of abdominal distention* [vasopressin] 20 U/mL ⧄ Pitocin

Pitrex ⓒⒶⓃ cream OTC *topical antifungal* [tolnaftate] 1%

pituitary, anterior

pituitary, posterior USP *antidiuretic hormone*

pituxate INN

pivalate USAN, INN, BAN *combining name for radicals or groups*

pivampicillin INN *aminopenicillin antibiotic* [also: pivampicillin HCl]

pivampicillin HCl USAN *aminopenicillin antibiotic* [also: pivampicillin]

pivampicillin pamoate USAN *antibacterial*

pivampicillin probenate USAN *antibacterial*

pivenfrine INN

pivmecillinam INN, BAN *aminopenicillin antibiotic* [also: amdinocillin pivoxil; pivmecillinam HCl]

pivmecillinam HCl JAN *aminopenicillin antibiotic* [also: amdinocillin pivoxil; pivmecillinam]

pivopril USAN *antihypertensive*

pivoxazepam INN

pivoxetil USAN, INN *combining name for radicals or groups*

pivoxil USAN, INN *combining name for radicals or groups*

pivsulbactam BAN *β-lactamase inhibitor; penicillin/cephalosporin synergist* [also: sulbactam pivoxil]

pix pini [see: pine tar]

Pixykine ℞ *investigational second-generation colony stimulating factor for neutropenia and thrombocytopenia* [milodistim]

pizotifen INN, BAN *anabolic; antidepressant; serotonin inhibitor (migraine specific)* [also: pizotyline]

pizotyline USAN *anabolic; antidepressant; serotonin inhibitor (migraine specific)* [also: pizotifen]

placebo *an inert substance with no therapeutic value* [also: obecalp]

placebo effect [L. I will please] *a perceived therapeutic effect from an inert substance* [compare to: nocebo effect]

Placidyl capsules (discontinued 2004) ℞ *hypnotic* [ethchlorvynol] 200, 500, 750 mg ⊉ Pathocil

plafibride INN

plague vaccine USP *active bacterin for plague (Yersinia pestis)* $1.8–2.2 \times 10^8$ bacilli/mL IM injection

Plan B tablets (in packs of 2) ℞ in the U.S.; available from pharmacists without a prescription in Canada, the U.K., and much of Europe *emergency postcoital contraceptive (progestin only)* [levonorgestrel] 0.75 mg

planadalin [see: carbromal]

Plantago lanceolata; P. major **and other species** *medicinal herb* [see: plantain]

Plantago ovata **(psyllium)** *medicinal herb* [see: plantain]

plantago seed USP *laxative*

plantain (*Plantago lanceolata; P. major* **and other species**) leaves and seeds *medicinal herb for bed-wetting, bladder infections, blood poisoning, constipation, diarrhea, diverticulitis, edema, hyperlipidemia, kidney disorders, neuralgia, snake bites, sores, and topical inflammation*

Plaquase powder for injection ℞ *investigational (orphan) agent for Peyronie disease* [collagenase]

Plaquenil film-coated tablets ℞ *antimalarial; antirheumatic; lupus erythematosus suppressant* [hydroxychloroquine sulfate] 200 mg

Plaretase 8000 tablets ℞ *porcine-derived digestive enzymes* [lipase; protease; amylase] 8000•30 000•30 000 USP units

Plasbumin-5; Plasbumin-25 IV infusion ℞ *blood volume expander for shock, burns, and hypoproteinemia* [human albumin] 5%; 25%

plasma, antihemophilic human USP

plasma concentrate factor IX [see: factor IX complex]

plasma expanders *a class of therapeutic blood modifiers used to increase the volume of circulating blood* [also called: blood volume expanders]

plasma protein fraction USP *blood volume supporter*

plasma protein fraction, human [now: plasma protein fraction]

plasma protein fractions *a class of therapeutic blood modifiers used to regulate the volume of circulating blood*

plasma thromboplastin component (PTC) [see: factor IX]

Plasma-Lyte 56 IV infusion (discontinued 2001) ℞ *intravenous electrolyte therapy* [combined electrolyte solution]

Plasma-Lyte A pH 7.4; Plasma-Lyte R; Plasma-Lyte 148 IV infusion ℞ *intravenous electrolyte therapy* [combined electrolyte solution]

Plasma-Lyte M (R; 56; 148) and 5% Dextrose IV infusion ℞ *intravenous nutritional/electrolyte therapy* [combined electrolyte solution; dextrose]

Plasmanate IV infusion ℞ *blood volume expander for shock due to burns, trauma, and surgery* [plasma protein fraction] 5%

Plasma-Plex IV infusion ℞ *blood volume expander for shock due to burns, trauma, and surgery* [plasma protein fraction] 5%

Plasmatein IV infusion ℞ *blood volume expander for shock due to burns, trauma, and surgery* [plasma protein fraction] 5%

plasmin BAN [also: fibrinolysin, human]

Plateau Cap (trademarked dosage form) *controlled-release capsule*

platelet cofactor II [see: factor IX]

platelet concentrate USP *platelet replenisher*

Platinol-AQ IV injection ℞ *alkylating antineoplastic for metastatic testicular tumors, metastatic ovarian tumors, and advanced bladder cancer* [cisplatin] 1 mg/mL

platinum *element (Pt)*

cis-**platinum** [now: cisplatin]

cis-**platinum II** [now: cisplatin]

platinum diamminodichloride [see: cisplatin]

plaunotol INN

plauracin USAN, INN *veterinary growth stimulant*

Plavix coated tablets ℞ *platelet aggregation inhibitor for stroke, myocardial infarction, peripheral artery disease, and acute coronary syndrome* [clopidogrel bisulfate] 75 mg

Plax, Advanced Formula mouthwash/gargle OTC [sodium pyrophosphate]

pleconaril USAN *investigational (NDA filed) viral replication inhibitor for treatment of viral respiratory infection and viral meningitis*

Plegisol solution ℞ *cardioplegic solution* [calcium chloride; magnesium chloride; potassium chloride; sodium chloride] 17.6•325.3•119.3•643 mg/100 mL

Plenaxis powder for IM injection *GnRH antagonist to suppress LH and FSH, leading to the cessation of testosterone production (medical castration, androgen ablation); treatment for prostate cancer; investigational for uterine fibroids, endometriosis, and precocious puberty* [abarelix] 100 mg/vial

Plendil extended-release tablets ℞ *antihypertensive; calcium channel blocker* [felodipine] 2.5, 5, 10 mg

Pletal tablets ℞ *vasodilator and platelet aggregation inhibitor for intermittent claudication* [cilostazol] 50, 100 mg

pleurisy root (*Asclepias tuberosa*) *medicinal herb for asthma, bronchitis, dysentery, emphysema, fever, pleurisy, and pneumonia*

pleuromulin INN

Plexion topical liquid, cleansing cloths ℞ *acne treatment* [sulfacetamide sodium; sulfur] 10%•5%

Plexion SCT cream ℞ *acne treatment* [sulfacetamide sodium; sulfur] 10%•5%

Plexion TS topical suspension ℞ *acne treatment* [sulfacetamide sodium; sulfur] 10%•5%

Pliagel solution OTC *surfactant cleaning solution for soft contact lenses*

plicamycin USAN, USP, INN *antibiotic antineoplastic for malignant testicular tumors*

plomestane USAN *antineoplastic; aromatase inhibitor*

plum *(Prunus americana; P. domestica; P. spinosa)* fruit and bark *medicinal herb used as an anthelmintic, astringent, and laxative*

Plus Sinus ⓒⓐⓝ extended-release caplets (discontinued 2001) OTC *nasal decongestant* [pseudoephedrine HCl] 120 mg

plutonium *element (Pu)*

PM Caps ⓒⓐⓝ OTC *vitamin supplement* [multiple vitamins; folic acid] ± ●0.2 mg

pMDI (dosage form) *pressurized metered-dose inhaler*

PMMA (polymethylmethacrylate) [q.v.]

PMPA (phosphonomethoxypropyl-adenine) [see: tenofovir]

PMPA prodrug [see: tenofovir disoproxil fumarate]

PMS-Bezafibrate ⓒⓐⓝ tablets ℞ *antihyperlipidemic* [bezafibrate] 200 mg

PMS-Bromocriptine ⓒⓐⓝ tablets, capsules ℞ *dopamine agonist for Parkinson disease; lactation inhibitor; growth hormone suppressant for acromegaly* [bromocriptine mesylate] 2.5 mg; 5 mg

PMS-Captopril ⓒⓐⓝ tablets ℞ *antihypertensive; angiotensin-converting enzyme (ACE) inhibitor* [captopril] 12.5, 25, 50, 100 mg

PMS-Carbamazepine CR ⓒⓐⓝ controlled-release tablets ℞ *anticonvulsant; analgesic for trigeminal neuralgia; antimanic* [carbamazepine] 200, 400 mg

PMS-Conjugated Estrogens ⓒⓐⓝ tablets ℞ *estrogen replacement therapy for postmenopausal symptoms* [conjugated estrogens] 0.3, 0.625, 0.9, 1.25 mg

PMS-Desferoxamine ⓒⓐⓝ powder for IM, IV, or subcu injection ℞ *adjunct treatment for iron intoxication or overload* [deferoxamine mesylate] 500 mg

PMS-Dexamethasone ⓒⓐⓝ injection ℞ *corticosteroidal anti-inflammatory* [dexamethasone sodium phosphate] 4, 10 mg/mL

PMS-Dexamethasone ⓒⓐⓝ tablets, elixir, eye drops, ear drops ℞ *corticosteroidal anti-inflammatory* [dexamethasone] 0.5, 0.75, 4 mg; 0.5 mg/5 mL; 0.1%; 0.1%

PMS-Dicitrate ⓒⓐⓝ oral solution ℞ *urinary alkalinizing agent* [sodium citrate; citric acid] 500●334 mg/5 mL

PMS-Diclofenac ⓒⓐⓝ tablets, suppositories ℞ *analgesic; antiarthritic; nonsteroidal anti-inflammatory drug (NSAID)* [diclofenac sodium] 25, 50 mg; 25, 50 mg

PMS-Diclofenac SR ⓒⓐⓝ slow-release tablets ℞ *analgesic; antiarthritic; nonsteroidal anti-inflammatory drug (NSAID)* [diclofenac sodium] 75, 100 mg

PMS-Dipivefrin ⓒⓐⓝ eye drops ℞ *topical antiglaucoma agent* [dipivefrin HCl] 0.1%

PMS-Fenofibrate Micro ⓒⓐⓝ capsules ℞ *antihyperlipidemic* [fenofibrate, micronized] 200 mg

PMS-Fluorometholone ⓒⓐⓝ eye drops ℞ *topical ophthalmic corticosteroidal anti-inflammatory* [fluorometholone] 0.1%

PMS-Fluphenazine Decanoate ⓒⓐⓝ subcu or IM injection ℞ *conventional (typical) phenothiazine antipsychotic for schizophrenia and psychotic disorders; used for prolonged parenteral neuroleptic therapy* [fluphenazine decanoate] 25, 100 mg/mL

PMS-Fluvoxamine ⓒⓐⓝ film-coated tablets ℞ *selective serotonin reuptake inhibitor (SSRI) for depression and obsessive-compulsive disorder (OCD)* [fluvoxamine maleate] 50, 100 mg

PMS-Gabapentin ⓒⓐⓝ capsules ℞ *anticonvulsant for partial-onset seizures* [gabapentin] 100, 300, 400 mg

PMS-Haloperidol LA ⓒⓐⓝ IM injection ℞ *conventional (typical) butyrophenone antipsychotic; antispasmodic/antidyskinetic for Tourette syndrome; treatment for severe pediatric behavioral disorders such as aggression, combativeness, hyperexcitability, and poor impulse control* [haloperidol decanoate] 50, 100 mg/mL

PMS-Indapamide ⓒⓐⓝ tablets ℞ *antihypertensive; diuretic* [indapamide] 1.25, 2.5 mg

PMS-Levobunolol ⒸⒶⓃ eye drops ℞ *topical antiglaucoma agent* [levobunolol HCl] 5 mg/mL

PMS-Lithium Carbonate ⒸⒶⓃ capsules ℞ *antipsychotic for manic episodes* [lithium carbonate] 150, 300, 600 mg

PMS-Lithium Citrate ⒸⒶⓃ syrup ℞ *antipsychotic for manic episodes* [lithium citrate] 300 mg/5 mL

PMS-Minocycline ⒸⒶⓃ capsules ℞ *tetracycline antibiotic* [minocycline HCl] 50, 100 mg

PMS-Moclobemide ⒸⒶⓃ tablets ℞ *antidepressant* [moclobemide] 100, 150 mg

PMS-Nizatidine ⒸⒶⓃ capsules ℞ *histamine H_2 antagonist for treatment of gastric and duodenal ulcers* [nizatidine] 150, 300 mg

PMS-Oxybutynin ⒸⒶⓃ tablets, syrup ℞ *urinary antispasmodic* [oxybutynin chloride] 2.5, 5 mg; 5 mg/5 mL

PMS-Pindolol ⒸⒶⓃ tablets ℞ *antihypertensive; antianginal* [pindolol] 5, 10, 15, 80, 160 mg

PMS-Polytrimethoprim ⒸⒶⓃ eye drops ℞ *topical ophthalmic antibiotic* [polymyxin B sulfate; trimethoprim sulfate] 10 000 U•1 mg per mL

PMS-Ranitidine ⒸⒶⓃ film-coated tablets ℞ *histamine H_2 antagonist for gastric and duodenal ulcers* [ranitidine HCl] 150, 300 mg

PMS-Sotalol ⒸⒶⓃ tablets ℞ *antiarrhythmic* [sotalol HCl] 80, 160 mg

PMS-Sucralfate ⒸⒶⓃ tablets ℞ *cytoprotective agent for gastric ulcers* [sucralfate]

PMS-Tamoxifen ⒸⒶⓃ tablets ℞ *antiestrogen antineoplastic for breast cancer* [tamoxifen citrate] 10, 20 mg

PMS-Terazosin ⒸⒶⓃ tablets ℞ *antihypertensive (α-blocker); treatment for benign prostatic hyperplasia (BPH)* [terazosin HCl] 1, 2, 5, 10 mg

PMS-Terbinafine ⒸⒶⓃ tablets ℞ *systemic allylamine antifungal* [terbinafine HCl] 250 mg

PMS-Ticlopidine ⒸⒶⓃ film-coated tablets ℞ *platelet aggregation inhibitor for stroke* [ticlopidine HCl] 250 mg

PMS-Tobramycin ⒸⒶⓃ eye drops ℞ *topical antibiotic* [tobramycin] 0.3%

P-MVAC (Platinol, methotrexate, vinblastine, Adriamycin, carboplatin) *chemotherapy protocol*

Pneumo 23 ⒸⒶⓃ subcu or IM injection ℞ *active immunization against 23 strains of* Streptococcus pneumoniae [pneumococcal vaccine, polyvalent] 0.5 mL

pneumococcal vaccine, 7-valent (PCV7) *active bacterin for pneumococcal pneumonia (polysaccharide isolates of seven strains of* Streptococcus pneumoniae: *4, 6B, 9V, 14, 18C, 19F, and 23F)*

pneumococcal vaccine, polyvalent *active bacterin for pneumococcal pneumonia (polysaccharide isolates of 23 strains of* Streptococcus pneumoniae)

Pneumomist sustained-release tablets (discontinued 2002) ℞ *expectorant* [guaifenesin] 600 mg

Pneumotussin caplets ℞ *narcotic antitussive; expectorant* [hydrocodone bitartrate; guaifenesin] 2.5•300 mg

Pneumotussin 2.5 Cough syrup ℞ *narcotic antitussive; expectorant* [hydrocodone bitartrate; guaifenesin] 5•400 mg/10 mL

Pneumotussin HC syrup (discontinued 2002) ℞ *narcotic antitussive; expectorant* [hydrocodone bitartrate; guaifenesin] 5•100 mg/5 mL

Pneumovax 23 subcu or IM injection ℞ *active immunization against 23 strains of* Streptococcus pneumoniae [pneumococcal vaccine, polyvalent] 25 μg of each strain per 0.5 mL dose

Pnu-Imune 23 subcu or IM injection (discontinued 2002) ℞ *active immunization against 23 strains of* Streptococcus pneumoniae [pneumococcal vaccine, polyvalent] 25 μg of each strain per 0.5 mL dose

pobilukast edamine USAN *antiasthmatic*

POC (procarbazine, Oncovin, CCNU) *chemotherapy protocol for pediatric brain tumors*

POCA (prednisone, Oncovin, cytarabine, Adriamycin) *chemotherapy protocol*

POCC (procarbazine, Oncovin, cyclophosphamide, CCNU) *chemotherapy protocol*

Pockethaler (trademarked delivery device) *nasal inhalation aerosol*

pod pepper *medicinal herb* [see: cayenne]

podilfen INN

Podocon-25 topical liquid ℞ *keratolytic for genital warts* [podophyllum resin] 25%

podofilox USAN *topical antimitotic for genital warts* [also: podophyllotoxin] 0.5% topical

Podofin topical liquid ℞ *keratolytic for genital warts* [podophyllum resin] 25% ⊇ podophyllin

podophyllin [see: podophyllum resin] ⊇ Podofin

podophyllotoxin BAN *topical antimitotic* [also: podofilox]

podophyllotoxins *a class of mitotic-inhibiting antineoplastics derived from podophyllotoxin*

podophyllum USP *caustic; cytotoxic agent for genital warts*

Podophyllum peltatum *medicinal herb* [see: mandrake]

podophyllum resin USP *caustic; cytotoxic agent for genital warts*

poinsettia (*Euphorbia pulcherrima; E. poinsettia; Poinsettia pulcherrima*) *plant and sap medicinal herb for fever, pain relief, stimulating lactation, toothache, and warts; also used as an antibacterial and depilatory*

Point-Two oral rinse ℞ *topical dental caries preventative* [sodium fluoride; alcohol 6%] 0.2%

poison, dog *medicinal herb* [see: dog poison]

Poison Antidote Kit (discontinued 2002) OTC *emergency treatment for various poisons* [syrup of ipecac; charcoal suspension] 30•60 mL

poison ash *medicinal herb* [see: fringe tree]

poison flag *medicinal herb* [see: blue flag]

poison hemlock (*Conium maculatum*) *plant medicinal herb that has been used for analgesia and sedation and as a method of execution; it is extremely poisonous*

poison ivy extract, alum precipitated USAN *ivy poisoning counteractant*

poison oak (*Tocicodendron diversilobum*) *extract medicinal herb used in homeopathic remedies for osteoarthritis*

poison oak extract USAN *antiallergic*

Poison Oak-N-Ivy Armor lotion (discontinued 2003) OTC *poison ivy protectant*

poke root (*Phytolacca decandra*) *medicinal herb* [see: pokeweed]

pokeweed (*Phytolacca americana; P. decandra; P. rigida*) *root and young shoots medicinal herb for arthritis, blood cleansing, bowel evacuation, dysmenorrhea, mucous membrane inflammation and discharge, mumps, pain, rheumatism, ringworm, scabies, syphilis, and tonsillitis; not generally regarded as safe and effective*

polacrilex [see: nicotine polacrilex]

polacrilin USAN, INN *pharmaceutic aid*

polacrilin potassium USAN, NF *tablet disintegrant*

Polaramine tablets, Repetabs (repeat-action tablets), syrup (discontinued 2002) ℞ *antihistamine* [dexchlorpheniramine maleate] 2 mg; 4, 6 mg; 2 mg/5 mL

Polaramine Expectorant oral liquid ℞ *decongestant; antihistamine; expectorant* [pseudoephedrine sulfate; dexchlorpheniramine maleate; guaifenesin; alcohol 7.2%] 20•2•100 mg/5 mL

poldine methylsulfate USAN, USP *anticholinergic* [also: poldine metilsulfate]

poldine metilsulfate INN *anticholinergic* [also: poldine methylsulfate]

polecat weed *medicinal herb* [see: skunk cabbage]

policapram USAN, INN *tablet binder*

policosanol *natural supplement from sugar cane plants; enhanced extract of octacosanol (q.v.) used for hypercholesterolemia; therapeutic effects are* *similar to statin drugs but without side effects such as liver dysfunction and muscle atrophy*

policresulen INN

polidexide sulfate INN

polidocanol INN, JAN, DCF *polyethylene glycol monododecyl ether*

polifeprosan INN *pharmaceutic aid; implantable, biodegradable drug carrier* [also: polifeprosan 20]

polifeprosan 20 USAN *pharmaceutic aid; implantable, biodegradable drug carrier* [also: polifeprosan]

poligeenan USAN, INN *dispersing agent*

poliglecaprone 25 USAN *absorbable surgical suture material*

poliglecaprone 90 USAN *absorbable surgical suture coating*

poliglusam USAN *antihemorrhagic*

polignate sodium USAN *pepsin enzyme inhibitor*

polihexanide INN [also: polyhexanide]

poliomyelitis vaccine [now: poliovirus vaccine, inactivated]

poliovirus vaccine, enhanced inactivated (eIPV) *active immunizing agent for poliomyelitis*

poliovirus vaccine, inactivated (IPV) USP *active immunizing agent for poliomyelitis*

poliovirus vaccine, live oral (OPV) USP *active immunizing agent for poliomyelitis*

polipropene 25 USAN *tablet excipient*

polisaponin INN

politef INN *prosthetic aid* [also: polytef]

polixetonium chloride USAN, INN *preservative*

Polocaine injection ℞ *injectable local anesthetic* [mepivacaine HCl] 1%, 2%, 3%

Polocaine MPF injection ℞ *injectable local anesthetic* [mepivacaine HCl] 1%, 1.5%, 2%

Polocaine with levonordefrin injection ℞ *injectable local anesthetic* [mepivacaine HCl; levonordefrin] 2%•1:20 000

polonium *element (Po)*

poloxalene USAN, INN, BAN *surfactant*

poloxamer USAN, NF, INN, BAN *ointment and suppository base; tablet binder*

poloxamer 124 USAN *surfactant; emulsifier; solubilizer; stabilizer*

poloxamer 188 USAN *surfactant; emulsifier; solubilizer; investigational (Phase III, orphan) for sickle cell crisis; investigational (orphan) for severe burns and vasospasm following cerebral aneurysm repair*

poloxamer 237 USAN *surfactant; emulsifier; solubilizer; stabilizer*

poloxamer 331 *investigational (orphan) for toxoplasmosis of AIDS*

poloxamer 338 USAN *surfactant; emulsifier; solubilizer; stabilizer*

poloxamer 407 USAN *surfactant; emulsifier; solubilizer; stabilizer*

poly I: poly C12U *investigational (Phase III, orphan) antiviral/immunomodulator for HIV, renal cell carcinoma, metastatic melanoma, and chronic fatigue syndrome*

polyamine-methylene resin

polyanhydroglucose [see: dextran]

polyanhydroglucuronic acid [see: dextran]

polybenzarsol INN

polybutester USAN *surgical suture material*

polybutilate USAN *surgical suture coating*

polycarbokane [see: polycarbophil]

polycarbophil USP, INN, BAN *bulk laxative; antidiarrheal*

Polycitra syrup ℞ *urinary alkalinizing agent* [potassium citrate; sodium citrate; citric acid] 550•500•334 mg/5 mL

Polycitra-K oral solution, crystals for oral solution ℞ *urinary alkalizing agent* [potassium citrate; citric acid] 1100•334 mg/5 mL; 3300•1002 mg/pkt.

Polycitra-LC solution ℞ *urinary alkalizing agent* [potassium citrate; sodium citrate; citric acid] 550•500•334 mg/5 mL

Polycose oral liquid, powder for oral liquid OTC *carbohydrate caloric supplement* [glucose polymers]

polydextrose USAN *food additive*

polydimethylsiloxane *surgical aid (retinal tamponade) for retinal detachment*

Polydine ointment, scrub, solution OTC *broad-spectrum antimicrobial* [povidone-iodine]

polydioxanone USAN *absorbable surgical suture material*

polyelectrolyte 211 [see: sodium alginate]

polyenes *a class of antifungals produced by a species of* Streptomyces *that damage fungal cell membranes*

polyestradiol phosphate INN, BAN *antineoplastic; estrogen*

polyetadene INN *antacid* [also: polyethadene]

polyethadene USAN *antacid* [also: polyetadene]

polyethylene excipient NF *stiffening agent*

polyethylene glycol (PEG) NF *ophthalmic moisturizer; ointment and suppository base; solvent*

polyethylene glycol *n* (*n* refers to the molecular weight: 300, 1000, etc.)

polyethylene glycol *n* **dioleate** (*n* refers to the molecular weight: 300, 400, 1000, etc.)

polyethylene glycol 8 monostearate [see: polyoxyl 8 stearate]

polyethylene glycol 1000 monocetyl ether [see: cetomacrogol 1000]

polyethylene glycol 1540 NF

polyethylene glycol 3350 *laxative* 255, 527 g oral

polyethylene glycol 4000 USP [also: macrogol 4000]

polyethylene glycol 6000 USP

polyethylene glycol–electrolyte solution (PEG-ES) *pre-procedure bowel evacuant* [contains PEG 3350]

polyethylene glycol monoleyl ether [see: polyoxyl 10 oleyl ether]

polyethylene glycol monomethyl ether NF *excipient*

polyethylene glycol monostearate [see: polyoxyl 40 & 50 stearate]

polyethylene glycol-superoxide dismutase (PEG-SOD) [see: pegorgotein]

polyethylene oxide NF *suspending and viscosity agent; tablet binder*

polyferose USAN *hematinic*

Polygala senega *medicinal herb* [see: senega]

Polygam powder for IV infusion (discontinued 2001; replaced by Polygam S/D) ℞ *passive immunizing agent for HIV* [immune globulin] 50 mg/mL

Polygam S/D freeze-dried powder for IV infusion ℞ *passive immunizing agent for HIV, idiopathic thrombocytopenic purpura, and B-cell chronic lymphocytic leukemia* [immune globulin, solvent/detergent treated] 50 mg/mL

polygeline INN, BAN

polyglactin 370 USAN *absorbable surgical suture coating*

polyglactin 910 USAN *absorbable surgical suture material*

polyglycolic acid USAN, INN *surgical suture material*

polyglyconate USAN, BAN *absorbable surgical suture material*

Polygonatum multiflorum; P. odoratum *medicinal herb* [see: Solomon's seal]

Polygonum aviculare; P. hydropiper; P. persicaria; P. punctatum *medicinal herb* [see: knotweed]

Polygonum bistorta *medicinal herb* [see: bistort]

Polygonum multiflorum *medicinal herb* [see: fo-ti; ho-shou-wu]

polyhexanide BAN [also: polihexanide]

Poly-Histine elixir ℞ *antihistamine for allergic and vasomotor rhinitis, allergic conjunctivitis, and mild urticaria* [pheniramine maleate; pyrilamine maleate; phenyltoloxamine citrate] 4•4•4 mg/5 mL

Poly-Histine CS syrup (discontinued 2002) ℞ *narcotic antitussive; decongestant; antihistamine* [codeine phosphate; phenylpropanolamine HCl; brompheniramine maleate] 10•12.5•2 mg/5 mL

Poly-Histine DM syrup (discontinued 2002) ℞ *antitussive; decongestant; antihistamine* [dextromethorphan hydrobromide; phenylpropanolamine HCl; brompheniramine maleate] 10•12.5•2 mg/5 mL

Poly-Histine-D sustained-release capsules, elixir (discontinued 2001) ℞ *decongestant; antihistamine* [phenylpropanolamine HCl; phenyltoloxamine citrate; pyrilamine maleate; pheniramine maleate] 50•16•16•16 mg; 12.5•4•4•4 mg/5 mL

Poly-Histine-D Ped Caps sustained-release capsules (discontinued 2001) ℞ *pediatric decongestant and antihistamine* [phenylpropanolamine HCl; phenyltoloxamine citrate; pyrilamine maleate; pheniramine maleate] 25•8•8•8 mg

poly-ICLC *investigational (orphan) for primary brain tumors*

poly-L-lactic acid *synthetic polymer for the correction of facial lipoatrophy due to HIV infections*

polyloxyl 8 stearate USAN *surfactant*

polymacon USAN *hydrophilic contact lens material*

polymanoacetate [now: acemannan]

polymeric oxygen [see: oxygen, polymeric]

polymetaphosphate P 32 USAN *radioactive agent*

polymethyl methacrylate (PMMA) *rigid hydrophobic polymer used for hard contact lenses*

polymixin E [see: colistin sulfate]

polymonine

polymyxin BAN *bactericidal antibiotic* [also: polymyxin B sulfate; polymyxin B]

polymyxin B INN *bactericidal antibiotic* [also: polymyxin B sulfate; polymyxin]

polymyxin B sulfate USP *bactericidal antibiotic* [also: polymyxin B; polymyxin] 500 000 U/vial eye drops or injection

polymyxin B sulfate & bacitracin zinc *topical antibiotic* 10 000•500 U/g ophthalmic

polymyxin B sulfate & bacitracin zinc & neomycin sulfate *topical antibiotic* 10 000 U•400 U•5 mg per g ophthalmic

polymyxin B sulfate & gramicidin & neomycin sulfate *topical antibiotic* 10 000 U•0.025 mg•1.75 mg per mL eye drops

polymyxin B sulfate & neomycin sulfate & dexamethasone *topical ophthalmic antibiotic and corticosteroidal anti-inflammatory* 10 000 U/mL•0.35%•0.1% eye drops

polymyxin B sulfate & neomycin sulfate & hydrocortisone *topical ophthalmic antibiotic and corticosteroidal anti-inflammatory* 10 000 U/mL•0.35%•1% eye drops

polymyxin B sulfate & trimethoprim sulfate *topical ophthalmic antibiotic* 10 000 U•1 mg per mL eye drops

polymyxin B₁ [see: polymyxin B]
polymyxin B₂ [see: polymyxin B]
polymyxin B₃ [see: polymyxin B]
polymyxin E [see: colistin sulfate]

polynoxylin INN, BAN

polyolprepolymer *topical base for gels and creams*

polyoxyethylene 20 sorbitan monolaurate [see: polysorbate 20]

polyoxyethylene 20 sorbitan monooleate [see: polysorbate 80]

polyoxyethylene 20 sorbitan monopalmitate [see: polysorbate 40]

polyoxyethylene 20 sorbitan monostearate [see: polysorbate 60]

polyoxyethylene 20 sorbitan trioleate [see: polysorbate 85]

polyoxyethylene 20 sorbitan tristearate [see: polysorbate 65]

polyoxyethylene 50 stearate [now: polyoxyl 50 stearate]

polyoxyethylene glycol 1000 monocetyl ether [see: cetomacrogol 1000]

polyoxyethylene nonyl phenol *surfactant/wetting agent*

polyoxyl 10 oleyl ether NF *surfactant*

polyoxyl 20 cetostearyl ether NF *surfactant*

polyoxyl 35 castor oil NF *emulsifying agent; surfactant*

polyoxyl 40 hydrogenated castor oil NF *emulsifying agent; surfactant*

polyoxyl 40 stearate USAN, NF *surfactant*

polyoxyl 50 stearate NF *surfactant; emulsifying agent*

polyoxypropylene 15 stearyl ether USAN *solvent*

polyphosphoric acid, sodium salt [see: sodium polyphosphate]

Polypodium vulgare medicinal herb [see: female fern]

Poly-Pred eye drop suspension ℞ *corticosteroidal anti-inflammatory; antibiotic* [prednisolone acetate; neomycin sulfate; polymyxin B sulfate] 0.5%•0.35%•10 000 U per mL

polypropylene glycol NF

polyribonucleotide [see: poly I: poly C12U]

polysaccharide-iron complex *hematinic; iron supplement* 150 mg Fe oral

Polysorb Hydrate cream OTC *moisturizer; emollient*

polysorbate 20 USAN, NF, INN *surfactant/wetting agent*

polysorbate 40 USAN, NF, INN *surfactant*

polysorbate 60 USAN, NF, INN *surfactant*

polysorbate 65 USAN, INN *surfactant*

polysorbate 80 USAN, NF, INN *surfactant/wetting agent; viscosity-increasing agent*

polysorbate 85 USAN, INN *surfactant*

Polysporin ointment, topical powder OTC *antibiotic* [polymyxin B sulfate; bacitracin zinc] 10 000•500 U/g

Polysporin ophthalmic ointment OTC *topical ophthalmic antibiotic* [polymyxin B sulfate; bacitracin zinc] 10 000•500 U/g

Polytabs-F chewable tablets ℞ *pediatric vitamin supplement and dental caries preventative* [multiple vitamins; fluoride; folic acid] ±•1•0.3 mg

Polytar shampoo, soap OTC *antiseborrheic; antipsoriatic; antipruritic; antibacterial* [coal tar (solution includes pine tar and juniper tar)] 0.5% (4.5%); 0.5% (2.5%)

Polytar Bath oil (discontinued 2003) OTC *antipsoriatic; antiseborrheic; antipruritic; antibacterial* [coal tar (solution includes pine tar and juniper tar)] 0.5% (25%)

polytef USAN *prosthetic aid* [also: politef]

polytetrafluoroethylene (PTFE) [see: polytef]

polythiazide USAN, USP, INN *diuretic; antihypertensive*

Polytrim eye drops (discontinued 2003) ℞ *antibiotic* [polymyxin B sulfate; trimethoprim] 10 000 U•1 mg per mL

Poly-Tussin syrup ℞ *narcotic antitussive; decongestant; antihistamine* [hydrocodone bitartrate; phenylephrine HCl; chlorpheniramine maleate] 5•5•2 mg/5 mL

polyurethane foam USAN *internal bone splint*

polyvalent Crotaline antivenin [see: antivenin (Crotalidae) polyvalent]

polyvalent gas gangrene antitoxin [see: gas gangrene antitoxin, pentavalent]

polyvidone INN *dispersing, suspending and viscosity-increasing agent* [also: povidone]

Poly-Vi-Flor chewable tablets ℞ *pediatric vitamin supplement and dental caries preventative* [multiple vitamins; sodium fluoride; folic acid] ±•0.25•0.3, ±•0.5•0.3, ±•1•0.3 mg

Poly-Vi-Flor drops ℞ *pediatric vitamin supplement and dental caries preventative* [multiple vitamins; sodium fluoride] ±•0.25, ±•0.5 mg/mL

Poly-Vi-Flor with Iron chewable tablets ℞ *pediatric vitamin/iron supplement and dental caries preventative* [multiple vitamins & minerals; sodium fluoride; iron; folic acid] ±•0.25•12•0.3, ±•0.5•12•0.3, ±•1•12•0.3 mg

Poly-Vi-Flor with Iron drops ℞ *pediatric vitamin/iron supplement and dental caries preventative* [multiple vitamins & minerals; sodium fluoride; iron] ±•0.25•10, ±•0.5•10 mg/mL

polyvinyl acetate phthalate NF *coating agent*

polyvinyl alcohol (PVA) USP *ophthalmic moisturizer; viscosity-increasing agent*

polyvinyl chloride, radiopaque *oral radiopaque contrast medium for severe constipation*

polyvinylpyrrolidone [now: povidone]

Poly-Vi-Sol chewable tablets OTC *vitamin supplement* [multiple vitamins; folic acid] ± •0.3 mg

Poly- drops OTC *vitamin supplement* [multiple vitamins]

Poly-Vi-Sol with Iron chewable tablets OTC *vitamin/iron supplement* [multiple vitamins; iron; folic acid] ± •12•0.3 mg

Poly-Vi-Sol with Iron drops OTC *vitamin/iron supplement* [multiple vitamins; iron] ± •10 mg/mL

Poly-Vitamin drops OTC *vitamin supplement* [multiple vitamins]

Polyvitamin Fluoride chewable tablets ℞ *pediatric vitamin supplement and dental caries preventative* [multiple vitamins; fluoride; folic acid] ± •0.5•0.3, ± •1•0.3 mg

Polyvitamin Fluoride drops ℞ *pediatric vitamin supplement and dental caries preventative* [multiple vitamins; fluoride] ± •0.25, ± •0.5 mg/mL

Polyvitamin Fluoride with Iron chewable tablets ℞ *pediatric vitamin/iron supplement and dental caries preventative* [multiple vitamins & minerals; fluoride; iron; folic acid] ± •1• 12•0.3 mg

Poly-Vitamin with Iron drops OTC *vitamin/iron supplement* [multiple vitamins; iron] ± •10 mg/mL

Polyvitamin with Iron and Fluoride drops ℞ *pediatric vitamin/iron supplement and dental caries preventative* [multiple vitamins; iron; fluoride] ± •10•0.25 mg/mL

Polyvitamins with Fluoride and Iron chewable tablets ℞ *pediatric vitamin/iron supplement and dental caries preventative* [multiple vitamins; fluoride; iron; folic acid] ± •0.5•12•0.3 mg

pomegranate *(Punica granatum)* seeds and fruit rind *medicinal herb used as an anthelmintic and astringent*

POMP (prednisone, Oncovin, methotrexate, Purinethol) *chemotherapy protocol*

ponalrestat USAN, INN, BAN *aldose reductase inhibitor*

ponfibrate INN

Ponstel capsules ℞ *analgesic; nonsteroidal anti-inflammatory drug (NSAID)* [mefenamic acid] 250 mg ⚕ Pronestyl

Pontocaine cream OTC *topical local anesthetic* [tetracaine HCl] 1%

Pontocaine ointment OTC *topical local anesthetic* [tetracaine; menthol] 0.5%•0.5%

Pontocaine HCl injection, powder for injection ℞ *local anesthetic for spinal anesthesia* [tetracaine HCl] 0.2%, 0.3%, 1%; 20 mg

Pontocaine HCl Mono-Drop (eye drops) ℞ *local anesthetic* [tetracaine HCl] 0.5%

Pontocaine HCl solution ℞ *nose/ throat anesthetic to abolish laryngeal and esophageal reflex* [tetracaine HCl; chlorobutanol] 2%•0.4%

poplar *(Populus tremuloides)* bark and buds *medicinal herb used as an antiperiodic, balsamic, febrifuge, and stomachic*

poplar, balsam *medicinal herb* [see: balm of Gilead]

poplar, black *medicinal herb* [see: black poplar]

Po-Pon-S sugar-coated tablets OTC *vitamin/mineral supplement* [multiple vitamins & minerals]

Populus balsamifera; P. candicans *medicinal herb* [see: balm of Gilead]

Populus nigra; P. tremula *medicinal herb* [see: black poplar]

Populus tremuloides *medicinal herb* [see: poplar]

poractant alfa BAN *porcine lung extract containing 90% phospholipids for emergency rescue and treatment of respiratory distress syndrome (RDS) in premature infants (orphan)*

Porcelana cream (discontinued 2003) OTC *hyperpigmentation bleaching agent* [hydroquinone] 2%

Porcelana with Sunscreen cream (discontinued 2003) OTC *hyperpigmentation bleaching agent* [hydroquinone (in a sunscreen base)] 2%

porcine islet preparation, encapsulated *investigational (orphan) antidiabetic for type 1 patients on immunosuppression*

porfimer sodium USAN, INN *laser light–activated antineoplastic for photodynamic therapy (PDT) of esophageal (orphan) and non–small cell lung cancers; used for ablation of high-grade dysplasia in Barrett esophagus (BE) patients; investigational (orphan) for bladder cancer*

porfiromycin USAN, INN, BAN *antibacterial; investigational (Phase III, orphan) antineoplastic for head, neck, and cervical cancers*

Porites spp. *natural material* [see: coral]

porofocon A USAN *hydrophobic contact lens material*

porofocon B USAN *hydrophobic contact lens material*

Portagen powder OTC *enteral nutritional therapy* [lactose-free formula]

Portia film-coated tablets (in packs of 21 or 28) ℞ *monophasic oral contraceptive; emergency postcoital contraceptive* [levonorgestrel; ethinyl estradiol] 0.15 mg•30 μg

posaconazole USAN *antifungal; investigational (Phase III) treatment for AIDS-related fungal infections*

posatirelin INN

posedrine [see: benzchlorpropamid]

poskine INN, BAN

posterior pituitary [see: pituitary, posterior]

Posture tablets OTC *calcium supplement* [calcium phosphate, tribasic] 600 mg Ca

Posture-D film-coated tablets OTC *dietary supplement* [calcium phosphate, tribasic; vitamin D] 600 mg•125 IU

Potaba tablets, capsules, Envules (powder for oral solution) ℞ *water-soluble vitamin; "possibly effective" for scleroderma and other skin diseases and Peyronie disease* [aminobenzoate potassium] 500 mg; 500 mg; 2 g

Potable Aqua tablets (discontinued 2002) OTC *emergency disinfectant for drinking water* [tetraglycine hydroperiodide (source of iodine)] 16.7% (6.68%)

Potasalan oral liquid ℞ *potassium supplement* [potassium chloride; alcohol 4%] 20 mEq K/15 mL

potash, sulfurated USP *source of sulfides*

potassic saline, lactated NF

potassium *element (K)*

potassium acetate USP *electrolyte replenisher* 2, 4 mEq/mL injection

potassium acid phosphate *urinary acidifier*

potassium alpha-phenoxyethyl penicillin [see: phenethicillin potassium]

potassium alum [see: alum, potassium]

potassium aminobenzoate [see: aminobenzoate potassium]

potassium aspartate [see: L-aspartate potassium]

potassium aspartate & magnesium aspartate USAN *nutrient*

potassium benzoate NF *preservative*

potassium benzyl penicillin [see: penicillin G potassium]

potassium bicarbonate USP *pH buffer; electrolyte replacement*

potassium bitartrate USAN

potassium borate *pH buffer*

potassium canrenoate JAN *aldosterone antagonist* [also: canrenoate potassium; canrenoic acid]

potassium carbonate USP *alkalizing agent*

potassium chloride (KCl) USP *electrolyte replenisher* 600, 750, 1500 mg oral; 20, 40 mEq/15 mL oral; 20 mEq/pkt oral; 2, 10, 20, 30, 40, 60, 90 mEq/mL injection

potassium chloride K 42 USAN *radioactive agent*

potassium citrate USP *electrolyte replacement; urinary alkalizer for nephrolithiasis and hypocitruria prevention (orphan)*

potassium clavulanate & amoxicillin [see: amoxicillin]

potassium clavulanate & ticarcillin [see: ticarcillin disodium]

potassium dichloroisocyanurate [see: troclosene potassium]

potassium gamma hydroxybutyrate (KGHB) [see: gamma hydroxybutyrate (GHB)]

potassium glucaldrate USAN, INN *antacid*

potassium gluconate USP *electrolyte replenisher* 500, 595 mg oral; 20 mEq/15 mL oral

potassium guaiacolsulfonate USP *expectorant* [also: sulfogaiacol]

potassium hydroxide (KOH) NF *alkalizing agent*

potassium hydroxymethoxybenzenesulfonate hemihydrate [see: potassium guaiacolsulfonate]

potassium iodate *prevents the uptake of radioactive iodine by the thyroid gland after a nuclear accident or attack*

potassium iodide USP *antifungal; expectorant; dietary iodine supplement; thyroid agent; prevents the uptake of radioactive iodine by the thyroid gland after a nuclear accident or attack* 1 g/mL oral

potassium mercuric iodide NF

potassium metabisulfite NF *antioxidant*

potassium metaphosphate NF *buffering agent*

potassium nitrate *tooth desensitizer*

potassium nitrazepate INN

potassium para-aminobenzoate (PAB) [see: aminobenzoate potassium]

potassium penicillin G [see: penicillin G potassium]

potassium perchlorate *radioimaging adjunct*

potassium permanganate USP *topical anti-infective*

potassium phosphate, dibasic USP *calcium regulator; phosphorus replacement; pH buffer*

potassium phosphate, monobasic NF *pH buffer; phosphorus replacement*

potassium sodium tartrate USP *laxative*

potassium sorbate NF *antimicrobial agent*

potassium tetraborate *pH buffer*

potassium thiocyanate NF

potassium-sparing diuretics *a class of diuretic agents that interfere with sodium reabsorption, thus decreasing potassium secretion*

potato, wild; wild sweet potato vine *medicinal herb* [see: wild jalap]

Potentilla anserina; P. canadensis; P. reptans medicinal herb [see: cinquefoil]

Potentilla tormentilla medicinal herb [see: tormentil]

Povidine ointment, scrub, solution OTC *broad-spectrum antimicrobial* [povidone-iodine] 10%, 5%, 10%

povidone USAN, USP *dispersing, suspending and viscosity-increasing agent* [also: polyvidone]

povidone I 125 USAN *radioactive agent*

povidone I 131 USAN *radioactive agent*

povidone-iodine USP, BAN *broad-spectrum antimicrobial* 10% topical

powdered cellulose [see: cellulose, powdered]

powdered ipecac [see: ipecac, powdered]

powdered opium [see: opium, powdered]

PowerMate tablets OTC *vitamin/mineral supplement* [multiple vitamins & minerals]

PowerSleep tablets OTC *vitamin/mineral supplement; nonprescription sleep aid* [multiple vitamins & minerals; 5-hydroxytryptophan; L-glutamine; melatonin; valerian] ≜•250•25•0.25•75 mg

PowerVites tablets OTC *vitamin/mineral supplement* [multiple vitamins & minerals; folic acid; biotin] ≜•150•25 μg

PPA (phenylpropanolamine) [q.v.]

PPAR (peroxisome proliferator–activated receptor) agonists *a class of agents that increase insulin receptor sensitivity in type 2 diabetes; PPAR-alpha is associated with lower triglyceride and higher HDL levels; PPAR-gamma is associated with lower blood glucose levels*

PPD (purified protein derivative [of tuberculin]) [see: tuberculin]

PPG-15 stearyl ether [now: polyoxypropylene 15 stearyl ether]

PPIs (proton pump inhibitors) [q.v.]

practolol USAN, INN *antiadrenergic (β-receptor)*

prajmalium bitartrate INN, BAN

pralidoxime chloride USAN, USP *cholinesterase reactivator for organophosphate poisoning and anticholinesterase overdose* ② *pyridoxine; pramoxine*

pralidoxime iodide USAN, INN *cholinesterase reactivator* ② *pyridoxine; pramoxine*

pralidoxime mesylate USAN *cholinesterase reactivator* ② *pyridoxine; pramoxine*

pralmorelin dihydrochloride USAN *growth hormone secretagogue*

PrameGel gel OTC *local anesthetic* [pramoxine HCl; menthol] 1%•0.5%

Pramilet FA Filmtabs (film-coated tablets) ℞ *prenatal vitamin/mineral/calcium/iron supplement* [multiple vitamins & minerals; calcium; iron; folic acid] ±•250•40•1 mg

pramipexole USAN, INN *dopamine agonist; antiparkinsonian; investigational for depression and schizophrenia*

pramipexole dihydrochloride USAN *dopamine agonist; antiparkinsonian; investigational for depression and schizophrenia*

pramiracetam INN *cognition adjuvant* [also: pramiracetam HCl]

pramiracetam HCl USAN *cognition adjuvant* [also: pramiracetam]

pramiracetam sulfate USAN *cognition adjuvant*

pramiverine INN, BAN

pramlintide USAN *antihyperglycemic; synthetic amylin analogue to slow gastric emptying*

pramlintide acetate USAN *synthetic amylin analogue to slow gastric emptying; antihyperglycemic for use with insulin for type 1 and type 2 diabetes*

pramocaine INN *topical anesthetic* [also: pramoxine HCl; pramoxine]

pramocaine HCl [see: pramoxine HCl]

Pramosone cream, lotion, ointment ℞ *corticosteroidal anti-inflammatory; local anesthetic* [hydrocortisone acetate; pramoxine] 1%•1%, 2.5%•1%; 2.5%•1%; 2.5%•1% ② *pramoxine*

pramoxine BAN *topical local anesthetic* [also: pramoxine HCl; pramocaine] ② *pralidoxime; Pramosone*

Pramoxine HC anorectal aerosol foam, cream ℞ *corticosteroidal anti-inflammatory; local anesthetic* [hydrocortisone acetate; pramoxine HCl] 1%•1%; 2.5%•1%

pramoxine HCl USP *topical local anesthetic* [also: pramocaine; pramoxine]

prampine INN, BAN

Prandase ⒸⒶⓃ tablets ℞ *alpha-glucosidase inhibitor for type 2 diabetes* [acarbose] 50, 100 mg

Prandin tablets ℞ *oral antidiabetic agent that stimulates the release of insulin from the pancreas for type 2 diabetes* [repaglinide] 0.5, 1, 2 mg

pranidipine INN

pranlukast INN, BAN *investigational treatment for asthma*

pranolium chloride USAN, INN *antiarrhythmic*

pranoprofen INN

pranosal INN

praseodymium *element (Pr)*

prasterone INN *synthetic dehydroepiandrosterone (DHEA); investigational (NDA filed) agent to increase bone density in patients with systemic lupus erythematosus (SLE) on corticosteroid therapy*

prasugrel *investigational (Phase III) adenosine phosphate inhibitor to block* *platelet aggregation in patients with acute coronary syndrome (ACS)*

Pravachol tablets ℞ *HMG-CoA reductase inhibitor for hyperlipidemia, hypertriglyceridemia, atherosclerosis, coronary procedures, and recurrent myocardial infarctions* [pravastatin sodium] 10, 20, 40, 80 mg ② Primacor

pravadoline INN *analgesic* [also: pravadoline maleate]

pravadoline maleate USAN *analgesic* [also: pravadoline]

pravastatin INN, BAN *HMG-CoA reductase inhibitor for hyperlipidemia, atherosclerosis, coronary procedures, and recurrent myocardial infarctions* [also: pravastatin sodium]

pravastatin sodium USAN, JAN *HMG-CoA reductase inhibitor for hyperlipidemia, atherosclerosis, coronary procedures, and recurrent myocardial infarctions* [also: pravastatin]

Pravigard PAC combo pack (1 tablet of each per dose) ℞ *antihyperlipidemic; HMG-CoA reductase inhibitor; antiplatelet nonsteroidal anti-inflammatory drug (NSAID)* [pravastatin sodium; bufered aspirin] 20•81, 20•325, 40•81, 40•325, 80•81, 80•325 mg

Prax lotion, cream OTC *local anesthetic* [pramoxine HCl] 1%

praxadine INN

prazarelix acetate USAN *gonadotropin-releasing hormone (GnRH) antagonist for uterine fibroids, endometriosis, and prostate cancer*

prazepam USAN, USP, INN *sedative; anxiolytic* 5 mg oral ② prazepine; prazosin

prazepine INN ② prazepam

praziquantel USAN, USP, INN, BAN *anthelmintic for schistosomiasis (flukes)*

prazitone INN, BAN

prazocillin INN

prazosin INN, BAN *alpha₁-adrenergic blocker for hypertension* [also: prazosin HCl] ② prazepam

prazosin HCl USAN, USP, JAN *alpha₁-adrenergic blocker for hypertension* [also: prazosin] 1, 2, 5 mg oral

Pre-Attain oral liquid OTC *enteral nutritional therapy* [lactose-free formula]

prebiotics *a class of natural foods, such as inulin and other fructo-oligosaccharides (FOS), that enhances or supports the growth of probiotic (beneficial) bacteria in the digestive system, thereby suppressing the growth of harmful bacteria* [compare to: probiotics]

PreCare Conceive film-coated tablets ℞ *pre-conception vitamin/mineral/calcium/iron supplement* [multiple vitamins & minerals; calcium; iron; folic acid] ≛•200•30•1 mg

PreCare Prenatal film-coated caplet ℞ *vitamin/mineral/calcium/iron supplement for pregnancy and lactation* [multiple vitamins & minerals; calcium; iron; folic acid] ≛•250•40•1 mg

precatory bean *(Abrus precatorius)* plant *medicinal herb for eye inflammation, hastening labor, and stimulating abortion; not generally regarded as safe and effective as it is highly toxic and ingestion may be fatal*

Precedex IV infusion ℞ *sedative for intubated and ventilated patients in an intensive care setting; premedication to anesthesia* [dexmedetomidine HCl] 100 µg/mL

precipitated calcium carbonate JAN *antacid; dietary calcium supplement* [also: calcium carbonate]

precipitated chalk [see: calcium carbonate]

precipitated sulfur [see: sulfur, precipitated]

Precision High Nitrogen Diet powder OTC *enteral nutritional therapy* [lactose-free formula]

Precision LR Diet powder OTC *enteral nutritional therapy* [lactose-free formula]

preclamol INN

Precose tablets ℞ *antidiabetic agent for type 2 diabetes; alpha-glucosidase inhibitor that delays the digestion of dietary carbohydrates* [acarbose] 25, 50, 100 mg

Pred Mild; Pred Forte eye drop suspension ℞ *corticosteroidal anti-inflam-*

matory [prednisolone acetate] 0.12%; 1%

Predalone 50 IM injection (discontinued 2005) ℞ *corticosteroid; anti-inflammatory* [prednisolone acetate] 50 mg/mL

Predcor-50 IM injection ℞ *corticosteroid; anti-inflammatory* [prednisolone acetate] 50 mg/mL

Pred-G eye drop suspension ℞ *topical ophthalmic corticosteroidal anti-inflammatory; antibiotic* [prednisolone acetate; gentamicin sulfate] 1%•0.3%

Pred-G S.O.P. ophthalmic ointment ℞ *ophthalmic topical corticosteroidal anti-inflammatory; antibiotic* [prednisolone acetate; gentamicin sulfate; chlorobutanol] 0.6%•0.3%•0.5%

prednazate USAN, INN *anti-inflammatory*

prednazoline INN

prednicarbate USAN, INN *corticosteroid; anti-inflammatory*

Prednicen-M tablets ℞ *corticosteroid; anti-inflammatory; immunosuppressant* [prednisone] 5 mg

prednimustine USAN, INN *antineoplastic; investigational for malignant non-Hodgkin lymphomas; orphan status withdrawn 1998*

Prednisol TBA intra-articular, intralesional, or soft tissue injection ℞ *corticosteroid; anti-inflammatory* [prednisolone tebutate] 20 mg/mL

prednisolamate INN, BAN

prednisolone USP, INN *corticosteroidal anti-inflammatory* 5 mg oral; 15 mg/5 mL oral ② prednisone

prednisolone acetate USP, BAN *corticosteroidal anti-inflammatory* 1% eye drops; 25, 50 mg/mL injection

prednisolone hemisuccinate USP *corticosteroidal anti-inflammatory*

prednisolone sodium phosphate USP *corticosteroidal anti-inflammatory* (base=74.25%) 5, 15 mg/5 mL oral; 0.125%, 1% eye drops

prednisolone sodium succinate USP *corticosteroidal anti-inflammatory*

prednisolone steaglate INN, BAN *corticosteroidal anti-inflammatory*

prednisolone tebutate USP *corticosteroidal anti-inflammatory* 20 mg/mL injection

prednisone USP, INN *corticosteroid; anti-inflammatory; immunosuppressant* 1, 2.5, 5, 20 mg oral ② prednisolone

prednival USAN *corticosteroid; anti-inflammatory*

prednylidene INN, BAN

prefenamate INN

Prefest tablets (in packs of 30) ℞ *hormone replacement therapy for postmenopausal symptoms* [estradiol; norgestimate] 1•0 mg × 3 days; 1•0.09 mg × 3 days; repeat without interruption

Prefill (dosage form) *prefilled applicator*

Preflex Daily Cleaner Especially for Sensitive Eyes solution OTC *surfactant cleaning solution for soft contact lenses*

Prefrin Liquifilm eye drops OTC *topical ophthalmic decongestant* [phenylephrine HCl] 0.12%

pregabalin USAN *gabamimetic anticonvulsant; agent for the management of neuropathic pain from diabetic peripheral neuropathy (DPN) and postherpetic neuralgia (PHN); investigational (Phase III) for generalized anxiety disorder (GAD)*

pregelatinized starch [see: starch, pregelatinized]

Pregestimil powder OTC *hypoallergenic infant food for severe malabsorption disorders* [enzymatically hydrolyzed protein formula]

pregnandiol JAN

pregneninolone [see: ethisterone]

pregnenolone INN *natural hormone precursor* [also: pregnenolone succinate]

pregnenolone succinate USAN *hormone precursor* [also: pregnenolone]

Pregnosis slide test for home use *in vitro diagnostic aid; urine pregnancy test* [latex agglutination test]

Pregnyl powder for IM injection ℞ *gonad-stimulating hormone for prepubertal cryptorchidism and hypogonadism; ovulation stimulant* [chorionic gonadotropin] 1000 U/mL

Prehist sustained-release capsules ℞ *decongestant; antihistamine* [phenylephrine HCl; chlorpheniramine maleate] 20•8 mg

Prehist D sustained-release capsules (discontinued 2002) ℞ *decongestant; antihistamine; anticholinergic to dry mucosal secretions* [phenylephrine HCl; chlorpheniramine maleate; methscopolamine nitrate] 20•8•2.5 mg

Pre-Hist-D sustained-release tablets ℞ *decongestant; antihistamine; anticholinergic to dry mucosal secretions* [phenylephrine HCl; chlorpheniramine maleate; methscopolamine nitrate] 20•8•2.5 mg

Prelone syrup ℞ *corticosteroid; antiinflammatory* [prednisolone; alcohol 5%] 15 mg/5 mL

Prelu-2 timed-release capsules ℞ *anorexiant; CNS stimulant* [phendimetrazine tartrate] 105 mg

premafloxacin USAN, INN *veterinary antibacterial*

Premarin tablets ℞ *hormone replacement therapy for the treatment of postmenopausal symptoms and prevention of postmenopausal osteoporosis; palliative therapy for prostate and breast cancer; investigational (Phase III) for Alzheimer disease* [conjugated estrogens (equine estrogen mixture)] 0.3, 0.45, 0.625, 0.9, 1.25 mg

Premarin Intravenous IV or IM injection ℞ *treatment of abnormal uterine bleeding due to hormonal imbalance* [conjugated estrogens (equine estrogen mixture)] 25 mg/vial

Premarin Vaginal cream ℞ *a mixture of equine estrogens; hormone replacement for postmenopausal atrophic vaginitis* [conjugated estrogens] 0.625 mg/g

premazepam INN, BAN

PremesisRx tablets ℞ *prenatal vitamin/mineral supplement* [vitamin B$_6$; vitamin B$_{12}$; folic acid; calcium carbonate] 75 mg•12 μg•1 mg•200 mg

Premphase tablets (in packs of 28) ℞ *equine/synthetic hormones; hormone replacement therapy for postmenopausal symptoms* [Phase 1 (14 days): conjugated estrogens; Phase 2 (14 days): conjugated estrogens; medroxyprogesterone acetate] 0.625 mg; 0.625•5 mg

Prempro tablets ℞ *equine/synthetic hormones; hormone replacement therapy for postmenopausal symptoms* [conjugated estrogens; medroxyprogesterone acetate] 0.3•1.5, 0.45•1.5, 0.625•2.5, 0.625•5 mg

Prēmsyn PMS caplets OTC *analgesic; antipyretic; diuretic; antihistaminic sleep aid* [acetaminophen; pamabrom; pyrilamine maleate] 500•25•15 mg

prenalterol INN, BAN *adrenergic* [also: prenalterol HCl]

prenalterol HCl USAN *adrenergic* [also: prenalterol]

Prenatabs RX film-coated tablets ℞ *vitamin/mineral/calcium/iron supplement* [multiple vitamins & minerals; calcium; iron; folic acid; biotin] ±•200•29•1•0.03 mg

Prenatal 19 tablets, chewable tablets ℞ *vitamin/mineral/calcium/iron supplement* [multiple vitamins & minerals; calcium; iron; folic acid] ±•200•29•1 mg

Prenatal AD tablets ℞ *vitamin/mineral/calcium/iron supplement* [multiple vitamins & minerals; calcium; iron; folic acid] ±•200•90•1 mg

Prenatal H.P. tablets ℞ *vitamin/calcium/iron supplement* [multiple vitamins; calcium; iron; folic acid] ±•50•30•0.8 mg

Prenatal Maternal tablets ℞ *vitamin/mineral/calcium/iron supplement* [multiple vitamins & minerals; calcium; iron; folic acid; biotin] ±•250•60•1•0.03 mg

Prenatal MR 90 delayed-release film-coated tablets ℞ *vitamin/calcium/iron supplement* [multiple vitamins; calcium; iron; folic acid] ±•250•90•1 mg

Prenatal PC 40 film-coated caplets ℞ *vitamin/mineral/calcium/iron supplement* [multiple vitamins and miner-

als; calcium; iron; folic acid] ± •
250•40•1 mg

**Prenatal Plus; Prenatal Plus
Improved** tablets ℞ *vitamin/calcium/
iron supplement* [multiple vitamins;
calcium; iron; folic acid] ± •200•
65•1 mg

Prenatal Plus Iron tablets ℞ *vitamin/
calcium/iron supplement* [multiple
vitamins; calcium; iron; folic acid]
± •200•27•1 mg

Prenatal Plus with Betacarotene
tablets (discontinued 2004) ℞ *vita-
min/calcium/iron supplement* [multiple
vitamins; calcium; iron; folic acid]
± •200•65•1 mg

Prenatal Rx tablets ℞ *vitamin/calcium/
iron supplement* [multiple vitamins;
calcium; iron; folic acid] ± •175•
29.5•1 mg

Prenatal Rx with Betacarotene tablets ℞ *vitamin/calcium/iron supplement* [multiple vitamins; calcium;
iron; folic acid; biotin] ± •200•60•
1•0.03 mg

Prenatal with Folic Acid tablets OTC
vitamin/calcium/iron supplement [mul-
tiple vitamins; calcium; iron; folic
acid] ± •200•60•0.8 mg

Prenatal Z delayed-release film-coated
tablets ℞ *vitamin/calcium/iron supplement* [multiple vitamins; calcium;
iron; folic acid] ± •300•65•1 mg

Prenatal-1 + Iron tablets ℞ *vitamin/
calcium/iron supplement* [multiple
vitamins; calcium; iron; folic acid]
± •200•65•1 mg

Prenatal-H capsules ℞ *vitamin/min-
eral/iron supplement* [multiple vitamins & minerals; iron; folic acid] ±
•106.5•1 mg

Prenatal-S tablets OTC *vitamin/calcium/
iron supplement* [multiple vitamins;
calcium; iron; folic acid] ± •200•
60•0.8 mg

Prenate Advance; Prenate 90
delayed-release film-coated tablets ℞
*prenatal vitamin/calcium/iron supple-
ment* [multiple vitamins; calcium;

iron; folic acid] ± •200•90•1 mg; ±
•250•90•1 mg

Prenate GT delayed-release gel-
coated tablets (discontinued 2004)
℞ *prenatal vitamin/calcium/iron supplement* [multiple vitamins; calcium;
iron; folic acid] ± •200•90•1 mg

Prenavite tablets OTC *vitamin/calcium/
iron supplement* [multiple vitamins;
calcium; iron; folic acid] ± •200•
60•0.8 mg

prenisteine INN

prenoverine INN

prenoxdiazine INN

prenylamine USAN, INN *coronary
vasodilator*

Preos subcu injection ℞ *investigational
(Phase III) recombinant human parathyroid hormone for postmenopausal
osteoporosis in women*

Preparation H anorectal cream, anorectal ointment OTC *temporary relief
of hemorrhoidal symptoms* [shark liver
oil; phenylephrine HCl] 3%•0.25%

Preparation H cleansing tissues OTC
*moisturizer and cleanser for external
rectal/vaginal areas* [propylene glycol]

Preparation H rectal suppositories
OTC *temporary relief of hemorrhoidal
symptoms* [shark liver oil] 3%

Preparation H Cooling Gel OTC *temporary relief of hemorrhoidal symptoms*
[phenylephrine HCl; hamamelis
water; alcohol 7.5%] 0.25%•50%

prepared chalk [see: calcium carbon-
ate]

Prepcat oral suspension ℞ *radiopaque
contrast medium for gastrointestinal
imaging* [barium sulfate] 1.5%

Pre-Pen solution for dermal scratch
test ℞ *diagnostic aid for penicillin
hypersensitivity* [benzylpenicilloyl
polylysine] 0.25 mL

Pre-Pen/MDM solution for dermal
scratch test ℞ *investigational (orphan)
agent for penicillin hypersensitivity
assessment* [benzylpenicillin]

Prepidil gel ℞ *prostaglandin for cervical
ripening at term* [dinoprostone] 0.5 mg

Prepulsid Ⓒ🄰🄽 tablets, oral suspension (discontinued 2001) ℞ *treatment for nocturnal heartburn due to gastro-esophageal reflux disease (GERD)* [cisapride] 5, 10, 20 mg; 1 mg/mL

Prestara ℞ *investigational (NDA filed) agent to increase bone density in patients with systemic lupus erythematosus (SLE) on corticosteroid therapy* [prasterone]

pretamazium iodide INN, BAN

prethcamide

prethrombin [see: prothrombin complex, activated]

pretiadil INN

Pretts Diet-Aid chewable tablets OTC *diet aid* [sodium carboxymethylcellulose; alginic acid; sodium bicarbonate] 100•200•70 mg

Pretty Feet & Hands cream OTC *moisturizer; emollient*

Pretz solution OTC *nasal moisturizer* [sodium chloride (saline solution)] 0.6%

Pretz Irrigating solution OTC *for postoperative irrigation* [sodium chloride (saline solution); glycerin; eriodictyon] 0.75%

Pretz Moisturizing nose drops OTC *nasal moisturizer* [sodium chloride (saline solution); glycerin; eriodictyon] 0.75%

Pretz-D nasal spray OTC *nasal decongestant* [ephedrine sulfate] 0.25%

PretzPak ointment (discontinued 2004) OTC *antimicrobial postoperative nasal pack* [benzyl alcohol; polyethylene glycol; carboxymethylcellulose; urea; allantoin]

Prevacid delayed-release enteric-coated granules in capsules ℞ *proton pump inhibitor for gastric and duodenal ulcers, erosive esophagitis, gastroesophageal reflux disease (GERD), and other gastroesophageal disorders* [lansoprazole] 15, 30 mg

Prevacid delayed-release enteric-coated granules in orally disintegrating tablets ℞ *proton pump inhibitor for gastric and duodenal ulcers, erosive*

esophagitis, gastroesophageal reflux disease (GERD), and other gastroesophageal disorders [lansoprazole] 15, 30 mg

Prevacid delayed-release enteric-coated granules for oral suspension ℞ *proton pump inhibitor for gastric and duodenal ulcers, erosive esophagitis, gastroesophageal reflux disease (GERD), and other gastroesophageal disorders* [lansoprazole] 15, 30 mg

Prevacid I.V. powder for infusion ℞ *proton pump inhibitor for erosive esophagitis in hospitalized patients* [lansoprazole] 30 mg/dose

Prevacid NapraPAC capsules + tablets in 7-day dose packs ℞ *proton pump inhibitor; nonsteroidal anti-inflammatory; treatment for gastric and duodenal ulcers* [lansoprazole (capsules); naproxen (tablets)] 15•375, 15•500 mg

Prevacid SoluTab (delayed-release orally disintegrating tablets) ℞ *proton pump inhibitor for gastric and duodenal ulcers, erosive esophagitis, gastroesophageal reflux disease (GERD), and other gastroesophageal disorders* [lansoprazole] 15, 30 mg

Prevalite powder for oral suspension ℞ *cholesterol-lowering antihyperlipidemic; also used for biliary obstruction* [cholestyramine resin] 4 g/dose

Preven kit (4 film-coated tablets + pregnancy test) ℞ *(available from pharmacists without a prescription in some states) emergency postcoital contraceptive* [levonorgestrel; ethinyl estradiol] 0.25•0.05 mg ② Preveon

Prevent-X powder for oral solution OTC *dietary supplement* [multiple vitamins & minerals; multiple amino acids]

PreviDent dental gel (for self-application) ℞ *topical caries preventative* [sodium fluoride] 1.1%

PreviDent 5000 Plus dental cream (for self-application) ℞ *topical caries preventative* [sodium fluoride] 1.1%

PreviDent Rinse oral solution ("swish and spit") ℞ *dental caries preventative* [sodium fluoride] 0.2%

Prevnar IM injection ℞ *active immunization against seven strains of* Streptococcus pneumoniae *in infants and toddlers; investigational (Phase III) for adults over 50 years* [pneumococcal vaccine, 7-valent] 2–4 μg of each strain per 0.5 mL dose

Prevpac three-drug daily pack ℞ *triple therapy for* H. pylori*: an antisecretory and two antibiotics* [lansoprazole; clarithromycin; amoxicillin] 2 × 30 mg; 2 × 500 mg; 4 × 500 mg

PreVue B. burgdorferi Antibody Detection Assay reagent kit for professional use *in vitro diagnostic aid for Lyme disease*

Prexige ℞ *investigational (Phase III) antiarthritic for osteoarthritis; analgesic for acute pain; COX-2 inhibitor; nonsteroidal anti-inflammatory drug (NSAID)* [lumiracoxib] 100 mg

prezatide copper acetate USAN, INN *immunomodulator; investigational (Phase II) wound-healing gel for venous leg ulcers*

Prialt intrathecal infusion ℞ *calcium-channel blocker; non-narcotic analgesic for intractable pain of cancer or AIDS; investigational epidural administration for spinal cord injury* [ziconotide acetate] 25, 100 μg/mL

pribecaine INN

prickly ash (Xanthoxylum americanum; X. fraxineum) bark *medicinal herb for fever, mouth sores, poor circulation, ulcers, and wounds*

prickly juniper (Juniperus oxycedrus) *medicinal herb* [see: juniper]

prickly pear *medicinal herb* [see: nopal]

pride of China (Melia azedarach) root bark and fruit *medicinal herb used as an anthelmintic, astringent, bitter tonic, emetic, emmenagogue, and purgative*

pride weed *medicinal herb* [see: fleabane; horseweed]

pridefine INN *antidepressant* [also: pridefine HCl]

pridefine HCl USAN *antidepressant* [also: pridefine]

prideperone INN

pridinol INN

priest's crown *medicinal herb* [see: dandelion]

prifelone USAN, INN *dermatologic anti-inflammatory*

prifinium bromide INN

Priftin film-coated tablets ℞ *antibacterial for tuberculosis (orphan); investigational (orphan) for AIDS-related* Mycobacterium avium *complex* [rifapentine] 150 mg

prifuroline INN

priliximab USAN, INN *monoclonal antibody to treat autoimmune lymphoproliferative diseases and in organ transplants; investigational (orphan) for multiple sclerosis*

prilocaine USAN, INN, BAN *topical local anesthetic*

prilocaine HCl USAN, USP *topical local anesthetic* [also: propitocaine HCl]

prilocaine & lidocaine *local anesthetic* 2.5%•2.5% topical

Prilosec delayed-release enteric-coated granules in capsules ℞ *proton pump inhibitor for gastric and duodenal ulcers, erosive esophagitis, GERD, and other gastroesophageal disorders* [omeprazole] 10, 20, 40 mg ⧖ Prozac

Prilosec OTC delayed-release tablets OTC *proton pump inhibitor for frequent heartburn* [omeprazole magnesium] 20.6 mg (=20 mg base)

primachine phosphate [see: primaquine phosphate]

Primacor IV infusion ℞ *vasodilator for congestive heart failure* [milrinone lactate] 0.2, 1 mg/mL ⧖ Pravachol

Primacor in 5% Dextrose IV infusion ℞ *vasodilator for congestive heart failure* [milrinone lactate; dextrose] 200 μg/mL; 5% ⧖ Pravachol

primaperone INN

primaquine INN *antimalarial* [also: primaquine phosphate]

primaquine phosphate USP *antimalarial; prevention of malarial relapse* [also: primaquine] 26.3 mg oral

primaquine phosphate & clindamycin HCl *investigational (orphan) for AIDS-associated* Pneumocystis carinii *pneumonia*

Primatene tablets OTC *bronchodilator; decongestant; expectorant* [ephedrine HCl; guaifenesin] 12.5●200 mg

Primatene Mist inhalation aerosol OTC *sympathomimetic bronchodilator* [epinephrine] 0.2 mg/dose

Primatuss Cough Mixture 4 oral liquid (discontinued 2002) OTC *antitussive; antihistamine* [dextromethorphan hydrobromide; chlorpheniramine maleate; alcohol 10% 15●2 mg/5 mL

Primatuss Cough Mixture 4D oral liquid (discontinued 2002) OTC *antitussive; decongestant; expectorant* [dextromethorphan hydrobromide; pseudoephedrine HCl; guaifenesin; alcohol 10%] 10●20●67 mg/5 mL

Primaxin I.M. powder for injection ℞ *carbapenem antibiotic* [imipenem; cilastatin sodium] 500●500, 750●750 mg

Primaxin I.V. powder for injection ℞ *carbapenem antibiotic* [imipenem; cilastatin sodium] 250●250, 500●500 mg

primidolol USAN, INN *antihypertensive; antianginal; antiarrhythmic*

primidone USP, INN, BAN *anticonvulsant for grand mal, psychomotor, or focal epileptic seizures* 50, 250 mg oral

Primobolan *brand name for methenolone acetate, a European anabolic steroid abused as a street drug*

Primobolan Depot *brand name for methenolone enanthate, a European anabolic steroid abused as a street drug*

Primsol oral solution ℞ *antibiotic for otitis media in children and urinary tract infections in adults* [trimethoprim HCl] 50 mg/5 mL

primycin INN

prince's pine *medicinal herb* [see: pipsissewa]

Principen capsules, powder for oral suspension ℞ *aminopenicillin antibiotic* [ampicillin] 250, 500 mg; 125, 250 mg/5 mL

Prinivil tablets ℞ *antihypertensive; angiotensin-converting enzyme (ACE) inhibitor; adjunctive treatment for CHF* [lisinopril] 2.5, 5, 10, 20, 40 mg

prinodolol [see: pindolol]

prinomastat USAN *investigational (Phase III) matrix metalloprotease inhibitor for advanced non–small cell lung cancer (NSCLC) and prostate cancer (clinical trials discontinued 2000); investigational (Phase II) for age-related macular degeneration*

prinomide INN *antirheumatic* [also: prinomide tromethamine]

prinomide tromethamine USAN *antirheumatic* [also: prinomide]

prinoxodan USAN, INN *cardiotonic*

Prinzide tablets ℞ *antihypertensive; angiotensin-converting enzyme (ACE) inhibitor; diuretic* [hydrochlorothiazide; lisinopril] 12.5●10 mg

Prinzide 12.5; Prinzide 25 tablets ℞ *antihypertensive; angiotensin-converting enzyme (ACE) inhibitor; diuretic* [hydrochlorothiazide; lisinopril] 12.5●20 mg; 25●20 mg

Priorix ⓒⒶⓃ injection ℞ *active immunizing agent* [measles, mumps, and rubella virus vaccine, live attenuated] 0.5 mL

Priscoline HCl IV injection (discontinued 2002) ℞ *antiadrenergic; peripheral vasodilator for neonatal persistent pulmonary hypertension* [tolazoline HCl] 25 mg/mL ② Apresoline

pristinamycin INN, BAN

privet, Egyptian *medicinal herb* [see: henna (Lawsonia)]

Privine nasal spray, nose drops OTC *nasal decongestant* [naphazoline HCl] 0.05%

prizidilol INN, BAN *antihypertensive* [also: prizidilol HCl]

prizidilol HCl USAN *antihypertensive* [also: prizidilol]

PRO 542 *investigational (Phase I/II) recombinant fusion protein, antigen-binding agent, and HIV attachment inhibitor for HIV infection*

PRO 2000 *investigational (Phase II) antiviral and microbicide gel for HIV infection*

Pro Fem cream OTC *natural progesterone from soy; hormone replacement therapy; postmenopausal osteoporosis preventative* [progesterone USP (in a liposomal base)] 2.5%

Pro Skin capsules OTC *vitamin/zinc supplement* [vitamins A, B$_5$, C, and E; zinc] 6250 IU•10 mg•100 mg• 100 IU•10 mg

Proact Ŗ *investigational (Phase III) immunomodulator for sarcoma*

proadifen INN *non-specific synergist* [also: proadifen HCl]

proadifen HCl USAN *non-specific synergist* [also: proadifen]

ProAmatine tablets Ŗ *vasopressor for orthostatic hypotension (orphan)* [midodrine HCl] 2.5, 5, 10 mg

proanthocyanidins *natural free radical scavenger found in grape seed extract and pine bark extract* [also: procyanidolic oligomers (PCOs); procyanidins]

Pro-Banthīne tablets Ŗ *GI antispasmodic; peptic ulcer treatment adjunct; antisecretory* [propantheline bromide] 7.5, 15 mg

probarbital sodium NF, INN

Probax gel OTC *relief from minor oral irritations* [propolis] 2%

Probec-T tablets OTC *vitamin supplement* [multiple B vitamins; vitamin C] ± •600 mg

probenecid USP, INN, BAN *uricosuric for gout* 500 mg oral

probicromil calcium USAN *prophylactic antiallergic* [also: ambicromil]

Pro-Bionate capsules, powder OTC *probiotic; dietary supplement; fever blister treatment; not generally regarded as safe and effective as an antidiarrheal* [*Lactobacillus acidophilus*] 2 billion CFU; 2 billion CFU/g

probiotics *a class of natural bacteria, such as* Lactobacillus acidophilus, *that favorably alter the microflora balance in the digestive system; an abundance of probiotic bacteria inhibit the growth of harmful bacteria and promote good digestion* [compare to: prebiotics]

probucol USAN, USP, INN *antihyperlipidemic; investigational (Phase II) antiviral for HIV and AIDS*

probutate USAN *combining name for radicals or groups* [also: buteprate]

procainamide INN *antiarrhythmic* [also: procainamide HCl]

procainamide HCl USP *antiarrhythmic* [also: procainamide] 250, 375, 500, 750, 1000 mg oral; 500 mg/mL injection

procaine INN *injectable local anesthetic* [also: procaine borate] 2 Procan

procaine borate NF *injectable local anesthetic* [also: procaine] 2 Procan

procaine HCl USP *injectable local anesthetic; sometimes used as a treatment for the overall effects of aging such as alopecia, arthritis, cerebral atherosclerosis, hypertension, progressive dementia, and sexual dysfunction; investigational (Phase II) for HIV infections* 1%, 2% 2 Procan

procaine penicillin BAN *bactericidal antibiotic* [also: penicillin G procaine] 2 Procan

ProcalAmine IV infusion Ŗ *peripheral parenteral nutrition* [multiple essential and nonessential amino acids; electrolytes]

Procanbid film-coated extended-release tablets Ŗ *twice-daily antiarrhythmic* [procainamide HCl] 500, 1000 mg

procarbazine INN *antineoplastic* [also: procarbazine HCl] 2 dacarbazine

procarbazine HCl USAN, USP *antineoplastic for Hodgkin disease* [also: procarbazine]

Procardia capsules Ŗ *antianginal; antihypertensive; calcium channel blocker* [nifedipine] 10 mg

Procardia XL film-coated sustained-release tablets Ŗ *antianginal; antihypertensive; calcium channel blocker* [nifedipine] 30, 60, 90 mg

procaterol INN, BAN *bronchodilator* [also: procaterol HCl]

procaterol HCl USAN *bronchodilator* [also: procaterol]

Prochieve vaginal gel ℞ *natural progestin; hormone replacement for secondary amenorrhea; hormone supplementation for assisted reproductive technology treatments* [progesterone] 4%, 8%

prochlorperazine USP, INN *conventional (typical) phenothiazine antipsychotic for schizophrenia; anxiolytic; antiemetic for nausea and vomiting; also used for acute treatment of migraine headaches* 25 mg suppositories

prochlorperazine bimaleate *conventional (typical) phenothiazine antipsychotic for schizophrenia; anxiolytic; antiemetic for nausea and vomiting; also used for acute treatment of migraine headaches*

prochlorperazine edisylate USP *conventional (typical) phenothiazine antipsychotic for schizophrenia; anxiolytic; antiemetic for nausea and vomiting; also used for acute treatment of migraine headaches* 5 mg/mL injection

prochlorperazine ethanedisulfonate [see: prochlorperazine edisylate]

prochlorperazine maleate USP *conventional (typical) phenothiazine antipsychotic for schizophrenia; anxiolytic; antiemetic for nausea and vomiting; also used for acute treatment of migraine headaches* 5, 10 mg oral

prochlorperazine mesylate *conventional (typical) phenothiazine antipsychotic for schizophrenia; anxiolytic; antiemetic for nausea and vomiting; also used for acute treatment of migraine headaches*

procinolol INN

procinonide USAN, INN *adrenocortical steroid*

Proclim ⒸⒶⓃ tablets (discontinued 2001) ℞ *progestin* [medroxyprogesterone acetate] 2.5, 5, 10 mg

proclonol USAN, INN *anthelmintic; antifungal*

procodazole INN

proconvertin [see: factor VII]

Procort cream, spray OTC *topical corticosteroidal anti-inflammatory* [hydrocortisone] 1%

Procrit IV or subcu injection ℞ *hematopoietic to stimulate RBC production for anemia of chronic renal failure, HIV, and chemotherapy (orphan) and to reduce the need for blood transfusions in surgery* [epoetin alfa] 2000, 3000, 4000, 10 000, 20 000, 40 000 U/mL

Proctocort anorectal cream, suppositories ℞ *topical corticosteroidal anti-inflammatory* [hydrocortisone] 1%; 30 mg

ProctoCream-HC 2.5% anorectal cream ℞ *corticosteroidal anti-inflammatory* [hydrocortisone acetate] 2.5%

Proctodan-HC ⒸⒶⓃ anorectal ointment, suppositories ℞ *topical corticosteroidal anti-inflammatory, local anesthetic, and astringent* [hydrocortisone acetate; pramoxine HCl; zinc sulfate] 0.5%•1%•0.5%; 10•20•10 mg

ProctoFoam NS anorectal aerosol foam OTC *topical local anesthetic* [pramoxine HCl] 1%

Proctofoam-HC anorectal aerosol foam ℞ *topical corticosteroidal anti-inflammatory; local anesthetic* [hydrocortisone acetate; pramoxine HCl] 1%•1%

Pro-Cute lotion OTC *moisturizer; emollient*

procyanidolic oligomers (PCOs) *natural free radical scavenger found in grape seed extract and pine bark extract* [also: proanthocyanidins; procyanidins]

ProCycle Gold tablets OTC *vitamin/mineral/iron supplement* [multiple vitamins & minerals; iron; folic acid; biotin] ≟•3•0.067•≟ mg

procyclidine HCl USP *anticholinergic; antiparkinsonian; skeletal muscle relaxant* [also: procyclidine]

procymate INN

prodeconium bromide INN

Proderm aerosol OTC *topical wound spray for decubitus ulcers* [castor oil; peruvian balsam] 650•72.5 mg/0.82 mL

prodilidine INN *analgesic* [also: prodilidine HCl]

prodilidine HCl USAN *analgesic* [also: prodilidine]

prodipine INN

Prodium tablets OTC *urinary analgesic* [phenazopyridine HCl] 95 mg

prodolic acid USAN, INN *anti-inflammatory*

pro-drugs *a class of agents which metabolize into a therapeutic or more potent form in the body*

profadol INN *analgesic* [also: profadol HCl]

profadol HCl USAN *analgesic* [also: profadol]

Profasi powder for IM injection Rx *gonad-stimulating hormone for prepubertal cryptorchidism and hypogonadism; ovulation stimulant* [chorionic gonadotropin] 500, 1000 U/mL

Pro-Fast HS; Pro-Fast SR capsules Rx *anorexiant; CNS stimulant* [phentermine HCl] 18.75 mg; 37.5 mg

Pro-Fast SA tablets Rx *anorexiant; CNS stimulant* [phentermine HCl] 8 mg

Profen II; Profen Forte extended-release tablets Rx *decongestant; expectorant* [pseudoephedrine HCl; guaifenesin] 45•800 mg; 90•800 mg

Profen II DM extended-release caplets Rx *antitussive; decongestant; expectorant* [dextromethorphan hydrobromide; pseudoephedrine HCl; guaifenesin] 30•45•800 mg

Profen II DM oral liquid (discontinued 2004) Rx *antitussive; decongestant; expectorant* [dextromethorphan hydrobromide; pseudoephedrine HCl; guaifenesin] 10•15•200 mg/5 mL

Profen Forte DM sustained-release caplets Rx *antitussive; decongestant; expectorant* [dextromethorphan hydrobromide; pseudoephedrine HCl; guaifenesin] 60•90•800 mg

Profen LA timed-release tablets (discontinued 2002) Rx *decongestant; expectorant* [phenylpropanolamine HCl; guaifenesin] 75•600 mg

Profenal Drop-Tainers (eye drops) Rx *ocular nonsteroidal anti-inflammatory*

drug (NSAID); intraoperative miosis inhibitor [suprofen] 1%

profenamine INN *antiparkinsonian* [also: ethopropazine HCl; ethopropazine]

profenamine HCl [see: ethopropazine HCl]

profexalone INN

Profiber oral liquid OTC *enteral nutritional therapy* [lactose-free formula]

Profilnine SD powder for IV injection Rx *anticoagulant to correct factor IX deficiency (hemophilia B; Christmas disease)* [coagulation factor IX concentrate, solvent/detergent treated]

Proflavanol C ⓒ tablets OTC *vitamin C supplement* [vitamin C as mixed ascorbates] 100 mg

proflavine INN [also: proflavine dihydrochloride]

proflavine dihydrochloride NF [also: proflavine]

proflavine sulfate NF

proflazepam INN

ProFree/GP Weekly Enzymatic Cleaner tablets OTC *enzymatic cleaner for rigid gas permeable contact lenses* [papain]

progabide USAN, INN *anticonvulsant; muscle relaxant*

Progestasert IUD Rx *intrauterine contraceptive* [progesterone] 38 mg

progesterone USP, INN *natural progestin; intrauterine contraceptive; hormone replacement for secondary amenorrhea; hormone supplementation for assisted reproductive technology (ART) treatments; investigational (orphan) for in vitro fertilization and embryo transfer* 50 mg/mL injection

progestins *a class of sex hormones that cause a sloughing of the endometrial lining, also used as a hormonal antineoplastic*

proglumetacin INN

proglumide USAN, INN, BAN, JAN *anticholinergic*

Proglycem capsules, oral suspension Rx *emergency antihypertensive; vasodilator; glucose-elevating agent* [diazoxide] 50 mg; 50 mg/mL

Prograf capsules, IV infusion ℞ *immunosuppressant for liver and kidney transplants; investigational for other transplants* [tacrolimus] 0.5, 1, 5 mg; 5 mg/mL

proguanil INN, BAN, DCF *antimalarial; dihydrofolate reductase inhibitor* [also: chloroguanide HCl]

proguanil HCl [see: chloroguanide HCl]

ProHance injection ℞ *MRI contrast media for brain and spine imaging* [gadoteridol] 279.3 mg/mL

proheptazine INN

proinsulin human USAN *antidiabetic*

Prolastin powder for IV infusion ℞ *enzyme replacement therapy for hereditary alpha₁-proteinase inhibitor deficiency, which leads to progressive panacinar emphysema (orphan)* [alpha₁-proteinase inhibitor] ≥ 20 mg/mL (500, 1000 mg/vial)

Proleukin powder for IV infusion ℞ *antineoplastic for metastatic melanoma and renal cell carcinoma (orphan); investigational (Phase III, orphan) for immunodeficiency diseases and acute myelogenous leukemia (AML); investigational (Phase II) for non-Hodgkin lymphoma* [aldesleukin] 18 million IU/mL

Prolex DH oral liquid ℞ *narcotic antitussive; expectorant* [hydrocodone bitartrate; potassium guaiacolsulfonate] 4.5•300 mg/5 mL

proligestone INN

proline (L-proline) USAN, USP, INN *nonessential amino acid; symbols: Pro, P* ⑨ Prolene

prolintane INN *antidepressant* [also: prolintane HCl]

prolintane HCl USAN *antidepressant* [also: prolintane]

Prolixin tablets, elixir, oral concentrate, IM injection (discontinued 2002) ℞ *conventional (typical) phenothiazine antipsychotic for schizophrenia and psychotic disorders* [fluphenazine HCl] 1, 2.5, 5, 10 mg; 2.5 mg/5 mL; 5 mg/mL; 2.5 mg/mL

Prolixin Decanoate subcu or IM injection ℞ *conventional (typical) phenothiazine antipsychotic for schizophrenia and psychotic disorders; used for prolonged parenteral neuroleptic therapy* [fluphenazine decanoate] 25 mg/mL

Prolixin Decanoate Unimatic (prefilled) syringe (discontinued 2003) ℞ *conventional (typical) phenothiazine antipsychotic for schizophrenia and psychotic disorders; used for prolonged parenteral neuroleptic therapy* [fluphenazine decanoate] 25 mg/mL

Prolixin Enanthate subcu or IM injection (discontinued 2002) ℞ *conventional (typical) phenothiazine antipsychotic for schizophrenia and psychotic disorders* [fluphenazine enanthate] 25 mg/mL

prolonium iodide INN

Proloprim tablets ℞ *anti-infective; antibacterial* [trimethoprim] 100, 200 mg

ProMACE (prednisone, methotrexate [with leucovorin rescue], Adriamycin, cyclophosphamide, etoposide) *chemotherapy protocol for non-Hodgkin lymphoma*

ProMACE/cytaBOM (ProMACE [above], cytarabine, bleomycin, Oncovin, mitoxantrone) *chemotherapy protocol for non-Hodgkin lymphoma*

ProMACE/MOPP (full course of ProMACE, followed by MOPP) *chemotherapy protocol for non-Hodgkin lymphoma*

Promacet tablets ℞ *sedative; barbiturate analgesic* [butalbital; acetaminophen] 50•650 mg

promazine INN *phenothiazine antipsychotic* [also: promazine HCl] ⑨ Promethazine

promazine HCl USP *phenothiazine antipsychotic* [also: promazine]

Promega Pearls (softgels) OTC *dietary supplement* [omega-3 fatty acids; multiple vitamins & minerals] 600• ±, 1000•± mg

promegestone INN

promelase INN

promestriene INN

Prometh VC Plain syrup ℞ *deconges-tant; antihistamine* [phenylephrine HCl; promethazine HCl; alcohol 7%] 5•6.25 mg/5 mL

Prometh VC with Codeine syrup ℞ *narcotic antitussive; decongestant; antihistamine* [codeine phosphate; phen-ylephrine HCl; promethazine HCl; alcohol 7%] 10•5•6.25 mg/5 mL

Prometh with Codeine syrup ℞ *nar-cotic antitussive; antihistamine* [codeine phosphate; promethazine HCl; alcohol 7%] 10•6.25 mg/5 mL

Prometh with Dextromethorphan syrup ℞ *antitussive; antihistamine* [dextromethorphan hydrobromide; promethazine HCl; alcohol 7%] 15• 6.25 mg/5 mL

promethazine INN *phenothiazine anti-histamine; antiemetic; antidopaminer-gic; motion sickness relief* [also: pro-methazine HCl]

Promethazine DM syrup (discontin-ued 2002) ℞ *antitussive; antihista-mine* [dextromethorphan hydrobro-mide; promethazine HCl; alcohol] 15•6.25 mg/5 mL

promethazine HCl USP *phenothiazine antihistamine; antiemetic; antidopamin-ergic; motion sickness relief* [also: pro-methazine] 12.5, 25, 50 mg oral; 6.25 mg/5 mL oral; 12.5, 25, 50 mg sup-positories; 25, 50 mg/mL injection

promethazine HCl & codeine phosphate *antihistamine; narcotic antitussive* 6.25•10 mg/5 mL oral

promethazine HCl & phenyleph-rine HCl *antihistamine; decongestant* 6.25•5 mg/5 mL oral

promethazine teoclate INN *phenothia-zine antihistamine*

Promethazine VC syrup (discontin-ued 2002) ℞ *decongestant; antihista-mine* [phenylephrine HCl; prometh-azine HCl] 5•6.25 mg/5 mL

Promethazine VC Plain syrup (dis-continued 2002) ℞ *decongestant; antihistamine* [phenylephrine HCl; promethazine HCl; alcohol 7%] 5• 6.25 mg/5 mL

Promethazine VC with Codeine syrup ℞ *narcotic antitussive; deconges-tant; antihistamine* [codeine phos-phate; phenylephrine HCl; pro-methazine HCl; alcohol 7.1%] 10• 5•6.25 mg/5 mL

Promethazine with Dextromethor-phan Cough syrup ℞ *antitussive; antihistamine* [dextromethorphan hydrobromide; promethazine HCl; alcohol 7%] 15•6.25 mg/5 mL

promethestrol [see: methestrol]

Promethist with Codeine syrup (dis-continued 2002) ℞ *narcotic antitus-sive; decongestant; antihistamine* [codeine phosphate; phenylephrine HCl; promethazine HCl; alcohol] 10•5•6.25 mg/5 mL

promethium *element (Pm)*

Prometrium capsules ℞ *natural pro-gestin for secondary amenorrhea and to prevent endometrial hyperplasia* [pro-gesterone, micronized] 100, 200 mg

Prominol tablets ℞ *analgesic; antipy-retic; sedative* [acetaminophen; butal-bital] 650•50 mg

Promit IV injection ℞ *monovalent hap-ten for prevention of dextran-induced anaphylactic reactions; investigational (orphan) for cystic fibrosis* [dextran 1] 150 mg/mL

ProMod powder OTC *oral protein supple-ment* [D-whey protein concentrate; soy lecithin]

promolate INN

promoxolane INN

prompt insulin zinc [see: insulin zinc, prompt]

Pronemia Hematinic capsules ℞ *hematinic* [ferrous fumarate; cyanoco-balamin; ascorbic acid; intrinsic fac-tor concentrate; folic acid] 115 mg• 15 μg•150 mg•75 mg•1 mg

Pronestyl capsules, tablets, IV or IM injection (discontinued 2003) ℞ *antiarrhythmic* [procainamide HCl] 250, 375, 500 mg; 250, 375, 500 mg; 100, 500 mg/mL ⧉ Ponstel

Pronestyl-SR sustained-release tablets (discontinued 2003) ℞ *antiarrhythmic* [procainamide HCl] 500 mg

pronetalol INN [also: pronethalol]

pronethalol BAN [also: pronetalol]

Pronto shampoo OTC *pediculicide for lice* [pyrethrins; piperonyl butoxide] 0.33%•4%

Propac powder OTC *oral protein supplement* [whey protein; lactose]

Propacet 100 film-coated tablets ℞ *narcotic analgesic* [propoxyphene napsylate; acetaminophen] 100•650 mg

propacetamol INN

propafenone INN, BAN *antiarrhythmic* [also: propafenone HCl]

propafenone HCl USAN *antiarrhythmic* [also: propafenone] 150, 225, 300 mg oral

Propagest tablets (discontinued 2001) OTC *nasal decongestant* [phenylpropanolamine HCl] 25 mg

propamidine INN, BAN, DCF

propamidine isethionate *investigational (orphan) eye drops for* Acanthamoeba *keratitis*

propaminodiphen [see: pramiverine]

propane NF *aerosol propellant*

1,2-propanediol [see: propylene glycol]

propanidid USAN, INN *intravenous anesthetic*

propanocaine INN

propanoic acid, sodium salt hydrate [see: sodium propionate]

2-propanol [see: isopropyl alcohol]

2-propanone [see: acetone]

propantheline bromide USP, INN *GI antispasmodic; peptic ulcer adjunct* 15 mg oral

PROPApH Acne cream OTC *keratolytic for acne* [salicylic acid] 2%

PROPApH Astringent Cleanser topical liquid OTC *keratolytic for acne* [salicylic acid; alcohol 55%] 2%

PROPApH Cleansing; PROPApH Cleansing for Sensitive Skin; PROPApH Cleansing Maximum Strength pads OTC *keratolytic for acne* [salicylic acid] 0.5%; 0.5%; 2%

PROPApH Cleansing for Normal/ Combination Skin; PROPApH Cleansing for Oily Skin lotion OTC *keratolytic for acne* [salicylic acid] 0.5%

PROPApH Foaming Face Wash topical liquid ℞ *keratolytic cleanser for acne* [salicylic acid] 2%

PROPApH Peel-Off Acne Mask OTC *keratolytic for acne* [salicylic acid] 2%

proparacaine HCl USP *topical ophthalmic anesthetic* [also: proxymetacaine] 0.5% eye drops

proparacaine HCl & fluorescein sodium *topical ophthalmic anesthetic; corneal disclosing agent* 0.5%•0.25%

propatyl nitrate USAN *coronary vasodilator* [also: propatylnitrate]

propatylnitrate INN *coronary vasodilator* [also: propatyl nitrate]

propazolamide INN

Propecia film-coated tablets ℞ *androgen hormone inhibitor for androgenic alopecia in men* [finasteride] 1 mg

1-propene homopolymer [see: polipropene 25]

propenidazole INN

propentofylline INN

p-**propenylanisole** [see: anethole]

propenzolate HCl USAN *anticholinergic* [also: oxyclipine]

propericiazine [see: periciazine]

properidine INN, BAN

propetamide INN

propetandrol INN

prophenamine HCl [see: ethopropazine HCl]

Pro-Phree powder OTC *supplement to breast milk* [protein-free formula with vitamins & minerals]

Prophyllin ointment OTC *topical antifungal; vulnerary; wound deodorant* [sodium propionate; chlorophyll derivatives] 5%•0.0125%

propicillin INN, BAN

propikacin USAN, INN *antibacterial*

Propimex-1 powder OTC *formula for infants with propionic or methylmalonicacidemia*

Propimex-2 powder OTC *enteral nutritional therapy for propionic or methylmalonic acidemia*

Propine eye drops ℞ *topical antiglaucoma agent* [dipivefrin HCl] 0.1%

propinetidine INN

propiodal [see: prolonium iodide]

propiolactone (β-propiolactone) USAN, INN *disinfectant*

propiomazine USAN, INN *preanesthetic sedative*

propiomazine HCl USP *sedative; analgesic adjunct*

propionic acid NF *antimicrobial; acidifying agent*

propionyl erythromycin lauryl sulfate [see: erythromycin estolate]

propipocaine INN

propiram INN, BAN *narcotic agonist-antagonist analgesic* [also: propiram fumarate]

propiram fumarate USAN *investigational (Phase III) narcotic agonist-antagonist analgesic* [also: propiram]

propisergide INN

propitocaine HCl JAN *topical local anesthetic* [also: prilocaine HCl]

propiverine INN

propizepine INN

Proplex T IV infusion ℞ *antihemophilic to correct factor VII, VIII (hemophilia A), and IX (hemophilia B; Christmas disease) deficiencies* [coagulation factors II, VII, IX, and X, heat treated] 30 mL

propofol USAN, INN, BAN *rapid-acting general anesthetic* 1% injection

propolis *natural resin collected from the buds of certain trees by bees and used as an antibiotic, anti-inflammatory, antioxidant, antineoplastic, fungicide, immune system stimulant, and vulnerary*

propoxate INN

propoxycaine INN *local anesthetic* [also: propoxycaine HCl]

propoxycaine HCl USP *local anesthetic* [also: propoxycaine]

propoxyphene HCl USAN, USP *narcotic analgesic* [also: dextropropoxyphene HCl] 65 mg oral

propoxyphene napsylate USAN, USP *narcotic analgesic*

propranolol INN, BAN *antianginal; antiarrhythmic; antihypertensive; antiadrenergic (β-blocker); migraine preventative* [also: propranolol HCl]

propranolol HCl USAN, USP *antianginal; antiarrhythmic; antihypertensive; antiadrenergic (β-blocker); migraine preventative* [also: propranolol] 10, 20, 40, 60, 80, 90, 120, 160 mg oral; 4, 8 mg/mL oral; 1 mg/mL injection

Propranolol Intensol oral solution ℞ *antianginal; antiarrhythmic; antihypertensive; antiadrenergic (β-blocker); migraine preventative* [propranolol HCl] 80 mg/mL

propyl p-aminobenzoate [see: risocaine]

propyl docetrizoate INN, BAN

propyl gallate NF *antioxidant*

propyl p-hydroxybenzoate [see: propylparaben]

propyl p-hydroxybenzoate, sodium salt [see: propylparaben sodium]

N-propylajmalinium tartrate [see: prajmalinum bitartrate]

propylene carbonate NF *gelling agent*

propylene glycol USP *humectant; solvent; suspending and viscosity-increasing agent*

propylene glycol alginate NF *suspending agent; viscosity-increasing agent*

propylene glycol diacetate NF *solvent*

propylene glycol ether of methylcellulose [see: hydroxypropyl methylcellulose]

propylene glycol monostearate NF *emulsifying agent*

propylhexedrine USP, INN, BAN *vasoconstrictor; nasal decongestant*

propyliodone USP, INN *radiopaque contrast medium* (56.7% iodine)

propylorvinol [see: etorphine]

propylparaben USAN, NF *antifungal agent; preservative*

propylparaben sodium USAN, NF *antimicrobial preservative*

2-propylpentanoic acid [see: valproic acid]

propylthiouracil (PTU) USP, INN *thyroid inhibitor*
2-propylvaleramide [see: valpromide]
propylvaleric acid [see: valproic acid]
propyperone INN
propyphenazone INN, BAN
propyromazine bromide INN
Pro-Q foam OTC *skin protectant* [dimethicone; glycerin; parabens]
Proquad ℞ *investigational (NDA filed) measles, mumps, rubella, and varicella vaccine* [measles, mumps, and rubella virus vaccine, live; varicella virus vaccine]
proquamezine BAN [also: aminopromazine]
proquazone USAN, INN *anti-inflammatory*
Proquin XR film-coated extended-release tablets ℞ *broad-spectrum fluoroquinolone antibiotic* [ciprofloxacin] 500 mg
proquinolate USAN, INN *coccidiostat for poultry*
prorenoate potassium USAN, INN *aldosterone antagonist*
proroxan INN *antiadrenergic (α-receptor)* [also: proroxan HCl]
proroxan HCl USAN *antiadrenergic (α-receptor)* [also: proroxan]
Proscar film-coated tablets ℞ *androgen hormone inhibitor for benign prostatic hyperplasia (BPH)* [finasteride] 5 mg ⑨ Posicor
proscillaridin USAN, INN *cardiotonic*
proscillaridin A [see: proscillaridin]
Prosed/DS sugar-coated tablets ℞ *urinary antibiotic; antiseptic; analgesic; antispasmodic* [methenamine; phenyl salicylate; methylene blue; benzoic acid; atropine sulfate; hyoscyamine sulfate] 81.6•36.2•10.8•9•0.06•0.06 mg
ProSight Lutein capsules OTC *dietary supplement* [calcium; vitamins C and E; zinc; copper (but no lutein)] 22 mg•60 mg•30 IU•15 mg•2 mg
ProSobee oral liquid, powder for oral liquid OTC *hypoallergenic infant food* [soy protein formula]
ProSobee LIPIL oral liquid, powder for oral liquid OTC *hypoallergenic infant food fortified with omega-3 fatty acids* [soy protein formula]
ProSol 20% IV infusion ℞ *total parenteral nutrition* [multiple essential and nonessential amino acids] 20 g
ProSom tablets ℞ *benzodiazepine sedative and hypnotic* [estazolam] 1, 2 mg
Prosorba Column for dialysis ℞ *treatment for rheumatoid arthritis* [protein A]
prospidium chloride INN
prostacyclin [now: epoprostenol]
prostaglandin agonists *a class of antiglaucoma agents that reduce intraocular pressure (IOP) by increasing the outflow of aqueous humor*
prostaglandin E_1 (PGE_1) [now: alprostadil]
prostaglandin E_1 enol ester *investigational (orphan) for advanced chronic critical limb ischemia*
prostaglandin E_2 (PGE_2) [see: dinoprostone]
prostaglandin $F_{2\alpha}$ ($PGF_{2\alpha}$) [see: dinoprost]
prostaglandin I_2 (PGI_2) [now: epoprostenol]
prostaglandin X (PGX) [now: epoprostenol]
prostaglandins *a class of agents that stimulate uterine contractions, used for abortions, cervical ripening, and postpartum hemorrhage*
prostalene USAN, INN *prostaglandin*
ProstaScint *imaging agent for prostate cancer and its metastases* [capromab pendetide]
Pro-Stat 64; Pro-Stat 101 oral liquid OTC *enteral nutritional therapy* [collagen hydrolysate formula] 500 g protein per 946 mL
ProStep transdermal patch (discontinued 2001) ℞ *smoking deterrent; nicotine withdrawal aid* [nicotine] 11, 22 mg/day
Prostigmin subcu or IM injection ℞ *cholinergic urinary stimulant for postsurgical urinary retention; treatment for myasthenia gravis; antidote to neuromuscular blockers* [neostigmine

methylsulfate] 1:1000 (1 mg/mL), 1:2000 (0.5 mg/mL), 1:4000 (0.25 mg/mL) (1:400 [2.5 mg/mL] available in Canada) ☑ physostigmine

Prostigmin tablets ℞ *myasthenia gravis treatment; antidote for neuromuscular blockers* [neostigmine bromide] 15 mg

Prostin E2 vaginal suppository ℞ *prostaglandin-type abortifacient* [dinoprostone] 20 mg

Prostin VR Pediatric IV injection ℞ *vasodilator; platelet aggregation inhibitor* [alprostadil] 500 μg/mL

prosulpride INN

prosultiamine INN

ProSure oral liquid OTC *enteral nutritional therapy for cancer patients* 8 oz.

protactinium *element (Pa)*

protamine sulfate USP, INN *antidote to heparin overdose* [also: protamine sulphate] 10 mg/mL IV infusion

protamine sulphate BAN *antidote to heparin overdose* [also: protamine sulfate]

protamine zinc insulin (PZI) INN *antidiabetic* [also: insulin, protamine zinc; insulin zinc protamine]

protargin, mild [see: silver protein, mild]

protease *digestive enzyme (digests protein)* [100 IU/mg in pancrelipase; 25 IU/mg in pancreatin]

protease inhibitors *a class of antivirals that block HIV replication*

proteasome inhibitors *a class of antineoplastics*

ProTech First Aid Stick topical liquid OTC *antiseptic; analgesic* [lidocaine; povidone-iodine] 2.5%•10%

Protectol Medicated topical powder OTC *antifungal* [calcium undecylenate] 15%

Protegra softgels OTC *vitamin/mineral supplement* [multiple vitamins & minerals]

protein A *treatment for rheumatoid arthritis*

protein C concentrate *investigational (orphan) anticoagulant for protein C deficiency*

protein hydrolysate USP *fluid and nutrient replenisher*

protein kinase C-beta inhibitor *investigational (Phase II/III) treatment for diabetic neuropathy, retinopathy, and macular edema*

α₁-proteinase inhibitor [see: alpha₁-proteinase inhibitor]

Protenate IV infusion ℞ *blood volume expander for shock due to burns, trauma, and surgery* [plasma protein fraction] 5%

proterguride INN

protheobromine INN

Prothiaden ℞ *investigational (NDA filed) tricyclic antidepressant* [dothiepin HCl]

prothionamide BAN [also: protionamide]

prothipendyl INN

prothipendyl HCl [see: prothipendyl]

prothixene INN

prothrombin complex, activated BAN

Protilase capsules containing entericcoated spheres (discontinued 2002) ℞ *digestive enzymes* [lipase; protease; amylase] 4000•25 000•20 000 USP units

ProTime test kit for home use *in vitro diagnostic aid for the management of anticoagulation therapy*

protiofate INN

protionamide INN [also: prothionamide]

protirelin USAN, INN, BAN *prothyrotropin; diagnostic aid for thyroid function; investigational (orphan) for infant respiratory distress syndrome of prematurity*

protizinic acid INN

protokylol HCl

proton pump inhibitors (PPIs) *a class of gastric antisecretory agents that inhibit the ATPase "proton pump" within the gastric parietal cell* [also called: ATPase inhibitors; substituted benzimidazoles]

Protonix enteric-coated delayed-release tablets ℞ *proton pump inhibitor for erosive esophagitis associated with gastroesophageal reflux disease (GERD) and Zollinger-Ellison syndrome* [pantoprazole sodium] 20, 40 mg

Protonix I.V. powder for infusion ℞ *proton pump inhibitor for erosive esophagitis associated with gastroesophageal reflux disease (GERD) and Zollinger-Ellison syndrome* [pantoprazole sodium] 40 mg/vial

Protopam Chloride IV injection ℞ *antidote for organophosphate poisoning and anticholinesterase overdose* [pralidoxime chloride] 1 g ⑨ Protamine

Protopic ointment ℞ *topical treatment of eczema* [tacrolimus] 0.03%, 0.1%

Protostat tablets ℞ *antibiotic; antiprotozoal; amebicide* [metronidazole] 250, 500 mg

protoveratrine A

Protovir ℞ *investigational (Phase I) antiviral for AIDS-related cytomegalovirus* [sevirumab]

protriptyline INN *tricyclic antidepressant* [also: protriptyline HCl]

protriptyline HCl USAN, USP *tricyclic antidepressant* [also: protriptyline] 5, 10 mg oral

Protropin powder for IM or subcu injection ℞ *growth hormone for congenital growth failure due to lack of endogenous growth hormone (orphan)* [somatrem] 5, 10 mg (15, 30 IU) per vial

Protuss oral liquid (discontinued 2005) ℞ *narcotic antitussive; expectorant* [hydrocodone bitartrate; potassium guaiacolsulfonate] 5•300 mg/5 mL

Protuss DM sustained-release tablets (discontinued 2004) ℞ *antitussive; decongestant; expectorant* [dextromethorphan hydrobromide; pseudoephedrine HCl; guaifenesin] 30•60•600 mg

Protuss-D oral liquid (discontinued 2005) ℞ *narcotic antitussive; decongestant; expectorant* [hydrocodone bitartrate; pseudoephedrine HCl; potassium guaiacolsulfonate] 5•30•300 mg/5 mL

prourokinase [see: saruplase]

Provenge ℞ *investigational (Phase III) theraccine for prostate cancer*

Proventil inhalation aerosol ℞ *sympathomimetic bronchodilator* [albuterol] 90 μg/dose

Proventil Repetabs (extended-release tablets) (discontinued 2004) ℞ *sympathomimetic bronchodilator* [albuterol sulfate] 4 mg

Proventil tablets, syrup, solution for inhalation ℞ *sympathomimetic bronchodilator* [albuterol sulfate] 2, 4 mg; 4 mg; 2 mg/5 mL; 0.083%, 0.5%

Proventil HFA inhalation aerosol with a CFC-free propellant ℞ *sympathomimetic bronchodilator* [albuterol sulfate] 90 μg/dose

Provera tablets ℞ *synthetic progestin for secondary amenorrhea, abnormal uterine bleeding, and endometrial hyperplasia* [medroxyprogesterone acetate] 2.5, 5, 10 mg ⑨ Covera; Provir; Trovert

Provigil caplets ℞ *analeptic for excessive daytime sleepiness due to narcolepsy (orphan), obstructive sleep apnea, or shift work sleep disorder (SWSD); also used for fatigue associated with multiple sclerosis* [modafinil] 100, 200 mg

Proviron brand name for mesterolone, an androgen abused with anabolic steroid street drugs

ProVisc prefilled syringes ℞ *cohesive viscoelastic agent for ophthalmic surgery* [hyaluronate sodium] 0.55, 0.85 mL

provitamin A [see: beta carotene]

Provocholine powder for inhalation solution ℞ *bronchoconstrictor for in vivo pulmonary function challenge test* [methacholine chloride] 100 mg/5 mL

proxazole USAN, INN *smooth muscle relaxant; analgesic; anti-inflammatory*

proxazole citrate USAN *smooth muscle relaxant; analgesic; anti-inflammatory*

proxetil INN *combining name for radicals or groups*

proxibarbal INN

proxibutene INN

proxicromil USAN, INN *antiallergic*

proxifezone INN

Proxigel (discontinued 2002) OTC *topical oral anti-inflammatory and anti-infective for braces* [carbamide peroxide] 10%

proxorphan INN *analgesic; antitussive* [also: proxorphan tartrate]

proxorphan tartrate USAN *analgesic; antitussive* [also: proxorphan]

proxymetacaine INN, BAN *topical ophthalmic anesthetic* [also: proparacaine HCl]

proxymetacaine HCl [see: proparacaine HCl]

proxyphylline INN, BAN

Prozac tablets, Pulvules (capsules), oral solution Ɍ *selective serotonin reuptake inhibitor (SSRI) for major depression, obsessive-compulsive disorder, bulimia nervosa, and panic disorder; investigational (orphan) for autism* [fluoxetine HCl] 10 mg; 10, 20, 40 mg; 20 mg/5 mL ☒ Prilosec

Prozac Weekly enteric-coated delayed-release pellets in capsules Ɍ *selective serotonin reuptake inhibitor (SSRI) for major depression, obsessive-compulsive disorder, and bulimia nervosa; once-weekly dosing for maintenance* [fluoxetine HCl] 90 mg

prozapine INN

Prozine-50 IM injection Ɍ *conventional (typical) antipsychotic* [promazine HCl] 50 mg/mL

prucalopride HCl USAN *investigational (Phase III) prokinetic agent for post-ileus and opioid-induced constipation*

prucalopride succinate USAN *investigational (Phase III) prokinetic agent for post-ileus and opioid-induced constipation*

Prunella vulgaris medicinal herb [see: woundwort]

Prunus africana medicinal herb [see: pygeum]

Prunus americana; P. domestica; P. spinosa medicinal herb [see: plum]

Prunus amygdalus medicinal herb [see: almond]

Prunus armeniaca medicinal herb [see: apricot]

Prunus persica medicinal herb [see: peach]

Prunus serotina medicinal herb [see: wild black cherry]

Prunus virginiana medicinal herb [see: wild cherry]

Prussian blue [see: ferric hexacyanoferrate]

PSE (pseudoephedrine HCl) [q.v.]

PSE 120/MSC 2.5 sustained-release tablets Ɍ *decongestant; anticholinergic to dry mucosal secretions* [pseudoephedrine HCl; methscopolamine nitrate] 120•2.5 mg

PSE CPM chewable tablets Ɍ *pediatric decongestant and antihistamine* [pseudoephedrine HCl; chlorpheniramine maleate] 15•2 mg

Pseudo oral liquid (discontinued 2002) OTC *nasal decongestant* [pseudoephedrine HCl] 30 mg/5 mL

Pseudo-Car DM syrup (discontinued 2002) Ɍ *antitussive; decongestant; antihistamine* [dextromethorphan hydrobromide; pseudoephedrine HCl; carbinoxamine maleate] 15•60•4 mg/5 mL

Pseudo-Chlor sustained-release capsules (discontinued 2002) Ɍ *decongestant; antihistamine* [pseudoephedrine HCl; chlorpheniramine maleate] 120•8 mg

pseudoephedrine INN, BAN *vasoconstrictor; nasal decongestant* [also: pseudoephedrine HCl]

pseudoephedrine HCl USAN, USP *vasoconstrictor; nasal decongestant* [also: pseudoephedrine] 30, 60 mg oral; 30 mg/5 mL oral

pseudoephedrine HCl & brompheniramine maleate *decongestant; antihistamine* 60•4 mg/5 mL oral

pseudoephedrine HCl & carbinoxamine maleate *nasal decongestant; antihistamine* 60•4 mg/5 mL oral; 25•2 mg/mL oral

pseudoephedrine HCl & carbinoxamine maleate & hydrocodone bitartrate *nasal decongestant; antihistamine; antitussive* 30•2•50 mg/5 mL oral

pseudoephedrine HCl & chlorpheniramine maleate *decongestant; antihistamine* 120•8 mg oral

pseudoephedrine HCl & guaifene-sin decongestant; expectorant 48•595, 60•600, 85•795 mg oral

pseudoephedrine HCl & triproli-dine HCl decongestant; antihistamine 60•2.5 mg oral

pseudoephedrine polistirex USAN nasal decongestant

pseudoephedrine sulfate USAN, USP bronchodilator; nasal decongestant

pseudoephedrine tannate bronchodilator; nasal decongestant

pseudoephedrine tannate & chlor-pheniramine tannate decongestant; antihistamine 4.5•75 mg/5 mL oral

Pseudofrin ⒸⒶⓃ tablets OTC decongestant [pseudoephedrine HCl] 60 mg

Pseudo-Gest tablets (discontinued 2002) OTC nasal decongestant [pseudoephedrine HCl] 30, 60 mg

Pseudo-Gest Plus tablets (discontinued 2002) OTC decongestant; antihistamine [pseudoephedrine HCl; chlorpheniramine maleate] 60•4 mg

Pseudomonas aeruginosa **purified extract** investigational (orphan) agent to increase platelet count in immune thrombocytopenic purpura

Pseudomonas **immune globulin** [see: mucoid exopolysaccharide *Pseudomonas* hyperimmune globulin]

pseudomonic acid A [see: mupirocin]

Pseudostat ℞ investigational (Phase II) theraccine for chronic bronchitis

Pseudovent sustained-release capsules ℞ decongestant; expectorant [pseudoephedrine HCl; guaifenesin] 120•250 mg

Pseudovent-PED sustained-release pediatric capsules ℞ decongestant; expectorant [pseudoephedrine HCl; guaifenesin] 60•300 mg

psilocin a hallucinogenic street drug closely related to psilocybin

psilocybin BAN a hallucinogenic street drug derived from the Psilocybe mexicana mushroom [also: psilocybine]

psilocybine INN, DCF a hallucinogenic street drug derived from the Psilocybe mexicana mushroom [also: psilocybin]

psoralens a class of oral or topical skin photosensitizing agents used with ultraviolet A light (320–400 nm wavelength) for the treatment of severe recalcitrant psoriasis

Psor-a-set bar OTC keratolytic skin cleanser [salicylic acid] 2%

Psorcon E cream, ointment ℞ topical corticosteroidal anti-inflammatory [diflorasone diacetate] 0.05%

Psoriatec cream ℞ antipsoriatic [anthralin] 1%

PsoriGel OTC antipsoriatic; antiseborrheic; antiseptic [coal tar solution; alcohol 28.3%] 7.5%

psyllium (Plantago ovata) medicinal herb [see: plantain]

psyllium husk USP bulk laxative

psyllium hydrocolloid bulk laxative

psyllium hydrophilic mucilloid bulk laxative

psyllium seed [see: plantago seed]

P-Tanna 12 pediatric oral suspension ℞ decongestant; antihistamine [phenylephrine tannate; pyrilamine tannate] 5•30 mg/5 mL

PTC (plasma thromboplastin component) [see: factor IX]

P.T.E.-4; P.T.E.-5 IV injection ℞ intravenous nutritional therapy [multiple trace elements (metals)]

pterins a class of investigational antineoplastics

pteroyldiglutamic acid (PDGA)

pteroylglutamic acid (PGA) [see: folic acid]

PTFE (polytetrafluoroethylene) [see: polytef]

PTU (propylthiouracil) [q.v.]

Pt/VM (Platinol, VM-26) chemotherapy protocol for pediatric neuroblastoma

ptyalagogues a class of agents that stimulate the secretion of saliva [also called: sialagogues]

puccoon, yellow medicinal herb [see: goldenseal]

Pueraria lobata; P. thunbergiana medicinal herb [see: kudzu]

puffball medicinal herb [see: dandelion]

Pulmicort Respules (single-dose ampule for inhalation) ℞ *corticosteroidal anti-inflammatory for chronic asthma in children* [budesonide] 0.25, 0.5 mg

Pulmicort Turbuhaler (dry powder in a metered-dose inhaler) ℞ *corticosteroidal anti-inflammatory for chronic asthma* [budesonide] 160 µg/dose

Pulmocare ready-to-use oral liquid OTC *enteral nutritional therapy for pulmonary problems*

Pulmonaria officinalis medicinal herb [see: lungwort]

pulmonary surfactant replacement, porcine [now: poractant alfa]

Pulmozyme solution for nebulization ℞ *reduces respiratory viscoelasticity of sputum in cystic fibrosis* (orphan) [dornase alfa] 1 mg/mL

pulse VAC *chemotherapy protocol for sarcomas* [see: VAC pulse]

pulse VAC (vincristine, Adriamycin, cyclophosphamide) *chemotherapy protocol* [also: VAC]

PulsePak (trademarked dosage form) *one-week dosage pack*

Pulvule (trademarked dosage form) *bullet-shaped capsule*

pumice USP *dental abrasive*

pumitepa INN

Punctum Plug ℞ *blocks the puncta and canaliculus to eliminate tear loss in keratitis sicca* [silicone plug]

Punica granatum medicinal herb [see: pomegranate]

Puralube ophthalmic ointment OTC *ocular moisturizer/lubricant* [white petrolatum; mineral oil]

Puralube Tears eye drops OTC *ophthalmic moisturizer/lubricant* [polyvinyl alcohol; polyethylene glycol 400] 1%•1%

Puregon ⓒᴬᴺ subcu or IM injection ℞ *recombinant follicle-stimulating hormone (FSH) for the induction of ovulation and development of multiple follicles for assisted reproductive technology (ART)* [follitropin beta] 50, 100 IU

purgatives *a class of agents that cause vigorous evacuation of the bowels by*

increasing bulk, stimulating peristaltic action, etc. [also called: cathartics]

Purge oral liquid OTC *stimulant laxative* [castor oil] 95%

purified cotton [see: cotton, purified]

purified protein derivative (PPD) of tuberculin [see: tuberculin]

purified rayon [see: rayon, purified]

purified siliceous earth [see: siliceous earth, purified]

purified water [see: water, purified]

H-purin-6-amine [see: adenine]

Purinethol tablets ℞ *antimetabolite antineoplastic for acute lymphocytic, lymphoblastic, myelogenous, and myelomonocytic leukemias* [mercaptopurine] 50 mg

puromycin USAN, INN *antineoplastic; antiprotozoal* (*Trypanosoma*)

puromycin HCl USAN *antineoplastic; antiprotozoal* (*Trypanosoma*)

purple angelica medicinal herb [see: angelica]

purple boneset medicinal herb [see: boneset]

purple cone flower medicinal herb [see: echinacea]

purple leptandra medicinal herb [see: Culver root]

Purpose Alpha Hydroxy Moisture lotion, cream OTC *moisturizer; emollient; exfoliant* [glycolic acid] 8%

Purpose Dry Skin cream OTC *moisturizer; emollient*

Purpose Soap bar OTC *therapeutic skin cleanser*

purshiana bark medicinal herb [see: cascara sagrada]

purslain, water medicinal herb [see: brooklime]

purvain medicinal herb [see: blue vervain]

pussywillow medicinal herb [see: willow]

PUVA *an acronym for psoralens (P) and ultraviolet A (UVA) light, used as a treatment for severe recalcitrant psoriasis* [see: psoralens; methoxsalen]

PVA (polyvinyl alcohol) [q.v.]

PVA (prednisone, vincristine, asparaginase) *chemotherapy protocol for acute lymphocytic leukemia (ALL)*

PVB (Platinol, vinblastine, bleomycin) *chemotherapy protocol for testicular cancer and adenocarcinoma*

PVC (polyvinyl chloride) [see: polyvinyl chloride, radiopaque]

PVDA (prednisone, vincristine, daunorubicin, asparaginase) *chemotherapy protocol for acute lymphocytic leukemia (ALL)*

PVP; PVP-16 (Platinol, VP-16) *chemotherapy protocol*

PVS Basics ℞ *hydrophobic contact lens material* [paflufocon E]

P-V-Tussin caplets ℞ *narcotic antitussive; antihistamine* [hydrocodone bitartrate; pseudoephedrine HCl] 5•60 mg

P-V-Tussin syrup ℞ *narcotic antitussive; decongestant; antihistamine* [hydrocodone bitartrate; pseudoephedrine HCl; chlorpheniramine maleate; alcohol 5%] 5•60•4 mg/10 mL

Pycnanthemum virginianum medicinal herb [see: wild hyssop]

Pycnogenol *natural free radical scavenger; a registered trade name for pine bark extract* [see: pine bark extract]

pygeum (Prunus africana; Pygeum africanum) bark *medicinal herb for prostate gland enlargement and urinary disorders*

Pylori-Check *test kit for professional use in vivo diagnostic aid for* H. pylori *in the breath*

Pylorid Ⓒᴬᴺ *film-coated tablets* (discontinued 2001) ℞ *histamine* H_2 *antagonist for duodenal ulcers with* H. pylori *infection* [ranitidine bismuth citrate] 400 mg

Pyloriset *reagent kit for professional use in vitro diagnostic aid for GI disorders*

pyrabrom USAN *antihistamine*

pyradone [see: aminopyrine]

pyrantel INN *anthelmintic for ascariasis (roundworm) and enterobiasis (pinworm)* [also: pyrantel pamoate]

pyrantel pamoate USAN, USP *anthelmintic for ascariasis (roundworm) and enterobiasis (pinworm)* [also: pyrantel]

pyrantel tartrate USAN *anthelmintic*

pyrathiazine HCl [see: parathiazine]

pyrazinamide (PZA) USP, INN, BAN *bactericidal; primary tuberculostatic* 500 mg oral

pyrazinecarboxamide [see: pyrazinamide]

pyrazofurin USAN *antineoplastic* [also: pirazofurin]

pyrazoline [see: antipyrine]

pyrazolopyrimidines *a class of sedative/hypnotics with rapid onset and short duration of action, used in the short-term treatment of insomnia*

pyrbenzindole [see: benzindopyrine HCl]

pyrbuterol HCl [see: pirbuterol HCl]

pyrethrins *a class of natural pesticides derived from pyrethrum flowers, especially* Chrysanthemum cinerariaefolium *and* C. coccineum

Pyrethrum parthenium medicinal herb [see: feverfew]

pyribenzamine (PBZ) [see: tripelennamine]

pyricarbate INN

pyridarone INN

Pyridiate; Pyridate No. 2 tablets ℞ *urinary analgesic* [phenazopyridine HCl] 100 mg; 200 mg

4-pyridinamine [see: fampridine]

2-pyridine aldoxime methylchloride (2-PAM) [see: pralidoxime chloride]

3-pyridinecarboxamide [see: niacinamide]

3-pyridinecarboxylic acid [see: niacin]

4-pyridinecarboxylic acid hydrazide [see: isoniazid]

3-pyridinecarboxylic acid methyl ester [see: methyl nicotinate]

3-pyridinemethanol [see: nicotinyl alcohol]

2-pyridinemethanol [see: piconol]

3-pyridinemethanol tartrate [see: nicotinyl tartrate]

Pyridium tablets ℞ *urinary analgesic* [phenazopyridine HCl] 100, 200 mg ⌧ Dyrenium; pyridoxine; pyrithione; pyritidium

Pyridium Plus tablets ℞ *urinary analgesic; antispasmodic; sedative* [phenazopyridine HCl; hyoscyamine hydrobromide; butabarbital] 150•0.3•15 mg

pyridofylline INN

pyridostigmine bromide USP, INN *cholinergic/anticholinesterase muscle stimulant* 60 mg oral ⌧ physostigmine

pyridoxal-5′-phosphate [see: pyridoxine HCl]

pyridoxamine [see: pyridoxine HCl]

pyridoxine (vitamin B₆) INN *water-soluble vitamin; enzyme cofactor* [also: pyridoxine HCl] ⌧ pralidoxime; Pyridium

pyridoxine HCl (vitamin B₆) USP *water-soluble vitamin; enzyme cofactor* [also: pyridoxine] 50, 100, 250, 500 mg oral; 100 mg/mL injection ⌧ pralidoxime; Pyridium

β-pyridylcarbinol [see: nicotinyl alcohol]

pyridylmethanol *me+* [see: nicotinyl alcohol]

pyrilamine maleate USP *anticholinergic; antihistamine; sleep aid* [also: mepyramine]

pyrilamine tannate & phenylephrine tannate & chlorpheniramine tannate *antihistamine; decongestant* 12.5•5•2 mg/5 mL oral

pyrimethamine USP, INN *folic acid antagonist for malaria suppression and transmission control; toxoplasmosis treatment adjunct*

pyrimethamine & sulfadiazine *treatment for* Toxoplasma gondii *encephalitis (orphan)*

pyrimidinedione [see: uracil]

pyrimitate INN, BAN

Pyrinex Pediculicide shampoo (discontinued 2003) OTC *pediculicide for lice* [pyrethrins; piperonyl butoxide; deodorized kerosene] 0.2%•2%•0.8%

pyrinoline USAN, INN *antiarrhythmic*

Pyrinyl topical liquid (discontinued 2003) OTC *pediculicide for lice* [pyrethrins; piperonyl butoxide; deodorized kerosene] 0.2%•2%•0.8%

Pyrinyl II topical liquid (discontinued 2003) OTC *pediculicide for lice* [pyrethrins; piperonyl butoxide] 0.3%•3%

Pyrinyl Plus shampoo OTC *pediculicide for lice* [pyrethrins; piperonyl butoxide] 0.3%•4%

pyrithen [see: chlorothen citrate]

pyrithione sodium USAN *topical antimicrobial* ⌧ Pyridium

pyrithione zinc USAN, INN, BAN *antibacterial; antifungal; antiseborrheic*

pyrithyldione INN

pyritidium bromide INN ⌧ Pyridium

pyritinol INN, BAN

pyrodifenium bromide [see: prifinium bromide]

pyrogallic acid [see: pyrogallol]

pyrogallol NF

pyrophendane INN

pyrophenindane [see: pyrophendane]

pyrovalerone INN *CNS stimulant* [also: pyrovalerone HCl]

pyrovalerone HCl USAN *CNS stimulant* [also: pyrovalerone]

pyroxamine INN *antihistamine* [also: pyroxamine maleate]

pyroxamine maleate USAN *antihistamine* [also: pyroxamine]

pyroxylin USP, INN *pharmaceutic necessity for collodion*

pyrrobutamine phosphate USP

pyrrocaine USAN, INN *local anesthetic*

pyrrocaine HCl NF

pyrrolifene INN *analgesic* [also: pyrroliphene HCl]

pyrrolifene HCl [see: pyrroliphene HCl]

pyrroliphene HCl USAN *analgesic* [also: pyrrolifene]

pyrrolnitrin USAN, INN *antifungal*

pyrroxane [now: proroxan HCl]

Pyrroxate capsules (discontinued 2001) OTC *decongestant; antihistamine; analgesic* [phenylpropanolamine HCl; chlorpheniramine maleate; acetaminophen] 25•4•650 mg

Pyrus malus *medicinal herb* [see: apple]
pyrvinium chloride INN
pyrvinium embonate [see: pyrvinium pamoate]
pyrvinium pamoate USP *anthelmintic* [also: viprynium embonate]
pytamine INN

PYtest reagent kit for professional use *in vitro diagnostic aid for* H. pylori *in the breath* [carbon C 14 urea] 1 mCi
PYY (peptide YY) [q.v.]
PZA (pyrazinamide) [q.v.]
PZI (protamine zinc insulin) [q.v.]

Qdall sustained-release capsules ℞ *decongestant; antihistamine* [pseudoephedrine HCl; chlorpheniramine maleate] 100•12 mg
Qdall AR dual-release capsules ℞ *antihistamine* [chlorpheniramine maleate] 12 mg (2 mg immediate release; 10 mg sustained release)
QTest test stick for home use (discontinued 2004) *in vitro diagnostic aid; urine pregnancy test*
QTest Ovulation test kit for professional use *in vitro diagnostic aid to predict ovulation time*
Quad Tann caplets ℞ *antitussive; decongestant; antihistamine* [carbetapentane tannate; phenylephrine tannate; ephedrine tannate; chlorpheniramine tannate] 60•10•10•5 mg
quadazocine INN, BAN *opioid antagonist* [also: quadazocine mesylate]
quadazocine mesylate USAN *opioid antagonist* [also: quadazocine]
Quadra-Hist D; Quadra-Hist D Ped extended-release capsules ℞ *decongestant; antihistamine* [pseudoephedrine HCl; phenyltoloxamine citrate; pyrilamine maleate; pheniramine maleate] 80•16•16•16 mg; 40•8•8•8 mg
Quadramet IV injection ℞ *radiopharmaceutical for treatment of bone pain from osteoblastic metastatic tumors* [samarium Sm 153 lexidronam] 1850 MBq/mL (50 mCi/mL)
quadrosilan INN
quaking aspen *medicinal herb* [see: poplar]

Quantaffirm reagent kit for professional use *in vitro diagnostic aid for mononucleosis*
Quarzan capsules (discontinued 2001) ℞ *anticholinergic; peptic ulcer treatment* [clidinium bromide] 2.5, 5 mg ⊞ Questran
quassia (Picrasma excelsa; Quassia amara) bark *medicinal herb used as an anthelmintic, antimalarial, appetizer, digestive aid, febrifuge, insecticide, pediculicide, and tonic*
quatacaine INN
quaternium-18 bentonite [see: bentoquatam]
quazepam USAN, INN *benzodiazepine sedative and hypnotic*
quazinone USAN, INN *cardiotonic*
quazodine USAN, INN *cardiotonic; bronchodilator*
quazolast USAN, INN *antiasthmatic; mediator release inhibitor*
Queen Anne's lace *medicinal herb* [see: carrot]
queen of the meadow *medicinal herb* [see: boneset; meadowsweet]
queen of the meadow (Eupatorium purpureum) leaves *medicinal herb for bursitis, gallstones, kidney infections and stones, neuralgias, rheumatism, ringworm, urinary disorders, and water retention*
Quelicin IV or IM injection ℞ *neuromuscular blocker* [succinylcholine chloride] 20, 50, 100 mg/mL
Quelidrine Cough syrup (discontinued 2002) OTC *antitussive; deconges-*

tant; *antihistamine; expectorant* [dextromethorphan hydrobromide; ephedrine HCl; phenylephrine HCl; chlorpheniramine maleate; ammonium chloride; ipecac; alcohol 2%] 10 mg•5 mg•5 mg•2 mg•40 mg•0.005 mL per 5 mL

quercetin *natural flavonoid used to protect capillary walls; antioxidant; active flavonol of rutin*

Quercetin tablets OTC *dietary supplement* [eucalyptus bioflavonoids] 50, 250 mg

Quercus alba medicinal herb [see: white oak]

Questran; Questran Light powder for oral suspension Ŗ *cholesterol-lowering antihyperlipidemic; also used for biliary obstruction* [cholestyramine resin] 4 g/dose

quetiapine fumarate USAN *novel (atypical) dibenzothiazepine antipsychotic for schizophrenia and manic episodes of a bipolar disorder; also used for agitation or psychosis due to Parkinson disease, Alzheimer disease, or various dementias*

Quibron; Quibron-300 capsules Ŗ *antiasthmatic; bronchodilator; expectorant* [theophylline; guaifenesin] 150•90 mg; 300•180 mg

Quibron-T Dividose (multiple-scored tablets) Ŗ *antiasthmatic; bronchodilator* [theophylline] 300 mg

Quibron-T/SR sustained-release Dividose (multiple-scored tablets) Ŗ *antiasthmatic; bronchodilator* [theophylline] 300 mg

Quick AC Enema Kit concentrated rectal suspension (discontinued 2001) Ŗ *radiopaque contrast medium for gastrointestinal imaging* [barium sulfate] 150%

Quick Care solutions OTC *two-step chemical disinfecting system for soft contact lenses* [hydrogen peroxide-based]

Quick Pep tablets (discontinued 2001) OTC *CNS stimulant; analeptic* [caffeine] 150 mg

Quicklets (trademarked dosage form) *quickly dissolving tablets*

Quickscreen test kit for home use *in vitro diagnostic aid for detection of multiple illicit drugs in the urine*

quick-set *medicinal herb* [see: hawthorn]

QuickVue H. pylori gII test kit for professional use *in vitro diagnostic aid for H. pylori in serum or plasma*

QuickVue Influenza Test for professional use *in vitro diagnostic aid for detection of influenza A and B from nasal excretions*

QuickVue Pregnancy Test cassettes for professional use *in vitro diagnostic aid; urine pregnancy test*

quifenadine INN

quiflapon sodium USAN *leukotriene biosynthesis inhibitor for asthma and inflammatory bowel disease*

Quilimmune-M Ŗ *investigational (Phase II) vaccine against malaria*

quillaia (*Quillaja saponaria***)** bark *medicinal herb for bronchitis and cough; also used topically for dandruff and scalp itchiness*

quillifoline INN

quilostigmine USAN *cholinesterase inhibitor for Alzheimer disease*

quinacainol INN

quinacillin INN, BAN

quinacrine HCl USP *antimalarial; anthelmintic for giardiasis and cestodiasis (tapeworm)* [also: mepacrine] ⧄ quinidine

Quinaglute Dura-Tabs (sustained-release tablets) (discontinued 2003) Ŗ *antiarrhythmic* [quinidine gluconate] 324 mg

quinalbarbitone sodium BAN *hypnotic; sedative* [also: secobarbital sodium]

quinaldine blue USAN *obstetric diagnostic aid*

quinambicide [see: clioquinol]

quinapril INN, BAN *angiotensin-converting enzyme (ACE) inhibitor; antihypertensive; adjunct to CHF therapy* [also: quinapril HCl]

quinapril HCl USAN *antihypertensive; angiotensin-converting enzyme (ACE) inhibitor; adjunctive treatment for CHF* [also: quinapril] 5, 10, 20, 40 mg

quinapril HCl & hydrochlorothiazide *antihypertensive; angiotensin-converting enzyme (ACE) inhibitor; diuretic* 10•12.5, 20•12.5, 20•25 mg oral

quinaprilat USAN, INN *antihypertensive; angiotensin-converting enzyme (ACE) inhibitor*

Quinaretic film-coated tablets ℞ *antihypertensive; angiotensin-converting enzyme (ACE) inhibitor; diuretic* [quinapril HCl; hydrochlorothiazide] 10•12.5, 20•12.5, 20•25 mg

quinazosin INN *antihypertensive* [also: quinazosin HCl]

quinazosin HCl USAN *antihypertensive* [also: quinazosin]

quinbolone USAN, INN *anabolic*

quincarbate INN

quindecamine INN *antibacterial* [also: quindecamine acetate]

quindecamine acetate USAN *antibacterial* [also: quindecamine]

quindonium bromide USAN, INN *antiarrhythmic*

quindoxin INN, BAN

quinelorane INN *antihypertensive; antiparkinsonian* [also: quinelorane HCl]

quinelorane HCl USAN *antihypertensive; antiparkinsonian* [also: quinelorane]

quinestradol INN, BAN

quinestrol USAN, USP, INN, BAN *estrogen replacement therapy for postmenopausal disorders*

quinetalate INN *smooth muscle relaxant* [also: quinetolate]

quinethazone USP, INN *diuretic; antihypertensive*

quinetolate USAN *smooth muscle relaxant* [also: quinetalate]

quinezamide INN

quinfamide USAN, INN *antiamebic*

quingestanol INN *progestin* [also: quingestanol acetate]

quingestanol acetate USAN *progestin* [also: quingestanol]

quingestrone USAN, INN *progestin*

Quinidex Extentabs (extended-release tablets) (discontinued 2004) ℞ *antiarrhythmic* [quinidine sulfate] 300 mg

quinidine NF, BAN *antiarrhythmic* 🄳 clonidine; quinacrine; Quinatime; quinine

quinidine gluconate USP *antiarrhythmic; antimalarial* (base=62%) 324 mg oral; 80 mg/mL injection

quinidine polygalacturonate *antiarrhythmic* (base=80%)

quinidine sulfate USP *antiarrhythmic* (base=83%) 200, 300 mg oral

quinine (*Cinchona calisaya; C. ledgeriana; C. succirubra*) NF, BAN bark *medicinal herb for cancer, fever, hemorrhoids, indigestion, inducing abortion, jaundice, malaria, mouth and throat diseases, parasites, stimulation of hair growth, and varicose veins* 🄳 quinidine

quinine ascorbate USAN *smoking deterrent*

quinine biascorbate [now: quinine ascorbate]

quinine bisulfate NF

quinine dihydrochloride NF *investigational anti-infective for pernicious malaria*

quinine ethylcarbonate NF

quinine glycerophosphate NF

quinine HCl NF

quinine hydrobromide NF

quinine hypophosphite NF

quinine monohydrobromide [see: quinine hydrobromide]

quinine monohydrochloride [see: quinine HCl]

quinine monosalicylate [see: quinine salicylate]

quinine phosphate NF

quinine phosphinate [see: quinine hypophosphite]

quinine salicylate NF

quinine sulfate USP *cinchona alkaloid; antimalarial for chloroquine-resistant falciparum malaria; also used to treat nocturnal leg cramps* 200, 260, 325 mg oral

quinine sulfate dihydrate [see: quinine sulfate]

quinine tannate USP

Quinine-Odan 🄰🄼 capsules OTC *antimalarial* [quinine sulfate] 200, 300 mg

quinisocaine INN [also: dimethisoquin HCl; dimethisoquin]

quinocide INN

8-quinolinol [see: oxyquinoline]

8-quinolinol benzoate [see: benzoxiquine]

quinolizidines *a class of antibiotics based on the quinolizidine (norlupinane) structure* [also called: norlupinanes]

quinolones [see: fluoroquinolones]

Quinora tablets (discontinued 2003) ℞ *antiarrhythmic* [quinidine sulfate] 300 mg

quinoxyl [see: chiniofon]

quinpirole INN *antihypertensive* [also: quinpirole HCl]

quinpirole HCl USAN *antihypertensive* [also: quinpirole]

quinprenaline INN *bronchodilator* [also: quinterenol sulfate]

quinprenaline sulfate [see: quinterenol sulfate]

Quinsana Plus powder OTC *topical antifungal* [tolnaftate] 1%

quinsy berry *medicinal herb* [see: currant]

Quintabs tablets OTC *vitamin supplement* [multiple vitamins; folic acid] ≛ •0.1 mg

Quintabs-M tablets OTC *vitamin/mineral/iron supplement* [multiple vitamins & minerals; iron; folic acid] ≛ •18•0.4 mg

quinterenol sulfate USAN *bronchodilator* [also: quinprenaline]

quintiofos INN, BAN

3-quinuclidinol benzoate [see: benzoclidine]

quinuclium bromide USAN, INN *antihypertensive*

quinupramine INN

quinupristin USAN, INN *streptogramin antibiotic; bacteriostatic to gram-positive infections*

quipazine INN *antidepressant; oxytocic* [also: quipazine maleate]

quipazine maleate USAN *antidepressant; oxytocic* [also: quipazine]

quisultazine INN

quisultidine [see: quisultazine]

Quixin eye drops ℞ *fluoroquinolone antibiotic for bacterial conjunctivitis* [levofloxacin] 0.5%

Qvar pressurized metered-dose inhaler (pMDI) with a CFC-free propellant ℞ *antiasthmatic* [beclomethasone dipropionate] 40, 80 μg/puff

R & C shampoo (discontinued 2003) OTC *pediculicide for lice* [pyrethrins; piperonyl butoxide] 0.3%•3%

R & D Calcium Carbonate/600 ℞ *investigational (orphan) agent for hyperphosphatemia of end-stage renal disease* [calcium carbonate]

RA Lotion OTC *topical acne treatment* [resorcinol; alcohol 43%] 3%

RabAvert IM injection ℞ *rabies vaccine for pre-exposure vaccination or post-exposure prophylaxis* [rabies vaccine, chick embryo cell] 2.5 IU

rabeprazole INN *proton pump inhibitor for duodenal ulcers, erosive or ulcera-* *tive gastroesophageal reflux disease (GERD), and other gastroesophageal disorders* [also: rabeprazole sodium]

rabeprazole sodium USAN *proton pump inhibitor for duodenal ulcers, erosive or ulcerative gastroesophageal reflux disease (GERD), H. pylori infection, and other gastroesophageal disorders* [also: rabeprazole]

rabies immune globulin (RIG) USP *passive immunizing agent for use after rabies exposure*

rabies vaccine USP *active immunizing agent* Challenge Virus Standard (CVS)

rabies vaccine, adsorbed (RVA)
[see: rabies vaccine]

rabies vaccine, DCO (diploid cell origin) [see: rabies vaccine]

rabies vaccine, HDCV (human diploid cell vaccine) [see: rabies vaccine]

race ginger *medicinal herb* [see: ginger]

racecadotril [see: acetorphan]

racefemine INN

racefenicol INN *antibacterial* [also: racephenicol]

racemethadol [see: dimepheptanol]

racemethionine USAN, USP *urinary acidifier* [also: methionine (the DL- form)]

racemethorphan INN, BAN

racemetirosine INN

racemic [def.] *A chemical compound with equal parts of* (+) *(formerly d- or dextro-) and* (−) *(formerly l- or levo-) enantiomers. Designated by the prefix* (±) *(formerly dl-).* [see also: isomer; enantiomer]

racemic amphetamine phosphate

racemic amphetamine sulfate [see: amphetamine sulfate]

racemic calcium pantothenate [see: calcium pantothenate, racemic]

racemoramide INN, BAN

racemorphan INN

racephedrine HCl USAN

racephenicol USAN *antibacterial* [also: racefenicol]

racepinefrine INN *sympathomimetic bronchodilator* [also: racepinephrine]

racepinephrine USP *sympathomimetic bronchodilator* [also: racepinefrine]

racepinephrine HCl USP *sympathomimetic bronchodilator*

raclopride INN, BAN

raclopride C 11 USAN *radiopharmaceutical*

racoonberry *medicinal herb* [see: mandrake]

ractopamine INN *veterinary growth stimulant* [also: ractopamine HCl]

ractopamine HCl USAN *veterinary growth stimulant* [also: ractopamine]

radio-chromated serum albumin [see: albumin, chromated]

radio-iodinated I 125 serum albumin [see: albumin, iodinated]

radio-iodinated I 131 serum albumin [see: albumin, iodinated]

radiomerisoprol ^{197}Hg [see: merisoprol Hg 197]

radioselenomethionine ^{75}Se [see: selenomethionine Se 75]

radiotolpovidone I 131 INN *hypoalbuminemia test; radioactive agent* [also: tolpovidone I 131]

radish (Raphanus sativus) *root medicinal herb used as an antispasmodic, astringent, cholagogue, and diuretic*

radium *element (Ra)*

radon *element (Rn)*

rAd/p53 gene therapy *investigational (Phase I) therapy for cancer*

rafoxanide USAN, INN *anthelmintic*

ragged cup (Silphium perfoliatum) root and gum *medicinal herb used as an antispasmodic, diaphoretic, and stimulant*

ragwort *medicinal herb* [see: life root]

ralitoline USAN, INN *anticonvulsant*

Ralivia ER controlled-release tablets ℞ *once-daily central analgesic* [tramadol HCl] 100, 200, 300 mg

raloxifene INN *antiestrogen; selective estrogen receptor modulator (SERM) for the prevention for postmenopausal osteoporosis; investigational (Phase III) for breast cancer* [also: raloxifene HCl]

raloxifene HCl USAN *antiestrogen; selective estrogen receptor modulator (SERM) for the prevention and treatment of postmenopausal osteoporosis* [also: raloxifene]

raltitrexed USAN *antimetabolite antineoplastic; investigational (Phase III) thymidylate synthase inhibitor for advanced colorectal cancer*

raluridine USAN *antiviral*

rambufaside [see: meproscillarin]

ramciclane INN

ramelton *melatonin MT-1 and MT-2 receptor antagonist for insomnia due to difficulty with sleep onset; investigational (Phase II) for circadian rhythm sleep disorder*

ramifenazone INN

ramipril USAN, INN, BAN *angiotensin-converting enzyme (ACE) inhibitor for hypertension, myocardial infarction, CHF, and stroke*

ramiprilat INN

ramixotidine INN

ramnodigin INN

ramoplanin USAN, INN *investigational (Phase III) broad-spectrum glycolipodepsipeptide antibiotic for vancomycin-resistant Enterococcus faecium (VREF) and other vancomycin-resistant enterococci (VRE)*

Ramses vaginal jelly (discontinued 2002) OTC *spermicidal contraceptive* [nonoxynol 9] 5%

Ramses Extra premedicated condom (discontinued 2002) OTC *spermicidal/barrier contraceptive* [nonoxynol 9] 15%

Ranexa ℞ *investigational (NDA filed) antianginal for chronic unstable angina* [ranolazine HCl]

Raniclor chewable tablets ℞ *cephalosporin antibiotic* [cefaclor] 125, 187, 250, 375 mg

ranimustine INN

ranimycin USAN, INN *antibacterial*

ranitidine USAN, INN, BAN *histamine H₂ antagonist for gastric ulcers* 150, 300 mg oral

ranitidine bismuth citrate USAN *histamine H₂ antagonist for gastric ulcers with H. pylori infection* [also: ranitidine bismutrex]

ranitidine bismutrex BAN *histamine H₂ antagonist for gastric ulcers with H. pylori infection* [also: ranitidine bismuth citrate]

ranitidine HCl USP, JAN *histamine H₂ antagonist for gastric ulcers* 75, 150 300 mg oral; 15 mg/mL oral

ranolazine INN *antianginal* [also: ranolazine HCl]

ranolazine HCl USAN *investigational (NDA filed) antianginal for chronic stable angina* [also: ranolazine]

ranpirnase USAN, INN *investigational (Phase III) adjunct to chemotherapy*

for pancreatic, breast, colorectal, prostate, and small cell lung cancers

Ranunculus acris; R. bulbosus; R. scleratus *medicinal herb* [see: buttercup]

rapacuronium bromide USAN *neuromuscular blocker; adjunct to general anesthesia*

Rapamune tablets, oral solution ℞ *immunosuppressant for renal transplantation* [sirolimus] 1, 2 mg; 1 mg/mL

rapamycin [now: sirolimus]

Raphanus sativus *medicinal herb* [see: radish]

Rapid Anthrax Test reagents for use with LightCycler assay device *diagnostic aid for anthrax DNA in human and environmental samples* [polymerase chain reaction (PCR) test]

RapidVue test kit for home use *in vitro diagnostic aid; urine pregnancy test*

Rapimelt (trademarked delivery system) *orally disintegrating tablets*

Rapinex (name changed to **Zegerid** upon marketing release in 2004)

RapiTab (trademarked delivery system) *orally disintegrating tablets*

Raplon IV injection (discontinued 2001) ℞ *rapid-onset, short-acting neuromuscular blocker for skeletal muscle relaxation as an adjunct to general anesthesia* [rapacuronium bromide] 100, 200 mg

Raptiva powder for subcu injection ℞ *immunosuppressant for plaque psoriasis* [efalizumab] 125 mg/dose

rasagiline INN

rasagiline mesylate USAN *investigational (NDA filed) monoamine oxidase B (MAO-B) inhibitor for Parkinson disease*

rasburicase USAN, INN *antimetabolite antineoplastic for leukemia, lymphoma, and solid tumor malignancies*

raspberry, ground *medicinal herb* [see: goldenseal]

raspberry, red; wild red raspberry *medicinal herb* [see: red raspberry]

raspberry [syrup] USP

rathyronine INN

rattleroot *medicinal herb* [see: black cohosh]

rattlesnake antivenin [see: antivenin (Crotalidae) polyvalent]

rattlesnake root *medicinal herb* [see: birthroot; black cohosh; senega]

rattleweed *medicinal herb* [see: black cohosh]

rauwolfia serpentina USP *antihypertensive; peripheral antiadrenergic; antipsychotic*

Rauzide tablets ℞ *antihypertensive; diuretic* [bendroflumethiazide; rauwolfia serpentina] 4•50 mg

Ravocaine & Novocaine with Levophed injection (discontinued 2002) ℞ *injectable local anesthetic for dental procedures* [propoxycaine HCl; procaine; norepinephrine bitartrate] 7.2•36•0.12 mg/1.8 mL

rayon, purified USAN, USP *surgical aid*

Razadyne film-coated tablets, oral drops ℞ *acetylcholinesterase inhibitor to increase cognition in Alzheimer disease* [galantamine hydrobromide] 4, 8, 12 mg; 4 mg/mL

Razadyne ER extended-release capsules ℞ *acetylcholinesterase inhibitor to increase cognition in Alzheimer disease* [galantamine hydrobromide] 8, 16, 24 mg

razinodil INN

razobazam INN

razoxane INN, BAN

⁸⁶Rb [see: rubidium chloride Rb 86]

rBPI (bactericidal and permeability-increasing protein, recombinant) [q.v.]

rCD4 (recombinant soluble human CD4) [see: CD4, recombinant soluble human]

RCF oral liquid OTC *hypoallergenic infant formula* [soy protein formula, carbohydrate free]

Reabilan; Reabilan HN ready-to-use oral liquid OTC *enteral nutritional therapy* [lactose-free formula]

Reactine ⓒ film-coated tablets, syrup ℞ *once-daily antihistamine* [cetirizine HCl] 5, 10, 20 mg; 5 mg/5 mL

reactrol [see: clemizole HCl]

rebamipide INN

Rebetol capsules, oral solution ℞ *nucleoside antiviral; combination therapy for chronic hepatitis C virus (HCV) infection* [ribavirin] 200 mg; 40 mg/mL

Rebetron capsules + subcu or IM injection ℞ *combination treatment for chronic hepatitis C* [Rebetol (ribavirin capsules); Intron A (interferon alfa-2b injection)] 200 mg•3 million IU

Rebif ⓒ powder for subcu injection ℞ *immunomodulator for relapsing remitting multiple sclerosis and condylomata acuminata* [interferon beta-1a] 3, 12 MIU/vial

Rebif prefilled syringes for subcu injection ℞ *immunomodulator for relapsing remitting multiple sclerosis (orphan); investigational (orphan) for malignant melanoma, metastatic renal cell carcinoma, T-cell lymphoma, and Kaposi sarcoma* [interferon beta-1a] 22, 44 μg (6, 12 MIU)/0.5 mL syringe

reboxetine INN *investigational (NDA filed) fast-acting selective norepinephrine reuptake inhibitor for depression*

reboxetine mesylate USAN *investigational (NDA filed) fast-acting selective norepinephrine reuptake inhibitor for depression*

recainam INN, BAN *antiarrhythmic* [also: recainam HCl]

recainam HCl USAN *antiarrhythmic* [also: recainam]

recainam tosylate USAN *antiarrhythmic*

recanescin [see: deserpidine]

Receptin ℞ *investigational (Phase II) antiviral for AIDS; orphan status withdrawn 1997* [CD4, recombinant soluble human]

reclazepam USAN, INN *sedative*

Reclomide tablets ℞ *antidopaminergic; antiemetic for chemotherapy; peristaltic* [metoclopramide HCl] 10 mg

Recombigen HIV-1 LA Test reagent kit for professional use *in vitro diagnostic aid for HIV-1 antibodies in*

blood, serum, or plasma [latex agglutination test]

recombinant alpha₁ antitrypsin [see: alpha₁ antitrypsin, recombinant]

recombinant antihemophilic factor [see: antihemophilic factor, recombinant]

recombinant factor VIIa [see: factor VIIa, recombinant]

recombinant factor VIII [see: antihemophilic factor, recombinant]

recombinant human activated protein C (rhAPC) [see: drotrecogan alfa]

recombinant human CD4 immunoglobulin G [CD4 immunoglobulin G, recombinant human]

recombinant human deoxyribonuclease (rhDNase) [see: dornase alfa]

recombinant human erythropoietin [see: erythropoietin, recombinant human]

recombinant human growth hormone (rhGH) [see: somatropin]

recombinant human interferon beta [see: interferon beta, recombinant human]

recombinant human interleukin-1 receptor (rhIL-1R; rhu IL-1R) [see: interleukin-1 receptor]

recombinant human monoclonal antibodies to vascular endothelial growth factor (rhuMAb-VEGF) [now: bevacizumab]

recombinant human superoxide dismutase (SOD) [see: superoxide dismutase, recombinant human]

recombinant interferon alfa-2a [see: interferon alfa-2a, recombinant]

recombinant interferon alfa-2b [see: interferon alfa-2b, recombinant]

recombinant interferon beta [see: interferon beta, recombinant]

recombinant interleukin-2 [see: interleukin-2, recombinant]

recombinant methionyl granulocyte CSF [see: methionyl granulocyte CSF, recombinant]

recombinant methionyl human granulocyte CSF [see: methionyl human granulocyte CSF, recombinant]

recombinant soluble human CD4 (rCD4) [see: CD4, recombinant soluble human]

recombinant tissue plasminogen activator (rtPA; rt-PA) [see: alteplase]

Recombinate powder for IV injection ℞ *antihemophilic to correct coagulation deficiency* [antihemophilic factor concentrate, recombinant] 250, 500, 1000 IU

Recombivax HB adult IM injection, pediatric/adolescent IM injection, dialysis formulation ℞ *active immunizing agent for hepatitis B and D* [hepatitis B virus vaccine, recombinant] 10 μg/mL; 5 μg/0.5 mL; 40 μg/mL

Rectacort rectal suppositories ℞ *corticosteroidal anti-inflammatory* [hydrocortisone acetate] 10%

Rectagene rectal suppositories OTC *temporary relief of hemorrhoidal symptoms* [live yeast cell derivative; shark liver oil] 2000 SRF U/oz.

Rectagene Medicated Rectal Balm ointment OTC *temporary relief of hemorrhoidal symptoms* [shark liver oil; phenyl mercuric nitrate; live yeast cell derivative] 3%•1:10 000•66.67 U/g

Rectolax suppositories OTC *stimulant laxative* [bisacodyl] 10 mg

red bay; red laurel *medicinal herb* [see: magnolia]

red bearberry *medicinal herb* [see: uva ursi]

red blood cells [see: blood cells, red]

red bush tea (Aspalathus contaminata; A. linearis; Borbonia pinifolia) leaves and stems *medicinal herb used as a free radical scavenger; investigational antineoplastic; investigational for preventing brain damage caused by aging*

red clover (Trifolium pratense) flower *medicinal herb for blood cleansing, bronchitis, cancer, clearing toxins, nervous disorders, and spasms*

Red Cross Toothache topical liquid OTC *oral analgesic* [eugenol] 85%

red currant *(Ribes rubrum) medicinal herb* [see: currant]

red elm *medicinal herb* [see: slippery elm]

red ferric oxide [see: ferric oxide, red]

red ink berries; red ink plant *medicinal herb* [see: pokeweed]

red laurel; red bay *medicinal herb* [see: magnolia]

red legs *medicinal herb* [see: bistort]

red mulberry *(Morus rubra) medicinal herb* [see: mulberry]

red oak *(Quercus rubra) medicinal herb* [see: white oak]

red paint root *medicinal herb* [see: bloodroot]

red pepper; African red pepper; American red pepper *medicinal herb* [see: cayenne]

red pimpernel *(Anagallis arvensis)* plant *medicinal herb used as a cholagogue, diaphoretic, diuretic, expectorant, nervine, purgative, and stimulant*

red puccoon *medicinal herb* [see: bloodroot]

red raspberry *(Rubus idaeus; R. strigosus)* leaves *medicinal herb for childbirth afterpains, diarrhea and other bowel disorders, fever, flu, morning sickness, menstrual disorders, mouth sores, nausea, and vomiting*

red root *medicinal herb* [see: bloodroot; danshen; New Jersey tea]

red sarsaparilla *medicinal herb* [see: sarsaparilla]

Red Throat Spray; Green Throat Spray OTC *topical antipruritic/counterirritant; mild local anesthetic* [phenol] 1.4%

red veterinarian petrolatum (RVP) [see: petrolatum]

red weed *medicinal herb* [see: pokeweed]

redberry *medicinal herb* [see: ginseng]

Redi Vial (trademarked packaging form) *dual-compartment vial*

Rediject (trademarked delivery system) *prefilled disposable syringe*

Redipak (trademarked packaging form) *unit dose or unit-of-issue package*

RediTabs (trademarked dosage form) *rapidly disintegrating tablets*

redmond clay (montmorillonite) *natural remedy for bug bites and stings and other skin problems*

Redutemp tablets OTC *analgesic; antipyretic* [acetaminophen] 500 mg

Reese's Pinworm soft gel capsules, oral liquid OTC *anthelmintic for ascariasis (roundworm) and enterobiasis (pinworm)* [pyrantel pamoate] 180 mg; 50 mg/mL

ReFacto powder for injection *anticoagulant for long-term treatment of hemophilia A and for surgical procedures (orphan)* [antihemophilic factor, recombinant]

Refensen Plus Severe Strength Cough & Cold Medicine caplets OTC *decongestant; expectorant* [pseudoephedrine HCl; guaifenesin] 60•400 mg

Refludan powder for IV injection *anticoagulant for heparin-associated thrombocytopenia (HAT) (orphan)* [lepirudin] 50 mg

Refresh eye drops OTC *ophthalmic moisturizer/lubricant* [polyvinyl alcohol] 1.4%

Refresh Plus; Refresh Tears eye drops OTC *ophthalmic moisturizer/lubricant* [carboxymethylcellulose] 0.5%

Refresh P.M. ophthalmic ointment OTC *ocular moisturizer/lubricant* [white petrolatum; mineral oil; lanolin]

refrigerants *a class of agents that lower abnormal body heat (a term used in folk medicine)*

regadenoson *investigational (Phase III) myocardial perfusion imaging agent*

Rēgain snack bar OTC *enteral nutritional therapy for impaired renal function* [multiple essential amino acids] ⊠ Rogaine

Regitine IV or IM injection (discontinued 2004) ℞ *antihypertensive for pheochromocytoma; α-blocker* [phentolamine mesylate] 5 mg/mL

Reglan syrup (discontinued 2004) ℞ *antidopaminergic; antiemetic for chemotherapy; peristaltic* [metoclopramide HCl] 5 mg/5 mL ⊠ Regonol

Reglan tablets, IV infusion ℞ *antidopaminergic; antiemetic for chemotherapy; peristaltic* [metoclopramide HCl] 5, 10 mg; 5 mg/mL ⍰ Regonol

Regonol IM or IV injection (discontinued 2003) ℞ *cholinergic/anticholinesterase muscle stimulant; muscle relaxant reversal* [pyridostigmine bromide] 5 mg/mL ⍰ Reglan

regramostim USAN, INN *antineutropenic; hematopoietic stimulant; biologic response modifier; bone marrow stimulant*

Regranex gel ℞ *recombinant platelet-derived growth factor B for chronic diabetic foot ulcers* [becaplermin] 0.01%

Regroton tablets ℞ *antihypertensive; diuretic* [chlorthalidone; reserpine] 50•0.25 mg ⍰ Hygroton

Regular Iletin II vials for subcu injection (discontinued 2005) OTC *antidiabetic* [insulin (pork)] 100 U/mL

regulator, female *medicinal herb* [see: life root]

Regulax SS capsules OTC *laxative; stool softener* [docusate sodium] 100 mg

Reguloid powder OTC *bulk laxative* [psyllium hydrophilic mucilloid] 3.4 g/tsp.

Rehydralyte oral solution OTC *electrolyte replacement* [sodium, potassium, and chloride electrolytes]

reishi mushrooms body and stem *medicinal herb for AIDS, allergies, fatigue, heart problems, and insomnia*

Rejuva-A ⓒⒶⓃ cream ℞ *treatment for photodamaged skin* [tretinoin] 0.025%

Rejuvenex cream OTC *antioxidant, moisturizer, and sunscreen for the face*

Relafen film-coated tablets ℞ *antiarthritic; nonsteroidal anti-inflammatory drug (NSAID)* [nabumetone] 500, 750 mg

Relagesic tablets ℞ *analgesic; antihistaminic sleep aid* [acetaminophen; phenyltoloxamine citrate] 650•50 mg

relaxin *investigational (orphan) for progressive systemic sclerosis; investigational (Phase II/III) for scleroderma*

Release+ ⓒⒶⓃ capsules OTC *vitamin C/manganese supplement* [calcium ascorbate; manganese citrate] 30•1.25 mg

Release-Tabs (dosage form) *timed-release tablets*

Relenza Rotadisks (powder for oral inhalation, for use with Diskhaler device) *influenza neuraminidase inhibitor for the treatment of acute influenza types A and B* [zanamivir] 5 mg

Reliable Gentle Laxative delayed-release enteric-coated tablets, suppositories OTC *stimulant laxative* [bisacodyl] 5 mg; 10 mg

Relief eye drops OTC *topical ophthalmic decongestant* [phenylephrine HCl] 0.12%

relomycin USAN, INN *antibacterial*

Relora tablets, capsules OTC *dietary supplement to relieve stress and anxiety by reducing cortisol levels and increasing DHEA levels; adjunct to weight reduction* [Magnolia officinalis extract; Phellodendron amurense extract] 250 mg

Relpax film-coated tablets ℞ *vascular serotonin 5-HT$_{1B/1D/1F}$ receptor agonist for the acute treatment of migraine* [eletriptan hydrobromide] 24.2, 48.5 mg (=20, 40 mg base)

remacemide INN *neuroprotective anticonvulsant* [also: remacemide HCl]

remacemide HCl USAN *neuroprotective anticonvulsant* [also: remacemide]

Remeron coated tablets ℞ *tetracyclic antidepressant* [mirtazapine] 15, 30, 45 mg ⍰ Femiron

Remeron SolTabs (orally disintegrating tablets) ℞ *tetracyclic antidepressant* [mirtazapine] 15, 30, 45 mg

Remicade powder for IV infusion ℞ *anti-inflammatory for severe and fistulizing Crohn disease (orphan), rheumatoid and psoriatic arthritis, and ankylosing spondylitis; also used for psoriasis and juvenile arthritis* [infliximab] 100 mg

Remifemin Menopause tablets OTC *natural remedy for postmenopausal symptoms* [black cohosh (standardized extract)] 20 mg (1 mg triterpene glycosides)

remifentanil INN, BAN *short-acting narcotic analgesic for general anesthesia* [also: remifentanil HCl]

remifentanil HCl USAN *short-acting narcotic analgesic for general anesthesia* [also: remifentanil]

remikiren INN

Reminyl film-coated tablets, oral drops (name changed to **Razadyne** in 2005) ② Amaryl

remiprostol USAN, INN *antiulcerative*

Remodulin continuous subcu infusion, IV injection ℞ *prostacyclin analogue for pulmonary arterial hypertension (orphan) and peripheral vascular disease (PVD); investigational (Phase II) for critical limb ischemia (CLI)* [treprostinil sodium] 1, 2.5, 5, 10 mg/mL

remoxipride USAN, INN, BAN *antipsychotic*

remoxipride HCl USAN *antipsychotic*

Remular-S tablets ℞ *skeletal muscle relaxant* [chlorzoxazone] 250 mg

Remune ℞ *investigational (Phase III) immunostimulant theraccine adjunct for HIV* [HIV-1 immunogen, gp120-depleted, inactivated]

Renacidin powder for solution ℞ *bladder and catheter irrigant for apatite or struvite calculi (orphan)* [citric acid; D-gluconic acid lactone; magnesium hydroxycarbonate] 6.602•0.198•3.177 g/100 mL

Renacidin Irrigation solution ℞ *bladder and catheter irrigant for apatite or struvite calculi (orphan)* [citric acid; glucono-delta-lactone; magnesium carbonate]

Renagel capsules (discontinued 2004) ℞ *phosphate-binding polymer for hyperphosphatemia of end-stage renal disease (ESRD)* [sevelamer HCl] 403 mg

Renagel film-coated tablets ℞ *phosphate-binding polymer for hyperphosphatemia of end-stage renal disease (ESRD); also used for hyperuricemia in dialysis patients* [sevelamer HCl] 400, 800 mg

RenAmin IV infusion ℞ *nutritional therapy for renal failure* [multiple essential and nonessential amino acids; electrolytes]

renanolone INN

Renax film-coated caplets ℞ *nutritional therapy for azotemia (uremia)* [multiple vitamins & minerals; folic acid; biotin] ±•2.5•0.3 mg

Renese tablets (discontinued 2003) ℞ *diuretic; antihypertensive* [polythiazide] 1, 2, 4 mg

Renese-R tablets ℞ *antihypertensive; diuretic* [polythiazide; reserpine] 2•0.25 mg

rennet, cheese *medicinal herb* [see: bedstraw]

Reno-30 intracavitary instillation ℞ *radiopaque contrast medium for urological imaging* [diatrizoate meglumine (46.67% iodine)] 300 mg/mL (141 mg/mL)

RenoCal-76 injection ℞ *radiopaque contrast medium* [diatrizoate meglumine; diatrizoate sodium (48.7% total iodine)] 660•100 mg/mL (370 mg/mL)

Reno-Dip; Reno-60 injection ℞ *radiopaque contrast medium* [diatrizoate meglumine (46.67% iodine)] 300 mg/mL (141 mg/mL); 600 mg/mL (282 mg/mL)

Renografin-60 injection ℞ *radiopaque contrast medium* [diatrizoate meglumine; diatrizoate sodium (48.75% total iodine)] 520•80 mg/mL (292.5 mg/mL)

Renoquid tablets ℞ *broad-spectrum bacteriostatic* [sulfacytine] 250 mg

Renova cream ℞ *retinoid for photodamage, fine wrinkles, mottled hyperpigmentation, and roughness of facial skin* [tretinoin] 0.02%, 0.05%

Rentamine Pediatric oral suspension (discontinued 2002) ℞ *antitussive; decongestant; antihistamine* [carbetapentane tannate; phenylephrine tannate; ephedrine tannate; chlorpheniramine tannate] 30•5•5•4 mg/5 mL

rentiapril INN

ReNu solution OTC *rinsing/storage solution for soft contact lenses* [sodium chloride (preserved saline solution)]

ReNu Effervescent Enzymatic Cleaner; ReNu Thermal Enzymatic Cleaner tablets OTC *enzymatic cleaner for soft contact lenses* [subtilisin]

ReNu Multi-Purpose solution OTC *chemical disinfecting solution for soft contact lenses*

renytoline INN *anti-inflammatory* [also: paranyline HCl]

renytoline HCl [see: paranyline HCl]

renzapride INN, BAN

ReoPro IV injection ℞ *platelet aggregation inhibitor for PTCA and acute arterial occlusive disorders* [abciximab] 2 mg/mL

repaglinide USAN *oral antidiabetic agent that stimulates the release of insulin from the pancreas for type 2 diabetes*

Repan tablets ℞ *analgesic; barbiturate sedative* [acetaminophen; caffeine; butalbital] 325•40•50 mg ▣ Riopan

Repan CF caplets ℞ *analgesic; barbiturate sedative* [acetaminophen; butalbital] 650•50 mg

Repetab (trademarked dosage form) *extended-release tablet*

repirinast USAN, INN *antiallergic; antiasthmatic*

Replagal ℞ *investigational (NDA filed, orphan) enzyme replacement therapy for Fabry disease* [agalsidase alfa]

Replens vaginal gel OTC *lubricant* [glycerin; mineral oil]

Replete ready-to-use oral liquid OTC *enteral nutritional therapy* [lactose-free formula]

rEPO (recombinant erythropoietin) [see: epoetin alfa; epoetin beta]

Reposans-10 capsules (discontinued 2003) ℞ *benzodiazepine anxiolytic; sedative* [chlordiazepoxide HCl] 10 mg

repository corticotropin [see: corticotropin, repository]

Reprexain tablets ℞ *narcotic analgesic* [hydrocodone bitartrate; ibuprofen] 5•200 mg

repromicin USAN, INN *antibacterial*

Repronex powder for IM or subcu injection ℞ *ovulation stimulant for women; spermatogenesis stimulant for men* [menotropins] 75, 150 IU

reproterol INN, BAN *bronchodilator* [also: reproterol HCl]

reproterol HCl USAN *bronchodilator* [also: reproterol]

Requip film-coated tablets ℞ *dopamine agonist; antiparkinsonian; treatment for restless leg syndrome (RLS)* [ropinirole HCl] 0.25, 0.5, 1, 2, 4, 5 mg

Resaid sustained-release capsules (discontinued 2001) ℞ *decongestant; antihistamine* [phenylpropanolamine HCl; chlorpheniramine maleate] 75•12 mg

Rescaps-D S.R. sustained-release capsules (discontinued 2002) ℞ *antitussive; decongestant* [caramiphen edisylate; phenylpropanolamine HCl] 40•75 mg

rescimetol INN

rescinnamine NF, INN, BAN *antihypertensive; rauwolfia derivative*

Rescon oral liquid (discontinued 2001) OTC *decongestant; antihistamine* [phenylpropanolamine HCl; chlorpheniramine maleate] 12.5•2 mg/5 mL

Rescon 12-Hour sustained-release capsules (discontinued 2003) ℞ *decongestant; antihistamine* [pseudoephedrine HCl; chlorpheniramine maleate] 120•12 mg

Rescon-DM oral liquid OTC *antitussive; decongestant; antihistamine* [dextromethorphan hydrobromide; pseudoephedrine HCl; chlorpheniramine maleate] 30•60•4 mg/10 mL

Rescon-ED controlled-release capsules (discontinued 2002) ℞ *decongestant; antihistamine* [pseudoephedrine HCl; chlorpheniramine maleate] 120•8 mg

Rescon-GG oral liquid OTC *decongestant; expectorant* [phenylephrine HCl; guaifenesin] 10•200 mg/10 mL

Rescon-Jr. sustained-release pediatric caplets ℞ *decongestant; antihistamine*

[phenylephrine HCl; chlorpheniramine maleate] 20•4 mg

Rescon-MX sustained-release tablets
℞ *decongestant; antihistamine; anticholinergic to dry mucosal secretions*
[phenylephrine HCl; chlorpheniramine maleate; methscopolamine
nitrate] 40•8•2.5 mg

Rescriptor tablets ℞ *antiretroviral; non-
nucleoside reverse transcriptase inhibitor (NNRTI) for HIV-1 infection*
[delavirdine mesylate] 100, 200 mg

Rescue Pak (trademarked dosage
form) *unit dose package*

Rescula eye drops (discontinued 2005)
℞ *prostaglandin $F_{2\alpha}$ analogue for glaucoma and ocular hypertension* [uno-
prostone isopropyl] 0.15%

Resectisol solution ℞ *genitourinary
irrigant* [mannitol] 5 g/100 mL

reserpine USP, INN *antihypertensive;
peripheral antiadrenergic; rauwolfia
derivative* 0.1, 0.25 mg oral

resibufogenin [see: bufogenin]

Resinol ointment (discontinued 2003)
OTC *poison ivy treatment* [calamine;
zinc oxide; resorcinol] 6%•12%•2%

resocortol butyrate USAN *topical anti-
inflammatory*

Resol oral solution OTC *electrolyte
replacement* [sodium, potassium,
chloride, calcium, magnesium, and
phosphate electrolytes]

Resolve/GP solution OTC *cleaning
solution for hard or rigid gas permeable
contact lenses*

resorantel INN

resorcin [see: resorcinol]

resorcin acetate [see: resorcinol
monoacetate]

resorcin brown NF

resorcinol USP *keratolytic; antifungal*

resorcinol monoacetate USP *antiseborrheic; keratolytic*

**Resource; Resource Plus; Resource
Diabetic; Resource Just for Kids**
ready-to-use oral liquid OTC *enteral
nutritional therapy* [lactose-free formula]

ReSource Arginaid powder for oral
liquid OTC *arginine-rich enteral nutri-*

*tional therapy to speed recovery of pres-
sure ulcers, burns, or surgery*

Resource Fruit Beverage ready-to-
use oral liquid OTC *enteral nutritional
therapy* [whey protein–based] 237
mL/pkt.

Respa A.R. tablets ℞ *decongestant;
antihistamine; anticholinergic to dry
mucosal secretions* [pseudoephedrine
HCl; chlorpheniramine maleate; belladonna alkaloids] 90•8•0.024 mg

Respa-1st sustained-release tablets ℞
decongestant; expectorant [pseudo-
ephedrine HCl; guaifenesin] 58•600
mg

Respa-DM sustained-release tablets ℞
antitussive; expectorant [dextrometh-
orphan hydrobromide; guaifenesin]
28•600 mg

Respa-GF sustained-release tablets
(discontinued 2004) ℞ *expectorant*
[guaifenesin] 600 mg

Respahist sustained-release capsules ℞
decongestant; antihistamine [pseudo-
ephedrine HCl; brompheniramine
maleate] 60•6 mg

Respaire-60 SR; Respaire-120 SR
extended-release capsules ℞ *decongestant; expectorant* [pseudoephedrine
HCl; guaifenesin] 60•200 mg; 120•
250 mg

Respalor ready-to-use oral liquid OTC
*enteral nutritional therapy for pulmo-
nary problems*

Respbid sustained-release tablets (discontinued 2004) ℞ *antiasthmatic;
bronchodilator* [theophylline] 250,
500 mg

RespiGam IV infusion ℞ *preventative
for respiratory syncytial virus (RSV)
infections in high-risk infants (orphan);
investigational (orphan) treatment for
RSV* [respiratory syncytial virus
immune globulin (RSV-IG)] 2500
mg/dose (50 mg/mL)

Respihaler (trademarked delivery system) *oral inhalation aerosol*

RespiPak (trademarked packaging
form) *tablets in daily compliance packaging*

Respiracult-Strep culture paddles for professional use *in vitro diagnostic test for Group A streptococci from throat and nasopharyngeal sources*

respiratory syncytial virus immune globulin (RSV-IG) *preventative for respiratory syncytial virus (RSV) infections in high-risk infants (orphan); investigational (orphan) treatment for RSV*

Respirgard II (trademarked delivery system) *nebulizer*

Respules (trademarked delivery system) *single-dose ampule for inhalation*

Restasis eye drop emulsion ℞ *immunomodulator and anti-inflammatory to increase tear production in patients with Sjögren keratoconjunctivitis sicca (orphan)* [cyclosporine] 0.05%

restoratives a class of agents that promote a restoration of strength and vigor (a term used in folk medicine)

Restoril capsules ℞ *benzodiazepine sedative and hypnotic* [temazepam] 7.5, 15, 22.5, 30 mg ⊡ Risperdal; Vistaril; Zestril

Restylane subcu injection in prefilled syringes ℞ *dermal filler for deep wrinkles and facial folds* [hyaluronic acid] 20 mg/mL

Retaane eye drop suspension ℞ *investigational (NDA filed) angiostatic steroid for neovascularization of the eye to preserve vision in patients with wet age-related macular degeneration* [anecortave acetate]

Retavase powder for IV infusion ℞ *thrombolytic; tissue plasminogen activator (tPA) for acute myocardial infarction* [reteplase] 18.8 mg (10.8 IU)

retelliptine INN

reteplase USAN, INN *thrombolytic; tissue plasminogen activator (tPA) for acute myocardial infarction*

Retin-A cream, gel, topical liquid ℞ *keratolytic for acne* [tretinoin] 0.025%, 0.05%, 0.1% (0.01% available in Canada); 0.01%, 0.025%, 0.1%; 0.05%

Retin-A Micro gel ℞ *keratolytic for acne* [tretinoin] 0.04%, 0.1%

retinamide R-II *investigational (orphan) for myelodysplastic syndrome*

retinoic acid (all-*trans*-retinoic acid) [see: tretinoin]

9-*cis*-retinoic acid [see: alitretinoin]

13-*cis*-retinoic acid [see: isotretinoin]

retinoids a class of antineoplastics chemically related to vitamin A

Retinol cream OTC *moisturizer; emollient* [vitamin A] 100 000 IU

retinol INN, BAN *vitamin A₁*

Retinol-A cream OTC *moisturizer; emollient* [vitamin A palmitate] 10 000 IU/g

Retisert ocular implant ℞ *corticosteroidal anti-inflammatory for uveitis (orphan)* [fluocinolone acetonide] 0.59 mg

Retrovir film-coated tablets, capsules, syrup, IV injection ℞ *nucleoside antiviral for AIDS and AIDS-related complex (orphan), HIV infection, and to prevent maternal-fetal HIV transfer* [zidovudine] 300 mg; 100 mg; 50 mg/5 mL; 10 mg/mL

Revaproxyn (European name for U.S. product **Efaproxyn**)

Revatio tablets ℞ *phosphodiesterase type 5 (PDE5) inhibitor; selective vasodilator for pulmonary arterial hypertension (PAH)* [sildenafil citrate] 20 mg

Reveal Rapid HIV-1 Antibody Test kit for professional use *in vitro diagnostic aid for HIV-1 in blood*

revenast INN

Reversa UV with Cosmederm-7 ⒸⒶⓃ cream, lip balm OTC *moisturizer; emollient; exfoliant; anti-irritant* [glycolic acid; strontium chloride] 4%•⍰, 8%•⍰; 2%•⍰

reverse transcriptase (RT) inhibitors a class of antiretroviral drugs that inhibit the activity of reverse transcriptase in viral cells, preventing cell replication; subdivided into nucleoside (purine- or pyrimidine-based) and nonnucleoside types [reverse transcriptase is also known as DNA polymerase]

reversible proton pump inhibitors [see: proton pump inhibitors]

Reversol IV or IM injection ℞ *myasthenia gravis treatment; antidote to curare overdose* [edrophonium chloride] 10 mg/mL

Revex IV, IM, or subcu injection ℞ *narcotic antagonist; antidote to opioid overdose; postanesthesia "stir-up"* [nalmefene] 0.1, 1 mg/mL

Rēv-Eyes powder for eye drops ℞ *miotic to reverse iatrogenic mydriasis* [dapiprazole HCl] 0.5%

ReVia film-coated tablets ℞ *narcotic antagonist for opiate dependence or overdose (orphan) and alcoholism* [naltrexone HCl] 50 mg

Revimid ℞ *investigational (orphan) for multiple myeloma; investigational (Phase III) for malignant melanoma* [3-(4'-aminoisoindoline-1'-one)-1-piperidine-2,6-dione]

Revlimid ℞ *investigational (NDA filed) immunomodulator for blood transfusions in patients with myelodysplastic syndrome (MDS)* [lenalidomide]

revospirone INN, BAN

Rexigen Forte sustained-release capsules (discontinued 2001) ℞ *anorexiant; CNS stimulant* [phendimetrazine tartrate] 105 mg

Rexin-G IV injection ℞ *investigational (NDA filed, orphan) tumor-targeted gene therapy for pancreatic cancer*

Rexolate IM injection ℞ *analgesic; antipyretic; anti-inflammatory; antirheumatic* [sodium thiosalicylate] 50 mg/mL

Reyataz capsules ℞ *antiviral; protease inhibitor for HIV-1 infection* [atazanavir sulfate] 100, 150, 200 mg

Rezamid lotion OTC *topical acne treatment* [sulfur; resorcinol; alcohol] 5%•2%•28%

Rezipas ℞ *investigational (orphan) for ulcerative colitis* [aminosalicylic acid]

rGCR (recombinant glucocerebrosidase) [see: glucocerebrosidase, recombinant retroviral vector]

rG-CSF (recombinant granulocyte colony-stimulating factor) [see: lenograstim]

R-Gel OTC *topical analgesic* [capsaicin] 0.025%

R-Gen elixir ℞ *expectorant* [iodinated glycerol] 60 mg/5 mL

R-gene 10 IV injection ℞ *diagnostic aid for pituitary (growth hormone) function* [arginine HCl] 10% (950 mOsm/L)

RGG0853, E1A lipid complex *investigational (orphan) for advanced ovarian cancer*

rGM-CSF; rhGM-CSF; rhuGM-CSF (granulocyte-macrophage colony-stimulating factor) [q.v.]

Rhamnus cathartica; R. frangula medicinal herb [see: buckthorn]

Rhamnus purshiana medicinal herb [see: cascara sagrada]

rhAPC (recombinant human activated protein C) [see: drotrecogan alfa]

(rhATIII) recombinant human antithrombin III) [see: antithrombin III]

rHb1.1 (recombinant human hemoglobin) [see: hemoglobin, recombinant human]

rhDNase (recombinant human deoxyribonuclease) [see: dornase alfa]

Rheaban caplets (discontinued 2004) OTC *antidiarrheal; GI adsorbent* [activated attapulgite] 750 mg

rhenium *element (Re)*

Rheomacrodex IV infusion ℞ *plasma volume expander for shock due to hemorrhage, burns, or surgery* [dextran 40] 10%

rheotran (45) [see: dextran 45]

rhetinic acid [see: enoxolone]

Rheum palmatum medicinal herb [see: rhubarb]

Rheumatex slide tests for professional use *in vitro diagnostic aid for rheumatoid factor in the blood* ② Rheumatrex

rheumatism root *medicinal herb* [see: twin leaf; wild yam]

rheumatism weed *medicinal herb* [see: pipsissewa]

Rheumaton slide tests for professional use *in vitro diagnostic aid for rheumatoid factor in serum or synovial fluid*

Rheumatrex Dose Pack (tablets) ℞ *antimetabolite antineoplastic for leukemia; systemic antipsoriatic; antirheumatic; investigational (orphan) for juvenile rheumatoid arthritis* [methotrexate] 2.5 mg ⃞ Rheumatex

rhFSH (recombinant human follicle-stimulating hormone) [see: menotropins]

rhGH (recombinant human growth hormone) [see: somatropin]

rhIGF-1 (recombinant human insulin-like growth factor-1) [now: mecasermin]

rhIL-1R; rhu IL-1R (recombinant human interleukin-1 receptor) [see: interleukin-1 receptor]

rhIL-11 (recombinant human interleukin-11) [see: interleukin-11, recombinant human]

rhIL-12 (recombinant human interleukin-12) [see: interleukin-12]

Rhinall nasal spray, nose drops OTC *nasal decongestant* [phenylephrine HCl] 0.25%

Rhinaris Lubricating Mist nasal spray, nasal gel OTC *nasal moisturizer* [polyethylene glycol; propylene glycol] 15%•5%; 15%•20%

Rhinatate tablets (discontinued 2002) ℞ *decongestant; antihistamine* [phenylephrine tannate; chlorpheniramine tannate; pyrilamine tannate] 25•8•25 mg

Rhinatate Pediatric oral suspension ℞ *decongestant; antihistamine* [phenylephrine tannate; chlorpheniramine tannate; pyrilamine tannate] 5•2•12.5 mg/5 mL

Rhinatate-NF Pediatric oral suspension ℞ *decongestant; antihistamine* [phenylephrine tannate; chlorpheniramine tannate] 5•4.5 mg/5 mL

Rhinocaps capsules (discontinued 2001) OTC *decongestant; analgesic; antipyretic* [phenylpropanolamine HCl; acetaminophen; aspirin] 20•162•162 mg

Rhinocort nasal inhalation aerosol (discontinued 2004) ℞ *corticosteroidal*

anti-inflammatory for seasonal or perennial rhinitis [budesonide] 32 μg/dose

Rhinocort Aqua nasal spray ℞ *corticosteroidal anti-inflammatory for seasonal or perennial rhinitis* [budesonide] 32 μg/dose

Rhinolar-EX; Rhinolar-EX 12 sustained-release capsules (discontinued 2001) ℞ *decongestant; antihistamine* [phenylpropanolamine HCl; chlorpheniramine maleate] 75•8 mg; 75•12 mg

Rhinosyn; Rhinosyn-PD oral liquid (discontinued 2002) OTC *decongestant; antihistamine* [pseudoephedrine HCl; chlorpheniramine maleate; alcohol] 60•4 mg/5 mL; 30•2 mg/5 mL

Rhinosyn-DM oral liquid (discontinued 2002) OTC *antitussive; decongestant; antihistamine* [dextromethorphan hydrobromide; pseudoephedrine HCl; chlorpheniramine maleate; alcohol 1.4%] 15•30•2 mg/5 mL

Rhinosyn-DMX syrup (discontinued 2002) OTC *antitussive; expectorant* [dextromethorphan hydrobromide; guaifenesin] 15•100 mg/5 mL

Rhinosyn-X oral liquid (discontinued 2002) OTC *antitussive; decongestant; expectorant* [dextromethorphan hydrobromide; pseudoephedrine HCl; guaifenesin; alcohol 7.5%] 10•30•100 mg/5 mL

$Rh_O(D)$ immune globulin USP *passive immunizing agent; treatment for immune thrombocytopenic purpura (orphan)*

$Rh_O(D)$ immune human globulin [now: $Rh_O(D)$ immune globulin]

rhodine [see: aspirin]

rhodium *element (Rh)*

Rho-Fluphenazine ⓒᴀɴ subcu or IM injection ℞ *conventional (typical) phenothiazine antipsychotic for schizophrenia and psychotic disorders; used for prolonged parenteral neuroleptic therapy* [fluphenazine decanoate] 25, 100 mg/mL

RhoGAM IM injection, prefilled syringes ℞ *obstetric Rh factor immunity*

suppressant [Rh$_O$(D) immune globulin (gamma globulin)] 300 μg (5%)

Rhophylac IM injection in prefilled syringes ℞ *obstetric Rh factor immunity suppressant* [Rh$_O$(D) immune globulin (gamma globulin)] 1500 IU (300 μg)

Rhoxal-amiodarone ⓒ tablets ℞ *antiarrhythmic for acute ventricular tachycardia and fibrillation (orphan)* [amiodarone HCl] 200 mg

Rhoxal-diltiazem CD ⓒ (once daily) sustained-release capsules ℞ *antihypertensive; antianginal; antiarrhythmic; calcium channel blocker* [diltiazem HCl] 120, 180, 240, 300 mg

Rhoxal-famotidine ⓒ film-coated tablets ℞ *histamine H$_2$ antagonist for gastric and duodenal ulcers* [famotidine] 20, 40 mg

Rhoxal-fluoxetine ⓒ capsules ℞ *selective serotonin reuptake inhibitor (SSRI) for depression, obsessive-compulsive disorder (OCD), and bulimia nervosa* [fluoxetine HCl] 10, 20 mg

Rhoxal-minocycline ⓒ capsules ℞ *tetracycline antibiotic* [minocycline HCl] 50, 100 mg

Rhoxal-orphenadrine ⓒ sustained-release tablets ℞ *skeletal muscle relaxant* [orphenadrine citrate] 100 mg

Rhoxal-oxaprozin ⓒ film-coated caplets ℞ *antiarthritic; nonsteroidal anti-inflammatory drug (NSAID)* [oxaprozin] 600 mg

Rhoxal-ranitidine ⓒ film-coated tablets ℞ *histamine H$_2$ antagonist for gastric and duodenal ulcers* [ranitidine HCl] 150, 300 mg

Rhoxal-ticlopidine ⓒ film-coated tablets ℞ *platelet aggregation inhibitor for stroke* [ticlopidine HCl] 250 mg

Rhoxal-timolol ⓒ eye drops ℞ *topical antiglaucoma agent (β-blocker)* [timolol maleate] 0.25%, 0.5%

Rhoxal-valproic ⓒ capsules, enteric-coated capsules ℞ *anticonvulsant* [valproic acid] 250 mg; 500 mg

rhubarb *(Rheum palmatum)* root *medicinal herb for colon and liver disorders*

Rhuli gel (discontinued 2003) OTC *poison ivy treatment* [benzyl alcohol; menthol; camphor] 2%•0.3%•0.3%

Rhuli spray (discontinued 2003) OTC *poison ivy treatment* [benzocaine; calamine; camphor] 5%•13.8%•0.7%

rhuMAb-E25 (recombinant human monoclonal antibodies E25) [now: omalizumab]

rhuMAb-VEGF (recombinant human monoclonal antibodies to vascular endothelial growth factor) [now: bevacizumab]

Rhus glabra medicinal herb [see: sumach]

Riba 3.0 SIA reagent kit for professional use *in vitro diagnostic aid for hepatitis C* [strip immunoblot assay (SIA)]

ribaminol USAN, INN *memory adjuvant*

Ribasphere pellet-filled capsules ℞ *nucleoside antiviral; combination therapy for chronic hepatitis C infection* [ribavirin] 200 mg

ribavirin USP, INN *nucleoside antiviral for severe lower respiratory tract infections; combination therapy for chronic hepatitis C infection; investigational (orphan) for hemorrhagic fever with renal syndrome* [also: tribavirin] 200 mg oral

Ribes nigrum; R. rubrum medicinal herb [see: currant]

ribgrass; ribwort medicinal herb [see: plantain]

riboflavin (vitamin B$_2$) USP, INN *water-soluble vitamin; enzyme cofactor* 50, 100 mg oral

riboflavin 5′-phosphate sodium USP *vitamin*

riboflavine [see: riboflavin]

riboprine USAN, INN *antineoplastic*

ribostamycin INN, BAN

riboxamide [see: tiazofurin]

ricainide [see: indecainide HCl]

rice bran oil (gamma oryzanol) extract *medicinal herb used as a hypolipidemic and to treat gastrointestinal and menopausal symptoms*

richweed *medicinal herb* [see: black cohosh; stone root]

ricin (blocked) conjugated murine monoclonal antibodies (MAb) (anti-MY9 MAb) *investigational (orphan) for myeloid leukemia (including AML), ex vivo treatment of autologous bone marrow in AML, and blast crisis in CML*

ricin (blocked) conjugated murine monoclonal antibodies (MAb) (CD6 MAb) *investigational (orphan) for T-cell leukemias, lymphomas, and other mature T-cell malignancies*

ricin (blocked) conjugated murine monoclonal antibodies (MAb) (N901 MAb) *investigational (orphan) for small cell lung cancer*

RID *shampoo, mousse (aerosol foam)* OTC *pediculicide for lice* [pyrethrins; piperonyl butoxide] 0.33%•4%

RID *topical liquid (discontinued 2003)* OTC *pediculicide for lice* [pyrethrins; piperonyl butoxide; petroleum distillate] 0.3%•3•1.2%

RID Pure Alternative *gel* OTC *pediculicide for lice* [dimethicone] 100%

Rid-A-Pain *gel* OTC *topical oral anesthetic* [benzocaine] 10%

Rid-A-Pain-HP *cream* OTC *analgesic; counterirritant* [capsaicin] 0.075%

Ridaura *capsules* ℞ *antirheumatic* [auranofin] 3 mg

ridazolol INN

RIDD (recombinant interleukin-2, dacarbazine, DDP) *chemotherapy protocol*

Ridenol *elixir* OTC *analgesic; antipyretic* [acetaminophen] 80 mg/5 mL

ridogrel USAN, INN, BAN *thromboxane synthetase inhibitor*

rifabutin USAN, INN *antiviral; antibacterial; for prevention of* Mycobacterium avium *complex (MAC) in advanced HIV patients (orphan)*

Rifadin *capsules, powder for IV injection* ℞ *tuberculostatic (orphan)* [rifampin] 150, 300 mg; 600 mg ⧉ Ritalin

rifalazil USAN *investigational (Phase II) rifampin derivative for* Mycobacterium

avium *complex (MAC) and* Mycobacterium tuberculosis

Rifamate *capsules* ℞ *tuberculostatic* [rifampin; isoniazid] 300•150 mg

rifametane USAN, INN *antibacterial*

rifamexil USAN *antibacterial*

rifamide USAN, INN *antibacterial*

rifampicin INN, BAN, JAN *antibacterial* [also: rifampin]

rifampin USAN, USP *antibacterial; antituberculosis agent (orphan)* [also: rifampicin] 150, 300 mg oral; 600 mg injection

rifampin & isoniazid & pyrazinamide *short-course treatment of tuberculosis (orphan)*

rifamycin INN, BAN

rifamycin diethylamide [see: rifamide]

rifamycin M-14 [see: rifamide]

rifapentine USAN, INN, BAN *antibacterial for tuberculosis (orphan); investigational (orphan) for AIDS-related* Mycobacterium avium *complex (MAC)*

Rifater *tablets* ℞ *short-course treatment for tuberculosis (orphan)* [rifampin; isoniazid; pyrazinamide] 120•50•300 mg

rifaxidin [see: rifaximin]

rifaximin USAN, INN *broad-spectrum rifamycin antibiotic for traveler's diarrhea; investigational (orphan) for hepatic encephalopathy*

rIFN-A (recombinant interferon alfa) [see: interferon alfa-2a, recombinant]

rIFN-α2 (recombinant interferon alfa-2) [see: interferon alfa-2b, recombinant]

rIFN-B (recombinant interferon beta) [see: interferon beta-1b, recombinant]

rIFN-beta *investigational (orphan) for malignant melanoma, metastatic renal cell carcinoma, T-cell lymphoma, and Kaposi sarcoma*

rifomycin [see: rifamycin]

RIG (rabies immune globulin) [q.v.]

rilapine INN

rilmazafone INN

rilmenidine INN

rilopirox INN

rilozarone INN

Rilutek film-coated tablets ℞ *amyotrophic lateral sclerosis (ALS) treatment (orphan); investigational (orphan) for Huntington disease; investigational (Phase III) for Parkinson disease* [riluzole] 50 mg

riluzole USAN, INN *amyotrophic lateral sclerosis (ALS) treatment (orphan); investigational (orphan) for Huntington disease; investigational (Phase III) for Parkinson disease*

Rimactane capsules ℞ *tuberculostatic* [rifampin] 300 mg

rimantadine INN *antiviral* [also: rimantadine HCl]

rimantadine HCl USAN *antiviral* [also: rimantadine]

rimazolium metilsulfate INN

rimcazole INN *antipsychotic* [also: rimcazole HCl]

rimcazole HCl USAN *antipsychotic* [also: rimcazole]

rimexolone USAN, INN, BAN *ophthalmic corticosteroidal anti-inflammatory*

rimiterol INN *bronchodilator* [also: rimiterol hydrobromide]

rimiterol hydrobromide USAN *bronchodilator* [also: rimiterol]

rimonabant *investigational (NDA filed) selective cannabinoid CB-1 blocker for smoking cessation, weight loss, increasing HDL, increasing insulin sensitivity, and decreasing C-reactive protein levels*

rimoprogin INN

Rimso-50 solution for bladder instillation ℞ *anti-inflammatory for symptomatic relief of interstitial cystitis* [dimethyl sulfoxide (DMSO)] 50%

Rinade B.I.D. sustained-release capsules (discontinued 2004) ℞ *decongestant; antihistamine* [pseudoephedrine HCl; chlorpheniramine maleate] 120•8 mg

Ringer injection USP *fluid and electrolyte replenisher* [also: compound solution of sodium chloride]

Ringer injection, lactated USP *fluid and electrolyte replenisher; systemic*

alkalizer [also: compound solution of sodium lactate]

Ringer irrigation USP *irrigation solution*

Ringer solution [now: Ringer irrigation]

riodipine INN

Riomet oral liquid ℞ *biguanide antidiabetic* [metformin HCl] 500 mg/5 mL

Riopan oral suspension OTC *antacid* [magaldrate] 540 mg/5 mL

Riopan Plus chewable tablets, oral suspension OTC *antacid; antiflatulent* [magaldrate; simethicone] 480•20, 1080•20 mg; 540•40, 1080•40 mg/5 mL

rioprostil USAN, INN *gastric antisecretory*

ripazepam USAN, INN *minor tranquilizer*

ripple grass *medicinal herb* [see: plantain]

Riquent ℞ *investigational (NDA filed, orphan) immunosuppressant for lupus-associated nephritis* [abetimus sodium]

risedronate sodium USAN *bisphosphonate bone resorption inhibitor for osteoporosis and Paget disease* 5, 30, 35 mg oral

rismorelin porcine USAN *growth stimulant for growth hormone deficiencies*

risocaine USAN, INN *local anesthetic*

risotilide HCl USAN *antiarrhythmic*

Risperdal tablets, M-Tabs (orally disintegrating tablets), oral drops ℞ *novel (atypical) benzisoxazole antipsychotic for schizophrenia and manic episodes of a bipolar disorder; also used for pediatric behavioral problems and autism, OCD, and agitation or psychosis due to Parkinson or Alzheimer disease* [risperidone] 0.25, 0.5, 1, 2, 3, 4 mg; 0.5, 1, 2 mg; 1 mg/mL ⊘ Restoril

Risperdal Consta long-acting injection ℞ *novel (atypical) benzisoxazole antipsychotic for schizophrenia; also used for pediatric behavioral problems and autism, OCD, and psychosis due to Parkinson or Alzheimer disease* [risperidone (encapsulated in polymer microspheres)] 25, 37.5, 50 mg ⊘ Restoril

risperidone USAN, INN, BAN *novel (atypical) benzisoxazole antipsychotic for schizophrenia and manic episodes of a bipolar disorder; also used for pedi-*

atric behavioral problems and autism, OCD, and agitation or psychosis due to Parkinson or Alzheimer disease

ristianol INN, BAN *immunoregulator* [also: ristianol phosphate]

ristianol phosphate USAN *immunoregulator* [also: ristianol]

ristocetin USP, INN, BAN

Ritadex (name changed to Focalin upon marketing release in 2001)

Ritalin tablets ℞ *CNS stimulant for attention-deficit hyperactivity disorder (ADHD) and narcolepsy; also abused as a street drug* [methylphenidate HCl] 5, 10, 20 mg ⑨ Ismelin; Rifadin

Ritalin LA dual-release capsules ℞ *CNS stimulant for attention-deficit hyperactivity disorder (ADHD)* [methylphenidate HCl] 10, 20, 30, 40 mg (50% immediate release, 50% delayed release)

Ritalin SR sustained-release tablets ℞ *CNS stimulant for attention-deficit hyperactivity disorder (ADHD) and narcolepsy* [methylphenidate HCl] 20 mg

ritanserin USAN, INN, BAN *investigational serotonin S_2 antagonist for various psychiatric illnesses and substance abuse*

ritiometan INN

ritodrine USAN, INN *smooth muscle relaxant*

ritodrine HCl USAN, USP *smooth muscle relaxant; uterine relaxant to arrest preterm labor* 10, 15 mg/mL injection

Ritodrine HCl in 5% Dextrose IV infusion in 500 mL LifeCare bags ℞ *uterine relaxant to arrest preterm labor* [ritodrine HCl; dextrose] 0.03% • 5%

ritolukast USAN, INN *antiasthmatic; leukotriene antagonist*

ritonavir USAN, INN *antiviral protease inhibitor for HIV infection*

ritropirronium bromide INN

ritrosulfan INN

Rituxan IV infusion ℞ *monoclonal antibody for non-Hodgkin B-cell lymphoma (orphan); investigational (Phase III) for rheumatoid arthritis and chronic lymphocytic leukemia* [rituximab] 10 mg/mL

rituximab USAN *monoclonal antibody for non-Hodgkin B-cell lymphoma (orphan); investigational (Phase III) for rheumatoid arthritis and chronic lymphocytic leukemia*

Riva-Diclofenac ⒸⒶⓃ enteric-coated tablets ℞ *analgesic; antiarthritic; nonsteroidal anti-inflammatory drug (NSAID)* [diclofenac sodium] 50 mg

Riva-Diclofenac-K ⒸⒶⓃ film-coated slow-release tablets ℞ *analgesic; antiarthritic; nonsteroidal anti-inflammatory drug (NSAID)* [diclofenac potassium] 75 mg

Riva-Loperamide ⒸⒶⓃ caplets OTC *antidiarrheal* [loperamide HCl] 2 mg

Riva-Lorazepam ⒸⒶⓃ tablets ℞ *benzodiazepine anxiolytic* [lorazepam] 0.5, 1, 2 mg

Riva-Naproxen ⒸⒶⓃ tablets ℞ *analgesic; antiarthritic; nonsteroidal anti-inflammatory drug (NSAID)* [naproxen] 250, 375, 500 mg

Riva-Norfloxacin ⒸⒶⓃ film-coated tablets ℞ *broad-spectrum fluoroquinolone antibiotic* [norfloxacin] 400 mg

rivastigmine USAN *acetylcholinesterase inhibitor to increase cognition in Alzheimer disease*

rivastigmine tartrate *acetylcholinesterase inhibitor to increase cognition in Alzheimer disease*

rivoglitazone USAN *antidiabetic for type 2 diabetes*

rizatriptan benzoate USAN *vascular serotonin $5\text{-HT}_{1B/1D}$ receptor agonist for the acute treatment of migraine*

rizatriptan sulfate USAN *vascular serotonin $5\text{-HT}_{1B/1D}$ receptor agonist for the acute treatment of migraine*

rizolipase INN

r-metHuLeptin [see: metreleptin]

RMP-7 (receptor-mediated permeabilizer) [see: lobradimil]

RMS suppositories ℞ *narcotic analgesic* [morphine sulfate] 5, 10, 20, 30 mg

rNPA (recombinant novel plasminogen activator) [see: novel plasminogen activator]

rob elder *medicinal herb* [see: elder-berry]

Robafen AC Cough syrup (discontinued 2002) ℞ *narcotic antitussive; expectorant* [codeine phosphate; guaifenesin; alcohol 3.5%] 10•100 mg/5 mL

Robafen CF oral liquid (discontinued 2002) OTC *antitussive; decongestant; expectorant* [dextromethorphan hydrobromide; phenylpropanolamine HCl; guaifenesin] 10•12.5•100 mg/5 mL

Robafen DAC syrup (discontinued 2002) ℞ *narcotic antitussive; decongestant; expectorant* [codeine phosphate; pseudoephedrine HCl; guaifenesin; alcohol 1.4%] 10•30•100 mg/5 mL

Robafen DM syrup (discontinued 2002) OTC *antitussive; expectorant* [dextromethorphan hydrobromide; guaifenesin; alcohol 1.4%] 10•100 mg/5 mL

Robafen PE oral liquid OTC *decongestant; expectorant* [pseudoephedrine HCl; guaifenesin] 60•200 mg/10 mL

RoBathol Bath Oil OTC *bath emollient*

Robaxin tablets, IV or IM injection ℞ *skeletal muscle relaxant* [methocarbamol] 500, 750 mg; 100 mg/mL

Robaxisal tablets (discontinued 2004) ℞ *skeletal muscle relaxant; analgesic* [methocarbamol; aspirin] 400•325 mg ⧉ Robaxacet

robenidine INN *coccidiostat for poultry* [also: robenidine HCl]

robenidine HCl USAN *coccidiostat for poultry* [also: robenidine]

Robicap (trademarked dosage form) *capsule*

Robinul tablets, IV or IM injection ℞ *GI antispasmodic; anticholinergic; peptic ulcer treatment adjunct; antisecretory* [glycopyrrolate] 1 mg; 0.2 mg/5 mL

Robinul Forte tablets ℞ *GI antispasmodic; anticholinergic; peptic ulcer treatment adjunct; antisecretory* [glycopyrrolate] 2 mg

Robitab (trademarked dosage form) *tablet*

Robitussin oral liquid OTC *expectorant* [guaifenesin] 100 mg/5 mL

Robitussin A-C syrup (discontinued 2002) ℞ *narcotic antitussive; expectorant* [codeine phosphate; guaifenesin; alcohol 3.5%] 10•100 mg/5 mL

Robitussin Allergy & Cough oral liquid OTC *antitussive; decongestant; antihistamine* [dextromethorphan hydrobromide; pseudoephedrine HCl; brompheniramine maleate] 20•60•4 mg/10 mL

Robitussin Cold, Cold & Congestion caplets, softgels OTC *antitussive; decongestant; expectorant* [dextromethorphan hydrobromide; pseudoephedrine HCl; guaifenesin] 10•30•200 mg

Robitussin Cold, Cold & Cough softgels OTC *antitussive; decongestant; expectorant* [dextromethorphan hydrobromide; pseudoephedrine HCl; guaifenesin] 10•30•200 mg

Robitussin Cold, Multi-Symptom Cold & Flu caplets, softgels OTC *antitussive; decongestant; expectorant; analgesic* [dextromethorphan hydrobromide; pseudoephedrine HCl; guaifenesin; acetaminophen] 10•30•200•325 mg; 10•30•100•250 mg

Robitussin Cold, Sinus & Congestion caplets OTC *decongestant; expectorant; analgesic* [pseudoephedrine HCl; guaifenesin; acetaminophen] 30•200•325 mg

Robitussin Cough oral liquid OTC *antitussive* [dextromethorphan hydrobromide; alcohol 1.4%] 15 mg/5 mL

Robitussin Cough Calmers lozenges (discontinued 2002) OTC *antitussive* [dextromethorphan hydrobromide] 5 mg

Robitussin Cough & Cold infant oral drops OTC *antitussive; decongestant; expectorant* [dextromethorphan hydrobromide; pseudoephedrine HCl; guaifenesin] 5•15•100 mg/2.5 mL

Robitussin Cough & Cold; Robitussin Honey Cough & Cold; Robitussin Pediatric Cough & Cold Formula oral liquid OTC *antitussive;*

decongestant [dextromethorphan hydrobromide; pseudoephedrine HCl] 30•60 mg/10 mL; 30•60 mg/ 15 mL; 7.5•15 mg/5 mL

Robitussin Cough & Congestion Formula oral liquid OTC *antitussive; expectorant* [dextromethorphan hydrobromide; guaifenesin] 20•400 mg/10 mL

Robitussin Cough Drops lozenge OTC *analgesic; mild local anesthetic* [menthol] 7.4, 10 mg

Robitussin CoughGels liquid-filled gelcaps OTC *antitussive* [dextromethorphan hydrobromide] 15 mg

Robitussin Flu oral liquid OTC *antitussive; decongestant; antihistamine; analgesic* [dextromethorphan hydrobromide; pseudoephedrine HCl; chlorpheniramine maleate; acetaminophen] 20•60•4•640 mg/20 mL

Robitussin Honey Cough DM ⒸⒶⓃ honey-based syrup OTC *antitussive* [dextromethorphan hydrobromide] 10 mg/5 mL

Robitussin Honey Flu Multi-Symptom Relief oral liquid OTC *antitussive; decongestant; analgesic* [dextromethorphan hydrobromide; pseudoephedrine HCl; acetaminophen] 20•60•500 mg/15 mL

Robitussin Honey Flu Nighttime syrup OTC *antitussive; decongestant; antihistamine; analgesic* [dextromethorphan hydrobromide; pseudoephedrine HCl; chlorpheniramine maleate; acetaminophen] 20•60•4•500 mg/pouch

Robitussin Honey Flu Non-Drowsy syrup for oral solution OTC *antitussive; decongestant; analgesic* [dextromethorphan hydrobromide; pseudoephedrine HCl; acetaminophen] 20•60•500 mg/pouch

Robitussin Liquid Center Cough Drops lozenges OTC *topical analgesic; counterirritant; mild local anesthetic* [menthol] 10 mg

Robitussin Night Relief oral liquid OTC *antitussive; decongestant; antihis-*

tamine; analgesic [dextromethorphan hydrobromide; pseudoephedrine HCl; pyrilamine maleate; acetaminophen] 30•60•50•650 mg/30 mL

Robitussin Pediatric Cough oral liquid OTC *antitussive* [dextromethorphan hydrobromide] 7.5 mg/5 mL

Robitussin Pediatric Night Relief Cough & Cold; Robitussin PM Cough & Cold oral liquid OTC *antitussive; decongestant; antihistamine* [dextromethorphan hydrobromide; pseudoephedrine HCl; chlorpheniramine maleate] 15•30•2 mg/10 mL

Robitussin Severe Congestion Liqui-Gels (liquid-filled softgels) OTC *decongestant; expectorant* [pseudoephedrine HCl; guaifenesin] 30•200 mg

Robitussin Sugar Free Cough oral liquid OTC *antitussive; expectorant* [dextromethorphan hydrobromide; guaifenesin] 20•200 mg/10 mL

Robitussin-CF oral liquid (discontinued 2002) OTC *antitussive; decongestant; expectorant* [dextromethorphan hydrobromide; phenylpropanolamine HCl; guaifenesin; alcohol 4.75%] 10•12.5•100 mg/5 mL

Robitussin-DAC syrup (discontinued 2002) ℞ *narcotic antitussive; decongestant; expectorant* [codeine phosphate; pseudoephedrine HCl; guaifenesin; alcohol 1.9%] 10•30•100 mg/5 mL

Robitussin-DM oral liquid, infants' oral drops OTC *antitussive; expectorant* [dextromethorphan hydrobromide; guaifenesin] 20•200 mg/10 mL; 5• 100 mg/2.5 mL

Robitussin-PE oral liquid OTC *decongestant; expectorant* [pseudoephedrine HCl; guaifenesin; alcohol 1.4%] 60• 200 mg/10 mL

Rocaltrol capsules, oral solution ℞ *vitamin D therapy for hypoparathyroidism and hypocalcemia of chronic renal dialysis; decreases severity of psoriatic lesions* [calcitriol] 0.25, 0.5 μg; 1 μg/mL

rocastine INN *antihistamine* [also: rocastine HCl]

rocastine HCl USAN *antihistamine* [also: rocastine]

Rocephin powder or frozen premix for IV or IM injection ℞ *cephalosporin antibiotic* [ceftriaxone sodium] 0.25, 0.5, 1, 2, 10 g

rochelle salt [see: potassium sodium tartrate]

rociverine INN

rock brake; rock polypod *medicinal herb* [see: female fern]

rock elm *medicinal herb* [see: slippery elm]

rock parsley *medicinal herb* [see: parsley]

rock rose *(Helianthemum canadense)* plant *medicinal herb used as an astringent and tonic*

Rocky Mountain grape *medicinal herb* [see: Oregon grape]

Rocky Mountain spotted fever vaccine USP

rocuronium bromide USAN, INN, BAN *nondepolarizing neuromuscular blocking agent; muscle relaxant; adjunct to general anesthesia*

rodocaine USAN, INN *local anesthetic*

rodorubicin INN

rofecoxib *analgesic; antiarthritic; antipyretic; COX-2 inhibitor; nonsteroidal anti-inflammatory drug (NSAID); treatment for acute migraine; withdrawn by the manufacturer in 2004 due to safety concerns*

rofelodine INN

Roferon-A subcu or IM injection in prefilled syringes ℞ *antineoplastic/antiviral for hairy cell leukemia, hepatitis C, Kaposi sarcoma (orphan), and chronic myelogenous leukemia (orphan); investigational (orphan) for renal cell carcinoma* [interferon alfa-2a] 3, 6, 9 million IU

roflumilast *investigational (Phase III) agent for chronic obstructive pulmonary disease (COPD) and asthma*

roflurane USAN, INN *inhalation anesthetic*

Rogaine for Men; Rogaine for Women topical solution OTC *hair growth stimulant* [minoxidil] 2%, 5%; 2% ⧉ Rēgain

rogletimide USAN, INN, BAN *antineoplastic; aromatase inhibitor*

Rohypnol (banned in the U.S.) ℞ *sedative and hypnotic; smuggled into the U.S. as a street drug, commonly called "roofies" or "the date rape drug"* [flunitrazepam]

rokitamycin INN

Rolaids; Calcium Rich Rolaids chewable tablets OTC *antacid* [magnesium hydroxide; calcium carbonate] 110•550, 135•675 mg; 80•412 mg

Rolaids Multi-Symptom chewable tablets OTC *antacid* [magnesium hydroxide; calcium carbonate; simethicone] 135•675•60 mg

Rolaids Softchews OTC *antacid; calcium supplement* [calcium carbonate] 1177 mg

Rolatuss Expectorant oral liquid (discontinued 2002) ℞ *narcotic antitussive; decongestant; antihistamine; expectorant* [codeine phosphate; phenylephrine HCl; chlorpheniramine maleate; ammonium chloride; alcohol 5%] 9.85•5•2•33.3 mg/5 mL

Rolatuss Plain oral liquid (discontinued 2002) OTC *decongestant; antihistamine* [phenylephrine HCl; chlorpheniramine maleate; alcohol 5%] 5•2 mg/5 mL

Rolatuss with Hydrocodone oral liquid (discontinued 2002) ℞ *narcotic antitussive; decongestant; antihistamine* [hydrocodone bitartrate; phenylpropanolamine HCl; phenylephrine HCl; pyrilamine maleate; pheniramine maleate] 1.7•3.3•5•3.3•3.3 mg/5 mL

Rolazar (name changed to **Alimta** upon marketing release in 2004)

roletamide USAN, INN *hypnotic*

rolgamidine USAN, INN, BAN *antidiarrheal*

rolicton [see: amisometradine]

rolicyclidine INN

rolicypram BAN *antidepressant* [also: rolicyprine]

rolicyprine USAN, INN *antidepressant* [also: rolicypram] rolipram USAN, INN *tranquilizer*

rolitetracycline USAN, USP, INN *antibacterial*

rolitetracycline nitrate USAN *antibacterial*

rolodine USAN, INN *skeletal muscle relaxant*

rolziracetam INN, BAN

Roman camomile *medicinal herb* [see: chamomile]

Roman laurel *medicinal herb* [see: laurel]

romazarit USAN, INN, BAN *anti-inflammatory; antirheumatic*

Romazicon IV injection ℞ *benzodiazepine antagonist to reverse anesthesia or treat overdose* [flumazenil] 0.1 mg/mL

rometin [see: clioquinol]

romifenone INN

romifidine INN

Romilar AC oral liquid ℞ *narcotic antitussive; expectorant* [codeine phosphate; guaifenesin] 20•200 mg/10 mL

romurtide INN

ronactolol INN

Rondamine-DM pediatric oral drops (discontinued 2002) ℞ *antitussive; decongestant; antihistamine* [dextromethorphan hydrobromide; pseudoephedrine HCl; carbinoxamine maleate] 4•25•2 mg/5 mL

Rondamine-DM syrup ℞ *pediatric antitussive, decongestant, and antihistamine* [dextromethorphan hydrobromide; pseudoephedrine HCl; brompheniramine maleate] 15•60•4 mg/5 mL

Rondec chewable tablets (discontinued 2002) ℞ *decongestant; antihistamine* [pseudoephedrine HCl; brompheniramine maleate] 60•4 mg

Rondec syrup ℞ *decongestant; antihistamine* [pseudoephedrine HCl; brompheniramine maleate] 45•4 mg/5 mL

Rondec tablets, pediatric oral drops ℞ *decongestant; antihistamine* [pseudoephedrine HCl; carbinoxamine maleate] 60•4 mg; 15•1 mg/mL

Rondec-DM pediatric oral drops ℞ *antitussive; decongestant; antihistamine* [dextromethorphan hydrobromide; pseudoephedrine HCl; carbinoxamine maleate] 4•15•1 mg/mL

Rondec-DM syrup ℞ *antitussive; decongestant; antihistamine* [dextromethorphan hydrobromide; pseudoephedrine HCl; brompheniramine maleate] 15•45•4 mg/5 mL

Rondec-TR timed-release tablets ℞ *decongestant; antihistamine* [pseudoephedrine HCl; carbinoxamine maleate] 120•8 mg

ronidazole USAN, INN *antiprotozoal*

ronifibrate INN

ronipamil INN

ronnel USAN *systemic insecticide* [also: fenclofos; fenchlorphos]

ropinirole INN, BAN *dopamine agonist; antiparkinsonian* [also: ropinirole HCl]

ropinirole HCl USAN *dopamine agonist; antiparkinsonian; treatment for restless leg syndrome (RLS)* [also: ropinirole]

ropitoin INN *antiarrhythmic* [also: ropitoin HCl]

ropitoin HCl USAN *antiarrhythmic* [also: ropitoin]

ropivacaine INN *long-acting injectable local anesthetic*

ropivacaine HCl *long-acting local or regional anesthetic for surgery; epidural block for cesarean section*

ropizine USAN, INN *anticonvulsant*

roquinimex USAN, INN *investigational (Phase II) immunomodulator for HIV; investigational for bone marrow transplant for leukemia*

Rosa acicularis; R. canina; R. rugosa and other species *medicinal herb* [see: rose]

Rosac cream ℞ *acne treatment* [sulfacetamide sodium; sulfur] 10%•5%

rosamicin [now: rosaramicin]

rosamicin butyrate [now: rosaramicin butyrate]

rosamicin propionate [now: rosaramicin propionate]

rosamicin sodium phosphate [now: rosaramicin sodium phosphate]

rosamicin stearate [now: rosaramicin stearate]

Rosanil cleanser ℞ *acne treatment* [sulfacetamide sodium; sulfur] 10%•5%
rosaprostol INN
rosaramicin USAN, INN *antibacterial*
rosaramicin butyrate USAN *antibacterial*
rosaramicin propionate USAN *antibacterial*
rosaramicin sodium phosphate USAN *antibacterial*
rosaramicin stearate USAN *antibacterial*
rosary pea *medicinal herb* [see: precatory bean]
rose (*Rosa acicularis; R. canina; R. rugosa* and other species) *flowers and hips medicinal herb for blood cleansing, cancer, colds, flu, infections, and sore throat; also used as a diuretic, mild laxative, and source of vitamin C*
rose, sun *medicinal herb* [see: rock rose]
rose bengal *diagnostic aid for corneal injury and pathology* 1.3 mg/strip
rose bengal sodium (^{131}I) INN *hepatic function test; radioactive agent* [also: rose bengal sodium I 131]
rose bengal sodium I 125 USAN *radioactive agent*
rose bengal sodium I 131 USAN, USP *hepatic function test; radioactive agent* [also: rose bengal sodium (^{131}I)]
rose laurel *medicinal herb* [see: mountain laurel]
rose oil NF *perfume*
rose petal aqueous infusion *ocular emollient*
rose water, stronger NF *perfume*
rose water ointment USP *emollient; ointment base*
rosemary (*Rosmarinus officinalis*) *leaves medicinal herb for flatulence, gastrointestinal spasm, halitosis, heart tonic, inducing diaphoresis, migraine headache, promoting menstrual flow, stimulating abortion, and stomach disorders*
Rosets *ophthalmic strips* OTC *diagnostic aid for corneal injury and pathology* [rose bengal] 1.3 mg
rosiglitazone maleate USAN *thiazolidinedione antidiabetic; increases cellular response to insulin without increasing insulin secretion* 2, 4, 8 mg oral

rosin USP
rosoxacin USAN, INN *antibacterial* [also: acrosoxacin]
rostaporfin USAN *investigational (Phase III) treatment for wet age-related macular degeneration (AMD) and other ophthalmic conditions*
rosterolone INN
Rosula *gel* ℞ *treatment for acne, rosacea, and seborrheic dermatitis* [sulfacetamide sodium; sulfur; urea] 10%•5%•10%
Rosula Aqueous Cleanser *topical liquid* ℞ *treatment for acne and rosacea* [sulfacetamide sodium; sulfur; urea] 10%•5%•10%
Rosula NS *cleansing pads* ℞ *treatment for acne and rosacea* [sulfacetamide sodium; urea] 10%•10%
rosuvastatin calcium USAN *HMG-CoA reductase inhibitor for hypercholesterolemia, mixed dyslipidemia, and hypertriglyceridemia*
Rotacaps (trademarked form) *encapsulated powder for inhalation*
Rotadisk (trademarked dosage form) *powder for inhalation* [used in a Diskhaler]
rotamicillin INN
Rotamune ℞ *investigational oral rotavirus vaccine*
RotateQ ℞ *investigational (NDA filed) live oral immunization against gastroenteritis* [rotavirus vaccine]
rotigotine *investigational (NDA filed) transdermal dopamine D$_2$ agonist for Parkinson disease and restless leg syndrome*
rotoxamine USAN, INN *antihistamine*
rotoxamine tartrate NF
rotraxate INN
round-leaved plantain *medicinal herb* [see: plantain]
rovelizumab USAN, INN *immunomodulator; investigational (Phase III) cell adhesion inhibitor for ischemic stroke, acute myocardial infarction, and trauma-induced hemorrhagic shock*
Rowasa *suppositories, rectal suspension enema* ℞ *anti-inflammatory for active*

ulcerative colitis, proctosigmoiditis, and proctitis [mesalamine (5-aminosalicylic acid)] 500 mg; 4 g/60 mL

roxadimate USAN, INN *sunscreen*

Roxanol; Roxanol T; Roxanol 100 oral concentrate R *narcotic analgesic* [morphine sulfate] 20 mg/mL; 20 mg/mL; 100 mg/5 mL

Roxanol Rescudose; Roxanol UD oral solution (discontinued 2001) R *narcotic analgesic* [morphine sulfate] 10 mg/2.5 mL; 10 mg/2.5 mL, 20 mg/5 mL, 30 mg/1.5 mL

roxarsone USAN, INN *antibacterial*

roxatidine INN, BAN *histamine H_2 antagonist for gastric and duodenal ulcers* [also: roxatidine acetate HCl]

roxatidine acetate HCl USAN *investigational (NDA filed) histamine H_2 antagonist for gastric and duodenal ulcers* [also: roxatidine]

roxibolone INN

Roxicet tablets, oral solution R *narcotic analgesic* [oxycodone HCl; acetaminophen] 5•325 mg; 5•325 mg/5 mL

Roxicet 5/500 caplets R *narcotic analgesic* [oxycodone HCl; acetaminophen] 5•500 mg

Roxicodone tablets, oral solution, Intensol (concentrated oral solution) R *narcotic analgesic* [oxycodone HCl] 5, 15, 30 mg; 5 mg/5 mL; 20 mg/mL ▣ oxycodone

roxifiban acetate USAN *antithrombotic; fibrinogen receptor antagonist*

Roxilox capsules R *narcotic analgesic* [oxycodone HCl; acetaminophen] 5•500 mg

Roxin R *investigational (NDA filed) histamine H_2 antagonist for duodenal and gastric ulcers* [roxatidine acetate HCl]

roxindole INN

Roxiprin tablets R *narcotic analgesic* [oxycodone HCl; oxycodone terephthalate; aspirin] 4.5•0.38•325 mg

roxithromycin USAN, INN *macrolide antibiotic*

roxolonium metilsulfate INN

roxoperone INN

royal jelly *natural remedy for improving fertility and increasing longevity*

Rozerem tablets R *melatonin MT-1 and MT-2 receptor antagonist for insomnia due to difficulty with sleep onset* [ramelteon] 8 mg

rPA; r-PA (recombinant plasminogen activator) *more properly called "recombinant tissue plasminogen activator" (rtPA)* [see: alteplase; anistreplase; lanoteplase; monteplase; reteplase; saruplase; tenecteplase]

R/S lotion OTC *topical acne treatment* [sulfur; resorcinol; alcohol] 5%•2%•28%

RSV-IG (respiratory syncytial virus immune globulin) [q.v.]

RT (reverse transcriptase) inhibitors [q.v.]

R-Tanna caplets R *decongestant; antihistamine* [phenylephrine tannate; chlorpheniramine tannate] 25•9 mg

R-Tanna 12 pediatric oral suspension R *decongestant; antihistamine* [phenylephrine tannate; pyrilamine tannate] 5•30 mg/5 mL

R-Tanna S Pediatric oral suspension R *decongestant; antihistamine* [phenylephrine tannate; chlorpheniramine tannate] 5•4.5 mg/5 mL

R-Tannamine tablets, pediatric oral suspension (discontinued 2002) R *decongestant; antihistamine* [phenylephrine tannate; chlorpheniramine tannate; pyrilamine tannate] 25•8•25 mg; 5•2•12.5 mg/5 mL

R-Tannate tablets, pediatric oral suspension (discontinued 2002) R *decongestant; antihistamine* [phenylephrine tannate; chlorpheniramine tannate; pyrilamine tannate] 25•8•25 mg; 5•2•12.5 mg/5 mL

R-Tannic-S A/D pediatric oral suspension (discontinued 2004) R *decongestant; antihistamine* [phenylephrine tannate; pyrilamine tannate] 5•30 mg/5 mL

rtPA; rt-PA (recombinant tissue plasminogen activator) [see: alteplase; anistreplase; lanoteplase; monteplase; reteplase; saruplase; tenecteplase]

Rubazyme reagent kit for professional use *in vitro diagnostic aid for rubella virus IgG antibodies in serum* [enzyme immunoassay (EIA)]

rubbing alcohol [see: alcohol, rubbing]

rubbing isopropyl alcohol [see: isopropyl alcohol, rubbing]

rubefacients *a class of gentle local irritants that redden the skin by producing active or passive hyperemia*

rubella & mumps virus vaccine, live *active immunizing agent for rubella and mumps*

rubella virus vaccine, live USP *active immunizing agent for rubella*

rubeola vaccine [see: measles virus vaccine, live]

Rubex powder for IV injection (discontinued 2004) ℞ *anthracycline antibiotic antineoplastic* [doxorubicin HCl] 100 mg

rubidium *element (Rb)*

rubidium chloride Rb 82 USAN *radioactive diagnostic aid for cardiac disease*

rubidium chloride Rb 86 USAN *radioactive agent*

rubitecan USAN *topoisomerase I inhibitor; investigational (Phase III, orphan) for pancreatic cancer and pediatric HIV/AIDS infections*

Rubramin PC IM or subcu injection ℞ *hematinic; vitamin B_{12} supplement* [cyanocobalamin] 100, 1000 μg/mL

Rubus fructicosus; R. villosus medicinal herb [see: blackberry]

Rubus idaeus; R. strigosus medicinal herb [see: red raspberry]

rue (*Ruta bracteosa; R. graveolens; R. montana***)** plant *medicinal herb for cramps, hypertension, hysteria, muscle strains, neuralgia, nervous disorders, sciatica, stimulation of abortion and menstruation, tendon strains, and trauma*

rufinamide USAN, INN *anticonvulsant*

rufloxacin INN

rufocromomycin INN, BAN *antineoplastic* [also: streptonigrin]

Ru-lets M 500 film-coated tablets OTC *vitamin/mineral supplement* [multiple vitamins & minerals]

Rulid Ⓔ tablets ℞ *macrolide antibiotic* [roxithromycin] 150 mg

RuLox oral suspension OTC *antacid* [aluminum hydroxide; magnesium hydroxide] 225•200 mg/5 mL

RuLox #1; RuLox #2 chewable tablets (discontinued 2004) OTC *antacid* [aluminum hydroxide; magnesium hydroxide] 200•200 mg; 400•400 mg

RuLox Plus chewable tablets, oral suspension OTC *antacid; antiflatulent* [aluminum hydroxide; magnesium hydroxide; simethicone] 200•200•25 mg; 500•450•40 mg/5 mL

rum cherry medicinal herb [see: wild black cherry]

Rumex acetosa medicinal herb [see: sorrel]

Rumex crispus medicinal herb [see: yellow dock]

Rumex hymenosepalus medicinal herb [see: canaigre]

Rum-K oral liquid ℞ *potassium supplement* [potassium chloride] 30 mEq K/15 mL

ruplizumab USAN *treatment for immune thrombocytopenic purpura and systemic lupus erythematosus (SLE) (orphan)*

Ruscus aculeatus medicinal herb [see: butcher's broom]

rush, sweet medicinal herb [see: calamus]

Ruta bracteosa; R. graveolens; R. montana medicinal herb [see: rue]

rutamycin USAN, INN *antifungal*

ruthenium *element (Ru)*

rutin NF *a bioflavonoid (q.v.)* [also: rutoside]

rutoside INN [also: rutin]

ruvazone INN

RVA (rabies vaccine, adsorbed) [see: rabies vaccine]

RVP (red veterinarian petrolatum) [see: petrolatum]

RxPak; ℞Pak (trademarked form) *prescription package*

Rymed capsules (discontinued 2002) ℞ *decongestant; expectorant* [pseudoephedrine HCl; guaifenesin] 30•250 mg

Rymed oral liquid (discontinued 2002) OTC *decongestant; expectorant*

[pseudoephedrine HCl; guaifenesin; alcohol 1.4%] 30•100 mg/5 mL

Rymed-TR long-acting caplets (discontinued 2002) ℞ *decongestant; expectorant* [phenylpropanolamine HCl; guaifenesin] 75•400 mg

Ryna oral liquid OTC *decongestant; antihistamine* [pseudoephedrine HCl; chlorpheniramine maleate] 60•4 mg/10 mL

Ryna-12 caplets ℞ *decongestant; antihistamine* [phenylephrine tannate; pyrilamine tannate] 25•60 mg

Ryna-12 S pediatric oral suspension ℞ *decongestant; antihistamine* [phenylephrine tannate; pyrilamine tannate] 5•30 mg/5 mL

Ryna-12D S oral suspension ℞ *pediatric antitussive, decongestant, and antihistamine* [carbetapentane tannate; phenylephrine tannate; pyrilamine tannate] 30•5•30 mg/5 mL

Ryna-C oral liquid ℞ *narcotic antitussive; decongestant; antihistamine* [codeine phosphate; pseudoephedrine HCl; chlorpheniramine maleate] 20•60•4 mg/10 mL

Ryna-CX oral liquid (discontinued 2002) ℞ *narcotic antitussive; decongestant; expectorant* [codeine phosphate; pseudoephedrine HCl; guaifenesin] 10•30•100 mg/5 mL

Rynatan pediatric oral suspension ℞ *decongestant; antihistamine* [phenylephrine tannate; chlorpheniramine tannate; pyrilamine tannate] 5•2•12.5 mg/5 mL

Rynatan caplets ℞ *decongestant; antihistamine* [phenylephrine tannate; chlorpheniramine tannate] 25•9 mg

Rynatan-12 S oral suspension ℞ *pediatric decongestant and antihistamine* [phenylephrine tannate; pyrilamine tannate] 5•30 mg/5 mL

Rynatan-S oral suspension (discontinued 2002) ℞ *pediatric decongestant and antihistamine* [phenylephrine tannate; chlorpheniramine tannate; pyrilamine tannate] 5•2•12.5 mg/5 mL

Rynatuss tablets, pediatric oral suspension ℞ *antitussive; decongestant; antihistamine* [carbetapentane tannate; phenylephrine tannate; ephedrine tannate; chlorpheniramine tannate] 60•10•10•5 mg; 30•5•5•4 mg/5 mL

Rythmol film-coated tablets, extended-release capsules ℞ *antiarrhythmic* [propafenone HCl] 150, 225, 300 mg; 225, 325, 425 mg

S

S-2 solution for inhalation OTC *sympathomimetic bronchodilator* [racepinephrine HCl] 2.25%

35S [see: sodium sulfate S 35]

SA (salicylic acid) [q.v.]

SA (serum albumin) [see: albumin, human]

Sabatia angularis medicinal herb [see: American centaury]

Sab-Betaxolol Ⓒ eye drops ℞ *topical antiglaucoma agent (β-blocker)* [betaxolol HCl] 0.5%

sabcomeline HCl USAN *muscarinic receptor agonist for Alzheimer disease*

Sab-Cortimyxin Ⓒ ophthalmic ointment ℞ *topical ophthalmic corticosteroidal anti-inflammatory; antibiotic* [hydrocortisone; neomycin sulfate; polymyxin B sulfate] 1%•0.35%•10 000 U per mL

sabeluzole USAN, INN, BAN *anticonvulsant; antihypoxic*

Sabin vaccine [see: poliovirus vaccine, live oral]

Sabril (approved in 40 foreign countries) ℞ *investigational (NDA filed) anticonvulsant; investigational treat-*

*ment for cocaine and methamphet-
amine addictions* [vigabatrin]

saccharated ferric oxide JAN *hematinic* [also: iron sucrose]

**saccharated iron; saccharated iron
oxide** [see: iron sucrose; saccharated
ferric oxide]

saccharin NF *flavoring agent*

saccharin calcium USP *non-nutritive
sweetener*

saccharin sodium USP *non-nutritive
sweetener*

sacred bark *medicinal herb* [see: cascara sagrada]

sacrosidase USAN *enzyme replacement
therapy for congenital sucrase-isomaltase deficiency (orphan)*

S-adenosyl-ʟ-methionine (SAMe)
*natural amino acid derivative used to
treat depression and protect the liver
from toxic overload; regenerates liver
function and restores hepatic glutathione levels when taken with vitamins
B_6, B_{12}, and folic acid*

Saf-Clens spray OTC *wound cleanser*

Safe Tussin oral liquid OTC *antitussive;
expectorant* [dextromethorphan
hydrobromide; guaifenesin] 30•200
mg/10 mL

safflower (Cahamus tinctorius) *flowers medicinal herb for delirium, digestive disorders, fever, gout, inducing
sweating, jaundice, liver disorders, lowering cholesterol, promoting expectoration, uric acid build-up, and urinary
disorders*

safflower oil USP *oleaginous vehicle;
essential fatty acid supplement*

saffron (Crocus sativus) *flowers
medicinal herb for fever, gout, inducing
sweating, measles, rheumatism, scarlet
fever, and sedation; also used as an
aphrodisiac and expectorant*

saffron, American; bastard saffron
medicinal herb [see: safflower]

safingol USAN *antipsoriatic; antineoplastic adjunct*

safingol HCl USAN *antipsoriatic; antineoplastic adjunct*

safrole USP

sagackhomi *medicinal herb* [see: uva ursi]

**sage (Salvia lavandulaefolia; S. lyrata;
S. officinalis)** *leaves medicinal herb
for cough, diarrhea, dysmenorrhea,
fever, gastritis, gum and mouth sores,
memory improvement, nausea, nervous
disorders, and sore throat*

sailor's tobacco *medicinal herb* [see:
mugwort]

St. Benedict thistle *medicinal herb*
[see: blessed thistle]

St. James weed; St. James wort
medicinal herb [see: shepherd's purse]

**St. John's wort (Hypericum perfora-
tum)** *plant medicinal herb for AIDS,
antiviral therapy, anxiety, bronchitis,
cancer, childbirth afterpains, depression,
gastritis, insomnia, and skin disorders*

St. Joseph Adult Chewable Aspirin
chewable tablets OTC *analgesic; antipyretic; anti-inflammatory* [aspirin] 81 mg

St. Joseph Cold Tablets for Children
chewable tablets (discontinued 2001)
OTC *pediatric decongestant and analgesic* [phenylpropanolamine HCl; acet-
aminophen] 3.125•80 mg

St. Joseph Cough Suppressant syrup
(discontinued 2002) OTC *antitussive*
[dextromethorphan hydrobromide]
7.5 mg/5 mL

St. Josephwort *medicinal herb* [see: basil]

Saizen powder for subcu or IM injection, cool.click (needle-free subcu
injector) ℞ *growth hormone for adults
or children with congenital or endogenous growth hormone deficiency, children with Turner syndrome or renal-
induced growth failure, or AIDS-
wasting syndrome (orphan)* [somatro-
pin] 5 mg (15 IU) per vial

SalAc topical liquid OTC *keratolytic
cleanser for acne* [salicylic acid] 2%

salacetamide INN

salacetin [see: aspirin]

Sal-Acid plaster OTC *keratolytic* [sali-
cylic acid in a collodion-like vehi-
cle] 40%

Salactic Film topical liquid OTC *keratolytic* [salicylic acid in a collodion-
like vehicle] 17%

salafibrate INN

Salagen film-coated tablets ℞ *treatment of xerostomia and keratoconjunctivitis sicca due to radiotherapy or Sjögren syndrome (orphan); also for dry mouth* [pilocarpine HCl] 5, 7.5 mg

salantel USAN, INN *veterinary anthelmintic*

salazodine INN

Salazopyrin (European name for U.S. product Azulfidine)

salazosulfadimidine INN [also: salazosulphadimidine]

salazosulfamide INN

salazosulfapyridine JAN *broad-spectrum bacteriostatic; anti-inflammatory for ulcerative colitis; antirheumatic* [also: sulfasalazine; sulphasalazine]

salazosulfathiazole INN

salazosulphadimidine BAN [also: salazosulfadimidine]

salbutamol INN, BAN *sympathomimetic bronchodilator* [also: albuterol]

Salbutamol Nebuamp ⊛ *solution for nebulization* ℞ *sympathomimetic bronchodilator* [salbutamol sulfate] 2.5 mL/ampule

salbutamol sulfate JAN *sympathomimetic bronchodilator* [also: albuterol sulfate]

salcatonin BAN *synthetic analogue of calcitonin (salmon); calcium regulator; investigational osteoporosis treatment* [also: calcitonin salmon (synthesis)]

salcetogen [see: aspirin]

Sal-Clens Acne Cleanser gel OTC *keratolytic for acne* [salicylic acid] 2%

salcolex USAN, INN *analgesic; anti-inflammatory; antipyretic*

SalEst test kit for professional use *in vitro diagnostic aid for estriol levels in saliva, used to predict spontaneous preterm labor and delivery*

saletamide INN *analgesic* [also: salethamide maleate]

saletamide maleate [see: salethamide maleate]

salethamide maleate USAN *analgesic* [also: saletamide]

saletin [see: aspirin]

Saleto tablets OTC *analgesic; antipyretic; anti-inflammatory* [acetaminophen; aspirin; salicylamide; caffeine] 115•210•65•16 mg

Saleto CF tablets (discontinued 2002) OTC *antitussive; decongestant; analgesic* [dextromethorphan hydrobromide; phenylpropanolamine; acetaminophen] 10•12.5•325 mg

Saleto-D capsules (discontinued 2001) OTC *decongestant; analgesic; antipyretic* [phenylpropanolamine HCl; acetaminophen; salicylamide; caffeine] 18•240•120•16 mg

Salex cream ℞ *keratolytic for acne* [salicylic acid] 6%

Salflex film-coated tablets OTC *analgesic; antipyretic; anti-inflammatory; antirheumatic* [salsalate] 500, 750 mg

salfluverine INN

salicain [now: salicyl alcohol]

salicin USP

salicin willow *medicinal herb* [see: willow]

salicyl alcohol USAN *local anesthetic*

salicylamide USP *analgesic*

salicylanilide NF

salicylate meglumine USAN *antirheumatic; analgesic*

salicylates *a class of drugs that have analgesic, antipyretic, and anti-inflammatory effects*

salicylazosulfapyridine [now: sulfasalazine]

salicylic acid (SA) USP *keratolytic; antiseborrheic; antipsoriatic*

salicylic acid, bimolecular ester [see: salsalate]

salicylic acid acetate [see: aspirin]

Salicylic Acid and Sulfur Soap bar OTC *medicated cleanser for acne* [salicylic acid; precipitated sulfur] 3%•10%

Salicylic Acid Cleansing bar OTC *medicated cleanser for acne* [salicylic acid] 2%

salicylic acid dihydrogen phosphate [see: fosfosal]

salicylsalicylic acid [see: salsalate]

saligenin [now: salicyl alcohol]

saligenol [now: salicyl alcohol]

salinazid INN, BAN

saline, lactated potassic [see: potassic saline, lactated]

saline laxatives *a subclass of laxatives that work by attracting and retaining water in the intestines to increase intraluminal pressure and cholecystokinin release* [see also: laxatives]

saline solution (SS) [also: normal saline]

SalineX nasal mist, nose drops OTC *nasal moisturizer* [sodium chloride (saline solution)] 0.4%

saliniazid [see: salinazid]

salinomycin INN, BAN

Saliva Substitute oral solution OTC *saliva substitute*

Salivart oral spray OTC *saliva substitute*

Salix lozenges (discontinued 2003) OTC *saliva substitute*

Salix alba; S. caprea; S. nigra; S. purpurea medicinal herb [see: willow]

salmaterol [see: salmeterol]

salmefamol INN, BAN

salmeterol USAN, INN, BAN *sympathomimetic bronchodilator*

salmeterol xinafoate USAN *adrenergic; sympathomimetic bronchodilator* (base=69%)

salmisteine INN

salmon calcitonin [see: salcatonin]

Salmonella typhi **vaccine** [see: typhoid vaccine]

Salmonine subcu or IM injection ℞ *calcium regulator for hypercalcemia, Paget disease, and postmenopausal osteoporosis* [calcitonin (salmon)] 200 IU/mL

salmotin [see: adicillin]

salnacedin USAN *topical anti-inflammatory*

Salofalk ⒸⒶⓃ enteric-coated tablets ℞ *anti-inflammatory for acute ulcerative colitis and the prevention of Crohn disease relapse following bowel resection* [mesalamine (5-aminosalicylic acid)] 250, 500 mg

Salofalk ⒸⒶⓃ suppositories, rectal suspension enema ℞ *anti-inflammatory*

for distal ulcerative colitis (DUC) and ulcerative proctitis [mesalamine (5-aminosalicylic acid)] 250, 500 mg; 2, 4 g/58 mL

Sal-Oil-T hair dressing ℞ *antipsoriatic; antiseborrheic; keratolytic* [coal tar; salicylic acid] 10%•6%

salol [see: phenyl salicylate]

Sal-Plant gel OTC *keratolytic* [salicylic acid in a collodion-like vehicle] 17%

salprotoside INN

salsalate USAN, USP, INN, BAN *analgesic; antipyretic; anti-inflammatory; antirheumatic* 500, 750 mg oral

Salsitab film-coated tablets ℞ *analgesic; antipyretic; anti-inflammatory; antirheumatic* [salsalate] 500, 750 mg

salt [def.] *The inactive part of a compound, made by combining an acid with an alkali. In naproxen sodium, for example, the base is* naproxen *(an acid) and the salt is* sodium *(from sodium hydroxide, an alkali).* [compare to: base]

Sal-Tropine tablets ℞ *GI/GU antispasmodic; antiparkinsonian; anticholinergic "drying agent" for the respiratory tract; antidote to insecticide poisoning* [atropine sulfate] 0.4 mg

Saluron tablets ℞ *diuretic; antihypertensive* [hydroflumethiazide] 50 mg

Salutensin; Salutensin-Demi tablets ℞ *antihypertensive* [hydroflumethiazide; reserpine] 50•0.125 mg; 25•0.125 mg ⑨ Diutensen

saluzide [see: opiniazide]

salvarsan [see: arsphenamine]

salverine INN

Salvia lavandulaefolia; S. lyrata; S. officinalis medicinal herb [see: sage]

Salvia miltiorrhiza medicinal herb [see: danshen]

samarium *element (Sm)*

samarium Sm 153 EDTMP (ethylenediaminetetramethylenephosphoric acid) [see: samarium Sm 153 lexidronam]

samarium Sm 153 lexidronam USAN *radiopharmaceutical for treat-*

ment of bone pain from osteoblastic metastatic tumors

Sambucus canadensis; S. ebulus; S. nigra; S. racemosa *medicinal herb* [see: elder flower; elderberry]

SAMe (S-adenosyl-L-methionine) [q.v.]

Sanchi ginseng (Panax pseudoginseng) *medicinal herb* [see: ginseng]

Sanctura film-coated tablets ℞ *urinary antispasmodic; muscarinic receptor antagonist for urinary frequency, urgency, and incontinence* [trospium chloride] 20 mg

sancycline USAN, INN *antibacterial*

sandalwood (Santalum album) oil *medicinal herb for headache, stomach ache, and urogenital disorders; also used topically as an antiseptic and astringent*

Sandimmune gelcaps, oral solution, IV injection ℞ *immunosuppressant for allogenic kidney, liver, and heart transplants (orphan)* [cyclosporine] 25, 100 mg; 100 mg/mL; 50 mg/mL

Sandimmune ophthalmic ointment ℞ *investigational (orphan) for keratoconjunctivitis sicca, keratoplasty graft rejection, and corneal melting syndrome* [cyclosporine] 2%

Sandimmune Neoral ⓐⓜ soft gels, oral solution [see: Neoral]

Sandoglobulin powder for IV infusion (discontinued 2003) ℞ *passive immunizing agent for HIV and idiopathic thrombocytopenic purpura (ITP)* [immune globulin] 1, 3, 6, 12 g

SandoPak (trademarked packaging form) *unit dose blister package*

Sandostatin subcu or IV injection ℞ *gastric antisecretory for acromegaly and severe diarrhea due to VIPomas and other tumors (orphan)* [octreotide acetate] 0.05, 0.1, 0.2, 0.5, 1 mg/mL ⑨ simvastatin; zinostatin

Sandostatin LAR Depot suspension for IM injection ℞ *gastric antisecretory for acromegaly and severe diarrhea due to VIPomas and other tumors (orphan)* [octreotide acetate]

sanfetrinem INN, BAN *antibacterial* [also: sanfetrinem sodium]

sanfetrinem cilexetil USAN *antibacterial*

sanfetrinem sodium USAN *antibacterial* [also: sanfetrinem]

SangCya oral solution (discontinued 2004) ℞ *immunosuppressive to prevent solid organ transplant rejection (orphan)* [cyclosporine; alcohol 10.5%] 100 mg/mL

Sanguinaria canadensis *medicinal herb* [see: bloodroot]

sanguinarine chloride [now: sanguinarium chloride]

sanguinarium chloride USAN, INN *antifungal; antimicrobial; anti-inflammatory*

sanicle (Sanicula europea; S. marilandica) root *medicinal herb used as an astringent, expectorant, discutient, depurative, nervine, and vulnerary*

Sani-Pak (trademarked packaging form) *sanitary dispensing box*

Sani-Supp suppositories OTC *hyperosmolar laxative* [glycerin]

Sanorex tablets (discontinued 2001) ℞ *anorexiant; CNS stimulant; investigational (orphan) treatment for Duchenne muscular dystrophy* [mazindol] 1, 2 mg

Sansert tablets (discontinued 2002) ℞ *agent for migraine and vascular headaches* [methysergide maleate] 2 mg

Santalum album *medicinal herb* [see: sandalwood]

santonin NF

Santyl ointment ℞ *topical enzyme for biochemical debridement* [collagenase] 250 U/g

saperconazole USAN, INN, BAN *antifungal*

Saponaria officinalis *medicinal herb* [see: soapwort]

saprisartan INN, BAN *antihypertensive; angiotensin II antagonist* [also: saprisartan potassium]

saprisartan potassium USAN *antihypertensive; angiotensin II antagonist* [also: saprisartan]

sapropterin INN

sapropterin HCl *investigational (Phase III) oral treatment for mild to moderate phenylketonuria*

saquinavir USAN, INN, BAN *antiretroviral protease inhibitor for HIV infection* [also: saquinavir mesylate]

saquinavir mesylate USAN *antiretroviral protease inhibitor for HIV infection* [also: saquinavir]

Sarafem capsules ℞ *selective serotonin reuptake inhibitor (SSRI) for premenstrual dysphoric disorder (PMDD)* [fluoxetine HCl] 10, 20 mg

sarafloxacin INN, BAN *anti-infective; DNA gyrase inhibitor* [also: sarafloxacin HCl]

sarafloxacin HCl USAN *anti-infective; DNA gyrase inhibitor* [also: sarafloxacin]

saralasin INN *antihypertensive* [also: saralasin acetate]

saralasin acetate USAN *antihypertensive; investigational (Phase I/II) mouthwash for oral candidiasis* [also: saralasin]

Sarasar *investigational (Phase III) antineoplastic for lung cancer* [lonafarnib]

Saratoga ointment OTC *astringent; antiseptic; wound protectant* [zinc oxide; boric acid; eucalyptol]

sarcolysin INN

L-sarcolysin [see: melphalan]

Sardo Bath & Shower oil OTC *bath emollient*

Sardoettes towelettes OTC *moisturizer; emollient*

sargramostim USAN, INN, BAN *antineutropenic for bone marrow transplant and graft delay (orphan); investigational (Phase III) cytokine for HIV infection*

sarmazenil INN

sarmoxicillin USAN, INN *antibacterial*

Sarmustine ℞ *investigational (orphan) for malignant glioma* [2-chloroethyl-3-sarcosinamide-1-nitrosourea]

Sarna Anti-Itch foam, lotion OTC *topical analgesic; counterirritant* [camphor; menthol] 0.5%•0.5%

saroten [see: amitriptyline]

Sarothamnus scoparius *medicinal herb* [see: broom]

sarpicillin USAN, INN *antibacterial*

Sarracenia purpurea *medicinal herb* [see: pitcher plant]

sarsaparilla (Smilax spp.) root *medicinal herb for blood cleansing (binding and expulsion of endotoxins), joint aches including arthritis and rheumatism, hormonal disorders, skin diseases including leprosy and psoriasis, and syphilis*

saruplase INN *investigational (Phase III) prourokinase (pro-UK) clot-dissolving agent for stroke*

sassafras (Sassafras albidum; S. officinale) root and bark *medicinal herb for acne, blood cleansing, insect bites and stings, obesity, psoriasis, skin diseases, and water retention; not generally regarded as safe and effective and banned by the FDA as a carcinogen with other serious side effects*

sassafras, swamp *medicinal herb* [see: magnolia]

SAStid Soap bar OTC *medicated cleanser for acne* [precipitated sulfur] 10%

saterinone INN

satinflower *medicinal herb* [see: chickweed]

satoribine [now: isatoribine]

satranidazole INN

Satraplatin ℞ *investigational (Phase III) platinum agent for prostate cancer*

satraplatin USAN *antineoplastic*

satumomab INN, BAN *radiodiagnostic monoclonal antibody for ovarian and colorectal carcinoma* [also: indium In 111 satumomab pendetide]

satumomab pendetide [see: indium In 111 satumomab pendetide]

Satureja hortensis *medicinal herb* [see: summer savory]

Satureja montana; S. obovata *medicinal herb* [see: winter savory]

savory *medicinal herb* [see: summer savory; winter savory]

savoxepin INN

Savvy vaginal gel ℞ *investigational (Phase I/II) microbicide and spermicide for HIV infection*

saw palmetto (*Serenoa repens; S. serrulata*) berries *medicinal herb for benign prostatic hypertrophy (BPH) and genitourinary, glandular, and reproductive disorders; also used to enlarge breasts, increase sperm production, promote weight gain, and enhance sexual vigor*

saxifrage, burnet; European burnet saxifrage; small burnet saxifrage; small saxifrage *medicinal herb* [see: burnet]

saxifrax *medicinal herb* [see: sassafras]

SBR-Lipocream OTC *emollient for dry skin* [oil-in-water emulsion] 70% oil•30• water

SC (succinylcholine) [see: succinylcholine chlorine]

SCA proteins (single-chain antigen-binding proteins) *a class of investigational antineoplastics*

scabicides *a class of agents effective against scabies*

scabwort *medicinal herb* [see: elecampane]

Scadan scalp lotion OTC *antiseptic; antiseborrheic* [myristyltrimethylammonium bromide; stearyl dimethyl benzyl ammonium chloride] 1%•0.1%

Scalpicin topical liquid OTC *antiseborrheic* [salicylic acid] 3%

scaly dragon's claw *medicinal herb* [see: coral root]

scammony, wild *medicinal herb* [see: wild jalap]

scandium *element (Sc)*

Scar Cream OTC *to reduce the appearance of surgical scars; sunscreens* [octinoxate; octisalate] 7.5%•5%

scarlet bergamot *medicinal herb* [see: Oswego tea]

scarlet berry *medicinal herb* [see: bittersweet nightshade]

scarlet fever streptococcus toxin

scarlet red NF *promotes wound healing*

Scarlet Red Ointment Dressings medication-impregnated gauze ℞ *wound dressing; vulnerary* [scarlet red] 5%

scarlet sumach *medicinal herb* [see: sumach]

SCCS (simethicone-coated cellulose suspension) [see: SonoRx]

sCD4-PE40 [see: alvircept sudotox]

Sceletium tortuosum *medicinal herb* [see: kanna]

SCF (stem cell factor) [q.v.]

Schamberg lotion OTC *topical analgesic; antiseptic; astringent; antifungal; counterirritant* [zinc oxide; menthol; phenol] 8.25%•0.25%•1.5%

Schick test [see: diphtheria toxin for Schick test]

Schick test control USP *dermal reactivity indicator*

Schirmer Tear Test ophthalmic strips *diagnostic tear flow test aid*

schizandra (*Schisandra arisanensis; S. chinensis; S. rubriflora; S. sphenanthera*) berries *medicinal herb for cough, gastrointestinal disorders, increasing energy and mental alertness, nervous disorders, respiratory illnesses, and stress; also used as a liver protectant*

Scleromate IV injection ℞ *sclerosing agent for varicose veins* [morrhuate sodium] 50 mg/mL

Sclerosol aerosol ℞ *treatment for malignant pleural effusion and pneumothorax via intrapleural thoracoscopy administration (orphan)* [talc, sterile]

Sclerosol ℞ *investigational (orphan) anti-inflammatory for the topical treatment for scleroderma* [dimethyl sulfoxide (DMSO)]

scoke *medicinal herb* [see: pokeweed]

Scopace tablets ℞ *GI antispasmodic; anticholinergic CNS depressant; motion sickness preventative* [scopolamine] 0.4 mg

scopafungin USAN *antibacterial; antifungal*

Scope mouthwash OTC *oral antiseptic* [cetylpyridinium chloride]

scopolamine *oral/transdermal motion sickness preventative; post-surgical antiemetic*

scopolamine hydrobromide USP *GI antispasmodic; anticholinergic CNS depressant; motion sickness preventative; cycloplegic; mydriatic* [also: hyoscine hydrobromide] 0.3, 0.4, 0.86, 1 mg/mL injection

scopolamine methyl nitrate [see: methscopolamine nitrate]

scopolamine methylbromide [see: methscopolamine bromide]

Scott's Emulsion OTC *vitamin supplement* [vitamins A and D] 1250•100 IU/5 mL

Scot-Tussin Allergy Relief Formula Clear oral liquid OTC *antihistamine* [diphenhydramine HCl] 12.5 mg/5 mL

Scot-Tussin DM oral liquid OTC *antitussive; antihistamine* [dextromethorphan hydrobromide; chlorpheniramine maleate] 30•4 mg/10 mL

Scot-Tussin DM Cough Chasers lozenges OTC *antitussive* [dextromethorphan hydrobromide] 5 mg

Scot-Tussin Expectorant oral liquid OTC *expectorant* [guaifenesin] 100 mg/5 mL

Scot-Tussin Original 5-Action Cold Formula syrup, sugar-free oral liquid OTC *decongestant; antihistamine; analgesic* [phenylephrine HCl; pheniramine maleate; sodium citrate; sodium salicylate; caffeine citrate] 4.2•13.3•83.3•83.3•25 mg

Scot-Tussin Senior Clear oral liquid OTC *antitussive; expectorant* [dextromethorphan hydrobromide; guaifenesin] 15•200 mg/5 mL

scrofula plant *medicinal herb* [see: figwort]

Scrophularia nodosa *medicinal herb* [see: figwort]

scullcap *medicinal herb* [see: skullcap]

Sculptra dermal injection R̲ *synthetic polymer for the correction of facial lipoatrophy due to HIV infections* [poly-L-lactic acid]

scuroforme [see: butyl aminobenzoate]

Scutellaria lateriflora *medicinal herb* [see: skullcap]

SD (streptodornase) [q.v.]

SDZ-ASM-981 *investigational (Phase III) nonsteroidal cream for atopic dermatitis*

⁷⁵Se [see: selenomethionine Se 75]

sea girdles *medicinal herb* [see: kelp (Laminaria)]

Sea Mist nasal spray (discontinued 2002) OTC *nasal moisturizer* [sodium chloride (saline solution)] 0.65%

Seale's Lotion Modified OTC *topical acne treatment* [sulfur] 6.4%

sealroot; sealwort *medicinal herb* [see: Solomon's seal]

Sea-Omega 30; Sea-Omega 50 softgels OTC *dietary supplement* [omega-3 fatty acids] 1200 mg; 1000 mg

Seasonale film-coated tablets (in packs of 91) R̲ *extended-cycle (3 months) monophasic oral contraceptive* [levonorgestrel; ethinyl estradiol] Phase 1 (84 days): 0.15 mg•30 μg; Counters (7 days)

Seasonique film-coated tablets (in packs of 91) R̲ *extended-cycle (3 months) biphasic oral contraceptive* [levonorgestrel; ethinyl estradiol] Phase 1 (84 days): 0.15 mg•30 μg; Phase 2 (7 days): 0•10 μg

seawrack *medicinal herb* [see: kelp (Fucus)]

Seba-Nil Cleansing Mask scrub OTC *abrasive cleanser for acne*

Seba-Nil Oily Skin Cleanser topical liquid OTC *cleanser for acne* [alcohol; acetone]

Sebasorb lotion OTC *keratolytic for acne* [salicylic acid; attapulgite] 2%•10%

Sebazole gel R̲ *investigational (Phase III) antifungal for seborrheic dermatitis* [ketoconazole]

Sebex shampoo OTC *antiseborrheic; keratolytic* [sulfur; salicylic acid] 2%•2%

Sebex-T shampoo OTC *antiseborrheic; antipsoriatic; keratolytic* [sulfur; salicylic acid; coal tar] 2%•2%•5%

Sebizon lotion (discontinued 2003) R̲ *antibiotic; antiseborrheic* [sulfacetamide sodium] 10%

Sebucare hair lotion (discontinued 2004) OTC *antiseborrheic; keratolytic* [salicylic acid; alcohol 61%] 1.8%

Sebulex with Conditioners shampoo OTC *antiseborrheic; keratolytic* [sulfur; salicylic acid] 2%•2%

secalciferol USAN, INN, BAN *calcium regulator; investigational (orphan) for familial hypophosphatemic rickets*

secbutabarbital sodium INN *sedative; hypnotic* [also: butabarbital sodium]

secbutobarbitone BAN *sedative; hypnotic* [also: butabarbital]

seclazone USAN, INN *anti-inflammatory; uricosuric*

secnidazole INN, BAN

secobarbital USP, INN *hypnotic; sedative*

secobarbital sodium USP, JAN *hypnotic; sedative; also abused as a street drug* [also: quinalbarbitone sodium] 100 mg oral; 50 mg/mL injection

Seconal Sodium Pulvules (capsules) R *sedative; hypnotic; also abused as a street drug* [secobarbital sodium] 100 mg

secoverine INN

Secran oral liquid OTC *vitamin supplement* [vitamins B₁, B₃, and B₁₂; alcohol 17%] 10 mg•10 mg•25 μg per 5 mL

SecreFlo powder for IV injection R *diagnostic aid for pancreatic function* [secretin] 16 μg/vial

secretin INN, BAN *diagnostic aid for pancreatic function*

Secretin Ferring powder for IV injection (name changed to SecreFlo in 2002)

secretory leukocyte protease inhibitor *investigational (orphan) for congenital alpha₁-antitrypsin deficiency, cystic fibrosis, and bronchopulmonary dysplasia*

Sectral capsules R *antihypertensive; antianginal; antiarrhythmic for premature ventricular contractions (PVCs); antiadrenergic (β-blocker)* [acebutolol HCl] 200, 400 mg

Secule (trademarked packaging form) *single-dose vial*

securinine INN

sedaform [see: chlorobutanol]

Sedapap caplets R *analgesic; barbiturate sedative* [acetaminophen; butalbital] 650•50 mg

sedatine [see: antipyrine]

sedatives *a class of soothing agents that reduce excitement, nervousness, distress, or irritation* [also called: calmatives]

sedecamycin USAN, INN *veterinary antibacterial*

sedeval [see: barbital]

sedge, sweet *medicinal herb* [see: calamus]

sedoxantrone trihydrochloride [now: ledoxantrone trihydrochloride]

seganserin INN, BAN

seglitide INN *antidiabetic* [also: seglitide acetate]

seglitide acetate USAN *antidiabetic* [also: seglitide]

selamectin USAN, INN *veterinary antiparasitic*

Selecor tablets R *investigational (NDA filed) antihypertensive; antianginal; β-blocker* [celiprolol HCl]

Select-A-Jet (trademarked delivery system) *syringe system*

selective estrogen receptor modulators (SERMs) *a class of osteoporosis prevention agents that reduce bone resorption and decrease overall bone turnover in postmenopausal women*

selective serotonin 5-HT₃ (hydroxytryptamine) blockers *a class of antiemetic and antinauseant agents used primarily after emetogenic cancer chemotherapy* [also called: 5-HT₃ receptor antagonists]

selective serotonin and norepinephrine reuptake inhibitors (SSNRIs) *a class of oral antidepressants that inhibit neuronal uptake of serotonin (5-HT) and norepinephrine, CNS neurotransmitters*

selective serotonin reuptake inhibitors (SSRIs) *a class of oral antidepressants that inhibit neuronal uptake of serotonin (5-HT), a CNS neurotransmitter*

selegiline INN, BAN *dopaminergic antiparkinsonian; investigational (Phase*

III) transdermal treatment for depression [also: selegiline HCl]

selegiline HCl USAN *dopaminergic antiparkinsonian (orphan)* [also: selegiline]

selenious acid USP *dietary selenium supplement (61% elemental selenium)* 65.4 μg/mL (40 μg Se/mL) injection

selenium *element (Se)*

selenium dioxide, monohydrated [see: selenious acid]

selenium sulfide USP *antiseborrheic; antipsoriatic; antifungal for tinea versicolor* 1%, 2.5% topical

selenomethionine (^{75}Se) INN *pancreas function test; radioactive agent* [also: selenomethionine Se 75]

selenomethionine Se 75 USAN, USP *pancreas function test; radioactive agent* [also: selenomethionine (^{75}Se)]

Sele-Pak IV injection ℞ *selenium supplement* [selenious acid (61% elemental selenium)] 65.4 μg/mL (40 μg Se/mL)

Selepen IV injection ℞ *selenium supplement* [selenious acid (61% elemental selenium)] 65.4 μg/mL (40 μg Se/mL)

selfotel USAN *NMDA (N-methyl-D-aspartate) antagonist for treatment of stroke-induced impairment*

Seloken (foreign name for U.S. product Lopressor)

Seloken ZOC (foreign name for U.S. product Toprol XL)

selprazine INN

Selsun lotion ℞ *antiseborrheic; antipsoriatic; antifungal for tinea versicolor* [selenium sulfide] 2.5%

Selsun Blue Medicated Treatment lotion/shampoo OTC *antiseborrheic; dandruff treatment* [selenium sulfide] 1%

Selsun Gold for Women lotion/shampoo (discontinued 2004) OTC *antiseborrheic; dandruff treatment* [selenium sulfide] 1%

sematilide INN *antiarrhythmic* [also: sematilide HCl]

sematilide HCl USAN *antiarrhythmic* [also: sematilide]

semduramicin USAN, INN *coccidiostat*

semduramicin sodium USAN *coccidiostat*

Semicid vaginal suppositories OTC *spermicidal contraceptive* [nonoxynol 9] 100 mg

semisodium valproate BAN *anticonvulsant; antipsychotic for manic episodes; migraine headache preventative; valproic acid derivative* [also: divalproex sodium; valproate semisodium]

semparatide acetate USAN *parathyroid hormone analogue to enhance fracture healing*

Semprex-D capsules ℞ *decongestant; antihistamine* [pseudoephedrine HCl; acrivastine] 60•8 mg

semustine USAN, INN *antineoplastic*

senecio, golden *medicinal herb* [see: life root]

Senecio aureus; S. jacoboea; S. vulgaris *medicinal herb* [see: life root]

senega (*Polygala senega*) *root medicinal herb used as an antitussive for asthma, chronic bronchitis, croup, lung congestion, and pneumonia*

Senexon tablets, oral liquid OTC *stimulant laxative* [sennosides] 8.6 mg; 8.8 mg/5 mL

Senilezol elixir ℞ *vitamin/iron supplement* [multiple B vitamins; ferric pyrophosphate] ≛•3.3 mg

senna USP *stimulant laxative*

senna (*Cassia acutifolia; C. angustifolia; C. senna*) *leaves medicinal herb for bowel evacuation before gastrointestinal procedures, constipation, edema, and expelling worms*

Senna Concentrate tablets OTC *stimulant laxative* [sennosides] 8.6 mg

Senna Plus tablets OTC *stimulant laxative; stool softener* [sennosides; docusate sodium] 8.6•50 mg

Senna-Gen tablets OTC *stimulant laxative* [sennosides] 8.6 mg

SennaPrompt capsules OTC *bulk/stimulant laxative* [psyllium; sennosides] 500•9 mg

sennosides USP *stimulant laxative*

Senokot tablets, granules, syrup OTC *stimulant laxative* [sennosides] 8.6 mg; 15 mg/5 mL; 8.8 mg/5 mL

Senokot-S tablets OTC *stimulant laxative; stool softener* [sennosides; docusate sodium] 8.6•50 mg

SenokotXtra tablets OTC *stimulant laxative* [sennosides] 17 mg

Sensability kit OTC *breast self-examination aid*

Sensipar film-coated tablets ℞ *calcimimetic agent for hypercalcemia due to parathyroid carcinoma (orphan) and secondary hyperparathyroidism (SHPT) due to chronic kidney disease* [cinacalcet HCl] 33, 66, 99 mg (=30, 60, 90 mg base)

Sensitive Eyes; Sensitive Eyes Plus solution OTC *rinsing/storage solution for soft contact lenses* [sodium chloride (preserved saline solution)]

Sensitive Eyes Daily Cleaner; Sensitive Eyes Saline/Cleaning Solution OTC *surfactant cleaning solution for soft contact lenses*

Sensitive Eyes Drops OTC *rewetting solution for soft contact lenses*

Sensitivity Protection Crest toothpaste OTC *tooth desensitizer; topical dental caries preventative* [potassium nitrate; sodium fluoride]

Sensodyne Cool Gel toothpaste OTC *tooth desensitizer; topical dental caries preventative* [potassium nitrate; sodium fluoride]

Sensodyne Fresh Mint toothpaste OTC *tooth desensitizer; dental caries preventative* [potassium nitrate; sodium monofluorophosphate]

Sensodyne-SC toothpaste OTC *tooth desensitizer* [strontium chloride hexahydrate] 10%

SensoGARD gel OTC *topical oral anesthetic* [benzocaine] 20%

Sensorcaine injection ℞ *injectable local anesthetic* [bupivacaine HCl] 0.25%, 0.5%

Sensorcaine injection ℞ *injectable local anesthetic* [bupivacaine HCl;

epinephrine] 0.25%•1:200 000; 0.5%•1:200 000

Sensorcaine MPF injection ℞ *injectable local anesthetic* [bupivacaine HCl] 0.25%, 0.5%, 0.75%

Sensorcaine MPF injection ℞ *injectable local anesthetic* [bupivacaine HCl; epinephrine] 0.25%•1:200 000, 0.5%•1:200 000, 0.75%•1:200 000

Sensorcaine MPF Spinal injection ℞ *injectable local anesthetic* [bupivacaine HCl] 0.75%

Sentinel test kit for professional use *urine test for HIV-1 antibodies* 🄬 fentanyl

sepazonium chloride USAN, INN *topical anti-infective*

seperidol HCl USAN *antipsychotic* [also: clofluperol]

Seprafilm hydrated gel film *to reduce the incidence, extent, and severity of postoperative adhesions* [hyaluronate sodium; carboxymethylcellulose]

seprilose USAN *antirheumatic*

seproxetine HCl USAN *antidepressant*

Septa ointment (discontinued 2001) OTC *topical antibiotic* [polymyxin B sulfate; neomycin sulfate; bacitracin] 5000 U•3.5 mg•400 U per g 🄬 Cipro; Septra

Septi-Soft solution ℞ *antiseptic; disinfectant* [triclosan] 0.25%

Septisol foam ℞ *bacteriostatic skin cleanser* [hexachlorophene; alcohol 56%] 0.23%

Septisol solution ℞ *antiseptic; disinfectant* [triclosan] 0.25%

Septocaine intraoral injection ℞ *local anesthetic for dentistry* [articaine HCl; epinephrine] 4%•1:100 000

septomonab [see: nebacumab]

Septopal polymethyl methacrylate (PMMA) beads on surgical wire ℞ *investigational (orphan) agent for chronic osteomyelitis* [gentamicin sulfate]

Septra tablets, oral suspension ℞ *anti-infective; antibacterial* [trimethoprim; sulfamethoxazole] 80•400 mg; 40•200 mg/5 mL 🄬 Cipro; Septa

Septra DS tablets ℞ *anti-infective; antibacterial* [trimethoprim; sulfamethoxazole] 160•800 mg

Septra IV infusion ℞ *anti-infective; antibacterial* [trimethoprim; sulfamethoxazole] 80•400 mg/5 mL

Sequels (trademarked dosage form) *sustained-release capsule or tablet*

sequential AC/paclitaxel (Adriamycin, cyclophosphamide; paclitaxel) *chemotherapy protocol for breast cancer*

sequential DOX → CMF (doxorubicin; cyclophosphamide, methotrexate, fluorouracil) *chemotherapy protocol for breast cancer*

sequifenadine INN

seractide INN *adrenocorticotropic hormone* [also: seractide acetate]

seractide acetate USAN *adrenocorticotropic hormone* [also: seractide]

Ser-Ap-Es tablets ℞ *antihypertensive; vasodilator; diuretic* [hydrochlorothiazide; reserpine; hydralazine HCl] 15•0.1•25 mg ☑ Catapres

seratrodast USAN, INN *anti-inflammatory; antiasthmatic; thromboxane receptor antagonist*

Serax capsules, tablets ℞ *benzodiazepine anxiolytic; sedative; alcohol withdrawal aid* [oxazepam] 10, 15, 30 mg; 15 mg ☑ Eurax; Urex; Xerac

serazapine HCl USAN *anxiolytic*

Serdolect (approved in Europe) ℞ *investigational (NDA filed) novel (atypical) antipsychotic; neuroleptic* [sertindole]

Sereine solution OTC *cleaning solution for hard contact lenses* [note: one of three different products with the same name]

Sereine solution OTC *wetting solution for hard contact lenses* [note: one of three different products with the same name]

Sereine solution OTC *wetting/soaking solution for hard contact lenses* [note: one of three different products with the same name]

Serenoa repens; S. serrulata *medicinal herb* [see: saw palmetto]

Serentil IM injection (discontinued 2003) ℞ *conventional (typical) phenothiazine antipsychotic for schizophrenia* [mesoridazine besylate] 25 mg/mL ☑ Surital

Serentil oral concentrate (discontinued 2004) ℞ *conventional (typical) phenothiazine antipsychotic for schizophrenia* [mesoridazine besylate] 25 mg/mL ☑ Surital

Serentil tablets (discontinued 2004) ℞ *conventional (typical) phenothiazine antipsychotic for schizophrenia* [mesoridazine besylate] 10, 50 mg ☑ Surital

Serevent oral metered dose inhaler (discontinued 2004) ℞ *twice-daily sympathomimetic bronchodilator for asthma and bronchospasm* [salmeterol xinafoate] 25 μg/dose

Serevent Diskus oral inhalation powder ℞ *twice-daily sympathomimetic bronchodilator for asthma and bronchospasm* [salmeterol xinafoate] 50 μg/dose

serfibrate INN

sergolexole INN *antimigraine* [also: sergolexole maleate]

sergolexole maleate USAN *antimigraine* [also: sergolexole]

serine (L-serine) USAN, USP, INN *nonessential amino acid; symbols: Ser, S*

L-serine diazoacetate [see: azaserine]

84-L-serineplasminogen activator [see: monteplase]

sermetacin USAN, INN *anti-inflammatory*

sermorelin INN, BAN *growth hormone deficiency diagnosis and treatment* [also: sermorelin acetate]

sermorelin acetate USAN *diagnostic aid for pituitary function; treatment for growth hormone deficiency (orphan), anovulation, and AIDS-related weight loss* [also: sermorelin]

SERMs (selective estrogen receptor modulators) [q.v.]

SeroJet (trademarked device) *needle-free subcutaneous injector for Serostim (somatropin)*

Seromycin Pulvules (capsules) ℞ *tuberculostatic* [cycloserine] 250 mg

Serophene tablets ℞ *ovulation stimulant* [clomiphene citrate] 50 mg

Seroquel film-coated tablets ℞ *novel (atypical) dibenzothiazepine antipsychotic for schizophrenia and manic episodes of a bipolar disorder; also used for agitation or psychosis due to Parkinson disease, Alzheimer disease, or various dementias* [quetiapine fumarate] 25, 100, 200, 300 mg

Serostim powder for subcu injection, prefilled one.click auto-injector syringe ℞ *growth hormone for adults or children with congenital or endogenous growth hormone deficiency, children with Turner syndrome or renal-induced growth failure, or AIDS-wasting syndrome (orphan)* [somatropin] 5, 6 mg (15, 18 IU) per vial; 8.8 mg (26.4 IU) per syringe

Serostim LQ subcu injection cartridges ℞ *growth hormone for adults or children with congenital or endogenous growth hormone deficiency, children with Turner syndrome or renal-induced growth failure, or AIDS-wasting syndrome (orphan)* [somatropin] 6 mg (18 IU) per 0.5 mL

serotonin (5-hydroxytriptamine$_1$; 5-HT$_1$) [see: selective serotonin reuptake inhibitors; vascular serotonin receptor antagonists]

Seroxat (European name for U.S. product Paxil)

SERPACWA (Skin Exposure Reduction Paste Against Chemical Warfare Agents) cream ℞ *to delay absorption of chemical warfare agents through the skin when applied before exposure; used in conjunction with MOPP (Mission Oriented Protective Posture) gear* [polytef; perfluoroalkylpolyether]

serrapeptase INN

Serratia marcescens extract (polyribosomes) *investigational (orphan) for primary brain malignancies*

sertaconazole INN *topical antifungal*

sertaconazole nitrate *topical antifungal*

sertindole USAN, INN *investigational (NDA filed) novel (atypical) antipsychotic; neuroleptic*

Sertoli cells, porcine *investigational (orphan) intracerebral implant for stage 4 and 5 Parkinson disease (for co-implantation with fetal neural cells)*

sertraline INN, BAN *selective serotonin reuptake inhibitor (SSRI) for depression, obsessive-compulsive disorder (OCD), panic disorder, post-traumatic stress disorder, premenstrual dysphoric disorder (PMDD), and social anxiety disorder* [also: sertraline HCl]

sertraline HCl USAN *selective serotonin reuptake inhibitor (SSRI) for depression, obsessive-compulsive disorder (OCD), panic disorder, post-traumatic stress disorder, premenstrual dysphoric disorder (PMDD), and social anxiety disorder* [also: sertraline]

serum albumin (SA) [see: albumin, human]

serum albumin, iodinated (^{125}I) human [see: albumin, iodinated I 125 serum]

serum albumin, iodinated (^{131}I) human [see: albumin, iodinated I 131 serum]

serum fibrinogen (SF) [see: fibrinogen, human]

serum globulin (SG) [see: globulin, immune]

serum gonadotrophin [see: gonadotrophin, serum]

serum gonadotropin [see: gonadotrophin, serum]

serum prothrombin conversion accelerator (SPCA) factor [see: factor VII]

Serutan granules OTC *bulk laxative* [psyllium] 2.5 g/tsp.

Serzone tablets (discontinued 2004 due to safety concerns) ℞ *antidepressant* [nefazodone HCl] 50, 100, 150, 200, 250 mg

Serzone-5HT$_2$ ⊛ tablets ℞ *antidepressant* [nefazodone HCl] 50, 100, 150, 200 mg

sesame oil NF *solvent; oleaginous vehicle*

Sesame Street Complete chewable tablets OTC *vitamin/mineral/calcium/ iron supplement* [multiple vitamins & minerals; calcium; iron; folic acid; biotin] ±•80•10•0.2•0.015 mg

Sesame Street Plus Extra C chewable tablets (discontinued 2004) OTC *vitamin supplement* [multiple vitamins; folic acid] ±•0.2 mg

Sesame Street Plus Iron chewable tablets OTC *vitamin/iron supplement* [multiple vitamins; iron; folic acid] ±•10•0.2 mg

setastine INN

setazindol INN

setiptiline INN

setoperone USAN, INN *antipsychotic*

setwall *medicinal herb* [see: valerian]

Seudotabs tablets (discontinued 2002) OTC *nasal decongestant* [pseudoephedrine HCl] 30 mg

sevelamer HCl USAN *phosphate-binding polymer for hyperphosphatemia of end-stage renal disease (ESRD); also used for hyperuricemia in dialysis patients*

7 + 3 protocol (cytarabine, daunorubicin) *chemotherapy protocol for acute myelocytic leukemia (AML)*

7 + 3 protocol (cytarabine, idarubicin) *chemotherapy protocol for acute myelocytic leukemia (AML)*

7 + 3 protocol (cytarabine, mitoxantrone) *chemotherapy protocol for acute myelocytic leukemia (AML)*

7 + 3 + 7 protocol (cytarabine, daunorubicin, etoposide) *chemotherapy protocol for acute myelocytic leukemia (AML)*

seven barks *medicinal herb* [see: hydrangea]

7E3 monoclonal antibodies (MAb) [see: abciximab]

Severe Congestion Tussin softgels OTC *decongestant; expectorant* [pseudoephedrine HCl; guaifenesin] 30•200 mg

sevirumab USAN, INN *investigational (Phase I) antiviral for AIDS; orphan status withdrawn 1996*

sevitropium mesilate INN

sevoflurane USAN, INN *inhalation general anesthetic*

sevopramide INN

sezolamide HCl USAN *carbonic anhydrase inhibitor*

SF (serum fibrinogen) [see: fibrinogen, human]

SFC lotion OTC *soap-free therapeutic skin cleanser*

sfericase INN

SG (serum globulin) [see: globulin, immune]

SG (soluble gelatin) [see: gelatin]

shamrock, Indian *medicinal herb* [see: birthroot]

shamrock, water *medicinal herb* [see: buckbean]

shark cartilage (derived from Sphyrna lewini, Squalus acanthias, and other species) *natural remedy for cancer* [also: squalamine]

shark liver oil *emollient/protectant*

shavegrass *medicinal herb* [see: horsetail]

sheep laurel *medicinal herb* [see: mountain laurel]

Sheik Elite premedicated condom OTC *spermicidal/barrier contraceptive* [nonoxynol 9] 8%

shell flower *medicinal herb* [see: turtlebloom]

shellac NF *tablet coating agent*

Shellgel intraocular injection R *viscoelastic agent for ophthalmic surgery* [hyaluronate sodium] 12 mg/mL

Shepard's Cream Lotion; Shepard's Skin Cream OTC *moisturizer; emollient*

shepherd's club *medicinal herb* [see: mullein]

shepherd's heart *medicinal herb* [see: shepherd's purse]

shepherd's purse (Capsella bursa-pastoris) plant *medicinal herb for bleeding, ear disease, hypertension, painful menstruation, and urinary bleeding*

shigoka *medicinal herb* [see: Siberian ginseng]

shiitake mushrooms (Lentinula edodes; Tricholomopsis edodes) stem and cap *medicinal herb for boosting the*

immune system, cancer, lowering cholesterol, and viral illnesses

Shohl solution, modified (sodium citrate & citric acid) urinary alka-lizer; compounding agent

short chain fatty acids investigational (orphan) for left-sided ulcerative colitis and chronic radiation proctitis

short-leaved buchu medicinal herb [see: buchu]

Shur-Clens solution OTC wound clean-ser [poloxamer 188] 20%

Shur-Seal vaginal gel OTC spermicidal contraceptive (for use with a diaphragm) [nonoxynol 9] 2%

siagoside INN

sialagogues a class of agents that stimu-late the secretion of saliva [also called: ptyalagogues]

Sibelium ℞ investigational (orphan) vasodilator for alternating hemiplegia [flunarizine HCl]

sibenadet HCl USAN treatment for chronic obstructive pulmonary disease (COPD)

Siberian ginseng (Acanthopanax senticosus; Eleutherococcus senti-cosus) an older (and incorrect) name for eleuthero; Siberian ginseng is not in the ginseng family [now: eleuthero; compare to: ginseng]

sibopirdine USAN cognition enhancer for Alzheimer disease; nootropic

sibrafiban USAN platelet inhibitor; fib-rinogen receptor antagonist; investiga-tional (Phase III) oral glycoprotein IIb/IIIa receptor antagonist for acute coro-nary syndrome

sibutramine INN, BAN anorexiant for the treatment of obesity; monoamine reuptake inhibitor antidepressant [also: sibutramine HCl]

sibutramine HCl USAN anorexiant for the treatment of obesity; monoamine reuptake inhibitor antidepressant [also: sibutramine]

siccanin INN

Sickledex test kit for professional use in vitro diagnostic aid for hemoglobin S (sickle cell)

sicklewort medicinal herb [see: wound-wort]

side-flowering skullcap medicinal herb [see: skullcap]

SigPak (trademarked packaging form) unit-of-use package

Sigtab tablets OTC vitamin supplement [multiple vitamins; folic acid] ≛•0.4 mg

Sigtab-M tablets OTC vitamin/mineral/calcium/iron supplement [multiple vitamins & minerals; calcium; iron; folic acid; biotin] ≛•200•18•0.4•0.045 mg

siguazodan INN, BAN

Silace syrup OTC laxative; stool softener [docusate sodium] 60 mg/15 mL

Silace-C syrup (discontinued 2003) OTC stimulant laxative; stool softener [casanthranol; docusate sodium; alcohol 10%] 30•60 mg/15 mL

Siladryl elixir OTC antihistamine [diphen-hydramine HCl] 12.5 mg/5 mL

Silafed syrup OTC decongestant; antihis-tamine [pseudoephedrine HCl; tri-prolidine HCl] 60•2.5 mg/10 mL

silafilcon A USAN hydrophilic contact lens material

silafocon A USAN hydrophobic contact lens material

Silaminic Cold syrup (discontinued 2002) OTC decongestant; antihistamine [phenylpropanolamine HCl; chlor-pheniramine maleate] 12.5•2 mg/5 mL

Silaminic Expectorant syrup (discon-tinued 2002) OTC decongestant; expec-torant [phenylpropanolamine HCl; guaifenesin; alcohol 5%] 12.5•100 mg/5 mL

silandrone USAN, INN androgen

Silapap, Children's oral liquid OTC analgesic; antipyretic [acetaminophen] 80 mg/2.5 mL

Silapap, Infant's drops OTC analgesic; antipyretic [acetaminophen] 100 mg/mL

Sildec-DM pediatric oral drops ℞ anti-tussive; decongestant; antihistamine [dextromethorphan hydrobromide;

pseudoephedrine HCl; carbinoxamine maleate] 4•15•2 mg/mL

Sildec-DM syrup ℞ *antitussive; decongestant; antihistamine* [dextromethorphan hydrobromide; pseudoephedrine HCl; brompheniramine maleate] 15•60•4 mg/5 mL

sildenafil citrate USAN *phosphodiesterase type 5 (PDE5) inhibitor; selective vasodilator for erectile dysfunction (ED) and pulmonary arterial hypertension (PAH)*

Sildicon-E pediatric oral drops (discontinued 2002) OTC *decongestant; expectorant* [phenylpropanolamine HCl; guaifenesin] 6.25•30 mg/mL

Silfedrine, Children's oral liquid OTC *nasal decongestant* [pseudoephedrine HCl] 30 mg/5 mL

silibinin INN

silica, dental-type NF *pharmaceutic aid*

silica gel [now: silicon dioxide]

siliceous earth, purified NF *filtering medium*

silicic acid, magnesium salt [see: magnesium trisilicate]

silicon *element (Si)*

silicon dioxide NF *dispersing and suspending agent*

silicon dioxide, colloidal NF *suspending agent; tablet and capsule diluent*

silicone

Silicone No. 2 ointment OTC *skin protectant* [silicone; hydrophobic starch derivative] 10%•?

silicone oil [see: polydimethylsiloxane]

silicristin INN

silidianin INN

silkweed *medicinal herb* [see: milkweed; pleurisy root]

silky swallow wort; Virginia silk *medicinal herb* [see: milkweed]

silodrate USAN *antacid* [also: simaldrate]

Silphen Cough syrup OTC *antihistamine; antitussive* [diphenhydramine HCl; alcohol 5%] 12.5 mg/5 mL

Silphen DM syrup OTC *antitussive* [dextromethorphan hydrobromide; alcohol 5%] 10 mg/5 mL

Silphium perfoliatum *medicinal herb* [see: ragged cup]

Siltapp with Dextromethorphan Cold & Cough elixir (discontinued 2002) ℞ *antitussive; decongestant; antihistamine* [dextromethorphan hydrobromide; phenylpropanolamine HCl; brompheniramine maleate] 10•12.5•2 mg/5 mL

Sil-Tex oral liquid (discontinued 2002) ℞ *decongestant; expectorant* [phenylpropanolamine HCl; phenylephrine HCl; guaifenesin; alcohol 5%] 20•5•100 mg/5 mL

Siltussin CF oral liquid (discontinued 2002) OTC *antitussive; decongestant; expectorant* [dextromethorphan hydrobromide; phenylpropanolamine HCl; guaifenesin; alcohol 4.75%] 10•12.5•100 mg/5 mL

Siltussin DAS oral liquid OTC *expectorant* [guaifenesin] 100 mg/5 mL

Siltussin DM Cough syrup OTC *antitussive; expectorant* [dextromethorphan hydrobromide; guaifenesin] 20•200 mg/10 mL

Siltussin SA oral liquid OTC *expectorant* [guaifenesin] 100 mg/5 mL

Silvadene cream ℞ *broad-spectrum bactericidal for adjunctive burn treatment* [silver sulfadiazine] 10 mg/g ⑨ Azulfidine

silver *element (Ag)*

silver nitrate USP *ophthalmic neonatal anti-infective; strong caustic* 1% eye drops; 10%, 25%, 50%, 75% topical

silver nitrate, toughened USP *caustic*

silver protein, mild NF *ophthalmic antiseptic; ophthalmic surgical aid*

silver sulfadiazine (SSD) USAN, USP *broad-spectrum bactericidal; adjunct to burn therapy* [also: sulfadiazine silver]

silverweed; silver cinquefoil *medicinal herb* [see: cinquefoil]

Silybum marianum *medicinal herb* [see: milk thistle]

Simaal Gel 2 oral liquid OTC *antacid; antiflatulent* [aluminum hydroxide; magnesium hydroxide; simethicone] 500•400•40 mg/5 mL

simaldrate INN *antacid* [also: silodrate]

Simdax (approved in several European countries) *investigational (Phase III) calcium sensitizer and vasodilator for decompensated heart failure* [levosimendan]

simethicone USAN, USP *antiflatulent; adjunct to gastrointestinal imaging* 80 mg oral; 40 mg/0.6 mL oral

simethicone-coated cellulose suspension (SCCS) [see: SonoRx]

simetride INN

simfibrate INN

Similac Advance with Iron ready-to-use oral liquid, powder for oral liquid OTC *infant formula fortified with omega-3 fatty acids*

Similac Human Milk Fortifier powder OTC *supplement to breast milk* 900 mg/pkt.

Similac Low Iron oral liquid, powder for oral liquid OTC *total or supplementary infant feeding*

Similac PM 60/40 Low-Iron oral liquid OTC *formula for infants predisposed to hypocalcemia* [whey formula with lowered mineral levels]

Similac with Iron oral liquid, powder for oral liquid OTC *total or supplementary infant feeding*

simple syrup [see: syrup]

Simpler's joy *medicinal herb* [see: blue vervain]

Simplet tablets OTC *decongestant; antihistamine; analgesic* [pseudoephedrine HCl; chlorpheniramine maleate; acetaminophen] 60•4•650 mg ☒ Singlet

Simply Cough oral liquid OTC *antitussive* [dextromethorphan hydrobromide] 5 mg/5 mL

Simply Saline nasal spray OTC *nasal moisturizer* [sodium chloride (saline solution)]

Simply Sleep tablets OTC *antihistaminic sleep aid* [diphenhydramine HCl] 25 mg

Simply Stuffy tablets, oral liquid OTC *nasal decongestant* [pseudoephedrine HCl] 30 mg; 15 mg/5 mL

Simron Plus capsules OTC *vitamin/iron supplement* [multiple vitamins; ferrous gluconate; folic acid] ±•10•0.1 mg

simtrazene USAN, INN *antineoplastic*

Simulect powder for IV infusion *immunosuppressant; IL-2 receptor antagonist for the prevention of acute rejection of renal transplants (orphan)* [basiliximab] 20 mg

simvastatin USAN, INN, BAN *HMG-CoA reductase inhibitor for hyperlipidemia, hypertriglyceridemia, and coronary heart disease* ☒ Sandostatin; zinostatin

Sinapils tablets (discontinued 2001) OTC *decongestant; antihistamine; analgesic* [phenylpropanolamine HCl; chlorpheniramine maleate; acetaminophen; caffeine] 12.5•2•325•32.5 mg

Sinapis alba *medicinal herb* [see: mustard]

sinapultide USAN *pulmonary surfactant for respiratory distress syndrome*

Sinarest; Sinarest Sinus tablets (discontinued 2002) OTC *decongestant; antihistamine; analgesic* [pseudoephedrine HCl; chlorpheniramine maleate; acetaminophen] 30•2•500 mg; 30•2•325 mg

Sinarest, No Drowsiness tablets (discontinued 2002) OTC *decongestant; analgesic; antipyretic* [pseudoephedrine HCl; acetaminophen] 30•500 mg

Sinarest 12 Hour nasal spray (discontinued 2002) OTC *nasal decongestant* [oxymetazoline HCl] 0.05%

sincalide USAN, INN *choleretic; diagnostic aid for gallbladder function*

Sine-Aid tablets, caplets, gelcaps (discontinued 2002) OTC *decongestant; analgesic; antipyretic* [pseudoephedrine HCl; acetaminophen] 30•500 mg

Sine-Aid IB caplets (discontinued 2002) OTC *decongestant; analgesic* [pseudoephedrine HCl; ibuprofen] 30•200 mg

sinefungin USAN, INN *antifungal*

Sinemet 10-100; Sinemet 25-100; Sinemet 25-250 tablets ℞ *antiparkinsonian; dopamine precursor; decar-*

boxylase inhibitor [carbidopa; levodopa] 10•100 mg; 25•100 mg; 25•250 mg

Sinemet CR sustained-release tablets ℞ *antiparkinsonian; dopamine precursor; decarboxylase inhibitor* [carbidopa; levodopa] 25•100, 50•200 mg

Sine-Off Night Time Formula Sinus, Cold, & Flu Medicine gelcaps OTC *decongestant; antihistamine; analgesic* [pseudoephedrine HCl; diphenhydramine HCl; acetaminophen] 30•25•500 mg

Sine-Off No Drowsiness Formula caplets OTC *decongestant; analgesic; antipyretic* [pseudoephedrine HCl; acetaminophen] 30•500 mg

Sine-Off Sinus Medicine caplets OTC *decongestant; antihistamine; analgesic* [pseudoephedrine HCl; chlorpheniramine maleate; acetaminophen] 30•2•500 mg

Sinequan capsules ℞ *tricyclic antidepressant; anxiolytic* [doxepin HCl] 10, 25, 50, 75, 100, 150 mg

Sinequan concentrate for oral solution (discontinued 2004) ℞ *tricyclic antidepressant; anxiolytic* [doxepin HCl] 10 mg/mL

Sinex 12-Hour Long Acting; Sinex 12-Hour Ultra Fine Mist for Sinus Relief nasal spray OTC *nasal decongestant* [oxymetazoline HCl] 0.05%

Sinex Ultra Fine Mist nasal spray OTC *nasal decongestant* [phenylephrine HCl] 0.5%

single-chain antigen-binding proteins (SCA proteins) *a class of investigational antineoplastics*

SingleJect (trademarked dosage form) *prefilled syringe*

Singlet for Adults tablets OTC *decongestant; antihistamine; analgesic* [pseudoephedrine HCl; chlorpheniramine maleate; acetaminophen] 60•4•650 mg ② Simplet

Singulair film-coated tablets, chewable tablets, granules for oral solution ℞ *leukotriene receptor inhibitor for allergic rhinitis and the prophylaxis and chronic treatment of asthma* [mon-

telukast sodium] 10 mg; 4, 5 mg; 4 mg/pkt.

Sinografin intracavitary instillation ℞ *radiopaque contrast medium for gynecological imaging* [diatrizoate meglumine; iodipamide meglumine (47.8% total iodine)] 727•268 mg/mL (380 mg/mL)

sinorphan [now: ecadotril]

sintropium bromide INN

Sinufed Timecelles (sustained-release capsules) (discontinued 2002) ℞ *decongestant; expectorant* [pseudoephedrine HCl; guaifenesin] 60•300 mg

Sinulin tablets (discontinued 2001) OTC *decongestant; antihistamine; analgesic* [phenylpropanolamine HCl; chlorpheniramine maleate; acetaminophen] 25•4•650 mg

Sinumist-SR sustained-release Capsulets (capsule-shaped tablet) (discontinued 2002) ℞ *expectorant* [guaifenesin] 600 mg

Sinupan controlled-release capsules (discontinued 2002) ℞ *decongestant; expectorant* [phenylephrine HCl; guaifenesin] 40•200 mg

Sinus Headache & Congestion tablets (discontinued 2002) OTC *decongestant; antihistamine; analgesic* [pseudoephedrine HCl; chlorpheniramine maleate; acetaminophen] 30•2•500 mg

Sinus Relief caplets OTC *decongestant; analgesic* [pseudoephedrine HCl; acetaminophen] 30•500 mg

Sinustop capsules OTC *nasal decongestant* [pseudoephedrine HCl] 60 mg

Sinutab Non-Drying liquid-filled capsules OTC *decongestant; expectorant* [pseudoephedrine HCl; guaifenesin] 30•200 mg

Sinutab Sinus Allergy caplets OTC *decongestant; antihistamine; analgesic* [pseudoephedrine HCl; chlorpheniramine maleate; acetaminophen] 30•2•500 mg

Sinutab Sinus Without Drowsiness tablets, caplets OTC *decongestant;*

analgesic; antipyretic [pseudoephedrine HCl; acetaminophen] 30•325 mg; 30•500 mg

SINUtuss DM caplets ℞ *antitussive; decongestant; expectorant* [dextromethorphan hydrobromide; phenylephrine HCl; guaifenesin] 30•15•60 mg

SINUvent long-acting tablets (discontinued 2002) ℞ *decongestant; expectorant* [phenylpropanolamine HCl; guaifenesin] 75•600 mg

SINUvent PE extended-release caplets ℞ *decongestant; expectorant* [phenylephrine HCl; guaifenesin] 15•600 mg

Sirdalud (foreign name for U.S. product **Zanaflex**)

sirolimus USAN *immunosuppressant for renal transplantation* ② temsirolimus

sisomicin USAN, INN *antibacterial* [also: sissomicin]

sisomicin sulfate USAN, USP *antibacterial*

sissomicin BAN *antibacterial* [also: sisomicin]

sitafloxacin USAN, INN *antibacterial; DNA-gyrase inhibitor*

sitalidone INN

sitaxsentan *investigational (NDA filed) antihypertensive for pulmonary arterial hypertension (PAH)*

sitofibrate INN

sitogluside USAN, INN *antiprostatic hypertrophy*

sitosterols NF

Sitzmarks capsules ℞ *radiopaque contrast medium for severe constipation* [polyvinyl chloride, radiopaque] 24 rings/capsule

666 Cold Preparation oral liquid OTC *antitussive; decongestant; analgesic* [dextromethorphan hydrobromide; pseudoephedrine HCl; acetaminophen] 20•60•650 mg/30 mL

sizofiran INN

SK (streptokinase) [q.v.]

Skeeter Stik topical liquid OTC *local anesthetic; counterirritant* [lidocaine; menthol] 4%•1%

Skelaxin tablets ℞ *skeletal muscle relaxant* [metaxalone] 800 mg

Skelid tablets ℞ *bisphosphonate bone resorption inhibitor for Paget disease* [tiludronate disodium] 240 mg

skin respiratory factor (SRF) *claimed to promote wound healing*

Skin Shield topical liquid OTC *skin protectant; local anesthetic* [dyclonine HCl; benzethonium chloride] 0.75%•0.2%

Skinoren (German name for U.S. product **Azelex**)

skullcap (*Scutellaria lateriflora*) plant *medicinal herb for convulsions, epilepsy, fever, hypertension, infertility, insomnia, nervous disorders, rabies, and restlessness*

skunk cabbage (*Symplocarpus foetidus*) root *medicinal herb used as an antispasmodic, diuretic, emetic, expectorant, pectoral, stimulant, and sudorific*

skunk weed *medicinal herb* [see: skunk cabbage]

SL (sodium lactate) [q.v.]

Sleep-Eze 3 tablets (discontinued 2003) OTC *antihistaminic sleep aid* [diphenhydramine HCl] 25 mg

Sleepinal capsules, soft gels OTC *antihistaminic sleep aid* [diphenhydramine HCl] 50 mg

Sleepwell 2-nite tablets OTC *antihistaminic sleep aid* [diphenhydramine HCl] 25 mg

Slidecase (packaging form) *patient compliance package for oral contraceptives*

Slim-Mint gum (discontinued 2001) OTC *decrease taste perception of sweetness* [benzocaine] 6 mg

slippery elm (*Ulmus fulva; U. rubra*) inner bark *medicinal herb for asthma, blackened or bruised eyes, boils, bronchitis, burns, cold sores, colitis, cough, diaper rash, diarrhea, indigestion, lung disorders, sore throat, and urinary tract inflammation*

slippery root *medicinal herb* [see: comfrey]

Slo-bid Gyrocaps (extended-release capsules) ℞ *antiasthmatic; bronchodilator* [theophylline] 50, 75, 100, 125, 200, 300 mg

Slocaps (trademarked form) *sustained-release capsules*

Slo-Niacin controlled-release tablets OTC *vitamin B₃ supplement; antihyperlipidemic* [niacin] 250, 500, 750 mg

Slonnon (Japanese name for U.S. product Acova)

Slo-phyllin Gyrocaps (extended-release capsules) (discontinued 2004) ℞ *antiasthmatic; bronchodilator* [theophylline] 60, 125, 250 mg

Slo-phyllin tablets, syrup ℞ *antiasthmatic; bronchodilator* [theophylline] 100, 200 mg; 80 mg/15 mL

Slo-phyllin GG capsules, syrup (discontinued 2004) ℞ *antiasthmatic; bronchodilator; expectorant* [theophylline; guaifenesin] 150•90 mg; 150•90 mg/15 mL

Slo-Salt-K slow-release tablets OTC *electrolyte replacement; dehydration preventative* [sodium chloride; potassium chloride] 410•150 mg

slow channel blockers *a class of coronary vasodilators that inhibit cardiac muscle contraction and slow cardiac electrical conduction velocity* [also called: calcium channel blockers; calcium antagonists]

Slow Fe slow-release tablets OTC *hematinic; iron supplement* [ferrous sulfate, dried (source of iron)] 160 mg (50 mg)

Slow Fe with Folic Acid slow-release tablets OTC *hematinic* [ferrous sulfate; folic acid] 50•0.4 mg

Slow-K controlled-release tablets (discontinued 2004) ℞ *potassium supplement* [potassium chloride] 600 mg (8 mEq K)

Slow-Mag delayed-release enteric-coated tablets OTC *magnesium supplement* [magnesium chloride] 535 mg ② Flomax; Zomig

Slow-Mag enteric-coated tablets OTC *magnesium supplement* [magnesium chloride hexahydrate] 64 mg Mg

Slow-Release Iron extended-release tablets OTC *hematinic; iron supplement* [ferrous fumarate, dried (source of iron)] 150 mg (50 mg)

SLT hair lotion (discontinued 2004) OTC *antiseborrheic; antipsoriatic; keratolytic; antiseptic* [coal tar; salicylic acid; lactic acid; alcohol 65%] 2%•3%•5%

small burnet saxifrage *medicinal herb* [see: burnet]

small pimpernel *medicinal herb* [see: burnet]

small saxifrage *medicinal herb* [see: burnet]

smallpox vaccine USP *active immunizing agent*

SMART anti-CD3 antibody *investigational (Phase I) immunosuppressant*

SMART anti-gpIIb/IIIa monoclonal antibody *investigational cardiovascular antiplatelet agent*

SMART anti-tac; humanized anti-tac [now: dacliximab]

SmartMist (trademarked form) *handheld inhalation device*

smartweed; water smartweed *medicinal herb* [see: knotweed]

SMF (streptozocin, mitomycin, fluorouracil) *chemotherapy protocol for pancreatic cancer*

Smilax **spp.** *medicinal herb* [see: sarsaparilla]

smooth sumach *medicinal herb* [see: sumach]

SMX; SMZ (sulfamethoxazole) [q.v.]

SMZ-TMP (sulfamethoxazole & trimethoprim) [q.v.]

SN (streptonigrin) [q.v.]

snake bite *medicinal herb* [see: birthroot]

snake head *medicinal herb* [see: turtlebloom]

snake lily *medicinal herb* [see: blue flag]

snake weed *medicinal herb* [see: bistort; plantain]

snakebite antivenin [see: antivenin, Crotalidae & Micrurus fulvius]

snakeroot *medicinal herb* [see: echinacea]

snakeroot, black *medicinal herb* [see: black cohosh; sanicle]

Snaplets-DM granules for pediatric oral solution (discontinued 2002) OTC *antitussive; decongestant* [dextromethorphan hydrobromide; phenyl-propanolamine HCl] 5•6.25 mg/pkt.

Snaplets-EX granules for pediatric oral solution (discontinued 2002) OTC *decongestant; expectorant* [phenylpropanolamine HCl; guaifenesin] 6.25•50 mg/pkt.

Snaplets-Multi granules for pediatric oral solution (discontinued 2002) OTC *antitussive; decongestant; antihistamine* [dextromethorphan hydrobromide; phenylpropanolamine HCl; chlorpheniramine maleate] 5•6.25• 1 mg/pkt.

snapping hazel *medicinal herb* [see: witch hazel]

SnapTab (trademarked dosage form) *scored tablet*

SnET2 (tin ethyl etiopurpurin) [see: rostaporfin]

Snooze Fast tablets OTC *antihistaminic sleep aid* [diphenhydramine HCl] 50 mg

Sno-Strips ophthalmic strips *diagnostic tear flow test aid*

snout, swine *medicinal herb* [see: dandelion]

snowball, wild *medicinal herb* [see: New Jersey tea]

snowdrop tree; snowflower *medicinal herb* [see: fringe tree]

Soac-Lens solution OTC *wetting/soaking solution for hard contact lenses*

soap, green USP *detergent*

soapwort (Saponaria officinalis) plant and roots *medicinal herb for acne, boils, eczema, poison ivy rash and psoriasis; also used in skin disinfectants and soaps*

SOD (superoxide dismutase) [see: orgotein]

soda lime NF *carbon dioxide absorbent*

sodium *element (Na)*

sodium acetate USP *dialysis aid; electrolyte replenisher; pH buffer 2, 4 mEq/mL (16.4%, 32.8%) injection*

sodium acetate trihydrate [see: sodium acetate]

sodium acetrizoate INN, BAN [also: acetrizoate sodium]

sodium acetylsalicylate *analgesic*

sodium acid phosphate *urinary acidifier*

sodium alginate NF *suspending agent*

sodium amidotrizoate INN *oral/rectal/parenteral radiopaque contrast medium (59.87% iodine)* [also: diatrizoate sodium; sodium diatrizoate]

sodium aminobenzoate [see: aminobenzoate sodium]

sodium amylopectin sulfate [see: sodium amylosulfate]

sodium amylosulfate USAN *enzyme inhibitor*

sodium anoxynaphthonate BAN *blood volume and cardiac output test* [also: anazolene sodium]

sodium antimony gluconate [see: sodium stibogluconate]

sodium antimonylgluconate BAN

sodium apolate INN, BAN *anticoagulant* [also: lyapolate sodium]

sodium arsenate, exsiccated NF

sodium arsenate As 74 USAN *radioactive agent*

sodium ascorbate (vitamin C) USP, INN *water-soluble vitamin; antiscorbutic*

sodium aurothiomalate INN *antirheumatic* [also: gold sodium thiomalate]

sodium aurotiosulfate INN [also: gold sodium thiosulfate]

sodium azodisalicylate [now: olsalazine sodium]

sodium benzoate USAN, NF, JAN *antihyperammonemic; antifungal agent; preservative*

sodium benzoate & caffeine *analeptic for respiratory depression due to an overdose of CNS depressants 250 mg/mL injection*

sodium benzoate & sodium phenylacetate *to prevent and treat hyperammonemia of urea cycle enzymopathy (orphan)*

sodium benzyl penicillin [see: penicillin G sodium]

sodium bicarbonate USP *electrolyte replenisher; systemic alkalizer; antacid 325, 600, 650 mg oral; 0.5, 0.6, 0.9, 1 mEq/mL (4.2%, 5%, 7.5%, 8.4%) injection*

sodium biphosphate *urinary acidifier; pH buffer*

sodium bisulfite NF *antioxidant*

sodium bitionolate INN *topical anti-infective* [also: bithionolate sodium]

sodium borate NF *alkalizing agent; antipruritic; bacteriostatic agent in cold creams, eye washes, and mouth rinses*

sodium borocaptate (^{10}B) INN *antineoplastic; radioactive agent* [also: borocaptate sodium B 10]

sodium cacodylate NF

sodium calcium edetate INN *heavy metal chelating agent* [also: edetate calcium disodium; sodium calcium-edetate; calcium disodium edetate]

sodium calciumedetate BAN *heavy metal chelating agent* [also: edetate calcium disodium; sodium calcium edetate; calcium disodium edetate]

sodium caprylate *antifungal*

sodium carbonate NF *alkalizing agent*

sodium chloride (NaCl) USP *ophthalmic hypertonic; electrolyte replacement; abortifacient* [sterile isotonic solution] 650, 1000, 2250 mg oral; 0.45%, 0.9%, 3%, 5%, 14.6%, 23.4% injection/diluent

0.45% sodium chloride (½ normal saline; ½ NS) *electrolyte replacement*

0.9% sodium chloride (normal saline; NS) *electrolyte replacement* [also: saline solution]

sodium chloride, compound solution of INN *fluid and electrolyte replenisher* [also: Ringer's injection]

sodium chloride Na 22 USAN *radioactive agent*

sodium chondroitin sulfate [see: chondroitin sulfate sodium]

sodium chromate (^{51}Cr) INN *blood volume test; radioactive agent* [also: sodium chromate Cr 51]

sodium chromate Cr 51 USAN *blood volume test; radioactive agent* [also: sodium chromate (^{51}Cr)]

sodium citrate USP *systemic alkalizer; pH buffer; antacid; investigational (orphan) adjunct to leukapheresis procedures*

sodium colistin methanesulfonate [see: colistimethate sodium]

sodium cromoglycate [see: cromolyn sodium]

sodium cyclamate NF, INN

sodium cyclohexanesulfamate [see: sodium cyclamate]

sodium dehydroacetate NF *antimicrobial preservative*

sodium dehydrocholate INN [also: dehydrocholate sodium]

sodium denyl [see: phenytoin sodium]

sodium diatrizoate BAN *oral/rectal/parenteral radiopaque contrast medium (59.87% iodine)* [also: diatrizoate sodium; sodium amidotrizoate]

sodium dibunate INN, BAN

sodium dicloroacetate (sodium DCA) USAN *pyruvate dehydrogenase activator; investigational (orphan) for acute head trauma and neurologic injury; investigational (orphan) for lactic acidosis and homozygous familial hypercholesterolemia*

sodium diethyldithiocarbamate [see: ditiocarb sodium]

sodium diiodomethanesulfonate [see: dimethiodal sodium]

sodium dioctyl sulfosuccinate INN *stool softener; surfactant* [also: docusate sodium]

sodium diphenylhydantoin [see: phenytoin sodium]

sodium diprotrizoate INN, BAN [also: diprotrizoate sodium]

Sodium Diuril powder for IV injection ℞ *diuretic* [chlorothiazide] 500 mg

sodium edetate [see: edetate sodium]

sodium estrone sulfate *estrogen replacement therapy for postmenopausal disorders* 0.625, 1.25, 2.5, 5 mg oral

sodium etasulfate INN *detergent* [also: sodium ethasulfate]

sodium ethasulfate USAN *detergent* [also: sodium etasulfate]

sodium feredetate INN [also: sodium ironedetate]

sodium ferric gluconate *hematinic for iron deficiency due to chronic hemodialysis with epoetin therapy*

sodium fluoride USP *fluoride replacement therapy; dental caries preventative* 1.1, 2.2 mg oral; 0.125, 0.5 mg/mL oral

sodium fluoride F 18 USP

sodium fluoride & phosphoric acid USP *dental caries prophylactic*

sodium formaldehyde sulfoxylate NF *preservative*

sodium gamma hydroxybutyrate (NaGHB) [see: gamma hydroxybutyrate (GHB); sodium oxybate]

sodium gammahydroxyburate [see: sodium oxybate]

sodium gentisate INN

sodium glucaspaldrate INN, BAN

sodium gluconate USP *electrolyte replenisher*

sodium glucosulfone USP

sodium glutamate

sodium glycerophosphate NF

sodium glycocholate [see: bile salts]

sodium gualenate INN [also: azulene sulfonate sodium]

sodium hyaluronate [see: hyaluronate sodium]

sodium hydroxide NF *alkalizing agent*

sodium hydroxybenzenesulfonate [see: phenolsulphonate sodium]

sodium 4-hydroxybutyrate [see: sodium oxybate]

sodium hypochlorite USP, JAN *disinfectant; bleach; used for utensils and equipment*

sodium hypochlorite, diluted NF [also: antiformin, dental]

sodium hypophosphite NF

sodium iodide USP *dietary iodine supplement (85% elemental iodine)*

sodium iodide (^{123}I) JAN *thyroid function test; radioactive agent* [also: sodium iodide I 123]

sodium iodide (^{125}I) INN *thyroid function test; radioactive agent* [also: sodium iodide I 125]

sodium iodide (^{131}I) JAN *antineoplastic for thyroid carcinoma; radioactive agent for hyperthyroidism* [also: sodium iodide I 131]

sodium iodide I 123 USP *diagnostic aid for thyroid function; radioactive*

agent [also: sodium iodide (^{123}I)] 3.7, 7.4 MBq oral

sodium iodide I 125 USAN, USP *thyroid function test; radioactive agent* [also: sodium iodide (^{125}I)]

sodium iodide I 131 USAN, USP, INN *antineoplastic for thyroid carcinoma; radioactive agent for hyperthyroidism* [also: sodium iodide (^{131}I)] 0.75–100 mCi, 3.5–150 mCi oral

sodium iodohippurate (^{131}I) INN, JAN *renal function test; radioactive agent* [also: iodohippurate sodium I 131]

sodium iodomethanesulfonate [see: methiodal sodium]

sodium iopodate JAN *oral radiopaque contrast medium for cholecystography (61.4% iodine)* [also: ipodate sodium; sodium ipodate]

sodium iotalamate (^{125}I) INN *radioactive agent* [also: iothalamate sodium I 125]

sodium iotalamate (^{131}I) INN *radioactive agent* [also: iothalamate sodium I 131]

sodium iothalamate BAN *parenteral radiopaque contrast medium (59.9% iodine)* [also: iothalamate sodium]

sodium ioxaglate BAN *radiopaque contrast medium* [also: ioxaglate sodium]

sodium ipodate INN, BAN *oral radiopaque contrast medium for cholecystography (61.4% iodine)* [also: ipodate sodium; sodium iopodate]

sodium ironedetate BAN [also: sodium feredetate]

sodium lactate (SL) USP *electrolyte replenisher* 167 mEq/L (1/6 molar) injection

sodium lactate, compound solution of INN *electrolyte and fluid replenisher; systemic alkalizer* [also: Ringer's injection, lactated]

sodium lauryl sulfate NF *surfactant/ wetting agent* [also: laurilsulfate]

sodium lignosulfonate [see: polignate sodium]

sodium metabisulfite NF *antioxidant*

sodium metrizoate INN *radiopaque contrast medium* [also: metrizoate sodium]

sodium monododecyl sulfate [see: sodium lauryl sulfate]

sodium monofluorophosphate USP *dental caries prophylactic*

sodium monomercaptoundecahydro-closo-dodecaborate *investigational (orphan) for boron neutron capture therapy (BNCT) for glioblastoma multiforme*

sodium morrhuate INN *sclerosing agent* [also: morrhuate sodium]

sodium nitrite USP *antidote to cyanide poisoning* 30 mg/mL injection

sodium nitroferricyanide [see: sodium nitroprusside]

sodium nitroferricyanide dihydrate [see: sodium nitroprusside]

sodium nitroprusside USP *emergency antihypertensive; vasodilator* 50 mg/dose injection

sodium noramidopyrine methanesulfonate [see: dipyrone]

sodium oxybate USAN *adjunct to anesthesia; CNS depressant for narcolepsy, cataplexy, sleep paralysis, and hypnagogic hallucinations (orphan)* [also known as: gamma hydroxybutyrate (GHB)]

sodium oxychlorosene [see: oxychlorosene sodium]

sodium paratoluenesulfan chloramide [see: chloramine-T]

sodium PCA; Na PCA (sodium pyrrolidone carboxylic acid) [q.v.]

sodium penicillin G [see: penicillin G sodium]

sodium pentosan polysulfate [see: pentosan polysulfate sodium]

sodium perborate *topical antiseptic/germicidal*

sodium perborate monohydrate USAN

sodium pertechnetate Tc 99m USAN, USP *radioactive agent*

sodium phenolate [see: phenolate sodium]

sodium phenylacetate USAN *antihyperammonemic*

sodium phenylacetate & sodium benzoate *to prevent and treat hyper-* *ammonemia of urea cycle enzymopathy (orphan)*

sodium phenylbutyrate USAN *antihyperammonemic for urea cycle disorders (orphan); investigational (orphan) for various sickling disorders*

sodium phosphate (^{32}P) INN *antineoplastic; antipolycythemic; neoplasm test* [also: sodium phosphate P 32]

sodium phosphate, dibasic USP *saline laxative; phosphorus replacement; pH buffer*

sodium phosphate, monobasic USP *saline laxative; phosphorus replacement; pH buffer*

sodium phosphate P 32 USAN, USP *antipolycythemic; radiopharmaceutical antineoplastic for various leukemias and skeletal metastases* [also: sodium phosphate (^{32}P)] 0.67 mCi/mL

sodium picofosfate INN

sodium picosulfate INN

sodium polyphosphate USAN *pharmaceutic aid*

sodium polystyrene sulfonate USP *potassium-removing ion-exchange resin for hyperkalemia* 15 g/60 mL oral

sodium propionate NF *preservative; antifungal*

sodium propionate hydrate [see: sodium propionate]

sodium 2-propylvalerate [see: valproate sodium]

sodium psylliate NF

sodium pyrophosphate USAN *pharmaceutic aid*

sodium pyrrolidone carboxylic acid (sodium PCA; Na PCA) *natural skin moisturizing factor; humectant*

sodium radiochromate [see: sodium chromate Cr 51]

sodium rhodanate [see: thiocyanate sodium]

sodium salicylate (SS) USP *analgesic; antipyretic; anti-inflammatory; antirheumatic* 325, 650 mg oral

sodium starch glycolate NF *tablet excipient*

sodium stearate NF *emulsifying and stiffening agent*

sodium stearyl fumarate NF *tablet and capsule lubricant*

sodium stibocaptate INN [also: stibocaptate]

sodium stibogluconate INN, BAN, DCF *investigational antiparasitic for leishmaniasis and trypanosomiasis*

Sodium Sulamyd eye drops, ophthalmic ointment ℞ *antibiotic* [sulfacetamide sodium] 10%, 30%; 10%

sodium sulfacetamide [see: sulfacetamide sodium]

sodium sulfate USP *calcium regulator*

sodium sulfate S 35 USAN *radioactive agent*

sodium sulfocyanate [see: thiocyanate sodium]

sodium taurocholate [see: bile salts]

sodium tetradecyl (STD) sulfate INN *sclerosing agent for varicose veins; investigational (orphan) for bleeding esophageal varices*

sodium thiomalate, gold [see: gold sodium thiomalate]

sodium thiosalicylate *analgesic; antipyretic; anti-inflammatory; antirheumatic* 50 mg/mL injection

sodium thiosulfate USP *antidote to cyanide poisoning; antiseptic; antifungal* 10%, 25% (100, 250 mg/mL) injection

sodium thiosulfate, gold [see: gold sodium thiosulfate]

sodium thiosulfate & hydroxocobalamin *investigational (orphan) for severe acute cyanide poisoning*

sodium thiosulfate pentahydrate [see: sodium thiosulfate]

sodium timerfonate INN *topical anti-infective* [also: thimerfonate sodium]

sodium trimetaphosphate USAN *pharmaceutic aid*

sodium tyropanoate INN *oral radiopaque contrast medium for cholecystography* (57.4% iodine) [also: tyropanoate sodium]

sodium valproate [see: valproate sodium]

Sodol Compound tablets ℞ *skeletal muscle relaxant; analgesic* [carisoprodol; aspirin] 200•325 mg

sofalcone INN

Sofenol 5 lotion (discontinued 2004) OTC *moisturizer; emollient*

Sof-lax softgels OTC *laxative; stool softener* [docusate sodium] 100 mg

Soft Mate Comfort Drops for Sensitive Eyes OTC *rewetting solution for soft contact lenses*

Soft Mate Consept solution + aerosol spray OTC *two-step chemical disinfecting system for soft contact lenses* [hydrogen peroxide based] 3%

Soft Mate Disinfecting for Sensitive Eyes solution OTC *chemical disinfecting solution for soft contact lenses*

Soft Mate Hands Off Daily Cleaner solution OTC *surfactant cleaning solution for soft contact lenses*

soft pine *medicinal herb* [see: white pine]

Soft Sense lotion OTC *moisturizer; emollient*

Softabs (trademarked dosage form) *chewable tablets*

softgels (dosage form) *soft gelatin capsules*

SoftWear solution OTC *rinsing/storage solution for soft contact lenses* [sodium chloride (preserved saline solution)]

Solagé topical solution ℞ *depigmenting agent for solar lentigines* [mequinol; tretinoin; alcohol 77.8%] 2%•0.01%

Solanum dulcamara *medicinal herb* [see: bittersweet nightshade]

solapsone BAN [also: solasulfone]

Solaquin cream OTC *hyperpigmentation bleaching agent* [hydroquinone in a sunscreen base] 2%

Solaquin Forte cream, gel ℞ *hyperpigmentation bleaching agent* [hydroquinone (in a sunscreen base)] 4%

Solaraze gel ℞ *topical treatment for actinic keratosis* [diclofenac potassium] 3%

Solarcaine aerosol spray, lotion OTC *topical local anesthetic; antiseptic* [benzocaine; triclosan] 20%•0.13%

Solarcaine Aloe Extra Burn Relief spray, gel, cream OTC *topical local anesthetic* [lidocaine] 0.5%

solasulfone INN [also: solapsone]

soldier's woundwort *medicinal herb* [see: yarrow]

Solfoton tablets, capsules ℞ *long-acting barbiturate sedative, hypnotic, and anticonvulsant* [phenobarbital] 16 mg

Solganal IM injection ℞ *antirheumatic* [aurothioglucose] 50 mg/mL

Solia tablets (in packs of 28) ℞ *monophasic oral contraceptive* [desogestrel; ethinyl estradiol] 0.15 mg•30 µg

Solidago nemoralis; S. odora; S. virgaurea medicinal herb [see: goldenrod]

solifenacin succinate *selective muscarinic M₃ receptor antagonist; antispasmodic for overactive bladder with urinary incontinence, urgency, and frequency*

Solomon's seal *(Polygonatum multiflorum; P. odoratum)* root *medicinal herb used as an astringent, demulcent, emetic, and expectorant*

solpecainol INN

SolTabs (trademarked dosage form) *orally disintegrating tablets*

Soltice Quick-Rub OTC *analgesic; counterirritant* [methyl salicylate; camphor; menthol; eucalyptus oil]

soluble complement receptor [see: complement receptor type I, soluble recombinant human]

soluble ferric pyrophosphate [see: ferric pyrophosphate, soluble]

soluble gelatin (SG) [see: gelatin]

Soluble T4 ℞ *investigational (orphan) treatment for AIDS* [CD4 human truncated 369 AA polypeptide]

Solu-Cortef powder for IV or IM injection ℞ *corticosteroid; anti-inflammatory* [hydrocortisone sodium succinate] 100, 250, 500, 1000 mg/vial

Solu-Medrol powder for IV or IM injection ℞ *corticosteroid; anti-inflammatory; immunosuppressant* [methylprednisolone sodium succinate] 40, 125, 500, 1000, 2000 mg/vial

Solumol OTC *ointment base*

Solurex intra-articular, intralesional, soft tissue, or IM injection ℞ *corticosteroid; anti-inflammatory* [dexamethasone sodium phosphate] 4 mg/mL

Solurex LA intralesional, intra-articular, soft tissue, or IM injection ℞ *corticosteroid; anti-inflammatory* [dexamethasone acetate] 8 mg/mL

Soluspan (trademarked form) *injectable suspension*

Soluvite C.T. chewable tablets ℞ *pediatric vitamin supplement and dental caries preventative* [multiple vitamins; fluoride; folic acid] ≛•1•0.3 mg

Soluvite-f drops ℞ *pediatric vitamin supplement and dental caries preventative* [vitamins A, C, and D; fluoride] 1500 IU•35 mg•400 IU•0.25 mg per 0.6 mL

Solvent-G OTC *liquid base*

Solvet (trademarked dosage form) *soluble tablet*

solypertine INN *antiadrenergic* [also: solypertine tartrate]

solypertine tartrate USAN *antiadrenergic* [also: solypertine]

Soma tablets ℞ *skeletal muscle relaxant* [carisoprodol] 350 mg

Soma Compound tablets ℞ *skeletal muscle relaxant; analgesic* [carisoprodol; aspirin] 200•325 mg

Soma Compound with Codeine tablets ℞ *skeletal muscle relaxant; narcotic antitussive; analgesic* [carisoprodol; aspirin; codeine phosphate] 200•325•16 mg

somagrebove USAN *veterinary galactopoietic agent*

somalapor USAN, INN, BAN *porcine growth hormone*

somantadine INN *antiviral* [also: somantadine HCl]

somantadine HCl USAN *antiviral* [also: somantadine]

somatomedin-C [see: mecasermin]

somatorelin INN *growth hormone-releasing factor (GH-RF)*

somatostatin (SS) INN, BAN *growth hormone-release inhibiting factor; investigational (orphan) for cutaneous* *gastrointestinal fistulas and bleeding esophageal varices*

SomatoTher ℞ *investigational (orphan) radiotherapeutic agent for somatostatin receptor–positive neuroendocrine tumors* [indium In 111 pentetreotide]

somatotropin, human [see: somatropin]

somatrem USAN, INN, BAN *growth hormone for congenital growth failure due to lack of endogenous growth hormone (orphan)*

somatropin USAN, INN, BAN, JAN *growth hormone for adults or children with congenital or endogenous growth hormone deficiency, children with Turner syndrome or renal-induced growth failure, short bowel syndrome, or AIDS-wasting syndrome (orphan); investigational (orphan) for severe burns* [also: human growth hormone]

somatropin & glutamine *investigational (orphan) for GI malabsorption due to short bowel syndrome*

Somavert subcu injection ℞ *growth hormone receptor antagonist for acromegaly (orphan)* [pegvisomant] 10, 15, 20 mg/dose

somavubove USAN, INN *veterinary galactopoietic agent*

somenopor USAN *porcine growth hormone*

sometribove USAN, INN, BAN *veterinary growth stimulant*

sometripor USAN, INN, BAN *veterinary growth stimulant*

somfasepor USAN *veterinary growth stimulant*

somidobove USAN, INN *synthetic bovine growth hormone*

Sominex tablets, caplets OTC *antihistaminic sleep aid* [diphenhydramine HCl] 25 mg; 50 mg

Sominex Pain Relief tablets OTC *antihistaminic sleep aid; analgesic* [diphenhydramine HCl; acetaminophen] 25•500 mg

Somnote capsules ℞ *nonbarbiturate sedative and hypnotic; also abused as a street drug* [chloral hydrate] 500 mg

Sonata capsules ℞ *rapid-onset, short-duration hypnotic for the short-term treatment of insomnia* [zaleplon] 5, 10 mg

sonepiprazole mesylate USAN *dopamine D_4 antagonist; antipsychotic*

SonoRx oral suspension ℞ *ultrasound imaging agent to reduce gas shadowing* [simethicone-coated cellulose] 7.5 mg/mL

SonoVue ℞ *investigational ultrasound imaging agent* [sulfur hexafluoride]

Soothaderm lotion OTC *local anesthetic; antihistamine; emollient* [pyrilamine maleate; benzocaine; zinc oxide] 2.07•2.08•41.35 mg/mL

sopecainol [see: solpecainol]

sopitazine INN

sopromidine INN

soproxil USAN *combining name for radicals or groups* [also: disoproxil]

soquinolol INN

sorb apple *medicinal herb* [see: mountain ash]

sorbic acid NF *antimicrobial agent; preservative*

sorbide nitrate [see: isosorbide dinitrate]

sorbimacrogol laurate 300 [see: polysorbate 20]

sorbimacrogol oleate 300 [see: polysorbate 80]

sorbimacrogol palmitate 300 [see: polysorbate 40]

sorbimacrogol stearate [see: polysorbate 60]

sorbimacrogol tristearate 300 [see: polysorbate 65]

sorbinicate INN

sorbinil USAN, INN, BAN *aldose reductase enzyme inhibitor*

sorbitan laurate INN *surfactant* [also: sorbitan monolaurate]

sorbitan monolaurate USAN, NF *surfactant* [also: sorbitan laurate]

sorbitan monooleate USAN, NF *surfactant* [also: sorbitan oleate]

sorbitan monopalmitate USAN, NF *surfactant* [also: sorbitan palmitate]

sorbitan monostearate USAN, NF *surfactant* [also: sorbitan stearate]

sorbitan oleate INN *surfactant* [also: sorbitan monooleate]

sorbitan palmitate INN *surfactant* [also: sorbitan monopalmitate]

sorbitan sesquioleate USAN, INN *surfactant*

sorbitan stearate INN *surfactant* [also: sorbitan monostearate]

sorbitan trioleate USAN, INN *surfactant*

sorbitan tristearate USAN, INN *surfactant*

sorbitol NF *flavoring agent; tablet excipient; urologic irrigant* 3%, 3.3%

sorbitol (solution) USP *flavoring agent; tablet excipient*

Sorbitrate sublingual tablets (discontinued 2004) ℞ *antianginal; vasodilator* [isosorbide dinitrate] 2.5, 5 mg

Sorbitrate tablets, chewable tablets (discontinued 2005) ℞ *antianginal; vasodilator* [isosorbide dinitrate] 5, 10, 20, 30, 40 mg; 5, 10 mg

Sorbsan pads *absorbent dressing for wet wounds* [calcium alginate fiber]

Sorbus americana; S. aucuparia *medicinal herb* [see: mountain ash]

Soriatane capsules ℞ *systemic antipsoriatic* [acitretin] 10, 25 mg

sorivudine USAN, INN, BAN *antiviral for varicella zoster and herpes zoster in immunocompromised patients; orphan status withdrawn 1997*

sornidipine INN

sorrel *(Rumex acetosa)* plant *medicinal herb used as an antiscorbutic, astringent, diuretic, laxative, refrigerant, and vermifuge*

sorrel, common; mountain sorrel; white sorrel *medicinal herb* [see: wood sorrel]

sorrel, Jamaica *medicinal herb* [see: hibiscus]

Sortis (European name for U.S. product **Lipitor**)

sotalol INN, BAN *antiarrhythmic; antiadrenergic (β-receptor)* [also: sotalol HCl]

sotalol HCl USAN *antiarrhythmic (β-blocker) for ventricular arrhythmias (orphan)* [also: sotalol] 80, 120, 160, 240 mg oral

Sotalol HCl AF tablets ℞ *antiarrhythmic (β-blocker) for atrial fibrillation or atrial flutter* [sotalol HCl] 80, 120, 160 mg

soterenol INN *adrenergic; bronchodilator* [also: soterenol HCl]

soterenol HCl USAN *adrenergic; bronchodilator* [also: soterenol]

Sotradecol IV injection, Dosette (unit-of-use injection) ℞ *sclerosing agent for varicose veins; investigational (orphan) for bleeding esophageal varices* [sodium tetradecyl sulfate] 10, 30 mg/mL

Sotret softgels ℞ *keratolytic for severe recalcitrant cystic acne* [isotretinoin] 10, 20, 30, 40 mg

sour dock *medicinal herb* [see: yellow dock]

sourberry; sowberry *medicinal herb* [see: barberry]

sourgrass *medicinal herb* [see: sorrel]

Southern ginseng *medicinal herb* [see: jiaogulan]

Soviet gramicidin [see: gramicidin S]

sowberry; sourberry *medicinal herb* [see: barberry]

soy; soya; soybean *(Glycine max) medicinal herb and food crop; isoflavone compounds provide phytoestrogens to alleviate menopausal symptoms, including osteoporosis, and provide antineoplastic, cardiovascular, and gastrointestinal benefits*

Soyalac; I-Soyalac oral liquid, powder for oral liquid OTC *hypoallergenic infant food* [soy protein formula]

soybean oil USP *pharmaceutic necessity*

spaglumic acid INN

Span C tablets OTC *vitamin C supplement with bioflavonoids* [ascorbic acid and rose hips; citrus bioflavonoids] 200•300 mg

Spancap No. 1 sustained-release capsules ℞ *CNS stimulant* [dextroamphetamine sulfate] 15 mg

Spancaps (dosage form) *timed-release capsules*

Spanish chestnut *medicinal herb* [see: horse chestnut]

Spanish pepper *medicinal herb* [see: cayenne]

Spansule (trademarked dosage form) *sustained-release capsule*

sparfloxacin (SPFX) USAN, INN, BAN *broad-spectrum fluoroquinolone antibiotic*

sparfosate sodium USAN *antineoplastic* [also: sparfosic acid]

sparfosic acid INN *antineoplastic* [also: sparfosate sodium]

Sparine tablets (discontinued 2001) ℞ *conventional (typical) antipsychotic* [promazine HCl] 25, 50 mg

Sparkles effervescent granules OTC *antacid; aid in endoscopic examination* [sodium bicarbonate; citric acid; simethicone] 2000•1500• ≟ mg/dose

sparsomycin USAN, INN *antineoplastic*

Spartaject ℞ *investigational (Phase II/ III) intravenous delivery device*

Spartaject Busulfan ℞ *investigational (orphan) alkylating antineoplastic for neoplastic meningitis and primary brain malignancies* [busulfan]

sparteine INN *oxytocic* [also: sparteine sulfate]

sparteine sulfate USAN *oxytocic* [also: sparteine]

Spasmolin tablets ℞ *GI antispasmodic; anticholinergic; sedative* [atropine sulfate; scopolamine hydrobromide; hyoscyamine hydrobromide; phenobarbital] 0.0194•0.0065•0.1037•16.2 mg

SPCA (serum prothrombin conversion accelerator) factor [see: factor VII]

spearmint NF

spearmint (Mentha spicata) leaves *medicinal herb for colds, colic, flu, gas, nausea, and vomiting*

spearmint oil NF

Spec-T lozenges OTC *topical oral anesthetic* [benzocaine] 10 mg

Spec-T Sore Throat/Cough Suppressant lozenges (discontinued 2002) OTC *topical oral anesthetic; antitussive* [benzocaine; dextromethorphan hydrobromide] 10•10 mg

Spec-T Sore Throat/Decongestant lozenges (discontinued 2001) OTC *decongestant; topical oral anesthetic* [phenylpropanolamine HCl; phenyl-

ephrine HCl; benzocaine] 10.5•5• 10 mg

Spectazole cream ℞ *antifungal* [econazole nitrate] 1%

spectinomycin INN *antibiotic* [also: spectinomycin HCl]

spectinomycin HCl USAN, USP *antibiotic for gonorrhea* [also: spectinomycin]

Spectracef capsules ℞ *broad-spectrum cephalosporin antibiotic* [cefditoren pivoxil] 200, 400 mg

Spectrobid film-coated tablets (discontinued 2002) ℞ *aminopenicillin antibiotic* [bacampicillin HCl] 400 mg

Spectrocin Plus ointment (discontinued 2005) OTC *antibiotic; local anesthetic* [polymyxin B sulfate; neomycin sulfate; bacitracin zinc; pramoxine HCl] 10 000 U•3.5 mg• 500 U•10 mg per g

Spectro-Jel topical liquid OTC *soapfree therapeutic skin cleanser*

speedwell (Veronica officinalis) flowering plant *medicinal herb used as a diuretic, expectorant, and stomachic*

speedwell, tall *medicinal herb* [see: Culver root]

spenbolic [see: methandriol]

spermaceti, synthetic [see: cetyl esters wax]

spermicides *a class of topical contraceptive agents that kill the male sperm*

Spexil ℞ *investigational (Phase III) broad-spectrum aminocyclitol antibiotic for respiratory, gynecologic, and abdominal infections* [trospectomycin]

SPFX (sparfloxacin) [q.v.]

Spheramine ℞ *investigational (Phase II, orphan) dopamine-producing brain implants for stage 3 and 4 Parkinson disease* [human retinal pigment epithelial (RPE) cells on spherical cell-coated microcarriers (CCM)]

Spherulin intradermal injection ℞ *diagnostic aid for coccidioidomycosis* [coccidioidin] 1:100, 1:10

spiceberry *medicinal herb* [see: wintergreen]

spiclamine INN

spiclomazine INN

spicy wintergreen *medicinal herb* [see: wintergreen]

spider bite antivenin [see: antivenin (Latrodectus mactans)]

spignet *medicinal herb* [see: spikenard]

spikenard (Aralia racemosa) root *medicinal herb for asthma, childbirth, cough, and rheumatism*

spindle tree *medicinal herb* [see: wahoo]

spiperone USAN, INN *antipsychotic*

spiradoline INN *analgesic* [also: spiradoline mesylate]

spiradoline mesylate USAN *analgesic* [also: spiradoline]

spiramide INN

spiramycin USAN, INN, BAN *macrolide antibiotic* [also: acetylspiramycin]

spirapril INN, BAN *angiotensin-converting enzyme (ACE) inhibitor* [also: spirapril HCl]

spirapril HCl USAN *angiotensin-converting enzyme (ACE) inhibitor* [also: spirapril]

spiraprilat USAN, INN *angiotensin-converting enzyme (ACE) inhibitor*

spirazine INN

spirazine HCl [see: spirazine]

spirendolol INN

spirgetine INN

spirilene INN, BAN

spirit of nitrous ether [see: ethyl nitrite]

Spiriva powder in capsules for inhalation (used with HandiHaler device) ℞ *once-daily bronchodilator for chronic obstructive pulmonary disease (COPD)* [tiotropium bromide] 18 μg/dose

spirobarbital sodium

spirofylline INN

spirogermanium INN, BAN *antineoplastic* [also: spirogermanium HCl]

spirogermanium HCl USAN *antineoplastic* [also: spirogermanium]

spirohydantoin mustard [now: spiromustine]

spiromustine USAN, INN *antineoplastic*

spironolactone USP, INN, BAN, JAN *antihypertensive; potassium-sparing diuretic; aldosterone antagonist* 25, 50, 100 mg oral

spiroplatin USAN, INN, BAN *antineoplastic*

spirorenone INN

spirotriazine HCl [see: spirazine]

spiroxamide [see: spiroxatrine]

spiroxasone USAN, INN *diuretic*

spiroxatrine INN

spiroxepin INN

spirulina (Spirulina pratensis) plant *medicinal herb for chronic disease, enhancing antibody production, lowering serum lipids and triglycerides, and reducing gastric secretory activity; also used as a blood builder and food supplement*

spizofurone INN

SPL (staphage lysate) [q.v.]

spoonwood *medicinal herb* [see: linden tree]

Sporanox capsules, PulsePak, IV infusion ℞ *systemic triazole antifungal* [itraconazole] 100 mg; 28 × 100 mg; 10 mg/mL

Sporanox oral solution ("swish and swallow") ℞ *antifungal for esophageal and oropharyngeal candidiasis* [itraconazole] 10 mg/mL

Sporidin-G ℞ *investigational (orphan) treatment of cryptosporidiosis-induced diarrhea in immunocompromised patients* [Cryptosporidium parvum bovine colostrum IgG concentrate]

Sports Spray OTC *analgesic; counterirritant; antiseptic* [methyl salicylate; menthol; camphor; alcohol 58%] 3.5%•10%•5%

Sportscreme OTC *topical analgesic* [trolamine salicylate] 10%

Sportscreme Ice gel OTC *topical analgesic; counterirritant* [trolamine; menthol] ≟•2%

spotted alder *medicinal herb* [see: witch hazel]

spotted-comfrey *medicinal herb* [see: lungwort]

spotted cranesbill *medicinal herb* [see: alum root]

spotted geranium *medicinal herb* [see: alum root]

spotted hemlock; spotted cowbane; spotted parsley *medicinal herb* [see: poison hemlock]

spotted lungwort *medicinal herb* [see: lungwort]

spotted thistle *medicinal herb* [see: blessed thistle]

spp. plural of *species*

SPP100 *investigational (Phase III) renin antagonist for hypertension*

SPPG (sulfated polysaccharide peptidoglycan) [see: tecogalan sodium]

Spray-U-Thin *oral spray* (discontinued 2001) OTC *diet aid* [phenylpropanolamine HCl] 6.58 mg

spring wintergreen *medicinal herb* [see: wintergreen]

Sprinkle Caps (trademarked form) *powder*

Sprintec *tablets* (in packs of 28) ℞ *monophasic oral contraceptive* [norgestimate; ethinyl estradiol] 0.25 mg• 35 μg

sprodiamide USAN *heart and CNS imaging aid for MRI*

spruce (Picea excelsa; P. mariana) young shoots *medicinal herb used as a calmative, diaphoretic, expectorant, and pectoral*

spruce, Norway *medicinal herb* [see: spruce]

spruce, weeping *medicinal herb* [see: hemlock]

SPS *oral suspension* ℞ *potassium-removing agent for hyperkalemia* [sodium polystyrene sulfonate] 15 g/60 mL

spurge laurel; spurge olive *medicinal herb* [see: mezereon]

squalamine *natural remedy; investigational (Phase III) angiogenesis inhibitor for the treatment of solid tumors; investigational (Phase II) for advanced non–small cell lung cancer (NSCLC)* [also: shark cartilage]

squalane NF *oleaginous vehicle*

square, carpenter's *medicinal herb* [see: figwort]

squaw balm; squaw mint *medicinal herb* [see: pennyroyal]

squaw root *medicinal herb* [see: black cohosh; blue cohosh]

squaw tea *medicinal herb* [see: ephedra]

squaw vine (Mitchella repens) plant *medicinal herb for easing childbirth, lactation, and menstruation and for uterine disorders*

squaw weed *medicinal herb* [see: life root]

squawberry *medicinal herb* [see: squaw vine]

squill (Urginea indica; U. maritima; U. scilla) bulb *medicinal herb for edema and inducing emesis and expectoration; also used as a rat poison*

squirrel pea, ground *medicinal herb* [see: twin leaf]

SR-57746 *investigational (Phase III) agent for Alzheimer disease*

^{85}**Sr** [see: strontium chloride Sr 85]

^{85}**Sr** [see: strontium nitrate Sr 85]

^{85}**Sr** [see: strontium Sr 85]

SRC Expectorant *oral liquid* (discontinued 2002) ℞ *narcotic antitussive; decongestant; expectorant* [hydrocodone bitartrate; pseudoephedrine HCl; guaifenesin; alcohol 12.5%] 5• 60•200 mg/5 mL

SRF (skin respiratory factor) [q.v.]

SS (saline solution)

SS (sodium salicylate) [q.v.]

SS (somatostatin) [q.v.]

SSD (silver sulfadiazine) [q.v.]

SSD; SSD AF *cream* ℞ *broad-spectrum bactericidal for adjunctive burn treatment* [silver sulfadiazine] 10 mg/g

SSKI *oral solution* ℞ *expectorant* [potassium iodide] 1 g/mL

SSNRIs (selective serotonin and norepinephrine reuptake inhibitors) [q.v.]

SSRIs (selective serotonin reuptake inhibitors) [q.v.]

S.S.S. High Potency Vitamin Tablets OTC *vitamin/mineral/iron supplement* [multiple vitamins & minerals; iron; biotin] ≚•27•0.0225 mg

S.S.S. Vitamin and Mineral Complex *oral liquid* OTC *vitamin/mineral/iron supplement* [multiple vitamins & minerals; iron; biotin; alcohol 6.6%] ≚•3•0.1 mg

S.T. 37 solution OTC *topical antiseptic* [hexylresorcinol] 0.1%

S·T Cort lotion ℞ *topical corticosteroidal anti-inflammatory* [hydrocortisone] 0.5%

S·T Forte syrup, oral liquid (discontinued 2002) ℞ *narcotic antitussive; decongestant; antihistamine; expectorant* [hydrocodone bitartrate; phenylephrine HCl; phenylpropanolamine HCl; pheniramine maleate; guaifenesin; alcohol 5%] 2.5•5•5• 13.33•80 mg/5 mL

S·T Forte 2 oral liquid ℞ *narcotic antitussive; antihistamine* [hydrocodone bitartrate; chlorpheniramine maleate] 2.5•2 mg/5 mL

Staarvisc intraocular injection ℞ *viscoelastic agent for ophthalmic surgery* [hyaluronate sodium]

stable factor [see: factor VII]

Stachys officinalis medicinal herb [see: betony]

Stadol IV or IM injection ℞ *narcotic agonist-antagonist analgesic* [butorphanol tartrate] 1, 2 mg/mL

Stadol NS nasal spray (discontinued 2004) ℞ *narcotic agonist-antagonist analgesic; antimigraine agent* [butorphanol tartrate] 10 mg/mL

staff vine *medicinal herb* [see: bittersweet nightshade]

Stagesic capsules ℞ *narcotic analgesic* [hydrocodone bitartrate; acetaminophen] 5•500 mg

staggerweed *medicinal herb* [see: turkey corn]

staghorn *medicinal herb* [see: club moss]

Stahist sustained-release tablets ℞ *decongestant; antihistamine; anticholinergic to dry mucosal secretions* [phenylephrine HCl; pseudoephedrine HCl; chlorpheniramine maleate; hyoscyamine sulfate; atropine sulfate; scopolamine hydrobromide] 25•40•8•0.19•0.04•0.01 mg

Stalevo 50; Stalevo 100; Stalevo 150 tablets ℞ *multi-modal antiparkinsonian: dopamine precursor + dopa-decarboxylase inhibitor + catechol-O-*methyltransferase (COMT) *inhibitor* [levodopa; carbidopa; entacapone] 50•12.5•200 mg; 100•25•200 mg; 150•37.5•200 mg

stallimycin INN *antibacterial* [also: stallimycin HCl]

stallimycin HCl USAN *antibacterial* [also: stallimycin]

Stamoist E sustained-release film-coated caplets ℞ *decongestant; expectorant* [pseudoephedrine HCl; guaifenesin] 120•500 mg

Stamoist LA sustained-release tablets (discontinued 2002) ℞ *decongestant; expectorant* [phenylpropanolamine HCl; guaifenesin] 75•400 mg

standard VAC *chemotherapy protocol for sarcomas* [see: VAC standard]

Stanford V (mechlorethamine, doxorubicin, vinblastine, vincristine, bleomycin, etoposide, prednisone) *chemotherapy protocol for Hodgkin lymphoma*

stannous chloride USAN *pharmaceutic aid*

stannous fluoride USP *dental caries prophylactic* 0.4%, 0.63% topical oral

stannous pyrophosphate USAN *skeletal imaging aid*

stannous sulfur colloid USAN *bone, liver and spleen imaging aid*

stannsoporfin USAN *investigational bilirubin inhibitor for neonatal hyperbilirubinemia*

stanolone BAN *investigational (orphan) for AIDS-wasting syndrome* [also: androstanolone]

stanozolol USAN, USP, INN, BAN *androgen; anabolic steroid for hereditary angioedema*

staphage lysate (SPL) *active bacterin for staphylococcal infections*

StaphVAX ℞ *investigational (Phase III) vaccine against* Staphylococcus aureus *infection of end-stage renal disease*

Staphylococcus aureus vaccine [see: staphage lysate]

star anise (*Illicium anisatum; I. verum***)** seeds *medicinal herb used as a carminative, stimulant, and stomachic;*

also added to other herbal medications to improve digestibility and taste

star chickweed; starweed *medicinal herb* [see: chickweed]

star grass (Aletris farinosa) root and rhizome *medicinal herb for diarrhea, dysmenorrhea and menstrual discomfort, gas and colonic cramps, and rheumatism*

star root *medicinal herb* [see: star grass]

starch NF *dusting powder; pharmaceutic aid*

starch, pregelatinized NF *tablet excipient*

starch, topical USP *dusting powder*

starch carboxymethyl ether, sodium salt [see: sodium starch glycolate]

starch glycerite NF

starch 2-hydroxyethyl ether [see: hetastarch; pentastarch]

Starlix tablets ℞ *antidiabetic agent that stimulates the release of insulin from the pancreas for type 2 diabetes* [nateglinide] 60, 120 mg

Starnoc ⓒᴬᴺ capsules ℞ *rapid-onset, short-duration hypnotic for the short-term treatment of insomnia* [zaleplon] 5, 10 mg

Star-Otic ear drops OTC *antibacterial; antifungal* [acetic acid; aluminum acetate; boric acid]

Starsis (Japanese name for U.S. product **Starlix**)

Starvisc [see: Staarvisc]

starwort; mealy starwort *medicinal herb* [see: chickweed; star grass]

Stat-Crit electrode device *for professional use in vitro diagnostic aid for hemoglobin/hematocrit measurement*

STATdose (trademarked device) *pre-filled syringes for self-administration*

Staticin topical solution (discontinued 2004) ℞ *antibiotic for acne* [erythromycin; alcohol 55%] 1.5%

"statins" *brief term for a class of antihyperlipidemics that include atorvastatin, cerivastatin, fluvastatin, lovastatin, pravastatin, rosuvastatin, and simvastatin* [properly called: HMG-CoA reductase inhibitors]

statolon USAN *antiviral* [also: vistatolon]

Stat-One gel (discontinued 2004) OTC *antiseptic* [hydrogen peroxide] 3%

Stat-One gel (discontinued 2004) OTC *antiseptic* [isopropyl alcohol] 70%

Stat-Pak (trademarked packaging form) *unit-dose package*

Statuss Expectorant oral liquid (discontinued 2002) ℞ *narcotic antitussive; decongestant; expectorant* [codeine phosphate; phenylpropanolamine HCl; guaifenesin; alcohol 5%] 10•12.5•100 mg/5 mL

Statuss Green oral liquid ℞ *narcotic antitussive; decongestant; antihistamine* [hydrocodone bitartrate; phenylephrine HCl; pseudoephedrine HCl; chlorpheniramine maleate; pyrilamine maleate] 5•10•6.6•4•6.6 mg/10 mL

staunch, blood *medicinal herb* [see: fleabane; horseweed]

stavudine USAN, INN *nucleoside reverse transcriptase inhibitor; antiviral for HIV-1 infection*

Stay Alert tablets (discontinued 2001) OTC *CNS stimulant; analeptic* [caffeine] 200 mg

Stay Awake tablets OTC *CNS stimulant; analeptic* [caffeine] 200 mg

Stay-Wet 3; Stay-Wet 4 solution OTC *disinfecting/wetting/soaking solution for rigid gas permeable contact lenses*

STD (sodium tetradecyl sulfate) [q.v.]

steaglate INN *combining name for radicals or groups*

STEAM (streptonigrin, thioguanine, cyclophosphamide, actinomycin, mitomycin) *chemotherapy protocol*

stearethate 40 [see: polyoxyl 40 stearate]

stearic acid NF *emulsion adjunct; tablet and capsule lubricant*

stearyl alcohol NF *emulsion adjunct*

stearyl dimethyl benzyl ammonium chloride

stearylsulfamide INN

Stedicor *investigational antiarrhythmic* [azimilide dihydrochloride]

steffimycin USAN, INN *antibacterial; antiviral*

Stelazine film-coated tablets (discontinued 2003) ℞ *conventional (typical) phenothiazine antipsychotic for schizophrenia; anxiolytic for nonpsychotic anxiety* [trifluoperazine HCl] 5 mg

Stelazine IM injection (discontinued 2003) ℞ *conventional (typical) phenothiazine antipsychotic for schizophrenia; anxiolytic for nonpsychotic anxiety* [trifluoperazine HCl] 2 mg/mL

Stelazine oral concentrate (discontinued 2002) ℞ *conventional (typical) phenothiazine antipsychotic for schizophrenia; anxiolytic for nonpsychotic anxiety* [trifluoperazine HCl] 10 mg/mL

Stellaria media medicinal herb [see: chickweed]

Stemetil ⓐ film-coated tablets ℞ *conventional (typical) phenothiazine antipsychotic for schizophrenia; anxiolytic; antiemetic for nausea and vomiting; also used for acute treatment of migraine headaches* [prochlorperazine bimaleate] 5, 10 mg

Stemetil ⓐ oral liquid, IV or IM injection ℞ *conventional (typical) phenothiazine antipsychotic for schizophrenia; anxiolytic; antiemetic for nausea and vomiting; also used for acute treatment of migraine headaches* [prochlorperazine mesylate] 5 mg/5 mL; 5 mg/mL

Stemetil ⓐ suppositories ℞ *conventional (typical) phenothiazine antipsychotic for schizophrenia; anxiolytic; antiemetic for nausea and vomiting; also used for acute treatment of migraine headaches* [prochlorperazine] 10 mg

Stemgen ⓐ powder for subcu injection ℞ *recombinant human stem cell factor; hematopoietic growth factor; adjunct to myelosuppressive and myeloablative therapy (investigational (NDA filed, orphan) in the U.S.)* [ancestim] 187.5 mg/vial

stenbolone INN *anabolic steroid; also abused as a street drug* [also: stenbolone acetate]

stenbolone acetate USAN *anabolic steroid; also abused as a street drug* [also: stenbolone]

Step 2 creme rinse (discontinued 2003) OTC *for use following a pediculicide shampoo to remove lice eggs from hair*

stepronin INN

Sterapred; Sterapred DS tablets, Unipak (dispensing pack) ℞ *corticosteroid; anti-inflammatory* [prednisone] 5 mg; 10 mg

Sterculia tragacantha; S. urens; S. villosa medicinal herb [see: karaya gum]

stercuronium iodide INN

Steri-Dose (trademarked delivery system) *prefilled disposable syringe*

SteriNail topical solution OTC *antifungal* [undecylenic acid; tolnaftate] ? • ?

Steri-Vial (trademarked packaging form) *ampule*

Sterules (trademarked dosage form) *solution for nebulization*

stevaladil INN

stevia (*Stevia rebaudiana*) leaves *medicinal herb used as a non-caloric sugar substitute; also used for diabetes, food cravings, hypertension, obesity, and tobacco cravings*

stibamine glucoside INN, BAN

stibocaptate BAN [also: sodium stibocaptate]

stibophen NF

stibosamine INN

stickwort; sticklewort medicinal herb [see: agrimony]

stigmata maidis (corn silk) medicinal herb [see: Indian corn]

stilbamidine isethionate [see: stilbamidine isetionate]

stilbamidine isetionate INN

stilbazium iodide USAN, INN *anthelmintic*

stilbestroform [see: diethylstilbestrol]

stilbestrol [see: diethylstilbestrol] ⓓ Stilphostrol

stilbestronate [see: diethylstilbestrol dipropionate]

stilboestroform [see: diethylstilbestrol]

stilboestrol BAN *estrogen* [also: diethylstilbestrol]

stilboestrol DP [see: diethylstilbestrol dipropionate]

stillingia (*Stillingia ligustina*) root *medicinal herb for acne, eczema, and other skin disorders, blood cleansing, liver disorders, respiratory illnesses, and syphilis*

Stilnoct; Stilnox (European name for U.S. product Ambien)

stilonium iodide USAN, INN *antispasmodic*

Stilphostrol tablets, IV injection (discontinued 2001) ℞ *hormonal antineoplastic for palliative therapy of advanced prostatic carcinoma* [diethylstilbestrol diphosphate] 50 mg; 250 mg ⍰ Disophrol; stilbestrol

stilronate [see: diethylstilbestrol dipropionate]

Stimate nasal spray ℞ *posterior pituitary hormone for hemophilia A and von Willebrand disease (orphan)* [desmopressin acetate] 150 μg (600 IU)/dose

stimulant laxatives *a subclass of laxatives that work by direct action on the intestinal mucosa and nerve plexus to increase peristaltic action* [see also: laxatives]

stimulants *a class of agents that excite the activity of physiological processes*

Sting-Eze concentrate OTC *topical antihistamine; antipruritic; anesthetic; bacteriostatic* [diphenhydramine HCl; camphor; phenol; benzocaine; eucalyptol]

stinging nettle *medicinal herb* [see: nettle]

Sting-Kill swabs OTC *topical local anesthetic* [benzocaine; menthol] 20% • 1%

stingless nettle *medicinal herb* [see: blind nettle]

stinking nightshade *medicinal herb* [see: henbane]

stirimazole INN, BAN

stiripentol USAN, INN *anticonvulsant*

stirocainide INN

stirofos USAN *veterinary insecticide*

stitchwort *medicinal herb* [see: chickweed]

Stoko Gard cream (discontinued 2003) OTC *protection from the effects of poison ivy*

stomachics *a class of agents that promote the functional activity of the stomach*

stone root (*Collinsonia canadensis*) roots and leaves *medicinal herb used as a diuretic and vulnerary*

Stool Softener capsules OTC *laxative; stool softener* [docusate sodium] 100, 250 mg

Stool Softener; Stool Softener DC capsules OTC *laxative; stool softener* [docusate calcium] 240 mg

stool-softening laxatives *a subclass of laxatives that work by increasing the amount of fat and water in the stool to ease its movement through the intestines* [see also: laxatives]

Stop gel ℞ *topical dental caries preventative* [stannous fluoride] 0.4%

storax USP

storax (*Liquidambar orientalis; L. styraciflua*) leaves and gum *medicinal herb for diarrhea, inducing expectoration, parasitic infections, promoting sweating and diuresis, skin sores and wounds, and sore throat*

Storzfen eye drops ℞ *topical ophthalmic decongestant and vasoconstrictor; mydriatic* [phenylephrine HCl] 2.5%

Storzine 2 eye drops ℞ *topical antiglaucoma agent; direct-acting miotic* [pilocarpine HCl] 2%

Storz-N-D eye drops ℞ *topical ophthalmic corticosteroidal anti-inflammatory; antibiotic* [dexamethasone sodium phosphate; neomycin sulfate] 0.1% • 0.35%

Storz-N-P-D eye drop suspension ℞ *topical ophthalmic corticosteroidal anti-inflammatory; antibiotic* [dexamethasone; neomycin sulfate; polymyxin B sulfate] 0.1% • 0.35% • 10 000 U/mL

Storz-Sulf eye drops ℞ *antibiotic* [sulfacetamide sodium] 10%

stramonium [see: jimsonweed]

Strattera capsules ℞ *non-stimulant treatment for attention-deficit hyperactivity disorder (ADHD); investigational (orphan) for Tourette syndrome* [atomoxetine HCl] 10, 18, 25, 40, 60 mg

strawberry (*Fragaria vesca*) leaves *medicinal herb for blood cleansing,* *diarrhea, eczema, intestinal disorders, preventing miscarriage, and stomach cleansing*

strawberry bush; strawberry tree *medicinal herb* [see: wahoo]

Strep Detect slide tests for professional use *in vitro diagnostic aid for streptococcal antigens in throat swabs*

Streptase powder for IV or intracoronary infusion ℞ *thrombolytic enzyme for lysis of thrombi and catheter clearance* [streptokinase] 250 000, 750 000, 1 500 000 IU ⧉ Streptonase

streptodornase (SD) INN, BAN

streptoduocin USP

streptogramins *a class of antibiotics, isolated from* Streptomyces pristinaespirales, *used for gram-positive infections*

streptokinase (SK) INN *thrombolytic enzymes for myocardial infarction, thrombosis or embolism* ⧉ Streptonase

streptomycin INN, BAN *aminoglycoside antibiotic; primary tuberculostatic* [also: streptomycin sulfate]

streptomycin sulfate USP *aminoglycoside antibiotic; primary tuberculostatic* [also: streptomycin] 1 g injection

Streptonase-B test kit for professional use *in vitro diagnostic test for DNAse-B streptococcal antigens in serum* ⧉ Streptase; streptokinase

streptoniazid INN *antibacterial* [also: streptonicozid]

streptonicozid USAN *antibacterial* [also: streptoniazid]

streptonigrin (SN) USAN *antineoplastic* [also: rufocromomycin]

streptovarycin INN

streptozocin USAN, INN *nitrosourea-type alkylating antineoplastic for metastatic islet cell carcinoma of the pancreas*

streptozotocin [see: streptozocin]

Streptozyme slide tests for professional use *in vitro diagnostic test for streptococcal extracellular antigens in blood, plasma, and serum*

Stress 600 with Zinc tablets OTC *vitamin/mineral supplement* [multiple vitamins & minerals; folic acid; biotin] ± • 400 • 45 μg

Stress B Complex tablets OTC *vitamin/mineral supplement* [multiple vitamins & minerals; folic acid; biotin] ± • 400 • 45 μg

Stress B Complex with Vitamin C timed-release tablets OTC *vitamin/mineral supplement* [multiple B vitamins; vitamin C; zinc] ± • 300 • 15 mg

Stress Formula 600 tablets OTC *vitamin supplement* [multiple vitamins; folic acid; biotin] ± • 400 • 45 μg

Stress Formula Vitamins capsules, tablets OTC *vitamin supplement* [multiple vitamins; folic acid; biotin] ± • 400 • 45 μg

Stress Formula with Iron film-coated tablets OTC *vitamin/iron supplement* [multiple B vitamins; vitamins C and E; ferrous fumarate; folic acid; biotin] ± • 500 mg • 30 IU • 27 mg • 0.4 mg • 45 μg

Stress Formula with Zinc tablets OTC *vitamin/iron supplement* [multiple B vitamins; vitamins C and E; multiple minerals; folic acid; biotin] ± • 500 mg • 30 IU • ± • 0.4 mg • 45 μg

StressForm "605" with Iron tablets (discontinued 2003) OTC *vitamin/iron supplement* [multiple B vitamins; vitamins C and E; iron; folic acid; biotin] ± • 605 mg • 30 IU • 27 mg • 0.4 mg • 45 μg

Stresstabs tablets OTC *vitamin supplement* [multiple vitamins; folic acid; biotin] ± • 400 • 45 μg

Stresstabs + Iron film-coated tablets OTC *vitamin/iron supplement* [multiple B vitamins; vitamins C and E; ferrous fumarate; folic acid; biotin] ± • 500 mg • 30 IU • 18 mg • 0.4 mg • 45 μg

Stresstabs + Zinc film-coated tablets OTC *vitamin/mineral supplement* [multiple vitamins & minerals; folic acid; biotin] ± • 400 • 45 μg

Stresstein powder OTC *enteral nutritional therapy for moderate to severe stress or trauma* [multiple branched chain amino acids]

Striant mucoadhesive buccal tablets ℞ *hormone replacement therapy for male hypogonadism* [testosterone] 30 mg

Stri-Dex pads OTC *keratolytic cleanser for acne* [salicylic acid; alcohol] 0.5%•28%, 2%•44%, 2%•54%

Stri-Dex Cleansing bar OTC *medicated cleanser for acne* [triclosan] 1%

Stri-Dex Clear gel OTC *keratolytic cleanser for acne* [salicylic acid; alcohol] 2%•9.3%

Stri-Dex Face Wash solution OTC *medicated cleanser for acne* [triclosan] 1%

strinoline INN

striped alder *medicinal herb* [see: winterberry; witch hazel]

Stromectol tablets ℞ *anthelmintic for strongyloidiasis and onchocerciasis* [ivermectin] 3, 6 mg

strong ammonia solution [see: ammonia solution, strong]

Strong Iodine solution, tincture ℞ *thyroid-blocking therapy; topical antimicrobial* [iodine; potassium iodide] 5%•10%; 7%•5%

stronger rose water [see: rose water, stronger]

StrongStart caplets ℞ *vitamin/mineral/calcium/iron supplement; stool softener* [multiple vitamins & minerals; calcium; iron; folic acid; docusate sodium] ≐•200•29•1•25 mg

StrongStart chewable tablets ℞ *vitamin/mineral/calcium/iron supplement* [multiple vitamins & minerals; calcium; iron; folic acid] ≐•200•29•1 mg

strontium *element (Sr)*

strontium chloride *topical anti-irritant*

strontium chloride Sr 85 USAN *radioactive agent*

strontium chloride Sr 89 USAN *radioactive agent; analgesic for metastatic bone pain*

strontium nitrate Sr 85 USAN *radioactive agent*

strontium salicylate NF

strontium Sr 85 USP

Strovite tablets ℞ *vitamin supplement* [multiple B vitamins; vitamin C; folic acid] ≐•500•0.5 mg

Strovite Advance; Strovite Forte; Strovite Plus caplets ℞ *geriatric vitamin/mineral therapy* [multiple vitamins & minerals; folic acid; biotin] ≐•1000•100 µg; ≐•1000•150 µg; ≐•800•150 µg

structum *natural remedy* [see: chondroitin sulfate]

strychnine NF *an extremely poisonous CNS stimulant; occasionally abused as a street drug in combination with LSD*

strychnine glycerophosphate NF

strychnine nitrate NF

strychnine phosphate NF

strychnine sulfate NF

strychnine valerate NF

Stuart Formula tablets OTC *vitamin/mineral/iron supplement* [multiple vitamins & minerals; iron; folic acid] ≐•18•0.1 mg

Stuart Prenatal tablets OTC *vitamin/calcium/iron supplement* [multiple vitamins; calcium; iron; folic acid] ≐•200•28•0.8 mg

StuartNatal Plus tablets (discontinued 2003) ℞ *vitamin/calcium/iron supplement* [multiple vitamins; calcium; iron; folic acid] ≐•200•65•1 mg

StuartNatal Plus 3 tablets ℞ *vitamin/calcium/iron supplement* [multiple vitamins; calcium; iron; folic acid] ≐•200•28•1 mg

stugeron [see: cinnarizine]

stutgin [see: cinnarizine]

Stye ophthalmic ointment OTC *emollient* [white petrolatum; mineral oil; boric acid]

styptics *a class of hemostatic agents that stop bleeding of the skin by astringent action* [see also: astringents; hemostatics]

Stypto-Caine solution OTC *to stop bleeding of minor cuts* [aluminum chloride; tetracaine HCl; oxyquinoline sulfate] 250•2.5•1 mg/g

styramate INN

styronate resins

subathizone INN

Subdue ⓒ oral liquid OTC *enteral nutritional therapy for patients with inflammatory bowel disease*

subendazole INN

Sublimaze IV or IM injection ℞ *narcotic analgesic; adjunct to anesthesia* [fentanyl citrate] 50 µg/mL

sublimed sulfur [see: sulfur, sublimed]

Sublingual B Total drops OTC *vitamin supplement* [multiple B vitamins; vitamin C] ± •60 mg/mL

Suboxone sublingual tablets ℞ *narcotic agonist-antagonist analgesic for outpatient maintenance of opiate dependence (orphan)* [buprenorphine HCl; naloxone HCl] 2•0.5, 8•2 mg

substance F [see: demecolcine]

substituted benzimidazoles *a class of gastric antisecretory agents that inhibit the ATPase "proton pump" within the gastric parietal cell* [also called: proton pump inhibitors; ATPase inhibitors]

Subutex sublingual tablets ℞ *narcotic agonist-antagonist analgesic for inpatient treatment of opiate dependence (orphan)* [buprenorphine HCl] 2, 8 mg

Suby G solution; Suby solution G (citric acid, magnesium oxide, sodium carbonate) *urologic irrigant to dissolve phosphatic calculi*

succimer USAN, INN, BAN *heavy metal chelating agent for lead poisoning (orphan); investigational (orphan) for mercury poisoning and cysteine kidney stones*

succinchlorimide NF

succinimides *a class of anticonvulsants*

succinylcholine chloride USP *neuromuscular blocker; muscle relaxant; anesthesia adjunct* [also: suxamethonium chloride] 20 mg/mL injection

succinyldapsone [see: succisulfone]

succinylsulfathiazole USP

succisulfone INN

succory *medicinal herb* [see: chicory]

Succus Cineraria Maritima eye drops ℞ *treatment for optic opacity caused by cataract* [senecio compositae; hamamelis water; boric acid]

suclofenide INN, BAN

Sucraid oral solution ℞ *enzyme replacement therapy for congenital sucrase-isomaltase deficiency (orphan)* [sacrosidase] 8500 IU/mL

sucralfate USAN, INN, BAN *cytoprotective agent for gastric ulcers; investigational (orphan) for oral mucositis and stomatitis following cancer radiation or chemotherapy* 1 g oral; 1 g/10 mL oral

sucralose BAN

sucralox INN, BAN

Sucrets throat spray OTC *antipruritic/counterirritant; mild local anesthetic* [dyclonine HCl] 0.1%

Sucrets Children's Sore Throat; Vapor Lemon Sucrets; Sucrets Maximum Strength lozenges OTC *antipruritic/counterirritant; mild local anesthetic* [dyclonine HCl] 1.2 mg; 2 mg; 3 mg

Sucrets Cough Control; Sucrets 4-Hour Cough lozenges (discontinued 2002) OTC *antitussive* [dextromethorphan hydrobromide] 5 mg; 15 mg

Sucrets Sore Throat lozenges OTC *oral antiseptic* [hexylresorcinol] 2.4 mg

sucrose NF *flavoring agent; tablet excipient* ⑨ sucrase

sucrose octaacetate NF *alcohol denaturant*

sucrosofate potassium USAN *antiulcerative*

Sudafed tablets OTC *nasal decongestant* [pseudoephedrine HCl] 30, 60 mg

Sudafed, Children's chewable tablets OTC *nasal decongestant* [pseudoephedrine HCl] 15 mg

Sudafed, Children's Non-Drowsy oral liquid OTC *nasal decongestant* [pseudoephedrine HCl] 15 mg/5 mL

Sudafed Children's Non-Drowsy Cold & Cough oral liquid OTC *antitussive; decongestant* [dextromethorphan hydrobromide; pseudoephedrine HCl] 5•15 mg/5 mL

Sudafed Cold & Allergy tablets OTC *decongestant; antihistamine* [pseudoephedrine HCl; chlorpheniramine maleate] 60•4 mg

Sudafed Cold & Sinus Non-Drowsy
Liqui-Caps (liquid-filled gelcaps)
OTC *decongestant; analgesic; antipyretic* [pseudoephedrine HCl; acetaminophen] 30•325 mg

Sudafed Multi-Symptom Cold & Cough liquid caps OTC *antitussive; decongestant; expectorant; analgesic* [dextromethorphan hydrobromide; pseudoephedrine HCl; guaifenesin; acetaminophen] 10•30•100•250 mg

Sudafed Non-Drowsy tablets OTC *nasal decongestant* [pseudoephedrine HCl] 30 mg

Sudafed Non-Drowsy 12 Hour Long Acting extended-release caplets OTC *nasal decongestant* [pseudoephedrine HCl] 120 mg

Sudafed Non-Drowsy 24 Hour Long Acting dual-release tablets OTC *nasal decongestant* [pseudoephedrine HCl] 240 mg (60 mg immediate release, 180 mg extended release)

Sudafed Non-Drowsy Non-Drying Sinus liquid-filled capsules OTC *decongestant; expectorant* [pseudoephedrine HCl; guaifenesin] 30•120 mg

Sudafed Non-Drowsy Severe Cold Formula caplets OTC *antitussive; decongestant; analgesic* [dextromethorphan hydrobromide; pseudoephedrine HCl; acetaminophen] 15•30•500 mg

Sudafed PE tablets OTC *nasal decongestant* [phenylephrine HCl] 10 mg

Sudafed Plus tablets (name changed to **Sudafed Cold & Allergy** in 2002)

Sudafed Severe Cold tablets (discontinued 2002) OTC *antitussive; decongestant; analgesic* [dextromethorphan hydrobromide; pseudoephedrine HCl; acetaminophen] 15•30•500 mg

Sudafed Sinus Advance ⒸⒶⓃ caplets OTC *decongestant; analgesic; antipyretic* [pseudoephedrine HCl; ibuprofen] 30•200 mg

Sudafed Sinus Headache Non-Drowsy tablets, caplets OTC *decongestant; analgesic; antipyretic* [pseudoephedrine HCl; acetaminophen] 30•500 mg

Sudafed Sinus Nighttime tablets OTC *decongestant; antihistamine* [pseudoephedrine HCl; triprolidine HCl] 60•2.5 mg

Sudafed Sinus Nighttime Plus Pain Relief caplets OTC *decongestant; antihistamine; analgesic* [pseudoephedrine HCl; diphenhydramine HCl; acetaminophen] 30•25•500 mg

Sudal 60/500 sustained-release caplets Ⓡ *decongestant; expectorant* [pseudoephedrine HCl; guaifenesin] 60•500 mg

Sudal-DM sustained-release tablets Ⓡ *antitussive; expectorant* [dextromethorphan hydrobromide; guaifenesin] 30•500 mg

sudexanox INN

sudismase INN

Sudodrin tablets OTC *nasal decongestant* [pseudoephedrine HCl] 30 mg

SudoGest tablets OTC *decongestant* [pseudoephedrine HCl] 60 mg

SudoGest Children's Syrup OTC *antitussive; decongestant* [dextromethorphan hydrobromide; pseudoephedrine HCl] 5•15 mg/5 mL

SudoGest Cold & Allergy tablets OTC *decongestant; antihistamine* [pseudoephedrine HCl; chlorpheniramine maleate] 60•4 mg

SudoGest Sinus tablets OTC *decongestant; analgesic; antipyretic* [pseudoephedrine HCl; acetaminophen] 30•500 mg

sudorifics *a class of agents that promote profuse perspiration* [also called: diaphoretics]

sudoxicam USAN, INN *anti-inflammatory*

Sufenta IV injection Ⓡ *narcotic analgesic; anesthetic* [sufentanil citrate] 50 μg/mL

sufentanil USAN, INN, BAN *narcotic analgesic; investigational (Phase III) for cancer-related pain*

sufentanil citrate USAN *narcotic analgesic* 50 μg/mL injection

sufosfamide INN

sufotidine USAN, INN, BAN *antagonist to histamine H₂ receptors*

sugar, compressible NF *flavoring agent; tablet excipient*

sugar, confectioner's NF *flavoring agent; tablet excipient*

sugar, invert (50% dextrose & 50% fructose) USP *fluid and nutrient replenisher; caloric replacement*

sugar spheres NF *solid carrier vehicle*

sulamserod HCl USAN *selective 5-HT₄ receptor antagonist; antiarrhythmic; treatment for urge incontinence*

Sulamyd [see: Sodium Sulamyd]

Sular extended-release tablets ℞ *calcium channel blocker for hypertension* [nisoldipine] 10, 20, 30, 40 mg

sulazepam USAN, INN *minor tranquilizer*

sulbactam INN, BAN *β-lactamase inhibitor; penicillin/cephalosporin synergist*

sulbactam benzathine USAN *β-lactamase inhibitor; penicillin/cephalosporin synergist*

sulbactam pivoxil USAN *β-lactamase inhibitor; penicillin/cephalosporin synergist* [also: pivsulbactam]

sulbactam sodium USAN, USP *β-lactamase inhibitor; penicillin/cephalosporin synergist*

sulbenicillin INN

sulbenox USAN, INN *veterinary growth stimulant*

sulbentine INN

sulbutiamine INN [also: bisibutiamine]

sulclamide INN

sulconazole INN, BAN *antifungal* [also: sulconazole nitrate]

sulconazole nitrate USAN, USP *topical antifungal* [also: sulconazole]

sulergine [see: disulergine]

sulesomab USAN *monoclonal antibody; diagnostic aid for infectious lesions* [also: technetium Tc 99m sulesomab]

Sulf-10 eye drops ℞ *ophthalmic antibiotic* [sulfacetamide sodium] 10% ② Sulten-10

sulfabenz USAN, INN *antibacterial; coccidiostat for poultry*

sulfabenzamide USAN, USP, INN *bacteriostatic antibiotic*

sulfabromomethazine sodium NF

sulfacarbamide INN [also: sulphaurea]

sulfacecole INN

sulfacetamide USP, INN *bacteriostatic antibiotic*

sulfacetamide sodium USP *bacteriostatic antibiotic* 10%, 30% eye drops

Sulfacet-R lotion ℞ *acne treatment* [sulfacetamide sodium; sulfur] 10%•5%

sulfachlorpyridazine INN

sulfachrysoidine INN

sulfacitine INN *antibacterial* [also: sulfacytine]

sulfaclomide INN

sulfaclorazole INN

sulfaclozine INN

sulfacombin [see: sulfadiazine]

sulfacytine USAN *broad-spectrum bacteriostatic* [also: sulfacitine]

sulfadiasulfone sodium INN *antibacterial; leprostatic* [also: acetosulfone sodium]

sulfadiazine USP, INN, JAN *broad-spectrum sulfonamide bacteriostatic* [also: sulphadiazine] 500 mg oral

sulfadiazine & pyrimethamine *oral* Toxoplasma gondii *encephalitis treatment (orphan)*

sulfadiazine silver JAN *broad-spectrum bactericidal; adjunct to burn therapy* [also: silver sulfadiazine]

sulfadiazine sodium USP, INN *antibacterial* [also: sulphadiazine sodium]

sulfadicramide INN, DCF

sulfadicrolamide [see: sulfadicramide]

sulfadimethoxine NF [also: sulphadimethoxine]

sulfadimidine INN, BAN *antibacterial* [also: sulfamethazine]

sulfadoxine USAN, USP *bacteriostatic; antimalarial adjunct*

sulfaethidole NF, INN [also: sulphaethidole]

sulfafurazole INN *broad-spectrum sulfonamide bacteriostatic* [also: sulfisoxazole; sulphafurazole]

sulfaguanidine NF, INN

sulfaguanole INN

sulfaisodimidine [see: sulfisomidine]

sulfalene USAN, INN *antibacterial* [also: sulfametopyrazine]

sulfaloxic acid INN [also: sulphaloxic acid]

sulfamates *a class of broad-spectrum anticonvulsants*

sulfamazone INN

sulfamerazine USP, INN *broad-spectrum bacteriostatic*

sulfamerazine sodium NF, INN

sulfameter USAN *antibacterial* [also: sulfametoxydiazine; sulfamethoxydiazine]

sulfamethazine USP *broad-spectrum bacteriostatic* [also: sulfadimidine]

sulfamethizole USP, INN, JAN *broad-spectrum sulfonamide bacteriostatic* [also: sulphamethizole] ⊉ sulfamethoxazole

sulfamethoxazole (SMX; SMZ) USAN, USP, INN, JAN *broad-spectrum sulfonamide antibiotic* [also: sulphamethoxazole; acetylsulfamethoxazole; sulfamethoxazole sodium] ⊉ sulfamethizole

sulfamethoxazole sodium JAN *broad-spectrum sulfonamide antibiotic* [also: sulfamethoxazole; sulphamethoxazole; acetylsulfamethoxazole]

sulfamethoxydiazine BAN *antibacterial* [also: sulfameter; sulfametoxydiazine]

sulfamethoxypyridazine USP, INN [also: sulphamethoxypyridazine]

sulfamethoxypyridazine acetyl

sulfametin [see: sulfameter]

sulfametomidine INN

sulfametopyrazine BAN *antibacterial* [also: sulfalene]

sulfametoxydiazine INN *antibacterial* [also: sulfameter; sulfamethoxydiazine]

sulfametrole INN, BAN

sulfamidothiodiazol [see: glybuzole]

sulfamonomethoxine USAN, INN, BAN *antibacterial*

sulfamoxole USAN, INN *antibacterial* [also: sulphamoxole]

p-sulfamoylbenzoic acid [see: carzenide]

4′-sulfamoylsuccinanilic acid [see: sulfasuccinamide]

Sulfamylon cream Ŗ *broad-spectrum bacteriostatic for second- and third-degree burns* [mafenide acetate] 85 mg/g

Sulfamylon powder for topical solution Ŗ *broad-spectrum bacteriostatic to prevent meshed autograft loss on second- and third-degree burns (orphan)* [mafenide acetate] 5%

sulfanilamide NF, INN *broad-spectrum sulfonamide antibiotic* 15% topical

sulfanilanilide [see: sulfabenz]

sulfanilate zinc USAN *antibacterial*

N-sulfanilylacetamide [see: sulfacetamide]

N-sulfanilylacetamide monosodium salt monohydrate [see: sulfacetamide sodium]

N-p-sulfanilylphenylglycine sodium [see: acediasulfone sodium]

N-sulfanilylstearamide [see: stearylsulfamide]

4′-sulfanilylsuccinanilic acid [see: succisulfone]

sulfanilylurea [see: sulfacarbamide]

sulfanitran USAN, INN, BAN *antibacterial; coccidiostat for poultry*

sulfaperin INN

sulfaphenazole INN [also: sulphaphenazole]

sulfaphtalythiazol [see: phthalylsulfathiazole]

sulfaproxyline INN [also: sulphaproxyline]

sulfapyrazole INN, BAN *antibacterial* [also: sulfazamet]

sulfapyridine USP, INN *investigational (orphan) dermatitis herpetiformis suppressant* [also: sulphapyridine]

sulfapyridine sodium NF

sulfaquinoxaline INN, BAN

sulfarsphenamine NF, INN

sulfasalazine USAN, USP, INN *broad-spectrum bacteriostatic; antirheumatic; anti-inflammatory for ulcerative colitis* [also: sulphasalazine; salazosulfapyridine] 500 mg oral

sulfasomizole USAN, INN *antibacterial* [also: sulphasomizole]

sulfastearyl [see: stearylsulfamide]

sulfasuccinamide INN

sulfasymazine INN

sulfated polysaccharide peptidoglycan (SPPG) [see: tecogalan sodium]

sulfathiazole USP, INN *bacteriostatic antibiotic* [also: sulphathiazole] ② sulfisoxazole

sulfathiazole sodium NF

sulfathiocarbamide [see: sulfathiourea]

sulfathiourea INN

sulfatolamide INN

Sulfatrim oral suspension ℞ *anti-infective; antibacterial* [trimethoprim; sulfamethoxazole] 40•200 mg/5 mL

sulfatroxazole INN

sulfatrozole INN

sulfazamet USAN *antibacterial* [also: sulfapyrazole]

sulfinalol INN *antihypertensive* [also: sulfinalol HCl]

sulfinalol HCl USAN *antihypertensive* [also: sulfinalol]

sulfinpyrazone USP, INN *uricosuric for gout* [also: sulphinpyrazone] 100, 200 mg oral

sulfiram INN [also: monosulfiram]

sulfisomidine [also: sulphasomidine]

sulfisoxazole USP, JAN *broad-spectrum sulfonamide antibiotic* [also: sulfafurazole; sulphafurazole] 500 mg oral ② sulfathiazole

sulfisoxazole acetyl USP *broad-spectrum sulfonamide antibiotic*

sulfisoxazole diolamine USAN, USP *broad-spectrum sulfonamide antibiotic*

Sulfoam shampoo OTC *antiseborrheic; keratolytic* [sulfur] 2%

sulfobenzylpenicillin [see: sulbenicillin]

sulfobromophthalein sodium USP *hepatic function test*

sulfobromphthalein sodium [see: sulfobromophthalein sodium]

sulfocon B USAN *hydrophobic contact lens material*

sulfogaiacol INN *expectorant* [also: potassium guaiacolsulfonate]

Sulfoil topical liquid (discontinued 2004) OTC *soap-free therapeutic skin cleanser* [sulfonated castor oil]

Sulfolax soft gels OTC *laxative; stool softener* [docusate calcium] 240 mg

sulfomyxin USAN, INN *antibacterial* [also: sulphomyxin sodium]

sulfonal [see: sulfonmethane]

sulfonamides *a class of broad-spectrum bacteriostatic antibiotics effective against both gram-positive and gram-negative organisms*

sulfonated hydrogenated castor oil [see: hydroxystearin sulfate]

sulfonethylmethane NF

sulfonmethane NF

sulfonterol INN *bronchodilator* [also: sulfonterol HCl]

sulfonterol HCl USAN *bronchodilator* [also: sulfonterol]

sulfonylureas *a class of antidiabetic agents that stimulate insulin production in the pancreas*

Sulforcin lotion OTC *topical acne treatment* [sulfur; resorcinol; alcohol] 5%•2%•11.65%

sulforidazine INN

sulfosalicylic acid

sulfoxone sodium USP *antibacterial; leprostatic* [also: aldesulfone sodium]

Sulfoxyl Regular; Sulfoxyl Strong lotion ℞ *keratolytic for acne* [benzoyl peroxide; sulfur] 5%•2%; 10%•5%

sulfur *element (S)* [see: sulfur, precipitated; sulfur, sublimed]

sulfur, precipitated USP *scabicide; topical antibacterial; topical exfoliant*

sulfur, sublimed USP *scabicide; topical antibacterial; topical exfoliant*

sulfur dioxide NF *antioxidant*

sulfur hexafluoride (SF$_6$) USAN *ultrasound imaging agent*

Sulfur Soap bar OTC *medicated cleanser for acne* [precipitated sulfur] 10%

sulfurated lime solution [see: lime, sulfurated]

sulfurated potash [see: potash, sulfurated]

sulfuric acid NF *acidifying agent*

sulfuric acid, aluminum ammonium salt, dodecahydrate [see: alum, ammonium]

sulfuric acid, aluminum potassium salt, dodecahydrate [see: alum, potassium]

sulfuric acid, aluminum salt, hydrate [see: aluminum sulfate]

sulfuric acid, barium salt [see: barium sulfate]

sulfuric acid, calcium salt [see: calcium sulfate]

sulfuric acid, copper salt pentahydrate [see: cupric sulfate]

sulfuric acid, disodium salt decahydrate [see: sodium sulfate]

sulfuric acid, magnesium salt [see: magnesium sulfate]

sulfuric acid, manganese salt [see: manganese sulfate]

sulfuric acid, zinc salt hydrate [see: zinc sulfate]

sulfurous acid, monosodium salt [see: sodium bisulfite]

sulglicotide INN [also: sulglycotide]

sulglycotide BAN [also: sulglicotide]

sulicrinat INN

sulindac USAN, USP, INN, BAN *antiarthritic; nonsteroidal anti-inflammatory drug (NSAID) for ankylosing spondylitis and acute bursitis/tendinitis* 150, 200 mg oral ⊉ Zoladex

sulisatin INN

sulisobenzone USAN, INN *ultraviolet screen*

sulmarin USAN, INN *hemostatic*

Sulmasque mask OTC *antibacterial and exfoliant for acne* [sulfur] 6.4%

sulmazole INN

sulmepride INN

sulnidazole USAN, INN *antiprotozoal (Trichomonas)*

sulocarbilate INN

suloctidil USAN, INN, BAN *peripheral vasodilator*

sulodexide INN *investigational (Phase III) glycosaminoglycan for diabetic nephropathy*

sulofenur USAN, INN *antineoplastic*

sulopenem USAN, INN *antibacterial*

sulosemide INN

sulotroban USAN, INN, BAN *treatment for glomerulonephritis*

suloxifen INN *bronchodilator* [also: suloxifen oxalate]

suloxifen oxalate USAN *bronchodilator* [also: suloxifen]

sulphabutin [see: busulfan]

sulphadiazine BAN *broad-spectrum bacteriostatic* [also: sulfadiazine]

sulphadiazine sodium BAN *antibacterial* [also: sulfadiazine sodium]

sulphadimethoxine BAN [also: sulfadimethoxine]

sulphaethidole BAN [also: sulfaethidole]

sulphafurazole BAN *broad-spectrum sulfonamide bacteriostatic* [also: sulfisoxazole; sulfafurazole]

sulphaloxic acid BAN [also: sulfaloxic acid]

sulphamethizole BAN *broad-spectrum sulfonamide bacteriostatic* [also: sulfamethizole]

sulphamethoxazole BAN *broad-spectrum sulfonamide bacteriostatic* [also: sulfamethoxazole; acetylsulfamethoxazole; sulfamethoxazole sodium]

sulphamethoxypyridazine BAN [also: sulfamethoxypyridazine]

sulphamoxole BAN *antibacterial* [also: sulfamoxole]

sulphan blue BAN *lymphangiography aid* [also: isosulfan blue]

sulphaphenazole BAN [also: sulfaphenazole]

sulphaproxyline BAN [also: sulfaproxyline]

sulphapyridine BAN *dermatitis herpetiformis suppressant* [also: sulfapyridine]

sulphasalazine BAN *broad-spectrum bacteriostatic; antirheumatic; anti-inflammatory for ulcerative colitis* [also: sulfasalazine; salazosulfapyridine]

sulphasomidine BAN [also: sulfisomidine]

sulphasomizole BAN *antibacterial* [also: sulfasomizole]

sulphathiazole BAN *antibacterial* [also: sulfathiazole]

sulphaurea BAN [also: sulfacarbamide]

sulphinpyrazone BAN *uricosuric for gout* [also: sulfinpyrazone]

sulphocarbolate sodium [see: phe-nolsulphonate sodium]

Sulpho-Lac cream, soap OTC *antibacterial and exfoliant for acne* [sulfur] 5%

Sulpho-Lac Acne Medication cream OTC *antibacterial; exfoliant* [sulfur; zinc sulfate] 5%•27%

sulphomyxin sodium BAN *antibacterial* [also: sulfomyxin]

sulphonal [see: sulfonmethane]

sulpiride USAN, INN *antidepressant*

sulprosal INN

sulprostone USAN, INN *prostaglandin*

sultamicillin USAN, INN, BAN *antibacterial*

sulthiame USAN *anticonvulsant* [also: sultiame]

sultiame INN *anticonvulsant* [also: sulthiame]

sultopride INN

sultosilic acid INN

Sultrin Triple Sulfa vaginal inserts, vaginal cream (discontinued 2001) ℞ *broad-spectrum antibiotic* [sulfathiazole; sulfacetamide; sulfabenzamide] 172.5•143.75•184 mg; 3.42%•2.86%•3.7%

sultroponium INN

sulukast USAN, INN *antiasthmatic; leukotriene antagonist*

sulverapride INN

suma (Pfaffia paniculata) bark and root *medicinal herb for circulatory disorders, chronic disease, fatigue, hormone regulation, immune system stimulation, lowering cholesterol levels, and stress; also used as a tonic*

Sumacal powder OTC *carbohydrate caloric supplement* [glucose polymers]

sumacetamol INN, BAN

sumach (Rhus glabra) bark, leaves, and berries *medicinal herb used as an antiseptic, astringent, diaphoretic, diuretic, emmenagogue, febrifuge, and refrigerant*

sumarotene USAN, INN *keratolytic*

sumatriptan INN, BAN *vascular serotonin 5-HT$_1$ receptor agonist for the acute treatment of migraine headaches* [also: sumatriptan succinate]

sumatriptan succinate USAN *vascular serotonin 5-HT$_1$ receptor agonist for the acute treatment of migraine and cluster headaches* [also: sumatriptan]

sumetizide INN

summer savory (Calamintha hortensis; Satureja hortensis) leaves and stems *medicinal herb for diarrhea, nausea, promoting expectoration, relieving gas and flatulence, and stimulation of menstruation; also used as an aphrodisiac*

Summer's Eve Disposable Douche solution OTC *antifungal; vaginal cleanser and deodorizer; acidity modifier* [sodium benzoate; citric acid]

Summer's Eve Disposable Douche; Summer's Eve Disposable Douche Extra Cleansing solution OTC *vaginal cleanser and deodorizer; acidity modifier* [vinegar (acetic acid)]

Summer's Eve Feminine Bath topical liquid OTC *for external perivaginal cleansing*

Summer's Eve Feminine Powder OTC *absorbs vaginal moisture* [cornstarch; benzethonium chloride]

Summer's Eve Feminine Wash topical liquid, wipes OTC *for external perivaginal cleansing*

Summer's Eve Medicated Disposable Douche solution OTC *antiseptic/germicidal; vaginal cleanser and deodorizer* [povidone-iodine] 0.3%

Summer's Eve Post-Menstrual Disposable Douche solution OTC *vaginal cleanser and deodorizer; acidity modifier* [monosodium phosphate; disodium phosphate]

Summit Extra Strength coated caplets OTC *analgesic; antipyretic; anti-inflammatory* [acetaminophen; aspirin; caffeine] 250•250•65 mg

Sumycin syrup ℞ *broad-spectrum antibiotic* [tetracycline HCl] 125 mg/5 mL

Sumycin '250'; Sumycin '500' capsules, tablets ℞ *broad-spectrum antibiotic* [tetracycline HCl] 250 mg; 500 mg

sun rose *medicinal herb* [see: rock rose]

sunagrel INN

suncillin INN *antibacterial* [also: suncillin sodium]

suncillin sodium USAN *antibacterial* [also: suncillin]

sunepitron HCl USAN *anxiolytic; antidepressant*

sunitinib malate *investigational (NDA filed) receptor tyrosine kinase (RTK) antineoplastic for gastrointestinal stromal tumor (GIST) and metastatic renal carcinoma*

SunKist Multivitamins Complete, Children's chewable tablets OTC *vitamin/mineral/iron supplement* [multiple vitamins & minerals; iron; folic acid; biotin] $\pm \bullet 18$ mg$\bullet 400$ μg$\bullet 40$ μg

SunKist Multivitamins + Extra C chewable tablets OTC *vitamin supplement* [multiple vitamins; folic acid] $\pm \bullet 0.3$ mg

SunKist Multivitamins + Iron, Children's chewable tablets (discontinued 2004) OTC *vitamin/iron supplement* [multiple vitamins; iron; folic acid] $\pm \bullet 15 \bullet 0.3$ mg

SunKist Vitamin C chewable tablets OTC *vitamin C supplement* [ascorbic acid and sodium ascorbate] 60, 250, 500 mg

Supartz intra-articular injection in prefilled syringes ℞ *viscoelastic lubricant and "shock absorber" for osteoarthritis and TMJ syndrome* [hyaluronate sodium] 25 mg/2.5 mL 🄂 *sports*

Super 2 Daily softgels OTC *vitamin/mineral supplement* [multiple vitamins & minerals; fish oil concentrate; lecithin; phosphatidyl choline; bioflavonoids; lutein] $\pm \bullet 385 \bullet 30 \bullet 25 \bullet 12.5 \bullet 0.025$ mg

Super CalciCaps tablets OTC *dietary supplement* [dibasic calcium phosphate; calcium gluconate; calcium carbonate; vitamin D] 400 mg (Ca)$\bullet 42$ mg (P)$\bullet 133$ IU

Super CalciCaps M-Z tablets OTC *dietary supplement* [vitamins A and D; multiple minerals] 1667 mg$\bullet 133$ IU$\bullet \pm$

Super Calcium '1200' softgels OTC *dietary supplement* [calcium; vitamin D] 600 mg$\bullet 200$ IU

Super Carnosine capsules OTC *anti-aging supplement* [carnosine] 500 mg

Super D Perles (capsules) OTC *vitamin supplement* [vitamins A and D] 10 000$\bullet 400$ IU

Super Flavons; Super Flavons-300 tablets OTC *dietary supplement* [mixed bioflavonoids] 300 mg

Super Hi Potency tablets OTC *vitamin/mineral supplement* [multiple vitamins & minerals; folic acid; biotin] $\pm \bullet 0.4$ mg$\bullet 0.075$ mg

Super Ivy-Dry lotion OTC *poison ivy treatment* [zinc acetate; benzyl alcohol; isopropanol] 2%$\bullet 10\% \bullet 35\%$

Super MiraForte with Chrysin capsules OTC *natural supplement to increase free testosterone levels in men* [chrysin; muira puama; maca; nettle; ginger; piperine; zinc] 375$\bullet 212.5 \bullet 80 \bullet 70.5 \bullet 12.5 \bullet 3.75 \bullet 3.75$ mg

Super Quints-50 tablets OTC *vitamin supplement* [multiple B vitamins; folic acid; biotin] $\pm \bullet 400 \bullet 50$ μg

Superdophilus powder OTC *probiotic; dietary supplement; fever blister treatment; not generally regarded as safe and effective as an antidiarrheal* [Lactobacillus acidophilus] 2 billion CFU/g

SuperEPA 1200; SuperEPA 2000 softgels OTC *dietary supplement* [omega-3 fatty acids] 1200 mg; 1000 mg

superoxide dismutase (SOD) [see: orgotein]

Superplex-T tablets OTC *vitamin supplement* [multiple B vitamins; vitamin C] $\pm \bullet 500$ mg

supidimide INN

Suplena ready-to-use oral liquid OTC *enteral nutritional therapy for renal failure* [multiple essential amino acids]

Supprelin subcu injection (discontinued 2004) ℞ *LHRH agonist for treatment of central precocious puberty (orphan)* [histrelin acetate] 120, 300, 600 μg/0.6 mL

Suppress lozenges (discontinued 2002) OTC *antitussive* [dextromethorphan hydrobromide] 7.5 mg

Supprette (trademarked dosage form) *suppository*

Suprane liquid for vaporization ℞ *inhalation general anesthetic* [desflurane]

Suprax film-coated tablets, powder for oral suspension ℞ *cephalosporin antibiotic* [cefixime] 200, 400 mg; 100 mg/5 mL

Suprefact ⒸⒶⓃ nasal solution ℞ *LHRH analogue; hormonal antineoplastic for prostatic cancer and endometriosis* [buserelin acetate] 1 mg/mL

Suprefact; Suprefact Depot ⒸⒶⓃ subcu injection ℞ *LHRH analogue; hormonal antineoplastic for prostatic cancer and endometriosis* [buserelin acetate] 1 mg/mL; 6.6 mg/dose

suproclone USAN, INN *sedative*

suprofen USAN, INN, BAN *ocular nonsteroidal anti-inflammatory drug (NSAID); antimiotic*

Supule (trademarked dosage form) *suppository*

suramin hexasodium USAN *investigational (NDA filed, orphan) growth factor antagonist for prostate cancer*

suramin sodium USP, BAN *antiparasitic for African trypanosomiasis and onchocerciasis*

Surbex Filmtabs (film-coated tablets) OTC *vitamin supplement* [multiple B vitamins]

Surbex 750 with Iron Filmtabs (film-coated tablets) OTC *vitamin/iron supplement* [multiple B vitamins; vitamins C and E; ferrous sulfate, dried; folic acid] ≛•750 mg•30 IU•27 mg•0.4 mg

Surbex 750 with Zinc Filmtabs (film-coated tablets) OTC *vitamin/zinc supplement* [multiple vitamins; zinc sulfate; folic acid] ≛•22.5•0.4 mg

Surbex-T; Surbex with C Filmtabs (film-coated tablets) OTC *vitamin supplement* [multiple B vitamins; vitamin C] ≛•500 mg; ≛•250 mg

Surbu-Gen-T film-coated tablets OTC *vitamin supplement* [multiple B vitamins; vitamin C] ≛•500 mg

Sure Cell Chlamydia Test reagent kit for professional use *in vitro diagnostic aid for* Chlamydia trachomatis [monoclonal antibody-based enzyme-linked immunosorbent assay]

Sure Cell Herpes (HSV) Test reagent kit for professional use *in vitro diagnostic aid for herpes simplex virus in genital, rectal, oral, or dermal swabs* [monoclonal antibody-based enzyme-linked immunosorbent assay (ELISA)]

Sure Cell Pregnancy test kit for professional use *in vitro diagnostic aid; urine pregnancy test* [monoclonal/polyclonal antibody ELISA test]

Sure Cell Streptococci test kit for professional use *in vitro diagnostic aid for Group A streptococcal antigens in blood and throat swabs* [enzyme-linked immunosorbent assay (ELISA)]

SureLac chewable tablets OTC *digestive aid for lactose intolerance* [lactase enzyme] 3000 U

surface active extract of saline lavage of bovine lungs [see: beractant]

surfactant laxatives *a subclass of laxatives that work by increasing the amount of fat and water in the stool to ease its movement through the intestines* [more commonly called stool softeners]

surfactant TA [see: beractant]

surfactant TA, modified bovine lung surfactant extract [see: beractant]

Surfak Liquigels (capsules) OTC *laxative; stool softener* [docusate calcium] 240 mg

surfilcon A USAN *hydrophilic contact lens material*

Surfol Post-Immersion Bath Oil OTC *bath emollient*

surfomer USAN, INN *hypolipidemic*

Surgel vaginal gel OTC *lubricant* [propylene glycol; glycerin]

surgibone USAN *internal bone splint*

surgical catgut [see: suture, absorbable surgical]

surgical gut [see: suture, absorbable surgical]

Surgicel strips, Nu-knit pads ℞ *topical local hemostat for surgery* [cellulose, oxidized]

suricainide INN *antiarrhythmic* [also: suricainide maleate]

suricainide maleate USAN, INN *antiarrhythmic* [also: suricainide]

suriclone INN, BAN

Surinam wood *medicinal herb* [see: quassia]

suritozole USAN, INN *antidepressant*

Surmontil capsules ℞ *tricyclic antidepressant* [trimipramine maleate] 25, 50, 100 mg

Surodex intraocular injection ℞ *investigational (Phase II) corticosteroidal anti-inflammatory* [dexamethasone]

suronacrine INN *cholinesterase inhibitor* [also: suronacrine maleate]

suronacrine maleate USAN *cholinesterase inhibitor* [also: suronacrine]

Surpass chewing gum OTC *antacid; calcium supplement* [calcium carbonate] 300, 450 mg

Survanta suspension for intratracheal instillation ℞ *pulmonary surfactant for neonatal respiratory distress syndrome or respiratory failure (orphan)* [beractant] 25 mg/mL

Susano elixir ℞ *GI antispasmodic; anticholinergic; sedative* [atropine sulfate; scopolamine hydrobromide; hyoscyamine hydrobromide; phenobarbital] 0.0194•0.0065•0.1037•16.2 mg/5 mL

Sus-Phrine subcu injection (discontinued 2001) ℞ *sympathomimetic bronchodilator for bronchial asthma, bronchospasm, and COPD; vasopressor for shock* [epinephrine] 1:200 (5 mg/mL)

Sustacal powder OTC *enteral nutritional therapy* [milk-based formula]

Sustacal pudding OTC *enteral nutritional therapy* [milk-based formula]

Sustacal ready-to-use oral liquid OTC *enteral nutritional therapy* [lactose-free formula]

Sustacal Basic; Sustacal Plus ready-to-use oral liquid OTC *enteral nutritional therapy* [lactose-free formula]

Sustagen powder OTC *enteral nutritional therapy* [milk-based formula]

Sustain tablets ℞ *electrolyte replacement; dehydration preventative* [sodium chloride; potassium chloride; calcium carbonate] 220•15•18 mg

Sustaire timed-release tablets (discontinued 2004) ℞ *antiasthmatic; bronchodilator* [theophylline] 100, 300 mg

Sustiva capsules, film-coated caplets ℞ *antiviral non-nucleoside reverse transcriptase inhibitor (NNRTI) for HIV infection* [efavirenz] 50, 100, 200 mg; 600 mg

Sutent ℞ *investigational (NDA filed) receptor tyrosine kinase (RTK) antineoplastic for gastrointestinal stromal tumor (GIST) and metastatic renal carcinoma* [sunitinib malate]

sutilains USAN, USP, INN, BAN *topical proteolytic enzymes for necrotic tissue debridement*

sutoprofen [see: suprofen]

suture, absorbable surgical USP *surgical aid*

suture, nonabsorbable surgical USP *surgical aid*

Su-Tuss DM oral liquid ℞ *antitussive; expectorant* [dextromethorphan hydrobromide; guaifenesin; alcohol 5%] 20•200 mg/5 mL

Su-Tuss HD elixir ℞ *narcotic antitussive; decongestant; expectorant* [hydrocodone bitartrate; pseudoephedrine HCl; guaifenesin] 5•60•200 mg/10 mL

suxamethone [see: succinylcholine chloride]

suxamethonium chloride INN, BAN *neuromuscular blocking agent* [also: succinylcholine chloride]

suxemerid INN *antitussive* [also: suxemerid sulfate]

suxemerid sulfate USAN *antitussive* [also: suxemerid]

suxethonium chloride INN

suxibuzone INN

swallow wort, orange *medicinal herb* [see: pleurisy root]

swallow wort, silky *medicinal herb* [see: milkweed]

swamp cabbage *medicinal herb* [see: skunk cabbage]

swamp laurel; swamp sassafras *medicinal herb* [see: magnolia]

sweet, mountain *medicinal herb* [see: New Jersey tea]

sweet, winter *medicinal herb* [see: marjoram]

sweet anise; sweet chervil *medicinal herb* [see: sweet cicely]

sweet balm *medicinal herb* [see: lemon balm]

sweet basil *medicinal herb* [see: basil]

sweet bay *medicinal herb* [see: laurel]

sweet birch *medicinal herb* [see: birch]

sweet birch oil [see: methyl salicylate]

sweet cicely (*Osmorhiza longistylis*) root *medicinal herb used as a carminative, expectorant, and stomachic*

sweet clover *medicinal herb* [see: melilot]

sweet dock *medicinal herb* [see: bistort]

sweet elder *medicinal herb* [see: elderberry]

sweet elm *medicinal herb* [see: slippery elm]

sweet fennel *medicinal herb* [see: fennel]

sweet flag *medicinal herb* [see: calamus]

sweet grass *medicinal herb* [see: calamus]

sweet leaf *medicinal herb* [see: stevia]

sweet magnolia *medicinal herb* [see: magnolia]

sweet marjoram *medicinal herb* [see: marjoram]

sweet myrtle *medicinal herb* [see: calamus]

sweet orange peel tincture [see: orange peel tincture, sweet]

sweet potato vine, wild *medicinal herb* [see: wild jalap]

sweet root *medicinal herb* [see: calamus]

sweet rush *medicinal herb* [see: calamus]

sweet sedge *medicinal herb* [see: calamus]

sweet spirit of nitre [see: ethyl nitrite]

sweet vernal grass (*Anthoxanthum odoratum*) *natural flavoring banned by* the FDA *as it is not generally regarded as safe and effective*

sweet violet *medicinal herb* [see: violet]

sweet water lily; sweet-scented water lily *medicinal herb* [see: white pond lily]

sweet weed *medicinal herb* [see: marsh mallow]

sweet woodruff (*Asperula odorata; Galium odoratum*) plant *medicinal herb for diuresis, inducing expectoration, liver disorders, promoting wound healing, relieving gastrointestinal spasms, and sedation*

Sweet'n Fresh Clotrimazole-7 cream, vaginal suppositories (discontinued 2001) OTC *antifungal* [clotrimazole] 1%; 100 mg

sweet-scented pond lily; sweet-scented water lily *medicinal herb* [see: white pond lily]

sweetwood *medicinal herb* [see: licorice]

Swim-Ear ear drops OTC *antiseptic* [isopropyl alcohol] 95%

swine snout *medicinal herb* [see: dandelion]

Syllact powder OTC *bulk laxative* [psyllium husks] 3.3 g/tsp.

Symax-SL sublingual tablets ℞ *GI/GU antispasmodic; antiparkinsonian; anticholinergic "drying agent" for allergic rhinitis and hyperhidrosis* [hyoscyamine sulfate] 0.125 mg

Symax-SR sustained-release caplets ℞ *GI/GU antispasmodic; antiparkinsonian; anticholinergic "drying agent" for allergic rhinitis and hyperhidrosis* [hyoscyamine sulfate] 0.375 mg

Symbicort 100; Symbicort 200 ⓒᴬᴺ Turbuhaler (dry powder in a metered-dose inhaler) ℞ *corticosteroidal anti-inflammatory and bronchodilator combination for chronic asthma* [budesonide; formoterol] 100•6 μg; 200•6 μg

Symbyax capsules ℞ *antipsychotic plus selective serotonin reuptake inhibitor (SSRI) for depressive episodes of a bipolar disorder* [olanzapine; fluoxetine HCl] 6•25, 6•50, 12•25, 12•50 mg

symclosene USAN, INN *topical anti-infective*

symetine INN *antiamebic* [also: symetine HCl]

symetine HCl USAN *antiamebic* [also: symetine]

Symlin subcu injection ℞ *synthetic amylin analogue to slow gastric emptying; antihyperglycemic for use with insulin for type 1 and type 2 diabetes* [pramlintide acetate] 0.6 mg/mL

Symmetrel tablets, syrup ℞ *antiviral for influenza A infections; dopaminergic antiparkinson agent* [amantadine HCl] 100 mg; 50 mg/5 mL

sympatholytics *a class of cardiovascular drugs that block the passage of impulses through the sympathetic nervous system* [also called: antiadrenergics]

sympathomimetics *a class of bronchodilators that relax the bronchial muscles, reducing bronchospasm; a class of cardiac agents that increase myocardial contractility, causing a vasopressor effect to counteract shock (inadequate tissue perfusion)* [also called: adrenergic agonists]

Symphytum officinale; S. tuberosum medicinal herb [see: comfrey]

Symplocarpus foetidus medicinal herb [see: skunk cabbage]

Synacol CF tablets (discontinued 2002) OTC *antitussive; expectorant* [dextromethorphan hydrobromide; guaifenesin] 15•200 mg

Synacort cream ℞ *topical corticosteroidal anti-inflammatory* [hydrocortisone] 1%, 2.5%

Synagis IM injection, powder for IM injection ℞ *monoclonal antibody for prophylaxis of respiratory syncytial virus (RSV) in infants* [palivizumab] 100 mg/mL; 50, 100 mg/vial

Synalar cream, ointment, topical solution ℞ *topical corticosteroidal anti-inflammatory* [fluocinolone acetonide] 0.01, 0.25%; 0.025%; 0.01%

Synalar-HP cream ℞ *topical corticosteroidal anti-inflammatory* [fluocinolone acetonide] 0.2%

Synalgos-DC capsules ℞ *narcotic analgesic* [dihydrocodeine bitartrate; aspirin; caffeine] 16•356.4•30 mg

Synarel nasal spray ℞ *gonadotropin-releasing hormone for central precocious puberty (orphan) and endometriosis* [nafarelin acetate] 2 mg/mL (200 μg/spray)

SynBiotics-3 capsules OTC *dietary supplement; fever blister treatment; not generally regarded as safe and effective as an antidiarrheal* [Bifidobacterium longum; Lactobacillus rhamnosus A; L. plantarum; Saccharomyces boulardii] 4.5 billion CFU

Synemol cream ℞ *corticosteroidal anti-inflammatory* [fluocinolone acetonide] 0.025%

Synercid powder for IV infusion ℞ *semi-synthetic streptogramin antibiotic for life-threatening infections* [quinupristin; dalfopristin] 150•350 mg/10 mL

synestrin [see: diethylstilbestrol]

synnematin B [see: adicillin]

Synophylate-GG syrup ℞ *antiasthmatic; bronchodilator; expectorant* [theophylline; guaifenesin; alcohol 10%] 150•100 mg/15 mL

Syn-Rx controlled-release tablets (14-day, 56-tablet treatment regimen) (discontinued 2002) ℞ *decongestant; expectorant* [pseudoephedrine HCl; guaifenesin] 60•600 mg

Synsorb Cd ℞ *investigational (Phase III) antidiarrheal for AIDS-related diarrhea due to* Clostridium difficile *infection*

Syntest D.S. sugar-coated tablets (discontinued 2004) ℞ *hormone replacement therapy for postmenopausal symptoms* [esterified estrogens; methyltestosterone] 1.25•2.5 mg

Syntest H.S. sugar-coated tablets (discontinued 2004) ℞ *hormone replacement therapy for postmenopausal symptoms* [esterified estrogens; methyltestosterone] 0.625•1.25 mg

synthestrin [see: diethylstilbestrol]

synthetic conjugated estrogens [see: estrogens, synthetic conjugated (A and B)]

synthetic lung surfactant [see: colfosceril palmitate]

synthetic monosaccharides *a class of investigational synthetic carbohydrates with immunomodulatory and anti-inflammatory effects being evaluated for the treatment of rheumatic arthritis*

synthetic paraffin [see: paraffin, synthetic]

synthetic spermaceti [now: cetyl esters wax]

synthoestrin [see: diethylstilbestrol]

Synthroid tablets, powder for injection ℞ *synthetic thyroid hormone (T_4 fraction only)* [levothyroxine sodium] 25, 50, 75, 88, 100, 112, 125, 137, 150, 175, 200, 300 μg; 200, 500 μg

synvinolin [now: simvastatin]

Synvisc intra-articular injection ℞ *viscoelastic lubricant and "shock absorber" for osteoarthritis and TMJ syndrome* [hylan G-F 20] 16 mg/2 mL

Syprine capsules ℞ *copper chelating agent for Wilson disease (orphan)* [trientine HCl] 250 mg

Syracol CF tablets (discontinued 2002) OTC *antitussive; expectorant* [dextromethorphan hydrobromide; guaifenesin] 15 • 200 mg

syrosingopine NF, INN, BAN

syrup NF *flavoring agent*

syrupus cerasi [see: cherry juice]

Syrvite oral liquid OTC *vitamin supplement* [multiple vitamins]

Systane eye drops OTC *moisturizer; lubricant* [polyethylene glycol 400; polypropylene glycol] 0.4% • 0.3%

Syzygium aromaticum *medicinal herb* [see: cloves]

(S)-zopiclone [see: esopiclone]

T-2 protocol (dactinomycin, doxorubicin, vincristine, cyclophosphamide, radiation) *chemotherapy protocol*

T_3 (liothyronine sodium) [q.v.]

T_4 (levothyroxine sodium) [q.v.]

T4 endonuclease V (T4N5), liposome encapsulated *investigational (orphan) for prevent cutaneous neoplasms in xeroderma pigmentosum*

T-10 protocol (methotrexate, doxorubicin, cisplatin, bleomycin, cyclophosphamide, dactinomycin) *chemotherapy protocol*

T-67 *investigational (Phase III) tubulin antagonist for liver cancer*

T-1249 *investigational (Phase I/II) fusion inhibitor for HIV infection*

Tab-A-Vite tablets OTC *vitamin supplement* [multiple vitamins; folic acid] ± • 0.4 mg

Tab-A-Vite + Iron tablets OTC *vitamin/iron supplement* [multiple vitamins; iron; folic acid] ± • 18 • 0.4 mg

Tabebuia avellanedae; T. impetiginosa *medicinal herb* [see: pau d'arco]

Tabernanthe iboga *street drug* [see: iboga]

tabilautide INN

Tabloid (trademarked dosage form) *tablet with raised lettering*

Tabloid tablets ℞ *antimetabolite antineoplastic for acute nonlymphocytic leukemias (ANLL)* [thioguanine] 40 mg

Tabules (dosage form) *tablets*

Tac-3 IM, intra-articular, intrabursal, intradermal injection ℞ *corticosteroid; anti-inflammatory* [triamcinolone acetonide] 3 mg/mL

Tac-40 suspension for injection ℞ *corticosteroid; anti-inflammatory* [triamcinolone acetonide] 40 mg/mL

taclamine INN *minor tranquilizer* [also: taclamine HCl]

taclamine HCl USAN *minor tranquilizer* [also: taclamine]

tacmahac *medicinal herb* [see: balm of Gilead]

tacrine INN, BAN *reversible cholinesterase inhibitor; cognition adjuvant for Alzheimer dementia* [also: tacrine HCl]

tacrine HCl USAN *reversible cholinesterase inhibitor; cognition adjuvant for Alzheimer dementia* [also: tacrine]

tacrolimus USAN, INN *immunosuppressant for liver and kidney transplants; topical treatment for eczema; investigational (Phase III) treatment for rheumatoid arthritis*

TAD (thioguanine, ara-C, daunorubicin) *chemotherapy protocol for acute myelocytic leukemia (AML)* [also: DAT; DCT]

tadalafil *phosphodiesterase type 5 (PDE5) inhibitor; selective vasodilator for erectile dysfunction (ED); investigational (Phase III) for pulmonary arterial hypertension; investigational (Phase II) for benign prostatic hyperplasia; investigational for female sexual dysfunction*

taeniacides *a class of agents that destroy tapeworms* [see also: anthelmintics; vermicides; vermifuges]

Tagamet film-coated tablets ℞ *histamine H_2 antagonist for gastric and duodenal ulcers and gastric hypersecretory conditions* [cimetidine] 300, 400, 800 mg ⑨ Tegopen

Tagamet oral liquid, IV or IM injection, premixed injection (discontinued 2005) ℞ *histamine H_2 antagonist for gastric and duodenal ulcers and gastric hypersecretory conditions* [cimetidine HCl] 300 mg/5 mL; 300 mg/2 mL; 300 mg/vial

Tagamet 100 (100 mg strength available in Europe)

Tagamet HB film-coated tablets, oral suspension (discontinued 2005) OTC *histamine H_2 antagonist for episodic heartburn and acid indigestion* [cimetidine] 100 mg; 200 mg

Tagamet HB 200 film-coated tablets OTC *histamine H_2 antagonist for episodic heartburn and acid indigestion* [cimetidine] 200 mg

taglutimide INN

taheebo *medicinal herb* [see: pau d'arco]

tail, colt's; cow's tail; horse tail; mare's tail *medicinal herb* [see: fleabane; horseweed]

tail, lion's *medicinal herb* [see: motherwort]

tailed cubebs; tailed pepper *medicinal herb* [see: cubeb]

TAK-603 *investigational (orphan) for Crohn disease*

Talacen caplets ℞ *narcotic agonist-antagonist analgesic; antipyretic* [pentazocine HCl; acetaminophen] 25•650 mg

talampicillin INN *antibacterial* [also: talampicillin HCl]

talampicillin HCl USAN *antibacterial* [also: talampicillin]

talastine INN

talbutal USP, INN *sedative; hypnotic*

talc USP, JAN *dusting powder; tablet and capsule lubricant*

talc, sterile aerosol *treatment for malignant pleural effusion and pneumothorax via intrapleural thoracoscopy administration (orphan)*

taleranol USAN, INN *gonadotropin enzyme inhibitor*

talinolol INN

talipexole INN

talisomycin USAN, INN *antineoplastic*

tall speedwell *medicinal herb* [see: Culver root]

tall veronica *medicinal herb* [see: Culver root]

tallimustine INN *investigational antineoplastic for leukemia and solid tumors*

tallow shrub *medicinal herb* [see: bayberry]

tallysomycin A [now: talisomycin]

talmetacin USAN, INN *analgesic; anti-inflammatory; antipyretic*

talmetoprim INN

talnetant HCl USAN *NK_3 receptor antagonist for urinary frequency, urgency, and incontinence*

talniflumate USAN, INN *anti-inflammatory; analgesic*

talopram INN *catecholamine potentiator* [also: talopram HCl]

talopram HCl USAN *catecholamine potentiator* [also: talopram]

talosalate USAN, INN *analgesic; anti-inflammatory*

Taloxa (foreign name for U.S. product Felbatol)

taloximine INN, BAN

talsaclidine INN

talsaclidine fumarate USAN *muscarinic M_1 agonist for Alzheimer disease*

talsupram INN

taltibride [see: metibride]

taltrimide INN

taludipine [see: teludipine]

taludipine HCl [see: teludipine HCl]

Talwin IV, IM, or subcu injection, Carpuject (prefilled syringes) ℞ *narcotic agonist-antagonist analgesic for moderate to severe pain; adjunct to surgical anesthesia; also abused as a street drug* [pentazocine lactate] 30 mg/mL; 60 mg

Talwin Compound caplets ℞ *narcotic agonist-antagonist analgesic; antipyretic; also abused as a street drug* [pentazocine HCl; aspirin] 12.5•325 mg

Talwin NX tablets ℞ *narcotic agonist-antagonist analgesic; also abused as a street drug* [pentazocine HCl; naloxone HCl] 50•0.5 mg

tamarind *(Tamarindus indica)* fruit and leaves *medicinal herb used as an anthelmintic, laxative, and refrigerant*

Tambocor tablets ℞ *antiarrhythmic* [flecainide acetate] 50, 100, 150 mg

tameridone USAN, INN, BAN *veterinary sedative*

tameticillin INN

tametraline INN *antidepressant* [also: tametraline HCl]

tametraline HCl USAN *antidepressant* [also: tametraline]

Tamiflu capsules, powder for oral suspension ℞ *antiviral for the prophylaxis and treatment of influenza A and B infections* [oseltamivir phosphate] 75 mg; 12 mg/mL

Tamine S.R. sustained-release tablets (discontinued 2001) ℞ *decongestant; antihistamine* [phenylpropanolamine HCl; phenylephrine HCl; brompheniramine maleate] 15•15•12 mg

tamitinol INN

tamoxifen INN, BAN *antiestrogen antineoplastic for breast cancer* [also: tamoxifen citrate]

tamoxifen citrate USAN, USP, JAN *antiestrogen antineoplastic for breast cancer; also for breast cancer prevention in high-risk patients* [also: tamoxifen] 10, 20 mg oral

tamoxifen & DTIC *chemotherapy protocol for malignant melanoma*

tamoxifen & epirubicin *chemotherapy protocol for breast cancer*

tampramine INN *antidepressant* [also: tampramine fumarate]

tampramine fumarate USAN *antidepressant* [also: tampramine]

Tamp-R-Tel (trademarked packaging form) *tamper-evident cartridge-needle unit*

tamsulosin INN *alpha$_1$-adrenergic blocker for benign prostatic hyperplasia (BPH)* [also: tamsulosin HCl]

tamsulosin HCl USAN, JAN *alpha$_1$-adrenergic blocker for benign prostatic hyperplasia (BPH)* [also: tamsulosin]

Tanac gel OTC *oral anesthetic; vulnerary* [dyclonine HCl; allantoin] 1%•0.5%

Tanac topical liquid OTC *oral anesthetic; antiseptic* [benzocaine; benzalkonium chloride] 10%•0.12%

Tanac Dual Core stick OTC *topical oral anesthetic; antiseptic; astringent* [benzocaine; benzalkonium chloride; tannic acid] 7.5%•0.12%•6%

Tanacetum parthenium *medicinal herb* [see: feverfew]

Tanacetum vulgare *medicinal herb* [see: tansy]

Tanafed oral suspension (discontinued 2003) ℞ *decongestant; antihistamine* [pseudoephedrine tannate; chlorpheniramine tannate] 150•9 mg/10 mL

Tanafed DM pediatric oral suspension (discontinued 2003) ℞ *decongestant; antihistamine; antitussive* [pseudoephedrine tannate; chlorpheniramine tannate; dextromethorphan tannate] 75•4.5•25 mg/5 mL

Tanafed DMX pediatric oral suspension ℞ *decongestant; antihistamine; antitussive* [pseudoephedrine tannate; dexchlorpheniramine tannate; dextromethorphan tannate] 75•2.5•25 mg/5 mL

Tanafed DP pediatric oral suspension ℞ *decongestant; antihistamine* [pseudoephedrine tannate; dexchlorpheniramine tannate] 75•2.5 mg/5 mL

tanaproget *investigational (Phase III) oral progesterone receptor antagonist contraceptive that inhibits ovulation*

tandamine INN *antidepressant* [also: tandamine HCl]

tandamine HCl USAN *antidepressant* [also: tandamine]

tandospirone INN, BAN *anxiolytic* [also: tandospirone citrate]

tandospirone citrate USAN *anxiolytic* [also: tandospirone]

taniplon INN

tannic acid USP, JAN *astringent; topical mucosal protectant*

tannic acid acetate [see: acetyltannic acid]

Tannic-12 caplets ℞ *antitussive; antihistamine* [carbetapentane tannate; chlorpheniramine tannate] 60•5 mg

Tannic-12 pediatric oral suspension ℞ *antitussive; decongestant; antihistamine* [carbetapentane tannate; phenylephrine tannate; chlorpheniramine tannate] 30•5•4 mg/5 mL

tannin [see: tannic acid]

tannyl acetate [see: acetyltannic acid]

Tanoral tablets (discontinued 2002) ℞ *decongestant; antihistamine* [phenylephrine tannate; chlorpheniramine tannate; pyrilamine tannate] 25•8•25 mg

tansy (Chrysanthemum vulgare; Tanacetum vulgare) leaves and seeds *medicinal herb for inducing diaphoresis,* *promoting wound healing, relieving spasms, stimulating menstruation, and treating worm infections*

tantalum *element (Ta)*

Tantum ℞ *investigational (orphan) radioprotectant for oral mucosa following radiation therapy for head and neck cancer* [benzydamine HCl]

Tao capsules (discontinued 2004) ℞ *macrolide antibiotic* [troleandomycin] 250 mg

taoryi edisylate [see: caramiphen edisylate]

Tapanol tablets, caplets, gelcaps OTC *analgesic; antipyretic* [acetaminophen] 325, 500 mg; 500 mg; 500 mg

Tapazole tablets ℞ *antithyroid agent* [methimazole] 5, 10 mg

tape, adhesive USP *surgical aid*

taprostene INN

tar [see: coal tar]

tarweed *medicinal herb* [see: yerba santa]

Tarabine PFS subcu, intrathecal, or IV injection ℞ *antimetabolite antineoplastic for various leukemias* [cytarabine] 20 mg/mL

Taraphilic ointment OTC *antipsoriatic; antiseborrheic* [coal tar] 1%

Taraxacum officinale *medicinal herb* [see: dandelion]

Tarceva film-coated tablets ℞ *antineoplastic for advanced or metastatic non–small cell lung cancer (NSCLC) and pancreatic cancer; investigational (Phase III) for breast cancer; investigational (orphan) for non-Hodgkin lymphoma* [erlotinib HCl] 25, 100, 150 mg

targeted monoclonal antibody vehicles (T-MAVs) *a class of agents that deliver a cytotoxic drug or radioactivity directly to the targeted tissue, usually a cancerous tumor; T-MAVs are not therapeutic per se, but transport the therapeutic agent (effector molecule) to a specific site*

Targocid (approved in 13 foreign countries) ℞ *investigational (NDA filed) glycopeptide antibiotic* [teicoplanin]

Targretin capsules, gel ℞ *synthetic retinoid analogue antineoplastic for*

*cutaneous T-cell lymphoma (orphan);
investigational (Phase III) for lung cancer* [bexarotene] 75 mg; 1% ?
Tegopen; Tegrin

tariquidar *investigational (Phase III)
p-glycoprotein pump inhibitor for lung
cancer*

Tarka film-coated dual-release tablets
℞ *once-daily antihypertensive; angiotensin-converting enzyme (ACE)
inhibitor; calcium channel blocker*
[trandolapril (immediate release);
verapamil HCl (extended release)]
2•180, 1•240, 2•240, 4•240 mg

Tarlene hair lotion OTC *antiseborrheic;
antipsoriatic; keratolytic* [salicylic
acid; coal tar] 2.5%•2%

Taro-Desoximetasone Ⓒᴬᴺ cream, gel
(name changed to Desoxi in 2001)

Taro-Warfarin Ⓒᴬᴺ tablets ℞ *coumarin-
derivative anticoagulant* [warfarin
sodium] 1, 2, 2.5, 3, 4, 5, 6, 7.5, 10 mg

tarragon *(Artemisia dracunculus)*
flowering plant *medicinal herb used as
a diuretic, emmenagogue, hypnotic,
and stomachic*

Tarsum shampoo OTC *antipsoriatic;
antiseborrheic; keratolytic* [coal tar;
salicylic acid] 10%•5%

tartar emetic [see: antimony potassium tartrate]

tartaric acid NF *buffering agent*

Tasmar film-coated tablets ℞ COMT
*inhibitor; adjunct to carbidopa and levo-
dopa for Parkinson disease* [tolcapone]
100, 200 mg

tasosartan USAN, INN *antihypertensive;
angiotensin II antagonist*

tasuldine INN

TAT antagonist *investigational (Phase
I/II) antiviral for HIV infection*

taurine INN [also: aminoethylsulfonic
acid]

taurocholate sodium [see: sodium
taurocholate]

taurolidine INN, BAN *investigational
antitoxin for the treatment of sepsis*

tauromustine INN *investigational treatment for renal cancer and multiple sclerosis*

tauroselcholic acid INN, BAN

taurultam INN, BAN

Tavist tablets, syrup (discontinued
2002) ℞ *antihistamine* [clemastine
fumarate] 2.68 mg; 0.67 mg/5 mL

Tavist Allergy tablets OTC *antihistamine* [clemastine fumarate] 1.34 mg

Tavist Allergy/Sinus/Headache caplets OTC *decongestant; antihistamine;
analgesic* [pseudoephedrine HCl;
clemastine fumarate; acetamino-
phen] 30•0.335•500 mg

Tavist ND tablets OTC *nonsedating antihistamine for allergic rhinitis and chronic
idiopathic urticaria* [loratadine] 10 mg

Tavist Sinus caplets OTC *decongestant;
analgesic; antipyretic* [pseudoephedrine
HCl; acetaminophen] 30•500 mg

Tavist-D film-coated sustained-release
tablets (discontinued 2001) OTC
decongestant; antihistamine [phenyl-
propanolamine HCl; clemastine
fumarate] 75•1.34 mg

taxanes; taxoids *a class of antineoplastics
that inhibits cancer cell mitosis by dis-
rupting the cells' microtubular network*

Taxol IV infusion ℞ *antineoplastic for
AIDS-related Kaposi sarcoma (orphan),
breast and ovarian cancers, and non–
small cell lung cancer (NSCLC)*
[paclitaxel] 6 mg/mL

Taxoprexin ℞ *investigational (orphan)
taxane for hormone-refractory prostate
cancer, pancreatic cancer, malignant
melanoma, and adenocarcinoma of the
GI tract; investigational (Phase III) for
breast cancer* [docosahexaenoic acid
(DHA); paclitaxel]

Taxotere IV infusion ℞ *antineoplastic
for advanced or metastatic breast, prostate, and non–small cell lung cancer
(NSCLC); investigational (Phase III)
for head and neck cancers* [docetaxel]
20, 80 mg/vial

Taxus bacatta and other species
medicinal herb [see: yew]

tazadolene INN *analgesic* [also: tazadolene succinate]

tazadolene succinate USAN *analgesic*
[also: tazadolene]

tazanolast INN

tazarotene USAN, INN *retinoid prodrug; topical keratolytic for acne and psoriasis; adjuvant treatment for facial wrinkles, hyper- and hypopigmentation, and benign lentigines*

tazasubrate INN, BAN

tazeprofen INN

Tazicef powder or frozen premix for IV or IM injection ℞ *cephalosporin antibiotic* [ceftazidime] 1, 2, 6 g

Tazidime powder for IV or IM injection ℞ *cephalosporin antibiotic* [ceftazidime] 0.5, 1, 2, 6 g

tazifylline INN *antihistamine* [also: tazifylline HCl]

tazifylline HCl USAN *antihistamine* [also: tazifylline]

taziprinone INN

tazobactam USAN, INN, BAN *β-lactamase inhibitor; penicillin synergist*

tazobactam sodium USAN *β-lactamase inhibitor; penicillin synergist*

Tazocin (European name for U.S. product **Zosyn**)

tazofelone USAN *investigational (Phase II) treatment for ulcerative colitis and Crohn disease*

tazolol INN *cardiotonic* [also: tazolol HCl]

tazolol HCl USAN *cardiotonic* [also: tazolol]

tazomeline citrate USAN *cholinergic agonist for Alzheimer disease*

Tazorac cream, gel ℞ *retinoid pro-drug; keratolytic for acne and psoriasis* [tazarotene] 0.05%, 0.1%

Taztia XT extended-release capsules ℞ *antihypertensive; calcium channel blocker* [diltiazem HCl] 120, 180, 240, 300, 360 mg

TBC-3B *investigational (Phase I) vaccine for AIDS*

TBZ (thiabendazole) [q.v.]

TC (thioguanine, cytarabine) *chemotherapy protocol*

3TC [now: lamivudine]

⁹⁹ᵐ**Tc** [see: macrosalb (⁹⁹ᵐTc)]

⁹⁹ᵐ**Tc** [see: sodium pertechnetate Tc 99m]

⁹⁹ᵐ**Tc** [see: technetium Tc 99m albumin]

⁹⁹ᵐ**Tc** [see: technetium Tc 99m albumin aggregated]

⁹⁹ᵐ**Tc** [see: technetium Tc 99m albumin colloid]

⁹⁹ᵐ**Tc** [see: technetium Tc 99m albumin microaggregated]

⁹⁹ᵐ**Tc** [see: technetium Tc 99m antimony trisulfide colloid]

⁹⁹ᵐ**Tc** [see: technetium Tc 99m biciromab]

⁹⁹ᵐ**Tc** [see: technetium Tc 99m bicisate]

⁹⁹ᵐ**Tc** [see: technetium Tc 99m disofenin]

⁹⁹ᵐ**Tc** [see: technetium Tc 99m etidronate]

⁹⁹ᵐ**Tc** [see: technetium Tc 99m exametazine]

⁹⁹ᵐ**Tc** [see: technetium Tc 99m ferpentetate]

⁹⁹ᵐ**Tc** [see: technetium Tc 99m furifosmin]

⁹⁹ᵐ**Tc** [see: technetium Tc 99m gluceptate]

⁹⁹ᵐ**Tc** [see: technetium Tc 99m lidofenin]

⁹⁹ᵐ**Tc** [see: technetium Tc 99m mebrofenin]

⁹⁹ᵐ**Tc** [see: technetium Tc 99m medronate]

⁹⁹ᵐ**Tc** [see: technetium Tc 99m medronate disodium]

⁹⁹ᵐ**Tc** [see: technetium Tc 99m mertiatide]

⁹⁹ᵐ**Tc** [see: technetium Tc 99m oxidronate]

⁹⁹ᵐ**Tc** [see: technetium Tc 99m pentetate]

⁹⁹ᵐ**Tc** [see: technetium Tc 99m pentetate calcium trisodium]

⁹⁹ᵐ**Tc** [see: technetium Tc 99m (pyro- & trimeta-) phosphates]

⁹⁹ᵐ**Tc** [see: technetium Tc 99m pyrophosphate]

⁹⁹ᵐ**Tc** [see: technetium Tc 99m red blood cells]

⁹⁹ᵐ**Tc** [see: technetium Tc 99m sestamibi]

⁹⁹ᵐ**Tc** [see: technetium Tc 99m siboroxime]

99mTc [see: technetium Tc 99m succimer]

99mTc [see: technetium Tc 99m sulfur colloid]

99mTc [see: technetium Tc 99m teboroxime]

99mTc [see: technetium Tc 99m tetrofosmin]

99mTc [see: technetium Tc 99m tiatide]

TCC (trichlorocarbanilide) [see: triclocarban]

TCF (Taxol, cisplatin, fluorouracil) *chemotherapy protocol for esophageal cancer*

TCI Ovulation Tester test kit for home use OTC *in vitro diagnostic aid to predict ovulation time from a saliva sample*

TD; Td (tetanus & diphtheria [toxoids]) *the designation TD (or DT) denotes the pediatric vaccine; Td denotes the adult vaccine* [see: diphtheria & tetanus toxoids, adsorbed]

tea, Canada; mountain tea; redberry tea *medicinal herb* [see: wintergreen]

tea tree oil (Melaleuca alternifolia) *medicinal herb for acne, boils, burns, Candida infections, cold sores, joint pain, skin disorders, staphylococcal and streptococcal infections, and sunburn; also used as a douche for trichomonal cervicitis and vaginal candidiasis*

TEAB (tetraethylammonium bromide) [see: tetrylammonium bromide]

teaberry oil [see: methyl salicylate]

TEAC (tetraethylammonium chloride) [q.v.]

teamster's tea *medicinal herb* [see: ephedra]

TearGard eye drops OTC *ocular moisturizer/lubricant* [hydroxyethylcellulose]

Teargen eye drops OTC *ophthalmic moisturizer/lubricant* [polyvinyl alcohol]

Tearisol eye drops OTC *ophthalmic moisturizer/lubricant* [hydroxypropyl methylcellulose] 0.5%

Tears Naturale; Tears Naturale II; Tears Naturale Free eye drops OTC *ophthalmic moisturizer/lubricant* [hydroxypropyl methylcellulose] 0.3%

Tears Naturale Forte eye drops OTC *ophthalmic moisturizer/lubricant* [hydroxypropyl methylcellulose; glycerin] 0.3%•0.2%

Tears Naturale P.M. ⒸⒶⒹ ophthalmic ointment OTC *ocular moisturizer/lubricant* [white petrolatum; mineral oil; lanolin]

Tears Plus eye drops OTC *ophthalmic moisturizer/lubricant* [polyvinyl alcohol] 1.4%

Tears Renewed eye drops OTC *ophthalmic moisturizer/lubricant* [hydroxypropyl methylcellulose] 0.3%

Tears Renewed ophthalmic ointment OTC *ocular moisturizer/lubricant* [white petrolatum; mineral oil]

TearSaver Punctum Plugs ℞ *blocks the puncta and canaliculus to eliminate tear loss in keratitis sicca* [silicone plug]

Tebamide suppositories, pediatric suppositories ℞ *anticholinergic; post-surgical antiemetic* [trimethobenzamide HCl; benzocaine] 200 mg•2%; 100 mg•2%

tebatizole INN

tebethion [see: thioacetazone; thiacetazone]

tebufelone USAN, INN *analgesic; anti-inflammatory*

tebuquine USAN, INN *antimalarial*

tebutate USAN, INN *combining name for radicals or groups*

TEC (thiotepa, etoposide, carboplatin) *chemotherapy protocol*

tecadenoson *investigational (Phase III) agent for paroxysmal supraventricular tachycardia (PSVT)*

teceleukin USAN, INN, BAN *immunostimulant; investigational (orphan) for metastatic renal cell carcinoma and metastatic malignant melanoma*

teceleukin & interferon alfa-2a *investigational (orphan) for metastatic renal cell carcinoma and metastatic malignant melanoma*

technetium *element (Tc)*

technetium (99mTc) dimercaptosuccinic acid JAN *diagnostic aid for renal* *function testing* [also: technetium Tc 99m succimer]

technetium (^{99m}Tc) human serum albumin JAN *radioactive agent*

technetium (^{99m}Tc) labeled macro-aggregated human albumin JAN [also: macrosalb (^{99m}Tc)]

technetium (^{99m}Tc) methylenedi-phosphonate JAN *radioactive diagnostic aid for skeletal imaging* [also: technetium Tc 99m medronate]

technetium (^{99m}Tc) phytate JAN *radioactive agent*

technetium Tc 99m albumin USP *radioactive agent*

technetium Tc 99m albumin aggregated USAN, USP *radioactive diagnostic aid for lung imaging*

technetium Tc 99m albumin colloid USAN, USP *radioactive agent*

technetium Tc 99m albumin microaggregated USAN *radioactive agent*

technetium Tc 99m antimelanoma murine monoclonal antibodies (MAb) *investigational (orphan) for diagnostic imaging agent for metastases of malignant melanoma*

technetium Tc 99m antimony trisulfide colloid USAN *radioactive agent*

technetium Tc 99m apcitide *radiopharmaceutical diagnostic aid for acute venous thrombosis*

technetium Tc 99m arcitumomab USAN *radiopharmaceutical diagnostic aid for recurrent or metastatic thyroid and colorectal cancers*

technetium Tc 99m bectumomab *monoclonal antibody; investigational (Phase III, orphan) diagnostic aid for non-Hodgkin B-cell lymphoma, AIDS-related lymphomas, and other acute and chronic B-cell leukemias* [also: bectumomab]

technetium Tc 99m biciromab *radioactive diagnostic aid for deep vein thrombosis*

technetium Tc 99m bicisate USAN, INN, BAN *radioactive diagnostic aid for brain imaging*

technetium Tc 99m disofenin USP *radioactive diagnostic aid for hepatobiliary function testing*

technetium Tc 99m DMSA (dimer-captosuccinic acid) [see: technetium Tc 99m succimer]

technetium Tc 99m DTPA (diethylenetriaminepentaacetic acid) [see: technetium Tc 99m pentetate]

technetium Tc 99m etidronate USP *radioactive agent*

technetium Tc 99m exametazine USAN *radioactive agent*

technetium Tc 99m ferpentetate USP *radioactive agent*

technetium Tc 99m furifosmin USAN, INN *radioactive agent; diagnostic aid for cardiac disease*

technetium Tc 99m gluceptate USP *radioactive agent*

technetium Tc 99m HSA (human serum albumin) [see: technetium Tc 99m albumin]

technetium Tc 99m iron ascorbate pentetic acid complex [now: technetium Tc 99m ferpentetate]

technetium Tc 99m lidofenin USAN, USP *radioactive agent*

technetium Tc 99m MAA (microaggregated albumin) [see: technetium Tc 99m albumin aggregated]

technetium Tc 99m MDP (methylenediphosphonate) [see: technetium Tc 99m medronate]

technetium Tc 99m mebrofenin USAN, USP *radioactive agent*

technetium Tc 99m medronate USP *radioactive diagnostic aid for skeletal imaging* [also: technetium (^{99m}Tc) methylenediphosphonate]

technetium Tc 99m medronate disodium USAN *radioactive agent*

technetium Tc 99m mertiatide USAN *radioactive diagnostic aid for renal function testing*

technetium Tc 99m murine monoclonal antibodies (MAb) to human alpha-fetoprotein (AFP) *investigational (orphan) diagnostic aid* *for AFP-producing tumors, hepatoblastoma, and hepatocellular carcinoma*

technetium Tc 99m murine monoclonal antibodies (MAb) to human chorionic gonadotropin (hCG) *investigational (orphan) diagnostic aid for hCG-producing tumors*

technetium Tc 99m murine monoclonal antibodies (MAb) IgG₂a to B cell [now: technetium Tc 99m bectumomab]

technetium Tc 99m oxidronate USP *radioactive diagnostic aid for skeletal imaging*

technetium Tc 99m pentetate USP *radioactive agent* [also: human serum albumin diethylenetriaminepentaacetic acid technetium (^{99m}Tc)]

technetium Tc 99m pentetate calcium trisodium USAN *radioactive agent*

technetium Tc 99m pentetate sodium [now: technetium Tc 99m pentetate]

technetium Tc 99m (pyro- and trimeta-) phosphates USP *radioactive agent*

technetium Tc 99m pyrophosphate USP, JAN *radioactive agent*

technetium Tc 99m red blood cells USAN *radioactive agent*

technetium Tc 99m sestamibi USAN, INN, BAN *radioactive/radiopaque diagnostic aid for cardiac perfusion imaging and mammography*

technetium Tc 99m siboroxime USAN, INN *radioactive diagnostic aid for brain imaging*

technetium Tc 99m sodium gluceptate [now: technetium Tc 99m gluceptate]

technetium Tc 99m succimer USP *diagnostic aid for renal function testing* [also: technetium (^{99m}Tc) dimercaptosuccinic acid]

technetium Tc 99m sulesomab *monoclonal antibody; diagnostic aid for infectious lesions* [also: sulesomab]

technetium Tc 99m sulfur colloid (TSC) USAN, USP *radioactive agent*

technetium Tc 99m teboroxime USAN, INN, BAN *radioactive/radiopaque diagnostic aid for cardiac perfusion imaging*

technetium Tc 99m tetrofosmin *radioactive agent for cardiovascular imaging*

technetium Tc 99m tiatide BAN

technetium Tc 99m TSC (technetium sulfur colloid) [see: technetium Tc 99m sulfur colloid]

technetium Tc 99m-labeled CEA scan [see: arcitumomab]

teclothiazide INN, BAN

teclozan USAN, INN *antiamebic*

Tecnu Outdoor Skin Cleanser lotion OTC *for the removal of toxic oils from poison ivy, oak, or sumac; use before or as soon as rash appears; can also be used to clean clothing and equipment* [deodorized mineral spirits; propylene glycol; fatty acid soap]

Tecnu Poison Oak-N-Ivy topical liquid (name changed to **Tecnu Outdoor Skin Cleanser** in 2003)

tecogalan sodium USAN *antiangiogenic antineoplastic*

Teczem film-coated extended-release tablets ℞ *antihypertensive; angiotensin-converting enzyme (ACE) inhibitor; calcium channel blocker* [diltiazem maleate; enalapril maleate] 180•5 mg

tedisamil INN *investigational calcium channel blocker for ischemic heart disease and arrhythmias*

Tedrigen tablets OTC *antiasthmatic; bronchodilator; decongestant; sedative* [theophylline; ephedrine HCl; phenobarbital] 120•22.5•7.5 mg

tefazoline INN

tefenperate INN

tefludazine INN

teflurane USAN, INN *inhalation anesthetic*

teflutixol INN

tegafur USAN, INN, BAN *antineoplastic; prodrug of fluorouracil*

tegaserod USAN *selective serotonin 5-HT₄ receptor antagonist for irritable bowel syndrome (IBS)*

tegaserod maleate *selective serotonin 5-HT₄ receptor antagonist for irritable bowel syndrome (IBS) with chronic constipation in women and chronic idiopathic constipation in all*

Tegison capsules (discontinued 2002) ℞ *systemic antipsoriatic* [etretinate] 10, 25 mg

Tegretol chewable tablets, tablets, oral suspension ℞ *anticonvulsant; analgesic for trigeminal neuralgia; antimanic* [carbamazepine] 100 mg; 200 mg; 100 mg/5 mL ⊇ Tegrin

Tegretol-XR extended-release tablets ℞ *twice-daily anticonvulsant; antimanic* [carbamazepine] 100, 200, 400 mg

Tegrin for Psoriasis cream, lotion, soap (discontinued 2003) OTC *antipsoriatic; antiseborrheic; antiseptic* [coal tar solution] 5% ⊇ Targretin; Tegopen; Tegretol

Tegrin Medicated gel shampoo, lotion shampoo (discontinued 2003) OTC *antiseborrheic; antipsoriatic; antipruritic; antibacterial* [coal tar] 5%

Tegrin Medicated Extra Conditioning; Advanced Formula Tegrin shampoo (discontinued 2003) OTC *antiseborrheic; antipsoriatic; antipruritic; antibacterial* [coal tar] 7%

Tegrin-HC ointment OTC *topical corticosteroidal anti-inflammatory* [hydrocortisone] 1%

Tegrin-LT shampoo/conditioner (discontinued 2003) OTC *pediculicide for lice* [pyrethrins; piperonyl butoxide technical] 0.33%•3.15%

teholamine [see: aminophylline]

TEIB (triethyleneiminobenzoquinone) [see: triaziquone]

teicoplanin USAN, INN, BAN *investigational (NDA filed) glycopeptide antibiotic*

teicoplanin A₂₋₁, A₂₋₂, A₂₋₃, A₂₋₄, A₂₋₅, and A₃₋₁ *components of teicoplanin*

Teladar cream ℞ *corticosteroidal anti-inflammatory* [betamethasone dipropionate] 0.05%

telbermin USAN *angiogenic growth factor; vascular endothelial growth factor, recombinant human (rhVEGF); investigational (Phase II, orphan) for peripheral vascular disease and coronary artery disease*

telbivudine *investigational (Phase II) treatment for hepatitis B infection*

Telcyta ℞ *investigational (Phase III) antineoplastic for ovarian cancer*

Teldrin 12-Hour Allergy Relief sustained-release capsules (discontinued 2001) OTC *decongestant; antihistamine* [phenylpropanolamine HCl; chlorpheniramine maleate] 75•8 mg

Tel-E-Amp (trademarked packaging form) *unit dose ampule*

Tel-E-Dose (trademarked packaging form) *unit dose package*

Tel-E-Ject (trademarked delivery system) *prefilled disposable syringe*

telenzepine INN

Tel-E-Pack (trademarked packaging form) *packaging system*

Telepaque tablets ℞ *radiopaque contrast medium for cholecystography* [iopanoic acid (66.68% iodine)] 500 mg (333.4 mg)

Tel-E-Vial (trademarked packaging form) *unit dose vial*

telinavir USAN *antiviral; HIV protease inhibitor*

telithromycin *broad-spectrum ketolide antibiotic for respiratory tract infections*

tellurium *element (Te)*

telmisartan USAN *long-acting antihypertensive; angiotensin II receptor antagonist*

teloxantrone INN *antineoplastic* [also: teloxantrone HCl]

teloxantrone HCl USAN *antineoplastic* [also: teloxantrone]

teludipine INN *antihypertensive; calcium channel antagonist* [also: teludipine HCl]

teludipine HCl USAN *antihypertensive; calcium channel antagonist* [also: teludipine]

Telzir (European name for U.S. product **Lexiva**)

temafloxacin INN, BAN *antibacterial; microbial DNA topoisomerase inhibitor* [also: temafloxacin HCl]

temafloxacin HCl USAN *antibacterial; microbial DNA topoisomerase inhibitor* [also: temafloxacin]

temarotene INN

tematropium methylsulfate USAN *anticholinergic* [also: tematropium metilsulfate]

tematropium metilsulfate INN *anticholinergic* [also: tematropium methylsulfate]

temazepam USAN, INN *benzodiazepine sedative and hypnotic* 15, 30 mg oral

Temazin Cold syrup (discontinued 2001) OTC *decongestant; antihistamine* [phenylpropanolamine HCl; chlorpheniramine maleate] 12.5•2 mg/5 mL

Tembid (trademarked dosage form) *sustained-action capsule*

temefos USAN, INN *veterinary ectoparasiticide*

temelastine USAN, INN, BAN *antihistamine*

temocapril HCl USAN *antihypertensive*

temocillin USAN, INN, BAN *antibacterial*

Temodal ⓒᴬᴺ capsules Ŗ *alkylating antineoplastic for refractory anaplastic astrocytoma and recurrent malignant glioma* [temozolomide] 5, 20, 100, 250 mg

Temodar capsules Ŗ *alkylating antineoplastic for refractory anaplastic astrocytoma (AA) and recurrent glioblastoma multiforme (GBM); investigational (NDA filed) for metastatic malignant melanoma* [temozolomide] 5, 20, 100, 250 mg

temodox USAN, INN *veterinary growth stimulant*

temoporfin USAN, INN, BAN *photosensitizer for photodynamic cancer therapy; investigational (NDA filed) for head and neck cancer*

Temovate ointment, gel, cream, scalp application Ŗ *corticosteroidal anti-inflammatory* [clobetasol propionate] 0.05%

Temovate Emollient cream Ŗ *corticosteroidal anti-inflammatory* [clobetasol propionate in an emollient base] 0.05%

temozolomide INN, BAN *alkylating antineoplastic for refractory anaplastic astrocytoma (AA) and recurrent glioblastoma multiforme (GBM); investigational (NDA filed) for metastatic malignant melanoma*

TEMP (tamoxifen, etoposide, mitoxantrone, Platinol) *chemotherapy protocol*

Temp Tab tablets OTC *electrolyte replacement* [sodium, potassium, and chloride electrolytes] 180•15•287 mg

Tempium Ŗ *investigational treatment for Alzheimer disease* [lazabemide HCl]

Tempo chewable tablets OTC *antacid; antiflatulent* [aluminum hydroxide; magnesium hydroxide; calcium carbonate; simethicone] 133•81•414•20 mg

Tempra ⓒᴬᴺ chewable tablets, syrup, oral drops OTC *pediatric analgesic and antipyretic* [acetaminophen] 80 mg; 80, 160 mg/5 mL; 80 mg/mL

Tempra 1 drops OTC *analgesic; antipyretic* [acetaminophen] 100 mg/mL

Tempra 2 syrup OTC *analgesic; antipyretic* [acetaminophen] 160 mg/5 mL

Tempra 3 chewable tablets OTC *analgesic; antipyretic* [acetaminophen] 80, 160 mg

Tempra FirsTabs ⓒᴬᴺ (quick dissolving tablets) OTC *pediatric analgesic and antipyretic* [acetaminophen] 160 mg

Tempra Quicklets (quickly dissolving tablets) OTC *analgesic; antipyretic* [acetaminophen] 80, 160 mg

Tempule (trademarked dosage form) *timed-release capsule or tablet*

temsirolimus *investigational (Phase III) antineoplastic for renal cell carcinoma, metastatic breast cancer, and mantle cell lymphoma; investigational (Phase II) immunosuppressant for rheumatoid arthritis and multiple sclerosis* ② *sirolimus*

temurtide USAN, INN, BAN *vaccine adjuvant*

10 Benzagel; 5 Benzagel gel Ŗ *topical keratolytic for acne* [benzoyl peroxide] 10%; 5%

10% LMD IV injection ℞ *plasma volume expander for shock due to hemorrhage, burns, or surgery* [dextran 40] 10%

tenamfetamine INN

Tencet capsules ℞ *analgesic; antipyretic; sedative* [acetaminophen; caffeine; butalbital] 325•40•50 mg

Tencon capsules (discontinued 2004) ℞ *analgesic; barbiturate sedative* [acetaminophen; butalbital] 650•50 mg

tendamistat INN

tenecteplase USAN *genetically engineered mutation of tissue plasminogen activator (tPA); thrombolytic/fibrinolytic for acute myocardial infarction (AMI)*

Tenex tablets ℞ *antihypertensive; antiadrenergic* [guanfacine HCl] 1, 2 mg ⊡ Xanax

tenidap USAN, INN *investigational (NDA filed) anti-inflammatory for osteoarthritis and rheumatoid arthritis; cytokine inhibitor*

tenidap sodium USAN *anti-inflammatory for osteoarthritis and rheumatoid arthritis*

tenilapine INN

teniloxazine INN

tenilsetam INN

teniposide USAN, INN, BAN *antineoplastic for refractory childhood acute lymphocytic leukemia (orphan)*

Ten-K controlled-release tablets ℞ *potassium supplement* [potassium chloride] 750 mg (10 mEq K)

tenoate INN *combining name for radicals or groups*

tenocyclidine INN

tenofovir USAN *antiviral; nucleotide reverse transcriptase inhibitor (NRTI)*

tenofovir disoproxil fumarate (tenofovir DF) *oral antiviral; nucleotide reverse transcriptase inhibitor for HIV-1 infection (base=82%)*

tenonitrozole INN

Tenoretic 50; Tenoretic 100 tablets ℞ *antihypertensive; β-blocker; diuretic* [chlorthalidone; atenolol] 25•50 mg; 25•100 mg

Tenormin tablets, IV injection ℞ *antianginal; antihypertensive; β-blocker* [atenolol] 25, 50, 100 mg; 5 mg/10 mL

Tenovil ℞ *investigational immunomodulator for Crohn disease, ulcerative colitis, rheumatoid arthritis (RA), and psoriasis* [ilodecakin]

tenoxicam USAN, INN, BAN *anti-inflammatory*

Tensilon IV or IM injection ℞ *myasthenia gravis treatment; antidote to curare overdose* [edrophonium chloride] 10 mg/mL

Ten-Tab (trademarked dosage form) *controlled-release tablet*

Tenuate tablets, Dospan (controlled-release tablets) ℞ *anorexiant; CNS stimulant* [diethylpropion HCl] 25 mg; 75 mg

tenylidone INN

teoclate INN *combining name for radicals or groups* [also: theoclate]

teopranitol INN

teoprolol INN

tepirindole INN

tepoxalin USAN, INN *antipsoriatic*

teprenone INN

teprosilate INN *combining name for radicals or groups*

teprotide USAN, INN *angiotensin-converting enzyme (ACE) inhibitor*

Tequin film-coated tablets, powder for oral suspension, IV infusion ℞ *broad-spectrum fluoroquinolone antibiotic* [gatifloxacin] 200, 400 mg; 200 mg/5 mL; 200, 400 mg/vial

Tera-Gel shampoo OTC *antiseborrheic; antipsoriatic; antipruritic; antibacterial* [coal tar] 0.5%

Terak with Polymyxin B Sulfate ophthalmic ointment ℞ *topical ophthalmic antibiotic* [oxytetracycline HCl; polymyxin B sulfate] 5 mg•10 000 U per g

Terazol 3 vaginal suppositories, vaginal cream in prefilled applicator ℞ *antifungal* [terconazole] 80 mg; 0.8%

Terazol 7 vaginal cream in prefilled applicator ℞ *antifungal* [terconazole] 0.4%

terazosin INN, BAN *alpha₁-adrenergic blocker for hypertension and benign prostatic hyperplasia (BPH)* [also: terazosin HCl]

terazosin HCl USAN *alpha₁-adrenergic blocker for hypertension and benign prostatic hyperplasia (BPH)* [also: terazosin] 1, 2, 5, 10 mg oral

terbinafine USAN, INN, BAN *systemic allylamine antifungal* [also: terbinafine HCl]

terbinafine HCl JAN *allylamine antifungal* [also: terbinafine] 250 mg oral

terbium *element (Tb)*

terbogrel USAN *platelet aggregation inhibitor*

terbucromil INN

terbufibrol INN

terbuficin INN

terbuprol INN

terbutaline INN, BAN *sympathomimetic bronchodilator* [also: terbutaline sulfate]

terbutaline sulfate USAN, USP *sympathomimetic bronchodilator* [also: terbutaline] 2.5, 5 mg oral

terciprazine INN

terconazole USAN, INN, BAN *topical antifungal* 0.4%, 0.8% vaginal

terfenadine USAN, USP, INN, JAN *piperidine antihistamine*

terflavoxate INN

terfluranol INN

terguride INN *investigational dopamine agonist for central nervous system disorders*

teriparatide USAN, INN *human parathyroid hormone, recombinant; osteoporosis treatment that stimulates new bone formation; diagnostic aid for parathyroid-induced hypocalcemia*

teriparatide acetate USAN, JAN *diagnostic aid for parathyroid-induced hypocalcemia (orphan)*

terizidone INN

terlakiren USAN *antihypertensive; renin inhibitor*

terlipressin INN, BAN *investigational (orphan) for bleeding esophageal varices*

ternidazole INN

terodiline INN, BAN, JAN *coronary vasodilator* [also: terodiline HCl]

terodiline HCl USAN *coronary vasodilator; investigational agent for urinary incontinence* [also: terodiline]

terofenamate INN

teroxalene INN *antischistosomal* [also: teroxalene HCl]

teroxalene HCl USAN *antischistosomal* [also: teroxalene]

teroxirone USAN, INN *antineoplastic*

terpin hydrate USP *(disapproved for use as an expectorant in 1991)*

terpinol [see: terpin hydrate]

terrafungine [see: oxytetracycline]

Terramycin capsules (discontinued 2003) ℞ *broad-spectrum tetracycline antibiotic* [oxytetracycline HCl] 250 mg ⃝ Garamycin; Theramycin

Terramycin IM or IV injection ℞ *broad-spectrum tetracycline antibiotic* [oxytetracycline; lidocaine] 100 mg•2%, 250 mg•2% per 2 mL dose

Terramycin with Polymyxin B ophthalmic ointment ℞ *ophthalmic antibiotic* [oxytetracycline HCl; polymyxin B sulfate] 5 mg•10 000 U per g

Terrell liquid for vaporization ℞ *inhalation general anesthetic* [isoflurane]

Tersaseptic shampoo/cleanser OTC *soap-free therapeutic cleanser*

tertatolol INN, BAN

tertiary amyl alcohol [see: amylene hydrate]

tert-pentyl alcohol [see: amylene hydrate]

tesaglitazar *investigational (Phase III) peroxisome proliferator–activated receptor (PPAR) agonist for type 2 diabetes*

Tesamone IM injection (discontinued 2001) ℞ *androgen replacement for delayed puberty or breast cancer* [testosterone] 100 mg/mL

tesicam USAN, INN *anti-inflammatory*

tesimide USAN, INN *anti-inflammatory*

Teslac tablets ℞ *adjunctive hormonal chemotherapy for advanced postmenopausal breast carcinoma* [testolactone] 50 mg

Teslascan IV injection ℞ *MRI contrast medium for liver imaging* [mangofodipir trisodium] 37.9 mg/mL (50 μmol/mL)

tesmilifene HCl USAN *antihistamine; chemopotentiator for adjunctive treatment of malignant tumors*

TESPA (triethylenethiophosphoramide) [see: thiotepa]

Tessalon Perles (capsules) ℞ *antitussive* [benzonatate] 100, 200 mg

Test Pack kit for professional use *in vitro diagnostic aid for Group A streptococcal antigens in throat swabs* [enzyme immunoassay]

Testandro IM injection (discontinued 2001) ℞ *androgen replacement for delayed puberty or breast cancer* [testosterone] 100 mg/mL

Testim gel ℞ *hormone replacement therapy for male hypogonadism* [testosterone; alcohol 74%] 1% (50 mg/pkt.)

Testoderm; Testoderm with Adhesive transdermal patch (for scrotal area) (discontinued 2005) ℞ *hormone replacement therapy for male hypogonadism* [testosterone] 4, 6 mg/day (10, 15 mg total)

Testoderm TTS transdermal patch (for nonscrotal skin) (discontinued 2003) ℞ *hormone replacement therapy for hypogonadism* [testosterone] 5 mg/day

testolactone USAN, USP, INN *antineoplastic; androgen hormone* ⊡ testosterone

Testopel pellets for subcu implantation ℞ *hormone replacement therapy for hypogonadism* [testosterone] 75 mg

testosterone USP, INN, BAN *androgen for hypogonadism and testosterone deficiency in men; investigational (Phase II, orphan) for AIDS-wasting syndrome and delay of growth and puberty in boys* ⊡ testolactone

Testosterone Aqueous IM injection ℞ *androgen for hypogonadism, delayed puberty, and androgen-responsive metastatic cancers* [testosterone] 25, 50, 100 mg/mL

testosterone cyclopentanepropionate [see: testosterone cypionate]

testosterone cyclopentylpropionate [see: testosterone cypionate]

testosterone cypionate USP *parenteral androgen; sometimes abused as a street drug* 100, 200 mg/mL injection

testosterone enanthate USP *parenteral androgen for testosterone deficiency in men, delayed puberty in boys, and metastatic breast cancer in women; sometimes abused as a street drug*

testosterone heptanoate [see: testosterone enanthate]

testosterone ketolaurate USAN, INN *androgen*

testosterone 3-oxododecanoate [see: testosterone ketolaurate]

testosterone phenylacetate USAN *androgen*

testosterone propionate USP *parenteral androgen; investigational (orphan) for vulvar dystrophies* 100 mg/mL injection

TestPack [see: Abbott TestPack]

Testred capsules ℞ *androgen for hypogonadism or testosterone deficiency in men, delayed puberty in boys, and metastatic breast cancer in women; also abused as a street drug* [methyltestosterone] 10 mg

tetanus antitoxin USP *passive immunizing agent*

tetanus & gas gangrene antitoxins NF

tetanus & gas gangrene polyvalent antitoxin [see: tetanus & gas gangrene antitoxins]

tetanus immune globulin (TIG) USP *passive immunizing agent*

tetanus immune human globulin [now: tetanus immune globulin]

tetanus toxoid USP *active immunizing agent*

tetanus toxoid, adsorbed USP *active immunizing agent*

tetanus toxoid & diphtheria toxoid & acellular pertussis (TDaP; Tdap) vaccine *active immunizing* *agent for tetanus, diphtheria, and pertussis; vaccine booster for adolescents (10–18 years)*

tetiothalein sodium [see: iodophthalein sodium]

tetnicoran [see: nicofurate]

tetrabarbital INN

tetrabenazine INN, BAN *investigational (NDA filed, orphan) selective dopamine depletor for Huntington disease and severe tardive dyskinesia*

TetraBriks (trademarked delivery form) *ready-to-use liquid containers*

tetracaine USP, INN *topical local anesthetic* [also: amethocaine]

tetracaine HCl USP, JAN *topical local anesthetic; injectable local anesthetic for spinal anesthesia* [also: amethocaine HCl]

Tetracap capsules (discontinued 2003) ℞ *broad-spectrum antibiotic* [tetracycline HCl] 250 mg

tetrachlorodecaoxide *investigational (Phase III) immunomodulator and growth factor for HIV and AIDS*

tetrachloroethylene USP

tetrachloromethane [see: carbon tetrachloride]

tetracosactide INN *adrenocorticotropic hormone* [also: cosyntropin; tetracosactrin]

tetracosactrin BAN *adrenocorticotropic hormone* [also: cosyntropin; tetracosactide]

tetracyclics *a class of antidepressants which enhance noradrenergic and serotonergic activity by blocking norepinephrine or serotonin uptake*

tetracycline USP, INN, BAN *bacteriostatic antibiotic; antirickettsial*

tetracycline HCl USP *bacteriostatic antibiotic; antirickettsial* 250, 500 mg oral

tetracycline phosphate complex USP, BAN *antibacterial*

tetracyclines *a class of bacteriostatic, antimicrobial antibiotics*

tetradecanoic acid, methylethyl ester [see: isopropyl myristate]

tetradonium bromide INN

tetraethylammonium bromide (TEAB) [see: tetrylammonium bromide]

tetraethylammonium chloride (TEAC)

tetraethylthiuram disulfide [see: disulfiram]

tetrafilcon A USAN *hydrophilic contact lens material*

Tetra-Formula lozenges OTC *antitussive; topical oral anesthetic* [dextromethorphan hydrobromide; benzocaine] 10•15 mg

tetraglycine hydroperiodide *source of iodine for disinfecting water*

tetrahydroacridinamine (THA) [see: tacrine HCl]

tetrahydroaminoacridine (THA) [see: tacrine HCl]

tetrahydrocannabinol (THC) [see: dronabinol]

tetrahydrolipstatin [see: orlistat]

tetrahydrozoline BAN *vasoconstrictor; nasal decongestant; topical ophthalmic decongestant* [also: tetrhydrozoline HCl; tetryzoline]

tetrahydrozoline HCl USP *vasoconstrictor; nasal decongestant; topical ophthalmic decongestant* [also: tetryzoline; tetrahydrozoline] 0.05% eye drops

tetraiodophenolphthalein sodium [see: iodophthalein sodium]

tetrallobarbital [see: butalbital]

tetramal [see: tetrabarbital]

tetrameprozine [see: aminopromazine]

tetramethrin INN

tetramethylene dimethanesulfonate [see: busulfan]

tetramisole INN *anthelmintic* [also: tetramisole HCl]

tetramisole HCl USAN *anthelmintic* [also: tetramisole]

Tetramune IM injection (discontinued 2001) ℞ *pediatric vaccine for diphtheria, pertussis, tetanus and Haemophilus influenzae type b* [diphtheria & tetanus toxoids & whole-cell pertussis (DTwP) vaccine; Hemophilus b conjugate vaccine] 0.5 mL

tetranitrol [see: erythrityl tetranitrate]

tetrantoin

TetraPaks (trademarked delivery form) *ready-to-use open system containers*

Tetrasine; Tetrasine Extra eye drops OTC *topical ophthalmic decongestant and vasoconstrictor* [tetrahydrozoline HCl] 0.05%

tetrasodium ethylenediaminetetraacetate [see: edetate sodium]

tetrasodium pyrophosphate [see: sodium pyrophosphate]

tetrazepam INN

tetrazolast INN *antiallergic; antiasthmatic* [also: tetrazolast meglumine]

tetrazolast meglumine USAN *antiallergic; antiasthmatic* [also: tetrazolast]

tetridamine INN *analgesic; anti-inflammatory* [also: tetrydamine]

tetriprofen INN

tetrofosmin USAN, INN, BAN *diagnostic aid*

tetronasin INN, BAN *veterinary growth promoter* [also: tetronasin sodium; tetronasin 5930]

tetronasin 5930 INN *veterinary growth promoter* [also: tetronasin sodium; tetronasin]

tetronasin sodium USAN *veterinary growth promoter* [also: tetronasin; tetronasin 5930]

tetroquinone USAN, INN *systemic keratolytic*

tetroxoprim USAN, INN *antibacterial*

tetrydamine USAN *analgesic; anti-inflammatory* [also: tetridamine]

tetrylammonium bromide INN

tetryzoline INN *vasoconstrictor; nasal decongestant; topical ocular decongestant* [also: tetrahydrozoline HCl; tetrahydrozoline]

tetryzoline HCl [see: tetrahydrozoline HCl]

tetterwort *medicinal herb* [see: bloodroot; celandine]

Teveten film-coated caplets *antihypertensive; angiotensin II receptor antagonist* [eprosartan mesylate] 600 mg

Teveten HCT film-coated caplets ℞ *antihypertensive; angiotensin II receptor antagonist; diuretic* [eprosartan mesylate; hydrochlorothiazide] 600•12.5, 600•25 mg

Tev-Tropin powder for subcu injection ℞ *growth hormone for adults or children with congenital or endogenous growth hormone deficiency, children with Turner syndrome or renal-induced growth failure* [somatropin] 5 mg (15 IU) per vial

Texacort solution ℞ *topical corticosteroidal anti-inflammatory* [hydrocortisone] 1%

texacromil INN

tezacitabine USAN *antineoplastic for colon and rectal cancers*

tezosentan *investigational (Phase III) parenteral vasoconstrictor and endothelin receptor antagonist for acute heart failure, pulmonary edema, and hepatorenal syndrome*

6-TG (6-thioguanine) [see: thioguanine]

TG (thyroglobulin) [q.v.]

T-Gen suppositories, pediatric suppositories ℞ *anticholinergic; post-surgical antiemetic* [trimethobenzamide HCl; benzocaine] 200 mg•2%; 100 mg•2%

T-Gesic capsules ℞ *narcotic analgesic* [hydrocodone bitartrate; acetaminophen] 5•500 mg

αTGI (α-triglycidyl isocyanurate) [see: teroxirone]

TH (theophylline) [q.v.]

TH (thyroid hormone) [see: levothyroxine sodium]

THA (tetrahydroaminoacridine or tetrahydroacridinamine) [see: tacrine HCl]

thalidomide USAN, INN, BAN *immunomodulator for erythema nodosum leprosum (ENL) (orphan) and multiple myeloma; investigational (Phase III, orphan) for graft vs. host disease, AIDS-wasting syndrome, lupus, and mycobacterial infections; investigational (Phase II/III, orphan) for various cancers; investigational (Phase III) for aphthous ulcers*

Thalitone tablets ℞ *antihypertensive; diuretic* [chlorthalidone] 15, 25 mg

thallium *element (Tl)* ⊡ Valium

thallous chloride Tl 201 USAN, USP *radiopaque contrast medium; radioactive agent*

Thalomid capsules ℞ *immunomodulator for erythema nodosum leprosum (ENL; orphan) and multiple myeloma; investigational (Phase III, orphan) for graft vs. host disease, AIDS-wasting syndrome, lupus, and mycobacterial infections; investigational (Phase II/III, orphan) for various cancers; investigational (Phase III) for aphthous ulcers* [thalidomide] 50, 100, 200 mg

Tham IV infusion ℞ *systemic alkalizer; corrects acidosis associated with cardiac bypass surgery or cardiac arrest* [tromethamine] 18 g/500 mL (150 mEq/ 500 mL)

thaumatin BAN

THC (tetrahydrocannabinol) [see: dronabinol]

THC (thiocarbanidin)

theanine (L-theanine) *natural extract of green tea that produces calming and relaxing effects without drowsiness; effective in controlling PMS symptoms; increases brain levels of the neurotransmitters GABA and dopamine, which increase alpha brain wave activity*

thebacon INN, BAN

theine [see: caffeine]

Thelin ℞ *investigational (Phase III) antihypertensive for pulmonary arterial hypertension (PAH)* [sitaxsentan]

thenalidine INN

thenium closilate INN *veterinary anthelmintic* [also: thenium closylate]

thenium closylate USAN *veterinary anthelmintic* [also: thenium closilate]

thenyldiamine INN

thenylpyramine HCl [see: methapyrilene HCl]

Theo-24 timed-release capsules ℞ *antiasthmatic; bronchodilator* [theophylline] 100, 200, 300 mg

Theobid Duracaps (sustained-release capsules) (discontinued 2004) ℞ *antiasthmatic; bronchodilator* [theophylline] 260 mg

theobromine NF

theobromine calcium salicylate NF

theobromine sodium acetate NF

theobromine sodium salicylate NF

Theobromo cacao medicinal herb [see: cocoa]

Theochron extended-release tablets ℞ *antiasthmatic; bronchodilator* [theophylline] 100, 200, 300, 450 mg

theoclate BAN *combining name for radicals or groups* [also: teoclate]

Theoclear L.A. extended-release capsules (discontinued 2004) ℞ *antiasthmatic; bronchodilator* [theophylline] 130, 260 mg

Theoclear-80 oral solution (discontinued 2004) ℞ *antiasthmatic; bronchodilator* [theophylline] 80 mg/15 mL ⊡ Theolair

theodrenaline INN, BAN

Theodrine tablets OTC *antiasthmatic; bronchodilator; decongestant* [theophylline; ephedrine HCl] 120•22.5 mg

Theo-Dur extended-release tablets (discontinued 2003) ℞ *antiasthmatic; bronchodilator* [theophylline] 100, 200, 300, 450 mg

theofibrate USAN *antihyperlipoproteinemic* [also: etofylline clofibrate]

Theolair oral liquid (discontinued 2004) ℞ *antiasthmatic; bronchodilator* [theophylline] 80 mg/15 mL

Theolair tablets ℞ *antiasthmatic; bronchodilator* [theophylline] 125 mg ⊡ Theoclear; Thyrolar

Theolair-SR sustained-release tablets ℞ *antiasthmatic; bronchodilator* [theophylline] 200, 250, 300, 500 mg

Theolate oral liquid ℞ *antiasthmatic; bronchodilator; expectorant* [theophylline; guaifenesin] 150•90 mg/15 mL

Theomax DF pediatric syrup ℞ *antiasthmatic; bronchodilator; decongestant; antihistamine* [theophylline; ephedrine sulfate; hydroxyzine HCl; alcohol 5%] 97.5•18.75•7.5 mg/15 mL

theophyldine [see: aminophylline]

theophyllamine [see: aminophylline]

Theophyllin KI elixir ℞ *antiasthmatic; bronchodilator; expectorant* [theophylline; potassium iodide] 80•130 mg/15 mL

theophylline (TH) USP, BAN *bronchodilator* 100, 125, 200, 300, 400, 450, 600 mg oral

theophylline aminoisobutanol [see: ambuphylline]

theophylline calcium salicylate *bronchodilator*

theophylline ethylenediamine [now: aminophylline]

theophylline monohydrate [see: theophylline]

theophylline olamine USP

theophylline sodium acetate NF

theophylline sodium glycinate USP *smooth muscle relaxant*

Theo-Sav controlled-release tablets (discontinued 2004) R *antiasthmatic; bronchodilator* [theophylline] 100, 200, 300 mg

Theospan-SR timed-release capsules (discontinued 2003) R *antiasthmatic; bronchodilator* [theophylline] 130, 260 mg

Theostat 80 syrup (discontinued 2003) R *antiasthmatic; bronchodilator* [theophylline; alcohol 1%] 80 mg/15 mL

Theovent timed-release capsules (discontinued 2004) R *antiasthmatic; bronchodilator* [theophylline] 125, 250 mg

Theo-X controlled-release tablets (discontinued 2004) R *antiasthmatic; bronchodilator* [theophylline] 100, 200, 300 mg

Thera Hematinic tablets OTC *hematinic; vitamin supplement* [ferrous fumarate; multiple vitamins; folic acid] 66.7•≛•0.33 mg

Thera Multi-Vitamin oral liquid OTC *vitamin supplement* [multiple vitamins]

Therabid tablets OTC *vitamin supplement* [multiple vitamins]

Therac lotion (discontinued 2004) OTC *acne treatment* [colloidal sulfur] 10%

theraccines *a class of vaccines with therapeutic action, usually used to help prevent the spread of cancer*

TheraCys powder for intravesical instillation R *antineoplastic for urinary bladder cancer* [BCG vaccine, live] 81 mg (1.8–19.2 × 10^8 CFU)

TheraFlu Cold & Cough Night Time; TheraFlu Flu, Cold & Cough powder for oral solution OTC *antitussive; decongestant; antihistamine; analgesic* [dextromethorphan hydrobromide; pseudoephedrine HCl; chlorpheniramine maleate; acetaminophen] 20•60•4•650 mg/pkt. ⃟ Thera-Flur

TheraFlu Flu, Cold & Cough; TheraFlu Flu & Chest Congestion Non-Drowsy powder for oral solution OTC *antitussive; decongestant; expectorant; analgesic* [dextromethorphan hydrobromide; pseudoephedrine HCl; guaifenesin; acetaminophen] 30•60•400•1000 mg/pkt

TheraFlu Flu, Cold & Cough Night Time; TheraFlu Flu, Cold & Cough, and Sore Throat; TheraFlu Flu & Cough Night Time; TheraFlu Severe Cold & Congestion powder for oral solution OTC *antitussive; decongestant; antihistamine; analgesic* [dextromethorphan hydrobromide; pseudoephedrine HCl; chlorpheniramine maleate; acetaminophen] 20•60•4•1000 mg/pkt. ⃟ Thera-Flur

TheraFlu Flu & Cold Medicine for Sore Throat; TheraFlu Flu & Sore Throat; TheraFlu Flu & Sore Throat Night Time powder for oral solution OTC *decongestant; antihistamine; analgesic* [pseudoephedrine HCl; chlorpheniramine maleate; acetaminophen] 60•4•1000 mg/pkt.

TheraFlu Flu & Cold Medicine Original Formula powder for oral solution OTC *decongestant; antihistamine; analgesic* [pseudoephedrine HCl; chlorpheniramine maleate; acetaminophen] 60•4•650 mg/pkt.

TheraFlu Flu & Congestion Non-Drowsy powder for oral solution (name changed to **Theraflu Flu &**

Chest Congestion Non-Drowsy in 2005)

TheraFlu NightTime Formula Flu, Cold, & Cough Medicine caplets OTC *antitussive; decongestant; antihistamine; analgesic* [dextromethorphan hydrobromide; pseudoephedrine HCl; chlorpheniramine maleate; acetaminophen] 15•30•2•500 mg

TheraFlu Non-Drowsy Flu, Cold & Cough; TheraFlu Severe Cold & Congestion Non-Drowsy powder for oral solution OTC *antitussive; decongestant; analgesic* [dextromethorphan hydrobromide; pseudoephedrine HCl; acetaminophen] 30•60•100 mg/pkt.

TheraFlu Non-Drowsy Formula caplets OTC *antitussive; decongestant; analgesic* [dextromethorphan hydrobromide; pseudoephedrine HCl; acetaminophen] 15•30•500 mg

Theraflu Thin Strips Long Acting Cough orally disintegrating film OTC *antitussive* [dextromethorphan hydrobromide] 15 mg

Theraflu Thin Strips Multi Symptom orally disintegrating film OTC *antitussive; antihistamine; sleep aid* [diphenhydramine HCl] 25 mg

TheraFlu Vapor Stick OTC *topical counterirritant* [camphor; menthol] 4.8%•2.6%

Thera-Flur; Thera-Flur-N gel (for self-application) ℞ *topical dental caries preventative* [sodium fluoride] 1.1% ⊡ TheraFlu

Thera-Gesic cream OTC *analgesic; counterirritant* [methyl salicylate; menthol] 15%• ±

Theragran caplets OTC *vitamin supplement* [multiple vitamins; folic acid; biotin] ± •400•30 μg ⊡ Theragyn

Theragran oral liquid OTC *vitamin supplement* [multiple vitamins] ⊡ Phenergan

Theragran AntiOxidant softgels OTC *vitamin/mineral supplement* [vitamins A, C, and E; multiple minerals] 5000 IU•250 mg•200 IU• ±

Theragran Hematinic tablets (discontinued 2003) ℞ *hematinic; vitamin/mineral supplement* [ferrous fumarate; multiple vitamins & minerals; folic acid] 66.7• ± •0.33 mg

Theragran Stress Formula tablets OTC *vitamin/iron supplement* [multiple B vitamins; vitamins C and E; ferrous fumarate; folic acid; biotin] ± •600 mg•30 IU•27 mg•0.4 mg•45 μg

Theragran-M caplets (discontinued 2005) OTC *vitamin/mineral/calcium/iron supplement* [multiple vitamins & minerals; calcium; iron; folic acid; biotin] ± •40•27•0.4•0.03 mg

Thera-Hist Cold & Allergy pediatric syrup OTC *decongestant; antihistamine* [pseudoephedrine HCl; chlorpheniramine maleate] 30•2 mg/10 mL

Thera-Hist Cold & Cough pediatric syrup OTC *antitussive; decongestant; antihistamine* [dextromethorphan hydrobromide; pseudoephedrine HCl; chlorpheniramine maleate] 10•30•2 mg/10 mL

Thera-Hist Expectorant Chest Congestion pediatric oral liquid OTC *decongestant; expectorant* [pseudoephedrine HCl; guaifenesin] 15•50 mg/5 mL

Thera-Ject (trademarked delivery system) *prefilled disposable syringe*

Thera-M tablets OTC *vitamin/mineral/iron supplement* [multiple vitamins & minerals; iron; folic acid; biotin] ± •27 mg•0.4 mg•35 μg

Theramycin Z topical solution (discontinued 2003) ℞ *antibiotic for acne* [erythromycin] 2% ⊡ Garamycin; Terramycin

TheraPatch patch OTC *analgesic; counterirritant* [methyl salicylate; menthol; camphor]

TheraPatch Cold Sore patch OTC *topical local anesthetic and antipruritic* [lidocaine; camphor; aloe vera; eucalyptus oil] 4%•0.5%• ± • ±

TheraPatch Vapor Patch for Kids OTC *counterirritant; cough suppressant* [camphor; menthol] 4.7%•2.6%

Therapeutic tablets OTC *vitamin supplement* [multiple vitamins; folic acid; biotin] ± •400•30 μg

Therapeutic B with C capsules OTC *vitamin supplement* [multiple B vitamins; vitamin C] ± •300 mg

Therapeutic Bath lotion, oil OTC *moisturizer; emollient*

Therapeutic Mineral Ice; Therapeutic Mineral Ice Exercise Formula gel OTC *topical analgesic; counterirritant* [menthol] 2%; 4%

Therapeutic-H tablets OTC *hematinic; vitamin supplement* [ferrous fumarate; multiple vitamins; folic acid] 66.7• ± •0.33 mg

Therapeutic-M tablets OTC *vitamin/mineral/iron supplement* [multiple vitamins & minerals; iron; folic acid; biotin] ± •27 mg•0.4 mg•30 μg

Theraplex T shampoo (discontinued 2003) OTC *antiseborrheic; antipsoriatic; antipruritic; antibacterial* [coal tar] 1%

Theraplex Z shampoo (discontinued 2003) OTC *antiseborrheic; antibacterial; antifungal* [pyrithione zinc] 2%

TheraTears ophthalmic gel OTC *ocular moisturizer/lubricant* [carboxymethylcellulose sodium] 1%

Theravee tablets OTC *vitamin supplement* [multiple vitamins; folic acid; biotin] ± •400•15 μg

Theravee Hematinic tablets OTC *hematinic; vitamin supplement* [ferrous fumarate; multiple vitamins; folic acid] 66.7• ± •0.33 mg

Theravee-M tablets OTC *vitamin/mineral/iron supplement* [multiple vitamins & minerals; iron; folic acid; biotin] ± •27 mg•0.4 mg•15 μg

Theravim tablets OTC *vitamin supplement* [multiple vitamins; folic acid; biotin] ± •400•35 μg

Theravim-M tablets OTC *vitamin/mineral/iron supplement* [multiple vitamins & minerals; iron; folic acid; biotin] ± •27 mg•0.4 mg•30 μg

Theravite oral liquid OTC *vitamin supplement* [multiple vitamins] 𝔇 Theravac

Therems tablets OTC *vitamin supplement* [multiple vitamins; folic acid; biotin] ± •400•15 μg

Therems-M tablets OTC *vitamin/mineral/iron supplement* [multiple vitamins & minerals; iron; folic acid; biotin] ± •27 mg•0.4 mg•30 μg

Therevac-Plus disposable enema OTC *hyperosmotic laxative; stool softener; local anesthetic* [glycerin; docusate sodium; benzocaine] 275•283•20 mg 𝔇 Theravite

Therevac-SB disposable enema OTC *hyperosmotic laxative; stool softener* [glycerin; docusate sodium] 275•283 mg

Thermazene cream ℞ *broad-spectrum bactericidal for adjunctive burn treatment* [silver sulfadiazine] 10 mg/g

ThexForte caplets OTC *vitamin supplement* [multiple B vitamins; vitamin C] ± •500 mg

THF (thymic humoral factor) [q.v.]

thiabendazole (TBZ) USAN, USP *anthelmintic for strongyloidiasis (threadworm), larva migrans, and trichinosis* [also: tiabendazole]

thiabutazide [see: buthiazide]

thiacetarsamide sodium INN

thiacetazone BAN [also: thioacetazone]

thialbarbital INN [also: thialbarbitone]

thialbarbitone BAN [also: thialbarbital]

thialisobumal sodium [see: buthalital sodium]

thiamazole INN *thyroid inhibitor* [also: methimazole]

thiambutosine INN, BAN

Thiamilate enteric-coated tablets OTC *vitamin B_1 supplement* [thiamine HCl] 20 mg

thiamine (vitamin B_1) INN *water-soluble vitamin; enzyme cofactor* [also: thiamine HCl]

thiamine HCl (vitamin B_1) USP *water-soluble vitamin; enzyme cofactor* [also: thiamine] 50, 100, 250 mg oral; 100 mg/mL injection

thiamine mononitrate USP *vitamin B_1; enzyme cofactor*

thiamine propyl disulfide [see: prosultiamine]

thiaminogen *medicinal herb* [see: rice bran oil]

thiamiprine USAN *antineoplastic* [also: tiamiprine]

thiamphenicol USAN, INN, BAN *antibacterial*

thiamylal USP *barbiturate general anesthetic*

thiamylal sodium USP, JAN *barbiturate general anesthetic*

thiazesim HCl USAN *antidepressant* [also: tiazesim]

thiazides *a class of diuretic agents that increase urinary excretion of sodium and chloride in approximately equal amounts*

thiazinamium chloride USAN *antiallergic*

thiazinamium metilsulfate INN

4-thiazolidinecarboxylic acid [see: timonacic]

thiazolidinediones *a class of antidiabetic agents that increase insulin sensitivity and reduce plasma insulin levels*

thiazolidinediones (TZDs) *a class of antidiabetic agents that increase cellular response to insulin without increasing insulin secretion*

thiazolsulfone [see: thiazosulfone]

thiazosulfone INN

thiazothielite [see: antienite]

thiazothienol [see: antazonite]

thienamycins *a class of antibiotics*

thienobenzodiazepines *a class of novel (atypical) antipsychotic agents*

thiethylperazine USAN, INN *antiemetic; antidopaminergic*

thiethylperazine malate USP *antiemetic; antipsychotic*

thiethylperazine maleate USAN, USP *antiemetic*

thihexinol methylbromide NF, INN

thimbleberry *medicinal herb* [see: blackberry]

thimerfonate sodium USAN *topical anti-infective* [also: sodium timerfonate]

thimerosal USP *topical anti-infective; preservative (49% mercury)* [also: thiomersal] 1:1000 topical

thioacetazone INN, DCF [also: thiacetazone]

thiocarbanidin (THC)

thiocarlide BAN [also: tiocarlide]

thiocolchicine glycoside [see: thiocolchicoside]

thiocolchicoside INN

thioctan; thioctacid; thioctic acid *natural antioxidant* [see: alpha lipoic acid]

thiocyanate sodium NF

thiodiglycol INN

thiodiphenylamine [see: phenothiazine]

thiofuradene INN

thioguanine (6-TG) USAN, USP *antimetabolite antineoplastic for acute non-lymphocytic leukemias (ANLL)* [also: tioguanine]

thiohexallymal [see: thialbarbital]

thiohexamide INN

Thiola *sugar-coated tablets* ℞ *prevention of cystine nephrolithiasis in homozygous cystinuria (orphan)* [tiopronin] 100 mg

thiomebumal sodium [see: thiopental sodium]

thiomersal INN, BAN *topical anti-infective; preservative* [also: thimerosal]

thiomesterone BAN [also: tiomesterone]

thiomicid [see: thioacetazone; thiacetazone]

thioparamizone [see: thioacetazone; thiacetazone]

thiopental sodium USP, INN, JAN *barbiturate general anesthetic; anticonvulsant* [also: thiopentone sodium] 2%, 2.5% (20, 25 mg/mL) injection

thiopentone sodium BAN *general anesthetic; anticonvulsant* [also: thiopental sodium]

thiophanate BAN

thiophosphoramide [see: thiotepa]

Thioplex *powder for IV, intracavitary, or intravesical injection* ℞ *alkylating antineoplastic for lymphomas and carcinoma of the breast, ovary, or bladder* [thiotepa] 15 mg

thiopropazate INN [also: thiopropazate HCl]

thiopropazate HCl NF [also: thiopropazate]

thioproperazine INN, BAN *phenothiazine antipsychotic* [also: thioproperazine mesylate]

thioproperazine mesylate *phenothiazine antipsychotic* [also: thioproperazine]

thioproperazine methanesulfonate [see: thioproperazine mesylate]

thioridazine USAN, USP, INN *conventional (typical) phenothiazine antipsychotic for schizophrenia; sedative*

thioridazine HCl USP *conventional (typical) phenothiazine antipsychotic for schizophrenia; sedative; also used for agitation or psychosis due to Alzheimer or other dementias* 10, 15, 25, 50, 100, 150, 200 mg oral

thiosalan USAN *disinfectant* [also: tiosalan]

Thiosulfil Forte tablets (discontinued 2001) ℞ *broad-spectrum sulfonamide bacteriostatic* [sulfamethizole] 500 mg

thiosulfuric acid, disodium salt pentahydrate [see: sodium thiosulfate]

thiotepa USP, INN, BAN, JAN *alkylating antineoplastic for lymphomas and carcinoma of the breast, ovary, or bladder* 15 mg/vial injection

thiotetrabarbital INN

thiothixene USAN, USP, BAN *conventional (typical) thioxanthene antipsychotic for schizophrenia* [also: tiotixene] 1, 2, 5, 10 mg oral

thiothixene HCl USAN, USP *conventional (typical) thioxanthene antipsychotic for schizophrenia*

thiouracil

thiourea *antioxidant*

thioxanthenes *a class of dopamine receptor antagonists with conventional (typical) antipsychotic activity*

thioxolone BAN [also: tioxolone]

thiphenamil HCl USAN *smooth muscle relaxant* [also: tifenamil]

thiphencillin potassium USAN *antibacterial* [also: tifencillin]

thiram USAN, INN *antifungal*

thistle, bitter; holy thistle; Saint Benedict thistle; spotted thistle *medicinal herb* [see: blessed thistle]

thistle, carline; ground thistle *medicinal herb* [see: carline thistle]

thonzonium bromide USAN, USP *detergent; surface-active agent* [also: tonzonium bromide]

thonzylamine HCl USAN, INN

Thorazine Spansules (capsules) (discontinued 2003) ℞ *conventional (typical) phenothiazine antipsychotic for schizophrenia and manic episodes of a bipolar disorder; antiemetic for nausea and vomiting* [chlorpromazine] 30, 75, 150 mg

Thorazine syrup, oral concentrate (discontinued 2003) ℞ *conventional (typical) phenothiazine antipsychotic for schizophrenia and manic episodes of a bipolar disorder; antiemetic for nausea and vomiting* [chlorpromazine] 10 mg/5 mL; 100 mg/mL

Thorazine tablets, IV or IM injection, suppositories ℞ *conventional antipsychotic for schizophrenia, manic episodes of a bipolar disorder, pediatric hyperactivity, and severe pediatric behavioral problems; treatment for acute intermittent porphyria, nausea/vomiting, and intractable hiccoughs* [chlorpromazine] 25, 50, 100, 200 mg; 25 mg/mL; 100 mg

thorium *element (Th)*

thorn, Egyptian *medicinal herb* [see: acacia]

thorn-apple *medicinal herb* [see: hawthorn; jimsonweed]

thousand-leaf; thousand seal *medicinal herb* [see: yarrow]

thozalinone USAN *antidepressant* [also: tozalinone]

THQ (tetrahydroxybenzoquinone) [see: tetroquinone]

THR (trishydroxyethyl rutin) [see: troxerutin]

Threamine DM syrup (discontinued 2002) OTC *antitussive; decongestant; antihistamine* [dextromethorphan hydrobromide; phenylpropanolamine HCl; chlorpheniramine maleate] 10•12.5•2 mg/5 mL

Threamine Expectorant oral liquid (discontinued 2002) OTC *deconges-*

tant; expectorant [phenylpropanol-
amine HCl; guaifenesin; alcohol
5%] 12.5•100 mg/5 mL

3 in 1 Toothache Relief topical liquid, gum, lotion/gel OTC *oral anesthetic* [benzocaine]

three-leaved nightshade *medicinal
herb* [see: birthroot]

3TC [now: lamivudine]

threonine (L-threonine) USAN, USP,
INN *essential amino acid; symbols:
Thr, T; investigational (orphan) for
familial spastic paraparesis and amyotrophic lateral sclerosis* 500 mg oral

Throat Discs lozenges OTC *analgesic;
counterirritant* [capsicum; peppermint
oil]

throatwort *medicinal herb* [see: figwort;
foxglove]

Thrombate III powder for IV infusion
℞ *for thrombosis and pulmonary emboli
of congenital AT-III deficiency (orphan)*
[antithrombin III] 500, 1000 IU

thrombin USP, INN *topical local hemostatic*

Thrombinar powder ℞ *topical local
hemostatic for surgery* [thrombin]
1000, 5000, 50 000 U

Thrombin-JMI powder (discontinued
2004) ℞ *topical hemostatic for surgery*
[thrombin] 10 000, 20 000, 50 000 U

thrombinogen (prothrombin)

Thrombogen powder ℞ *topical local
hemostatic for surgery* [thrombin]
1000, 5000, 10 000, 20 000 U

thrombolytics *a class of enzymes that
dissolve blood clots, used emergently to
treat stroke, pulmonary embolus, and
myocardial infarct*

thromboplastin USP

**thrombopoietin, recombinant
human** *investigational (orphan)
adjunct to hematopoietic stem cell
transplantation*

Thrombostat powder ℞ *topical local
hemostatic for surgery* [thrombin]
5000, 10 000, 20 000 U

throw-wort *medicinal herb* [see: moth-
erwort]

thulium *element (Tm)*

**thunder god vine *(Tripterygium wil-
fordii)*** plant *medicinal herb for abscesses, autoimmune diseases, boils, fever,
inflammation, tumors, and viruses;
also used as an insecticide to kill maggots or larvae and as a rat and bird poison* [also: triptolide]

thymalfasin USAN *vaccine enhancer for
hepatitis C, cancer, and infectious diseases; investigational (Phase III, orphan)
for chronic active hepatitis B; investigational (orphan) for DiGeorge syndrome
with immune defects; investigational
(orphan) for hepatocellular carcinoma*

**thyme *(Thymus serpyllum; T. vul-
garis)*** plant *medicinal herb for acute
bronchitis, colic, digestive disorders, gas,
gout, headache, laryngitis, lung congestion, sciatica, and throat disorders*

**thymic tissue for transplantation,
cultured, partially T-cell depleted**
*investigational (orphan) agent for pri-
mary immune deficiency due to athymia
associated with complete DiGeorge syndrome*

thymidylate synthase (TS) inhibitors
a class of folate-based antineoplastics

Thymitaq ℞ *thymidylate synthase
inhibitor that disrupts DNA replication;
investigational (Phase III) for inoperable primary liver cancer* [nolatrexed
dihydrochloride]

thymocartin INN

thymoctonan INN *investigational antiviral for HIV infection, genital herpes,
and chronic viral hepatitis*

Thymoglobulin powder for IV infusion ℞ *passive immunizing agent to
prevent allograft rejection of renal
transplants (orphan); investigational
(orphan) for myelodysplastic syndrome
(MDS)* [antithymocyte globulin,
rabbit] 25 mg

thymol NF *stabilizer; topical antiseptic*

thymol iodide NF

thymopentin USAN, INN, BAN *immunoregulator; investigational (Phase III)
for asymptomatic HIV infection*

thymopoietin 32-36 [now: thymo-
pentin]

thymosin alpha-1 [now: thymalfasin]

thymostimulin INN *investigational (Phase III) immunomodulator for AIDS*

thymotrinan INN

thymoxamine BAN [also: moxisylyte]

Thymus serpyllum; T. vulgaris medicinal herb [see: thyme]

Thypinone IV injection (discontinued 2003) ℞ *diagnostic aid for thyroid function* [protirelin] 500 μg/mL

Thyrel TRH IV injection (discontinued 2003) ℞ *diagnostic aid for thyroid function* [protirelin] 500 μg/mL

Thyro-Block tablets ℞ *thyroid-blocking therapy* [potassium iodide] 130 mg

thyrocalcitonin [see: calcitonin]

Thyrogen injection ℞ *recombinant human thyroid-stimulating hormone (rhTSH); diagnostic aid for thyroid cancer (orphan); investigational (NDA filed, orphan) treatment for thyroid cancer* [thyrotropin alfa] 1.1 mg

thyroglobulin (TG) USAN, USP, INN *thyroid hormone*

thyroid USP *natural thyroid hormone (a 4:1 mixture of T_4 and T_3)* 32.5, 65, 130, 195 mg oral

thyroid hormone (TH) [see: levothyroxine sodium]

thyroid-stimulating hormone (TSH) [see: thyrotropin]

Thyrolar tablets ℞ *synthetic thyroid hormone (a 4:1 mixture of T_4 and T_3)* [liotrix] 15, 30, 60, 120, 180 mg ⑨ Theolair; Thyrar

thyromedan HCl USAN *thyromimetic* [also: tyromedan]

thyropropic acid INN

Thyro-Tabs tablets ℞ *synthetic thyroid hormone (T_4 fraction only)* [levothyroxine sodium] 25, 50, 75, 88, 100, 112, 125, 150, 175, 200, 300 μg

thyrotrophic hormone [see: thyrotrophin]

thyrotrophin INN *thyroid-stimulating hormone* [also: thyrotropin]

thyrotropin *thyroid-stimulating hormone; in vivo diagnostic aid for thyroid function* [also: thyrotrophin]

thyrotropin alfa USAN *recombinant human thyroid-stimulating hormone (rhTSH); diagnostic aid for thyroid cancer (orphan); investigational (NDA filed, orphan) treatment for thyroid cancer*

thyrotropin-releasing hormone (TRH) [see: protirelin]

thyroxine BAN *synthetic thyroid hormone (T_4 fraction only)* [also: levothyroxine sodium]

D-thyroxine [see: dextrothyroxine sodium]

L-thyroxine [see: levothyroxine sodium]

thyroxine I 125 USAN *radioactive agent*

thyroxine I 131 USAN *radioactive agent*

Thytropar powder for IM or subcu injection (discontinued 2001) ℞ *thyroid-stimulating hormone (TSH); in vivo diagnostic aid for thyroid function* [thyrotropin] 10 IU

tiabendazole INN *anthelmintic* [also: thiabendazole]

tiacrilast USAN, INN *antiallergic*

tiacrilast sodium USAN *antiallergic*

tiadenol INN

tiafibrate INN

tiagabine INN *anticonvulsant adjunct for partial seizures*

tiagabine HCl USAN *anticonvulsant adjunct for partial seizures*

Tiamate extended-release film-coated tablets (discontinued 2002) ℞ *antihypertensive; antianginal; antiarrhythmic; calcium channel blocker* [diltiazem maleate] 120, 180, 240 mg

tiamenidine USAN, INN *antihypertensive*

tiamenidine HCl USAN *antihypertensive*

tiametonium iodide INN

tiamiprine INN *antineoplastic* [also: thiamiprine]

tiamizide INN *diuretic; antihypertensive* [also: diapamide]

tiamulin USAN, INN *veterinary antibacterial*

tiamulin fumarate USAN *veterinary antibacterial*

tianafac INN

tianeptine INN

tiapamil INN, BAN *antagonist to calcium* [also: tiapamil HCl]

tiapamil HCl USAN *antagonist to calcium* [also: tiapamil]

tiapirinol INN

tiapride INN

tiaprofenic acid INN *nonsteroidal anti-inflammatory drug (NSAID)*

tiaprost INN

tiaramide INN, BAN *antiasthmatic* [also: tiaramide HCl]

tiaramide HCl USAN *antiasthmatic* [also: tiaramide]

Tiazac extended-release capsules ℞ *antihypertensive; antianginal; antiarrhythmic; calcium channel blocker* [diltiazem HCl] 120, 180, 240, 300, 360, 420 mg ⚕ Dyazide; thiazides

tiazesim INN *antidepressant* [also: thiazesim HCl]

tiazesim HCl [see: thiazesim HCl]

tiazofurin USAN *investigational (Phase II/III, orphan) antineoplastic for chronic myelogenous leukemia* [also: tiazofurine]

tiazofurine INN *antineoplastic* [also: tiazofurin]

tiazuril USAN, INN *coccidiostat for poultry*

tibalosin INN

tibenelast sodium USAN *antiasthmatic; bronchodilator*

tibenzate INN

tibezonium iodide INN

tibolone USAN, INN, BAN *investigational (NDA filed) synthetic steroid for osteoporosis and other postmenopausal symptoms*

tibric acid USAN, INN *antihyperlipoproteinemic*

tibrofan USAN, INN *disinfectant*

ticabesone INN *corticosteroid; anti-inflammatory* [also: ticabesone propionate]

ticabesone propionate USAN *corticosteroid; anti-inflammatory* [also: ticabesone]

Ticar powder for IV or IM injection ℞ *extended-spectrum penicillin antibiotic* [ticarcillin disodium] 3 g/vial ⚕ Tigan

ticarbodine USAN, INN *anthelmintic*

ticarcillin INN *extended-spectrum penicillin antibiotic* [also: ticarcillin disodium]

ticarcillin cresyl sodium USAN *extended-spectrum penicillin antibiotic*

ticarcillin disodium USAN, USP *extended-spectrum penicillin antibiotic* [also: ticarcillin]

Tice BCG dermal puncture injection for TB, intravesical instillation for cancer ℞ *tuberculosis immunizing agent; antineoplastic for urinary bladder cancer* [BCG vaccine, Tice strain] 50 mg (1–8 × 10^8 CFU)

tickweed *medicinal herb* [see: pennyroyal]

ticlatone USAN, INN *antibacterial; antifungal*

Ticlid film-coated tablets ℞ *platelet aggregation inhibitor for stroke* [ticlopidine HCl] 250 mg

ticlopidine INN, BAN *platelet aggregation inhibitor* [also: ticlopidine HCl]

ticlopidine HCl USAN *platelet aggregation inhibitor for stroke* [also: ticlopidine] 250 mg oral

ticolubant USAN *leukotriene B$_4$ receptor antagonist for psoriasis*

Ticon IM injection (discontinued 2005) ℞ *anticholinergic; post-surgical antiemetic* [trimethobenzamide HCl] 100 mg/mL

ticrynafen USAN *diuretic; uricosuric; antihypertensive* [also: tienilic acid]

tidembersat USAN *antimigraine*

tidiacic INN

tiemonium iodide INN, BAN

tienilic acid INN *diuretic; uricosuric; antihypertensive* [also: ticrynafen]

tienocarbine INN

tienopramine INN

tienoxolol INN

tifacogin USAN *anticoagulant; lipoprotein-associated coagulation inhibitor (LACI); investigational (Phase III) recombinant tissue factor pathway inhibitor*

tifemoxone INN

tifenamil INN *smooth muscle relaxant* [also: thiphenamil HCl]

tifenamil HCl [see: thiphenamil HCl]

tifencillin INN *antibacterial* [also: thiphencillin potassium]

tifencillin potassium [see: thiphencillin potassium]

tiflamizole INN

tiflorex INN

tifluadom INN

tiflucarbine INN

Tifolar (name changed to Alimta upon marketing release in 2004)

tiformin INN [also: tyformin]

tifurac INN *analgesic* [also: tifurac sodium]

tifurac sodium USAN *analgesic* [also: tifurac]

TIG (tetanus immune globulin) [q.v.]

Tigan capsules, IM injection ℞ *anticholinergic; post-surgical antiemetic* [trimethobenzamide HCl] 300 mg; 100 mg/mL ⚕ Ticar; Triban

Tigan suppositories, pediatric suppositories ℞ *anticholinergic; post-surgical antiemetic* [trimethobenzamide HCl; benzocaine] 200 mg•2%; 100 mg•2% ⚕ Ticar; Triban

tigecycline *broad-spectrum glycylcycline antibiotic for intra-abdominal and complicated skin structure infections and methicillin-resistant* Staphylococcus aureus *(MRSA)*

tigemonam INN *antimicrobial* [also: tigemonam dicholine]

tigemonam dicholine USAN *antimicrobial* [also: tigemonam]

tigestol USAN, INN *progestin*

tigloidine INN, BAN

tiglyl*pseudo*tropine [see: tigloidine]

tiglyltropeine [see: tropigline]

Tikosyn capsules ℞ *antiarrhythmic; potassium channel blocker* [dofetilide] 125, 250, 500 μg

tilactase INN *digestive enzyme*

Tilad (Spanish name for U.S. product Tilade)

Tilade oral inhalation aerosol ℞ *respiratory anti-inflammatory; mast cell stabilizer; antiasthmatic; bronchodilator* [nedocromil sodium] 1.75 mg/dose

tilarginine acetate *investigational (Phase III) nitric oxide inhibitor for the treatment of cardiogenic shock*

tilbroquinol INN

tiletamine INN *anesthetic; anticonvulsant* [also: tiletamine HCl]

tiletamine HCl USAN *anesthetic; anticonvulsant* [also: tiletamine]

Tilia americana; T. cordata; T. europaea; T. platyphyllos *medicinal herb* [see: linden tree]

tilidate HCl BAN *analgesic* [also: tilidine HCl; tilidine]

tilidine INN *analgesic* [also: tilidine HCl; tilidate HCl]

tilidine HCl USAN *analgesic* [also: tilidine; tilidate HCl]

tiliquinol INN

tilisolol INN

tilmicosin USAN, INN, BAN *veterinary antibacterial*

tilmicosin phosphate USAN *veterinary antibacterial*

tilomisole USAN, INN *immunoregulator*

tilorone INN *antiviral* [also: tilorone HCl]

tilorone HCl USAN *antiviral* [also: tilorone]

tilozepine INN

tilsuprost INN

Tiltab (trademarked dosage form) *film-coated tablets*

tiludronate disodium USAN *bisphosphonate bone resorption inhibitor for Paget disease*

tiludronic acid INN

timcodar dimesylate USAN *antineoplastic adjunct to prevent emergence of multidrug-resistant tumors*

Timecap (trademarked dosage form) *sustained-release capsule*

Timecelle (trademarked dosage form) *timed-release capsule*

timefurone USAN, INN *antiatherosclerotic*

timegadine INN

Time-Hist sustained-release capsules ℞ *decongestant; antihistamine* [pseudoephedrine HCl; chlorpheniramine maleate] 120•8 mg

timelotem INN

Timentin powder or frozen premix for IV infusion ℞ *extended-spectrum penicillin antibiotic plus synergist* [ticarcillin

disodium; clavulanate potassium] 3•
0.1 g

timepidium bromide INN

Timespan (trademarked dosage form)
timed-release tablets

Timesules (dosage form) *sustained-release capsules*

timiperone INN

timobesone INN *topical adrenocortical steroid* [also: timobesone acetate]

timobesone acetate USAN *topical adrenocortical steroid* [also: timobesone]

timofibrate INN

Timolide 10·25 tablets ℞ *antihypertensive; β-blocker; diuretic* [timolol maleate; hydrochlorothiazide] 10•25 mg

timolol USAN, INN, BAN *topical antiglaucoma agent (β-blocker)* ⊘ atenolol

timolol hemihydrate *topical antiglaucoma agent (β-blocker)*

timolol maleate USAN, USP *antianginal; antihypertensive; antiadrenergic (β-receptor); topical antiglaucoma agent; migraine prophylaxis* 5, 10, 20 mg oral; 0.25%, 0.5% eye drops

timonacic INN

timoprazole INN

Timoptic Ocumeter (eye drops), Ocudose (single-use eye drop dispenser) ℞ *topical antiglaucoma agent (β-blocker)* [timolol maleate] 0.25%, 0.5%

Timoptic-XE gel-forming Ocumeter (eye drops) ℞ *topical once-daily antiglaucoma agent (β-blocker)* [timolol maleate] 0.25%, 0.5%

Timunox ℞ *investigational (Phase III) immunomodulator for asymptomatic HIV infection* [thymopentin]

tin *element (Sn)*

tin chloride dihydrate [see: stannous chloride]

tin ethyl etiopurpurin (SnET2) [see: rostaporfin]

tin fluoride [see: stannous fluoride]

tinabinol USAN, INN *antihypertensive*

Tinactin cream, powder, spray powder, spray liquid, topical solution OTC *antifungal* [tolnaftate] 1% ⊘ Taractan

Tinactin for Jock Itch cream, spray powder OTC *topical antifungal* [tolnaftate] 1%

tinazoline INN

TinBen tincture OTC *skin protectant* [benzoin; alcohol 75–83%]

Tincture of Green Soap topical liquid OTC *antiseptic cleanser* [green soap; alcohol 28–32%]

Tindamax film-coated tablets ℞ *antiprotozoal; amebicide; treatment for trichomoniasis* [tinidazole] 250, 500 mg

Tine Test OT [see: Tuberculin Tine Test, Old]

Tine Test PPD single-use intradermal puncture test device (discontinued 2002) *tuberculosis skin test* [tuberculin purified protein derivative] 5 U

Ting cream OTC *topical antifungal* [tolnaftate] 1%

Ting spray powder OTC *antifungal* [miconazole nitrate] 2%

tinidazole USAN, INN *antiprotozoal; amebicide; treatment for trichomoniasis*

tinisulpride INN

tinofedrine INN

tinoridine INN

Tinver lotion ℞ *antifungal; keratolytic; antipruritic; anesthetic* [sodium thiosulfate; salicylic acid; alcohol 10%] 25%•1%

tinzaparin sodium USAN, INN, BAN *a low molecular weight heparin–type anticoagulant and antithrombotic for the prevention of deep vein thrombosis (DVT)*

tiocarlide INN [also: thiocarlide]

tioclomarol INN

tioconazole USAN, USP, INN, BAN, JAN *topical antifungal*

tioctilate INN

tiodazosin USAN, INN *antihypertensive*

tiodonium chloride USAN, INN *antibacterial*

tiofacic [see: stepronin]

tioguanine INN *antineoplastic* [also: thioguanine]

tiomergine INN

tiomesterone INN [also: thiomesterone]

tioperidone INN *antipsychotic* [also: tioperidone HCl]

tioperidone HCl USAN *antipsychotic* [also: tioperidone]

tiopinac USAN, INN *anti-inflammatory; analgesic; antipyretic*

tiopronin INN *prevention of cystine nephrolithiasis in homozygous cystinuria (orphan)*

tiopropamine INN

tiosalan INN *disinfectant* [also: thiosalan]

tiosinamine [see: allylthiourea]

tiospirone INN *antipsychotic* [also: tiospirone HCl]

tiospirone HCl USAN *antipsychotic* [also: tiospirone]

tiotidine USAN, INN *antagonist to histamine H_2 receptors*

tiotixene INN *conventional (typical) thioxanthene antipsychotic for schizophrenia* [also: thiothixene]

tiotropium bromide *long-acting anticholinergic bronchodilator for chronic obstructive pulmonary disease (COPD)*

tioxacin INN

tioxamast INN

tioxaprofen INN

tioxidazole USAN, INN *anthelmintic*

tioxolone INN [also: thioxolone]

TIP (Taxol, isosfamide [with mesna rescue], Platinol) *chemotherapy protocol for head, neck, and esophageal cancers*

tipentosin INN, BAN *antihypertensive* [also: tipentosin HCl]

tipentosin HCl USAN *antihypertensive* [also: tipentosin]

tipepidine INN

tipetropium bromide INN

tipifarnib USAN *antineoplastic for advanced pancreatic, colorectal, and non–small cell lung cancers*

tipindole INN

tipranavir disodium USAN *antiviral protease inhibitor for HIV infection*

tipredane USAN, INN, BAN *topical adrenocortical steroid*

tiprenolol INN *antiadrenergic (β-receptor)* [also: tiprenolol HCl]

tiprenolol HCl USAN *antiadrenergic (β-receptor)* [also: tiprenolol]

tiprinast INN *antiallergic* [also: tiprinast meglumine]

tiprinast meglumine USAN *antiallergic* [also: tiprinast]

tipropidil INN *vasodilator* [also: tipropidil HCl]

tipropidil HCl USAN *vasodilator* [also: tipropidil]

tiprostanide INN, BAN

tiprotimod INN

tiqueside USAN, INN *antihyperlipidemic*

tiquinamide INN *gastric anticholinergic* [also: tiquinamide HCl]

tiquinamide HCl USAN *gastric anticholinergic* [also: tiquinamide]

tiquizium bromide INN

tirapazamine USAN, INN *antineoplastic; investigational (Phase III) for head, neck, and lung cancers*

tiratricol INN

tiratricol & levothyroxine sodium *investigational (orphan) to suppress thyroid-stimulating hormone (TSH) in thyroid cancer*

tirilazad INN, BAN *antioxidant; lipid peroxidation inhibitor; 21-aminosteroid (lazaroid)* [also: tirilazad mesylate]

tirilazad mesylate USAN *antioxidant; lipid peroxidation inhibitor; investigational (NDA filed) 21-aminosteroid (lazaroid) for subarachnoid hemorrhage (SAH), ischemic stroke, spinal cord and head injuries; investigational (Phase I/II) protease inhibitor for HIV infection* [also: tirilazad]

tirofiban HCl USAN *glycoprotein (GP) IIb/IIIa receptor antagonist; platelet aggregation inhibitor for acute coronary syndrome, unstable angina, myocardial infarction, and cardiac surgery*

tiropramide INN

tisilfocon A USAN *hydrophobic contact lens material*

Tisit *topical liquid, gel, shampoo* OTC *pediculicide for lice* [pyrethrins; piperonyl butoxide] 0.3%•2%; 0.3%•3%; 0.3%•4%

Tisit Blue *gel (discontinued 2003)* OTC *pediculicide for lice* [pyrethrins; piperonyl butoxide; petroleum distillate] 0.3%•3%•1.2%

tisocromide INN

TiSol solution OTC *anesthetic and anti-microbial throat irrigation* [benzyl alcohol; menthol] 1%•0.04%

tisopurine INN

tisoquone INN

tissue factor [see: thromboplastin]

tissue plasminogen activator (tPA; t-PA) [see: alteplase]

Tis-U-Sol solution ℞ *sterile irrigant* [physiological irrigating solution]

TIT (methotrexate, cytarabine, hydrocortisone) *chemotherapy protocol for CNS prophylaxis of pediatric acute lymphocytic leukemia; intrathecal (IT) administration*

Titan solution OTC *cleaning solution for hard contact lenses*

titanium *element (Ti)*

titanium dioxide USP *topical protectant; astringent*

titanium oxide [see: titanium dioxide]

Titradose (trademarked dosage form) *scored tablet*

Titralac chewable tablets OTC *antacid* [calcium carbonate] 420, 750 mg

Titralac Plus chewable tablets, oral liquid OTC *antacid; antiflatulent* [calcium carbonate; simethicone] 420•21 mg; 500•20 mg/5 mL

tivanidazole INN

tivazine [see: piperazine citrate]

tixadil INN

tixanox USAN *antiallergic* [also: tixanoxum]

tixanoxum INN *antiallergic* [also: tixanox]

tixocortol INN *topical anti-inflammatory* [also: tixocortol pivalate]

tixocortol pivalate USAN *topical anti-inflammatory* [also: tixocortol]

Tixogel VP *investigational topical skin protectant for allergic contact dermatitis* [bentoquatam]

tizabrin INN

tizanidine INN, BAN *antispasmodic; central* α_2 *agonist* [also: tizanidine HCl]

tizanidine HCl USAN, JAN *antispasmodic for multiple sclerosis and spinal cord injury (orphan); central* α_2 *agonist* [also: tizanidine] 2, 4 mg oral

tizolemide INN

tizoprolic acid INN

T-Koff oral liquid (discontinued 2002) ℞ *narcotic antitussive; decongestant; antihistamine* [codeine phosphate; phenylpropanolamine HCl; phenylephrine HCl; chlorpheniramine maleate] 10•20•20•5 mg/5 mL

^{201}Tl [see: thallous chloride Tl 201]

TLK286 *investigational (Phase III) antineoplastic for ovarian cancer*

T-lymphotrophic virus antigens [see: human T-lymphotropic virus type III (HTLV-III) gp-160 antigens]

T-MAVs (targeted monoclonal antibody vehicles) [q.v.]

TMB (trimedoxime bromide) [q.v.]

TMG (trimethylglycine) [q.v.]

TMP (trimethoprim) [q.v.]

TMP-SMZ (trimethoprim & sulfamethoxazole) [q.v.]

TNF (tumor necrosis factor) [q.v.]

TNKase powder for IV injection ℞ *thrombolytic/fibrinolytic for the treatment of acute myocardial infarction (AMI)* [tenecteplase] 50 mg/vial

TNK-tPA *a genetically engineered mutation of tissue plasminogen activator (tPA); "TNK" refers to the three specific sites of genetic modification* [see: tenecteplase]

TOAP (thioguanine, Oncovin, [cytosine] arabinoside, prednisone) *chemotherapy protocol*

tobacco *dried leaves of the* Nicotiana tabacum *plant; sedative narcotic; emetic; diuretic; heart depressant; antispasmodic* [also see: nicotine]

tobacco, British *medicinal herb* [see: coltsfoot]

tobacco, Indian; wild tobacco *medicinal herb* [see: lobelia]

tobacco, sailor's *medicinal herb* [see: mugwort]

tobacco wood *medicinal herb* [see: witch hazel]

TOBI solution for inhalation ℞ *antibiotic for* Pseudomonas aeruginosa *lung infections in cystic fibrosis patients (orphan); investigational (Phase II) for bronchiectasis and pulmonary tuberculosis* [tobramycin] 300 mg/5 mL

toborinone USAN *cardiotonic*

TobraDex eye drop suspension ℞ *topical ophthalmic corticosteroidal anti-inflammatory; antibiotic* [dexamethasone; tobramycin] 0.1%•0.3% ℞ Tobrex

TobraDex ophthalmic ointment ℞ *topical ophthalmic corticosteroidal anti-inflammatory; antibiotic* [dexamethasone; tobramycin; chlorobutanol] 0.1%•0.3%•0.5%

tobramycin USAN, USP, INN, BAN *aminoglycoside antibiotic; inhalant for* Pseudomonas aeruginosa *lung infections in cystic fibrosis patients (orphan)* 0.3% eye drops ℞ Trobicin

tobramycin sulfate USP *aminoglycoside antibiotic* 10, 40 mg/mL injection

Tobrex Drop-Tainers (eye drops), ophthalmic ointment ℞ *topical ophthalmic antibiotic* [tobramycin] 0.3%; 3 mg/g ℞ TobraDex

tobuterol INN

tocainide USAN, INN, BAN *antiarrhythmic*

tocainide HCl USP *antiarrhythmic*

tocamphyl USAN, INN *choleretic*

Tocicodendron diversilobum medicinal herb [see: poison oak]

tocladesine USAN *immunomodulator; antineoplastic*

tocofenoxate INN

tocofersolan INN *dietary vitamin E supplement* [also: tocophersolan]

tocofibrate INN

tocolytics *a class of drugs used to inhibit uterine contractions*

tocopherol, d-alpha [see: vitamin E]

tocopherol, dl-alpha [see: vitamin E]

tocopherols, mixed [see: vitamin E]

tocopherols excipient NF *antioxidant*

tocophersolan USAN *dietary vitamin E supplement* [also: tocofersolan]

tocopheryl acetate, d-alpha [see: vitamin E]

tocopheryl acetate, dl-alpha [see: vitamin E]

tocopheryl acid succinate, d-alpha [see: vitamin E]

tocopheryl acid succinate, dl-alpha [see: vitamin E]

tocopheryl polyethylene glycol succinate (TPGS) [see: tocophersolan]

Today vaginal sponge OTC *spermicidal/barrier contraceptive* [nonoxynol 9] 1 g

todralazine INN, BAN

tofenacin INN *anticholinergic* [also: tofenacin HCl]

tofenacin HCl USAN *anticholinergic* [also: tofenacin]

tofesilate INN *combining name for radicals or groups*

tofetridine INN

tofisoline

tofisopam INN

Tofranil sugar-coated tablets ℞ *tricyclic antidepressant; treatment for childhood enuresis* [imipramine HCl] 10, 25, 50 mg ℞ Tepanil

Tofranil-PM capsules ℞ *tricyclic antidepressant* [imipramine pamoate] 75, 100, 125, 150 mg

tolamolol USAN, INN *vasodilator; antiarrhythmic; antiadrenergic (β-receptor)*

tolazamide USAN, USP, INN, BAN *sulfonylurea antidiabetic* 100, 250, 500 mg oral

tolazoline INN *antiadrenergic; peripheral vasodilator for hypertension* [also: tolazoline HCl]

tolazoline HCl USP *antiadrenergic; peripheral vasodilator for neonatal persistent pulmonary hypertension* [also: tolazoline]

tolboxane INN

tolbutamide USP, INN, BAN *sulfonylurea antidiabetic* 500 mg oral

tolbutamide sodium USP *diagnostic aid for diabetes*

tolcapone USAN, INN *antiparkinsonian; catechol-O-methyltransferase (COMT) inhibitor*

tolciclate USAN, INN *antifungal*

tolclotide [see: disulfamide]

toldimfos INN, BAN

Tolectin 200; Tolectin 600 tablets ℞ *antiarthritic; nonsteroidal anti-inflammatory drug (NSAID) for ankylosing spondylitis and acute bursitis/tendinitis* [tolmetin sodium] 200 mg; 600 mg

Tolectin DS capsules ℞ *antiarthritic; nonsteroidal anti-inflammatory drug (NSAID) for ankylosing spondylitis and acute bursitis/tendinitis* [tolmetin sodium] 400 mg

Tolerex powder OTC *enteral nutritional therapy* [lactose-free formula]

tolfamide USAN, INN *urease enzyme inhibitor*

tolfenamic acid INN, BAN

Tolfrinic film-coated tablets OTC *hematinic* [ferrous fumarate; cyanocobalamin; ascorbic acid] 200 mg•25 μg•100 mg

tolgabide USAN, INN, BAN *anticonvulsant*

tolhexamide [see: glycyclamide]

tolimidone USAN, INN *antiulcerative*

Tolinase tablets ℞ *sulfonylurea antidiabetic* [tolazamide] 250 mg ⊡ Orinase

tolindate USAN, INN *antifungal*

toliodium chloride USAN, INN *veterinary food additive*

toliprolol INN

tolmesoxide INN

tolmetin USAN, INN *antiarthritic; nonsteroidal anti-inflammatory drug (NSAID) for ankylosing spondylitis and acute bursitis/tendinitis*

tolmetin sodium USAN, USP *antiarthritic; nonsteroidal anti-inflammatory drug (NSAID) for ankylosing spondylitis and acute bursitis/tendinitis* 200, 400, 600 mg oral

tolnaftate USAN, USP, INN, BAN *antifungal* 1% topical

tolnapersine INN

tolnidamine INN

toloconium metilsulfate INN

tolofocon A USAN *hydrophobic contact lens material*

tolonidine INN

tolonium chloride INN *blue dye used in histology; diagnostic aid for oral cancer*

toloxatone INN

toloxichloral [see: toloxychlorinol]

toloxychlorinol INN

tolpadol INN

tolpentamide INN, BAN

tolperisone INN, BAN

tolpiprazole INN, BAN

tolpovidone I 131 USAN *hypoalbuminemia test; radioactive agent* [also: radiotolpovidone I 131]

tolpronine INN, BAN

tolpropamine INN, BAN

tolpyrramide USAN, INN *antidiabetic*

tolquinzole INN

tolrestat USAN, INN, BAN *investigational (NDA filed) aldose reductase inhibitor for diabetic neuropathy*

tolterodine USAN *anticholinergic; muscarinic receptor antagonist for urinary frequency, urgency, and incontinence*

tolterodine tartrate USAN *anticholinergic; muscarinic receptor antagonist for urinary frequency, urgency, and incontinence*

toltrazuril USAN, INN, BAN *veterinary coccidiostat*

tolu balsam USP *pharmaceutic aid*

p-toluenesulfone dichloramine [see: dichloramine T]

tolufazepam INN

toluidine blue O [see: tolonium chloride]

toluidine blue O chloride [see: tolonium chloride]

Tolu-Sed DM oral liquid OTC *antitussive; expectorant* [dextromethorphan hydrobromide; guaifenesin; alcohol 10%] 10•100 mg/5 mL

tolycaine INN, BAN

tomelukast USAN, INN *antiasthmatic; leukotriene antagonist*

Tomocat concentrated oral suspension ℞ *radiopaque contrast medium for gastrointestinal imaging* [barium sulfate] 5%

tomoglumide INN

tomoxetine INN *antidepressant* [also: tomoxetine HCl]

tomoxetine HCl USAN *antidepressant* [also: tomoxetine]

tomoxiprole INN

Tom's of Maine Natural Cough & Cold Rub vaporizing ointment OTC *counterirritant; cough suppressant* [menthol; camphor] 4.8%•2.6%

Tomudex ℞ *antimetabolite antineoplastic; investigational (Phase III) thymidylate synthase inhibitor for colorectal cancer* [raltitrexed]

Tomycine ⓒ eye drops ℞ *topical antibiotic* [tobramycin] 0.3%

tonazocine INN *analgesic* [also: tonazocine mesylate]

tonazocine mesylate USAN *analgesic* [also: tonazocine]

tongue grass *medicinal herb* [see: chickweed]

tonics *a class of agents that restore normal tone to tissue and strengthen or invigorate organs (a term used in folk medicine)*

tonka bean *(Dipteryx odorata; D. oppositifolia)* fruit and seed *medicinal herb for cramps, nausea, and schistosomiasis*

Tonocard film-coated tablets (discontinued 2004) ℞ *antiarrhythmic* [tocainide HCl] 400, 600 mg

Tonopaque powder for oral suspension ℞ *radiopaque contrast medium for gastrointestinal imaging* [barium sulfate] 95%

tonzonium bromide INN *detergent; surface-active agent* [also: thonzonium bromide]

tooth, lion's *medicinal herb* [see: dandelion]

Toothache gel OTC *topical oral anesthetic* [benzocaine]

toothache bush; toothache tree *medicinal herb* [see: prickly ash]

Top Care Flu, Cold, & Cough Medicine Night Time powder for oral solution OTC *antitussive; decongestant; antihistamine; analgesic* [dextromethorphan hydrobromide; pseudoephedrine HCl; chlorpheniramine maleate; acetaminophen] 20•60•4•1000 mg/pkt.

Top Care Multi-Symptom Pain Relief Cold caplets OTC *antitussive; decongestant; analgesic* [dextromethor-

phan hydrobromide; pseudoephedrine HCl; acetaminophen] 15•30•325 mg

Top Care Multi-Symptom Pain Relief Cold caplets OTC *antitussive; decongestant; antihistamine; analgesic* [dextromethorphan hydrobromide; pseudoephedrine HCl; chlorpheniramine maleate; acetaminophen] 15•30•2•325 mg

Top Care Nite Time Multi-Symptom Cold/Flu Relief LiquiCaps (liquid-filled capsules) OTC *antitussive; decongestant; antihistamine; analgesic* [dextromethorphan hydrobromide; pseudoephedrine HCl; doxylamine succinate; acetaminophen] 10•30•6.25•250 mg

Top Care Soothing Cough & Head Congestion Relief D oral liquid OTC *antitussive; decongestant* [dextromethorphan hydrobromide; pseudoephedrine HCl; alcohol 5%] 30•60 mg/15 mL

Topamax coated tablets, sprinkle caps ℞ *broad-spectrum sulfamate anticonvulsant for partial-onset and generalized tonic-clonic seizures; migraine headache preventative; investigational (orphan) for Lennox-Gastaut syndrome* [topiramate] 25, 50, 100, 200 mg; 15, 25 mg

Topic gel OTC *topical analgesic; counterirritant* [benzyl alcohol; camphor; menthol; alcohol 30%] 5%•2̲•2̲ 2̱ Topicort

topical starch [see: starch, topical]

TopiCare (trademarked ingredient) *topical polyolprepolymer base for creams and gels*

Topicort ointment, cream, gel ℞ *corticosteroidal anti-inflammatory* [desoximetasone] 0.25%; 0.25%; 0.05% 2̱ Topic

Topicort LP cream ℞ *topical corticosteroidal anti-inflammatory* [desoximetasone] 0.05%

Topicycline solution (discontinued 2003) ℞ *antibiotic for acne* [tetracycline HCl] 2.2 mg/mL

topiramate USAN, INN, BAN *broad-spectrum sulfamate anticonvulsant for* *partial-onset and generalized tonic-clonic seizures; migraine headache preventative; investigational (orphan) for Lennox-Gastaut syndrome*

topo/CTX (topotecan, cyclophosphamide [with mesna rescue]) *chemotherapy protocol for pediatric bone and soft tissue sarcomas*

topoisomerase I inhibitors *a class of hormonal antineoplastics that prevent DNA replication of tumors by inhibiting the re-ligation of naturally occurring single-strand breaks*

Toposar IV injection ℞ *antineoplastic for testicular and small cell lung cancers* [etoposide; alcohol 30.5%] 20 mg/mL

topotecan INN, BAN *topoisomerase I inhibitor; antineoplastic for ovarian and small cell lung cancers* [also: topotecan HCl]

topotecan HCl USAN *topoisomerase I inhibitor; antineoplastic for ovarian and small cell lung cancers; investigational (Phase II) for AIDS-related progressive multifocal leukoencephalopathy (PML)* [also: topotecan]

toprilidine INN

Toprol-XL film-coated extended-release tablets ℞ *antihypertensive; long-term antianginal; antiadrenergic (β-blocker)* [metoprolol succinate] 25, 50, 100, 200 mg

topterone USAN, INN *antiandrogen*

TOPV (trivalent oral poliovirus vaccine) [see: poliovirus vaccine, live oral]

toquizine USAN, INN *anticholinergic*

Toradol film-coated tablets, Tubex (prefilled syringes) for IM or IV injection ℞ *nonsteroidal anti-inflammatory drug (NSAID); analgesic for acute, moderately severe, opioid-level pain* [ketorolac tromethamine] 10 mg; 15, 30 mg/mL

torasemide INN, BAN *antihypertensive; loop diuretic* [also: torsemide]

torbafylline INN

torcetrapib *investigational (Phase III) antihyperlipidemic; cholesterol ester*

transfer protein (CETP) inhibitor that raises HDL cholesterol

Torecan IM injection ℞ *antiemetic* [thiethylperazine maleate] 5 mg/mL

Torecan tablets (discontinued 2004) ℞ *antiemetic* [thiethylperazine maleate] 10 mg

toremifene INN, BAN *antiestrogen; antineoplastic* [also: toremifene citrate]

toremifene citrate USAN *antiestrogen antineoplastic for metastatic breast cancer in postmenopausal women (orphan); investigational (orphan) for desmoid tumors* [also: toremifene]

toripristone INN

tormentil (Potentilla tormentilla; Tormentilla erecta) root *medicinal herb used as an antiphlogistic, antiseptic, astringent, and hemostatic*

Tornalate oral inhalation aerosol, solution for inhalation (discontinued 2001) ℞ *sympathomimetic bronchodilator* [bitolterol mesylate] 0.8%; 0.2%

torsemide USAN *antihypertensive; loop diuretic* [also: torasemide] 5, 10, 20, 100 mg oral ⊅ furosemide

tosactide INN [also: octacosactrin]

tosifen USAN, INN *antianginal*

tosilate INN *combining name for radicals or groups* [also: tosylate]

tositumomab *cytotoxic monoclonal antibody to non-Hodgkin lymphoma (NHL)* [see also: iodine I 131 tositumomab]

tosufloxacin USAN, INN *antibacterial*

tosulur INN

tosylate USAN, BAN *combining name for radicals or groups* [also: tosilate]

tosylchloramide sodium INN [also: chloramine-T]

Totacillin capsules, powder for oral suspension (discontinued 2002) ℞ *aminopenicillin antibiotic* [ampicillin] 250, 500 mg; 125, 250 mg/5 mL

Total solution OTC *cleaning/soaking/wetting solution for hard contact lenses*

Total Formula; Total Formula-2 tablets OTC *vitamin/mineral/iron supplement* [multiple vitamins & minerals; iron; folic acid; biotin] ≛•20• 0.4•0.3 mg

Total Formula-3 without Iron tablets OTC *vitamin/mineral supplement* [multiple vitamins & minerals; folic acid; biotin] ±•0.4•0.3 mg

touch-me-not; pale touch-me-not *medicinal herb* [see: celandine; jewelweed; Siberian ginseng]

toughened silver nitrate [see: silver nitrate, toughened]

Touro Allergy sustained-release capsules ℞ *decongestant; antihistamine* [pseudoephedrine HCl; brompheniramine maleate] 60•5.75 mg

Touro CC sustained-release caplets ℞ *antitussive; decongestant; expectorant* [dextromethorphan hydrobromide; pseudoephedrine HCl; guaifenesin] 30•60•575 mg

Touro DM sustained-release tablets ℞ *antitussive; expectorant* [dextromethorphan hydrobromide; guaifenesin] 30•575 mg

Touro Ex sustained-release caplets (discontinued 2004) ℞ *expectorant* [guaifenesin] 575 mg

Touro LA sustained-release caplets ℞ *decongestant; expectorant* [pseudoephedrine HCl; guaifenesin] 120• 525 mg

toxoids *a class of drugs used for active immunization that produce endogenous antibodies to toxins*

toywort *medicinal herb* [see: shepherd's purse]

tozalinone INN *antidepressant* [also: thozalinone]

tPA; t-PA (tissue plasminogen activator) [see: alteplase; anistreplase; lanoteplase; monteplase; reteplase; saruplase; tenecteplase]

TPCH (thioguanine, procarbazine, CCNU, hydroxyurea) *chemotherapy protocol*

TPDCV (thioguanine, procarbazine, DCD, CCNU, vincristine) *chemotherapy protocol*

TPGS (tocopheryl polyethylene glycol succinate) [see: tocophersolan]

T-Phyl timed-release tablets ℞ *antiasthmatic; bronchodilator* [theophylline] 200 mg

TPM Test kit for professional use *in vitro diagnostic aid for* Toxoplasma gondii *antibodies in serum* [indirect hemagglutination test]

TPN Electrolytes; TPN Electrolytes II; TPN Electrolytes III IV admixture ℞ *intravenous electrolyte therapy* [combined electrolyte solution]

traboxopine INN

Trac Tabs 2X tablets ℞ *urinary antibiotic; analgesic; antispasmodic; acidifier* [methenamine; phenyl salicylate; atropine sulfate; hyoscyamine sulfate; benzoic acid; methylene blue] 120•30•0.06•0.03•7.5•6 mg

tracazolate USAN, INN, BAN *sedative*

Trace Metals Additive in 0.9% NaCl IV injection (name changed to **4 Trace Elements** in 2005)

Tracelyte; Tracelyte II; Tracelyte with Double Electrolytes; Tracelyte II with Double Electrolytes IV admixture (discontinued 2003) ℞ *intravenous nutritional therapy* [multiple trace elements (metals); electrolytes]

Tracleer film-coated tablets ℞ *endothelin receptor antagonist (ERA) for pulmonary arterial hypertension (orphan)* [bosentan] 62.5, 125 mg

Tracrium IV infusion ℞ *nondepolarizing neuromuscular blocker; adjunct to anesthesia* [atracurium besylate] 10 mg/mL

trafermin USAN *investigational (Phase II/III) fibroblast growth factor for stroke and coronary artery disease*

tragacanth NF *suspending agent*

tralonide USAN, INN *corticosteroid; anti-inflammatory*

tramadol INN *central analgesic* [also: tramadol HCl] ☑ trazodone

Tramadol ER extended-release tablets ℞ *central analgesic for moderate to severe chronic pain* [tramadol] 100, 200, 300 mg

tramadol HCl USAN *central analgesic* [also: tramadol] 50 mg oral ▣ trazodone

tramadol HCl & acetaminophen *central analgesic for acute pain* 37.5•325 mg oral

Tramadol ODT (orally disintegrating tablets) ℞ *central analgesic for moderate to severe pain* [tramadol] 50 mg

tramazoline INN *adrenergic* [also: tramazoline HCl]

tramazoline HCl USAN *adrenergic* [also: tramazoline]

Trandate film-coated tablets, IV injection ℞ *antihypertensive; antiadrenergic (α- and β-blocker)* [labetalol HCl] 100, 200, 300 mg; 5 mg/mL

trandolapril INN, BAN *antihypertensive; angiotensin converting enzyme (ACE) inhibitor; treatment for CHF*

trandolaprilat INN

tranexamic acid USAN, INN, BAN *systemic hemostatic; orphan status withdrawn 1996*

tranilast USAN, INN *antiasthmatic*

trans AMCHA (*trans*-aminomethyl cyclohexanecarboxylic acid) [see: tranexamic acid]

transcainide USAN, INN *antiarrhythmic*

transclomiphene [now: zuclomiphene]

Transderm Scōp transdermal patch ℞ *motion sickness preventative; post-surgical antiemetic* [scopolamine] 1.5 mg (1 mg dose over 3 days)

Transderm-Nitro transdermal patch ℞ *antianginal; vasodilator* [nitroglycerin] 12.5, 25, 50, 75, 100 mg (0.1, 0.2, 0.4, 0.6, 0.8 mg/hr.)

transforming growth factor beta 2 *investigational (orphan) growth stimulator for full-thickness macular holes*

trans-π-oxocamphor JAN *topical antipruritic; mild local anesthetic; counterirritant* [also: camphor]

trans-retinoic acid [see: tretinoin]

Trans-Ver-Sal Adult-Patch; Trans-Ver-Sal Pedia-Patch; Trans-Ver-Sal Plantar-Patch patch OTC *keratolytic* [salicylic acid] 15%

trantelinium bromide INN

Tranxene T-Tabs ("T"-imprinted tablets) ℞ *benzodiazepine anxiolytic; minor tranquilizer; alcohol withdrawal aid; anticonvulsant adjunct* [clorazepate dipotassium] 3.75, 7.5, 15 mg

Tranxene-SD; Tranxene-SD Half Strength extended-release tablets ℞ *benzodiazepine anxiolytic; minor tranquilizer; alcohol withdrawal aid; anticonvulsant adjunct* [clorazepate dipotassium] 22.5 mg; 11.25 mg

tranylcypromine INN, BAN *antidepressant; MAO inhibitor* [also: tranylcypromine sulfate]

tranylcypromine sulfate USP *antidepressant; MAO inhibitor* [also: tranylcypromine]

trapencaine INN

trapidil INN

trapymin [see: trapidil]

trastuzumab *antineoplastic monoclonal antibody to HER-2 (human epidermal growth factor receptor 2) protein for metastatic breast cancer*

trastuzumab & paclitaxel *chemotherapy protocol for breast cancer*

Trasylol IV infusion ℞ *systemic hemostatic for coronary artery bypass graft (CABG) surgery (orphan)* [aprotinin] 10 000 KIU/mL (kallikrein inhibitor units) ▣ Travasol

TraumaCal ready-to-use oral liquid OTC *enteral nutritional therapy for moderate to severe stress or trauma* [multiple branched chain amino acids]

Travasol 2.75% in 5% (10%, 25%) Dextrose; Travasol 4.25% in 5% (10%, 25%) Dextrose IV infusion ℞ *total parenteral nutrition; peripheral parenteral nutrition* [multiple essential and nonessential amino acids; dextrose] ▣ Trasylol

Travasol 3.5% (5.5%, 8.5%) with Electrolytes IV infusion ℞ *total parenteral nutrition (all except 3.5%); peripheral parenteral nutrition (all)* [multiple essential and nonessential amino acids; electrolytes]

Travasol 5.5% (8.5%, 10%) IV infusion ℞ *total parenteral nutrition; periph-*

eral parenteral nutrition [multiple essential and nonessential amino acids]

Travasorb HN; Travasorb MCT; Travasorb STD powder OTC *enteral nutritional therapy* [lactose-free formula]

Travatan Drop-Tainers (eye drops) ℞ *prostaglandin F$_{2\alpha}$ analogue for glaucoma and ocular hypertension* [travoprost] 0.004%

traveler's joy *medicinal herb* [see: blue vervain; woodbine]

5% Travert and Electrolyte No. 2; 10% Travert and Electrolyte No. 2 IV infusion ℞ *intravenous nutritional/electrolyte therapy* [combined electrolyte solution; invert sugar (50% dextrose + 50% fructose)]

travoprost USAN *topical prostaglandin F$_{2\alpha}$ analogue for glaucoma and ocular hypertension*

traxanox INN

traxoprodil mesylate USAN *selective NMDA receptor antagonist for traumatic brain injury*

Traypak (trademarked packaging form) *multivial carton*

trazitiline INN

trazium esilate INN

trazodone INN *triazolopyridine antidepressant for panic disorder, aggressive behavior, alcoholism, and cocaine withdrawal; serotonin uptake inhibitor* [also: trazodone HCl] ☒ tramadol

trazodone HCl USAN *triazolopyridine antidepressant for panic disorder, aggressive behavior, alcoholism, and cocaine withdrawal; serotonin uptake inhibitor* [also: trazodone] 50, 100, 150, 300 mg oral ☒ tramadol

trazolopride INN

trebenzomine INN *antidepressant* [also: trebenzomine HCl]

trebenzomine HCl USAN *antidepressant* [also: trebenzomine]

trecadrine INN

Trecator-SC tablets ℞ *tuberculostatic* [ethionamide] 250 mg

trecetilide fumarate USAN *antiarrhythmic*

trecovirsen sodium USAN *antisense antiviral for HIV and AIDS*

trefentanil HCl USAN *analgesic*

trefoil, bean; bitter trefoil; marsh trefoil *medicinal herb* [see: buckbean]

treloxinate USAN, INN *antihyperlipoproteinemic*

Trelstar Depot IM injection (once monthly) ℞ *gonadotropin-releasing hormone (GnRH) antineoplastic for palliative treatment of advanced prostate cancer* [triptorelin pamoate] 3.75 mg

Trelstar LA IM injection (three-month depot) ℞ *gonadotropin-releasing hormone (GnRH) agonist; antineoplastic for palliative treatment of advanced prostate cancer* [triptorelin pamoate] 11.25 mg

tremacamra USAN *antiviral; inhibits viral attachment to host cells*

trembling poplar; trembling tree *medicinal herb* [see: poplar]

trenbolone INN, BAN *veterinary anabolic steroid, also abused as a street drug* [also: trenbolone acetate]

trenbolone acetate USAN *veterinary anabolic steroid, also abused as a street drug* [also: trenbolone]

trenbolone hexahydrobenzylcarbonate *veterinary anabolic steroid, also abused as a street drug*

trengestone INN

trenizine INN

Trental film-coated controlled-release tablets ℞ *peripheral vasodilator to improve blood microcirculation in intermittent claudication* [pentoxifylline] 400 mg

treosulfan INN, BAN *investigational (orphan) for ovarian cancer*

trepibutone INN

trepipam INN *sedative* [also: trepipam maleate]

trepipam maleate USAN *sedative* [also: trepipam]

trepirium iodide INN

treprostinil sodium *prostacyclin analogue for pulmonary arterial hypertension (orphan) and peripheral vascular* *disease (PVD); investigational (Phase II) for critical limb ischemia*

treptilamine INN

trequinsin INN

trestolone INN *antineoplastic; androgen* [also: trestolone acetate]

trestolone acetate USAN *antineoplastic; androgen* [also: trestolone]

tretamine INN, BAN [also: triethylenemelamine]

trethinium tosilate INN

trethocanic acid INN

trethocanoic acid [see: trethocanic acid]

tretinoin USAN, USP, INN, BAN *topical keratolytic for acne; treatment for acute promyelocytic leukemia (APL; orphan); investigational (orphan) for other leukemias and ophthalmic squamous metaplasia; investigational (Phase II) for AIDS-related Kaposi sarcoma and non-Hodgkin lymphoma 0.01%, 0.025%, 0.05%, 0.1% topical*

tretoquinol INN

Trexall film-coated tablets ℞ *antimetabolite antineoplastic for leukemia; systemic antipsoriatic; antirheumatic* [methotrexate] 5, 7.5, 10, 15 mg

Trexima ℞ *investigational (Phase III) combination 5-HT$_{1B/1D}$ agonist and nonsteroidal anti-inflammatory drug (NSAID) for the acute treatment of migraine headaches* [sumatriptan; naproxen sodium]

TRH (thyrotropin-releasing hormone) [see: protirelin]

Tri Vit with Fluoride drops ℞ *pediatric vitamin supplement and dental caries preventative* [vitamins A, C, and D; fluoride] 1500 IU•35 mg•400 IU•0.25 mg, 1500 IU•35 mg•400 IU•0.5 mg per mL

TRIAC (triiodothyroacetic acid) [q.v.]

Triacet cream ℞ *topical corticosteroidal anti-inflammatory* [triamcinolone acetonide] 0.1%

triacetin USP, INN *antifungal*

triacetyloleandomycin BAN *macrolide antibiotic* [also: troleandomycin]

Triacin-C Cough syrup ℞ *narcotic antitussive; decongestant; antihistamine* [codeine phosphate; pseudoephedrine HCl; triprolidine HCl; alcohol 4.3%] 20•60•2.5 mg/10 mL

triaconazole [now: terconazole]

Triactin syrup (discontinued 2001) OTC *decongestant; antihistamine* [phenylpropanolamine HCl; chlorpheniramine maleate] 6.25•1 mg/5 mL

Triacting pediatric oral liquid OTC *decongestant; expectorant* [pseudoephedrine HCl; guaifenesin] 15•50 mg/5 mL

Triacting Cold & Allergy pediatric oral liquid OTC *decongestant; antihistamine* [pseudoephedrine HCl; chlorpheniramine maleate] 30•2 mg/10 mL

Tri-Acting Cold & Allergy pediatric syrup OTC *decongestant; antihistamine* [pseudoephedrine HCl; chlorpheniramine maleate] 30•2 mg/10 mL

Tri-Acting Cold & Cough pediatric syrup OTC *antitussive; decongestant; antihistamine* [dextromethorphan hydrobromide; pseudoephedrine HCl; chlorpheniramine maleate] 10•30•2 mg/10 mL

Triad capsules ℞ *sedative; barbiturate analgesic* [acetaminophen; caffeine; butalbital] 325•40•50 mg

Triafed with Codeine syrup (discontinued 2000) (discontinued 2002) ℞ *narcotic antitussive; decongestant; antihistamine* [codeine phosphate; pseudoephedrine HCl; triprolidine HCl] 10•30•1.25 mg/5 mL

triafungin USAN, INN *antifungal*

Trial AG (Anti-Gas) tablets OTC *antacid; antiflatulent* [aluminum hydroxide; magnesium hydroxide; simethicone] 200•200•25 mg

Trial Antacid tablets OTC *antacid; calcium supplement* [calcium carbonate] 420 mg

Triam Forte IM injection ℞ *corticosteroid; anti-inflammatory* [triamcinolone diacetate] 40 mg/mL

Triam-A IM, intra-articular, intrabursal, intradermal injection ℞ *cortico-*

steroid; anti-inflammatory [triamcinolone acetonide] 40 mg/mL

triamcinolone USP, INN, BAN, JAN *corticosteroid* 4 mg oral ⧠ Triaminicin

triamcinolone acetonide USP, JAN *corticosteroidal anti-inflammatory; treatment for chronic asthma and rhinitis* 0.025%, 0.1%, 0.5% topical; 40 mg/mL injection

triamcinolone acetonide sodium phosphate USAN *corticosteroid*

triamcinolone benetonide INN *corticosteroid*

triamcinolone diacetate USP, JAN *corticosteroid* 40 mg/mL injection

triamcinolone furetonide INN *corticosteroid*

triamcinolone hexacetonide USAN, USP, INN, BAN *corticosteroid*

Triaminic pediatric syrup (discontinued 2001) OTC *decongestant; antihistamine* [phenylpropanolamine HCl; chlorpheniramine maleate] 6.25•0.5 mg; 6.25•1 mg/5 mL ⧠ Triaminicin; TriHemic

Triaminic Allerchews orally disintegrating tablets OTC *nonsedating antihistamine for allergic rhinitis and chronic idiopathic urticaria* [loratadine] 10 mg

Triaminic Allergy; Triaminic Cold tablets (discontinued 2001) OTC *decongestant; antihistamine* [phenylpropanolamine HCl; chlorpheniramine maleate] 25•4 mg; 12.5•2 mg

Triaminic Allergy, Sinus, & Headache Softchews (pediatric chewable tablets) OTC *decongestant; analgesic; antipyretic* [pseudoephedrine HCl; acetaminophen] 15•150 mg

Triaminic Allergy Congestion Softchews (chewable tablets), pediatric oral liquid OTC *nasal decongestant* [pseudoephedrine HCl] 15 mg; 15 mg/5 mL

Triaminic AM Decongestant Formula syrup (discontinued 2002) OTC *decongestant* [pseudoephedrine HCl] 15 mg/5 mL

Triaminic AM Non-Drowsy Cough & Decongestant pediatric oral liquid OTC *antitussive; decongestant* [dextromethorphan hydrobromide; pseudoephedrine HCl] 7.5•15 mg/5 mL

Triaminic Chest & Nasal Congestion pediatric oral liquid OTC *decongestant; expectorant* [pseudoephedrine HCl; guaifenesin] 15•50 mg/5 mL

Triaminic Cold & Allergy pediatric oral liquid OTC *decongestant; antihistamine* [pseudoephedrine HCl; chlorpheniramine maleate] 6.25•1 mg/5 mL

Triaminic Cold & Cough pediatric oral liquid OTC *antitussive; decongestant; antihistamine* [dextromethorphan hydrobromide; pseudoephedrine HCl; chlorpheniramine maleate] 10•30•2 mg/10 mL

Triaminic Cold & Cough; Triaminic Cough pediatric soft chews OTC *antitussive; decongestant; antihistamine* [dextromethorphan hydrobromide; pseudoephedrine HCl; chlorpheniramine maleate] 5•15•1 mg

Triaminic Cough pediatric oral liquid OTC *antitussive; decongestant* [dextromethorphan hydrobromide; pseudoephedrine HCl] 7.5•15 mg/5 mL

Triaminic Cough & Sore Throat pediatric oral liquid OTC *antitussive; decongestant; analgesic* [dextromethorphan hydrobromide; pseudoephedrine HCl; acetaminophen] 7.5•15•160 mg/5 mL

Triaminic Decongestant oral infant drops OTC *pediatric decongestant* [pseudoephedrine HCl] 7.5 mg/0.8 mL

Triaminic DM syrup (discontinued 2002) OTC *antitussive; decongestant* [dextromethorphan hydrobromide; phenylpropanolamine HCl] 5•6.25 mg/5 mL

Triaminic Expectorant oral liquid (discontinued 2002) OTC *decongestant; expectorant* [phenylpropanolamine HCl; guaifenesin] 6.25•50 mg/5 mL

Triaminic Expectorant DH oral liquid (discontinued 2002) ℞ *narcotic antitussive; decongestant; antihistamine; expectorant* [hydrocodone bitartrate; phenylpropanolamine HCl; pyrilamine maleate; pheniramine maleate; guaifenesin; alcohol 5%] 1.67•12.5•6.25•6.25•100 mg/5 mL

Triaminic Expectorant with Codeine oral liquid (discontinued 2002) ℞ *narcotic antitussive; decongestant; expectorant* [codeine phosphate; phenylpropanolamine HCl; guaifenesin; alcohol 5%] 10•12.5•100 mg/5 mL

Triaminic Flu, Cough, & Fever pediatric oral liquid OTC *antitussive; decongestant; antihistamine; analgesic; antipyretic* [dextromethorphan hydrobromide; pseudoephedrine HCl; chlorpheniramine maleate; acetaminophen] 15•30•2•320 mg/10 mL

Triaminic Night Time Cough & Cold pediatric oral liquid OTC *antitussive; decongestant; antihistamine* [dextromethorphan hydrobromide; pseudoephedrine HCl; chlorpheniramine maleate] 15•30•2 mg/10 mL

Triaminic Nite Light pediatric oral liquid (name changed to **Triaminic Cold & Night Time Cough** in 2002)

Triaminic Severe Cold & Fever pediatric oral liquid (name changed to **Triaminic Cold, Cough, & Fever** in 2002)

Triaminic Softchews (pediatric chewable tablets) OTC *decongestant; antihistamine* [pseudoephedrine HCl; chlorpheniramine maleate] 15•1 mg
🄐 Triaminicin; TriHemic

Triaminic Softchews Cold & Sore Throat (pediatric chewable tablets) OTC *antitussive; decongestant; analgesic* [dextromethorphan hydrobromide; pseudoephedrine HCl; acetaminophen] 5•15•160 mg

Triaminic Sore Throat Spray OTC *topical antipruritic/counterirritant; mild local anesthetic* [phenol] 0.5%

Triaminic Thin Strips Cough & Runny Nose orally disintegrating film OTC *antitussive; antihistamine; sleep aid* [diphenhydramine HCl] 12.5 mg

Triaminic Thin Strips Long Acting Cough orally disintegrating film OTC *antitussive* [dextromethorphan hydrobromide] 7.5 mg

Triaminic Throat Pain & Cough pediatric soft chews OTC *antitussive; decongestant; analgesic* [dextromethorphan hydrobromide; pseudoephedrine HCl; acetaminophen] 5•15•160 mg

Triaminic Vapor Patch OTC *counterirritant; cough suppressant* [camphor; menthol] 4.7%•2.6%

Triaminic-12 sustained-release tablets (discontinued 2001) OTC *decongestant; antihistamine* [phenylpropanolamine HCl; chlorpheniramine maleate] 75•12 mg

Triaminicin Cold, Allergy, Sinus Medicine tablets OTC *decongestant; antihistamine; analgesic* [pseudoephedrine HCl; chlorpheniramine maleate; acetaminophen] 60•4•650 mg
🄐 triamcinolone; Triaminic

Triaminicol Multi-Symptom Cough and Cold tablets (discontinued 2002) OTC *antitussive; decongestant; antihistamine* [dextromethorphan hydrobromide; phenylpropanolamine HCl; chlorpheniramine maleate] 10•12.5•2 mg

Triaminicol Multi-Symptom Relief oral liquid (discontinued 2002) OTC *antitussive; decongestant; antihistamine* [dextromethorphan hydrobromide; phenylpropanolamine HCl; chlorpheniramine maleate] 10•12.5•2 mg/5 mL

Triaminicol Multi-Symptom Relief Colds with Cough pediatric oral liquid (discontinued 2002) OTC *antitussive; decongestant; antihistamine* [dextromethorphan hydrobromide; phenylpropanolamine HCl; chlorpheniramine maleate] 5•6.25•1 mg/5 mL

Triamolone 40 IM injection ℞ *corticosteroid; anti-inflammatory* [triamcinolone diacetate] 40 mg/mL

Triamonide 40 IM, intra-articular, intrabursal, intradermal injection ℞

corticosteroid; anti-inflammatory [triamcinolone acetonide] 40 mg/mL

triampyzine INN *anticholinergic* [also: triampyzine sulfate]

triampyzine sulfate USAN *anticholinergic* [also: triampyzine]

triamterene USAN, USP, INN, BAN, JAN *antihypertensive; potassium-sparing diuretic* ⊡ trimipramine

triamterene & hydrochlorothiazide *antihypertensive; potassium-sparing diuretic* 37.5•25 mg oral

trianisestrol [see: chlorotrianisene]

Triapine ℞ *investigational (Phase I) anticancer agent* ⊡ Triaprim

Triavil tablets (discontinued 2004) ℞ *conventional (typical) phenothiazine antipsychotic for schizophrenia and psychotic disorders; antidepressant* [perphenazine; amitriptyline HCl] 2•10 mg; 2•25 mg; 4•10 mg; 4•25 mg

Triavil 4-50 tablets (discontinued 2000) ℞ *conventional (typical) phenothiazine antipsychotic for schizophrenia and psychotic disorders; antidepressant* [perphenazine; amitriptyline HCl] 4•50 mg

Tri-A-Vite F drops ℞ *pediatric vitamin supplement and dental caries preventative* [vitamins A, C, and D; fluoride] 1500 IU•35 mg•400 IU•0.5 mg per mL

Triaz gel, topical liquid (discontinued 2003) ℞ *keratolytic for acne* [benzoyl peroxide] 3%, 6%, 9%, 10%

Triaz lotion ℞ *keratolytic for acne* [benzoyl peroxide] 3%, 6%, 10%

Triaz skin cleanser (discontinued 2003) ℞ *keratolytic for acne* [benzoyl peroxide] 9%, 10%

triaziquone INN, BAN

triazolam USAN, USP, INN *benzodiazepine sedative and hypnotic* 0.125, 0.25 mg oral

Triban; Pediatric Triban suppositories ℞ *anticholinergic; post-surgical antiemetic* [trimethobenzamide HCl; benzocaine] 200 mg•2%; 100 mg•2% ⊡ Tigan

tribasic calcium phosphate [see: calcium phosphate, tribasic]

tribavirin BAN *antiviral for severe lower respiratory tract infections* [also: ribavirin]

tribendilol INN

tribenoside USAN, INN *sclerosing agent*

Tribiotic Plus ointment (discontinued 2001) OTC *topical antibiotic; anesthetic* [polymyxin B sulfate; bacitracin; neomycin sulfate; lidocaine] 5000 U•500 U•3.5 mg•40 mg per g

Tri-Biozene ointment OTC *antibiotic; local anesthetic* [polymyxin B sulfate; neomycin sulfate; bacitracin zinc; pramoxine HCl] 10 000 U•3.5 mg•500 U•10 mg per g

tribromoethanol NF

tribromomethane [see: bromoform]

tribromsalan USAN, INN *disinfectant*

tribuzone INN

tricalcium phosphate [see: calcium phosphate, tribasic]

tricarbocyanine dye [see: indocyanine green]

tricetamide USAN *sedative*

Trichinella extract USP

Tri-Chlor topical liquid ℞ *cauterant; keratolytic* [trichloroacetic acid] 80%

trichlorethoxyphosphamide [see: defosfamide]

trichlorfon USP *veterinary anthelmintic; investigational (NDA filed) acetylcholinesterase inhibitor for Alzheimer dementia* [also: metrifonate; metriphonate]

trichlorisobutylalcohol [see: chlorobutanol]

trichlormethiazide USP, INN *diuretic; antihypertensive* 4 mg oral

trichlormethine INN [also: trimustine]

trichloroacetic acid USP *strong keratolytic/cauterant*

trichlorocarbanilide (TCC) [see: triclocarban]

trichloroethylene NF, INN

trichlorofluoromethane [see: trichloromonofluoromethane]

trichlorofon [see: metrifonate]

trichloromonofluoromethane NF *aerosol propellant; topical anesthetic*

trichlorphon [see: metrifonate]

Tricholomopsis edodes *medicinal herb*
[see: shiitake mushrooms]

Trichophyton extract *diagnosis and treatment of Trichophyton-induced skin infections*

trichorad [see: acinitrazole]

Trichosanthes kirilowii *medicinal herb*
[see: Chinese cucumber]

Trichotine Douche powder OTC *antiseptic/germicidal; vaginal cleanser and deodorizer; acidity modifier* [sodium perborate]

Trichotine Douche solution OTC *antiseptic/germicidal; vaginal cleanser and deodorizer; acidity modifier* [sodium borate]

triciribine INN *antineoplastic* [also: triciribine phosphate]

triciribine phosphate USAN *antineoplastic* [also: triciribine]

tricitrates (sodium citrate, potassium citrate, and citric acid) USP *systemic alkalizer; urinary alkalizer; antiurolithic*

triclabendazole INN

triclacetamol INN

triclazate INN

triclobisonium chloride NF, INN

triclocarban USAN, INN *disinfectant*

triclodazol INN

triclofenate INN *combining name for radicals or groups*

triclofenol piperazine USAN, INN *anthelmintic*

triclofos INN *hypnotic; sedative* [also: triclofos sodium]

triclofos sodium USAN *hypnotic; sedative* [also: triclofos]

triclofylline INN

triclonide USAN, INN *anti-inflammatory*

triclosan USAN, INN, BAN *disinfectant/antiseptic*

Tricodene Cough and Cold oral liquid R *narcotic antitussive; antihistamine* [codeine phosphate; pyrilamine maleate] 16.4•25 mg/10 mL

Tricodene Forte; Tricodene NN oral liquid (discontinued 2002) OTC *antitussive; decongestant; antihistamine* [dextromethorphan hydrobromide; phenylpropanolamine HCl;

chlorpheniramine maleate] 10•12.5•2 mg/5 mL

Tricodene Pediatric Cough & Cold oral liquid (discontinued 2002) OTC *antitussive; decongestant* [dextromethorphan hydrobromide; phenylpropanolamine HCl] 10•12.5 mg/5 mL

Tricodene Sugar Free oral liquid OTC *antitussive; antihistamine* [dextromethorphan hydrobromide; chlorpheniramine maleate] 20•4 mg/10 mL

TriCor capsules (discontinued 2002) R *antihyperlipidemic for primary hypercholesterolemia (types IIa and IIb hyperlipidemia), hypertriglyceridemia (types IV and V hyperlipidemia), and mixed dyslipidemia* [fenofibrate] 67, 134, 200 mg

TriCor tablets R *antihyperlipidemic for primary hypercholesterolemia (types IIa and IIb hyperlipidemia), hypertriglyceridemia (types IV and V hyperlipidemia), and mixed dyslipidemia; also used for hyperuricemia* [fenofibrate] 48, 145 mg

tricosactide INN

Tricosal film-coated tablets R *analgesic; antipyretic; antirheumatic* [choline magnesium trisalicylate] 500, 750, 1000 mg

tricyclamol chloride INN

Tri-Cyclen [see: Ortho Tri-Cyclen]

tricyclics *a class of antidepressants that inhibit reuptake of amines, norepinephrine, and serotonin*

Triderm cream R *topical corticosteroidal anti-inflammatory* [triamcinolone acetonide] 0.1%

Tridesilon cream, ointment R *corticosteroidal anti-inflammatory* [desonide] 0.05%

Tridesilon Otic [see: Otic Tridesilon]

tridihexethyl chloride USP *peptic ulcer treatment adjunct*

tridihexethyl iodide INN

Tridil IV infusion (discontinued 2004) R *antianginal; vasodilator; perioperative antihypertensive; for congestive heart failure with myocardial infarction* [nitroglycerin] 0.5, 5 mg/mL

Tridione capsules, Dulcets (chewable tablets) (discontinued 2004) ℞ *anticonvulsant for absence (petit mal) seizures* [trimethadione] 300 mg; 150 mg

tridolgosir HCl USAN *chemoprotectant for solid tumor chemotherapy*

Tridrate Bowel Cleansing System oral solution + 3 tablets + 1 suppository OTC *pre-procedure bowel evacuant* [magnesium citrate (solution); bisacodyl (tablets and suppository)] 300 mL; 5 mg; 10 mg

trientine INN *copper chelating agent* [also: trientine HCl; trientine dihydrochloride]

trientine dihydrochloride BAN *copper chelating agent* [also: trientine HCl; trientine]

trientine HCl USAN, USP *copper chelating agent for Wilson disease (orphan)* [also: trientine; trientine dihydrochloride]

triest; triestrogen [see: estriol]

triethanolamine [now: trolamine]

triethyl citrate NF *plasticizer*

triethyleneiminobenzoquinone (TEIB) [see: triaziquone]

triethylenemelamine NF [also: tretamine]

triethylenethiophosphoramide (TSPA; TESPA) [see: thiotepa]

Trifed·C Cough syrup (discontinued 2002) ℞ *narcotic antitussive; decongestant; antihistamine* [codeine phosphate; pseudoephedrine HCl; triprolidine HCl; alcohol 4.4%] 10•30• 1.25 mg/5 mL

trifenagrel USAN, INN *antithrombotic*

trifezolac INN

triflocin USAN, INN *diuretic*

Tri-Flor-Vite with Fluoride drops ℞ *pediatric vitamin supplement and dental caries preventative* [vitamins A, C, and D; fluoride] 1500 IU•35 mg• 400 IU•0.25 mg per mL

triflubazam USAN, INN *minor tranquilizer*

triflumidate USAN, INN *anti-inflammatory*

trifluomeprazine INN, BAN

trifluoperazine INN *conventional (typical) phenothiazine antipsychotic for schiz-* *ophrenia; anxiolytic for nonpsychotic anxiety* [also: trifluoperazine HCl]

trifluoperazine HCl USP *conventional (typical) phenothiazine antipsychotic for schizophrenia; anxiolytic for nonpsychotic anxiety* [also: trifluoperazine] 1, 2, 5, 10 mg oral

trifluorothymidine [see: trifluridine]

trifluperidol USAN, INN *antipsychotic*

triflupromazine USP, INN *phenothiazine antipsychotic; antiemetic*

triflupromazine HCl USP *phenothiazine antipsychotic; antiemetic*

trifluridine USAN, INN *ophthalmic antiviral* 1% eye drops

triflusal INN *investigational treatment for stroke and vascular dementia*

triflutate USAN, INN *combining name for radicals or groups*

Trifolium pratense medicinal herb [see: red clover]

trigevolol INN

Triglide tablets ℞ *antihyperlipidemic for primary hypercholesterolemia (types IIa and IIb hyperlipidemia), hypertriglyceridemia (types IV and V hyperlipidemia), and mixed dyslipidemia* [fenofibrate] 50, 160 mg

α-triglycidyl isocyanurate (αTGI) [see: teroxirone]

Trigonella foenum-graecum medicinal herb [see: fenugreek]

TriHemic 600 film-coated tablets ℞ *hematinic* [ferrous fumarate; cyanocobalamin; ascorbic acid; vitamin E; intrinsic factor concentrate; docusate sodium; folic acid] 115 mg•25 μg•600 mg•30 IU•75 mg•50 mg• 1 mg ⑨ Triaminic

Trihexy-2; Trihexy-5 tablets ℞ *anticholinergic; antiparkinsonian* [trihexyphenidyl HCl] 2 mg; 5 mg

trihexyphenidyl INN *anticholinergic; antiparkinsonian* [also: trihexyphenidyl HCl; benzhexol]

trihexyphenidyl HCl USP *anticholinergic; antiparkinsonian* [also: trihexyphenidyl; benzhexol] 2, 5 mg oral; 2 mg/5 mL oral

TriHIBit IM injection ℞ *active immunizing agent for diphtheria, tetanus, pertussis, and* Haemophilus influenzae *type b* [diphtheria & tetanus toxoids & acellular pertussis (DTaP) vaccine; Hemophilus B conjugate vaccine] supplied as separate 0.5 mL vials of Tripedia (q.v.) and ActHib (q.v.)

Tri-Hydroserpine tablets ℞ *antihypertensive; vasodilator; diuretic* [hydrochlorothiazide; reserpine; hydralazine HCl] 15•0.1•25 mg

Tri-Immunol IM injection (discontinued 2001) ℞ *active immunizing agent for diphtheria, tetanus and pertussis* [diphtheria & tetanus toxoids & whole-cell pertussis (DTwP) vaccine, adsorbed] 12.5 LfU•5 LfU•4 U/0.5 mL

3,5,3′-triiodothyroacetate *investigational (orphan) for thyroid carcinoma*

triiodothyroacetic acid (TRIAC) *thyroid hormone analogue*

triiodothyronine sodium, levo [see: liothyronine sodium]

Tri-K oral liquid ℞ *potassium supplement* [potassium acetate; potassium bicarbonate; potassium citrate] 45 mEq K/15 mL

trikates USP *electrolyte replenisher*

Trikof-D sustained-release tablets (discontinued 2002) OTC *antitussive; decongestant; expectorant* [dextromethorphan hydrobromide; phenylpropanolamine HCl; guaifenesin] 30•37.5•600 mg

Tri-Kort IM, intra-articular, intrabursal, or intradermal injection ℞ *corticosteroid; anti-inflammatory* [triamcinolone acetonide] 40 mg/mL

Trilafon coated tablets, IV or IM injection (discontinued 2003) ℞ *conventional (typical) phenothiazine antipsychotic for schizophrenia and psychotic disorders; treatment for nausea and vomiting* [perphenazine] 2, 4, 8, 16 mg; 5 mg/mL

Trilafon oral concentrate (discontinued 2002) ℞ *conventional (typical) phenothiazine antipsychotic for schizophrenia and psychotic disorders; treatment for nausea and vomiting* [perphenazine] 2, 4, 8, 16 mg; 16 mg/5 mL; 5 mg/mL

Trileptal film-coated tablets, oral suspension ℞ *anticonvulsant for partial seizures* [oxcarbazepine] 150, 300, 600 mg; 300 mg/5 mL

triletide INN

Tri-Levlen film-coated tablets (in Slidecases of 21 or 28) ℞ *triphasic oral contraceptive; emergency postcoital contraceptive* [levonorgestrel; ethinyl estradiol]
Phase 1 (6 days): 50•30 μg;
Phase 2 (5 days): 75•40 μg;
Phase 3 (10 days): 125•30 μg

Trilisate tablets, oral liquid (discontinued 2004) ℞ *analgesic; antipyretic; anti-inflammatory; antirheumatic* [choline salicylate; magnesium salicylate] 750, 1000 mg; 500 mg/5 mL

trilithium citrate tetrahydrate [see: lithium citrate]

Trillium erectum; T. grandiflorum; T. pendulum medicinal herb [see: birthroot]

Trilog IM, intra-articular, intrabursal, intradermal injection ℞ *corticosteroid; anti-inflammatory* [triamcinolone acetonide] 40 mg/mL

Trilone IM injection ℞ *corticosteroid; anti-inflammatory* [triamcinolone diacetate] 40 mg/mL

trilostane USAN, INN, BAN *adrenocortical suppressant; antisteroidal antineoplastic*

Tri-Luma cream ℞ *short-term treatment for melasma of the face* [hydroquinone; fluocinolone acetonide; tretinoin] 4%•0.01%•0.05%

TriLyte powder for oral solution ℞ *pre-procedure bowel evacuant* [polyethylene glycol–electrolyte solution (PEG 3350)]

Trimazide suppositories, pediatric suppositories ℞ *anticholinergic; post-surgical antiemetic* [trimethobenzamide HCl] 200 mg; 100 mg

trimazosin INN, BAN *antihypertensive* [also: trimazosin HCl]

trimazosin HCl USAN *antihypertensive* [also: trimazosin]

trimebutine INN *GI antispasmodic*

trimecaine INN

trimedoxime bromide INN

trimegestone USAN *progestin for postmenopausal hormone deficiency*

trimeperidine INN, BAN

trimeprazine BAN *phenothiazine antihistamine; antipruritic* [also: trimeprazine tartrate; alimemazine; alimemazine tartrate] ⓘ trimipramine

trimeprazine tartrate USP *phenothiazine antihistamine; antipruritic* [also: alimemazine; trimeprazine; alimemazine tartrate]

trimeproprimine [see: trimipramine]

trimetamide INN

trimetaphan camsilate INN *antihypertensive* [also: trimethaphan camsylate; trimetaphan camsylate]

trimetaphan camsylate BAN *antihypertensive* [also: trimethaphan camsylate; trimetaphan camsilate]

trimetazidine INN, BAN

trimethadione USP, INN *oxazolidinedione anticonvulsant for absence (petit mal) seizures* [also: troxidone]

trimethamide [see: trimetamide]

trimethaphan camphorsulfonate [see: trimethaphan camsylate] ⓘ trimethoprim

trimethaphan camsylate USP *emergency antihypertensive* [also: trimetaphan camsilate; trimetaphan camsylate]

trimethidinium methosulfate NF, INN

trimethobenzamide INN *anticholinergic; post-surgical antiemetic* [also: trimethobenzamide HCl]

trimethobenzamide HCl USP *anticholinergic; post-surgical antiemetic* [also: trimethobenzamide] 300 mg oral; 100, 200 mg suppositories; 100 mg/mL injection

trimethoprim (TMP) USAN, USP, INN, BAN *antibacterial antibiotic* 100, 200 mg oral ⓘ trimethaphan

trimethoprim sulfate USAN *antibiotic*

trimethoprim sulfate & polymyxin B sulfate *topical ophthalmic antibiotic* 1 mg•10 000 U per mL eye drops

trimethoquinol [see: tretoquinol]

trimethylammonium chloride carbamate [see: bethanechol chloride]

3,3,5-trimethylcyclohexyl salicylate [see: homosalate]

trimethylene [see: cyclopropane]

trimethylglycine (TMG) *natural methylation agent used to prevent cardiovascular disease by lowering homocysteine levels, to boost neurological function by remyelinating nerve cells, and to slow cellular aging by protecting DNA; precursor to SAMe (q.v.)*

trimethyltetradecylammonium bromide [see: tetradonium bromide]

trimetozine USAN, INN *sedative*

trimetrexate USAN, INN, BAN *antimetabolic antineoplastic; systemic antiprotozoal*

trimetrexate glucuronate USAN *antimetabolic antineoplastic; antiprotozoal for AIDS-related* Pneumocystis carinii pneumonia *(orphan); investigational (orphan) for multiple cancers*

trimexiline INN

Triminol Cough syrup (discontinued 2002) OTC *antitussive; decongestant; antihistamine* [dextromethorphan hydrobromide; phenylpropanolamine HCl; chlorpheniramine maleate] 10•12.5•2 mg/5 mL

trimipramine USAN, INN *tricyclic antidepressant* ⓘ imipramine; triamterene; trimeprazine

trimipramine maleate USAN *tricyclic antidepressant*

trimolide [see: trimetozine]

trimopam maleate [now: trepipam maleate]

trimoprostil USAN, INN *gastric antisecretory*

Trimo-San vaginal jelly OTC *antibacterial; astringent; antipruritic* [oxyquinoline sulfate; boric acid; sodium borate] 0.025%•1%•0.7%

Trimox chewable tablets, capsules, powder for oral suspension ℞ *aminopenicil-*

lin antibiotic [amoxicillin] 125, 250 mg; 250, 500 mg; 125, 250 mg/5 mL

Trimox pediatric drops (discontinued 2002) ℞ *aminopenicillin antibiotic* [amoxicillin] 50 mg/mL

trimoxamine INN *antihypertensive* [also: trimoxamine HCl]

trimoxamine HCl USAN *antihypertensive* [also: trimoxamine]

Trimpex tablets ℞ *anti-infective; antibacterial* [trimethoprim] 100 mg

trimustine BAN [also: trichlormethine]

Trinalin Repetabs (sustained-release tablets) ℞ *decongestant; antihistamine* [pseudoephedrine sulfate; azatadine maleate] 120•1 mg

Trinam reservoir delivery device ℞ *investigational (Phase II, orphan) gene-based therapy for neointimal hyperplasia disease* [vascular endothelial growth factor (VEGF)]

Tri-Nasal nasal spray (discontinued 2002) ℞ *once-daily corticosteroidal anti-inflammatory for chronic allergic rhinitis* [triamcinolone acetonide] 50 μg/spray

Trinate tablets ℞ *vitamin/mineral/calcium/iron supplement* [multiple vitamins & minerals; calcium; iron; folic acid] ≛•200•28•1 mg

trinecol (pullus) USAN *collagen derivative for treatment of rheumatoid arthritis*

Tri-Nefrin tablets (discontinued 2001) OTC *decongestant; antihistamine* [phenylpropanolamine HCl; chlorpheniramine maleate] 25•4 mg

TriNessa tablets (in packs of 28) ℞ *triphasic oral contraceptive* [norgestimate; ethinyl estradiol]
Phase 1 (7 days): 180•35 μg;
Phase 2 (7 days): 215•35 μg;
Phase 3 (7 days): 250•35 μg

Trinipatch ⓒᴬᴺ transdermal patch ℞ *antianginal; vasodilator* [nitroglycerin] 22.4, 44.8, 67.2 mg (0.2, 0.4, 0.6 mg/hr.)

trinitrin [see: nitroglycerin]

trinitrophenol NF

Tri-Norinyl tablets (in Wallettes of 28) ℞ *triphasic oral contraceptive* [norethindrone; ethinyl estradiol]

Phase 1 (7 days): 500•35 μg;
Phase 2 (9 days): 1000•35 μg;
Phase 3 (5 days): 500•35 μg

Trinsicon capsules ℞ *hematinic* [ferrous fumarate; cyanocobalamin; ascorbic acid; intrinsic factor concentrate; folic acid] 110 mg•15 μg•75 mg•240 mg•0.5 mg

2′,3′,5′-tri-o-acetyluridine *investigational (orphan) treatment for mitochondrial disease*

Triofed syrup (discontinued 2002) OTC *decongestant; antihistamine* [pseudoephedrine HCl; triprolidine HCl] 30•1.25 mg/5 mL

triolein I 125 USAN *radioactive agent*

triolein I 131 USAN *radioactive agent*

trional [see: sulfonethylmethane]

Trionate caplets ℞ *antitussive; antihistamine* [carbetapentane tannate; chlorpheniramine tannate] 60•5 mg

Triostat IV injection ℞ *synthetic thyroid hormone (T_3 fraction only) for myxedema coma or precoma (orphan)* [liothyronine sodium] 10 μg/mL ⑨ Threostat

Triotann tablets (discontinued 2002) ℞ *decongestant; antihistamine* [phenylephrine tannate; chlorpheniramine tannate; pyrilamine tannate] 25•8•25 mg

Triotann Pediatric; Triotann-S Pediatric oral suspension ℞ *decongestant; antihistamine* [phenylephrine tannate; chlorpheniramine tannate; pyrilamine tannate] 5•2•12.5 mg/5 mL

Tri-Otic ear drops ℞ *topical corticosteroidal anti-inflammatory; topical local anesthetic; antiseptic* [hydrocortisone; pramoxine HCl; chloroxylenol] 10•10•1 mg/mL

trioxifene INN *antiestrogen* [also: trioxifene mesylate]

trioxifene mesylate USAN *antiestrogen* [also: trioxifene]

trioxsalen USAN, USP *systemic psoralens for repigmentation of idiopathic vitiligo; also used to enhance pigmentation and increase tolerance to sunlight* [also: trioxysalen]

trioxyethylrutin [see: troxerutin]

trioxymethylene [see: paraformaldehyde]

trioxysalen INN *systemic psoralens for repigmentation of idiopathic vitiligo; also used to enhance pigmentation and increase tolerance to sunlight* [also: trioxsalen]

Tri-P oral infant drops (discontinued 2001) ℞ *decongestant; antihistamine* [phenylpropanolamine HCl; pyrilamine maleate; pheniramine maleate] 20•10•10 mg/mL

tripamide USAN, INN *antihypertensive; diuretic*

triparanol INN *(withdrawn from market)*

Tripedia IM injection ℞ *active immunizing agent for diphtheria, tetanus, and pertussis* [diphtheria & tetanus toxoids & acellular pertussis (DTaP) vaccine, adsorbed] 6.7 LfU•5 LfU•46.8 μg per 0.5 mL dose

tripelennamine INN *ethylenediamine antihistamine* [also: tripelennamine citrate]

tripelennamine citrate USP *ethylenediamine antihistamine* [also: tripelennamine]

tripelennamine HCl USP *ethylenediamine antihistamine*

Triphasil tablets (in packs of 21 or 28) ℞ *triphasic oral contraceptive; emergency postcoital contraceptive* [levonorgestrel; ethinyl estradiol]
Phase 1 (6 days): 50•30 μg;
Phase 2 (5 days): 75•40 μg;
Phase 3 (10 days): 125•30 μg

Tri-Phen-Chlor syrup, pediatric syrup, pediatric drops (discontinued 2001) ℞ *decongestant; antihistamine* [phenylpropanolamine HCl; phenylephrine HCl; chlorpheniramine maleate; phenyltoloxamine citrate] 20•5•2.5•7.5 mg/5 mL; 5•1.25•0.5•2 mg/5 mL; 5•1.25•0.5•2 mg/mL

Tri-Phen-Chlor T.R. timed-release tablets (discontinued 2002) ℞ *decongestant; antihistamine* [phenylpropanolamine HCl; phenylephrine HCl;

chlorpheniramine maleate; phenyltoloxamine citrate] 40•10•5•15 mg

Tri-Phen-Mine syrup, oral drops (discontinued 2001) ℞ *pediatric decongestant and antihistamine* [phenylpropanolamine HCl; phenylephrine HCl; chlorpheniramine maleate; phenyltoloxamine citrate] 5•1.25•0.5•2 mg/5 mL; 5•1.25•0.5•2 mg/mL

Tri-Phen-Mine S.R. timed-release tablets (discontinued 2002) ℞ *decongestant; antihistamine* [phenylpropanolamine HCl; phenylephrine HCl; chlorpheniramine maleate; phenyltoloxamine citrate] 40•10•5•15 mg

Triphenyl syrup (discontinued 2001) OTC *decongestant; antihistamine* [phenylpropanolamine HCl; chlorpheniramine maleate] 6.25•1 mg/5 mL

Triphenyl Expectorant oral liquid (discontinued 2002) OTC *decongestant; expectorant* [phenylpropanolamine HCl; guaifenesin; alcohol 5%] 12.5•100 mg/5 mL

Triple Antibiotic ointment OTC *antibiotic* [polymyxin B sulfate; neomycin sulfate; bacitracin] 5000 U•3.5 mg•400 U per g

Triple Antibiotic Plus ointment (discontinued 2003) OTC *antibiotic; local anesthetic* [polymyxin B sulfate; neomycin sulfate; bacitracin zinc; pramoxine HCl] 10 000 U•3.5 mg•500 U•10 mg per g

Triple Sulfa vaginal cream (discontinued 2001) ℞ *broad-spectrum antibiotic* [sulfathiazole; sulfacetamide; sulfabenzamide] 3.42%•2.86%•3.7%

triple sulfa (sulfathiazole, sulfacetamide, and sulfabenzamide) [q.v.]

Triple Vitamin ADC with Fluoride drops ℞ *pediatric vitamin supplement and dental caries preventative* [vitamins A, C, and D; fluoride] 1500 IU•35 mg•400 IU•0.5 mg per mL

Triple X Kit topical liquid + shampoo (discontinued 2003) OTC *pediculicide for lice* [pyrethrins; piperonyl butoxide; petroleum distillate] 0.3%•3%• ≟

Triposed tablets, syrup (discontinued 2002) OTC *decongestant; antihistamine* [pseudoephedrine HCl; triprolidine HCl] 60•2.5 mg; 30•1.25 mg/5 mL

tripotassium citrate monohydrate [see: potassium citrate]

Tri-Previfem tablets (in packs of 28) ℞ *triphasic oral contraceptive* [norgestimate; ethinyl estradiol]
Phase 1 (7 days): 180•35 μg;
Phase 2 (7 days): 215•35 μg;
Phase 3 (7 days): 250•35 μg

triproamylin [see: pramlintide]

triprolidine INN *antihistamine* [also: triprolidine HCl]

triprolidine HCl USP *antihistamine* [also: triprolidine]

triprolidine HCl & pseudoephedrine HCl *antihistamine; decongestant* 2.5•60 mg oral

Tripterygium wilfordii medicinal herb [see: thunder god vine]

Triptone long-acting caplets OTC *antinauseant; antiemetic; antivertigo; motion sickness preventative* [dimenhydrinate] 50 mg

triptorelin USAN, INN *gonadotropin-releasing hormone (GnRH) antineoplastic*

triptorelin pamoate *gonadotropin-releasing hormone (GnRH) antineoplastic for palliative treatment of advanced prostate cancer*

trisaccharides A & B *investigational (orphan) for newborn hemolytic disease and ABO blood incompatibility of organ or bone marrow transplants*

Trisan ⓒⒶⓃ foaming gel OTC *medicated cleanser for acne* [triclosan] 0.25%

Trisenox injection ℞ *antineoplastic for acute promyelocytic leukemia (orphan); investigational (NDA filed) for renal cell carcinoma; investigational (orphan) for multiple myeloma and myelodysplastic syndromes* [arsenic trioxide] 10 mg/10 mL

trisodium citrate [see: sodium citrate]

trisodium citrate dihydrate [see: sodium citrate]

trisodium hydrogen ethylenediaminetetraacetate [see: edetate trisodium]

Trisoralen tablets (discontinued 2003) ℞ *systemic psoralens for repigmentation of idiopathic vitiligo; also used to enhance pigmentation and increase tolerance to sunlight* [trioxsalen] 5 mg

Tri-Sprintec tablets (in packs of 28) ℞ *triphasic oral contraceptive* [norgestimate; ethinyl estradiol]
Phase 1 (7 days): 180•35 μg;
Phase 2 (7 days): 215•35 μg;
Phase 3 (7 days): 250•35 μg

Tri-Statin II cream ℞ *topical corticosteroidal anti-inflammatory; antifungal* [triamcinolone acetonide; nystatin] 0.1%•100 000 U per g

Tristoject IM injection ℞ *corticosteroid; anti-inflammatory* [triamcinolone diacetate] 40 mg/mL

trisulfapyrimidines USP (a mixture of sulfadiazine, sulfamerazine, and sulfamethazine) *broad-spectrum bacteriostatic*

Tri-Super Flavons 1000 tablets OTC *dietary supplement* [mixed bioflavonoids] 1000 mg

Tritan tablets (discontinued 2002) ℞ *decongestant; antihistamine* [phenylephrine tannate; chlorpheniramine tannate; pyrilamine tannate] 25•8• 25 mg

Tri-Tannate tablets, pediatric oral suspension (discontinued 2002) ℞ *decongestant; antihistamine* [phenylephrine tannate; chlorpheniramine tannate; pyrilamine tannate] 25•8• 25 mg; 5•2•12.5 mg/5 mL

Tri-Tannate Plus Pediatric oral suspension (discontinued 2002) ℞ *antitussive; decongestant; antihistamine* [carbetapentane tannate; phenylephrine tannate; ephedrine tannate; chlorpheniramine tannate] 30•5• 5•4 mg/5 mL

Tritec film-coated tablets (discontinued 2004) ℞ *histamine H_2 antagonist for duodenal ulcers with H. pylori infection* [ranitidine bismuth citrate] 400 mg

tritheon [see: acinitrazole]

tritiated water USAN *radioactive agent*

Triticum repens *medicinal herb* [see: couch grass]

tritiozine INN

tritoqualine INN

Triva Douche powder (discontinued 2003) OTC *antiseptic/germicidal; vaginal cleanser and deodorizer* [oxyquinoline sulfate] 2%

Trivagizole 3 vaginal cream OTC *topical antifungal for yeast infections* [clotrimazole] 2%

trivalent oral poliovirus vaccine (TOPV) [see: poliovirus vaccine, live oral]

Tri-Vi-Flor chewable tablets, drops ℞ *pediatric vitamin supplement and dental caries preventative* [vitamins A, C, and D; sodium fluoride] 2500 IU•60 mg•400 IU•1 mg; 1500 IU•35 mg•400 IU•0.25 mg, 1500 IU•35 mg•400 IU•0.5 mg per mL

Tri-Vi-Flor with Iron drops ℞ *pediatric vitamin/iron supplement and dental caries preventative* [vitamins A, C, and D; iron; sodium fluoride] 1500 IU•35 mg•400 IU•0.25 mg per mL

Tri-Vi-Sol drops OTC *pediatric vitamin supplement* [vitamins A, C, and D] 1500 IU•35 mg•400 IU per mL

Tri-Vi-Sol with Iron drops OTC *vitamin/iron supplement* [vitamins A, C, and D; ferrous sulfate] 1500 IU•35 mg•400 IU•10 mg per mL

Trivitamin Fluoride chewable tablets, drops ℞ *pediatric vitamin supplement and dental caries preventative* [vitamins A, C, and D; fluoride] 2500 IU•60 mg•400 IU•1 mg; 1500 IU•35 mg•400 IU•0.25 mg, 1500 IU•35 mg•400 IU•0.5 mg per mL

Tri-Vitamin Infants' Drops OTC *vitamin supplement* [vitamins A, C, and D] 1500 IU•35 mg•400 IU per mL

Tri-Vitamin with Fluoride drops ℞ *pediatric vitamin supplement and dental caries preventative* [vitamins A, C, and D; fluoride] 1500 IU•35 mg•400 IU•0.5 mg per mL

Trivora tablets (in packs of 28) ℞ *triphasic oral contraceptive* [levonorgestrel; ethinyl estradiol]
Phase 1 (6 days): 50•30 μg;
Phase 2 (5 days): 75•40 μg;
Phase 3 (10 days): 125•30 μg

trixolane INN

Trizivir film-coated caplets ℞ *antiretroviral nucleoside reverse transcriptase inhibitor (NRTI) for HIV infection* [abacavir sulfate; zidovudine; lamivudine] 300•300•150 mg

trizoxime INN

Trizyme (ingredient) OTC *digestive enzymes* [amylolytic, proteolytic, and cellulolytic enzymes (amylase; protease; cellulase)]

Trobicin powder for IM injection ℞ *antibiotic for gonorrhea* [spectinomycin HCl] 400 mg/mL ⑨ tobramycin

Trocade ℞ *matrix metalloproteinase inhibitor; investigational cartilage protective agent for rheumatoid arthritis* [cipemastat]

Trocaine lozenges OTC *topical oral anesthetic* [benzocaine] 10 mg

Trocal lozenges OTC *antitussive* [dextromethorphan hydrobromide] 7.5 mg

trocimine INN

troclosene potassium USAN, INN *topical anti-infective*

trofosfamide INN

troglitazone USAN, INN *thiazolidinedione antidiabetic; increases cellular response to insulin without increasing insulin secretion*

trolamine USAN, NF *alkalizing agent; analgesic*

trolamine polypeptide oleate-condensate *cerumenolytic to emulsify and disperse ear wax*

trolamine salicylate *topical analgesic*

troleandomycin USAN, USP *macrolide antibiotic; investigational (orphan) for severe asthma* [also: triacetyloleandomycin]

trolnitrate INN

trolnitrate phosphate [see: trolnitrate]

tromantadine INN

trometamol INN, BAN *alkalizer for cardiac bypass surgery* [also: tromethamine]

tromethamine USAN, USP *alkalizer for cardiac bypass surgery* [also: trometamol]

Tronolane anorectal cream OTC *topical local anesthetic* [pramoxine HCl] 1% 🔃 Tronothane

Tronolane rectal suppositories OTC *astringent; emollient* [zinc oxide] 11%

Tronothane HCl cream OTC *topical local anesthetic* [pramoxine HCl] 1% 🔃 Tronolane

tropabazate INN

Tropaeolum majus medicinal herb [see: Indian cress]

tropanserin INN, BAN *migraine-specific serotonin receptor antagonist* [also: tropanserin HCl]

tropanserin HCl USAN *migraine-specific serotonin receptor antagonist* [also: tropanserin]

tropapride INN

tropatepine INN

tropenziline bromide INN

TrophAmine 6%; TrophAmine 10% IV infusion R *total parenteral nutrition; peripheral parenteral nutrition* [multiple essential and nonessential amino acids]

Trophite + Iron oral liquid OTC *hematinic* [ferric pyrophosphate; vitamins B_1 and B_{12}] 60 mg•30 mg•75 μg per 15 mL

trophosphamide [see: trofosfamide]

Tropicacyl eye drops R *cycloplegic; mydriatic* [tropicamide] 0.5%, 1%

tropicamide USAN, USP, INN *ophthalmic anticholinergic; cycloplegic; short-acting mydriatic*

tropigline INN, BAN

tropirine INN

tropisetron INN, BAN *investigational treatment for nausea and vomiting related to chemotherapy*

Tropi-Storz eye drops R *cycloplegic; mydriatic* [tropicamide] 0.5%, 1%

tropodifene INN

troquidazole INN

trospectomycin INN, BAN *investigational (Phase III) broad-spectrum aminocyclitol antibiotic* [also: trospectomycin sulfate]

trospectomycin sulfate USAN *broad-spectrum aminocyclitol antibiotic* [also: trospectomycin]

trospium chloride INN *muscarinic receptor antagonist for urinary frequency, urgency, and incontinence*

trovafloxacin mesylate USAN *broad-spectrum fluoroquinolone antibiotic*

Trovan film-coated tablets R *broad-spectrum fluoroquinolone antibiotic* [trovafloxacin mesylate] 100, 200 mg

Trovan IV infusion R *broad-spectrum fluoroquinolone antibiotic* [alatrofloxacin mesylate] 5 mg/mL 🔃 Atrovent

Trovan/Zithromax Compliance Pak R *single-dose antibiotic treatment for sexually transmitted diseases* [Trovan (trovafloxacin mesylate); Zithromax (azithromycin)] 100 mg tablet; 1 g pkt. of powder for oral suspension

troxacitabine USAN, INN *antineoplastic for various leukemias and solid tumors*

troxerutin INN, BAN *vitamin P_4*

troxidone BAN *anticonvulsant* [also: trimethadione]

troxipide INN

troxolamide INN

troxonium tosilate INN [also: troxonium tosylate]

troxonium tosylate BAN [also: troxonium tosilate]

troxundate INN *combining name for radicals or groups*

troxypyrrolium tosilate INN [also: troxypyrrolium tosylate]

troxypyrrolium tosylate BAN [also: troxypyrrolium tosilate]

true ivy medicinal herb [see: English ivy]

T.R.U.E. Test patch *diagnostic aid for contact dermatitis* [skin test antigens (23 different) plus 1 negative control]

Trugene genetic testing system for professional use *in vitro diagnostic aid for HIV mutations that cause resistance to anti-AIDS drugs; used to determine* which treatment regimen is most effective in individual patients

Truphylline suppositories ℞ antiasthmatic; bronchodilator [aminophylline] 250, 500 mg

Trusopt eye drops ℞ carbonic anhydrase inhibitor for glaucoma [dorzolamide HCl] 2%

Truvada film-coated caplets ℞ once-daily nucleoside reverse transcriptase inhibitor (NRTI) antiviral combination for HIV infections [emtricitabine; tenofovir disoproxil fumarate] 200•300 mg

truxicurium iodide INN

truxipicurium iodide INN

Trycet film-coated caplets ℞ narcotic analgesic [propoxyphene napsylate; acetaminophen] 100•325 mg

trypaflavine [see: acriflavine HCl]

trypan blue surgical aid for staining the anterior capsule of the lens

tryparsamide USP, INN

trypsin, crystallized USP topical proteolytic enzyme; necrotic tissue debridement

tryptizol [see: amitriptyline]

tryptizol HCl [see: amitriptyline HCl]

tryptophan (L-tryptophan) USAN, USP, INN essential amino acid; serotonin precursor (The FDA has banned all OTC tryptophan supplements.)

Trysul vaginal cream (discontinued 2001) ℞ broad-spectrum antibiotic [sulfathiazole; sulfacetamide; sulfabenzamide] 3.42%•2.86%•3.7%

TSC (technetium sulfur colloid) [see: technetium Tc 99m sulfur colloid]

T/Scalp topical liquid OTC corticosteroidal anti-inflammatory [hydrocortisone] 1%

TSH (thyroid-stimulating hormone) [see: thyrotropin]

TSPA (triethylenethiophosphoramide) [see: thiotepa]

TST (tuberculin skin test) [see: tuberculin]

T-Stat topical solution, medicated pads (discontinued 2004) ℞ antibiotic for acne [erythromycin; alcohol 71.2%] 2%

Tsuga canadensis medicinal herb [see: hemlock]

T-Tabs (trademarked form) tablets with a "T" imprint

tuaminoheptane USP, INN adrenergic; vasoconstrictor

tuaminoheptane sulfate USP

tuberculin USP tuberculosis skin test

tuberculin, crude [see: tuberculin]

tuberculin, old (OT) [see: tuberculin]

tuberculin purified protein derivative (PPD) [see: tuberculin]

Tuberculin Tine Test, Old single-use intradermal puncture test device (discontinued 2002) tuberculosis skin test [old tuberculin] 5 U

tuberculosis vaccine [see: BCG vaccine]

Tubersol intradermal injection ℞ tuberculosis skin test [tuberculin purified protein derivative] 5 U/0.1 mL

Tubex (trademarked delivery system) cartridge-needle unit

tubocurarine chloride USP, INN, BAN neuromuscular blocker; muscle relaxant 3 mg (20 U)/mL injection

tubocurarine chloride HCl pentahydrate [see: tubocurarine chloride]

tubulozole INN antineoplastic; microtubule inhibitor [also: tubulozole HCl]

tubulozole HCl USAN, INN antineoplastic; microtubule inhibitor [also: tubulozole]

tucaresol INN, BAN investigational (Phase II) immunopotentiator for HIV infection

Tucks; Tucks Take-Alongs cleansing pads OTC moisturizer and cleanser for the perineal area; astringent [witch hazel; glycerin] 50%•10%

Tucks Clear gel OTC astringent [hamamelis water; glycerin] 50%•10%

tuclazepam INN

Tuinal Pulvules (capsules) ℞ sedative; hypnotic; also abused as a street drug [amobarbital sodium; secobarbital sodium] 50•50, 100•100 mg ② Luminal; Tylenol

tulobuterol INN, BAN, JAN [also: tulobuterol HCl]

tulobuterol HCl JAN [also: tulobuterol]

tulopafant INN

tumeric root *medicinal herb* [see: goldenseal]

tumor necrosis factor-binding protein I and II *investigational (orphan) for symptomatic AIDS patients*

Tums; Tums E-X; Tums Ultra; Tums Calcium for Life PMS; Tums Calcium for Life Bone Health chewable tablets OTC *antacid; calcium supplement* [calcium carbonate] 500 mg (200 mg Ca); 750 mg (300 mg Ca); 1 g (400 mg Ca); 750 mg (300 mg Ca); 1250 mg (500 mg Ca)

Tums Smooth Dissolve (orally disintegrating tablets) OTC *antacid; calcium supplement* [calcium carbonate] 750 mg (300 mg Ca)

tung seed (Aleurites cordata; A. moluccana) seed and oil *medicinal herb for asthma, bowel evacuation, and tumors; not generally regarded as safe and effective as it is highly toxic*

tungsten *element (W)*

Turbinaire (trademarked delivery system) *nasal inhalation aerosol*

Turbuhaler (trademarked delivery system) *dry powder in a metered-dose inhaler*

turkey corn (Corydalis formosa) root *medicinal herb used as an antisyphilitic, bitter tonic, and diuretic*

turkey pea; wild turkey pea *medicinal herb* [see: turkey corn]

turmeric (Curcuma domestica; C. longa) rhizomes *medicinal herb for flatulence, hemorrhage, hepatitis and jaundice, topical analgesia, and ringworm*

Turnera aphrodisiaca; T. diffusa; T. microphylla *medicinal herb* [see: damiana]

turosteride INN

turpentine (Pinus palustris) gum *natural treatment for colds, cough, and toothache; also used topically as a counterirritant for muscle pain and rheumatic disorders*

turtlebloom (Chelone glabra) leaves *medicinal herb used as an anthelmintic, aperient, cholagogue, and detergent*

Tusibron syrup (discontinued 2002) OTC *expectorant* [guaifenesin; alcohol 3.5%] 100 mg/5 mL ⊘ Tussigon

Tusibron-DM syrup (discontinued 2002) OTC *antitussive; expectorant* [dextromethorphan hydrobromide; guaifenesin] 15•100 mg/5 mL

Tusquelin syrup (discontinued 2002) ℞ *antitussive; decongestant; antihistamine; analgesic* [dextromethorphan hydrobromide; phenylpropanolamine HCl; phenylephrine HCl; chlorpheniramine maleate; alcohol 5%] 15•5•5•2 mg/5 mL

Tussafed pediatric oral drops (discontinued 2002) ℞ *antitussive; decongestant; antihistamine* [dextromethorphan hydrobromide; pseudoephedrine HCl; carbinoxamine maleate; menthol] 4•25•2 mg/mL ⊘ Tussafin

Tussafed syrup ℞ *antitussive; decongestant; antihistamine* [dextromethorphan hydrobromide; pseudoephedrine HCl; carbinoxamine maleate; menthol] 15•60•4 mg/5 mL ⊘ Tussafin

Tussafed HC syrup ℞ *narcotic antitussive; decongestant; expectorant* [hydrocodone bitartrate; phenylephrine HCl; guaifenesin] 5•15•100 mg/10 mL

Tussafed-LA sustained-release caplets ℞ *antitussive; decongestant; expectorant* [dextromethorphan hydrobromide; pseudoephedrine HCl; guaifenesin] 30•60•600 mg

Tussafin Expectorant oral liquid (discontinued 2002) ℞ *narcotic antitussive; decongestant; expectorant* [hydrocodone bitartrate; pseudoephedrine HCl; guaifenesin; alcohol 12.5%] 5•60•200 mg/5 mL ⊘ Tussafed

Tuss-Allergine Modified T.D. capsules (discontinued 2002) ℞ *antitussive; decongestant* [caramiphen edisylate; phenylpropanolamine HCl] 40•75 mg

Tussanil DH syrup (discontinued 2002) ℞ *narcotic antitussive; decongestant; antihistamine* [hydrocodone bitartrate; phenylephrine HCl; chlorpheniramine maleate; alcohol 5%] 2.5•10•4 mg/5 mL

Tussanil DH tablets (discontinued 2002) ℞ *narcotic antitussive; decongestant; expectorant; analgesic* [hydrocodone bitartrate; phenylpropanolamine HCl; guaifenesin; salicylamide] 1.66•25•100•300 mg

Tussar DM syrup (discontinued 2002) OTC *antitussive; decongestant; antihistamine* [dextromethorphan hydrobromide; pseudoephedrine HCl; chlorpheniramine maleate] 15•30•2 mg/5 mL

Tussar SF; Tussar-2 oral liquid (discontinued 2002) ℞ *narcotic antitussive; antihistamine; expectorant* [codeine phosphate; pseudoephedrine HCl; guaifenesin; alcohol 2.5%] 10•30•100 mg/5 mL

Tuss-DM tablets OTC *antitussive; expectorant* [dextromethorphan hydrobromide; guaifenesin] 10•200 mg

Tussend caplets ℞ *narcotic antitussive; decongestant; antihistamine* [hydrocodone bitartrate; pseudoephedrine HCl; chlorpheniramine maleate] 5•60•4 mg

Tussend syrup ℞ *narcotic antitussive; decongestant; antihistamine* [hydrocodone bitartrate; pseudoephedrine HCl; chlorpheniramine maleate; alcohol 5%] 5•60•4 mg/10 mL

Tussex Cough syrup (discontinued 2002) OTC *antitussive; decongestant; expectorant* [dextromethorphan hydrobromide; phenylephrine HCl; guaifenesin] 10•5•100 mg/5 mL ⊠ Tussionex; Tussirex

Tussi-12 caplets, pediatric oral suspension ℞ *antitussive; antihistamine* [carbetapentane tannate; chlorpheniramine tannate] 60•5 mg; 30•4 mg/5 mL

Tussi-12 D caplets ℞ *decongestant; antihistamine; antitussive* [phenylephrine tannate; pyrilamine tannate; carbetapentane tannate] 10•40•60 mg

Tussi-12D S oral suspension ℞ *decongestant; antihistamine; antitussive* [phenylephrine tannate; pyrilamine tannate; carbetapentane tannate] 5•30•30 mg/5 mL

Tussi-bid sustained-release caplets ℞ *antitussive; expectorant* [dextromethorphan hydrobromide; guaifenesin] 60•1200 mg

Tussigon tablets ℞ *narcotic antitussive; anticholinergic* [hydrocodone bitartrate; homatropine methylbromide] 5•1.5 mg ⊠ Tusibron

Tussilago farfara medicinal herb [see: coltsfoot]

Tussionex Pennkinetic extended-release oral suspension ℞ *narcotic antitussive; antihistamine* [hydrocodone polistirex; chlorpheniramine polistirex] 10•8 mg/5 mL ⊠ Tussex; Tussirex

Tussi-Organidin DM NR oral liquid ℞ *antitussive; expectorant* [dextromethorphan hydrobromide; guaifenesin] 20•200 mg/10 mL

Tussi-Organidin NR; Tussi-Organidin-S NR oral liquid (S includes a 10 mL oral syringe) ℞ *narcotic antitussive; expectorant* [codeine phosphate; guaifenesin] 20•200 mg/10 mL

Tussi-Pres oral liquid ℞ *antitussive; decongestant; expectorant* [dextromethorphan hydrobromide; phenylephrine HCl; guaifenesin] 15•5•200 mg/5 mL

Tussirex syrup, sugar-free oral liquid (discontinued 2002) ℞ *narcotic antitussive; decongestant; antihistamine; expectorant; analgesic* [codeine phosphate; phenylephrine HCl; pheniramine maleate; sodium citrate; sodium salicylate; caffeine citrate] 10•4.17•13.33•83.3•83.33•25 mg/5 mL ⊠ Tussex; Tussionex

Tussizone-12 RF caplets, pediatric oral suspension ℞ *antitussive; antihistamine* [carbetapentane tannate;

chlorpheniramine tannate] 60•5 mg; 30•4 mg/5 mL

Tuss-LA sustained-release tablets (discontinued 2002) ℞ *decongestant; expectorant* [pseudoephedrine HCl; guaifenesin] 120•500 mg

Tusso-DM oral liquid (discontinued 2002) ℞ *antitussive; expectorant* [dextromethorphan hydrobromide; iodinated glycerol] 10•30 mg/5 mL

Tussogest extended-release capsules (discontinued 2002) ℞ *antitussive; decongestant* [caramiphen edisylate; phenylpropanolamine HCl] 40•75 mg

Tuss-Tan tablets, pediatric oral suspension ℞ *antitussive; decongestant; antihistamine* [carbetapentane tannate; phenylephrine tannate; ephedrine tannate; chlorpheniramine tannate] 60•10•10•5 mg; 30•5•5•4 mg/5 mL

Tusstat syrup ℞ *antihistamine* [diphenhydramine HCl; alcohol 5%] 12.5 mg/5 mL

tuvatidine INN

tuvirumab USAN, INN *investigational (Phase II) antiviral monoclonal antibody for hepatitis B*

T-Vites tablets OTC *vitamin/mineral supplement* [multiple vitamins & minerals; biotin] ±•30 µg

12 Hour nasal spray OTC *nasal decongestant* [oxymetazoline HCl] 0.05%

12 Hour Cold sustained-release tablets (discontinued 2002) OTC *decongestant; antihistamine* [pseudoephedrine sulfate; dexbrompheniramine maleate] 120•6 mg

Twelve Resin-K tablets OTC *vitamin B_{12} supplement* [cyanocobalamin on resin] 1000 µg

Twice-A-Day 12-Hour nasal spray OTC *nasal decongestant* [oxymetazoline HCl] 0.05%

Twilite caplets OTC *antihistaminic sleep aid* [diphenhydramine HCl] 50 mg

twin leaf (*Jeffersonia diphylla*) root *medicinal herb used as an antirheumatic, antispasmodic, antisyphilitic, diuretic, emetic, and expectorant*

Twinject injection ℞ *sympathomimetic bronchodilator for bronchial asthma, bronchospasm, and COPD; vasopressor for shock* [epinephrine HCl]

Twin-K oral liquid ℞ *potassium supplement* [potassium gluconate; potassium citrate] 20 mEq K/15 mL

Twinrix IM injection ℞ *immunizing agent for hepatitis A, B, and D in adults* [hepatitis A vaccine, inactivated; hepatitis B virus vaccine, recombinant] 720 EL.U.•20 µg per mL

TwoCal HN ready-to-use oral liquid OTC *enteral nutritional therapy* [lactose-free formula]

tybamate USAN, NF, INN, BAN *minor tranquilizer*

tyformin BAN [also: tiformin]

Tygacil powder for IV infusion ℞ *broad-spectrum glycylcycline antibiotic for intra-abdominal and complicated skin structure infections and methicillin-resistant* Staphylococcus aureus (MRSA) [tigecycline] 50 mg/vial

tylcalsin [see: calcium acetylsalicylate]

tylemalum [see: carburbarb]

Tylenol tablets, caplets, gelcaps, oral liquid OTC *analgesic; antipyretic* [acetaminophen] 325, 500 mg; 325, 650 mg; 500 mg; 500 mg/15 mL 𝕫 Tuinal

Tylenol, Children's chewable tablets, oral liquid OTC *analgesic; antipyretic* [acetaminophen] 80 mg; 160 mg/5 mL

Tylenol, Children's Ⓖ oral suspension OTC *analgesic; antipyretic* [acetaminophen] 32 mg/mL

Tylenol 8 Hour extended-release geltabs, extended-release caplets OTC *analgesic; antipyretic* [acetaminophen] 650 mg

Tylenol Allergy Complete Multi-Symptom caplets, gelcaps, geltabs OTC *decongestant; antihistamine; analgesic* [pseudoephedrine HCl; chlorpheniramine maleate; acetaminophen] 30•2•500 mg

Tylenol Allergy Complete Night-Time caplets OTC *decongestant; antihistamine; analgesic* [pseudoephedrine

HCl; diphenhydramine HCl; aceta-
minophen] 30•25•500 mg

Tylenol Allergy Sinus caplets, gelcaps, geltabs (name changed to
Tylenol Complete Multi-Symptom
in 2005)

Tylenol Allergy Sinus NightTime
caplets (name changed to **Tylenol
Allergy Complete NightTime** in
2005)

Tylenol Arthritis Extended Relief
extended-release caplets OTC *analgesic;
antipyretic* [acetaminophen] 650 mg

Tylenol Children's Cold chewable
tablets, oral liquid OTC *decongestant;
antihistamine; analgesic* [pseudo-
ephedrine HCl; chlorpheniramine
maleate; acetaminophen] 7.5•0.5•
80 mg; 15•1•160 mg/10 mL

Tylenol Children's Cold Plus Cough
chewable tablets, oral suspension
OTC *antitussive; decongestant; antihistamine; analgesic* [dextromethorphan
hydrobromide; pseudoephedrine
HCl; chlorpheniramine maleate;
acetaminophen] 2.5•7.5•0.5•80
mg; 10•30•2•320 mg/10 mL

Tylenol Children's Flu oral suspension OTC *antitussive; decongestant;
antihistamine; analgesic* [dextometh-
orphan hydrobromide; pseudoephedrine HCl; chlorpheniramine maleate; acetaminophen] 15•30•2•320
mg/10 mL

Tylenol Children's Plus Cold oral
suspension OTC *decongestant; analgesic; antipyretic* [pseudoephedrine HCl;
acetaminophen] 15•160 mg/5 mL

Tylenol Children's Sinus oral suspension (name changed to **Tylenol
Children's Plus Cold** in 2005)

Tylenol Cold, Children's chewable
tablets, oral liquid OTC *pediatric decongestant, antihistamine and analgesic*
[pseudoephedrine HCl; chlorpheniramine maleate; acetaminophen] 7.5•
0.5•80 mg; 15•1•160 mg/5 mL

Tylenol Cold Day Non-Drowsy caplets, gelcaps OTC *antitussive; decongestant; analgesic* [dextromethorphan

hydrobromide; pseudoephedrine HCl;
acetaminophen] 15•30•325 mg

**Tylenol Cold Night Time Complete
Formula** caplets OTC *antitussive;
decongestant; antihistamine; analgesic*
[dextromethorphan hydrobromide;
pseudoephedrine HCl; chlorpheniramine maleate; acetaminophen] 15•
30•2•325 mg

Tylenol Cold Severe Congestion
caplets OTC *antitussive; decongestant;
expectorant; analgesic* [dextromethor-
phan hydrobromide; pseudoephedrine HCl; guaifenesin; acetamino-
phen] 15•30•200•325 mg

Tylenol Cough, Multi-Symptom
oral liquid (discontinued 2002) OTC
antitussive; analgesic [dextromethor-
phan hydrobromide; acetaminophen;
alcohol 5%] 10•216.7 mg/5 mL

**Tylenol Cough with Decongestant,
Multi-Symptom** oral liquid (discontinued 2002) OTC *antitussive;
decongestant; analgesic* [dextometh-
orphan hydrobromide; pseudoephedrine HCl; acetaminophen; alcohol
5%] 10•20•200 mg/5 mL

Tylenol Flu, Tylenol Flu Night Time
gelcaps OTC *decongestant; antihistamine; analgesic* [pseudoephedrine
HCl; diphenhydramine HCl; aceta-
minophen] 30•25•500 mg

Tylenol Flu Night Time oral liquid
OTC *antitussive; decongestant; antihistamine; analgesic* [dextromethorphan
hydrobromide; pseudoephedrine HCl;
doxylamine succinate; acetamino-
phen] 30•60•12.5•1000 mg/30 mL

Tylenol Flu NightTime powder for
oral solution (discontinued 2002)
OTC *decongestant; antihistamine; analgesic* [pseudoephedrine HCl; diphenhydramine HCl; acetaminophen]
60•50•1000 mg/pkt.

Tylenol Flu Non-Drowsy gelcaps
OTC *antitussive; decongestant; analgesic* [dextromethorphan hydrobromide; pseudoephedrine HCl; aceta-
minophen] 15•30•500 mg

Tylenol Fruit; Tylenol Junior Fruit
ⓒᴬᴺ chewable tablets OTC *analgesic;
antipyretic* [acetaminophen] 80 mg;
160 mg

Tylenol Infant's Cold concentrated
oral drops (name changed to **Tylenol
Infant's Drops Plus Cold** in 2005)

**Tylenol Infants' Cold, Decongestant, & Fever Reducer Plus
Cough** concentrated oral drops OTC
*antitussive; decongestant; analgesic;
antipyretic* [dextromethorphan hydrobromide; pseudoephedrine HCl; acetaminophen] 5•15•160 mg/1.6 mL

Tylenol Infants' Drops ⓒᴬᴺ oral suspension OTC *analgesic; antipyretic*
[acetaminophen] 80 mg/mL

Tylenol Infants' Drops solution OTC
analgesic; antipyretic [acetaminophen]
100 mg/mL

Tylenol Infant's Drops Plus Cold
OTC *decongestant; analgesic; antipyretic* [pseudoephedrine HCl; acetaminophen] 15•160 mg/1.6 mL

Tylenol Junior Strength chewable
tablets OTC *analgesic; antipyretic*
[acetaminophen] 160 mg

Tylenol Menstrual ⓒᴬᴺ tablets OTC
analgesic; diuretic; antihistamine [acetaminophen; pamabrom; pyrilamine
maleate] 500•25•15 mg

**Tylenol Multi-Symptom Cold
Severe Congestion** caplets (name
changed to **Tylenol Cold Severe
Congestion** in 2005)

Tylenol Multi-Symptom Hot Medication powder for oral solution (discontinued 2002) OTC *antitussive;
decongestant; antihistamine; analgesic*
[dextromethorphan hydrobromide;
pseudoephedrine HCl; chlorpheniramine maleate; acetaminophen] 30•
60•4•650 mg/pkt.

**Tylenol Multi-Symptom Menstrual
Relief, Women's** caplets OTC *analgesic; diuretic* [acetaminophen; pamabrom] 500•25 mg

Tylenol No. 2, No. 3, and No. 4
[see: Tylenol with Codeine]

Tylenol PM tablets, caplets, gelcaps
OTC *analgesic; antihistaminic sleep aid*
[acetaminophen; diphenhydramine
HCl] 500•25 mg

Tylenol Severe Allergy caplets OTC
antihistamine; analgesic [diphenhydramine HCl; acetaminophen] 12.5•
500 mg

Tylenol Sinus Night Time caplets
OTC *decongestant; antihistamine; analgesic* [pseudoephedrine HCl; doxylamine succinate; acetaminophen]
30•6.25•500 mg

Tylenol Sinus Non-Drowsy caplets,
geltabs, gelcaps OTC *decongestant;
analgesic; antipyretic* [pseudoephedrine
HCl; acetaminophen] 30•500 mg

Tylenol Sinus Severe Congestion
caplets OTC *decongestant; expectorant;
analgesic* [pseudoephedrine HCl;
guaifenesin; acetaminophen] 30•
200•325 mg

Tylenol Sore Throat oral liquid OTC
analgesic; antipyretic [acetaminophen]
1000 mg/30 mL

Tylenol with Codeine elixir ℞ *narcotic antitussive; analgesic* [codeine
phosphate; acetaminophen] 12•120
mg/5 mL

**Tylenol with Codeine No. 2, No. 3,
and No. 4** tablets ℞ *narcotic antitussive; analgesic; sometimes abused as a
street drug* [codeine phosphate; acetaminophen] 15•300 mg; 30•300
mg; 60•300 mg

tylosin INN, BAN

Tylox capsules ℞ *narcotic analgesic*
[oxycodone HCl; acetaminophen]
5•500 mg

tyloxapol USAN, USP, INN, BAN *detergent; wetting agent; cleaner/lubricant
for artificial eyes; investigational
(orphan) for cystic fibrosis*

Tympagesic ear drops ℞ *topical local
anesthetic; analgesic; decongestant*
[benzocaine; antipyrine; phenylephrine HCl] 5%•5%•0.25%

Typherix ⓒᴬᴺ IM injection in prefilled
syringe ℞ *typhoid vaccine for adults
and children over 2 years* [typhoid

vaccine (Ty-2), Vi polysaccharide] 25 µg/0.5 mL

Typhim Vi IM injection ℞ *typhoid vaccine for adults and children over 2 years* [typhoid vaccine (Ty-2), Vi polysaccharide] 25 µg/0.5 mL dose

typhoid vaccine USP *active bacterin for typhoid fever (Salmonella typhi Ty21a, attenuated)*

Typhoid Vaccine (AKD) subcu injection by jet injectors only ℞ *typhoid vaccine for military use only* [typhoid vaccine (Ty-2), acetone-killed and dried] 8 U/mL

Typhoid Vaccine (H-P) subcu injection (discontinued 2003) ℞ *typhoid vaccine for adults and children* [typhoid vaccine (Ty-2), heat- and phenol-inactivated] 8 U/mL

typhoid Vi capsular polysaccharide vaccine *active bacterin for typhoid fever (Salmonella typhi Ty-2, inactivated)*

typhus vaccine USP

"typical" antipsychotics [see: conventional antipsychotics]

Tyrex-2 powder OTC *enteral nutritional therapy for tyrosinemia type II*

Tyrodone oral liquid (discontinued 2002) ℞ *antitussive; decongestant* [hydrodocone bitartrate; pseudoephedrine HCl; alcohol 5%] 5•60 mg/5 mL

tyromedan INN *thyromimetic* [also: thyromedan HCl]

tyromedan HCl [see: thyromedan HCl]

Tyromex-1 powder OTC *formula for infants with tyrosinemia type I*

tyropanoate sodium USAN, USP *oral radiopaque contrast medium for cholecystography (57.4% iodine)* [also: sodium tyropanoate]

tyrosine (L-tyrosine) USAN, USP, INN *nonessential amino acid; symbols: Tyr, Y*

Tyrosum Cleanser topical liquid, packets OTC *cleanser for acne* [isopropanol; acetone] 50%•10%

tyrothricin USP, INN *antibacterial*

Tysabri IV infusion ℞ *humanized monoclonal antibody (huMAb) anti-inflammatory for treatment of multiple sclerosis; investigational (Phase III) for Crohn disease and rheumatoid arthritis; withdrawn from the market in 2005 due to safety concerns* [natalizumab] 300 mg/15 mL dose

Tyzine nasal spray, nose drops, pediatric nose drops ℞ *nasal decongestant* [tetrahydrozoline HCl] 0.1%; 0.1%; 0.05%

TZDs (thiazolidinediones) *a class of antidiabetic agents that increase cellular response to insulin without increasing insulin secretion*

UAA sugar-coated tablets ℞ *urinary antibiotic; analgesic; antispasmodic; acidifier* [methenamine; phenyl salicylate; atropine sulfate; methylene blue; hyoscyamine sulfate; benzoic acid] 40.8•18.1•0.03•5.4•0.03•4.5 mg

UAD Otic ear drop suspension ℞ *topical corticosteroidal anti-inflammatory; antibiotic* [hydrocortisone; neomycin sulfate; polymyxin B sulfate] 1%•5 mg•10 000 U per mL

ubenimex INN

ubidecarenone USAN, INN

ubiquinone [see: coenzyme Q10]

ubisindine INN

UBT Breath Test for H. pylori test for professional use *diagnostic aid for the detection of ulcers*

Ucephan oral solution ℞ *to prevent and treat hyperammonemia of urea cycle enzymopathy (orphan)* [sodium benzoate; sodium phenylacetate] 10•10 g/100 mL

UCG Beta Slide Monoclonal II slide tests for professional use *in vitro diagnostic aid; urine pregnancy test*

UCG Slide tests for professional use *in vitro diagnostic aid; urine pregnancy test* [latex agglutination test]

U-Cort cream ℞ *corticosteroidal anti-inflammatory* [hydrocortisone acetate] 1%

UDIP (trademarked packaging form) *unit-dose identification package*

Udo's Choice Oil oral liquid OTC *a blend of natural seed oils that supply a balance of essential fatty acids* [omega-3 oils; omega-6 oils; omega-9 oils; medium-chain triglycerides] 6.4•3.2•3•0.231 g/15 mL

Uendex ℞ *investigational (orphan) inhalant for cystic fibrosis* [dextran sulfate]

ufenamate INN

ufiprazole INN

U-Ject (trademarked delivery system) *prefilled disposable syringe*

Ulcerease mouth rinse OTC *topical antipruritic/counterirritant; mild local anesthetic* [phenol] 0.6%

uldazepam USAN, INN *sedative*

ulinastatin INN

Ulmus fulva; U. rubra medicinal herb [see: slippery elm]

ulobetasol INN *topical corticosteroidal anti-inflammatory* [also: halobetasol propionate]

ULR-LA long-acting tablets (discontinued 2002) ℞ *decongestant; expectorant* [phenylpropanolamine HCl; guaifenesin] 75•400 mg

Ultane liquid for vaporization ℞ *inhalation general anesthetic* [sevoflurane]

Ultiva powder for IV infusion ℞ *short-acting narcotic analgesic for general anesthesia* [remifentanil HCl] 1, 2, 5 mg/mL

Ultra Derm lotion, bath oil (discontinued 2004) OTC *moisturizer; emollient*

Ultra KLB6 tablets OTC *dietary supplement* [vitamin B₆; multiple food supplements] 16.7•≟ mg

Ultra Mide 25 lotion OTC *moisturizer; emollient; keratolytic* [urea] 25%

Ultra Tears eye drops OTC *ophthalmic moisturizer/lubricant* [hydroxypropyl methylcellulose] 1%

Ultra Vent (trademarked delivery system) *jet nebulizer*

Ultra Vita Time tablets OTC *dietary supplement* [multiple vitamins & minerals; multiple food products; iron; folic acid; biotin] ≟•6•0.4•1 mg

UltraBrom extended-release capsules ℞ *decongestant; antihistamine* [pseudoephedrine HCl; brompheniramine maleate] 120•12 mg

UltraBrom PD extended-release pediatric capsules ℞ *decongestant; antihistamine* [pseudoephedrine HCl; brompheniramine maleate] 60•6 mg

Ultracal oral liquid OTC *enteral nutritional therapy* [lactose-free formula]

Ultra-Care solution + tablets OTC *two-step chemical disinfecting system for soft contact lenses* [hydrogen peroxide-based] 3%

Ultracet film-coated caplets ℞ *central analgesic for acute pain* [tramadol HCl; acetaminophen] 37.5•325 mg

Ultra-Freeda; Ultra Freeda, Iron Free tablets OTC *geriatric vitamin/mineral supplement* [multiple vitamins & minerals; folic acid; biotin] ≟•270•100 μg

UltraJect prefilled syringe ℞ *narcotic analgesic* [morphine sulfate]

Ultralan oral liquid OTC *enteral nutritional therapy* [lactose-free formula]

Ultram film-coated caplets ℞ *central analgesic* [tramadol HCl] 50 mg

Ultram XL ℞ *investigational (Phase III) extended-release formulation* [tramadol HCl]

UltraMide 25 ⒸⒶⓃ lotion OTC *moisturizer; emollient* [urea] 25%

Ultra-NatalCare tablets ℞ *vitamin/mineral/iron supplement for pregnancy and lactation* [multiple vitamins & minerals; carbonyl iron; folic acid] ≟•90 mg iron•1 mg

Ultrase; Ultrase MT 12; Ultrase MT 18; Ultrase MT 20 capsules containing enteric-coated microspheres

℞ porcine-derived digestive enzymes [lipase; protease; amylase] 4500•25 000•20 000; 12 000•39 000•39 000; 18 000•58 500•58 500; 20 000•65 000•65 000 USP units

Ultravate ointment, cream ℞ topical corticosteroidal anti-inflammatory [halobetasol propionate] 0.05%

Ultravist IV injection ℞ radiopaque contrast medium for imaging of the head, heart, peripheral vascular system, and genitourinary tract [iopromide (39% iodine)] 311.7, 498.72, 623.4, 768.86 mg/mL (150, 240, 300, 370 mg/mL)

Ultrazyme Enzymatic Cleaner effervescent tablets OTC enzymatic cleaner for soft contact lenses [subtilisin A]

Ultrex gel in unit-dose packs OTC hydrogel wound dressing [acemannan]

Umecta emulsion, topical suspension ℞ moisturizer; emollient; keratolytic [urea] 40%

umespirone INN

uña de gato medicinal herb [see: cat's claw]

UN-Aspirin tablets OTC analgesic; antipyretic [acetaminophen] 500 mg

Unasyn powder for IV or IM injection ℞ aminopenicillin antibiotic plus synergist [ampicillin sodium; sulbactam sodium] 1•0.5, 2•1, 10•5 g ⑨ Anacin; Unisom

Uncaria guianensis; U. tomentosa medicinal herb [see: cat's claw]

10-undecenoic acid [see: undecylenic acid]

10-undecenoic acid, calcium salt [see: calcium undecylenate]

undecoylium chloride-iodine

undecylenic acid USP antifungal

Unguentine cream OTC local anesthetic; antifungal [benzocaine; resorcinol] 5%•2%

Unguentine ointment OTC minor burn treatment [phenol; zinc oxide; eucalyptus oil] 1%• ² • ²

Unguentine Plus cream OTC topical local anesthetic [lidocaine HCl; phenol] 2%•0.5%

Unguentum Bossi cream (discontinued 2003) ℞ topical antipsoriatic; anti-infective; bactericidal [ammoniated mercury; methenamine sulfosalicylate; coal tar] 5%•2%•2%

Uni-Ace drops OTC analgesic; antipyretic [acetaminophen] 100 mg/mL

Uni-Amp (trademarked packaging form) single-dose ampule

Unibase OTC ointment base

Uni-Bent Cough syrup (discontinued 2002) OTC antihistamine; antitussive [diphenhydramine HCl; alcohol 5%] 12.5 mg/5 mL

Unicap capsules, tablets OTC vitamin supplement [multiple vitamins; folic acid] ± •0.4 mg

Unicap Jr. chewable tablets OTC vitamin supplement [multiple vitamins; folic acid] ± •0.4 mg

Unicap M; Unicap T tablets OTC vitamin/mineral/iron supplement [multiple vitamins & minerals; iron; folic acid] ± •18•0.4 mg

Unicap Plus Iron tablets OTC vitamin/iron supplement [multiple vitamins; iron; folic acid] ± •22.5•0.4 mg

Unicap Sr. tablets OTC vitamin/mineral/iron supplement [multiple vitamins & minerals; iron; folic acid] ± •10•0.4 mg

Unicomplex T & M tablets OTC vitamin/mineral/iron supplement [multiple vitamins & minerals; iron; folic acid] ± •18•0.4 mg

Uni-Decon sustained-release tablets (discontinued 2001) ℞ decongestant; antihistamine [phenylpropanolamine HCl; phenylephrine HCl; chlorpheniramine maleate; phenyltoloxamine citrate] 40•10•5•15 mg

Unidet ⑭ extended-release capsules ℞ anticholinergic; muscarinic receptor antagonist for urinary frequency, urgency, and incontinence [tolterodine tartrate] 2, 4 mg

Uni-Dur extended-release tablets (discontinued 2003) ℞ once-daily anti-asthmatic/bronchodilator [theophylline] 400, 600 mg

Unifed oral liquid oTc *nasal decongestant* [pseudoephedrine HCl] 30 mg/5 mL

Unifiber powder oTc *bulk laxative* [cellulose powder]

unifocon A USAN *hydrophobic contact lens material*

Unimatic (trademarked delivery system) *prefilled disposable syringe*

Uni-nest (trademarked packaging form) *ampule*

Unipak (packaging form) *dispensing pack*

Unipen capsules (discontinued 2002) R̸ *penicillinase-resistant penicillin antibiotic* [nafcillin sodium] 250 mg ⸬ Omnipen

Uniphyl timed-release tablets R̸ *antiasthmatic; bronchodilator* [theophylline] 400, 600 mg

Uniprost (name changed to **Remodulin** for the NDA in 2001)

Uniquin (foreign name for U.S. product **Maxaquin**)

Uniretic tablets R̸ *antihypertensive; angiotensin-converting enzyme (ACE) inhibitor; diuretic* [moexipril HCl; hydrochlorothiazide] 7.5•12.5, 15•12.5, 15•25 mg

Uni-Rx (trademarked packaging form) *unit-dose containers and packages*

Unisert (trademarked dosage form) *suppository*

Unisol; Unisol 4 solution oTc *rinsing/storage solution for soft contact lenses* [sodium chloride (saline solution)]

Unisol Plus aerosol solution oTc *rinsing/storage solution for soft contact lenses* [sodium chloride (saline solution)]

Unisom Natural Source Ⓐ gel capsules oTc *herbal sleep aid* [valerian extract (from valerian root)] 100 mg (400 mg)

Unisom Nighttime Sleep-Aid tablets oTc *antihistaminic sleep aid* [doxylamine succinate] 25 mg ⸬ Anacin; Unasyn

Unisom SleepGels (capsules) oTc *antihistaminic sleep aid* [diphenhydramine HCl] 50 mg ⸬ Anacin; Unasyn

Unisom with Pain Relief tablets oTc *antihistaminic sleep aid; analgesic* [diphenhydramine citrate; acetaminophen] 50•650 mg ⸬ Anacin; Unasyn

Unistep hCG test kit for professional use *in vitro diagnostic aid; urine pregnancy test*

Unithroid tablets R̸ *synthetic thyroid hormone (T_4 fraction only)* [levothyroxine sodium] 25, 50, 75, 88, 100, 112, 125, 150, 175, 200, 300 μg

Unitrol timed-release capsules (discontinued 2001) oTc *diet aid* [phenylpropanolamine HCl] 75 mg

Unituss HC syrup (discontinued 2002) R̸ *narcotic antitussive; decongestant; antihistamine* [hydrocodone bitartrate; phenylephrine HCl; chlorpheniramine maleate] 2.5•5•2 mg/5 mL

Uni-Tussin syrup (discontinued 2002) oTc *expectorant* [guaifenesin; alcohol 3.5%] 100 mg/5 mL

Uni-Tussin DM syrup (discontinued 2002) oTc *antitussive; expectorant* [dextromethorphan hydrobromide; guaifenesin] 10•100 mg/5 mL

Univasc tablets R̸ *antihypertensive; angiotensin-converting enzyme (ACE) inhibitor* [moexipril HCl] 7.5, 15 mg

Univial (trademarked form) *single-dose vials*

Unna's boot [see: Dome-Paste bandage]

unoprostone isopropyl *topical prostaglandin $F_{2\alpha}$ analogue for glaucoma and ocular hypertension*

Uracid capsules R̸ *urinary acidifier to control ammonia production* [racemethionine] 200 mg ⸬ uracil; Urised; Urocit

uracil USAN *antineoplastic potentiator for tegafur (not available separately; combined with tegafur in a 1:4 ratio)*

uracil mustard USAN, USP *nitrogen mustard-type alkylating antineoplastic* [also: uramustine] ⸬ Uracel; Uracid

Uracyst-S; Uracyst-S Concentrate Ⓐ liquid for bladder instillation R̸ *glycosaminoglycan temporary replacement* [chondroitin sulfate sodium] 2 mg/mL; 20 mg/mL

uradal [see: carbromal]

uralenic acid [see: enoxolone]

uramustine INN, BAN *nitrogen mustard-type alkylating antineoplastic* [also: uracil mustard]

uranin [see: fluorescein sodium]

uranium *element (U)*

urapidil INN, BAN

urea USP *osmotic diuretic; keratolytic; emollient* 35%, 40% topical

urea peroxide [see: carbamide peroxide]

Ureacin-10 lotion OTC *moisturizer; emollient; keratolytic* [urea] 10%

Ureacin-20 cream OTC *moisturizer; emollient; keratolytic* [urea] 20%

Ureaphil IV infusion ℞ *osmotic diuretic* [urea] 40 g/150 mL

Urecholine subcu injection (discontinued 2001) ℞ *cholinergic urinary stimulant for postsurgical and postpartum urinary retention* [bethanechol chloride] 5 mg/mL

Urecholine tablets ℞ *cholinergic urinary stimulant for postsurgical and postpartum urinary retention* [bethanechol chloride] 25 mg

uredepa USAN, INN *antineoplastic*

uredofos USAN, INN *veterinary anthelmintic*

urefibrate INN

p-**ureidobenzenearsonic acid** [see: carbarsone]

Urelle sugar-coated tablets ℞ *urinary antibiotic; antiseptic; analgesic; antispasmodic* [methenamine; sodium phosphate; phenyl salicylate; methylene blue; hyoscyamine sulfate] 81•40.8•32.4•10.8•0.12 mg

urethan NF [also: urethane]

urethane INN, BAN [also: urethan]

urethane polymers [see: polyurethane foam]

Uretron D/S sugar-coated tablets ℞ *urinary antibiotic; antiseptic; analgesic; antispasmodic* [methenamine; sodium biphosphate; phenyl salicylate; methylene blue; hyoscyamine sulfate] 120•40.8•36.2•10.8•0.12 mg

Urex tablets ℞ *urinary antibiotic* [methenamine hippurate] 1 g ⧉ Eurax; Serax

Urginea indica; U. maritima; U. scilla medicinal herb [see: squill]

Uricult culture paddles for professional use *in vitro diagnostic aid for nitrate, uropathogens, or bacteria in the urine*

uridine 5′-triphosphate *investigational (Phase I/II, orphan) for cystic fibrosis and primary ciliary dyskinesia*

Uridon Modified sugar-coated tablets ℞ *urinary antibiotic; analgesic; antispasmodic; acidifier* [methenamine; phenyl salicylate; atropine sulfate; methylene blue; hyoscyamine sulfate; benzoic acid] 40.8•18.1•0.03•5.4•0.03•4.5 mg

Urimar-T tablets ℞ *urinary antibiotic; antiseptic; analgesic; antispasmodic* [methenamine; sodium biphosphate; phenyl salicylate; methylene blue; hyoscyamine sulfate] 81.6•40.8•36.2•10.8•0.12 mg

Urimax film-coated tablets ℞ *urinary antibiotic; analgesic; antispasmodic; acidifier* [methenamine; phenyl salicylate; methylene blue; hyoscyamine sulfate; sodium biphosphate] 81.6•36.2•10.8•0.12•40.8 mg

Urinary Antiseptic No. 2 tablets ℞ *urinary antibiotic; analgesic; antispasmodic; acidifier* [methenamine; phenyl salicylate; atropine sulfate; methylene blue; hyoscyamine sulfate; benzoic acid] 40.8•18.1•0.03•5.4•0.03•4.5 mg

Urised sugar-coated tablets ℞ *urinary antibiotic; analgesic; antispasmodic; acidifier* [methenamine; phenyl salicylate; atropine sulfate; methylene blue; hyoscyamine sulfate; benzoic acid] 40.8•18.1•0.03•5.4•0.03•4.5 mg ⧉ Uracel; Uracid; Urispas

Urisedamine tablets ℞ *urinary antibiotic; antispasmodic* [methenamine mandelate; hyoscyamine] 500•0.15 mg

Uriseptic film-coated tablets ℞ *urinary antibiotic; antiseptic; analgesic; antispasmodic* [methenamine; phenyl salicylate; methylene blue; benzoic acid; atropine sulfate; hyoscyamine sulfate] 40.8•18.1•5.4•4.5•0.03•0.03 mg

Urispas film-coated tablets ℞ *urinary antispasmodic* [flavoxate HCl] 100 mg (200 mg available in Canada) ⑨ Urised

Uristat tablets ℞ *urinary analgesic* [phenazopyridine HCl] 95 mg

Uristix; Uristix 4 reagent strips *in vitro diagnostic aid for multiple urine products*

UriSym capsules ℞ *urinary antibiotic; antiseptic; analgesic; antispasmodic* [methenamine; sodium biphosphate; phenyl salicylate; methylene blue; hyoscyamine sulfate] 100•40.8•40•10.8•0.12 mg

Uritact DS caplets ℞ *urinary antibiotic; analgesic; antispasmodic; acidifier* [methenamine; phenyl salicylate; atropine sulfate; methylene blue; hyoscyamine sulfate; benzoic acid] 81.6•36.2•0.06•10.8•0.06•9 mg

Uritin tablets ℞ *urinary antibiotic; analgesic; antispasmodic; acidifier* [methenamine; phenyl salicylate; atropine sulfate; methylene blue; hyoscyamine sulfate; benzoic acid] 40.8•18.1•0.03•5.4•0.03•4.5 mg

Uro Blue sugar-coated tablets ℞ *urinary antibiotic; antiseptic; analgesic; antispasmodic* [methenamine; sodium biphosphate; phenyl salicylate; methylene blue; hyoscyamine sulfate] 120•40.8•36.2•10.8•0.12 mg

Urobak tablets (discontinued 2001) ℞ *broad-spectrum bacteriostatic* [sulfamethoxazole] 500 mg

urocidin *investigational (Phase III) mycobacterial cell wall complex (MCC) for bladder cancer*

Urocit-K tablets ℞ *urinary alkalizer for nephrolithiasis and hypocitruria prevention (orphan)* [potassium citrate] 5, 10 mEq K ⑨ Uracid

urofollitrophin BAN *follicle-stimulating hormone (FSH)* [also: urofollitropin]

urofollitropin USAN, INN *follicle-stimulating hormone (FSH); ovulation stimulant for polycystic ovarian disease (orphan) and assisted reproductive technologies (ART); investigational (orphan)*

for spermatogenesis in hormone-deficient males [also: urofollitrophin]

urogastrone *investigational (orphan) for recovery from corneal transplant surgery*

Urogesic tablets ℞ *urinary analgesic* [phenazopyridine HCl] 100 mg

Urogesic Blue sugar-coated tablets ℞ *urinary antibiotic; antiseptic; analgesic; antispasmodic* [methenamine; sodium biphosphate; phenyl salicylate; methylene blue; hyoscyamine sulfate] 81.6•40.8•36.2•10.8•0.12 mg

urokinase USAN, INN, BAN, JAN *plasminogen activator; thrombolytic enzyme*

urokinase alfa USAN *plasminogen activator; thrombolytic enzyme*

Uro-KP-Neutral film-coated caplets ℞ *urinary acidifier; phosphorus supplement* [sodium phosphate; potassium phosphate; monobasic sodium phosphate] 250 mg P

Urolene Blue tablets ℞ *urinary anti-infective and antiseptic; antidote to cyanide poisoning* [methylene blue] 65 mg

Uro-Mag capsules OTC *antacid; magnesium supplement* [magnesium oxide] 140 mg (84.5 mg Mg)

uronal [see: barbital]

Uro-Phosphate film-coated tablets ℞ *urinary antibiotic; acidifier* [methenamine; sodium biphosphate] 300•434.78 mg

Uroqid-Acid No. 2 film-coated tablets ℞ *urinary antibiotic; acidifier* [methenamine mandelate; sodium acid phosphate] 500•500 mg

Uroxatral extended-release tablets ℞ α_1-*adrenergic blocker for benign prostatic hyperplasia (BPH)* [alfuzosin HCl] 10 mg

Ursinus Inlay-Tabs (tablets) (discontinued 2002) OTC *decongestant; analgesic; antipyretic* [pseudoephedrine HCl; aspirin] 30•325 mg

Urso 250; Urso Forte tablets ℞ *naturally occurring bile acid for primary biliary cirrhosis (orphan)* [ursodiol] 250 mg; 500 mg

ursodeoxycholic acid INN, BAN *natu-rally occurring bile acid; anticholelitho-genic* [also: ursodiol]
ursodiol USAN *naturally occurring bile acid for primary biliary cirrhosis (orphan); gallstone preventative and dissolving agent* [also: ursodeoxy-cholic acid] 300 mg oral
ursulcholic acid INN
Urtica dioica; U. urens *medicinal herb* [see: nettle]
uva ursi (Arbutus uva ursi; Arcto-staphylos uva ursi) *leaves medicinal herb for bladder and kidney infections, Bright disease, constipation, diabetes, gonorrhea, nephritis, spleen disorders, urethritis, and uterine ulcerations*
Uvadex *extracorporeal solution (leuko-cytes are collected, photoactivated with the UVAR Photopheresis Sys-tem, then reinfused)* ℞ *palliative treat-ment for cutaneous T-cell lymphoma (CTCL); investigational (orphan) treat-ment of diffuse systemic sclerosis and to prevent rejection of cardiac allografts* [methoxsalen] 20 μg/mL

VA (vincristine, actinomycin D) *chemotherapy protocol*
VAAP (vincristine, asparaginase, Adriamycin, prednisone) *chemo-therapy protocol*
VAB; VAB-I (vinblastine, actinomy-cin D, bleomycin) *chemotherapy protocol*
VAB-II (vinblastine, actinomycin D, bleomycin, cisplatin) *chemotherapy protocol*
VAB-III (vinblastine, actinomycin D, bleomycin, cisplatin, chloram-bucil, cyclophosphamide) *chemo-therapy protocol*
VAB-V (vinblastine, actinomycin D, bleomycin, cyclophosphamide, cisplatin) *chemotherapy protocol*
VAB-6 (vinblastine, actinomycin D, bleomycin, cyclophosphamide, cisplatin) *chemotherapy protocol for testicular cancer*
VABCD (vinblastine, Adriamycin, bleomycin, CCNU, DTIC) *chemo-therapy protocol*
VAC (vincristine, Adriamycin, cis-platin) *chemotherapy protocol*
VAC (vincristine, Adriamycin, cyclophosphamide) *chemotherapy protocol for small cell lung cancer (SCLC)* [also: CAV]

VAC pediatric (vincristine, actino-mycin D, cyclophosphamide) *che-motherapy protocol for pediatric sarcomas*
VAC pulse; VAC standard (vincris-tine, actinomycin D, cyclophos-phamide) *chemotherapy protocol for sarcomas*
VACA (vincristine, actinomycin D, cyclophosphamide, Adriamycin) *chemotherapy protocol*
VACAD (vincristine, actinomycin D, cyclophosphamide, Adriamy-cin, dacarbazine) *chemotherapy pro-tocol*
VACAdr (vincristine, actinomycin D, cyclophosphamide, Adriamy-cin) *chemotherapy protocol for pedi-atric bone and soft tissue sarcomas*
vaccines *a class of drugs used for active immunization that consist of antigens that induce endogenous production of antibodies*
vaccinia immune globulin (VIG) USP *passive immunizing agent*
vaccinia immune human globulin [now: vaccinia immune globulin] .
vaccinia virus vaccine for human papillomavirus (HPV), recombi-nant *investigational (orphan) for cervi-cal cancer*

Vaccinium edule; V. erythrocarpum; V. macrocarpon; V. oxycoccos; V. vitis *medicinal herb* [see: cranberry]

Vaccinium myrtillus *medicinal herb* [see: bilberry]

VACP (VePesid, Adriamycin, cyclophosphamide, Platinol) *chemotherapy protocol*

VAD (vincristine, Adriamycin, dactinomycin) *chemotherapy protocol for pediatric Wilms tumor*

VAD (vincristine, Adriamycin, dexamethasone) *chemotherapy protocol for multiple myeloma and acute lymphocytic leukemia (ALL)*

Vademin-Z capsules OTC *vitamin/mineral supplement* [multiple vitamins & minerals]

vadocaine INN

VAdrC (vincristine, Adriamycin, cyclophosphamide) *chemotherapy protocol*

VAD/V (vincristine, Adriamycin, dexamethasone, verapamil) *chemotherapy protocol*

VAFAC (vincristine, amethopterin, fluorouracil, Adriamycin, cyclophosphamide) *chemotherapy protocol*

Vagifem film-coated vaginal tablets ℞ *synthetic estrogen; hormone replacement for postmenopausal atrophic vaginitis* [estradiol hemihydrate] 25.8 μg (=25 mg base)

Vagi-Gard; Vagi-Gard Advanced Sensitive Formula vaginal cream OTC *topical local anesthetic; keratolytic; antifungal* [benzocaine; resorcinol] 20%•3%; 5%•2%

Vaginex vaginal cream OTC *topical antihistamine* [tripelennamine HCl]

Vagisec Douche solution ℞ *vaginal cleanser and deodorizer*

Vagisec Plus vaginal suppositories ℞ *antibacterial* [aminacrine HCl] 6 mg

Vagisil cream OTC *topical local anesthetic; antipruritic; antifungal* [benzocaine; resorcinol] 5%•2%

Vagisil powder OTC *absorbs vaginal moisture* [cornstarch; aloe]

Vagistat-1 vaginal ointment in pre-filled applicator OTC *antifungal* [tioconazole] 6.5%

Vagistat-3 Combination Pack vaginal inserts + cream OTC *antifungal* [miconazole nitrate] 200 mg + 2%

VAI (vincristine, actinomycin D, ifosfamide) *chemotherapy protocol*

valaciclovir INN *oral antiviral for herpes simplex virus types 1 and 2 (HSV-1, cold sores; HSV-2, genital herpes) and herpes zoster (shingles) infections; suppressive therapy for recurrent outbreaks* [also: valacyclovir HCl]

valacyclovir HCl USAN *oral antiviral for herpes simplex virus types 1 and 2 (HSV-1, cold sores; HSV-2, genital herpes) and herpes zoster (shingles) infections; suppressive therapy for recurrent outbreaks* [also: valaciclovir]

valconazole INN

Valcyte tablets ℞ *nucleoside analogue antiviral for AIDS-related cytomegalovirus (CMV) retinitis; CMV prevention in organ transplants* [valganciclovir HCl] 450 mg

valdecoxib USAN *COX-2 inhibitor; nonsteroidal anti-inflammatory drug (NSAID) for osteoarthritis (OA), rheumatoid arthritis (RA), and menstrual pain; withdrawn from the market in 2005 due to safety concerns*

valdetamide INN

valdipromide INN

valepotriate [see: valtrate]

Valergen 20; Valergen 40 IM injection (discontinued 2003) ℞ *estrogen replacement therapy for the treatment of postmenopausal symptoms; hormonal antineoplastic for prostate cancer* [estradiol valerate in oil] 20 mg/mL; 40 mg/mL

valerian (Valeriana officinalis) root *medicinal herb for convulsions, hypertension, hysteria, hypochondria, nervousness, pain, and sedation*

valerian, false *medicinal herb* [see: life root]

Valertest No. 1 IM injection (discontinued 2003) ℞ *hormone replacement* *therapy for postmenopausal symptoms* [estradiol valerate; testosterone enanthate] 4•90 mg/mL

valethamate bromide NF

valganciclovir HCl USAN *nucleoside analogue antiviral for AIDS-related cytomegalovirus (CMV) retinitis; CMV prevention in organ transplants; oral prodrug of ganciclovir*

valine (L-valine) USAN, USP, INN, JAN *essential amino acid; symbols: Val, V*

valine & isoleucine & leucine *investigational (orphan) for hyperphenylalaninemia*

Valisone ointment, cream, lotion ℞ *topical corticosteroidal anti-inflammatory* [betamethasone valerate] 0.1%

Valisone Reduced Strength cream ℞ *topical corticosteroidal anti-inflammatory* [betamethasone valerate] 0.01%

Valium IV or IM injection, Tel-E-Ject syringes (discontinued 2003) ℞ *benzodiazepine sedative; anxiolytic; skeletal muscle relaxant; anticonvulsant; alcohol withdrawal aid; also abused as a street drug* [diazepam] 5 mg/mL; 10 mg ⊡ thallium; Valpin

Valium tablets ℞ *benzodiazepine sedative; anxiolytic; skeletal muscle relaxant; anticonvulsant; alcohol withdrawal aid; also abused as a street drug* [diazepam] 2, 5, 10 mg ⊡ thallium; Valpin

valnoctamide USAN, INN *tranquilizer*

valofane INN

valomaciclovir stearate USAN *DNA polymerase inhibitor; antiviral for herpes zoster infections*

valperinol INN

valproate pivoxil INN

valproate semisodium INN *anticonvulsant; antipsychotic for manic episodes; migraine headache preventative; valproic acid derivative* [also: divalproex sodium; semisodium valproate]

valproate sodium USAN *anticonvulsant; investigational for migraine relief* 250 mg/5 mL oral; 500 mg injection

valproic acid USAN, USP, INN, BAN *anticonvulsant* 250 mg oral

valpromide INN

valrubicin USAN *anthracycline antibiotic antineoplastic for bladder cancer (orphan)*

valsartan USAN, INN *angiotensin II receptor antagonist; antihypertensive; treatment for congestive heart failure (CHF)* 40, 80, 160, 320 mg oral

valspodar USAN, INN *investigational (Phase III) cyclosporine-derived P-glycoprotein (P-gp) inhibitor for multidrug-resistant (MDR) cancers, including acute myelogenous leukemia (AML), multiple myeloma, and ovarian cancer*

Valstar intravesical solution (discontinued 2004) ℞ *anthracycline antibiotic antineoplastic for bladder cancer (orphan)* [valrubicin] 40 mg/mL

Valtaxin ⊛ intravesical solution ℞ *anthracycline antibiotic antineoplastic for bladder cancer (orphan)* [valrubicin] 40 mg/mL

valtrate INN

Valtrex film-coated caplets ℞ *antiviral for herpes simplex virus types 1 and 2 (HSV-1, cold sores; HSV-2, genital herpes) and herpes zoster (shingles) infections; suppressive therapy for recurrent outbreaks* [valacyclovir HCl] 500, 1000 mg

VAM (vinblastine, Adriamycin, mitomycin) *chemotherapy protocol*

VAM (VP-16-213, Adriamycin, methotrexate) *chemotherapy protocol*

VAMP (vincristine, actinomycin, methotrexate, prednisone) *chemotherapy protocol*

VAMP (vincristine, Adriamycin, methylprednisolone) *chemotherapy protocol*

VAMP (vincristine, amethopterin, mercaptopurine, prednisone) *chemotherapy protocol*

vanadium *element (V)*

Vanamide cream ℞ *keratolytic for the removal of dystrophic nails* [urea] 40%

Vancenase Pockethaler (nasal inhalation aerosol) (discontinued 2004) ℞ *corticosteroidal anti-inflammatory for* *seasonal or perennial rhinitis* [beclomethasone dipropionate] 42 µg/dose

Vancenase AQ nasal spray (discontinued 2004) ℞ *corticosteroidal anti-inflammatory for seasonal or perennial rhinitis* [beclomethasone dipropionate] 0.084% (100 µg/dose)

Vanceril; Vanceril Double Strength oral inhalation aerosol (discontinued 2002) ℞ *corticosteroidal anti-inflammatory for chronic asthma* [beclomethasone dipropionate] 42 µg/dose; 84 µg/dose

Vancocin Pulvules (capsules), powder for oral solution, powder for IV or IM injection ℞ *tricyclic glycopeptide antibiotic* [vancomycin HCl] 125, 250 mg; 1, 10 g; 0.5, 1, 10 g

Vancoled powder for IV or IM injection ℞ *tricyclic glycopeptide antibiotic* [vancomycin HCl] 0.5, 1, 5 g

vancomycin INN, BAN *tricyclic glycopeptide antibiotic* [also: vancomycin HCl]

vancomycin HCl USP *tricyclic glycopeptide antibiotic* [also: vancomycin] 1 g oral; 0.5, 1, 5, 10 g/vial injection

vaneprim INN

Vanex Expectorant oral liquid (discontinued 2002) ℞ *narcotic antitussive; decongestant; expectorant* [hydrocodone bitartrate; pseudoephedrine HCl; guaifenesin; alcohol 5%] 2.5•30•100 mg/5 mL

Vanex Forte sustained-release caplets (discontinued 2001) ℞ *decongestant; antihistamine* [phenylpropanolamine HCl; phenylephrine HCl; chlorpheniramine maleate; pyrilamine maleate] 50•10•4•25 mg

Vanex Forte-R sustained-release capsules (discontinued 2001) ℞ *decongestant; antihistamine* [phenylpropanolamine HCl; chlorpheniramine maleate] 75•12 mg

Vanex HD oral liquid ℞ *narcotic antitussive; decongestant; antihistamine* [hydrocodone bitartrate; phenylephrine HCl; chlorpheniramine maleate] 3.33•10•4 mg/10 mL

Vanicream OTC *cream base*

vanilla NF *flavoring agent*

vanilla *(Vanilla fragrans; V. planifolia; V. tahitensis)* bean *medicinal herb for CNS stimulation, fever, and flatulence; also used as an aphrodisiac*

vanillin NF *flavoring agent*

N-vanillylnonamide [see: nonivamide]

N-vanillyloleamide [see: olvanil]

Vaniqa cream ℞ *hair growth inhibitor for unwanted facial hair on women* [eflornithine HCl] 13.9%

vanitiolide INN

Vanlev ℞ *vasopeptidase inhibitor (VPI); investigational (NDA filed) endopeptidase and angiotensin-converting enzyme (ACE) inhibitor for hypertension and congestive heart failure* [omapatrilat]

Vanocin lotion ℞ *acne treatment* [sulfacetamide sodium; sulfur] 10%•5%

Vanos cream ℞ *corticosteroidal anti-inflammatory* [fluocinonide] 0.1%

Vanoxide lotion (discontinued 2003) OTC *keratolytic for acne* [benzoyl peroxide] 5%

Vanoxide-HC lotion ℞ *topical corticosteroidal anti-inflammatory and keratolytic for acne* [benzoyl peroxide; hydrocortisone] 5%•0.5%

Vanquish caplets OTC *analgesic; antipyretic; anti-inflammatory* [acetaminophen; aspirin (buffered with magnesium hydroxide and aluminum hydroxide); caffeine] 194•227•(50•25)•33 mg

Vansil capsules (discontinued 2001) ℞ *anthelmintic for schistosomiasis (flukes)* [oxamniquine] 250 mg

Vantas once-yearly subcu implant ℞ *LHRH agonist for palliative treatment of advanced prostate cancer* [histrelin acetate] 50 mg

Vanticon (German name for U.S. product **Accolate**)

Vantin film-coated tablets, granules for suspension ℞ *broad-spectrum cephalosporin antibiotic* [cefpodoxime proxetil] 100, 200 mg; 50, 100 mg/5 mL ⍰ Banthine; Bantron

vanyldisulfamide INN

VAP (vinblastine, actinomycin D, Platinol) *chemotherapy protocol*

VAP (vincristine, Adriamycin, prednisone) *chemotherapy protocol*

VAP (vincristine, Adriamycin, procarbazine) *chemotherapy protocol*

VAP (vincristine, asparaginase, prednisone) *chemotherapy protocol*

vapiprost INN, BAN *antagonist to thromboxane A_2* [also: vapiprost HCl]

vapiprost HCl USAN *antagonist to thromboxane A_2* [also: vapiprost]

Vaporole (trademarked dosage form) *crushable ampule for inhalation*

vapreotide USAN *antineoplastic*

Vaqta adult IM injection, pediatric IM injection R *immunization against hepatitis A virus (HAV)* [hepatitis A vaccine, inactivated] 50 U/mL; 25 U/0.5 mL

vardenafil HCl USAN *phosphodiesterase type 5 (PDE5) inhibitor; selective vasodilator for erectile dysfunction (ED)*

varenicline *investigational (Phase III) nicotine receptor antagonist for smoking cessation*

varicella virus vaccine *live, attenuated vaccine for chickenpox*

varicella-zoster immune globulin (VZIG) USP *passive immunizing agent* 10%–18% (125 U/2.5 mL)

Varivax powder for subcu injection R *vaccine for chickenpox* [varicella virus vaccine, live attenuated] 1350 PFU/0.5 mL

Varoniscastrum virgincum medicinal herb [see: Culver root]

Vascor film-coated tablets (discontinued 2003) R *antianginal* [bepridil HCl] 200, 300 mg

Vascoray injection (discontinued 2001) R *radiopaque contrast medium* [iothalamate meglumine; iothalamate sodium (51.3% total iodine)] 520•260 mg/mL (400 mg/mL)

vascular endothelial growth factor (VEGF) *investigational (Phase II, orphan) gene-based therapy for neointimal hyperplasia disease*

vascular serotonin 5-HT$_1$ receptor agonists *a class of antimigraine agents that constrict cranial blood vessels and inhibit the release of inflammatory neuropeptides*

Vaseretic 5-12.5; Vaseretic 10-25 tablets R *antihypertensive; angiotensin-converting enzyme (ACE) inhibitor; diuretic* [enalapril maleate; hydrochlorothiazide] 5•12.5 mg; 10•25 mg

vasoactive intestinal polypeptide (VIP) *investigational (NDA filed) treatment for male sexual dysfunction; investigational (orphan) for acute esophageal food impaction*

Vasocidin eye drops R *corticosteroidal anti-inflammatory; antibiotic* [prednisolone sodium phosphate; sulfacetamide sodium] 0.25%•10% ⊡ Vasodilan

Vasocidin ophthalmic ointment (discontinued 2002) R *corticosteroidal anti-inflammatory; antibiotic* [prednisolone acetate; sulfacetamide sodium] 0.5%•10%

Vasocine ophthalmic ointment (discontinued 2003) R *corticosteroidal anti-inflammatory; antibiotic* [prednisolone acetate; sulfacetamide sodium] 0.5%•10% ⊡ Vaseline

VasoClear eye drops OTC *decongestant; lubricant* [naphazoline HCl; polyvinyl alcohol; polyethylene glycol 400] 0.02%•0.25%•1% ⊡ VasoCare

VasoClear A eye drops OTC *decongestant; astringent* [naphazoline HCl; zinc sulfate] 0.02%•0.25%

Vasocon Regular eye drops R *topical ophthalmic decongestant and vasoconstrictor* [naphazoline HCl] 0.1%

Vasocon-A eye drops R *ophthalmic decongestant and antihistamine* [naphazoline HCl; antazoline phosphate] 0.05%•0.5%

vasoconstrictors *a class of cardiovascular drugs that narrow the blood vessels*

Vasodilan tablets R *peripheral vasodilator* [isoxsuprine HCl] 10, 20 mg ⊡ Vasocidin

vasodilators *a class of cardiovascular drugs that dilate the blood vessels*

Vasoflux ℞ *investigational (Phase II) anticoagulant for use in acute myocardial infarction patients* ② Vasoprost; Vasosulf

vasopressin (VP) USP, INN *posterior pituitary hormone; antidiuretic* 20 U/mL injection

vasopressin tannate USP *posterior pituitary hormone; antidiuretic*

vasopressors *a class of posterior pituitary hormones that raise blood pressure by causing contraction of capillaries and arterioles; a class of sympathomimetic agents that raise blood pressure by increasing myocardial contractility* [also called: vasopressins]

Vasosulf eye drops ℞ *antibiotic; ophthalmic decongestant* [sulfacetamide sodium; phenylephrine HCl] 15%• 0.125% ② Velosef; Vasoflux

Vasotate HC ear drops ℞ *topical corticosteroidal anti-inflammatory; antibacterial; antifungal* [hydrocortisone; acetic acid] 1%•2%

Vasotec tablets ℞ *antihypertensive; angiotensin-converting enzyme (ACE) inhibitor; treatment for CHF* [enalapril maleate] 2.5, 5, 10, 20 mg

Vasotec I.V. injection (discontinued 2003) ℞ *antihypertensive; angiotensin-converting enzyme (ACE) inhibitor* [enalaprilat] 1.25 mg/mL

Vasoxyl IV or IM injection (discontinued 2001) ℞ *vasopressor for hypotensive shock during surgery* [methoxamine HCl] 20 mg/mL

VAT (vinblastine, Adriamycin, thiotepa) *chemotherapy protocol*

vatalanib *investigational (Phase III) tyrosine kinase inhibitor for cervical cancer*

VATD; VAT-D (vincristine, ara-C, thioguanine, daunorubicin) *chemotherapy protocol*

VATH (vinblastine, Adriamycin, thiotepa, Halotestin) *chemotherapy protocol for breast cancer*

Vatronol [see: Vicks Vatronol]

VAV (VP-16-213, Adriamycin, vincristine) *chemotherapy protocol*

Vaxigrip ⓒ IM injection ℞ *flu vaccine* [influenza split-virus vaccine] 0.5 mL/dose

VaZol oral liquid ℞ *antihistamine* [brompheniramine tannate] 2 mg/5 mL

VB (vinblastine, bleomycin) *chemotherapy protocol*

VBA (vincristine, BCNU, Adriamycin) *chemotherapy protocol*

VBAP (vincristine, BCNU, Adriamycin, prednisone) *chemotherapy protocol for multiple myeloma*

VBC (VePesid, BCNU, cyclophosphamide) *chemotherapy protocol*

VBC (vinblastine, bleomycin, cisplatin) *chemotherapy protocol*

VBCMP (vincristine, BCNU, cyclophosphamide, melphalan, prednisone) *chemotherapy protocol for multiple myeloma*

VBD (vinblastine, bleomycin, DDP) *chemotherapy protocol*

VBM (vincristine, bleomycin, methotrexate) *chemotherapy protocol*

VBMCP (vincristine, BCNU, melphalan, cyclophosphamide, prednisone) *chemotherapy protocol*

VBMF (vincristine, bleomycin, methotrexate, fluorouracil) *chemotherapy protocol*

VBP (vinblastine, bleomycin, Platinol) *chemotherapy protocol*

VC (VePesid, carboplatin) *chemotherapy protocol*

VC (vincristine) [q.v.]

VC (vinorelbine, cisplatin) *chemotherapy protocol for non–small cell lung cancer (NSCLC)*

VCAP (vincristine, cyclophosphamide, Adriamycin, prednisone) *chemotherapy protocol for multiple myeloma*

V-CAP III (VP-16-213, cyclophosphamide, Adriamycin, Platinol) *chemotherapy protocol*

VCF (vaginal contraceptive film) OTC *spermicidal contraceptive* [nonoxynol 9] 28%

VCF (vincristine, cyclophospha-mide, fluorouracil) *chemotherapy protocol*

VCMP (vincristine, cyclophospha-mide, melphalan, prednisone) *chemotherapy protocol for multiple myeloma* [also: VMCP]

VCP (vincristine, cyclophospha-mide, prednisone) *chemotherapy protocol*

VCR (vincristine) [q.v.]

VD (vinorelbine, doxorubicin) *chemotherapy protocol for breast cancer*

V-Dec-M sustained-release tablets ℞ *decongestant; expectorant* [pseudo-ephedrine HCl; guaifenesin] 120•500 mg

VDP (vincristine, daunorubicin, prednisone) *chemotherapy protocol*

Vectrin capsules (discontinued 2003) ℞ *tetracycline antibiotic* [minocycline HCl] 50, 100 mg

vecuronium bromide USAN, INN, BAN *nondepolarizing neuromuscular blocker; muscle relaxant; adjunct to anesthesia* 10, 20 mg injection

Veetids film-coated tablets, powder for oral solution ℞ *natural penicillin antibiotic* [penicillin V potassium] 250, 500 mg; 125, 250 mg/5 mL

vegetable oil, hydrogenated NF *tablet and capsule lubricant*

vegetable tallow; vegetable wax *medicinal herb* [see: bayberry]

VEGF (vascular endothelial growth factor) [see: telbermin]

Vehicle/N; Vehicle/N Mild OTC *lotion base*

VeIP (Velban, ifosfamide [with mesna rescue], Platinol) *chemotherapy protocol for genitourinary and testicular cancer*

Velac topical gel ℞ *investigational (NDA filed) antibiotic/keratolytic combination for acne* [clindamycin; tretinoin] 1%•0.025%

Velban powder for IV injection ℞ *antineoplastic for lung, breast, and testicular cancers, lymphomas, sarcomas,* *and neuroblastoma* [vinblastine sulfate] 10 mg/vial ⚕ Valpin

Velcade powder for IV injection ℞ *antineoplastic for multiple myeloma (orphan); investigational (Phase II) for mantle cell (non-Hodgkin) lymphoma* [bortezomib] 3.5 mg/vial

Veldona low-dose oral lozenge ℞ *investigational (Phase II) treatment for AIDS-related xerostomia; investigational (orphan) for oral human papillomavirus (HPV) warts in HIV-infected patients* [interferon alfa]

Veletri injection ℞ *investigational (Phase III) vasoconstrictor and endothelin receptor antagonist for acute heart failure, pulmonary edema, and hepatorenal syndrome* [tezosentan]

Velivet tablets (in packs of 28) ℞ *triphasic oral contraceptive; emergency postcoital contraceptive* [desogestrel; ethinyl estradiol]
Phase 1 (7 days): 100•25 µg;
Phase 2 (7 days): 125•25 µg;
Phase 3 (7 days): 150•25 µg

velnacrine INN, BAN *cholinesterase inhibitor* [also: velnacrine maleate]

velnacrine maleate USAN *cholinesterase inhibitor for Alzheimer disease* [also: velnacrine]

Velosef capsules, oral suspension ℞ *cephalosporin antibiotic* [cephradine] 250, 500 mg; 125, 250 mg/5 mL ⚕ Vasosulf

Velosef powder for IV or IM injection (discontinued 2004) ℞ *cephalosporin antibiotic* [cephradine] 250, 500, 1000, 2000 mg ⚕ Vasosulf

Velosulin BR vials for subcu injection (discontinued 2005) OTC *antidiabetic* [human insulin (rDNA)] 100 U/mL

Velvachol OTC *cream base*

Venice turpentine *medicinal herb* [see: larch]

venlafaxine INN, BAN *antidepressant; anxiolytic; selective serotonin and norepinephrine reuptake inhibitor (SSNRI)* [also: venlafaxine HCl]

venlafaxine HCl USAN *antidepressant; anxiolytic; selective serotonin and nor-*

Veramyst

epinephrine reuptake inhibitor (SSNRI) [also: venlafaxine]

Venofer IV injection ℞ *hematinic for iron deficiency due to chronic hemodialysis with erythropoietin therapy; also used in peritoneal dialysis and autologous blood donation* [iron sucrose] 20 mg Fe/mL

Venoglobulin-I powder for IV infusion (discontinued 2001; replaced by Venoglobulin-S) ℞ *passive immunizing agent for HIV and idiopathic thrombocytopenic purpura (ITP)* [immune globulin] 50 mg/mL

Venoglobulin-S powder for IV infusion (discontinued 2005) ℞ *passive immunizing agent for HIV and idiopathic thrombocytopenic purpura (ITP)* [immune globulin, solvent/detergent treated] 5%, 10%

Venomil subcu or IM injection ℞ *venom sensitivity testing (subcu); venom desensitization therapy (IM)* [extracts of honeybee, yellow jacket, yellow hornet, white-faced hornet, mixed vespid, and wasp venom]

Ventavis solution for inhalation ℞ *prostacyclin analogue for pulmonary arterial hypertension (PAH) (orphan)* [iloprost] 20 μg/2 mL dose

Ventolin ⒸⒶⓃ Diskus (inhalation powder device) ℞ *sympathomimetic bronchodilator* [albuterol sulfate] 200 μg/dose

Ventolin inhalation aerosol (discontinued 2003) ℞ *sympathomimetic bronchodilator* [albuterol] 90 μg/dose ② phentolamine

Ventolin Rotacap (encapsulated powder for inhalation), tablets, solution for inhalation, Nebules (unit-dose solution for inhalation), syrup (discontinued 2001) ℞ *sympathomimetic bronchodilator* [albuterol sulfate] 200 μg; 2, 4 mg; 0.05%; 0.083%; 2 mg/5 mL

Ventolin HFA inhalation aerosol with a CFC-free propellant ℞ *sympathomimetic bronchodilator* [albuterol] 90 μg/dose

VePesid IV injection, capsules ℞ *antineoplastic for testicular and small cell lung cancers* [etoposide] 20 mg/mL; 50 mg

veradoline INN *analgesic* [also: veradoline HCl]

veradoline HCl USAN *analgesic* [also: veradoline]

veralipride INN

verapamil USAN, INN, BAN *coronary vasodilator; calcium channel blocker*

verapamil HCl USAN, USP *antianginal; antiarrhythmic; antihypertensive; calcium channel blocker* 40, 80, 120, 180, 240 mg oral; 2.5 mg/mL injection

Veratrum **species** *medicinal herb* [see: hellebore]

veratrylidene-isoniazid [see: verazide]

verazide INN, BAN

Verazinc capsules OTC *zinc supplement* [zinc sulfate] 220 mg

Verbascum nigrum; V. phlomoides; V. thapsiforme; V. thapsus medicinal herb [see: mullein]

Verbena hastata medicinal herb [see: blue vervain]

Verelan sustained-release capsules ℞ *antihypertensive; antianginal; antiarrhythmic; calcium channel blocker* [verapamil HCl] 120, 180, 240, 360 mg

Verelan PM delayed-onset, extended-release capsules ℞ *antihypertensive; calcium channel blocker* [verapamil HCl] 100, 200, 300 mg

Vergon capsules (discontinued 2005) OTC *anticholinergic; antihistamine; antivertigo agent; motion sickness preventative* [meclizine HCl] 30 mg

Veridate (trademarked packaging form) *patient compliance package for oral contraceptives*

verilopam INN *analgesic* [also: verilopam HCl]

verilopam HCl USAN *analgesic* [also: verilopam]

verlukast USAN, INN *bronchodilator; antiasthmatic*

Verluma technetium Tc 99 prep kit ℞ *monoclonal antibody imaging agent for small cell lung cancer* [nofetumomab merpentan]

vermicides; vermifuges *a class of drugs effective against parasitic infections* [also called: anthelmintics]

Vermox chewable tablets R *anthelmintic for trichuriasis, enterobiasis, ascariasis, and uncinariasis* [mebendazole] 100 mg

verofylline USAN, INN *bronchodilator; antiasthmatic*

veronal [see: barbital]

veronal sodium [see: barbital sodium]

veronica, tall *medicinal herb* [see: Culver root]

Veronica beccabunga *medicinal herb* [see: brooklime]

Veronica officinalis *medicinal herb* [see: speedwell]

Versacaps sustained-release capsules R *decongestant; expectorant* [pseudoephedrine HCl; guaifenesin] 60•300 mg

Versed IV or IM injection, Tel-E-Ject syringes, pediatric syrup R *short-acting benzodiazepine general anesthetic adjunct for preoperative sedation* [midazolam HCl] 1, 5 mg/mL; 2 mg/mL

versetamide USAN *stabilizer; carrier agent for gadoversetamide*

Versiclear lotion R *antifungal; keratolytic; antipruritic; anesthetic* [sodium thiosulfate; salicylic acid; alcohol 10%] 25%•1%

verteporfin USAN *light-activated treatment for subfoveal choroidal neovascularization (CNV) due to age-related macular degeneration (AMD), pathologic myopia, or ocular histoplasmosis*

vervain *medicinal herb* [see: blue vervain]

Vesanoid capsules R *antineoplastic for acute promyelocytic leukemia (orphan); investigational (orphan) for other leukemias and ophthalmic squamous metaplasia* [tretinoin] 10 mg

vesicants *a class of agents that cause blisters*

VESIcare film-coated tablets R *once-daily antispasmodic for overactive bladder with urinary incontinence, urgency, and frequency* [solifenacin succinate] 5, 10 mg

vesnarinone USAN, INN *cardiotonic; inotropic for congestive heart failure*

vesperal [see: barbital]

Vesprin IV or IM injection (discontinued 2003) R *conventional (typical) antipsychotic; antiemetic* [triflupromazine HCl] 10, 20 mg/mL

Vestra tablets R *investigational (NDA filed) fast-acting selective norepinephrine reuptake inhibitor for depression* [reboxetine mesylate]

vetrabutine INN, BAN

Vetuss HC syrup (discontinued 2002) R *narcotic antitussive; decongestant; antihistamine* [hydrocodone bitartrate; phenylpropanolamine HCl; phenylephrine HCl; pyrilamine maleate; pheniramine maleate; alcohol 5%] 1.7•3.3•5•3.3•3.3 mg/5 mL

Vexol eye drop suspension R *topical ophthalmic corticosteroidal anti-inflammatory* [rimexolone] 1%

Vfend film-coated tablets, powder for oral suspension, powder for IV injection R *triazole antifungal for invasive aspergillosis, esophageal candidiasis, and other serious fungal infections* [voriconazole] 50, 200 mg; 40 mg/mL; 200 mg/vial

Viactiv chewable tablets OTC *calcium supplement* [calcium carbonate; vitamin D; vitamin K] 1.25 g•100 IU•40 μg

Viadur DUROS (once-yearly implant) R *antihormonal antineoplastic for the palliative treatment of advanced prostate cancer* [leuprolide acetate] 120 μg/day

Viaflex (trademarked form) *ready-to-use IV*

Viagra film-coated tablets R *phosphodiesterase type 5 (PDE5) inhibitor; selective vasodilator for erectile dysfunction (ED)* [sildenafil citrate] 25, 50, 100 mg

Vianain R *investigational (orphan) proteolytic enzymes for debridement of severe burns* [ananain; comosain; bromelains]

vibesate

Vibramycin capsules ℞ *tetracycline antibiotic* [doxycycline hyclate] 50, 100 mg

Vibramycin powder for oral suspension ℞ *tetracycline antibiotic* [doxycycline monohydrate] 25 mg/5 mL

Vibramycin syrup ℞ *tetracycline antibiotic* [doxycycline calcium] 50 mg/5 mL

Vibramycin I.V. powder for IV injection (discontinued 2003) ℞ *tetracycline antibiotic* [doxycycline hyclate] 100, 200 mg/vial

Vibra-Tabs film-coated tablets ℞ *tetracycline antibiotic* [doxycycline hyclate] 100 mg

Viburnum opulus medicinal herb [see: cramp bark]

VIC (VePesid, ifosfamide [with mesna rescue], carboplatin) *chemotherapy protocol for non–small cell lung cancer (NSCLC)* [also: CVI]

VIC (vinblastine, ifosfamide, CCNU) *chemotherapy protocol*

Vicam injection ℞ *parenteral vitamin therapy* [multiple B vitamins; vitamin C] ± • 50 mg/mL

Vicks 44 Cough Relief oral liquid OTC *antitussive* [dextromethorphan hydrobromide; alcohol 5%] 10 mg/5 mL

Vicks 44 Non-Drowsy Cold & Cough LiquiCaps (liquid-filled gelcaps) (discontinued 2002) OTC *antitussive; decongestant* [dextromethorphan hydrobromide; pseudoephedrine HCl] 30 • 60 mg

Vicks 44D Cough & Head Congestion Relief oral liquid OTC *antitussive; decongestant* [dextromethorphan hydrobromide; pseudoephedrine HCl; alcohol 5%] 30 • 60 mg/15 mL

Vicks 44E Cough & Chest Congestion Relief oral liquid OTC *antitussive; expectorant* [dextromethorphan hydrobromide; guaifenesin; alcohol 5%] 20 • 200 mg/15 mL

Vicks 44M Cold, Flu & Cough LiquiCaps (liquid-filled gelcaps) (discontinued 2002) OTC *antitussive; decongestant; antihistamine; analgesic* [dextromethorphan hydrobromide; pseudoephedrine HCl; chlorphenir-amine maleate; acetaminophen] 10 • 30 • 2 • 250 mg

Vicks 44M Cough, Cold, & Flu Relief oral liquid OTC *antitussive; decongestant; antihistamine; analgesic* [dextromethorphan hydrobromide; pseudoephedrine HCl; chlorphenir-amine maleate; acetaminophen; alcohol 10%] 30 • 60 • 4 • 650 mg/20 mL

Vicks Cough Drops; Vicks Menthol Cough Drops OTC *topical analgesic; counterirritant; mild local anesthetic* [menthol] 10 mg; 8.4 mg

Vicks Cough Silencers lozenges OTC *antitussive; topical oral anesthetic* [dextromethorphan hydrobromide; benzocaine] 2.5 • 1 mg

Vicks DayQuil products [see: DayQuil]

Vicks Dry Hacking Cough syrup (discontinued 2002) OTC *antitussive* [dextromethorphan hydrobromide; alcohol 10%] 15 mg/5 mL

Vicks Formula 44D Cough & Decongestant; Vicks Pediatric Formula 44d Cough & Decongestant oral liquid (discontinued 2002) OTC *antitussive; decongestant* [dextromethorphan hydrobromide; pseudoephedrine HCl] 10 • 20 mg/5 mL; 5 • 10 mg/5 mL

Vicks NyQuil products [see: NyQuil]

Vicks Pediatric 44d Dry Hacking Cough and Head Congestion syrup (discontinued 2002) OTC *antitussive* [dextromethorphan hydrobromide] 15 mg/15 mL

Vicks Pediatric 44e Cough & Chest Congestion Relief oral liquid OTC *antitussive; expectorant* [dextromethorphan hydrobromide; guaifenesin] 10 • 100 mg/15 mL

Vicks Pediatric 44m Cough & Cold Relief oral liquid OTC *antitussive; decongestant; antihistamine* [dextromethorphan hydrobromide; pseudoephedrine HCl; chlorpheniramine maleate] 15 • 30 • 2 mg/15 mL

Vicks Sinex products [see: Sinex]

Vicks Vapor inhaler OTC *nasal decongestant* [levmetamfetamine] 50 mg

Vicks VapoRub vaporizing ointment, cream OTC *counterirritant; cough suppressant* [camphor; menthol; eucalyptus oil] 5.2%•2.8%•1.2%

Vicks Vitamin C Drops (lozenges) OTC *vitamin C supplement* [ascorbic acid and sodium ascorbate] 25 mg

Vicodin; Vicodin ES; Vicodin HP tablets ℞ *narcotic analgesic* [hydrocodone bitartrate; acetaminophen] 5• 500 mg; 7.5•750 mg; 10•660 mg

Vicodin Tuss syrup ℞ *narcotic antitussive; expectorant* [hydrocodone bitartrate; guaifenesin] 5•100 mg/5 mL ⧉ Hycodan; Hycomine

Vicon Forte capsules ℞ *vitamin/mineral supplement* [multiple vitamins & minerals; folic acid] ±•1 mg

Vicon Plus capsules OTC *vitamin/mineral supplement* [multiple vitamins & minerals]

Vicon-C capsules OTC *vitamin/mineral supplement* [multiple B vitamins & minerals; vitamin C] ±•300 mg

Vicoprofen film-coated tablets ℞ *narcotic analgesic & antitussive* [hydrocodone bitartrate; ibuprofen] 7.5•200 mg

vicotrope [see: cosyntropin]

vidarabine USAN, USP, INN, BAN *antiviral* ⧉ cytarabine

vidarabine monohydrate [see: vidarabine]

vidarabine phosphate USAN *antiviral*

vidarabine sodium phosphate USAN *antiviral*

Vi-Daylin chewable tablets (discontinued 2003) OTC *vitamin supplement* [multiple vitamins; folic acid] ±•0.3 mg

Vi-Daylin ADC drops OTC *vitamin supplement* [vitamins A, C, and D] 1500 IU•35 mg•400 IU per mL

Vi-Daylin ADC Vitamins + Iron drops OTC *vitamin/iron supplement* [vitamins A, C, and D; ferrous gluconate] 1500 IU•35 mg•400 IU•10 mg per mL

Vi-Daylin Multivitamin oral liquid, drops OTC *vitamin supplement* [multiple vitamins]

Vi-Daylin Multivitamin + Iron chewable tablets (discontinued 2003) OTC *vitamin/iron supplement* [multiple vitamins; iron; folic acid] ±•12•0.3 mg

Vi-Daylin Multivitamin + Iron oral liquid, drops OTC *vitamin/iron supplement* [multiple vitamins; ferrous gluconate] ±•10 mg/5 mL; ±•10 mg/mL

Vi-Daylin/F ADC drops ℞ *pediatric vitamin supplement and dental caries preventative* [vitamins A, C, and D; sodium fluoride] 1500 IU•35 mg• 400 IU•0.25 mg per mL

Vi-Daylin/F ADC + Iron drops ℞ *pediatric vitamin/iron supplement and dental caries preventative* [vitamins A, C, and D; sodium fluoride; ferrous sulfate] 1500 IU•35 mg•400 IU• 0.25 mg•10 mg per mL

Vi-Daylin/F Multivitamin chewable tablets (discontinued 2004) ℞ *pediatric vitamin supplement and dental caries preventative* [multiple vitamins; sodium fluoride; folic acid] ±•1•0.3 mg

Vi-Daylin/F Multivitamin drops ℞ *pediatric vitamin supplement and dental caries preventative* [multiple vitamins; sodium fluoride] ±•0.25 mg/mL

Vi-Daylin/F Multivitamin + Iron chewable tablets ℞ *pediatric vitamin/iron supplement and dental caries preventative* [multiple vitamins; sodium fluoride; ferrous sulfate; folic acid] ± •1•12•0.3 mg

Vi-Daylin/F Multivitamin + Iron drops ℞ *pediatric vitamin/iron supplement and dental caries preventative* [multiple vitamins; sodium fluoride; ferrous sulfate] ±•0.25•10 mg/mL

Vidaza suspension for subcu injection ℞ *demethylating antineoplastic for myelodysplastic syndrome (orphan)* [azacitidine] 100 mg/vial

Videx chewable/dispersible tablets, powder for oral solution, powder for pediatric oral solution ℞ *antiviral for advanced HIV infection* [didanosine]

25, 50, 100, 200 mg; 100, 250 mg/
pkt.; 2, 4 g/bottle

Videx EC delayed-release capsules
with enteric-coated beads R̶ *antiviral
for advanced HIV infection* [didano-
sine] 200, 250, 500 mg

**VIE (vincristine, ifosfamide, etopo-
side)** *chemotherapy protocol*

vifilcon A USAN *hydrophilic contact lens
material*

vifilcon B USAN *hydrophilic contact lens
material*

Vi-Flor [see: Poly-Vi-Flor; Tri-Vi-Flor]

VIG (vaccinia immune globulin)
[q.v.]

vigabatrin USAN, INN, BAN *investigational (NDA filed) anticonvulsant;
investigational treatment for cocaine
and methamphetamine addictions*

Vigamox eye drops R̶ *broad-spectrum
fluoroquinolone antibiotic* [moxifloxa-
cin HCl] 0.5%

Vigomar Forte tablets OTC *vitamin/
mineral/iron supplement* [multiple
vitamins & minerals; iron] ≛•12 mg

Vigortol oral liquid OTC *geriatric vita-
min/mineral supplement* [multiple B
vitamins & minerals; alcohol 18%]

viloxazine INN, BAN *investigational
(NDA filed) bicyclic antidepressant;
investigational (orphan) for cataplexy
and narcolepsy* [also: viloxazine HCl]

viloxazine HCl USAN *bicyclic antidepressant* [also: viloxazine]

Viminate oral liquid OTC *geriatric vita-
min/mineral supplement* [multiple B
vitamins & minerals]

viminol INN

vinafocon A USAN *hydrophobic contact
lens material*

**Vinate Good Start Prenatal For-
mula** chewable tablets R̶ *prenatal
vitamin/mineral/calcium/iron supplement* [multiple vitamins & minerals;
calcium; iron; folic acid] ≛•200•
29•1 mg

Vinate GT tablets R̶ *prenatal vitamin/
mineral/calcium/iron supplement; stool
softener* [multiple vitamins & minerals; calcium; iron; folic acid; biotin;

docusate sodium] ≛•200•90•1•
0.03•50 mg

vinbarbital NF, INN [also: vinbarbitone]

vinbarbital sodium NF

vinbarbitone BAN [also: vinbarbital]

vinblastine INN *vinca alkaloid antineoplastic* [also: vinblastine sulfate]

vinblastine sulfate USAN, USP *vinca
alkaloid antineoplastic* [also: vinblas-
tine] 10 mg/vial, 1 mg/mL injection

vinblastine sulfate & estramustine
chemotherapy protocol for prostate cancer

vinburnine INN

vinca alkaloids *a class of natural antineoplastics*

Vinca major; V. minor *medicinal herb*
[see: periwinkle]

vincaleukoblastine sulfate [see: vinblastine sulfate]

vincamine INN, BAN

vincanol INN

vincantenate [see: vinconate]

vincantril INN

Vincasar PFS IV injection R̶ *antineoplastic* [vincristine sulfate] 1 mg/mL

vincofos USAN, INN *anthelmintic*

vinconate INN

vincristine (VC; VCR) INN *antineoplastic* [also: vincristine sulfate]

vincristine sulfate USAN, USP *antineoplastic* [also: vincristine] 1 mg/mL
injection

vindeburnol INN

vindesine USAN, INN, BAN *synthetic
vinca alkaloid antineoplastic*

vindesine sulfate USAN, JAN *investigational (NDA filed) synthetic vinca
alkaloid antineoplastic for leukemia,
melanoma, breast and lung cancers*

vinegar [see: acetic acid]

vinepidine INN *antineoplastic* [also:
vinepidine sulfate]

vinepidine sulfate USAN *antineoplastic*
[also: vinepidine]

vinformide INN

vinglycinate INN *antineoplastic* [also:
vinglycinate sulfate]

vinglycinate sulfate USAN *antineoplastic* [also: vinglycinate]

vinleurosine INN *antineoplastic* [also: vinleurosine sulfate]

vinleurosine sulfate USAN *antineoplastic* [also: vinleurosine]

vinmegallate INN

vinorelbine INN *antineoplastic* [also: vinorelbine tartrate]

vinorelbine & cisplatin *chemotherapy protocol for cervical cancer and non–small cell lung cancer (NSCLC)*

vinorelbine & doxorubicin *chemotherapy protocol for breast cancer*

vinorelbine & gemcitabine *chemotherapy protocol for non–small cell lung cancer (NSCLC)*

vinorelbine & paclitaxel *chemotherapy protocol for breast cancer*

vinorelbine tartrate USAN *antineoplastic* [also: vinorelbine] 10 mg/mL injection

vinpocetine USAN, INN *natural derivative of vincamine, an extract of the periwinkle plant; increases ATP levels in the brain, which increases memory and mental function by increasing the neuronal firing rate; also increases serotonin levels in the brain*

vinpoline INN

vinrosidine INN *antineoplastic* [also: vinrosidine sulfate]

vinrosidine sulfate USAN *antineoplastic* [also: vinrosidine]

vintiamol INN

vintoperol INN

vintriptol INN

vinyl alcohol polymer [see: polyvinyl alcohol]

vinyl ether USP

vinyl gamma-aminobutyric acid [see: vigabatrin]

vinylbital INN [also: vinylbitone]

vinylbitone BAN [also: vinylbital]

vinylestrenolone [see: norgesterone]

vinymal [see: vinylbital]

vinyzene [see: bromchlorenone]

vinzolidine INN *antineoplastic* [also: vinzolidine sulfate]

vinzolidine sulfate USAN *antineoplastic* [also: vinzolidine]

Vioform cream, ointment (discontinued 2000) OTC *topical antifungal; antibacterial* [clioquinol] 3%

Viogen-C capsules OTC *vitamin/mineral supplement* [multiple B vitamins & minerals; vitamin C] ± • 300 mg

Viokase powder ℞ *porcine-derived digestive enzymes* [lipase; protease; amylase] 16 800 • 70 000 • 70 000 USP units/¼ tsp.

Viokase 8; Viokase 16 tablets ℞ *porcine-derived digestive enzymes* [lipase; protease; amylase] 8000 • 30 000 • 30 000 USP units; 16 000 • 60 000 • 60 000 USP units

Viola odorata medicinal herb [see: violet]

Viola tricolor medicinal herb [see: pansy]

violet *(Viola odorata)* flowers and leaves *medicinal herb for asthma, bronchitis, cancer, colds, cough, sinus congestion, tumors, and ulcers*

violet, garden *medicinal herb* [see: pansy]

violetbloom *medicinal herb* [see: bittersweet nightshade]

viomycin INN [also: viomycin sulfate]

viomycin sulfate USP [also: viomycin]

viosterol in oil [see: ergocalciferol]

Vioxx tablets, oral suspension (withdrawn by the manufacturer in 2004 due to safety concerns) ℞ *analgesic; antiarthritic; antipyretic; COX-2 inhibitor; nonsteroidal anti-inflammatory drug (NSAID); treatment for acute migraine* [rofecoxib] 12.5, 25, 50 mg; 12.5, 25 mg/5 mL

Viozan ℞ *investigational treatment for chronic obstructive pulmonary disease (COPD)* [sibenadet HCl]

VIP (VePesid, ifosfamide [with mesna rescue], Platinol) *chemotherapy protocol for genitourinary cancers, testicular cancer, small cell lung cancer (SCLC), and non–small cell lung cancer (NSCLC)*

VIP (vinblastine, ifosfamide [with mesna rescue], Platinol) *chemotherapy protocol*

VIP-B (VP-16, ifosfamide, Platinol, bleomycin) *chemotherapy protocol*

Viprinex Ⓒⓐⓝ subcu injection, IV infusion ℞ *anticoagulant for deep vein thrombosis (DVT) and severe chronic peripheral circulatory disorders; investigational (orphan) in the U.S. for cardiopulmonary bypass in heparin-intolerant patients* [ancrod] 70 IU/mL

viprostol USAN, INN, BAN *hypotensive; vasodilator*

viprynium embonate BAN *anthelmintic* [also: pyrvinium pamoate]

viqualine INN

viquidil INN

Viquin Forte cream (discontinued 2003) ℞ *hyperpigmentation bleaching agent* [hydroquinone (in a sunscreen base)] 4%

Vira-A ophthalmic ointment (discontinued 2004) ℞ *antiviral for acute keratoconjunctivitis and recurrent epithelial keratitis due to herpes simplex virus infection* [vidarabine] 3%

Viracept film-coated tablets, powder for oral solution ℞ *antiretroviral; protease inhibitor for HIV-1 infection* [nelfinavir mesylate] 250, 650 mg; 50 mg/g

Viractin cream, gel (name changed to **Cēpacol Viractin** in 2001)

Viramune tablets, oral suspension ℞ *antiviral non-nucleoside reverse transcriptase inhibitor (NNRTI) for HIV-1 infections* [nevirapine] 200 mg; 50 mg/5 mL

Viravan-DM oral suspension, chewable tablets ℞ *pediatric antitussive, decongestant, and antihistamine* [dextromethorphan tannate; phenylephrine tannate; pyrilamine tannate] 25•12.5•30 mg/5 mL; 25•25•30 mg

Viravan-S pediatric oral suspension ℞ *decongestant antihistamine* [phenylephrine tannate; pyrilamine tannate] 12.5•30 mg/5 mL

Viravan-T pediatric chewable tablets ℞ *decongestant; antihistamine* [phenylephrine tannate; pyrilamine tannate] 25•30 mg

Virazole powder for inhalation aerosol ℞ *nucleoside antiviral for severe lower respiratory tract infections caused by respiratory syncytial virus (RSV);* investigational (orphan) for hemorrhagic fever with renal syndrome [ribavirin] 6 g/vial (20 mg/mL reconstituted)

Viread film-coated tablets ℞ *antiviral; nucleotide reverse transcriptase inhibitor (NRTI) for HIV-1 infection* [tenofovir disoproxil fumarate] 300 mg

Virginia mountain mint; Virginia thyme *medicinal herb* [see: wild hyssop]

Virginia silk *medicinal herb* [see: milkweed]

virginiamycin USAN, INN *antibacterial; veterinary food additive*

virginiamycin factor M₁ [see: virginiamycin]

virginiamycin factor S [see: virginiamycin]

virgin's bower *medicinal herb* [see: woodbine]

viridofulvin USAN, INN *antifungal*

Virilon capsules, IM injection ℞ *androgen for hypogonadism or testosterone deficiency in men, delayed puberty in boys, and metastatic breast cancer in women; also abused as a street drug* [methyltestosterone] 10 mg; 200 mg/mL

Virogen Herpes slide test for professional use *in vitro diagnostic aid for herpes simplex virus antigen in lesions or cell cultures* [latex agglutination test]

Virogen Rotatest slide test for professional use *in vitro diagnostic aid for fecal rotavirus* [latex agglutination test]

Viroptic Drop-Dose (eye drops) ℞ *ophthalmic antiviral for keratoconjunctivitis and epithelial keratitis due to herpes simplex virus infection* [trifluridine] 1%

viroxime USAN, INN *antiviral*

viroxime component A [see: zinviroxime]

viroxime component B [see: enviroxime]

Viroxyn oral gel OTC *germicide for cold sores/fever blisters* [benzalkonium chloride; isopropyl alcohol] 0.13%•70%

Virulizin *investigational (Phase III) macrophage activator for AIDS-related* *lymphomas, Kaposi sarcoma, and pancreatic cancer*

Viscoat prefilled syringes ℞ *viscoelastic agent for ophthalmic surgery* [hyaluronate sodium; chondroitin sulfate sodium] 30•40 mg/mL

Viscum album medicinal herb [see: mistletoe]

Visicol tablets ℞ *saline laxative; pre-procedure bowel evacuant* [sodium phosphate (monobasic and dibasic)] 1.5 g (1.102•0.398 g)

visilizumab USAN *investigational anti-CD3 monoclonal antibody for organ transplants, autoimmune diseases, and other T lymphocyte disorders*

visiluzumab [now: visilizumab]

Visine Allergy Relief eye drops OTC *topical ophthalmic decongestant and astringent* [tetrahydrozoline HCl; zinc sulfate] 0.05%•0.25%

Visine L.R. eye drops OTC *topical ophthalmic decongestant and vasoconstrictor* [oxymetazoline HCl] 0.025%

Visine Moisturizing eye drops OTC *topical ophthalmic decongestant, vasoconstrictor, and lubricant* [tetrahydrozoline HCl; polyethylene glycol 400] 0.05%•1%

Visine Pure Tears; Visine Tears; Visine Tears Preservative Free eye drops OTC *topical ophthalmic moisturizer and lubricant* [polyethylene glycol 400; glycerin; hypromellose] 1%•0.2%•0.2%

Visine-A eye drops OTC *topical ophthalmic decongestant and vasoconstrictor* [naphazoline HCl; pheniramine maleate] 0.025%•0.3%

Vision (trademarked device) OTC *needle-free insulin injection system*

Vision Care Enzymatic Cleaner tablets OTC *enzymatic cleaner for soft contact lenses* [pork pancreatin]

VisionBlue ophthalmic injection in prefilled syringes ℞ *surgical aid for staining the anterior capsule of the lens* [trypan blue] 0.06% in 0.5 mL syringes

Visipak (trademarked packaging form) *reverse-numbered package*

Visipaque 270; Visipaque 320 intra-arterial or IV injection ℞ *radiopaque contrast medium for CT, x-ray, and visceral digital subtraction angiography* [iodixanol (49.1% iodine)] 550 mg/mL (270 mg/mL); 652 mg/mL (320 mg/mL)

Visken tablets ℞ *antihypertensive; antianginal; β-blocker* [pindolol] 5, 10 mg

visnadine INN, BAN

visnafylline INN

Vi-Sol [see: Poly-Vi-Sol; Tri-Vi-Sol]

Vistaril capsules, oral suspension ℞ *anxiolytic; minor tranquilizer; antihistamine for allergic pruritus* [hydroxyzine pamoate] 25, 50, 100 mg; 25 mg/5 mL ⊘ Restoril

Vistaril deep IM injection ℞ *anxiolytic; antiemetic; antihistamine for allergic pruritus; adjunct to preoperative or prepartum analgesia* [hydroxyzine HCl] 25 mg/mL ⊘ Restoril; Zestril

vistatolon INN *antiviral* [also: statolon]

Vistazine 50 IM injection (discontinued 2003) ℞ *anxiolytic; antiemetic; antihistamine for allergic pruritus* [hydroxyzine HCl] 50 mg/mL

Vistide IV infusion ℞ *nucleoside antiviral for AIDS-related cytomegalovirus retinitis* [cidofovir] 75 mg/mL

Visual-Eyes ophthalmic solution OTC *extraocular irrigating solution* [sterile isotonic solution]

Visudyne powder for IV infusion ℞ *treatment for subfoveal choroidal neovascularization (CNV) due to age-related macular degeneration (AMD), pathologic myopia, or ocular histoplasmosis; activated with the Opal Photoactivator laser* [verteporfin] 2 mg/mL (15 mg/vial)

Vita-bee with C Captabs (capsule-shaped tablets) OTC *vitamin supplement* [multiple B vitamins; vitamin C] ≚•300 mg

Vita-Bob softgel capsules OTC *vitamin supplement* [multiple vitamins; folic acid] ≚•0.4 mg

Vita-C crystals oTc *vitamin C supplement* [ascorbic acid] 4 g/tsp.

VitaCarn oral solution (discontinued 2001) ℞ *dietary amino acid for primary and secondary genetic carnitine deficiency (orphan) and end-stage renal disease (orphan); investigational (orphan) for pediatric cardiomyopathy* [levocarnitine]

Vitafōl syrup ℞ *hematinic* [ferric pyrophosphate; multiple B vitamins; folic acid] 90● ± ●0.75 mg/15 mL

Vitafōl; Vitafōl-PN film-coated caplets ℞ *hematinic; vitamin supplement* [ferrous fumarate; multiple vitamins; folic acid] 65 mg● ± ● 1 mg

Vita-Kid chewable wafers oTc *vitamin supplement* [multiple vitamins; folic acid] ± ●0.3 mg

Vital B-50 timed-release tablets oTc *vitamin supplement* [multiple B vitamins; folic acid; biotin] ± ●100●50 μg

Vital High Nitrogen powder oTc *enteral nutritional therapy* [lactose-free formula] 79 g

Vitalets chewable tablets oTc *vitamin/mineral/iron supplement* [multiple vitamins & minerals; iron; biotin] ± ●10 mg●25 μg

Vitalize SF oral liquid oTc *hematinic* [ferric pyrophosphate; multiple B vitamins; lysine] 66● ± ●300 mg/15 mL

Vitalux ⒸⒶⒷ time-release tablet oTc *vitamin/antioxidant supplement* [multiple vitamins; multiple minerals]

vitamin A usp *fat-soluble vitamin; antixerophthalmic; topical emollient; essential for vision, dental development, growth, cortisone synthesis, epithelial tissue differentiation, embryonic development, reproduction, and mucous membrane maintenance* 10 000, 15 000, 25 000 IU oral

vitamin A acid [see: tretinoin]

vitamin A palmitate

vitamin A₁ [see: retinol]

Vitamin B Complex 100 injection ℞ *parenteral vitamin therapy* [multiple B vitamins]

vitamin B₁ [see: thiamine HCl]

vitamin B₁ mononitrate [see: thiamine mononitrate]

vitamin B₂ [see: riboflavin]

vitamin B₃ [see: niacin; niacinamide]

vitamin B₅ [see: calcium pantothenate]

vitamin B₆ [see: pyridoxine HCl]

vitamin B₈ [see: adenosine phosphate]

vitamin B₁₂ [now: cyanocobalamin; hydroxocobalamin]

vitamin B_c [see: folic acid]

vitamin B_t [see: carnitine]

vitamin C [see: ascorbic acid; calcium ascorbate; sodium ascorbate]

vitamin D *a family of fat-soluble vitamins consisting of ergocalciferol (vitamin D₂) and cholecalciferol (vitamin D₃), which is converted to calcitriol (the active form) in the body; considered a non-endogenous hormone* [see also: calcifediol; dihydrotachysterol; doxercalciferol; paricalcitol]

vitamin D₁ [see: dihydrotachysterol]

vitamin D₂ [see: ergocalciferol]

vitamin D₃ [see: cholecalciferol]

vitamin E usp *fat-soluble vitamin; antioxidant; platelet aggregation inhibitor; topical emollient* [note relative potencies at alpha tocopherol, et seq.] 100, 200, 400, 500, 800, 1000 IU oral; 15 IU/30 mL oral

Vitamin E with Mixed Tocopherols tablets oTc *vitamin supplement* [vitamin E] 100, 200, 400 IU

vitamin E-TPGS (tocopheryl polyethylene glycol succinate) [see: tocophersolan]

vitamin G [see: riboflavin]

vitamin H [see: biotin]

vitamin K₁ [see: phytonadione]

vitamin K₂ [see: menaquinone]

vitamin K₃ [see: menadione]

vitamin K₄ [see: menadiol sodium diphosphate]

vitamin M [see: folic acid]

vitamin P [see: bioflavonoids]

vitamin P₄ [see: troxerutin]

Vitamin-Mineral Supplement oral liquid oTc *vitamin/mineral supplement*

[multiple B vitamins & minerals; alcohol 18%]

Vitaneed oral liquid OTC *enteral nutritional therapy* [lactose-free formula]

Vita-Plus E softgels OTC *vitamin supplement* [vitamin E (as *d*-alpha tocopheryl acetate)] 400 IU

Vita-Plus G softgel capsules OTC *geriatric vitamin/mineral supplement* [multiple vitamins & minerals]

Vita-Plus H softgel capsules OTC *vitamin/mineral/iron supplement* [multiple vitamins & minerals; iron] ± • 13.4 mg

Vita-PMS; Vita-PMS Plus tablets OTC *vitamin/mineral supplement; digestive enzymes* [multiple vitamins & minerals; folic acid; biotin; amylase; protease; lipase; betaine acid HCl] ± • 0.33 mg • 10.4 μg • 2500 U • 2500 U • 200 U • 16.7 mg

Vitarex tablets OTC *vitamin/mineral/iron supplement* [multiple vitamins & minerals; iron] ± • 15 mg

Vite E cream OTC *emollient* [vitamin E] 50 mg/g

Vitec cream OTC *emollient* [vitamin E]

Vitelle Irospan capsules OTC *hematinic; vitamin/iron supplement* [ferrous sulfate, dried (source of iron); ascorbic acid] 200 (65) • 150 mg

Vitelle Irospan timed-release tablets (discontinued 2005) OTC *hematinic; vitamin/iron supplement* [ferrous sulfate, dried (source of iron); ascorbic acid] 200 (65) • 150 mg

Vitelle Lurline PMS tablets OTC *analgesic; antipyretic; diuretic; vitamin B$_6$* [acetaminophen; pamabrom; pyridoxine HCl] 500 • 25 • 50 mg

Vitelle Nesentials tablets OTC *vitamin/mineral supplement* [multiple vitamins & minerals]

Vitelle Nestabs OTC tablets OTC *prenatal vitamin/calcium/iron supplement* [multiple vitamins; calcium; iron; folic acid] ± • 200 • 29 • 0.8 mg

Vitelle Nestrex tablets OTC *vitamin B$_6$ supplement* [pyridoxine HCl] 25 mg

vitellin natural remedy [see: lecithin]

Vitex agnus-castus medicinal herb [see: chaste tree]

Vitinoin Ⓒ cream, gel (discontinued 2001) ℞ *keratolytic for acne* [tretinoin] 0.025%, 0.05%, 0.1%; 0.025%

Vitis coigetiae; V. vinifera medicinal herb [see: grape seed]

Vitrase powder for injection, solution for injection ℞ *adjuvant to increase the absorption and dispersion of injected drugs, hypodermoclysis, and subcutaneous urography; investigational (NDA filed) agent to clear vitreous hemorrhage; also used for diabetic retinopathy* [hyaluronidase (ovine)] 6200 U; 200 U/mL

Vitrasert intraocular implant (5–8 months' duration) ℞ *antiviral for AIDS-related CMV retinitis (orphan)* [ganciclovir] 4.5 mg

Vitravene intravitreal injection ℞ *ophthalmic antiviral for AIDS-related CMV retinitis* [fomivirsen sodium] 6.6 mg/mL

Vitron-C tablets OTC *hematinic; vitamin/iron supplement* [ferrous fumarate (source of iron); ascorbic acid] 200 (66) • 125 mg ⧉ Vytone

Vitussin syrup ℞ *narcotic antitussive; expectorant* [hydrocodone bitartrate; guaifenesin] 5 • 100 mg/5 mL

Vivactil film-coated tablets ℞ *tricyclic antidepressant* [protriptyline HCl] 5, 10 mg

Viva-Drops eye drops OTC *ocular moisturizer/lubricant*

Vivarin tablets OTC *CNS stimulant; analeptic* [caffeine] 200 mg

Vivelle; Vivelle-Dot transdermal patch ℞ *estrogen replacement therapy for the treatment of postmenopausal symptoms and prevention of postmenopausal osteoporosis* [estradiol] 37.5, 50, 75, 100 μg/day; 25, 37.5, 50, 75, 100 μg/day

Vivitrex extended-release injection ℞ *investigational (NDA filed) treatment for alcoholism; investigational (Phase I) treatment for opiate addiction* [naltrexone HCl]

Vivonex T.E.N. powder OTC *enteral nutritional therapy* [lactose-free formula]

Vivotif Berna enteric-coated capsules ℞ *typhoid fever vaccine* [typhoid vaccine (Ty21a), live attenuated] 2–6 × 10⁹ viable CFU + 5–50 × 10⁹ nonviable cells

Vi-Zac capsules OTC *vitamin/zinc supplement* [vitamins A, C, and E; zinc] 5000 IU•500 mg•50 mg•18 mg

VLP (vincristine, L-asparaginase, prednisone) *chemotherapy protocol*

VM (vinblastine, mitomycin) *chemotherapy protocol for breast cancer*

VM-26 [see: teniposide]

VM-26PP (teniposide, procarbazine, prednisone) *chemotherapy protocol*

VMAD (vincristine, methotrexate, Adriamycin, actinomycin D) *chemotherapy protocol*

VMCP (vincristine, melphalan, cyclophosphamide, prednisone) *chemotherapy protocol for multiple myeloma* [also: VCMP]

VMP (VePesid, mitoxantrone, prednimustine) *chemotherapy protocol*

VOCAP (VP-16-213, Oncovin, cyclophosphamide, Adriamycin, Platinol) *chemotherapy protocol*

Vofenal Ⓒᴬᴺ eye drops (discontinued 2001) ℞ *topical nonsteroidal anti-inflammatory drug (NSAID)* [diclofenac sodium] 0.1%

vofopitant dihydrochloride USAN *tachykinin NK₁ receptor antagonist; antiemetic*

voglibose USAN *investigational α-glucosidase inhibitor; antidiabetic*

volatile nitrites *amyl nitrite, butyl nitrite, and isobutyl nitrite vapors that produce coronary stimulant effects, abused as street drugs* [see also: nitrous oxide; petroleum distillate inhalants]

volazocine USAN, INN *analgesic*

Volmax extended-release tablets (discontinued 2004) ℞ *sympathomimetic bronchodilator* [albuterol sulfate] 4, 8 mg

Voltaren delayed-release tablets ℞ *analgesic; antiarthritic; nonsteroidal anti-inflammatory drug (NSAID) for ankylosing spondylitis* [diclofenac sodium] 25, 50, 75 mg

Voltaren eye drops ℞ *ocular nonsteroidal anti-inflammatory drug (NSAID) for postoperative treatment following cataract extraction or corneal refractive surgery* [diclofenac sodium] 0.1%

Voltaren Ⓒᴬᴺ suppositories ℞ *analgesic; antiarthritic; nonsteroidal anti-inflammatory drug (NSAID)* [diclofenac sodium] 50, 100 mg

Voltaren Ophtha Ⓒᴬᴺ eye drops ℞ *ocular nonsteroidal anti-inflammatory drug (NSAID) for postoperative treatment following cataract extraction* [diclofenac sodium] 0.1%

Voltaren Rapide Ⓒᴬᴺ tablets ℞ *analgesic; antiarthritic; nonsteroidal anti-inflammatory drug (NSAID)* [diclofenac potassium] 50 mg

Voltaren SR Ⓒᴬᴺ slow-release tablets ℞ *once-daily antiarthritic; nonsteroidal anti-inflammatory drug (NSAID)* [diclofenac sodium] 75, 100 mg

Voltaren XR extended-release tablets ℞ *once-daily antiarthritic; nonsteroidal anti-inflammatory drug (NSAID)* [diclofenac sodium] 100 mg

von Willebrand factor (VWF) *antihemophilic for von Willebrand disease*

Vopac caplets ℞ *narcotic analgesic; antitussive* [codeine phosphate; acetaminophen] 30•650 mg

voriconazole *triazole antifungal for invasive aspergillosis, esophageal candidiasis, and other serious fungal infections*

vorozole USAN, INN, BAN *antineoplastic; aromatase inhibitor*

vortel [see: clorprenaline HCl]

VōSol HC Otic ear drops ℞ *topical corticosteroidal anti-inflammatory; antibacterial; antifungal* [hydrocortisone; acetic acid] 1%•2%

VōSol Otic ear drops ℞ *antibacterial; antifungal* [acetic acid] 2%

VoSpire ER extended-release tablets ℞ *sympathomimetic bronchodilator* [albuterol sulfate] 4, 8 mg

votumumab USAN *monoclonal antibody for cancer imaging and therapy*

voxergolide INN

Voxsuprine tablets ℞ *peripheral vasodilator* [isoxsuprine HCl] 10, 20 mg

VP (vasopressin) [q.v.]

VP (VePesid, Platinol) *chemotherapy protocol for small cell lung cancer* (SCLC)

VP (vincristine, prednisone) *chemotherapy protocol*

VP + A (vincristine, prednisone, asparaginase) *chemotherapy protocol*

VP-16 [see: etoposide]

VPB (vinblastine, Platinol, bleomycin) *chemotherapy protocol*

VPBCPr (vincristine, prednisone, vinblastine, chlorambucil, procarbazine) *chemotherapy protocol*

VPCA (vincristine, prednisone, cyclophosphamide, ara-C) *chemotherapy protocol*

VPCMF (vincristine, prednisone, cyclophosphamide, methotrexate, fluorouracil) *chemotherapy protocol*

VP-L-asparaginase (vincristine, prednisone, L-asparaginase) *chemotherapy protocol*

VPP (VePesid, Platinol) *chemotherapy protocol*

V-TAD (VePesid, thioguanine, ara-C, daunorubicin) *chemotherapy protocol for acute myelocytic leukemia* (AML)

vulneraries *a class of agents that promote wound healing*

Vumon IV infusion ℞ *antineoplastic for acute lymphocytic leukemia (orphan) and bladder cancer* [teniposide] 50 mg (10 mg/mL)

V.V.S. vaginal cream (discontinued 2001) ℞ *broad-spectrum antibiotic* [sulfathiazole; sulfacetamide; sulfabenzamide] 3.42%•2.86%•3.7%

VWF (von Willebrand factor) [q.v.]

VX-175 *investigational (Phase III) protease inhibitor for HIV infections*

Vytone cream ℞ *topical corticosteroidal anti-inflammatory; antifungal; antibacterial* [hydrocortisone; iodoquinol] 1%•1% ☒ Hytone; Vitron

Vytorin 10/10; Vytorin 10/20; Vytorin 10/40; Vytorin 10/80 caplets ℞ *antihyperlipidemic for hypercholesterolemia; intestinal cholesterol absorption inhibitor; HMG-CoA reductase inhibitor* [ezetimibe; simvastatin] 10•10 mg; 10•20 mg; 10•40 mg; 10•80 mg

VZIG (varicella-zoster immune globulin) [q.v.]

wahoo (*Euonymus atropurpureus*) bark *medicinal herb used as a diuretic, expectorant, and laxative*

wakerobin *medicinal herb* [see: birthroot]

Wallette (trademarked packaging form) *patient compliance package for oral contraceptives*

wallflower; western wallflower *medicinal herb* [see: dogbane]

walnut (*Juglans* spp.) *medicinal herb* [see: black walnut; butternut; English walnut]

walnut, lemon; white walnut *medicinal herb* [see: butternut]

Walpole tea *medicinal herb* [see: New Jersey tea]

wandering milkweed *medicinal herb* [see: dogbane]

warfarin INN, BAN *coumarin-derivative anticoagulant* [also: warfarin potassium]

warfarin potassium USP *coumarin-derivative anticoagulant* [also: warfarin]

warfarin sodium USP *coumarin-derivative anticoagulant* 1, 2, 2.5, 3, 4, 5, 6, 7.5, 10 mg oral

Wart Remover topical liquid OTC *keratolytic* [salicylic acid in flexible collodion] 17%

Wartec ⓒᴬᴺ solution ℞ *antimitotic for external genital warts* [podofilox] 0.5%

Wart-Off topical liquid OTC *keratolytic* [salicylic acid in flexible collodion] 17%

water, purified USP *solvent*

water, tritiated [see: tritiated water]

water cabbage *medicinal herb* [see: white pond lily]

water dock (*Rumex aquaticus*) *medicinal herb* [see: yellow dock]

water eryngo (*Eryngium aquaticum*) root *medicinal herb used as a diaphoretic, diuretic, emetic, expectorant, and stimulant*

water fern *medicinal herb* [see: buckhorn brake]

water flag *medicinal herb* [see: blue flag]

water hemlock; water parsley *medicinal herb* [see: poison hemlock]

water lily *medicinal herb* [see: blue flag; white pond lily]

water lily, sweet; sweet-scented water lily; white water lily *medicinal herb* [see: white pond lily]

water moccasin snake antivenin [see: antivenin (Crotalidae) polyvalent]

water O 15 USAN *radioactive diagnostic aid for vascular disorders*

water pepper *medicinal herb* [see: knotweed]

water pimpernel; water purslain *medicinal herb* [see: brooklime]

water shamrock *medicinal herb* [see: buckbean]

water smartweed *medicinal herb* [see: knotweed]

[^{15}O]water [see: water O 15]

watercress (*Nasturtium officinale*) plant *medicinal herb for anemia, cramps, kidney and liver disorders, nervousness, and rheumatism*

water-d$_2$ [see: deuterium oxide]

wax, carnauba NF *tablet-coating agent*

wax, emulsifying NF *emulsifying and stiffening agent*

wax, microcrystalline NF *stiffening and tablet-coating agent*

wax, white NF *stiffening agent* [also: beeswax, white]

wax, yellow NF *stiffening agent* [also: beeswax, yellow]

wax cluster *medicinal herb* [see: wintergreen]

wax myrtle *medicinal herb* [see: bayberry]

weeping spruce *medicinal herb* [see: hemlock]

WelChol tablets ℞ *nonabsorbable cholesterol-lowering polymer for hyperlipidemia* [colesevelam HCl] 625 mg

Wellbutrin film-coated tablets ℞ *aminoketone antidepressant* [bupropion HCl] 75, 100 mg

Wellbutrin SR sustained-release film-coated tablets ℞ *aminoketone antidepressant* [bupropion HCl] 100, 150, 200 mg

Wellbutrin XL extended-release tablets ℞ *aminoketone antidepressant* [bupropion HCl] 150, 300 mg

Wellcovorin powder for IV infusion (discontinued 2002) ℞ *chemotherapy "rescue" agent (orphan)* [leucovorin calcium] 100 mg/vial

Wellcovorin tablets (discontinued 2002) ℞ *chemotherapy "rescue" agent (orphan); antidote to folic acid antagonist overdose* [leucovorin calcium] 5, 25 mg

Wellferon ⓒᴬᴺ subcu or IM injection (discontinued 2001) ℞ *biological response modifier for hairy cell leukemia, laryngeal papillomatosis, condylomata acuminata, and chronic hepatitis B and C* [interferon alfa-n1] 3, 5, 10 MU/mL (an MU or "megaunit" is 10^6 IU)

Westcort ointment, cream ℞ *corticosteroidal anti-inflammatory* [hydrocortisone valerate] 0.2%

western wallflower *medicinal herb* [see: dogbane]

Westhroid tablets ℞ *thyroid replacement therapy for hypothyroidism or thyroid* cancer [thyroid, desiccated (porcine)] 32.4, 64.8, 129.6, 194.4 mg

Wet-N-Soak solution OTC *rewetting solution for rigid gas permeable contact lenses*

Wet-N-Soak Plus solution OTC *disinfecting/wetting/soaking solution for rigid gas permeable contact lenses* [note: RGP contact indication different from hard contact indication for same product]

Wet-N-Soak Plus solution OTC *wetting/soaking solution for hard contact lenses* [note: hard contact indication different from RGP contact indication for same product]

Wetting solution OTC *wetting solution for hard contact lenses*

Wetting & Soaking solution OTC *disinfecting/wetting/soaking solution for rigid gas permeable contact lenses* [note: one of two different products with the same name]

Wetting & Soaking solution OTC *wetting/soaking solution for hard contact lenses* [note: one of two different products with the same name]

wheat germ oil (octacosanol) *natural dietary supplement for increasing muscle endurance*

WHF Lubricating Gel OTC *vaginal antimicrobial and lubricant* [chlorhexidine gluconate; glycerin]

white bay *medicinal herb* [see: magnolia]

white beeswax [see: beeswax, white]

White Cloverine Salve ointment OTC *skin protectant* [white petrolatum] 97%

White Cod Liver Oil Concentrate capsules, chewable tablets OTC *vitamin supplement* [vitamins A, D, and E] 10 000•400•2 IU; 4000•200•2 IU

White Cod Liver Oil Concentrate with Vitamin C chewable tablets OTC *vitamin supplement* [vitamins A, C, and D] 4000 IU•50 mg•200 IU

white cohosh (Actaea alba; A. pachypoda; A. rubra) plant and root *medicinal herb for arthritis, bowel evacuation, colds, cough, itching, promoting labor, reviving those near death,* *rheumatism, stimulating menses, stomach disorders, and urogenital disorders*

white endive *medicinal herb* [see: dandelion]

white fringe *medicinal herb* [see: fringe tree]

white hellebore (Veratrum album) [see: hellebore]

white horehound *medicinal herb* [see: horehound]

white lotion USP *astringent; topical protectant*

white mineral oil [see: petrolatum, white]

white mustard; white mustard seed *medicinal herb* [see: mustard]

white nettle *medicinal herb* [see: blind nettle]

white oak (Quercus alba) bark *medicinal herb for internal and external bleeding, menstrual disorders, mouth sores, skin irritation, toothache, strep throat, ulcers, and urinary bleeding*

white ointment [see: ointment, white]

white petrolatum [see: petrolatum, white]

white phenolphthalein [see: phenolphthalein]

white pine (Pinus strobus) bark *medicinal herb for bronchitis, dysentery, laryngitis, and mucous build-up*

white pond lily (Nymphaea odorata) root *medicinal herb used as an antiseptic, astringent, demulcent, discutient, and vulnerary*

white root *medicinal herb* [see: pleurisy root]

white sorrel *medicinal herb* [see: wood sorrel]

white walnut *medicinal herb* [see: butternut]

white water lily *medicinal herb* [see: white pond lily]

white wax [see: wax, white]

white willow (Salix alba) *medicinal herb* [see: willow]

whitethorn *medicinal herb* [see: hawthorn]

Whitfield's Ointment OTC *antifungal; keratolytic* [benzoic acid; salicylic acid] 6%•3%

Whitfield's ointment [see: benzoic & salicylic acids]

whole blood [see: blood, whole]

whole root rauwolfia [see: rauwolfia serpentina]

whole-cell pertussis vaccine [see: diphtheria & tetanus toxoids & whole-cell pertussis (DTwP) vaccine, adsorbed]

whorlywort *medicinal herb* [see: Culver root]

Wibi lotion OTC *moisturizer; emollient*

widow spider species antivenin [now: antivenin (*Latrodectus mactans*)]

Wigraine suppositories (discontinued 2005) ℞ *migraine-specific vasoconstrictor* [ergotamine tartrate; caffeine; tartaric acid] 2•100•21.5 mg

Wigraine tablets (discontinued 2005) ℞ *migraine-specific vasoconstrictor* [ergotamine tartrate; caffeine] 1•100 mg

wild bergamot (*Monarda fistulosa*) leaves *medicinal herb used as a carminative and stimulant*

wild black cherry (*Prunus serotina*) bark *medicinal herb used as an astringent, pectoral, sedative, and stimulant*

wild carrot *medicinal herb* [see: carrot]

wild cherry (*Prunus virginiana*) bark *medicinal herb for asthma, bronchitis, cough, fever, hypertension, and mucosal inflammation with discharge; also used as an expectorant*

wild cherry syrup USP

wild chicory *medicinal herb* [see: chicory]

wild clover *medicinal herb* [see: red clover]

wild cranesbill *medicinal herb* [see: alum root]

wild daisy (*Bellis perennis*) flowers and leaves *medicinal herb used as an analgesic, antispasmodic, demulcent, digestive, expectorant, laxative, and purgative*

wild endive *medicinal herb* [see: dandelion]

wild fennel *medicinal herb* [see: fennel]

wild geranium *medicinal herb* [see: alum root]

wild ginger (*Asarum canadense*) root *medicinal herb used as a carminative, diaphoretic, expectorant, and irritant; sometimes used as a substitute for ginger (*Zingiber*)*

wild hydrangea *medicinal herb* [see: hydrangea]

wild hyssop *medicinal herb* [see: blue vervain]

wild hyssop (*Pycnanthemum virginianum*) plant *medicinal herb used as an antispasmodic, carminative, diaphoretic, and stimulant*

wild indigo (*Baptisia tinctoria*) plant *medicinal herb used as an antiseptic, astringent, emetic, purgative, and stimulant*

wild jalap (*Ipomoea pandurata*) root *medicinal herb used as a strong cathartic*

wild lemon *medicinal herb* [see: mandrake]

wild lettuce (*Lactuca virosa*) leaves, flowers, and seeds *medicinal herb for asthma, bronchitis, chronic pain, circulatory disorders, cramps, laryngitis, nervous disorders, stimulating lactation, swollen genitals, and urinary tract infections*

wild marjoram *medicinal herb* [see: marjoram]

wild Oregon grape *medicinal herb* [see: Oregon grape]

wild pepper *medicinal herb* [see: mezereon; Siberian ginseng]

wild potato; wild scammony; wild sweet potato vine *medicinal herb* [see: wild jalap]

wild red raspberry *medicinal herb* [see: red raspberry]

wild senna *medicinal herb* [see: senna]

wild snowball *medicinal herb* [see: New Jersey tea]

wild strawberry *medicinal herb* [see: strawberry]

wild tobacco *medicinal herb* [see: lobelia]

wild turkey pea *medicinal herb* [see: turkey corn]

wild valerian, great *medicinal herb* [see: valerian]

wild woodbine *medicinal herb* [see: American ivy]

wild yam (Dioscorea villosa) root *medicinal herb for arthritis, bilious colic, bowel spasms, gas, menstrual cramps, morning sickness, and spasmodic asthma*

Willard water *natural remedy for acne, alopecia, anxiety, arthritis, hypertension, and stomach ulcers*

willow (Salix alba; S. caprea; S. nigra; S. purpurea) bark and buds *medicinal herb for analgesia, diuresis, eczema, fever, inducing diaphoresis, headache, nervousness, rheumatism, and ulcerations; also used as an anaphrodisiac, antiseptic, and astringent*

wind root *medicinal herb* [see: pleurisy root]

wineberry *medicinal herb* [see: currant]

winged elm *medicinal herb* [see: slippery elm]

WinRho SDF freeze-dried powder for IV or IM injection ℞ *obstetric Rh factor immunity suppressant; treatment for immune thrombocytopenic purpura (orphan)* [Rh₀(D) immune globulin, solvent/detergent treated] 600, 1500, 5000 IU (120, 300, 1000 μg)

Winstrol tablets (discontinued 2005) ℞ *anabolic steroid for hereditary angioedema* [stanozolol] 2 mg

winter bloom *medicinal herb* [see: witch hazel]

winter clover *medicinal herb* [see: squaw vine]

winter marjoram; winter sweet *medicinal herb* [see: marjoram]

winter savory (Calamintha montana; Satureja montana; S. obovata) leaves and stems *medicinal herb for diarrhea, nausea, promoting expectoration, relieving gas and flatulence, and stimulation of menstruation; also used as an aphrodisiac*

winterberry (Ilex verticillata) bark and fruit *medicinal herb used as an astringent, bitter tonic, and febrifuge*

wintergreen (Gaultheria procumbens) leaves and oil *medicinal herb for aches and pains, colds, gout, lumbago, and migraine headache; also used topically as an astringent and rubefacient*

wintergreen, bitter; false wintergreen *medicinal herb* [see: pipsissewa]

wintergreen oil [see: methyl salicylate]

winterlein *medicinal herb* [see: flaxseed]

Wintersteiner's compound F [see: hydrocortisone]

winterweed *medicinal herb* [see: chickweed]

witch hazel (Hamamelis virginiana) bark *medicinal herb for bruises, burns, colds, colitis, diarrhea, dysentery, eye irritations, hemorrhoids, internal and external bleeding, mucous membrane inflammation of mouth, gums, and throat, tuberculosis, and varicose veins*

withania (Withania somnifera) fruit and roots *medicinal herb for diuresis, inducing emesis, liver disorders, inflammation, sedation, tuberculosis, and tumors*

withe; withy *medicinal herb* [see: willow]

wolf claw *medicinal herb* [see: club moss]

Women's Daily Formula capsules OTC *vitamin/calcium/iron supplement* [multiple vitamins; calcium; iron; folic acid] ±•450•25•0.4 mg

Women's Gentle Laxative enteric-coated tablets OTC *stimulant laxative* [bisacodyl] 5 mg

Wonder Ice gel OTC *topical analgesic; counterirritant* [menthol] 5.25%

Wondra lotion OTC *moisturizer; emollient* [lanolin]

wood betony *medicinal herb* [see: betony]

wood creosote [see: creosote carbonate]

wood sanicle *medicinal herb* [see: sanicle]

wood sorrel (Oxalis acetosella) plant *medicinal herb used as an anodyne, diuretic, emmenagogue, irritant, and stomachic*

wood strawberry *medicinal herb* [see: strawberry]

woodbine *(Clematis virginiana)* leaves *medicinal herb for bowel evacuation, cancer, edema, fever, hypertension, inflammation, insomnia, itching, kidney disorders, skin cuts and sores, tuberculous cervical lymphadenitis, tumors, and venereal eruptions; not generally regarded as safe and effective*

woodbine; American woodbine; wild woodbine *medicinal herb* [see: American ivy]

woodruff *medicinal herb* [see: sweet woodruff]

woody nightshade *medicinal herb* [see: bittersweet nightshade]

Woolley's antiserotonin [see: benanserin HCl]

wooly parsnip *medicinal herb* [see: masterwort]

wormwood *(Artemisia absinthium)* plant and leaves *medicinal herb for aiding digestion, constipation, debility, fever, intestinal worms, jaundice, labor pains, menstrual cramps, and stomach and liver disorders; not generally regarded as safe and effective*

wound weed *medicinal herb* [see: goldenrod]

woundwort *(Prunella vulgaris)* plant *medicinal herb used as an antispasmodic, astringent, bitter tonic, diuretic, hemostatic, vermifuge, and vulnerary*

woundwort, soldier's *medicinal herb* [see: yarrow]

WOWtabs (trademarked dosage form) *quickly dissolving "without water" tablets*

Wyamine Sulfate IV or IM injection (discontinued 2005) ℞ *vasopressor for hypotensive shock* [mephentermine sulfate] 15, 30 mg/mL

Wyanoids Relief Factor rectal suppositories OTC *emollient* [cocoa butter; shark liver oil] 79%•3%

Wycillin IM, IV, intrapleural, or intrathecal injection, Tubex (cartridge-needle units) (discontinued 2003) ℞ *natural penicillin antibiotic* [penicillin G procaine] 600 000, 1 200 000 U/vial ☑ Bicillin; V-Cillin

Wydase IV or subcu injection, powder for injection (discontinued 2001) ℞ *adjuvant to increase absorption and dispersion of injected drugs* [hyaluronidase] 150 U/mL; 150, 1500 U/vial ☑ Lidex

Wygesic tablets (discontinued 2004) ℞ *narcotic analgesic* [propoxyphene HCl; acetaminophen] 65•650 mg

wymote *medicinal herb* [see: marsh mallow]

Wymox capsules, powder for oral suspension (discontinued 2002) ℞ *aminopenicillin antibiotic* [amoxicillin] 250, 500 mg; 125, 250 mg/5 mL

Wyseal (trademarked dosage form) *film-coated tablet*

Wytensin tablets ℞ *antihypertensive* [guanabenz acetate] 4, 8 mg

Xalatan eye drops ℞ *prostaglandin agonist for glaucoma and ocular hypertension* [latanoprost] 0.005% ☑ Dilantin

xamoterol USAN, INN, BAN *cardiac stimulant*

xamoterol fumarate USAN *cardiac stimulant*

Xanax tablets ℞ *benzodiazepine anxiolytic; sedative; treatment for panic disorders and agoraphobia* [alprazolam] 0.25, 0.5, 1, 2 mg ☑ Tenex; Zantac

Xanax XR extended-release tablets ℞ *benzodiazepine anxiolytic for panic disorder and agoraphobia* [alprazolam] 0.5, 1, 2, 3 mg

xanomeline USAN *cholinergic agonist for Alzheimer disease*

xanomeline tartrate USAN *cholinergic agonist for Alzheimer disease*

xanoxate sodium USAN *bronchodilator*

xanoxic acid INN

xanthan gum NF *suspending agent*

xanthines, xanthine derivatives *a class of bronchodilators*

xanthinol niacinate USAN *peripheral vasodilator* [also: xantinol nicotinate]

xanthiol INN

xanthiol HCl [see: xanthiol]

xanthocillin BAN [also: xantocillin]

Xanthorhiza simplicissima *medicinal herb* [see: yellow root]

xanthotoxin [see: methoxsalen]

Xanthoxylum americanum; X. fraxineum *medicinal herb* [see: prickly ash]

xantifibrate INN

xantinol nicotinate INN *peripheral vasodilator* [also: xanthinol niacinate]

xantocillin INN [also: xanthocillin]

xantofyl palmitate INN

Xatral (foreign name for U.S. product **Uroxatral**)

Xcytrin injection ℞ *investigational (Phase III) radiosensitizer for brain metastases* [motexafin gadolinium]

127Xe [see: xenon Xe 127]

133Xe [see: xenon Xe 133]

Xeloda film-coated tablets ℞ *antineoplastic for metastatic breast and colorectal cancer; investigational (Phase III) for pancreatic cancer* [capecitabine] 150, 500 mg

xemilofiban HCl USAN *antianginal*

xenalamine [see: xenazoic acid]

xenaldial [see: xenygloxal]

xenalipin USAN, INN *hypolipidemic*

xenazoic acid INN

xenbucin USAN, INN *antihypercholesterolemic*

xenbuficin [see: xenbucin]

Xenical capsules ℞ *lipase inhibitor for weight loss; preventative for type 2 diabetes* [orlistat] 120 mg

xenipentone INN

xenon *element* (Xe)

xenon (133Xe) INN *radioactive agent* [also: xenon Xe 133]

xenon Xe 127 USP *diagnostic aid; medicinal gas; radioactive agent*

xenon Xe 133 USAN, USP *radioactive agent* [also: xenon (133Xe)]

xenthiorate INN

xenygloxal INN

xenyhexenic acid INN

xenysalate INN, BAN *topical anesthetic; antibacterial; antifungal* [also: biphenamine HCl]

xenysalate HCl [see: biphenamine HCl]

xenytropium bromide INN

Xerac AC topical liquid ℞ *cleanser for acne* [aluminum chloride; alcohol] 6.25%•96%

Xerecept *investigational (Phase I/II, orphan) agent for peritumoral brain edema* [corticotropin-releasing factor]

xibenolol INN

xibornol INN, BAN

Xibrom eye drops ℞ *long-acting nonsteroidal anti-inflammatory drug (NSAID) for the treatment of ocular inflammation following cataract surgery* [bromfenac sodium] 0.09%

Xifaxan film-coated tablets ℞ *broadspectrum rifamycin antibiotic for traveler's diarrhea* [rifaximin] 200 mg

Xigris powder for IV infusion ℞ *antithrombotic; recombinant human activated protein C (rhAPC) for severe sepsis* [drotrecogin alfa] 5, 20 mg/vial

xilobam USAN, INN *muscle relaxant*

ximelagatran *investigational (NDA filed) oral anticoagulant and direct thrombin inhibitor for the prevention of stroke due to atrial fibrillation and the prevention and treatment of a venous thromboembolic event (VTE); prodrug of melagatran*

ximoprofen INN

xinafoate USAN, INN, BAN *combining name for radicals or groups*

xinidamine INN

Xinlay ℞ *investigational (NDA filed) endothelin-A (EtA; ETA; ET_A) receptor antagonist to retard the progression of metastatic prostate cancer by reducing its proliferative effects in bone and prostate tissue* [atrasentan HCl]

xinomiline INN

xipamide USAN, INN *antihypertensive; diuretic*

xipranolol INN

Xiral sustained-release caplets ℞ *decongestant; antihistamine; anticholinergic to dry mucosal secretions* [pseudoephedrine HCl; chlorpheniramine maleate; methscopolamine nitrate] 120•8•2.5 mg

Xolair powder for subcu injection ℞ *immunoglobulin E (IgE) blocker for moderate to severe asthma* [omalizumab] 75 mg/0.6 mL dose, 150 mg/ 1.2 mL dose

XomaZyme-791 *investigational (orphan) for metastatic colorectal adenocarcinoma* [anti-TAP-72 immunotoxin]

Xopenex inhalation solution, inhalation solution concentrate ℞ *sympathomimetic bronchodilator* [levalbuterol HCl] 0.31, 0.63, 1.25 mg/3 mL dose; 1.25 mg/0.5 mL dose

xorphanol INN *analgesic* [also: xorphanol mesylate]

xorphanol mesylate USAN *analgesic* [also: xorphanol]

X-Prep oral liquid OTC *pre-procedure bowel evacuant* [senna extract] 74 mL

X-Prep Bowel Evacuant Kit-1 oral liquid + 2 tablets + 1 suppository OTC *pre-procedure bowel evacuant* [X-Prep liquid (q.v.); Senokot-S tablets (q.v.); Rectolax suppository (q.v.)]

X-Prep Bowel Evacuant Kit-2 oral liquid + granules + 1 suppository (discontinued 2003) OTC *pre-procedure bowel evacuant* [X-Prep liquid (q.v.); Citralax granules (q.v.); Rectolax suppository (q.v.)]

XRT (x-ray therapy) *adjunct to chemotherapy* [not a pharmaceutical agent]

X-Seb shampoo OTC *antiseborrheic; keratolytic* [salicylic acid] 4%

X-Seb Plus shampoo OTC *antiseborrheic; keratolytic; antibacterial; antifungal* [salicylic acid; pyrithione zinc] 2%•1%

X-Seb T shampoo OTC *antiseborrheic; antipsoriatic; keratolytic* [coal tar; salicylic acid] 10%•4%

X-Seb T Plus shampoo OTC *antiseborrheic; antipsoriatic; keratolytic* [coal tar; salicylic acid; menthol] 10%•3%•1%

xylamidine tosilate INN *serotonin inhibitor* [also: xylamidine tosylate]

xylamidine tosylate USAN *serotonin inhibitor* [also: xylamidine tosilate]

xylazine INN *analgesic; veterinary muscle relaxant* [also: xylazine HCl]

xylazine HCl USAN *analgesic; veterinary muscle relaxant* [also: xylazine]

xylitol NF *sweetened vehicle*

Xylocaine subcu and IV injection ℞ *local anesthetic (subcu); antiarrhythmic for acute ventricular arrhythmias (IV)* [lidocaine HCl] 0.5%, 1%, 2%

Xylocaine topical liquid, topical solution, ointment, gel ℞ *mucous membrane anesthetic* [lidocaine HCl] 5%; 4%; 2.5%, 5%; 2%

Xylocaine 10% Oral spray ℞ *mucous membrane anesthetic* [lidocaine HCl] 10%

Xylocaine HCl injection ℞ *injectable local anesthetic* [lidocaine HCl; dextrose] 1.5%•7.5%

Xylocaine HCl injection ℞ *injectable local anesthetic* [lidocaine HCl; epinephrine] 0.5%•1:200 000, 1%• 1:100 000, 1%•1:200 000, 2%• 1:50 000, 2%•1:100 000, 2%• 1:200 000

Xylocaine HCl IV for Cardiac Arrhythmias IV injection, IV admixture ℞ *antiarrhythmic* [lidocaine HCl] 1%, 2%, 4%, 20%

Xylocaine MPF injection ℞ *injectable local anesthetic* [lidocaine HCl] 0.5%, 1%, 1.5%, 2%, 4%

Xylocaine MPF injection ℞ *injectable local anesthetic* [lidocaine HCl; epinephrine] 1%•1:200 000, 1.5%• 1:200 000, 2%•1:200 000

Xylocaine MPF injection ℞ *injectable local anesthetic* [lidocaine HCl; glucose] 5%•7.5%

Xylocaine Viscous solution ℞ *mucous membrane anesthetic* [lidocaine HCl] 2%

xylocoumarol INN

xylofilcon A USAN *hydrophilic contact lens material*

xylometazoline INN, BAN *vasoconstrictor; nasal decongestant* [also: xylometazoline HCl]

xylometazoline HCl USP *vasoconstrictor; nasal decongestant* [also: xylometazoline]

Xylo-Pfan tablets (discontinued 2004) OTC *diagnostic aid for intestinal function* [xylose] 25 g

xylose (D-xylose) USP *diagnostic aid for intestinal function*

xyloxemine INN

Xyotax ℞ *investigational (Phase III) taxane for lung cancer* [polyglutamate paclitaxel]

Xyrem oral solution ℞ *CNS depressant for cataplexy in narcoleptic patients* [sodium oxybate] 500 mg/mL

Xyvion ℞ *investigational (NDA filed) synthetic steroid for osteoporosis and other postmenopausal symptoms* [tibolone]

Xyzal (approved in Europe) ℞ *investigational (Phase III) nonsedating antihistamine for allergic rhinitis* [efletirizine]

yam *medicinal herb* [see: wild yam]

yarrow (Achillea millefolium) *flower medicinal herb for bowel hemorrhage, colds, fever, flu, hypertension, inducing sweating, measles, mucosal inflammation with discharge, nosebleed, reducing heavy menstrual bleeding and pain, thrombosis, and topical hemostasis*

Yasmin film-coated tablets (in packs of 28) ℞ *monophasic oral contraceptive* [drospirenone; ethinyl estradiol] 3 mg•30 μg

yatren [see: chiniofon]

[169]Yb [see: pentetate calcium trisodium Yb 169]

[169]Yb [see: ytterbium Yb 169 pentetate]

yeast, dried NF

yeast cell derivative *claimed to promote wound healing*

Yeast-Gard vaginal suppositories OTC *for vaginal irritations, itching, and burning* [pulsatilla 28x; Candida albicans 28x]

Yeast-Gard Medicated Disposable Douche Premix solution OTC *antifungal; vaginal cleanser and deodorizer; acidity modifier* [sodium benzoate; lactic acid]

Yeast-Gard Medicated Douche; Yeast-Gard Medicated Disposable Douche solution OTC *antiseptic/germicidal; vaginal cleanser and deodorizer* [povidone-iodine] 10%; 0.3%

Yeast-X vaginal suppositories OTC *for vaginal irritations, itching, and burning* [pulsatilla 28x]

Yelets tablets OTC *vitamin/mineral/iron supplement* [multiple vitamins & minerals; ferrous fumarate; folic acid] ±•20•0.1 mg

yellow bedstraw; yellow cleavers *medicinal herb* [see: bedstraw]

yellow beeswax [see: beeswax, yellow]

yellow dock (Rumex crispus) *root medicinal herb for anemia, blood cleansing, constipation, itching, liver congestion, rheumatism, skin problems, and eyelid ulcerations; also used as a dentifrice*

yellow ferric oxide [see: ferric oxide, yellow]

yellow fever vaccine USP *active immunizing agent for yellow fever*

yellow gentian *medicinal herb* [see: gentian]

yellow ginseng *medicinal herb* [see: blue cohosh]

yellow Indian paint *medicinal herb* [see: goldenseal]

yellow jessamine *medicinal herb* [see: gelsemium]

yellow mercuric oxide [see: mercuric oxide, yellow]

yellow ointment [see: ointment, yellow]

yellow paint root; yellow root *medicinal herb* [see: goldenseal]

yellow petrolatum JAN *ointment base; emollient/protectant* [also: petrolatum]

yellow phenolphthalein [see: phenolphthalein, yellow]

yellow precipitate [see: mercuric oxide, yellow]

yellow puccoon *medicinal herb* [see: goldenseal]

yellow root *(Xanthorhiza simplicissima) medicinal herb used for diabetes and hypertension*

yellow root; yellow paint root *medicinal herb* [see: goldenseal]

yellow wax [see: wax, yellow]

yellow wood; yellow wood berries *medicinal herb* [see: prickly ash]

Yentreve (approved in Europe) ℞ *investigational (Phase II) selective serotonin and norepinephrine reuptake inhibitor (SSNRI) for stress urinary incontinence* [duloxetine HCl]

yerba maté *(Ilex paraguariensis) leaves medicinal herb used as a CNS stimulant, diuretic, and purifier*

yerba santa *(Eriodictyon californicum) leaves medicinal herb for asthma, bronchial congestion, colds, hay fever, inducing expectoration, inflammation, rheumatic pain, and tuberculosis*

yew *(Taxus bacatta and other* **species)** *leaves medicinal herb for liver disorders, rheumatism, and urinary tract disorders*

YF-Vax subcu injection ℞ *yellow fever vaccine* [yellow fever vaccine] 0.5 mL

Yocon tablets ℞ *alpha₂-adrenergic blocker for impotence and orthostatic hypotension; sympatholytic; mydriatic; may have aphrodisiac activity; no FDA-approved indications* [yohimbine HCl] 5.4 mg

Yodoxin tablets, powder ℞ *amebicide for intestinal amebiasis* [iodoquinol] 210, 650 mg; 25 g

yohimbe *(Corynanthe johimbe; Pausinystalia johimbe) bark medicinal herb for angina, hypertension, and impotence and other sexual dysfunction; also used as an aphrodisiac*

yohimbic acid INN

yohimbine HCl *alpha₂-adrenergic blocker for impotence and orthostatic hypotension; sympatholytic; mydriatic; may have aphrodisiac activity; no FDA-sanctioned indications* 5.4 mg oral

Yohimex tablets (discontinued 2003) ℞ *alpha₂-adrenergic blocker for impotence; sympatholytic; mydriatic; may have aphrodisiac activity; no FDA-approved indications* [yohimbine HCl] 5.4 mg

Yondelis ℞ *investigational (Phase III) tetrahydroisoquinoline alkaloid for sarcoma* [ecteinascidin]

Your Choice Non-Preserved Saline solution OTC *rinsing/storage solution for soft contact lenses* [sodium chloride (saline solution)]

Your Choice Sterile Preserved Saline solution OTC *rinsing/storage solution for soft contact lenses* [sodium chloride (preserved saline solution)]

youthwort *medicinal herb* [see: masterwort]

ytterbium *element* (Yb)

ytterbium Yb 169 pentetate USP *radioactive agent*

yttrium *element* (Y)

yttrium Y 90 ibritumomab tiuxetan *radioimmunotherapy for non-Hodgkin B-cell lymphoma*

yttrium Y 90 murine monoclonal antibodies (2B8-MXDTPA) & indium In 111 murine monoclonal antibodies (2B8-MXDTPA) *investigational (orphan) for non-Hodgkin B-cell lymphoma*

yucca *(Yucca glauca) root medicinal herb for arthritis, colitis, hypertension, migraine headache, and rheumatism*

yuma *medicinal herb* [see: wild yam]

Yutopar IV infusion (discontinued 2003) ℞ *uterine relaxant to arrest pre-* *term labor* [ritodrine HCl] 10, 15 mg/mL

$$\boxed{Z}$$

zabicipril INN

zacopride INN *antiemetic; peristaltic stimulant* [also: zacopride HCl]

zacopride HCl USAN, INN *antiemetic; peristaltic stimulant* [also: zacopride]

Zacutex IV injection ℞ *investigational (Phase III) platelet activating factor (PAF) antagonist for acute pancreatitis* [lexipafant]

Zadaxin (approved in several countries) ℞ *investigational (Phase III) influenza vaccine and vaccine enhancer for lung cancer; investigational (Phase III, orphan) for chronic hepatitis B; investigational (orphan) for DiGeorge syndrome with immune defects; investigational (orphan) for hepatocellular carcinoma; investigational (Phase II) for AIDS* [thymalfasin]

Zaditen Ophthalmic (foreign name for U.S. product Zaditor)

Zaditor eye drops ℞ *ophthalmic antihistamine and mast cell stabilizer for allergic conjunctivitis* [ketotifen fumarate] 0.025%

zafirlukast USAN, INN, BAN *leukotriene receptor antagonist (LTRA) for prevention and chronic treatment of asthma*

zafuleptine INN

Zagam film-coated tablets ℞ *once-daily broad-spectrum fluoroquinolone antibiotic for community-acquired respiratory infections* [sparfloxacin] 200 mg

zalcitabine USAN *nucleoside reverse transcriptase inhibitor (NRTI); antiviral for advanced HIV infection* (orphan)

zaleplon USAN *pyrazolopyrimidine hypnotic for the short-term treatment of insomnia*

zalospirone INN *anxiolytic* [also: zalospirone HCl]

zalospirone HCl USAN *anxiolytic* [also: zalospirone]

zaltidine INN, BAN *antagonist to histamine H$_2$ receptors* [also: zaltidine HCl]

zaltidine HCl USAN *antagonist to histamine H$_2$ receptors* [also: zaltidine]

zamifenacin INN, BAN *investigational treatment for irritable bowel syndrome*

Zanaflex tablets, capsules ℞ *antispasmodic for multiple sclerosis and spinal cord injury* (orphan) [tizanidine HCl] 2, 4 mg; 2, 4, 6 mg

zanamivir USAN *influenza neuraminidase inhibitor for the treatment of acute influenza types A and B*

Zanfel cream, wash OTC *poison ivy treatment* [polyethylene granules]

zankiren HCl USAN *antihypertensive*

Zanosar powder for IV injection ℞ *nitrosourea-type alkylating antineoplastic for metastatic islet cell carcinoma of pancreas* [streptozocin] 1 g (100 mg/mL)

zanoterone USAN *antiandrogen*

Zantac film-coated tablets, syrup, IV or IM injection ℞ *histamine H$_2$ antagonist for gastric and duodenal ulcers* [ranitidine HCl] 150, 300 mg; 15 mg/mL; 1, 25 mg/mL 🔊 Xanax

Zantac 75; Zantac 150 tablets OTC *histamine H$_2$ antagonist for episodic heartburn* [ranitidine HCl] 75 mg; 150 mg

Zantac EFFERdose effervescent granules (discontinued 2005) ℞ *histamine H$_2$ antagonist for gastric and duodenal ulcers* [ranitidine HCl] 150 mg/pkt.

Zantac EFFERdose effervescent tablets ℞ *histamine H$_2$ antagonist for gastric and duodenal ulcers* [ranitidine HCl] 25, 150 mg

Zantac GELdose capsules ℞ *histamine H$_2$ antagonist for gastric and duodenal ulcers* [ranitidine HCl] 150, 300 mg

Zanthorhiza apiifolia *medicinal herb* [see: yellow root]

Zantryl capsules (discontinued 2001) ℞ *anorexiant; CNS stimulant* [phentermine HCl] 30 mg

Zanzibar aloe *medicinal herb* [see: aloe]

zapizolam INN

zaprinast INN, BAN

zardaverine INN

Zarontin capsules, syrup ℞ *anticonvulsant* [ethosuximide] 250 mg; 250 mg/5 mL ⑨ Zaroxolyn

Zaroxolyn tablets ℞ *antihypertensive; diuretic* [metolazone] 2.5, 5, 10 mg ⑨ Zarontin; Zeroxin

zatosetron INN, BAN *antimigraine* [also: zatosetron maleate]

zatosetron maleate USAN *antimigraine* [also: zatosetron]

Zavedos (European name for U.S. product **Idamycin**)

Zavesca capsules ℞ *treatment for type I Gaucher disease* [miglustat] 100 mg

Zazole vaginal cream ℞ *antifungal* [terconazole] 0.8%

Z-Bec tablets OTC *vitamin/zinc supplement* [multiple vitamins; zinc sulfate] ≛•22.5 mg

ZBT Baby topical powder (discontinued 2003) OTC *diaper rash treatment* [talc]

Z-Cof DM syrup ℞ *antitussive; decongestant; expectorant* [dextromethorphan hydrobromide; pseudoephedrine HCl; guaifenesin] 30•80•400 mg/10 mL

Z-Cof HC syrup ℞ *narcotic antitussive; decongestant; antihistamine* [hydrocodone bitartrate; phenylephrine HCl; chlorpheniramine maleate] 3.5•10•2.5 mg/5 mL

Z-Cof LA sustained-release tablets ℞ *antitussive; expectorant* [dextromethorphan hydrobromide; guaifenesin] 3•650 mg

ZDV (zidovudine) [q.v.]

ZE Caps soft capsules OTC *dietary supplement* [vitamin E; zinc gluconate] 200•9.6 mg

Zea mays *medicinal herb* [see: Indian corn]

Zeasorb AF Ⓒᴬᴺ topical solution OTC *topical antifungal* [tolnaftate] 10 mg/mL

Zeasorb-AF powder OTC *antifungal* [miconazole nitrate] 2%

zeaxanthin *natural carotenoid used to prevent and treat age-related macular degeneration (AMD), retinitis pigmentosa (RP), and other retinal dysfunction*

Zebeta film-coated tablets ℞ *antihypertensive; β-blocker* [bisoprolol fumarate] 5, 10 mg

Zee-Seltzer effervescent tablets OTC *antacid; analgesic* [sodium bicarbonate; citric acid; aspirin] 1916•1000•325 mg

Zefazone powder or frozen premix for IV injection ℞ *cephalosporin antibiotic* [cefmetazole sodium] 1, 2 g ⑨ cefazolin

Zegerid chewable tablets ℞ *investigational (NDA filed) doseform* [omeprazole]

Zegerid powder for oral suspension ℞ *proton pump inhibitor for gastric and duodenal ulcers, erosive esophagitis, GERD, upper GI bleeding, and other gastroesophageal disorders* [omeprazole] 20, 40 mg/pkt.

zein NF *coating agent*

Zeldox (European name for U.S. product **Geodon**)

Zelmac (name changed to **Zelnorm** upon marketing release in 2002)

Zelnorm tablets ℞ *selective serotonin receptor antagonist for irritable bowel syndrome (IBS) with chronic constipation in women and chronic idiopathic constipation in all* [tegaserod maleate] 2, 6 mg

Zemaira powder for IV infusion ℞ *enzyme replacement therapy for hereditary alpha₁-proteinase inhibitor deficiency, which leads to progressive panacinar emphysema* [alpha₁-proteinase inhibitor] 50 mg/mL (1000 mg/vial)

Zemplar capsules, parenteral injection during dialysis ℞ *synthetic vitamin D analogue for osteodystrophy and hyper-*

parathyroidism secondary to chronic renal failure [paricalcitol] 1, 2, 4 μg; 5 μg/mL

Zemuron IV injection ℞ nondepolarizing neuromuscular blocking agent; muscle relaxant; adjunct to general anesthesia [rocuronium bromide] 10 mg/mL

Zenapax injection ℞ immunosuppressant; monoclonal antibodies (MAb) to prevent acute rejection of organ and bone marrow transplants (orphan) [daclizumab] 25 mg/5 mL

zenarestat USAN investigational (Phase III) aldose reductase inhibitor for diabetic neuropathy

Zenate, Advanced Formula film-coated tablets ℞ vitamin/iron supplement [multiple vitamins; iron; folic acid] ±•65•1 mg

zenazocine mesylate USAN analgesic

Zendra ℞ investigational GABA (A) receptor modulator for acute ischemic stroke [clomethiazole edisylate]

zepastine INN

Zephiran Chloride tincture, tincture spray, aqueous solution, towelettes, disinfectant concentrate OTC topical antiseptic [benzalkonium chloride] 1:750; 1:750; 1:750; 1:750; 17%

zephirol [see: benzalkonium chloride]

Zephrex film-coated tablets ℞ decongestant; expectorant [pseudoephedrine HCl; guaifenesin] 60•400 mg

Zephrex LA extended-release tablets ℞ decongestant; expectorant [pseudoephedrine HCl; guaifenesin] 120•600 mg

zeranol USAN, INN anabolic

Zerit capsules, powder for oral solution ℞ antiviral for HIV infection [stavudine] 15, 20, 30, 40 mg; 1 mg/mL

Zerit XR extended-release capsules ℞ antiviral for HIV infection [stavudine] 37.5, 50, 75, 100 mg

Zestoretic tablets ℞ antihypertensive; angiotensin-converting enzyme (ACE) inhibitor; diuretic [hydrochlorothiazide; lisinopril] 12.5•10, 25•20 mg

Zestra oil OTC natural sexual lubricant; claimed to "increase female sexual sensation, arousal, and pleasure" when topically applied to the vaginal area [borage oil; evening primrose oil; angelica seed oil; coleus extract; vitamins C and E]

Zestril tablets ℞ antihypertensive; angiotensin-converting enzyme (ACE) inhibitor; adjunctive treatment for CHF [lisinopril] 2.5, 5, 10, 20, 30, 40 mg ▣ Restoril; Vistaril

Zetacet topical suspension, wash ℞ acne treatment [sulfacetamide sodium; sulfur] 10%•5%

Zetar shampoo OTC antiseborrheic; antipsoriatic; antipruritic; antibacterial [coal tar] 1%

Zetar Emulsion bath oil (discontinued 2003) ℞ antipsoriatic; antiseborrheic; antipruritic; emollient [coal tar] 30%

Zetia caplets ℞ antihyperlipidemic; intestinal cholesterol absorption inhibitor [ezetimibe] 10 mg

zetidoline INN, BAN

Zevalin powder for injection ℞ radioimmunotherapy carrier; radiolabeled with indium In 111 (step 1) and yttrium Y 90 (step 2) to treat non-Hodgkin B-cell lymphoma [ibritumomab tiuxetan]

Zevalin therapeutic regimen "kit" (complete package for a one-week course of treatment) ℞ multistep treatment protocol for non-Hodgkin B-cell lymphoma [rituximab; indium In 111 ibritumomab tiuxetan; yttrium Y 90 ibritumomab tiuxetan]

Z-gen tablets OTC vitamin/zinc supplement [multiple vitamins; zinc] ±•22.5 mg

Zhuzishen (Panax pseudoginseng) medicinal herb [see: ginseng]

Ziac tablets ℞ antihypertensive; β-blocker; diuretic [hydrochlorothiazide; bisoprolol fumarate] 6.25•2.5, 6.25•5, 6.25•10 mg

Ziagen film-coated caplets, oral solution ℞ antiviral nucleoside reverse transcriptase inhibitor for HIV infection [abacavir sulfate] 300 mg; 20 mg/mL

ziconotide USAN non-narcotic analgesic; calcium channel blocker

ziconotide acetate *calcium-channel blocker; non-narcotic analgesic for intractable pain of cancer or AIDS; investigational epidural administration for spinal cord injury*

zidapamide USAN, INN

zidometacin USAN, INN *anti-inflammatory*

zidovudine (ZDV) USAN, INN, BAN *nucleoside antiviral for AIDS and AIDS-related complex (orphan), HIV infection, and to prevent maternal-fetal HIV transmission*

zifrosilone USAN *acetylcholinesterase inhibitor for Alzheimer disease*

Ziks cream OTC *analgesic; counterirritant* [methyl salicylate; menthol; capsaicin] 12%•1%•0.025% ℞ Vicks

Zilactin Medicated gel OTC *astringent for oral canker and herpes lesions* [tannic acid; alcohol 80%] 7%

Zilactin-B Medicated gel OTC *topical oral anesthetic* [benzocaine; alcohol 76%] 10%

Zilactin-L topical liquid OTC *local anesthetic* [lidocaine] 2.5%

zilantel USAN, INN *anthelmintic*

zileuton USAN, INN, BAN *5-lipoxygenase inhibitor; leukotriene receptor inhibitor; for prophylaxis and chronic treatment of asthma*

zilpaterol INN

zimeldine INN, BAN *antidepressant* [also: zimeldine HCl]

zimeldine HCl USAN *antidepressant* [also: zimeldine]

zimelidine HCl [now: zimeldine HCl]

zimidoben INN

Zinacef powder or frozen premix for IV or IM injection ℞ *cephalosporin antibiotic* [cefuroxime sodium] 0.75, 1.5, 7.5 g

zinc *element (Zn)*

Zinc 15 tablets OTC *zinc supplement* [zinc sulfate] 66 mg

zinc acetate USP *copper blocking/complexing agent for Wilson disease (orphan)*

zinc acetate, basic INN

zinc acetate dihydrate [see: zinc acetate]

zinc bacitracin [see: bacitracin zinc]

zinc caprylate *antifungal*

zinc carbonate USAN *dietary zinc supplement*

zinc chloride USP *astringent; dentin desensitizer; dietary zinc supplement*

zinc chloride Zn 65 USAN *radioactive agent*

zinc citrate *dietary zinc supplement (34% elemental zinc)*

zinc complex bacitracins [see: bacitracin zinc]

zinc gelatin USP

zinc gluconate USP *dietary zinc supplement* 10, 15, 50, 78 mg oral

Zinc Lozenges OTC *topical anti-infective to relieve sore throat* [zinc citrate and zinc gluconate] 23 mg

zinc mesoporphyrin & hemin *investigational (orphan) for acute porphyric syndromes*

zinc oleate NF

zinc oxide USP, JAN *astringent; topical protectant; emollient; antiseptic* 20% topical

zinc peroxide, medicinal USP

zinc phenolsulfonate NF *not generally regarded as safe and effective as an antidiarrheal*

zinc propionate *antifungal*

zinc pyrithione [see: pyrithione zinc]

zinc stearate USP *dusting powder; tablet and capsule lubricant; antifungal*

zinc sulfate USP, JAN *ophthalmic astringent; dietary zinc supplement* 200, 220, 250 mg oral; 1, 5 mg/mL injection

zinc sulfate heptahydrate [see: zinc sulfate]

zinc sulfate monohydrate [see: zinc sulfate]

zinc sulfocarbolate [see: zinc phenolsulfonate]

zinc undecylenate USP *antifungal*

zinc valerate USP

Zinc-220 capsules OTC *zinc supplement* [zinc sulfate] 220 mg

Zinca-Pak IV injection ℞ *intravenous nutritional therapy* [zinc sulfate] 1, 5 mg/mL

Zincate capsules ℞ *zinc supplement* [zinc sulfate] 220 mg

zinc-eugenol USP

Zincfrin Drop-Tainers (eye drops) OTC *topical ocular decongestant and astringent* [phenylephrine HCl; zinc sulfate] 0.12%•0.25%

Zincon shampoo OTC *antiseborrheic; antibacterial; antifungal* [pyrithione zinc] 1%

Zincvit capsules ℞ *vitamin/mineral supplement* [multiple vitamins & minerals; folic acid] ±•1 mg

zindotrine USAN, INN *bronchodilator*

zindoxifene INN

Zinecard powder for IV drip or push ℞ *cardioprotectant for doxorubicin-induced cardiomyopathy (orphan)* [dexrazoxane] 250, 500 mg/vial

Zingiber officinale *medicinal herb* [see: ginger]

zinoconazole INN *antifungal* [also: zinoconazole HCl]

zinoconazole HCl USAN *antifungal* [also: zinoconazole]

zinostatin USAN, INN *antineoplastic* ⑨ Sandostatin; simvastatin

zinterol INN *bronchodilator* [also: zinterol HCl]

zinterol HCl USAN *bronchodilator* [also: zinterol]

zinviroxime USAN, INN *antiviral*

zipeprol INN

ziprasidone HCl *novel (atypical) dihydroindolone antipsychotic for schizophrenia and manic episodes of a bipolar disorder; also used for agitation or psychosis of Alzheimer disease; serotonin 5-HT$_2$ and dopamine D$_2$ antagonist*

ziprasidone mesylate USAN *dihydroindolone antipsychotic; serotonin 5-HT$_2$ and dopamine D$_2$ antagonist*

Ziradryl lotion OTC *topical antihistamine; astringent; antiseptic* [diphenhydramine HCl; zinc oxide; alcohol 2%] 1%•2%

zirconium *element (Zr)*

zirconium oxide *astringent*

Zithromax ⒼⓂ capsules, tablets, powder for oral suspension ℞ *macrolide*

antibiotic [azithromycin] 250 mg; 250 mg; 300, 600 mg/15 mL, 900 mg/22.5 mL

Zithromax film-coated tablets, Tri-Pak (3 tablets), Z-Pak (6 tablets), powder for oral suspension, powder for IV or IM injection ℞ *macrolide antibiotic* [azithromycin] 250, 500, 600 mg; 500 mg; 250 mg; 100, 200 mg/5 mL, 1 g/pkt.; 500 mg

Zixoryn ℞ *investigational (orphan) agent for neonatal hyperbilirubinemia* [flumecinol]

Zmax extended-release oral suspension ℞ *macrolide antibiotic* [azithromycin] 2 g

⁶⁵Zn [see: zinc chloride Zn 65]

Zn-DTPA (zinc pentetate) [see: pentetate zinc trisodium]

ZNP cleansing bar OTC *antiseborrheic; antibacterial; antifungal* [pyrithione zinc] 2%

zocainone INN

Zocor film-coated tablets ℞ *HMG-CoA reductase inhibitor for hyperlipidemia, hypertriglyceridemia, and coronary heart disease* [simvastatin] 5, 10, 20, 40, 80 mg

Zocor Heart-Pro film-coated tablets (available OTC in England) *HMG-CoA reductase inhibitor for hyperlipidemia, hypertriglyceridemia, and coronary heart disease* [simvastatin] 10 mg

Zodeac-100 tablets ℞ *hematinic; vitamin/mineral supplement* [ferrous fumarate; multiple vitamins & minerals; folic acid; biotin] 60 mg• ±•1 mg•300 μg

Zoderm gel, cream, liquid cleanser ℞ *keratolytic for acne* [benzoyl peroxide (in a urea base)] 4.5%, 6.5%, 8.5%

zofenopril INN, BAN *angiotensin-converting enzyme (ACE) inhibitor* [also: zofenopril calcium]

zofenopril calcium USAN *angiotensin-converting enzyme (ACE) inhibitor* [also: zofenopril]

zofenoprilat INN *antihypertensive* [also: zofenoprilat arginine]

zofenoprilat arginine USAN *antihypertensive* [also: zofenoprilat]

zoficonazole INN

Zofran film-coated tablets, oral solution, IV infusion, IM injection ℞ *serotonin 5-HT₃ antagonist; antiemetic for nausea following chemotherapy, radiation, or surgery* [ondansetron HCl] 4, 8, 24 mg; 4 mg/5 mL; 32 mg/50 mL; 2 mg/mL

Zofran ODT (orally disintegrating tablets) ℞ *serotonin 5-HT₃ receptor antagonist; antiemetic for nausea following chemotherapy, radiation, or surgery* [ondansetron HCl] 4, 8 mg

Zoladex subcu implant in preloaded syringe ℞ *hormonal antineoplastic for palliative treatment of prostatic carcinoma, breast cancer, and endometriosis* [goserelin acetate] 3.6 mg (1-month implant), 10.8 mg (3-month implant) ⑫ sulindac

Zoladex LA ⑭ subcu implant in preloaded syringe ℞ *hormonal antineoplastic for palliative treatment of prostatic carcinoma; LHRH agonist for endometriosis* [goserelin acetate] 10.8 mg (3-month implant)

zolamine INN *antihistamine; topical anesthetic* [also: zolamine HCl]

zolamine HCl USAN *antihistamine; topical anesthetic* [also: zolamine]

zolazepam INN, BAN *sedative* [also: zolazepam HCl]

zolazepam HCl USAN *sedative* [also: zolazepam]

zoledronate disodium USAN *bone resorption inhibitor for osteoporosis*

zoledronate trisodium USAN *bone resorption inhibitor for osteoporosis*

zoledronic acid USAN *bisphosphonate bone resorption inhibitor for hypercalcemia of malignancy (HCM), multiple myeloma, bone metastases, and metabolic bone disorders such as Paget disease*

zolenzepine INN

zolertine INN *antiadrenergic; vasodilator* [also: zolertine HCl]

zolertine HCl USAN *antiadrenergic; vasodilator* [also: zolertine]

Zolicef powder for IV or IM injection ℞ *cephalosporin antibiotic* [cefazolin sodium] 1 g

zolimidine INN

zolimomab aritox USAN *anti-T lymphocyte monoclonal antibody*

zoliprofen INN

zoliridine [see: zolimidine]

zolmitriptan USAN *vascular serotonin 5-HT₁ᵦ/₁ᴅ receptor agonist for the acute treatment of migraine*

Zoloft film-coated tablets, oral drops ℞ *selective serotonin reuptake inhibitor (SSRI) for depression, obsessive-compulsive disorder (OCD), panic disorder, post-traumatic stress disorder, premenstrual dysmorphic disorder (PMDD), and social anxiety disorder* [sertraline HCl] 25, 50, 100 mg; 20 mg/mL

zoloperone INN

zolpidem INN, BAN *imidazopyridine sedative/hypnotic* [also: zolpidem tartrate]

zolpidem tartrate USAN *imidazopyridine sedative/hypnotic* [also: zolpidem]

Zomaril ℞ *investigational (Phase III) selective serotonin and dopamine antagonist for schizophrenia* [iloperidone]

zomebazam INN

zomepirac INN, BAN *analgesic; anti-inflammatory* [also: zomepirac sodium]

zomepirac sodium USAN, USP *analgesic; anti-inflammatory* [also: zomepirac]

Zometa powder for IV infusion ℞ *bone resorption inhibitor for hypercalcemia of malignancy, multiple myeloma, bone metastases, and metabolic bone disorders such as Paget disease* [zoledronic acid] 4 mg

zometapine USAN *antidepressant*

Zomig film-coated tablets, nasal spray ℞ *vascular serotonin 5-HT₁ᵦ/₁ᴅ receptor agonist for the acute treatment of migraine* [zolmitriptan] 2.5, 5 mg; 5 mg/dose ⑫ Flomax; Slow-Mag

Zomig Rapimelt ⑭ (orally disintegrating tablets) ℞ *vascular serotonin 5-HT₁ᵦ/₁ᴅ receptor agonist for the acute treatment of migraine* [zolmitriptan] 2.5 mg

Zomig-ZMT orally disintegrating tablets ℞ *vascular serotonin* 5-$HT_{1B/1D}$ *receptor agonist for the acute treatment of migraine* [zolmitriptan] 2.5 mg ⑨ Flomax; Slow-Mag

Zonalon cream ℞ *antihistamine; antipruritic* [doxepin HCl] 5%

Zone-A Forte lotion ℞ *topical corticosteroidal anti-inflammatory; local anesthetic* [hydrocortisone acetate; pramoxine] 2.5%•1%

Zonegran capsules ℞ *sulfonamide anticonvulsant for partial seizures* [zonisamide] 25, 50, 100 mg

zoniclezole INN *anticonvulsant* [also: zoniclezole HCl]

zoniclezole HCl USAN *anticonvulsant* [also: zoniclezole]

zonisamide USAN, INN, BAN *sulfonamide anticonvulsant for partial seizures*

Zonite Douche solution concentrate OTC *antiseptic; antipruritic/counterirritant; vaginal cleanser and deodorizer* [benzalkonium chloride; menthol; thymol]

Zophren (European name for U.S. product **Zofran**)

zopiclone INN, BAN, JAN *sedative; hypnotic*

zopolrestat USAN *antidiabetic; aldose reductase inhibitor*

zorbamycin USAN *antibacterial*

Zorbtive powder for subcu injection ℞ *treatment for short bowel syndrome (SBS) in children* [somatropin (rDNA)] 4, 5, 6, 8.8 mg (12, 15, 18, 24.6 IU) per vial

ZORprin Zero Order Release tablets ℞ *analgesic; antipyretic; anti-inflammatory; antirheumatic* [aspirin] 800 mg

zorubicin INN *antineoplastic* [also: zorubicin HCl]

zorubicin HCl USAN *antineoplastic* [also: zorubicin]

Zostavax ℞ *investigational (NDA filed) vaccine for prevention of herpes zoster infections and post-herpetic neuralgia and for reducing shingles-associated pain in adults* [zoster vaccine, live]

zoster vaccine, live *investigational (NDA filed) vaccine for prevention of herpes zoster infections and post-herpetic neuralgia and for reducing shingles-associated pain in adults*

Zostrix; Zostrix-HP cream OTC *topical analgesic* [capsaicin] 0.025%; 0.075%

zosuquidar trihydrochloride *investigational (Phase III) p-glycoprotein inhibitor for acute myelogenous leukemia (AML)*

Zosyn powder or frozen premix for IV injection ℞ *extended-spectrum penicillin antibiotic plus synergist* [piperacillin sodium; tazobactam sodium] 2•0.25, 3•0.375, 4•0.5, 36•4.5 g

zotepine INN, JAN *investigational antipsychotic*

Zoto-HC ear drops ℞ *topical corticosteroidal anti-inflammatory; antibacterial; local anesthetic* [hydrocortisone; chloroxylenol; pramoxine HCl] 10%•1%•10%

Zovia 1/35E; Zovia 1/50E tablets (in packs of 21 or 28) ℞ *monophasic oral contraceptive* [ethynodiol diacetate; ethinyl estradiol] 1 mg•35 µg; 1 mg•50 µg

Zovirax capsules, tablets, oral suspension ℞ *antiviral for herpes simplex, herpes zoster, and adult-onset chickenpox* [acyclovir] 200 mg; 400, 800 mg; 200 mg/5 mL

Zovirax cream ℞ *antiviral for recurrent herpes labialis* [acyclovir] 5%

Zovirax ointment ℞ *antiviral for herpes genitalis and mucocutaneous herpes simplex infections* [acyclovir] 5%

Zovirax powder for IV infusion ℞ *antiviral for herpes infections* [acyclovir sodium] 500 mg/vial

zoxazolamine NF, INN

Z-Pak (trademarked packaging form) *6-tablet pack of Zithromax*

ZTuss Expectorant oral liquid ℞ *narcotic antitussive; decongestant; antihistamine; expectorant* [hydrocodone bitartrate; pseudoephedrine HCl; chlorpheniramine maleate; guaifenesin] 5•30•4•200 mg/10 mL

Zucapsaicin ℞ *investigational (orphan) agent for postherpetic neuralgia of the trigeminal nerve* [civamide]

zucapsaicin USAN *topical analgesic*

zuclomifene INN

zuclomiphene USAN

zuclopenthixol INN, BAN *thioxanthene antipsychotic*

Z-Xtra lotion OTC *local anesthetic; antihistamine; emollient* [pyrilamine maleate; benzocaine; zinc oxide] 2.07•2.08•41.35 mg/mL

Zyban sustained-release film-coated tablets ℞ *non-nicotine aid to smoking cessation* [bupropion HCl] 150 mg

Zyderm gel for subcu injection ℞ *dermal filler for fine-to-moderate scars and wrinkles* [collagen, purified bovine] 35, 65 mg/mL

Zydis (trademarked dosage form) *orally disintegrating tablets*

Zydone tablets, capsules ℞ *narcotic analgesic* [hydrocodone bitartrate; acetaminophen] 5•400, 7.5•400, 10•400 mg; 5•500 mg

Zyflo film-coated tablets ℞ *5-lipoxygenase inhibitor; leukotriene receptor inhibitor; prophylaxis and treatment for chronic asthma* [zileuton] 600 mg

Zylet eye drop suspension ℞ *corticosteroidal anti-inflammatory; aminoglycoside antibiotic* [loteprednol etabonate; tobramycin] 0.5%•0.3%

zylofuramine INN

Zyloprim tablets ℞ *xanthine oxidase inhibitor for gout and hyperuricemia; antineoplastic adjunct for reducing uric acid levels following chemotherapy for leukemia, lymphoma, and solid-tumor malignancies (orphan)* [allopurinol] 100, 300 mg

Zymacap capsules OTC *vitamin supplement* [multiple vitamins; folic acid] ±•0.4 mg

Zymar eye drops ℞ *broad-spectrum fluoroquinolone antibiotic* [gatifloxacin] 0.3%

Zymase capsules containing enteric-coated spheres (discontinued 2002) ℞ *digestive enzymes* [lipase; protease; amylase] 12 000•24 000•24 000 USP units

Zymine oral liquid ℞ *antihistamine* [triprolidine HCl] 1.25 mg/5 mL

Zyplast gel for subcu injection ℞ *dermal filler for deep scars and wrinkles* [collagen, purified bovine, cross-linked] 35 mg/mL

Zyprexa film-coated tablets, Zydis (orally disintegrating tablets) ℞ *novel (atypical) thienobenzodiazepine antipsychotic for schizophrenia and manic episodes of a bipolar disorder; also used for obsessive-compulsive disorder (OCD) and agitation or psychosis due to Alzheimer or other dementias* [olanzapine] 2.5, 5, 7.5, 10, 15, 20 mg; 5, 10, 15, 20 mg

Zyprexa IntraMuscular IM injection ℞ *novel (atypical) antipsychotic for manic episodes of a bipolar disorder* [olanzapine] 5 mg/mL (10 mg/vial)

Zyrtec film-coated tablets, chewable tablets, syrup ℞ *nonsedating antihistamine for allergic rhinitis and chronic idiopathic urticaria* [cetirizine HCl] 5, 10 mg; 5, 10 mg; 5 mg/5 mL

Zyrtec-D 12 Hour extended-release tablets ℞ *nonsedating antihistamine and decongestant for allergic rhinitis* [cetirizine HCl; pseudoephedrine HCl] 5•120 mg

Zyvox film-coated tablets, powder for oral suspension, IV infusion ℞ *oxazolidinone antibiotic for gram-positive bacterial infections* [linezolid] 400, 600 mg; 100 mg/5 mL; 200, 400, 600 mg/bag

Zyvoxam Ⓒ tablets, IV infusion ℞ *oxazolidinone antibiotic for gram-positive bacterial infections* [linezolid] 600 mg; 2 mg/mL

APPENDIX **A**
Sound-Alikes

Listed below are 672 drug names that may be confused in transcription, followed by one or more possible "sound-alike" names. The list is not all-inclusive, and we would appreciate hearing of any additions the reader might suggest. These sound-alikes have also been included in the main section of the book. Look for the "ear" icon (🔊).

Accurbron	Accutane
Accutane	Accurbron
Aciphex	AcuTect
Actifed	Actidil
actinomycin	Achromycin; Aureomycin
Actonel	atenolol
AcuTect	Aciphex
adrenaline	adrenalone
adrenalone	adrenaline
Advil	Avail
Afrin	aspirin
Agoral	Argyrol
Akne-Mycin	Ak-Mycin
Alamag	Alma-Mag
Alco-Gel	aloe gel
Aldactazide	Aldactone
Aldactone	Aldactazide
Aldoril	Elavil; Eldepryl; Enovil; Equanil; Mellaril
Allergan	allergen; Auralgan
aloe	Alco-Gel
ALOMAD	Alomide
Alomide	ALOMAD
Alustra	Lustra
Amaryl	Reminyl
Ambenyl	Aventyl
Amicar	Amikin
Amikin	Amicar
amitriptyline	nortriptyline
amoxapine	amoxicillin; Amoxil
amoxicillin	amoxapine
Amoxil	amoxapine
Amphojel	Amphocil
Anacin	Unisom; Unasyn
Anafranil	enalapril
Analpram-HC	Analbalm
Ancobon	Oncovin

Ansaid	NSAID
Anturane	Artane
Anusol	Aplisol
Aplisol	Anusol; Apresoline
Appedrine	aprindine; ephedrine
aprindine	Appedrine; ephedrine
ara-C	ERYC
Aralen	Arlidin
Aricept	Erycette
Artane	Anturane
aspirin	Afrin
Atacand	Ativan
Atarax	Marax
atenolol	Actonel; timolol
Ativan	Atacand; Adapin; Avitene
Atrovent	Trovan
Auralgan	Allergan; allergen
Avail	Advil
Aventyl	Ambenyl; Bentyl
Avita	Evista
Avitene	Ativan
Axid	Biaxin
azolimine	Azulfidine
Azulfidine	Silvadene
Bacid	Banacid
bacitracin	Bacitrin; Bactrim
Bactocill	Pathocil
Bactrim	bacitracin
BAL	Balneol
Balneol	BAL in Oil
Banophen	Barophen
Banthīne	Brethine; Vantin
Beminal	Benemid
Benadryl	Bentyl; Benylin; Caladryl
Benemid	Beminal
Benoxyl	PanOxyl
Bentyl	Aventyl; Benadryl; Bontril
Benylin	Benadryl
Betagan	Betagen
Betagen	Betagan
Biaxin	Axid
Bichloracetic acid	dichloroacetic acid
Bicillin	V-Cillin; Wycillin
bleomycin	Cleocin
Bonamine	Bonine
Bontril	Bentyl; Vontrol
Boyol	boil
Brethine	Banthine
Brevital	Bretylol
Bromfed	Bromphen

Bromophen	Bromphen
Broncholate	Brondelate
Brondelate	Broncholate
butabarbital	butalbital
butalbital	butabarbital; Butibel
Butibel	butalbital
Butisol	Butazolidin
Byclomine	Hycomine
Caladryl	Benadryl
Calamox	Camalox
Calan	kaolin; Kaon
calcitonin	calcitriol
calcitriol	calcitonin
Capastat	Cepastat
Capitrol	captopril
captopril	Capitrol
Cardene	Cardizem
Cardizem	Cardene
Catapres	Catarase; Combipres; Ser-Ap-Es
Cedax	Cidex
Cefadyl	Cefzil
cefazolin	cephalothin; Zefazone
cefotaxime	cefoxitin
cefoxitin	cefotaxime
ceftizoxime	cefuroxime
cefuroxime	ceftizoxime
Cefzil	Cefadyl; Kefzol
Celebrex	Celexa; Cerebyx
Celexa	Celebrex
Cēpastat	Capastat
cephalexin	cefazolin; cephalothin
cephalothin	cefazolin
cephapirin	cephradine
cephradine	cephapirin
Cerebyx	Celebrex
chlorpheniramine	chlorphentermine
chlorphentermine	chlorpheniramine
Cidex	Cedax
cimetidine	dimethicone
Cipro	Septa; Septra
Citracal	Citrucel
Citrucel	Citracal
clara	Clearasil
claretin-12	Claritin; Clarityne
clarithromycin	dirithromycin; erythromycin
Claritin	claretin; Clarityne
Clarityne	claretin; Claritin
Clearasil	clara cell
Cleocin	bleomycin; Lincocin
clioxanide	Clinoxide

clomiphene	clonidine
clonidine	clomiphene; Klonopin; quinidine
clotrimazole	co-trimoxazole
Codegest	Codehist
Codehist	Codegest
codeine	Kaodene
Colestid	colistin
colestipol	colistin
colistin	Colestid; colestipol
Combipres	Catapres
Cort-Dome	Cortone
Cortenema	quart enema
cortisone	Cortizone
Cortizone-5	cortisone
Cortone	Cort-Dome
Cotrim	Cortin
co-trimoxazole	clotrimazole
Coumadin	Kemadrin
Covera-HS	Provera
cytarabine	vidarabine
dacarbazine	Dicarbosil; procarbazine
Dalmane	Dialume
danthron	Dantrium
Dantrium	danthron
Daranide	Daraprim
Daraprim	Daranide
Darvocet-N	Darvon-N
Darvon	Diovan
daunorubicin	doxorubicin
Decadron	Decaderm; Percodan
Deconsal	Deconal
Delcort	Dilacor
Demulen	Demerol; Demolin
Dermacort	DermiCort
deserpidine	desipramine
Desferal	Disophrol
desipramine	deserpidine
desoximetasone	dexamethasone
Desoxyn	digitoxin; digoxin
dexamethasone	desoximetasone
Dexedrine	dextran
dextran	Dexedrine; dextrin
dextrin	dextran
Dialume	Dalmane
dichloroacetic	Bichloracetic acid
dicumarol	Demerol
digitoxin	Desoxyn; digoxin
digoxin	Desoxyn; digitoxin
Dilacor	Delcort
Dilantin	Milontin; Mylanta; Xalatan

Dimacol	dimercaprol
dimenhydrinate	diphenhydramine
dimercaprol	Dimacol
Dimetabs	Dimetane; Dimetapp
Dimetapp	Dimetabs
dimethicone	cimetidine
Diovan	Darvon
diphenhydramine	dimenhydrinate
Diphenylan	Diphenylin
dirithromycin	clarithromycin; erythromycin
Disophrol	Desferal; disoprofol; Stilphostrol
disoprofol	Disophrol
Ditropan	Intropin
Diutensen-R	Salutensin
dobutamine	dopamine
Donnagel	Donnatal
Donnatal	Donnagel
Donnazyme	Entozyme
dopamine	dobutamine; Dopram
Dopar	Dopram
Dopram	dopamine; Dopar
doxepin	Doxidan; Loxitane
doxorubicin	daunorubicin
Dramanate	Dommanate
Duranest	Duratest
Duratest	Duranest; Duratuss
Duratuss	Duratest
Dyazide	thiazides; Tiazac
Dymelor	Demerol; Pamelor
Dyrenium	Pyridium
Ecotrin	Edecrin
Edecrin	Ecotrin; Ethaquin
Elavil	Aldoril; Elidel; Eldepryl; Enovil; Equanil; Mellaril
Eldepryl	Aldoril; Elavil; Enovil; Equanil; Mellaril
Elidel	Elavil
emetine	Emetrol
Emetrol	emetine
Enbrel	Incel
Endal	Intal
Enduron	Imuran; Inderal
Enduronyl	Inderal
ephedrine	Appedrine; aprindine
Epifrin	epinephrine; EpiPen
Epinal	Epitol
epinephrine	Epifrin
EpiPen	Epifrin
Epitol	Epinal
Epogen	"amp and gent" (ampicillin & gentamicin)
Equanil	Aldoril; Elavil; Eldepryl; Enovil; Mellaril
ERYC	ara-C

Erycette	Aricept
erythromycin	clarithromycin; dirithromycin
Esidrix	Lasix
Esimil	Estinyl; Isomil
Estinyl	Esimil
Estraderm	Estradurin
Estratab	Ethatab
ethacridine	ethacrynic
ethacrynic	ethacridine
ethinamate	ethionamide
Ethiodol	ethynodiol
ethionamide	ethinamate
ethynodiol	Ethiodol
Eurax	Serax; Urex
Evac-Q-Kwik	Evac-Q-Kit
Evista	Avita
Femiron	Remeron
fentanyl	Sentinel
Feosol	Feostat; Fer-In-Sol; Festal
Feostat	Feosol
Feverall	Fiberall
Fioricet	Lorcet
Fiorinal	Florinef
Flexeril	Flaxedil
Flomax	Slow-Mag; Zomig
Florinef	Fiorinal
folacin	Fulvicin
Fostex	pHisoHex
Fulvicin	folacin; Furacin
Furacin	Fulvicin
furosemide	torsemide
Gabitril	Carbatrol
Garamycin	Gamastan; kanamycin; Terramycin; Theramycin
Gelfoam	Ger-O-Foam
Genatap	Genapap
Generet-500	Gentap
gentamicin	Jenamicin; kanamycin
glucose	Glutose
Glutose	glucose
Glycotuss	Glytuss
Glytuss	Glycotuss
Gonak	Gonic
Gonic	Gonak
guaifenesin	guanfacine
guanethidine	guanidine
guanfacine	guaifenesin
guanidine	guanethidine
Guiatuss	Guiatussin
Guiatussin	Guiatuss
Haldol	Halenol; Halog

Halog	Haldol
Halotestin	Halotex; Halotussin
Halotex	Halotestin
Halotussin	Halotestin
Hespan	Histatan
Hexadrol	Hexalol
Hexalen	Hexalol
Hycodan	Hycomine; Vicodin
Hycomine	Byclomine; Hycodan; Vicodin
Hydergine	Hydramine
Hydramine	Bydramine; Hydergine; Hydramyn; Hytramyn
Hygroton	Regroton
Hyperstat	Hyper-Tet; HyperHep
Hytone	Vytone
Ilosone	inosine
imipramine	Imferon; Norpramin; trimipramine
Imuran	Enduron; Imferon
Inderal	Enduron; Enduronyl; Inderide
Inderide	Inderal
Indocin	Lincocin; Minocin
INFeD	NSAID
inosine	Ilosone
insulin	inulin
Intal	Endal
Intropin	Ditropan; Isoptin
inulin	insulin
Ismelin	Ritalin
Isomil	Esimil
Isoptin	Intropin
Isopto Atropine	Isopto Carpine
Isopto Carpine	Isopto Atropine
Isordil	Isuprel
Isuprel	Isordil
kanamycin	Garamycin; gentamicin
Kaochlor	K-Lor
kaolin	Calan; Kaon
Kaon	Calan; kaolin
Kaopectate	Kapectalin
Kapectolin	Kaopectate
Kay Ciel	KCl
KCl	Kay Ciel
Keflex	Keflet; Keflin
Kefzol	Cefzil
Kemadrin	Coumadin
Kenalog	Ketalar
Ketalar	Kenalog
Klonopin	clonidine
K-Lor	Kaochlor
Klotrix	Liotrix
Koromex	Komex

Lasix	Esidrix; Lidex
levallorphan	levorphanol
levodopa	methyldopa
levorphanol	levallorphan
levothyroxine	liothyronine
Lidex	Lasix; Lidox; Wydase
Lincocin	Cleocin; Indocin
liothyronine	levothyroxine
liotrix	Klotrix
Loniten	clonidine
Lonox	Lovenox
Lorcet	Fioricet
Lotrimin	Otrivin
Lovenox	Lonox
Loxitane	doxepin
Luminal	Tuinal
Lupron	Mepron; Napron
Maalox	Marax
Mandol	nadolol
Marax	Atarax; Maalox
Marcaine	Narcan
Maxzide	Microzide
mazindol	mebendazole
Mebaral	Medrol
mebendazole	mazindol
Meclan	Meclomen; Mezlin
meclizine	mescaline
meclozine	mescaline
Medrol	Mebaral
Mellaril	Aldoril; Elavil; Eldepryl; Enovil; Equanil; Moderil
meperidine	meprobamate
mephenytoin	Mephyton
Mephyton	mephenytoin; methadone
meprobamate	meperidine
Mepron	Lupron; Napron
mescaline	meclizine
Mestinon	Mesantoin; Metatensin
Metahydrin	Metandren
metaproterenol	metoprolol
Metatensin	Mesantoin; Mestinon
metaxalone	metolazone
metesind	medicine
methadone	Mephyton
methenamine	methionine
methionine	methenamine
methixene	methoxsalen
methoxsalen	methixene
methyldopa	levodopa
metolazone	metaxalone
Metopirone	metyrapone

metoprolol	metaproterenol
metyrapone	Metopirone; metyrosine
metyrosine	metyrapone
Mezlin	Meclan
MICRhoGAM	microgram
Microzide	Maxzide
Midrin	Mydfrin
Milontin	Dilantin; Miltown; Mylanta
Miltown	Milontin
Minocin	Indocin; Mithracin; niacin
Mithracin	Minocin
mithramycin	mitomycin
mitomycin	mithramycin; Mutamycin
Moban	Mobidin; Modane
Mobidin	Moban
Modane	Moban; Mudrane
Modicon	Mylicon
Moi-Stir	moisture
Monocaps	Monoclate; Monoket
Monocid	Monocete
Monoclate	Monocaps; Monoket
Monoket	Monocete
Mudrane	Modane
Mutamycin	mitomycin
Myambutol	Nembutal
Mydfrin	Midrin; Myfedrine
Mylanta	Dilantin; Milontin
Myleran	Mylicon
Mylicon	Modicon; Myleran
nadolol	Nandol
Naldecon	Nalfon
Nalfon	Naldecon
Naprosyn	Meprospan; Natacyn
Narcan	Marcaine
Nardil	Norinyl
Nasarel	Nizoral
Natacyn	Naprosyn
Nembutal	Myambutal
Neomixin	neomycin
neomycin	Neomixin
Neovastat	Novastan
niacin	Minocin
Nilstat	Nitrostat; nystatin
Nitro-Bid	Nicobid
nitroglycerin	Nitroglyn
Nitroglyn	nitroglycerin
Nizoral	Nasarel
Norinyl	Nardil
Norpramin	imipramine
nortriptyline	amitriptyline

NSAIDs	InFeD
nystatin	Nilstat; Nitrostat
Omnipen	Unipen
Oncovin	Ancobon
Orabase	Orinase
orarsan	Oracin; Orasone
Orasone	Oracin; orarsan
Oretic	Oreton
Oreton	Oretic
Orinase	Orabase; Ornade; Ornex; Tolinase
Ornade	Orinase; Ornex
Ornex	Orex; Orinase; Ornade
Orthoclone	Ortho-Creme
Otobiotic	Urobiotic
Otrivin	Lotrimin
O-Vax	Ovarex
oxycodone	OxyContin, Roxicodone
oxymetazoline	oxymetholone
oxymetholone	oxymetazoline; oxymorphone
oxymorphone	oxymetholone
Pamelor	Dymelor; Panlor
Panasol	Panscol
Panlor	Pamelor
Panoxyl	Benoxyl
Panscol	Panasol
Parafon	Pantopon
paramethadione	paramethasone
paramethasone	paramethadione
Pathilon	Pathocil
Pathocil	Bactocill; Pathilon; Placidyl
Pavabid	Pavased
Pavulon	Paverolan
penicillamine	penicillin
penicillin	penicillamine; Polycillin
pentobarbital	phenobarbital
Pentothal	pentrinitrol
pentrinitrol	Pentothal
Percodan	Decadron
Perdiem	Pyridium
Periactin	Taractan
Persantine	Pertofrane
Phazyme	Pherazine
phenacetin	phenazocine
phenazocine	phenacetin
phenelzine	Phenazine; Phenylzin
Phenergan	Phenaphen; Theragran
phenobarbital	pentobarbital
Phenoxine	Phenazine
phentermine	phentolamine
phentolamine	phentermine; Ventolin

pHisoHex	Fostex
physostigmine	pyridostigmine; Prostigmin
piperacetazine	piperazine
piperazine	piperacetazine
piracetam	piroxicam
piroxicam	piracetam
Pitocin	Pitressin
Pitressin	Pitocin
Placidyl	Pathocil
Podofin	podophyllin
podophyllin	Podofin
Ponstel	Pronestyl
pralidoxime	pyridoxine; pramoxine
Pramosone	pramoxine
pramoxine	pralidoxime; Pramosone
Pravachol	Primacor
prazepam	prazepine; prazosin
prazepine	prazepam
prazosin	prazepam
prednisolone	prednisone
prednisone	prednisolone
Preven	Preveon
Prilosec	Prozac
Primacor	Pravachol
Priscoline	Apresoline
procaine	Procan
procarbazine	dacarbazine
proline	Prolene
promazine	Promethazine
Pronestyl	Ponstel
Proscar	Posicor
Prostigmin	physostigmine
Protopam	Protamine
Provera	Covera; Provir; Trovert
Prozac	Prilosec
Pyridium	Dyrenium; pyridoxine; pyrithione; pyritidium
pyridostigmine	physostigmine
pyridoxine	pralidoxime; Pyridium
pyrithione	Pyridium
pyritidium	Pyridium
Quarzan	Questran
quinacrine	quinidine
quinidine	clonidine; quinacrine; Quinatime; quinine
quinine	quinidine
Rēgain	Rogaine
Reglan	Regonol
Regonol	Reglan
Regroton	Hygroton
Remeron	Femiron
Reminyl	Amaryl

Repan	Riopan
Restoril	Risperdal; Vistaril; Zestril
Rheumatex	Rheumatrex
Rheumatrex	Rheumatex
Rifadin	Ritalin
Risperdal	Restoril
Ritalin	Ismelin; Rifadin
Robaxisal	Robaxacet
Rogaine	Rēgain
Roxicodone	oxycodone
Salutensin	Diutensen
Sandostatin	simvastatin; zinostatin
Sentinel	fentanyl
Septa	Cipro; Septra
Septra	Cipro; Septa
Ser-Ap-Es	Catapres
Serax	Eurax; Urex; Xerac
Serentil	Surital
Silvadene	Azulfidine
Simplet	Singlet
simvastatin	Sandostatin; zinostatin
Singlet	Simplet
sirolimus	temsirolimus
Slow-Mag	Flomax; Zomig
stilbestrol	Stilphostrol
Stilphostrol	Disophrol; stilbestrol
Streptase	Streptonase
streptokinase	Streptonase
Streptonase	Streptase; streptokinase
sucrose	sucrase
Sulf-10	Sulten-10
sulfamethizole	sulfamethoxazole
sulfamethoxazole	sulfamethizole
sulfathiazole	sulfisoxazole
sulfisoxazole	sulfathiazole
sulindac	Zoladex
Supartz	sports
Tagamet	Tegopen
Targretin	Tegopen; Tegrin
Tegretol	Tegrin
Tegrin	Targretin; Tegopen; Tegretol
temsirolimus	sirolimus
Tenex	Xanax
Terramycin	Garamycin; Theramycin
testolactone	testosterone
testosterone	testolactone
thallium	Valium
Theoclear	Theolair
Theolair	Theoclear; Thyrolar
TheraFlu	Thera-Flur

Thera-Flur	TheraFlu
Theragran	Theragyn; Phenergan
Theramycin	Garamycin; Terramycin
Theravite	Therevac
Therevac	Theravite
Thyrolar	Theolair; Thyrar
Tiazac	Dyazide; thiazides
Ticar	Tigan
Tigan	Ticar; Triban
timolol	atenolol
Tinactin	Taractan
TobraDex	Tobrex
tobramycin	Trobicin
Tobrex	TobraDex
Tofranil	Tepanil
Tolinase	Orinase
Topic	Topicort
Topicort	Topic
torsemide	furosemide
tramadol	trazodone
Trasylol	Travasol
Travasol	Trasylol
trazodone	tramadol
triamcinolone	Triaminicin
Triaminic	Triaminicin; TriHemic
Triaminicin	triamcinolone; Triaminic
triamterene	trimipramine
Triapine	Triaprim
Triban	Tigan
TriHemic	Triaminic
trimeprazine	trimipramine
trimethaphan	trimethoprim
trimethoprim	trimethaphan
trimipramine	imipramine; triamterene; trimeprazine
Triostat	Threostat
Trobicin	tobramycin
Tronolane	Tronothane
Tronothane	Tronolane
Trovan	Atrovent
Tuinal	Luminal; Tylenol
Tusibron	Tussigon
Tussafed	Tussafin
Tussafin	Tussafed
Tussex	Tussionex; Tussirex
Tussigon	Tusibron
Tussionex	Tussex; Tussirex
Tussirex	Tussex; Tussionex
Tylenol	Tuinal
Unasyn	Anacin; Unisom
Unipen	Omnipen

Unisom	Anacin; Unasyn
Uracid	uracil; Urised; Urocit
uracil	Uracel; Uracid
Urex	Eurax; Serax
Urised	Uracel; Uracid; Urispas
Urispas	Urised
Urocit	Uracid
Valium	thallium; Valpin
Vantin	Banthine; Bantron
Vasocidin	Vasodilan
Vasocine	Vaseline
VasoClear	VasoCare
Vasodilan	Vasocidin
Vasoflux	Vasoprost; Vasosulf
Vasosulf	Velosef; Vasoflux
Velban	Valpin
Velosef	Vasosulf
Ventolin	phentolamine
Vicodin	Hycodan; Hycomine
vidarabine	cytarabine
Vistaril	Restoril; Zestril
Vitron	Vytone
Vytone	Hytone; Vitron
Wycillin	Bicillin; V-Cillin
Wydase	Lidex
Xalatan	Dilantin
Xanax	Tenex; Zantac
Zantac	Xanax
Zarontin	Zaroxolyn
Zaroxolyn	Zarontin; Zeroxin
Zefazone	cefazolin
Zestril	Restoril; Vistaril
Ziks	Vicks
zinostatin	Sandostatin; simvastatin
Zoladex	sulindac
Zomig	Flomax; Slow-Mag

Abbreviations Used with Medications and Dosages

Abbreviation/Term	Literally	Meaning
a.c.	ante cibum	before meals or food
ad	ad	to, up to
A.D., AD	auris dextra	right ear
ad lib.	ad libitum	at pleasure
A.L.	auris laeva	left ear
a.m., A.M.	ante meridiem	morning
Aq.	aqua	water
A.S., AS	auris sinistra	left ear
A.U., AU*	auris uterque	each ear
b.i.d.	bis in die	twice daily
b.m.	bowel movement	
cc, cm³	cubic centimeter	
CFU	colony-forming unit(s)	
d.	die	day
EL.U.	ELISA unit(s)	
et	et	and
g	gram(s)	
gt. (plural gtt.)	gutta (plural guttae)	a drop (drops)
h.	hora	hour
HAU	hemagglutinating unit(s)	
h.s.	hora somni	at bedtime
IM†	intramuscular	
IU	international unit(s)	
IV†	intravenous	
LfU	limes flocculating unit(s)	
	limit of flocculation unit(s)	
mcg, μg	microgram(s)	
mg	milligram(s)	
mEq	milliequivalent(s)	
mkat	millikatal unit(s)	
mL, ml	milliliter(s)	
mU, mIU	milliunit(s)	
MU, MIU	megaunit(s)	one million (10^6) IU
μg, mcg	microgram(s)	
nkat	nanokatal unit(s)	
O.D.	oculus dexter	right eye
O.L.	oculus laevus	left eye
O.S.	oculus sinister	left eye
O.U.§	oculus uterque	each eye

Abbreviation/Term	Literally	Meaning
p.c.	post cibum	after meals
p.m., P.M.	post meridiem	afternoon or evening
p.o.	per os	by mouth
p.r.n.	pro re nata	as needed
q.d.	quaque die	every day
q.h.	quaque hora	every hour
q.i.d.	quater in die	four times a day
q.o.d.		every other day
q.s.	quantum satis	sufficient quantity
q.s. ad	quantum satis ad	a sufficient quantity to make
℞, Rx	recipe	take; a recipe
Sig.	signetur	label
s.o.s.	si opus sit	if there is need
stat	statim	at once, immediately
subcu, subq, SQ	subcutaneous	beneath the skin
t.i.d.	ter in die	three times a day
tsp.	teaspoonful	
μg, mcg	microgram(s)	

---

* Although some references have aures unitas (Latin, both ears), this cannot be justified by classical Latin.

† Some references suggest that IM and IV be typed with periods to distinguish from Roman numerals, but we believe context is sufficient to make this distinction.

§ Although some references have oculi unitas (Latin, both eyes), this cannot be justified by classical Latin.

Therapeutic Drug Levels

Drug	Class	Serum Levels metric units (SI units)
amantadine	antiviral	300 ng/mL
amikacin	aminoglycoside	16–32 μg/mL
amiodarone	antiarrhythmic	0.5–2.5 μg/mL
amitriptyline	antidepressant	110–250 ng/mL
amoxapine	antidepressant	200–500 ng/mL
amrinone	cardiotonic	3.7 μg/mL
bretylium	antiarrhythmic	0.5–1.5 μg/mL
bupropion	antidepressant	25–100 ng/mL
carbamazepine	anticonvulsant	4–12 μg/mL (17–51 μmol/L)
chloramphenicol	antibiotic	10–20 μg/mL (31–62 μmol/L)
chlorpromazine	antipsychotic	30–500 ng/mL
clomipramine	antidepressant	80–100 ng/mL
cyclosporine	immunosuppressive	250–800 ng/mL (whole blood, RIA*)
trough values:		50–300 ng/mL (plasma, RIA*)
desipramine	antidepressant	125–300 ng/mL
digitoxin	antiarrhythmic	9–25 μg/L (11.8–32.8 nmol/L)
digoxin	antiarrhythmic	0.5–2.2 ng/mL (0.6–2.8 nmol/L)
disopyramide	antiarrhythmic	2–8 μg/mL (6–18 μmol/L)
doxepin	antidepressant	100–200 ng/mL
flecainide	antiarrhythmic	0.2–1 μg/mL
fluphenazine	antipsychotic	0.13–2.8 ng/mL
gentamicin	aminoglycoside	4–8 μg/mL
haloperidol	antipsychotic	5–20 ng/mL
hydralazine	antihypertensive	100 ng/mL
imipramine	antidepressant	200–350 ng/mL
kanamycin	aminoglycoside	15–40 μg/mL
lidocaine	antiarrhythmic	1.5–6 μg/mL (4.5–21.5 μmol/L)
lithium	antipsychotic	0.5–1.5 mEq/L (0.5–1.5 mmol/L)
maprotiline	antidepressant	200–300 ng/mL
mexiletine	antiarrhythmic	0.5–2 μg/mL
netilmicin	aminoglycoside	6–10 μg/mL

Drug	Class	Serum Levels metric units (SI units)
nortriptyline	antidepressant	50–150 ng/mL
perphenazine	antipsychotic	0.8–1.2 ng/mL
phenobarbital	anticonvulsant	15–40 μg/mL (65–172 μmol/L)
phenytoin	anticonvulsant	10–20 μg/mL (40–80 μmol/L)
primidone	anticonvulsant	5–12 μg/mL (25–46 μmol/L)
procainamide	antiarrhythmic	4–8 μg/mL (17–34 μmol/L)
propranolol	antiarrhythmic	50–200 ng/mL (190–770 nmol/L)
protriptyline	antidepressant	100–200 ng/mL
quinidine	antiarrhythmic	2–6 μg/mL (4.6–9.2 μmol/L)
salicylate	analgesic	100–200 mg/L (725–1448 μmol/L)
streptomycin	aminoglycoside	20–30 μg/mL
sulfonamide	antibiotic	5–15 mg/dL
terbutaline	bronchodilator	0.5–4.1 ng/mL
theophylline	bronchodilator	10–20 μg/mL (55–110 μmol/L)
thiothixene	antipsychotic	2–57 ng/mL
tobramycin	aminoglycoside	4–8 μg/mL
tocainide	antiarrhythmic	4–10 μg/mL
trazodone	antidepressant	800–1600 ng/mL
valproic acid	anticonvulsant	50–100 μg/mL (350–700 μmol/L)
vancomycin	antibiotic	30–40 ng/mL (peak)
verapamil	antiarrhythmic	0.08–0.3 μg/mL

* radioimmunoassay

The Most Prescribed Drugs

Drug	Class/Indication(s)
Accupril (quinapril HCl)	antihypertensive, ACE inhibitor
acetaminophen with codeine	analgesic, anti-inflammatory
Aciphex (rabeprazole sodium)	proton pump inhibitor for GERD
Actonel (risedronate sodium)	osteoporosis prevention and treatment
Actos (pioglitazone HCl)	oral antidiabetic
acyclovir	antiviral
Adderall XR (mixed amphetamines)	CNS stimulant for ADHD
Advair Discus (salmeterol xinafoate, fluticasone propionate)	bronchodilator and corticosteroidal anti-inflammatory for asthma
albuterol; albuterol sulfate	bronchodilator for asthma
Allegra (fexofenadine HCl)	nonsedating antihistamine for allergy
Allegra-D 12-Hour (fexofenadine HCl, pseudoephedrine HCl)	nonsedating antihistamine and decongestant for allergy
allopurinol	treatment for gout and hyperuricemia
alprazolam	anxiolytic, sedative
Altace (ramipril)	antihypertensive, ACE inhibitor
Amaryl (glimepiride)	oral antidiabetic
Ambien (zolpidem tartrate)	sedative, hypnotic
amitriptyline HCl	tricyclic antidepressant
amoxicillin	aminopenicillin antibiotic
amoxicillin & clavulanate potassium	aminopenicillin antibiotic
Amoxil (amoxicillin trihydrate)	aminopenicillin antibiotic
Aricept (donepezil HCl)	cognition aid for Alzheimer disease
aspirin	analgesic, antipyretic, NSAID
atenolol	antihypertensive, antianginal
Avandia (rosiglitazone maleate)	antidiabetic; decreases insulin resistance
Avapro (irbesartan)	antihypertensive
Avelox (moxifloxacin HCl)	fluoroquinolone antibiotic
Aviane (levonorgestrel, ethinyl estradiol)	monophasic oral contraceptive
benazepril HCl	antihypertensive, ACE inhibitor
Benicar (olmesartan medoxomil)	antihypertensive, angiotensin II blocker
Bextra (valdecoxib)	antiarthritic, NSAID, COX-2 inhibitor
Biaxin; Biaxin XL (clarithromycin)	macrolide antibiotic
bisoprolol & hydrochlorothiazide	β-blocker and diuretic for hypertension
bupropion HCl	aminoketone antidepressant
buspirone HCl	anxiolytic
carisoprodol	skeletal muscle relaxant
Cartia XT (diltiazem HCl)	antihypertensive, antianginal
Celebrex (celecoxib)	antiarthritic, NSAID, COX-2 inhibitor
Celexa (citalopram hydrobromide)	SSRI antidepressant
cephalexin	cephalosporin antibiotic

Drug	Class/Indication(s)
ciprofloxacin	fluoroquinolone antibiotic
Clarinex (desloratadine)	nonsedating antihistamine for allergy
clindamycin	lincosamide antibiotic
clonazepam	anticonvulsant
clonidine	antihypertensive
clotrimazole & betamethasone dipropionate	broad-spectrum antifungal, cortico-steroidal anti-inflammatory
Combivent (ipratropium bromide, albuterol sulfate)	bronchodilator for COPD
Concerta (methylphenidate HCl)	CNS stimulant for ADHD
Coreg (carvedilol)	α- and β-blocker for hypertension and congestive heart failure
Cotrim (trimethoprim, sulfamethoxazole)	sulfonamide antibiotic
Coumadin (warfarin sodium)	anticoagulant
Cozaar (losartan potassium)	antihypertensive, angiotensin II blocker
Crestor (rosuvastatin potassium)	antihyperlipidemic
cyclobenzaprine HCl	skeletal muscle relaxant
Depakote (divalproex sodium)	anticonvulsant
Detrol LA (tolterodine tartrate)	treatment for urinary frequency
diazepam	anxiolytic, skeletal muscle relaxant
diclofenac sodium	antiarthritic, analgesic, NSAID
Diflucan (fluconazole)	systemic antifungal
Digitek (digoxin)	antiarrhythmic
digoxin	antiarrhythmic
Dilantin (phenytoin sodium)	anticonvulsant
diltiazem HCl	antihypertensive, antianginal
Diovan (valsartan)	antihypertensive, angiotensin II blocker
Diovan HCT (valsartan, hydrochloro-thiazide)	antihypertensive, angiotensin II blocker, diuretic
doxazosin mesylate	α-blocker for hypertension and BPH
doxycycline hyclate	tetracycline antibiotic
Duragesic (fentanyl)	narcotic analgesic transdermal patch
Effexor XR (venlafaxine)	SSNRI antidepressant, anxiolytic
Elidel (pimecrolimus)	topical NSAID for atopic dermatitis
enalapril maleate	antihypertensive, ACE inhibitor
Endocet (oxycodone HCl; aceta-minophen)	narcotic analgesic
estradiol	oral estrogen for postmenopausal HRT
Evista (raloxifene HCl)	postmenopausal osteoporosis treatment
famotidine	histamine antagonist for gastric ulcers
ferrous sulfate	hematinic, iron supplement
Flomax (tamsulosin HCl)	benign prostatic hypertrophy treatment
Flonase (fluticasone propionate)	steroidal anti-inflammatory
Flovent (fluticasone propionate)	steroidal anti-inflammatory
fluconazole	systemic antifungal
fluoxetine HCl	SSRI antidepressant
folic acid	hematopoietic, prevents birth defects
Fosamax (alendronate sodium)	postmenopausal osteoporosis treatment

Drug	Class/Indication(s)
fosinopril sodium	antihypertensive, ACE inhibitor
furosemide	diuretic, antihypertensive
gemfibrozil	antihyperlipidemic
glipizide; glipizide ER	oral antidiabetic
glyburide	oral antidiabetic
Humalog (insulin lispro)	parenteral antidiabetic
Humulin N; Humulin 70/30 (insulin)	parenteral antidiabetic
hydrochlorothiazide	diuretic, antihypertensive
hydrocodone & acetaminophen	antitussive, analgesic
hydroxyzine HCl	anxiolytic, minor tranquilizer
Hyzaar (losartan potassium, hydro-chlorothiazide)	antihypertensive, angiotensin II blocker, diuretic
ibuprofen	antiarthritic, analgesic, NSAID
Imitrex [oral] (sumatriptan succinate)	migraine headache treatment
isosorbide mononitrate	coronary vasodilator, antianginal
ketoconazole	systemic/topical antifungal
Klor-Con; Klor-Con M20 (potassium chloride)	potassium supplement
Lamictal (lamotrigine)	anticonvulsant, antimanic
Lanoxin (digoxin)	antiarrhythmic
Lantus (insulin glargine)	parenteral antidiabetic
Lescol XL (fluvastatin sodium)	antihyperlipidemic
Levaquin (levofloxacin)	fluoroquinolone antibiotic
Levothroid (levothyroxine sodium)	thyroid hormone
levothyroxine sodium	thyroid hormone
Levoxyl (levothyroxine sodium)	thyroid hormone
Lexapro (escitalopram oxalate)	SSRI antidepressant
Lipitor (atorvastatin calcium)	antihyperlipidemic
lisinopril	antihypertensive, ACE inhibitor
lisinopril & hydrochlorothiazide	antihypertensive, ACE inhibitor, diuretic
loratadine	nonsedating antihistamine for allergy
lorazepam	anxiolytic, tranquilizer
Lotrel (amlodipine besylate, benazepril HCl)	antihypertensive, ACE inhibitor, calcium channel blocker
lovastatin	antihyperlipidemic
meclizine HCl	antiemetic for motion sickness, vertigo
metformin HCl	oral antidiabetic
methotrexate	antineoplastic, antipsoriatic, anti-rheumatic
methylprednisolone	corticosteroidal anti-inflammatory
metoclopramide HCl	antiemetic for chemotherapy
metoprolol tartrate	antianginal, antihypertensive
metronidazole	oral antibiotic, antiprotozoal
minocycline HCl	broad-spectrum antibiotic
Miralax (polyethylene glycol 3350)	laxative, pre-procedure bowel evacuant
mirtazapine	tetracyclic antidepressant
Mobic (meloxicam)	analgesic, antiarthritic, NSAID

Drug	Class/Indication(s)
naproxen; naproxen sodium	analgesic, antiarthritic, NSAID
Nasacort AQ (triamcinolone acetonide)	nasal steroid for allergic rhinitis
Nasonex (mometasone furoate)	nasal steroid for allergic rhinitis
Necon 1/35 (norethindrone, ethinyl estradiol)	monophasic oral contraceptive
Neurontin (gabapentin)	anticonvulsant
Nexium (esomeprazole magnesium)	proton pump inhibitor for GERD
Niaspan (niacin)	vasodilator, antihyperlipidemic
Norvasc (amlodipine)	antianginal, antihypertensive
nystatin	systemic antifungal
omeprazole	proton pump inhibitor for GERD
Omnicef (cefdinir)	cephalosporin antibiotic
Ortho Evra (norelgestromin, ethinyl estradiol)	once-weekly contraceptive patch
Ortho Tri-Cyclen; Ortho Tri-Cyclen Lo (norgestimate, ethinyl estradiol)	triphasic oral contraceptive
oxycodone HCl & acetaminophen	narcotic analgesic, NSAID
OxyContin (oxycodone HCl)	narcotic analgesic
paroxetine HCl	SSRI antidepressant
Patanol (olopatadine HCl)	ophthalmic antihistamine for allergy
Paxil; Paxil CR (paroxetine HCl)	SSRI antidepressant
penicillin VK (penicillin V potassium)	natural antibiotic
Plavix (clopidogrel bisulfate)	platelet aggregation inhibitor
potassium chloride	potassium supplement
Pravachol (pravastatin sodium)	antihyperlipidemic
prednisone	corticosteroidal anti-inflammatory
Premarin (conjugated estrogens)	estrogen replacement
Prempro (conjugated estrogens, medroxyprogesterone acetate)	hormone replacement therapy
Prevacid (lansoprazole)	antisecretory, antiulcer
promethazine HCl	antihistamine, antiemetic
promethazine with codeine	narcotic antitussive, antihistamine
propoxyphene napsylate/acetaminophen	narcotic analgesic, NSAID
propranolol HCl	antihypertensive, antiarrhythmic
Protonix (pantoprazole sodium)	proton pump inhibitor for GERD
Pulmicort (budesonide)	steroidal inhalant for asthma
quinine sulfate	antimalarial
ranitidine HCl	histamine antagonist for gastric ulcers
Rhinocort Aqua (budesonide)	nasal steroid for allergic rhinitis
Risperdal (risperidone)	antipsychotic
Seroquel (quetiapine fumarate)	antipsychotic
Singulair (montelukast sodium)	antiasthmatic
Skelaxin (metaxalone)	skeletal muscle relaxant
spironolactone	antihypertensive, diuretic
Strattera (atomoxetine HCl)	nonstimulant ADHD treatment
sulfamethoxazole & trimethoprim	anti-infective, antibacterial
Synthroid (levothyroxine sodium)	thyroid replacement
temazepam	tranquilizer, hypnotic

Drug	Class/Indication(s)
terazosin HCl	α-blocker for hypertension and BPH
Topamax (topiramate)	anticonvulsant
Toprol XL (metoprolol succinate)	antihypertensive, antianginal
tramadol HCl	central analgesic
trazodone HCl	tetracyclic antidepressant
triamcinolone acetonide	topical steroidal anti-inflammatory
triamterene & hydrochlorothiazide	diuretic, antihypertensive
Tricor (fenofibrate)	antihyperlipidemic
trimethoprim & sulfamethoxazole	anti-infective, antibacterial
Trimox (amoxicillin trihydrate)	aminopenicillin antibiotic
Trinessa (norgestimate, ethinyl estradiol)	triphasic oral contraceptive
Tri-Sprintec (norgestimate, ethinyl estradiol)	triphasic oral contraceptive
Ultracet (tramadol HCl, acetaminophen)	central analgesic, NSAID
Valtrex (valacyclovir HCl)	antiviral for herpes infections
verapamil HCl [sustained-release form]	antianginal, antiarrhythmic, calcium channel blocker
Viagra (sildenafil citrate)	vasodilator for erectile dysfunction
Vioxx (rofecoxib)	antiarthritic, NSAID, COX-2 inhibitor
warfarin sodium	anticoagulant
Wellbutrin SR (bupropion HCl)	aminoketone antidepressant
Xalatan (latanoprost)	topical antiglaucoma agent
Yasmin (drospirenone, ethinyl estradiol)	monophasic oral contraceptive
Zetia (ezetimibe)	antihyperlipidemic
Zithromax (azithromycin dihydrate)	macrolide antibiotic
Zocor (simvastatin)	antihyperlipidemic
Zoloft (sertraline)	SSRI antidepressant
Zyprexa (olanzapine)	antipsychotic, antimanic
Zyrtec (cetirizine HCl)	antihistamine

Dropped from the previous year's list:

Alphagan P (brimonidine tartrate)	topical antiglaucoma agent
Apri (desogestrel, ethinyl estradiol)	monophasic oral contraceptive
Atacand (candesartan cilexetil)	antihypertensive, angiotensin II blocker
Atrovent (ipratropium bromide)	bronchodilator
Augmentin (amoxicillin trihydrate, clavulanate potassium)	aminopenicillin antibiotic
Avalide (irbesartan, hydrochlorothiazide)	antihypertensive, angiotensin II blocker, diuretic
Bactroban (mupirocin calcium)	topical antibiotic
Cefzil (cefprozil)	cephalosporin antibiotic
Cipro (ciprofloxacin)	fluoroquinolone antibiotic
Ditropan XL (oxybutynin chloride)	treatment for urinary frequency
Glucophage XR (metformin HCl)	oral antidiabetic
Glucotrol XL (glipizide)	oral antidiabetic
Glucovance (glyburide, metformin HCl)	oral antidiabetic
Inderal LA (propranolol HCl)	antihypertensive, antiarrhythmic

Drug	Class/Indication(s)
Kariva (desogestrel, ethinyl estradiol)	biphasic oral contraceptive
Lotensin (benazepril HCl)	antihypertensive, ACE inhibitor
Low-Ogestrel (norgestrel, ethinyl estradiol)	monophasic oral contraceptive
Macrobid (nitrofurantoin)	urinary antibiotic
Miacalcin (calcitonin salmon)	calcium regulator for osteoporosis
Microgestin Fe (norethindrone acetate, ethinyl estradiol, ferrous fumarate)	monophasic oral contraceptive, iron supplement
Monopril (fosinopril sodium)	antihypertensive, ACE inhibitor
Nifediac CC (nifedipine)	antianginal, antihypertensive
nifedipine [extended-release form]	antianginal, antihypertensive
Nitroquick (nitroglycerin)	antianginal, coronary vasodilator
Ortho-Novum 7/7/7 (norethindrone, ethinyl estradiol)	triphasic oral contraceptive
Percocet (oxycodone HCl, acetaminophen)	narcotic analgesic, NSAID
phenytoin	anticonvulsant
Plendil (felodipine)	antihypertensive
Prilosec (omeprazole)	proton pump inhibitor for GERD
Proscar (finasteride)	androgen inhibitor for BPH
Remeron (mirtazapine)	tetracyclic antidepressant
Roxicet (oxycodone HCl, acetaminophen)	narcotic analgesic, NSAID
timolol maleate	topical antiglaucoma agent
TobraDex (tobramycin, dexamethasone)	ophthalmic antibiotic and steroid
Trivora (levonorgestrel, ethinyl estradiol)	triphasic oral contraceptive
Tussionex (hydrocodone polistirex, chlorpheniramine polistirex)	narcotic antitussive, antihistamine
Zyrtec-D (cetirizine HCl, pseudoephedrine HCl)	antihistamine, nasal decongestant